S0-BEE-029

Hospital Infections

Fourth Edition

HOSPITAL INFECTIONS

FOURTH EDITION 1998

Edited by

John V. Bennett, M.D.
Director for Scientific Affairs
The Task Force for Child Survival and Development
Professor, Department of Epidemiology
Rollins School of Public Health
Emory University
Atlanta, Georgia

Philip S. Brachman, M.D.
Professor, Department of International Health
Rollins School of Public Health
Emory University
Atlanta, Georgia

Lippincott - Raven
PUBLISHERS
Philadelphia • New York

Acquisitions Editor: Ruth W. Weinberg
Developmental Editor: Judith E. Hummel
Manufacturing Manager: Dennis Teston
Production Manager: Jodi Borgenicht
Production Editor: Michele Downes
Cover Designer: Betty Sokol
Indexer: Lisa Mulleneaux
Compositor: Lippincott–Raven Electronic Production
Printer: Maple Press

© 1998, by Lippincott–Raven Publishers. All rights reserved. This book is protected by copyright. No part of it may be reproduced, stored in a retrieval system, or transmitted, in any form or by any means—electronic, mechanical, photocopy, recording, or otherwise—without the prior written consent of the publisher, except for brief quotations embodied in critical articles and reviews. For information write **Lippincott–Raven Publishers, 227 East Washington Square, Philadelphia, PA 19106-3780.**

Materials appearing in this book prepared by individuals as part of their official duties as U.S. Government employees are not covered by the above-mentioned copyright.

Printed in the United States of America

9 8 7 6 5 4 3 2 1

Library of Congress Cataloging-in-Publication Data

Hospital infections / edited by John V. Bennett and Philip S. Brachman.—4th ed.
p. cm.
Includes bibliographical references and index.
ISBN 0-316-08902-8
1. Nosocomial infections. 2. Nosocomial infections—Prevention.
I. Bennett, John V. II. Brachman, Philip S.
[DNLM: 1. Cross infection—prevention & control. 2. Cross Infection—etiology. WX 167 H8294 1997]
RA969.H64 1998
614.4'4—dc21
DNLM/DLC
for Library of Congress

Care has been taken to confirm the accuracy of the information presented and to describe generally accepted practices. However, the authors, editors, and publisher are not responsible for errors or omissions or for any consequences from application of the information in this book and make no warranty, express or implied, with respect to the contents of the publication.

The authors, editors, and publisher have exerted every effort to ensure that drug selection and dosage set forth in this text are in accordance with current recommendations and practice at the time of publication. However, in view of ongoing research, changes in government regulations, and the constant flow of information relating to drug therapy and drug reactions, the reader is urged to check the package insert for each drug for any change in indications and dosage and for added warnings and precautions. This is particularly important when the recommended agent is a new or infrequently employed drug.

Some drugs and medical devices presented in this publication have Food and Drug Administration (FDA) clearance for limited use in restricted research settings. It is the responsibility of the health care provider to ascertain the FDA status of each drug or device planned for use in their clinical practice.

Contents

Contributing Authors

Miriam J. Alter, Ph.D.
Hepatitis Branch
National Center for Infectious Diseases
Centers for Disease Control and Prevention
Mail Stop G-37
1600 Clifton Road, North East
Atlanta, Georgia 30333

Matthew J. Arduino, M.S., Dr. P.H.
Hospital Infections Program
National Center for Infectious Diseases
Centers for Disease Control and Prevention
Mail Stop C-01
1600 Clifton Road, North East
Atlanta, Georgia 30333

G. Scott Baity, J.D.
Staff Attorney
Baptist/St. Vincent's Health System, Incorporated
1325 San Marco Boulevard, Suite 902
Jacksonville, Florida 32207

Nancy H. Bean, Ph.D.
Chief, Surveillance and Epidemic Investigations Section
Biostatistics and Information Management Branch
Division of Bacterial and Mycotic Diseases
National Center for Infectious Diseases
Centers for Disease Control and Prevention
Mail Stop C-09
1600 Clifton Road, North East
Atlanta, Georgia 30333

David M. Bell, M.D.
Assistant to the Director of the National Center for Infectious Diseases
Office of the Director
Division of Antimicrobial Resistance
National Center for Infectious Diseases
Centers for Disease Control and Prevention
Mail Stop C-12
1600 Clifton Road, North East
Atlanta, Georgia 30333

John V. Bennett, M.D.
Director for Scientific Affairs
Task Force for Child Survival and Development
One Copenhill
Atlanta, Georgia 30307

Elizabeth A. Bolyard, R.N., M.P.H.
Epidemiologist, Hospital Infections Program
National Center for Infectious Diseases
Centers for Disease Control and Prevention
Mail Stop E-68
1600 Clifton Road, North East
Atlanta, Georgia 30333

Philip S. Brachman, M.D.
Professor, Department of International Health
Rollins School of Public Health
Emory University
1518 Clifton Road, North East, Seventh Floor
Atlanta, Georgia 30322

John P. Burke, M.D.
Chief, Department of Clinical Epidemiology and Infectious Diseases
LDS Hospital
1966 Yale Avenue
Salt Lake City, Utah 84108-1827

Mary E. Chamberland, M.D., M.P.H.
Assistant Director for Blood Safety
Division of Viral and Rickettsial Diseases
National Center for Infectious Diseases
Centers for Disease Control and Prevention
Mail Stop A-30
1600 Clifton Road, North East
Atlanta, Georgia 30333

Donald E. Craven, M.D.
Professor of Medicine Epidemiology
Department of Infectious Diseases
Clinical AIDS Program
Boston Medical Center
One Boston Medical Center Place
Dowling Building 3, North
Boston, Massachusetts 02118-2353

David H. Culver, Ph.D.
Hospital Infections Program
National Center for Infectious Diseases
Centers for Disease Control and Prevention
Mail Stop E-55
1600 Clifton Road, North East
Atlanta, Georgia 30333

Michael D. Decker, M.D., M.P.H.
Associate Professor
Department of Preventive Medicine
A-1116 Medical Center North
Vanderbilt University School of Medicine
Nashville, Tennessee 37232

E. Patchen Dellinger, M.D.
Professor and Vice Chairman
Department of Surgery
University of Washington School of Medicine
P.O. Box 35-6410
Division of General Surgery
University of Washington Medical Center
1959 North East Pacific, BB487
Seattle, Washington 98195-6410

Herbert L. DuPont, M.D.
Clinical Professor
Department of Internal Medicine
Baylor College of Medicine
University of Texas at Houston
Chief, Internal Medicine Service
St. Luke's Episcopal Hospital
6720 Bertner Avenue, MC 1-164
Houston, Texas 77030

Jonathan R. Edwards, M.D.
Hospital Infections Program
Centers for Disease Control and Prevention
Mail Stop E-55
1600 Clifton Road, North East
Atlanta, Georgia 30333

N. Joel Ehrenkranz, M.D.
Director, Florida Consortium for Infection Control
5901 South West 74 Street, Suite 300
South Miami, Florida 33143-5163

Theodore C. Eickhoff, M.D.
Professor of Medicine
B-168, Division of Infectious Diseases
University of Colorado Health Sciences Center
4200 East 9th Avenue
Denver, Colorado 80262

Barry M. Farr, M.D., M.Sc.
William S. Jordan, Jr. Professor of Medicine and Epidemiology
Department of Internal Medicine
University of Virginia Health Sciences Center
P.O. Box 473
Charlottesville, Virginia 22908

Martin S. Favero, Ph.D.
Director of Scientific Affairs
Advanced Sterilization Products
Johnson & Johnson Medical, Incorporated
33 Technology Drive
Irvine, California 92618

Jay A. Fishman, M.D.
Assistant Professor of Medicine
Department of Infectious Disease and Transplantation
Massachusetts General Hospital
55 Fruit Street
Boston, Massachusetts 02114

Jonathan Freeman, M.D.
Department of Epidemiology
Harvard School of Public Health
677 Huntington Avenue
Boston, Massachusetts 02115

Richard A. Garibaldi, M.D.
Professor of Medicine
Department of Medicine
University of Connecticut School of Medicine
Farmington, Connecticut 06032

Julia S. Garner, M.S.N.
Hospital Infections Program
National Center for Infectious Diseases
Centers for Disease Control and Prevention
Mail Stop A-07
1600 Clifton Road, North East
Atlanta, Georgia 30333

Robert P. Gaynes, M.D.
Chief, Nosocomial Infections Surveillance Activity
Hospital Infections Program
National Center for Infectious Diseases
Centers for Disease Control and Prevention
Mail Stop E-55
1600 Clifton Road, North East
Atlanta, Georgia 30333

Donald A. Goldmann, M.D.
Professor of Pediatrics
Children's Hospital
Harvard Medical School
300 Longwood Avenue
Boston, Massachusetts 02115

Joy Goulding, B.S.
Division of Bacterial and Mycotic Diseases
National Center for Infectious Diseases
Centers for Disease Control and Prevention
Mail Stop C-09
1600 Clifton Road, North East
Atlanta, Georgia 30333

Robert W. Haley, M.D.
Associate Professor of Medicine
Department of Internal Medicine
Division of Epidemiology and Preventive Medicine
University of Texas Southwestern Medical Center
5323 Harry Hines Boulevard
Dallas, Texas 75235-8874

Stephan J. Harbarth, M.D.
Fellow, Infection Control Program
Division of Infectious Diseases
Geneva University Hospital
24, rue Micheli-du-Crest
CH-1211 Geneva 14
Switzerland

Mary K. Hayden, M.D.
Assistant Professor of Medicine and Pathology
Department of Medicine
Section of Infectious Disease
Rush Medical College
Rush-Presbyterian-St. Luke's Medical Center
1653 West Congress Parkway
Chicago, Illinois 60612

Walter J. Hierholzer, Jr., M.D.
Professor of Medicine and Epidemiology
Department of Internal Medicine
Director, Hospital Epidemiology Program
Division of Infectious Disease
Yale University School of Medicine
Yale-New Haven Hospital
20 York Street, GB 326
New Haven, Connecticut 06504

Cynthia A. Hubbard, R.N., B.S.
Senior Consultant
Lerch Bates Hospital Group, Incorporated
8089 South Lincoln, Suite 205
Littleton, Colorado 80122

Marguerite McMillan Jackson, R.N., Ph.D.
Administrative Director
Epidemiology Unit
University of California at San Diego Medical Center
200 West Arbor Drive
San Diego, California 92103-8951

William R. Jarvis, M.D.
Acting Director, Hospital Infections Program
National Center for Infectious Diseases
Centers for Disease Control and Prevention
Mail Stop E-69
1600 Clifton Road, North East
Atlanta, Georgia 30333

Andrew M. Kaunitz, M.D.
Professor and Assistant Chair
Department of Obstetrics and Gynecology
University of Florida Health Science Center
1325 San Marco Boulevard, Suite 902
Jacksonville, Florida 32207

Karen Rose Koppel Kaunitz, J.D.
Associate General Counsel
Baptist/St. Vincent's Health System
1325 San Marco Boulevard, Suite 902
Jacksonville, Florida 32207

F. Marc LaForce, M.D.
Professor of Medicine
Department of Medicine
University of Rochester School of Medicine
Rochester, New York 14642

William Ledger, M.D.
Department of Obstetrics and Gynecology
The New York Hospital-Cornell Medical Center
525 East 68th Street
New York, New York 10021

Daniel P. Lew, M.D.
Chief, Division of Infectious Diseases
Professor of Medicine
Department of Internal Medicine
Geneva University Hospital
24, rue Micheli-du-Crest
CH-1211 Geneva 14
Switzerland

Patricia Lynch, R.N., M.B.A.
Epidemiology Associates
8237 4th Avenue, North East
Seattle, Washington 98115

Dennis G. Maki, M.D.
Ovid O. Meyer Professor of Medicine
Head, Section of Infectious Diseases
University of Wisconsin Medical School
Attending Physician, Center for Trauma and Life Support
Clinical Sciences Center, Room H4-574
600 Highland Avenue
Madison, Wisconsin 53792

Stanley M. Martin, M.S.
Chief, Biostatistics and Information Management Branch
Division of Bacterial and Mycotic Diseases
National Center for Infectious Diseases
Centers for Disease Control and Prevention
Mail Stop C-09
1600 Clifton Road, North East
Atlanta, Georgia 30333

William Martone, M.D.
National Foundation for Infectious Diseases
4733 Bethesda Avenue, Suite 750
Bethesda, Maryland 20814

John E. McGowan, Jr., M.D.
Department of Pathology
Emory University
Department of Laboratory Medicine
Grady Memorial Hospital
P.O. Box 26248
80 Butler Street
Atlanta, Georgia 30335

Albert T. McManus, Ph.D.
Senior Scientist
Microbiology Branch
U.S. Army Institute of Surgical Research
3400 Rawley East Chambers Avenue
Fort Sam Houston, Texas 78234-6315

Leonard A. Mermel, D.O., Sc.M., F.A.C.P.
Associate Professor
Department of Medicine
Brown University School of Medicine
Medical Director, Infection Control Department
Division of Infectious Diseases
Rhode Island Hospital
593 Eddy Street
Providence, Rhode Island 02903

David W. Mozingo, M.D.
Associate Professor of Surgery and Anesthesiology
Department of Surgery
Director, Shands Burn Center
University of Florida College of Medicine
P.O. Box 100286
1600 South West Archer Road
Gainesville, Florida 32610-0286

Ronald Lee Nichols, M.D., M.S., F.A.C.S.
William Henderson Professor of Surgery
Professor of Microbiolgy and Immunology
Department of Surgery (SL-22)
Tulane University School of Medicine
1430 Tulane Avenue
New Orleans, Louisiana 70112

Brenda A. Nurse, M.D.
Associate Professor of Clinical Medicine
University of Connecticut School of Medicine
Department of Infectious Diseases and Epidemiology
Hospital for Special Care
2150 Corbin Avenue
New Britain, Connecticut 06053

Didier Pittet, M.D., M.S.
Associate Professor of Medicine
Division of Infectious Diseases
Geneva University Hospital
24, rue Micheli-du-Crest
CH-1211 Geneva 14
Switzerland

Brian D. Plikaytis, M.Sc.
Chief, Biostatistics Section
Biostatistics and Information Management Branch
Division of Bacterial Diseases
National Center for Infectious Diseases
Centers for Disease Control and Prevention
Mail Stop C-09
1600 Clifton Road, North East
Atlanta, Georgia 30333

Samuel Ponce-de-León Rosales, M.D., M.Sc.
Professor of Medicine
Department of Hospital Epidemiology
Instituto Nacional de la Nutrición
Vasco de Quiroga 15, Tlalpan
Mexico City, 14000
Mexico

Basil A. Pruitt, Jr., M.D.
Professor, Department of Surgery
University of Texas Health Science Center at San Antonio
7703 Floyd Curl Drive
San Antonio, Texas 78284-7842

Gina Pugliese, R.N., M.S.
Associate Faculty
Rush University College of Nursing
1300 West Belmont Avenue, Suite 205
Chicago, Illinois 60657

M. Sigfrido Rangel-Frausto, M.D., M.Sc.
Assistant Professor
Division of Hospital Epidemiology
Instituto Nacional de la Nutrición
Vasco de Quiroga 15, Tlalpan
Mexico City, 14000
Mexico

L. Barth Reller, M.D.
Professor, Departments of Pathology and Medicine
Duke University School of Medicine and Medical Center
P.O. Box 3938
116 CARL Building
Research Drive
Durham, North Carolina 27710

Frank S. Rhame, M.D.
Adjunct Associate Professor
Division of Epidemiology
University of Minnesota School of Public Health
Research Director, Clinic 42
Abbott Northwestern Hospital
800 East 28th Street
Minneapolis, Minnesota 55407–3799

Bruce S. Ribner, M.D., M.P.H.
Associate Professor of Medicine
Medical University of South Carolina
Hospital Epidemiologist
Medical University Hospital
Center Epidemiologist
Ralph H. Johnson DVA Medical Center
109 Bee Street
Charleston, South Carolina 29401

Robert H. Rubin, M.D.
Gordon and Marjorie Osbourne Chair of Health Sciences and Technology
Director, Division of Human Pharmacology and Experimental Therapeutics
Harvard-Massachusetts Institute of Technology Division of Health Sciences and Technology
40 Ames Street
Cambridge, Massachusetts 02142

Kenneth E. F. Sands, M.D., M.P.H.
Instructor, Department of Medicine
Beth Israel Deaconess Medical Center
330 Brookline Avenue
Boston, Massachusetts 02215

Dennis R. Schaberg, M.D.
Professor and Chairman
Department of Internal Medicine
University of Tennessee at Memphis
956 Court Avenue, Room D-334
Memphis, Tennessee 38163

William Schaffner, M.D.
Professor and Chairman
Department of Preventive Medicine
Professor of Medicine (Infectious Diseases)
Vanderbilt University School of Medicine
Hospital Epidemiologist
Vanderbilt University Hospital
Nashville, Tennessee 37232

William E. Scheckler, M.D.
Professor, Department of Family Medicine
University of Wisconsin Medical School
777 South Mills Street
Madison, Wisconsin 53715

W. Michael Scheld, M.D.
Professor of Medicine and Neurosurgery
Associate Chair for Residency Programs
University of Virginia Health Sciences Center
300 Park Place
MR4 Building, Room 2122
Charlottesville, Virginia 22908

Craig W. Shapiro, M.D.
Division of Viral and Rickettsial Diseases
National Center for Infectious Diseases
Centers for Disease Control and Prevention
Mail Stop G-37
1600 Clifton Road, North East
Atlanta, Georgia 30333

Jane D. Siegel, M.D.
Professor, Department of Pediatrics
University of Texas Southwestern Medical Center
5323 Harry Hines Boulevard
Dallas, Texas 76236-9036

Bryan P. Simmons, M.D.
Clinical Associate Professor of Medicine
Department of Preventive Medicine
Division of Biostatistic and Epidemiology
University of Tennessee School of Medicine
188 South Bellevue, Suite 408
Memphis, Tennessee 38104

Laurence Slutsker, M.D., M.P.H.
Medical Epidemiologist
Foodborne and Diarrheal Diseases Branch
National Center for Infectious Diseases
Centers for Disease Control and Prevention
Mail Stop A-38
1600 Clifton Road, North East
Atlanta, Georgia 30333

Walter E. Stamm, M.D.
Head, Division of Allergy and Infectious Diseases
University of Washington School of Medicine
P.O. Box 356523
Seattle, Washington 98195

Kathleen A. Steger, R.N., M.P.H.
Assistant Professor of Public Health
Clinical AIDS Program
Boston Medical Center
One Boston Medical Center Place
Boston, Massachusetts 02118

Ofelia C. Tablan, M.D.
Hospital Infections Program
National Center for Infectious Diseases
Centers for Disease Control and Prevention
Mail Stop E-69
1600 Clifton Road, North East
Atlanta, Georgia 30333

Fred C. Tenover, Ph.D.
Chief, Nosocomial Pathogens Laboratory Branch
Hospital Infections Program
National Center for Infectious Diseases
Centers for Disease Control and Prevention
Mail Stop G-08
1600 Clifton Road, North East
Atlanta, Georgia 30333

Jerome I. Tokars, M.D., M.P.H.
Medical Epidemiologist
Hospital Infections Program
National Center for Infectious Diseases
Centers for Disease Control and Prevention
Mail Stop E-69
1600 Clifton Road, North East
Atlanta, Georgia 30333

William M. Valenti, M.D.
Clinical Associate Professor of Medicine
University of Rochester School of Medicine
Community Health Network
758 South Avenue
Rochester, New York 14620

Margarita E. Villarino, M.D.
Hospital Infections Program
National Center for Infectious Diseases
Centers for Disease Control and Prevention
Mail Stop E-10
1600 Clifton Road, North East
Atlanta, Georgia 30333

Francis A. Waldvogel, M.D.
Professor of Medicine
Chairman, Department of Internal Medicine
Geneva University Hospital
24, rue Micheli-du-Crest
CH-1211 Geneva 14
Switzerland

Jeffrey W. Weinstein, M.D.
Assistant Clinical Professor
Department of Internal Medicine
Wright State University School of Medicine
3640 Colonel Glenn Highway
Dayton, Ohio 45401

Robert A. Weinstein, M.D.
Professor of Medicine
Department of Medicine
Rush Medical College
Division of Infectious Diseases
Cook County Hospital
1835 West Harrison Street
Chicago, Illinois 60612-9985

Sharon F. Welbel, M.D.
Assistant Professor
Department of Medicine
Rush Medical College
Hospital Epidemiologist
Division of Infectious Disease
Cook County Hospital
1835 West Harrison Street
Chicago, Illinois 60612

Walter W. Williams, M.D., M.P.H.
Chief, Adult Vaccine Preventable Diseases Branch
Epidemiology and Surveillance Division
National Immunization Program
Centers for Disease Control and Prevention
Mail Stop E-61
1600 Clifton Road, North East
Atlanta, Georgia 30333

Michael L. Wilson, M.D.
Associate Professor of Pathology
University of Colorado School of Medicine
Medical Laboratories
 # 0224 DHMC
777 Bancock
Denver, Colorado 80204-4507

Foreword

In the Foreword to the First Edition of *Hospital Infections,* Dr. Maxwell Finland noted the history of hospital infection control began with an attempt to assist the poor by providing charitable institutions to care for the sick. As with many good intentions, a seemingly reasonable project went awry due to an inability to fully understand the possible risks. Collecting the sick in semi-closed populations resulted in the transmission of infections, which quickened the mortality rate of those already dying. These "pest house" conditions in hospitals continued up until the middle 1800s when healthcare professionals such as Holmes, Semmelweis, and Nightingale introduced hygienic and sanitation practices, thus significantly improving infection-reduction even before microorganisms and their causal relationships with infection and disease had been discovered. After slow acceptance, the strict application of routine handwashing and aseptic surgical techniques in medical care had become well supported, until the onset of penicillin. The success of this antibiotic in controlling the gram-positive bacteria—a common cause of purulent disease—was so convincing that it had raised expectations: infectious disease could now be controlled without dealing with the constraining details of previously essential methods. Moreover, infectious agents would be conquered and disappear.

Within two decades, however, the error of this thinking would surface; penicillin-resistant staphylococci resulted in the extensive hospital epidemics of the 1950s and 1960s. Newly built nurseries and surgical suites were closed, and healthcare workers identified as carriers of epidemic strains of microorganisms were indefinitely furloughed. The identification of hospitals as "pest houses" reappeared.

It could be said that modern infection control largely arose from the medical and public health responses to these epidemics. The development and support of the Hospital Infection Program at the Centers for Disease Control (CDC) in the United States, in addition to the Infection Control sister in Great Britain, were part of the concerted effort to control this modern plague. Strong educational course work and professional support at the CDC, as well as administrative support at the American Hospital Association and the Joint Commission on Accreditation of Hospitals fostered the first professionals in the field. The volume of scientific support for infection control increased exponentially, including the unique CDC-sponsored program evaluation effort known as the Study of the Efficacy of Nosocomial Infection Control or SENIC.

The First Edition of this book appeared during the SENIC project in 1979, shortly before the first SENIC publications and during the influential tenure of its editors at the CDC. In its initial edition, *Hospital Infections* included core chapters on the basic concepts of surveillance and control, the importance of supportive microbiology, the interplay with personnel health issues, and on many of the features of the subspecialty unit problems. A chapter on isolation was included, and the first of the four chapters on antibiotics and nosocomial infections was contributed by Dr. Theodore Eickhoff, an early co-worker with the editors at CDC. The successful control (or at least the disappearance) of the staphylococcal epidemic was reflected by the absence of a chapter on gram-positive infections, and the inclusion of a final chapter on the next wave of nosocomial organisms—the gram-negative rods. Despite the emergence of this second cycle of resistant bacteria, no chapter on resistance was included, although the importance of viral agents was acknowledged. One chapter was devoted to outpatient departments, and Dr. William Schaffner contributed the first of his chapters on the relationship between hospitals and their communities.

In 1986, the editors presented a Second Edition that had grown from 29 chapters to 38 chapters, with 6 additional contributors. The chapter on gram-negative infections disappeared, but chapters on the prime-gram positives, group A Streptococci and Staphylococci returned to the discussion. Two chapters were also devoted to resistance in microorganisms. The scientific growth of infection-control methodologies was discussed in a new chapter on Statistical Techniques, and the growing importance of nosocomial infections in non-hospital environments was addressed by a revised chapter on Ambulatory Care Settings and a new chapter on Infections in Nursing Homes.

In 1992, the Third Edition was modestly expanded by the contributions of 16 additional authors, adding 308 pages to the text. New topics included descriptions on the use of computers, the now well-recognized role of the Hospital Epidemiologist, and the appearance of the Human-Immunodeficiency-Virus-(HIV)–related Acquired Immunodeficiency Syndrome (AIDS). In response to the AIDS epidemic, the chapter on Isolation Systems included the description of a new set of practices (termed "Universal Precautions"), designed to protect healthcare workers. Furthermore, as a bell weather of change in medical care financing, the Third Edition had, for the first time, a chapter on the Costs and Benefits of Infection Control Programs.

Between the Second and Third Editions, ad hoc committees at the CDC had completed several formalized sets of recommendations or guidelines for the surveillance, control, and prevention of nosocomial infections. These included recommendations for prevention and care in the areas of urinary tract infections, pneumonias, intravascular infections, surgical wound infections, handwashing and environmental control, and isolation precautions. The details of these recommendations also found their way into the text of the Third Edition.

This current edition, with 4 new chapters and 20 additional contributors, has been revised and expanded during a time of remarkable resurgent interest in infectious diseases. Newly emerging and reemerging infectious diseases have solidly laid to rest the misconception that microbial agents are soon to be conquered, or even controlled (except with special circumstances and vigilance).

Resistance to antimicrobials, a core issue in reemergent infectious agents, is addressed in chapters on Multiple Drug-Resistant Pathogens, the Molecular Biology of Resistance, Antibiotics and Nosocomial Infections, and in the ever present chapter on Staphylococci and Group A Streptococci. Resistance in gram-positive bacteria is exemplified by the largely untreatable, plasmid-carrying vancomycin, aminoglycoside, and penicillin-resistant enterococcus. The potential for this resistance grouping to include methicillin-resistant staphylococci raises the spector of the reappearance of hospital infections with an untreatable, highly pathogenic, easily carried and transmissible agent—a possible reemergence and reprise of the staphylococcal epidemics of the 1950s and 1960s. As in the case of that earlier epidemic, the early appearance of new antibiotics with novel mechanisms to control these untreatable strains seems unlikely.

Multiple drug resistance has also been a factor in the reemergence of pulmonary tuberculosis, in association with the HIV epidemic. The significance of this problem is reflected in the addition of the chapter on Tuberculosis.

At the time of the First Edition, misuse of environmental testing had been brought to the fore of social consciousness, and appropriate recommendations to counter this trend were made. With time, these recommendations were interpreted by many to indicate that the role of the inanimate environment in nosocomial transmission was minimal or even non-existant. As a result, it had become expected that the importance of the environment would continue to diminish and perhaps even disappear from discussion. However, many factors led to the emergence or reemergernce of disease events in healthcare venues: legionella and cryptosporidium agents in potable water systems; legionella in air conditioning systems; the potential for the airborne transmission of resurgent, multi-drug resistant tuberculosis; the long term viability of Hepatitis B virus in dialysis units; the continuing potential for the transmission of foodborne agents in the large batch processing and distribution of foods over wide geographical areas; and the decline in quality of water and sewage systems. More recently, both vancomycin-resistant enterococci and Clostridium difficile have been shown to linger in the bedside environment, especially if housekeeping is less than pristine. Carriage and transmission from such contaminated environments to patients is common. Therefore, the role of the contaminated environment as a risk in hospital infections has reemerged with an enhanced appreciation of its importance.

The battle against the AIDS epidemic continues with a stronger hope for control and prevention, based on new antivirals. The risk of transmission of bloodborne pathogens between healthcare workers and patients appears to be, according to new studies, preventable by administering new devices to diminish sharps injuries; however, it remains primarily a political and ethical issue. The role of viruses in the etiology of nosocomial infections and its resistance to therapeutic antivirals has increased as quickly as they have for bacterial agents. The emergence of the viral and bacterial childhood disease agents in the AIDS- and other immunocompromised-patient populations appears to be a growing problem, as exemplified by influenza, RSV, adenovirus, CMV, Herpes simplex, and pertussis.

The addition of the chapter on professional groups and agencies shows the importance of not only infection control, but the increasing bureaucracy of medical care. Continued development of data on the high benefit—cost of infection control programs in the chapter devoted to that topic is necessary and reasonable when one takes into account the rough-and-tumble competition for program support in the current corporate development of medicine.

An additional chapter on the relationship between the hospital and the community, in addition to previous discussions on ambulatory and extended care, reflect a major change in the role of the hospital with regard to medical care offered in non-hospital healthcare venues. Managed care in the home, the clinic/office, extended care, and even the hospice are new and special features requiring infection control inputs.

The editors are to be congratulated for their careful shepherding of a growing body of material that documents the continuing importance of the science and the programs for the surveillance, control, and prevention of infection. Hospitals remain a central and core component of this discussion. And although the core has held, the relationships have expanded, and continue to do so. These dynamic changes are reflected in the new edition of this thorough and dedicated text.

Walter J. Hierholzer, Jr., M.D.
Professor of Medicine and Epidemiology
Internal Medicine
Yale University School of Medicine
Director, Epidemiology Program
Infectious Disease
Yale-New Haven Hospital

Preface

Nosocomial infections continue to be a major worldwide public health problem, despite advances in our understanding and control of these infections. Healthcare facilities and providers, in administering to the needs of patients, should consistently incorporate measures to prevent nosocomial infections in their patients and staff. Such measures may impact the community at large, since hospital microorganisms (especially antibiotic-resistant organisms) are carried into the community, resulting in further disease transmission. There is increasing concern over emerging and reemerging infections, and these may interactively involve both community and healthcare facilities.

Advances continue to be made in our knowledge of the epidemiologic and microbiologic aspects of nosocomial infections, as investigatory procedures become increasingly skilled and sophisticated. The increasing number of investigations reported from hospitals throughout the world shows a heightened recognition of and concern for nosocomial-infection problems. As our knowledge of the pathogenicity of infectious diseases expands and microorganisms are identified and differentiated in ever-greater detail, new approaches and new technology for control and prevention are being identified, thus improving our ability to identify routes of transmission. Epidemiologic studies have resulted in a clearer definition of risk factors, such that control efforts can be more efficiently focused at reducing the risks, including the re-design of equipment, when relevant. Additionally, educational efforts can be more specifically directed at newly determined risk factors in attempting to prevent the occurrence of such infections.

In spite of all the scientific advances made in our knowledge of the control and prevention of nosocomial infections (emphasis on education and training regarding infection control practices and the development and publication of guidelines for work practices in healthcare facilities). Nosocomial infections continue to thrive, due to a multiplicity of dynamic competing factors. The number of older patients with chronic diseases, as well as immunosuppressed patients with increased risks of infection, continues to increase. We also continue to develop new diagnostic and therapeutic technology that challenges the patients' defense mechanisms against infectious diseases. Healthcare workers may not consistently implement recommended infection control measures. The potential seriousness for patients, staff, and community of failing to implement measures is highlighted by transmission of multidrug-resistant tuberculosis organisms. The emergence of multi-resistant enterococci, whose resistance spectrum now commonly encompasses vancomycin, is another dynamic development adversely effecting control programs.

Other areas of concern remain. Infection control personnel are not always successful in effecting change in the behavior of hospital care personnel. There is often difficulty and reluctance to adopt new recommended procedures that have proven successful, and to eliminate procedures that have proven ineffective or counterproductive.

The broad spectrum of these problems is discussed in this Fourth Edition of *Hospital Infections.* All chapters have been revised and references updated. All chapters reflect new concepts and information. Just as previous editions incorporated new areas of emphasis and interest, the present edition now includes new chapters on The Practice of Epidemiology in Community Hospitals, The Role of Professional and Regulatory Organizations in Infection Control Programs, Infection Control in Developing Countries, and Tuberculosis.

This text is directed at health professionals and students with responsibilities or interest in hospital infections. Part I reviews the general considerations of hospital infections, Part II discusses the functional areas of concern, and Part III focuses on specific endemic and epidemic hospital infections. Epidemiologic principles are stressed throughout the book. Chapters are authored by individuals who have in-depth personal knowledge of the topics they have reviewed.

We are greatly indebted to the contributing authors for their willingness to distill and summarize a large amount of data and information into authoritative, succinct, and timely chapters for this Fourth

Edition. We also appreciate the efforts of authors who contributed to earlier editions; their contributions have invariably assisted in strengthening this edition. We acknowledge the support of our former publisher, Little, Brown and Company and the continued support of our current publisher, Lippincott-Raven Publishers.

John V. Bennett
Philip S. Brachman

Part I

General Considerations of Hospital Infections

Hospital Infections, Fourth Edition,
edited by John V. Bennett and Philip S. Brachman.
Lippincott–Raven Publishers, Philadelphia © 1998

CHAPTER 1

Epidemiology of Nosocomial Infections

Philip S. Brachman

BASIC CONSIDERATIONS

This chapter is a review of the basic principles of epidemiology with special emphasis on the relationship to nosocomial infections. An understanding of nosocomial infections is necessary for the development and implementation of effective and efficient control and prevention measures. Epidemiologic methods are used to define the factors related to the occurrence of disease, including the relations among the agent, its reservoir and source, the route of transmission, the host, and the environment. Once these relations have been defined for a specific disease, the most appropriate means of control and prevention should be discernible. Without defining each of these relations, control and prevention efforts are, at best, a gamble. Defining the epidemiologic relations introduces science into control and prevention and leads to more effective and economical use of all resources.

DEFINITIONS

Epidemiology

The term epidemiology is derived from the Greek epi (on or upon), demos (people or population), and logos (word or reason). Literally, it means "the study of things that happen to people"; historically, it has involved the study of epidemics. Epidemiology is the dynamic study of the determinants, occurrence, and distribution of health and disease in a population, which, for nosocomial infections, is the hospital population. Epidemiology defines the relation of disease to the population at risk and involves the determination, analysis, and interpretation of rates (see Chapters 6,7).

P. S. Brachman: Department of International Health, Rollins School of Public Health, Emory University, Atlanta, Georgia 30322.

The principles of epidemiology are also being applied to broaden knowledge of hospital-based occurrences other than infectious disease. Not only are noninfectious disease problems being studied using epidemiologic principles, but the broad area of patient care is being strengthened by the application of epidemiology to the many activities encompassed in quality assurance programs (see Chapter 2).

Infection

Infection entails the replication of organisms in the tissues of a host; the related development of overt clinical manifestations is known as disease; however, if the infection provokes an immune response only, without overt clinical disease, it is a subclinical or inapparent infection. Colonization implies the presence of a microorganism in or on a host, with growth and multiplication of the microorganism but without any overt clinical expression or detected immune reaction at the time it is isolated. Subclinical or inapparent infection refers to a relation between the host and microorganism in which the microorganism is present; there is no overt expression of the presence of the microorganism, but there is interaction between the host and microorganism that results in a detectable immune response, such as a serologic reaction, a skin test conversion, or a proliferative response of white blood cells to antigens from infecting organisms. Therefore, special tests to detect immune responses may be needed to differentiate colonization from subclinical infection. In the absence of such information, it is customary to employ the term colonization. A carrier (or colonized person) is an individual colonized with a specific microorganism and from whom the organism can be recovered (i.e., cultured) but who shows no overt expression of the presence of the microorganism at the time it is isolated; a carrier may have a history of previous disease due to that organism, such as typhoid. A carrier may disseminate the organism into the environment. The carrier state may be transient (or short-term), intermittent (or occasional), or chronic (long-term, persistent, or permanent). We have found, for example, in culture studies of hospital staff for nasal carriage of Staphylococcus aureus, that ~ 15% to 20% are noncarriers, 60% to 70% are intermittent carriers, and 10% to 15% are persistent carriers. Epidemiologically, the important consideration is whether the carrier is the source of the infection for another individual; any carrier who is disseminating or shedding the organism may subsequently infect another person. Also, the carrier may develop disease with the source of the organism being himself or herself (endogenous source).

Dissemination

Dissemination, or shedding of microorganisms, refers to the movement of organisms from a person carrying them into the immediate environment. To show this, one cultures samples of air or surfaces and swabs objects onto which microorganisms from the carrier may have been deposited. Shedding studies may be conducted in specially constructed chambers designed to quantitate dissemination. While shedding studies have occasionally been useful to document unusual dissemination, they have not generally been useful in identifying carriers whose dissemination has resulted in infection in other persons. In the hospital setting, dissemination is most effectively identified by means of surveillance, in which the occurrence of infection among contacts is noted. When infection is shown to result from dissemination of organisms from a person, that person is referred to as a dangerous disseminator.

The demonstration by culturing techniques that an individual is carrying a specific organism defines a potential problem, whereas epidemiologic demonstration by surveillance and investigative techniques defines the real problem. In some hospitals, routine culture surveys of all or selected asymptomatic staff may be conducted in an attempt to identify carriers of certain organisms, but such surveys lack practical relevance unless the results are related to specific cases or an outbreak of disease. This practice only identifies those who are culture-positive and does not in itself reliably separate colonized persons into disseminators as distinct from nondisseminators. Usually only a fraction of colonized persons are disseminating; thus nondisseminators are not associated with the actual spread of infection. If disease transmission has occurred and a human source of infection is suspected, culture surveys in conjunction with epidemiologic investigation to identify the potential source are realistic, and additional laboratory studies to confirm the presence of a dangerous disseminator may then be undertaken. Thus culture surveys and microbiologic studies of dissemination in the absence of disease problems are usually inappropriate and wasteful of resources.

In some instances, dissemination from a carrier has been reported to be influenced by the occurrence of an unrelated disease such as a second infection. One report, for example, suggested that infants carrying staphylococci in their nares disseminate staphylococci only after the onset of a viral respiratory infection. Such infants are called cloud babies (see Chapters 6, 41). In another instance, a physician disseminated staphylococci from his skin because of a reactivation of chronic dermatitis. Desquamation of his skin led to the transmission of staphylococci (probably by skin squames) to patients with whom he had contact. Dissemination has been reported of tetracycline-resistant Staphylococcus aureus from individuals carrying this organism who were treated with tetracycline. Dissemination may be constant or sporadic. If sporadic, it may result from the intermittent occurrence of some precipitating event, such as a second infection, or it may be due to other, unknown factors. The risk of dissemination is generally greater from individuals with disease caused by that organism than from individuals with subclinical infection or who are colonized with the organism.

Contamination refers to microorganisms that are transiently present on body surface (such as hands) without tissue invasion or physiologic reaction. Contamination also refers to the presence of microorganisms on or in an inanimate object.

NOSOCOMIAL INFECTIONS

Nosocomial infections are infections that develop within a hospital or are produced by microorganisms acquired during hospitalization. Nosocomial infections may involve not only patients but also anyone else who has contact with a hospital, including members of staff, volunteers, visitors, workers, salespersons, and delivery personnel. The majority of nosocomial infections become clinically apparent while the patients are still hospitalized; however, the onset of disease can occur after a patient has been discharged. As many as 25% of postoperative wound infections, for example, become symptomatic after the patient has been discharged (see Chapter 37). In these cases, the patient became colonized or infected while in the hospital, but the incubation period was longer than the patient's hospital stay. This sequence is also seen in some infections of newborns and in most breast abscesses of new mothers. Hepatitis B is an example of a nosocomial disease with a long incubation period; its clinical onset usually occurs long after the patient is discharged from the hospital.

Infections incubating at the time of the patient's admission to the hospital are not nosocomial; they are community-acquired, unless they result from a previous hospitalization. However, community-acquired infections can serve as a ready source of infection for other patients or personnel and thus must be considered in the total scope of hospital-related infections.

The term preventable infection implies that some event related to the infection could have been altered and that such alteration would have prevented the infection from occurring. A medical attendant who does not wash his or her hands between contacts with the urinary collection equipment of 2 patients, for example, may transmit gram-negative organisms from the first patient to the second, which may result in a urinary tract infection. Hand-washing might have prevented this infection from occurring. The identification of such an event in retrospect, however, is likely to be difficult; it is necessary to distinguish this situation from circumstances in which both patients developed infections from their own endogenous flora (e.g., from Escherichia coli). It is often impossible to identify the precise mode of acquisition of individual nosocomial infections. More than one mode may contribute to the development of the same infection, and not all modes may be preventable.

A nonpreventable infection is one that will occur despite all possible precautions for example, infection in an immunosuppressed patient due to endogenous flora. It has been estimated that ~ 30% of all reported nosocomial infections are preventable (see Chapter 4). Epidemics, especially common-vehicle epidemics, are potentially preventable; however, epidemics account for only a small number of the nosocomial infections that occur. Prompt investigation and the institution of rational control measures should reduce the number of cases involved in epidemics (see Chapter 6). Endemic infections account for the majority of nosocomial infections, and the consistent application of recognized, effective control and prevention measures for endemic infections is probably the single most important factor in reducing the overall level of nosocomial infections.

Source: Endogenous (Autogenous) or Exogenous

Organisms that cause nosocomial infections come from either endogenous (autogenous) or exogenous sources. Endogenous infections are caused by the patient's own flora; exogenous infections result from transmission of organisms from a source other than the patient. Either endogenous organisms are brought into the hospital by a patient (this represents colonization outside the hospital), or the patient becomes colonized after being admitted to the hospital. In either instance, the organisms colonizing the patient may subsequently cause a nosocomial infection. It may not always be possible to determine whether a particular organism isolated from the patient with an infection caused by that organism is exogenous or endogenous, and the term autogenous should be used in this situation. Autogenous infection indicates that the infection was derived from the flora of the patient, whether or not the infecting organism became part of the patient's flora subsequent to admission. Information about current disease problems in the community or in hospital contacts may be useful in differentiating the two sources. Microbiologic determinations of the characteristics of the organism such as phage typing, antibiograms, biochemical reactions, or genetic analysis may help identify strains of nosocomial origin (see Chapters 9,16).

Spectrum of Occurrence of Cases

To determine whether a nosocomial infection problem exists in a particular hospital, one must relate the current frequency of cases to the past history of the disease in that institution. To characterize a disease's frequency as sporadic, endemic, or epidemic, investigators must know something of the past occurrence of that disease in relation to time, place, and person. Sporadic means that cases occur occasionally and irregularly, without any specific pattern. Endemic means that the disease occurs with ongoing frequency in a specific geographic area in a finite population and over a defined time period. Hyperendemic refers to what appears to be a gradual increase in the occurrence of a disease in a defined area beyond the expected number of cases; however, it may not be certain whether the disease will occur at epidemic proportions. An epidemic is a definite increase in the incidence of a disease above its expected endemic occurrence. Outbreak is used interchangeably with epidemic; however, some people use outbreak to mean an increased rate of occurrence but not at levels as serious as an epidemic (see Chapter 5).

An occasional gas gangrene infection among postoperative patients is an example of a sporadic infection. An endemic nosocomial infection is represented by the regular occurrence of infections either in a particular site or at different sites that are due to the same organism, occur at a nearly constant rate, and are generally considered by the hospital staff to be within expected and acceptable limits. Surgical wound infections due to a single organism that follow operations classified as "contaminated surgery," for example, could represent the endemic level of postoperative wound infections.

An epidemic classically begins with a sudden increase in the occurrence of disease among susceptible persons who have had contact with a contaminated source, but the onset of disease occurs at an unusually high frequency relative to that expected. On the other hand, an epidemic may also result from prolonged exposure to the source of the organism, with cases occurring irregularly due to irregular dissemination or distribution of the agent, irregular contact between the agent and a susceptible host, or irregular presence of a susceptible host. Cases of salmonellosis, for example, may result from contact with a contaminated food to which patients and staff are exposed over a long period of time, possibly months before it is identified. Only an occasional case of salmonellosis may result from this exposure but, depending on the past history of salmonellosis in the institution, these cases may represent epidemic salmonellosis.

A characteristic sharp and abrupt increase in the number of cases may fail to occur with diseases having a long and variable incubation period. Many people may be exposed to hepatitis B virus at one particular time, for example, but the appearance of the resulting disease may be spread out over weeks, thereby obscuring the presence of an epidemic (see Chapter 6).

Incidence and Prevalence

Occurrence of infection is quantified by calculating its incidence and prevalence. Incidence is the number of new cases in a specific population in a defined time period. To determine the true incidence of a disease, culture or serologic surveys may be necessary. Prevalence is the total number of current cases of an infection in a defined population at one point in time (point prevalence) or over a longer period of time (period prevalence). The prevalence rate will include cases of recent onset as well as cases of earlier onset that are still clinically apparent (see Chapter 5).

EPIDEMIOLOGIC METHODS

There are generally three techniques used in epidemiologic studies—descriptive, analytic, and experimental—all of which may be used in investigating nosocomial infections. The basic epidemiologic method, descriptive epidemiology, is used in most investigations. Once the initial problem has been defined, however, additional studies using one of the other two methods can be conducted to develop more information about the problem, confirm initial impressions, prove and disprove hypotheses, and evaluate the effectiveness of control measures, prevention measures, or both. Additionally, the principles involved in these methods have application to surveillance; surveillance data are commonly analyzed by the descriptive method, and such analysis may suggest the need for analytic studies to identify certain features of a disease. Furthermore, analysis of surveillance data may lead to the development of experimental studies to deal with a specific disease.

Descriptive Epidemiology

Descriptive epidemiology describes the occurrence of disease in terms of time, place, and person; each case of a disease is first characterized by describing these three attributes (see Chapter 6). When data from the individual cases are combined and analyzed, the parameters of the epidemic or disease problem should be characterized.

Time

There are four time trends to consider: secular, periodic, seasonal, and acute. Secular trends are long-term trends in the occurrence of a disease—that is, variations that occur over a period of years. The gradual but steady reduction in the incidence of diphtheria in the United States over the past 50 years, for example, is the secular trend of that disease. The secular trend generally reflects the immunologic, socioeconomic, educational, and nutritional levels of the population from which the secular data have been reported. In a hospital, the secular trend of a disease may be difficult to portray due to the lack of adequate data concerning the occurrence of the disease over time.

Periodic trends are temporal interruptions of the secular trend and usually reflect changes in the overall susceptibility to the disease in the population. The upsurge in influenza A activity every 2 to 3 years, for instance, reflects the periodic trend of this disease and is generally the result of antigenic drift of the influenza A virus. The periodic trend can also reflect the variations in the herd immunity of a specific population (the herd).

Seasonal trends are the annual variations in disease incidence that are related in part to seasons. In general, the occurrence of a particular communicable disease increases when the circumstances that influence its transmission are favorable. The seasonal pattern of both community-acquired and nosocomial respiratory disease, for example, involves high incidence in the fall and winter months, when transmission through the air is enhanced because people are together in rooms with closed windows and are breathing unfiltered, recirculating air. Thus they have greater contact with one another and with droplets as well as droplet nuclei. There may also be agent and host factors that influence the seasonal trends. The seasonal trend of foodborne disease involves higher incidence in the summer months when ambient temperatures are elevated and refrigeration may be inadequate. Foods contaminated with what normally are non-disease-producing levels of microorganisms may be allowed to incubate, resulting in the attainment of infectious doses.

The fourth type of time variation is the acute or epidemic occurrence of a disease with its characteristic upsurge in incidence. The overall shape of the epidemic curve depends on the interaction of many factors: characteristics of the specific agent; its pathogenicity, concentration, and incubation period; the mode and ease of its transmission; the method of transmission; host factors, including the susceptibility and concentration of susceptible individuals; and environmental factors, such as temperature, humidity, movement of air, and general housekeeping.

An epidemic can be portrayed by an epidemic curve that is, a graphic representation of the number of cases of the disease plotted against time (see Chapter 6). The time scale will vary according to the incubation or latency period, ranging from minutes, as in an outbreak of disease following exposure to a toxin or a chemical, to months, as in a nosocomial epidemic of hepatitis B. The time scale (abscissa or horizontal scale) should be selected with three facts in mind: (1) The unit time interval should be less than the average incubation period (commonly one fourth to one third the probable incubation period) so that the true nature of the epidemic curve will be apparent (i.e., all the cases will not be bunched together); (2) the scale should be carried out far enough in time to allow all cases to be plotted; and (3) any cases that occurred before the epidemic should be plotted to give a basis for comparison with the epidemic experience [1].

If the epidemic curve starts with the index case (i.e., the first case in the outbreak), the time between the index case and onset of the next case reflects the incubation period if transmission was from the index case directly to the next case—that is, from person to person. The upslope in the curve is determined by the incubation period, the number and concentration of exposed susceptible persons, the number of infected sources, and the ease of transmission. The height of the peak of the curve is influenced by the total number of exposed susceptible individuals and the time interval over which they occur. The downslope of the curve is usually more gradual than the upslope; its gradual change reflects cases with longer incubation periods and the decreasing number of susceptible individuals. The initiation of control measures may contribute to the gradual decline or to a sudden decrease in the appearance of new cases. Cases resulting from secondary transmission-that is, resulting from contact with earlier cases in the epidemic-will also be represented on the downslope of the epidemic curve or, occasionally, by a second upswing, which reflects a second, distinct, and usually smaller wave or cluster of cases following the main outbreak. Consecutive clusters of cases may represent ongoing transmission from new focuses or from one focus that is intermittently or periodically infective or from which organisms are periodically disseminated. When consecutive clusters of cases occur resulting from transmission from one cluster to the next, we refer to each cluster as a generation-first generation of cases, second generation of cases, and so on. This may also be referred to as a propagated epidemic. In a common-vehicle epidemic in which contact with the common vehicle is limited to a defined period, the epidemic curve usually rises rather sharply and then gradually falls off. However, if the common vehicle is present consistently or sporadically over a prolonged period, then the epidemic curve will be prolonged over time. In a contact-spread epidemic (person-to-person), the epidemic curve usually rises gradually, has a flatter peak than the common-vehicle curve, and then falls off.

Place

The second feature of descriptive epidemiology is place. In an investigation, there may be three different places involved. The first is where the patient is when disease is diagnosed, and the second is where contact occurred between the patient and the agent. If a vehicle of infection is involved, the third place is where the vehicle became infected. To implement the most appropriate control and preventive measures, it is necessary to distinguish between these three geographic areas; certain actions may control additional spread from a specific focus but may not prevent new cases from occurring if the source continues to infect new vehicles. Several examples will help to emphasize the importance of carefully describing place or places involved in disease outbreaks.

In an outbreak of nosocomial salmonellosis, the patients were located on various wards throughout the hospital at the time they developed disease. Individual control measures were directed at each patient on the various wards; however, the place of infection was the radiology department, where barium used for gastrointestinal tract roentgenographic examinations was contaminated with salmonella. The barium had been contaminated in the radiology department, and thus preventive measures directed there resolved the problem..

Another example involves outbreaks of septicemia associated with intravenous fluids. In these instances, it is important to determine whether the fluid became contaminated in the process of manufacture (intrinsic contamination) or after the fluid had been bottled (extrinsic contamination). Extrinsic contamination can occur during shipment to the hospital, after being brought into the hospital, while being prepared for use, or during actual use. Delineation of the epidemiological parameters of this problem is important in order to be able to institute the most effective control and/or preventive measures to prevent further infections (see Chapter 44).

Person

The third major component of descriptive epidemiology is person. Careful evaluation of host factors related to the individual person includes consideration of age, sex, race, immunization status, competence of the immune system, and presence of underlying disease that may influence susceptibility (acute or chronic), therapeutic or diagnostic procedures, medications, and nutritional status (see Chapter 6). In essence, any host factor that can influence the development of disease must be considered and described. Those that increase the patient's chance of developing disease are known as risk factors.

Age sometimes influences the occurrence of diseases and also provides a clue regarding the cause of an outbreak. Persons at either end of the age spectrum-the young and the elderly-are generally more susceptible to disease. Such susceptibility may reflect levels of immunity, both active and passive, as well as the levels of less specific personal factors of protection against development of disease. Age can also be an important clue to the source of an outbreak of disease. If, in an apparent common-source outbreak, for example, all ages from infancy to old age are involved, then the source of the outbreak must have been available to patients scattered through at least several wards. On the other hand, if all the patients involved in an epidemic are women of childbearing age, then in attempting to identify the place of the exposure, the investigation can be narrowed to the obstetric or, possibly, the gynecologic ward.

Consideration of therapeutic procedures may be of similar importance. If all patients who developed bacteremia due to the same organism have received intravenous fluid therapy, then a common source of intravenous fluids would be suspected as the cause of the outbreak.

These few examples demonstrate that the description of individual host factors among involved patients may identify important information that may lead to a solution of the epidemic problem.

Analytic Epidemiology

The second method of epidemiologic investigation is analytic epidemiology, in which the determinants of disease distribution are evaluated in terms of possible causal relations. An hypothesis generated by a descriptive epidemiology study can be evaluated by an analytic epidemiology study. Two basic methods are used: case-control and cohort studies. In both instances, associations are sought that may identify causes and effects: the case-control method starts with the effect (cases) and searches for causative host and exposure factors: the cohort method starts with potential causative factors and evaluates the effect. The case-control and cohort methods have also been referred to as retrospective and prospective studies, respectively; both methods, however, can be either retrospective or prospective. These terms indicate the temporal frame of reference for the collection of specific data: in a retrospective study, data are collected after the event has occurred; in a prospective study, the data are collected as the event occurs.

Case-Control Study

The case-control method starts with an allocation of persons between a study group (those already affected with the disease) and a comparison control group or groups (see Chapters 6, 7). The comparison group should be selected from the same population that the case group came from and be similar to the case group except ideally they should not have had the disease or condition being investigated. The latter event may be difficult to ascertain. Questions are then asked of both groups pertaining to past events that may identify the causative factor. Any differences between these groups are then determined. In an outbreak of nosocomial urinary tract infections due to Proteus rettgeri, for example, a group of patients with this infection was compared to a group that did not have urinary tract infection due to P. rettgeri. It was shown that the infected patients were more likely than the comparison group patients to have had indwelling urinary tract catheters, to have been located in the same area of the hospital, and to have previously received systemic antibiotic therapy. Thus it was concluded that in this epidemic, indwelling urethral catheters, proximity of patients to one another, and previous systemic antibiotic therapy were directly related to the subsequent development of urinary tract infections due to P. rettgeri.

The case-control approach has the advantages of being inexpensive, relatively quick, and easily reproducible. It is used most often in acute disease investigations, since the epidemiologist arrives after a problem is recognized and often after the peak of the epidemic has passed. This approach, however, may introduce bias into the selection of the control group since it may be difficult retrospectively to reconstruct the involved and noninvolved populations. In selecting a comparison control group, bias may be introduced if one is unable to exclude patients who are asymptomatically infected with the causative agent being studied. A lesser problem, but a real one, is ascertaining in retrospect that a patient actually had disease and was not asymptomatically infected or colonized. This latter circumstance presents considerable difficulty in categorizing critically ill patients with manifestations that resemble those of infection but stem from other causes. Fortunately, the search for sources can be pursued by including all culture-positive persons in the case definition, and thus it need not be restricted to those with clinical disease. This approach does, however, jeopardize the search for important host factors related to disease occurrence. Another limitation is the memory of the involved patients for past events, the specification of which may be important to the investigation. Also, the hospital records may lack documentation of events important to the investigation. These limitations derive from the retrospective approach rather than deficiencies in the case-control approach per se. Indeed prospective case-control studies can be implemented, but usually they have little usefulness in outbreak investigations.

Cohort Study

In the cohort method, patients exposed to a factor are compared with a group not exposed to the factor to see what the effect will be. In the above outbreak of P. rettgeri urinary tract infections, for example, the importance of the proximity of patients with urethral catheter-an infectious risk-was prospectively analyzed by scattering certain patients with urethral catheters throughout the hospital. Inhibition of the nosocomial spread of infection was demonstrated by this cohort approach. Several cohorts may be followed, each representing a different level of exposure to a factor, thus allowing for the determination of a dose response.

The advantage of the cohort study is that it provides a direct estimate of the risk carried by a particular factor for disease occurrence, and this is relatively easy to accomplish when the incubation period is short. Although bias may still be a problem, it is less likely to be introduced in this type of study, which usually is conducted prospectively. The cohort study, however, is usually more difficult, more expensive, and more time-consuming than retrospective studies. For diseases with long incubation periods, the difficulties may be insurmountable.

Another technique of analytic epidemiology is a cross-sectional survey, which allows for collection of data over a specific limited period of time. It makes possible accessing the relation between two or more factors, the presence of which can be confirmed at the time of the survey.

Experimental Epidemiology

The third method of epidemiologic investigation is the experimental method, which is a definitive method of proving or disproving a hypothesis. The experimental method assumes that risk or protective factors are followed by effects on outcomes and that a deliberate manipulation of these factors is predictably followed by an alteration in the outcomes that could rarely be explained by chance. The two groups selected for study are ideally similar in all respects except for the presence of the study factor in one group. Either the case-control or the cohort method is used to evaluate the interaction between the cause and the effect.

An example of the experimental method is the evaluation of a new drug as treatment for a disease: A group of patients with the disease is randomly divided into two subgroups that are equal in all respects, except one of the subgroups is treated with the experimental drug and the other subgroup (the control group) is given a placebo or another agent known to be effective in treating or preventing the disease. If there is no other variation between the two groups, any differences in the course of the disease may be ascribed to the use of the drug.

The experimental method has less direct use in the investigation of outbreaks of nosocomial disease today than the other two methods. This method, however, does have usefulness in assessing general patient care practices and in evaluating new methods to control and prevent disease. Placebo controlled trials have less use in therapeutic studies because of the need for informed consent and the need to prevent placing the patient at an unjustified or greater risk in attempting to conduct a specific study.

CHAIN OF INFECTION

General Aspects

Infection results from the interaction between an infectious agent and a susceptible host. This interaction-called transmission-occurs by means of contact between the agent and the host. Three interrelated factors-the agent, transmission, and the host-represent the chain of infection.

The links interrelate in and are affected by the environment; this relation is referred to as the ecology of infection-that is, the relation of microorganisms to disease as affected by the factors of their environment. In attempting to control and/or prevent nosocomial infections, an attack on the chain of infection at its weakest link is generally the most effective procedure. With definition of the links in the chain for each nosocomial infection, future trends of the disease should be predictable, and it should be possible to develop effective control and prevention techniques. Defining the chain of infection leads to specific action, in contrast to the incorporation of nonspecific actions in an attempt to control a nosocomial infection problem.

Disease causation is multifactorial-that is, disease results from the interaction of many factors related to the agent, transmission, and host. The development of disease reflects the interaction of these factors as they affect a person. Thus some people exposed to an infectious agent develop disease and others do not. For example, among a group of people exposed to group A hemolytic streptococci, usually only some develop disease; this reflects the variability in the various factors related to susceptibility and the development of disease. Determination as to why some exposed persons did not develop disease may be useful in developing control/prevention measures for that disease.

Agent

The first link in the chain of infection is the microbial agent, which may be a bacterium, virus, fungus, or parasite. The majority of nosocomial infection problems are caused by bacteria and viruses; fungi are assuming a greater role, and parasites rarely cause nosocomial infections. There are a number of factors that help to portray the agent.

Infectiousness

The determination of the number of the susceptible individuals who become infected with an organism to which they are exposed is a measure of the infectiousness of that organism. Host factors can influence the infectiousness of an organism.

Pathogenicity

The measure of the ability of microorganisms to induce disease is referred to as pathogenicity, and it may be assessed by disease-colonization ratios. One organism with high pathogenicity is Yersinia pestis; it almost always causes clinical disease in a host. An organism with low pathogenicity is alpha-hemolytic streptococcus; it commonly colonizes in humans but only rarely causes clinical disease. The pathogenicity of an organism is additionally described by characterizing the organism's virulence and invasiveness.

Virulence is the measure of the severity of the disease. In epidemiologic studies, virulence is defined more specifically by assessing morbidity and mortality rates and the degree of communicability. The virulence of organisms ranges from slightly to highly virulent. Although some organisms are described as avirulent, it appears that any organism can cause disease under certain circumstances. It may be possible to reduce virulence by a deliberate manipulation of the organism (e.g., by repeated subculturing on a specific medium or by exposure to a certain drug or to radiation). Purposeful attempts to develop avirulent strains have been related to efforts to develop a microbial strain for vaccination purposes, such as the attenuated poliomyelitis virus used for oral vaccination. Under certain host-factor conditions, however, clinical poliomyelitis can result from oral vaccination with the attenuated strain. Some naturally occurring organisms have been considered avirulent or of low virulence; however, under certain conditions-such as high doses, host immunodeficiency, or both-disease has resulted from contact with these organisms. For years, Serratia marcescens, for example, was considered to be an avirulent organism; because of this and because certain strains produce easily recognizable red pigment, these organisms were used for environmental studies in hospitals. However, as hospitalized patients became more susceptible to developing infections due to advancing age, presence of chronic diseases, and the effects of new diagnostic and therapeutic measures-nosocomial disease due to S. marcescens organisms subsequently became recognized and reported. It became apparent that this organism could cause disease in individuals with compromised defense systems. Thus avirulence is a relative term; whether an organism is avirulent depends on many factors including agent factors such as dose and host factors such as responsiveness of the immune system, and the nutritional status.

Invasiveness describes the ability of microorganisms to invade tissues. Some organisms can penetrate the intact integument, whereas other microorganisms can enter only through a break in the skin or mucous membranes. An example of the former is Leptospira and of the latter, Clostridium tetani. Vibrio cholerae organisms are noninvasive: Once in the gastrointestinal tract, they do not invade the endothelium; rather, they elaborate a toxin that is absorbed. Shigella organisms are highly invasive and cause a symptomatic response by invading the submucosal tissue.

Dose

Another important agent factor is dose-that is, the number of organisms available to cause infection. The infective dose of an agent is that quantity of the agent necessary to cause infection. The number of organisms necessary to cause infection varies from organism to organism and from host to host, and it will be influenced by the mode of transmission. The relation of dose to the onset of typhoid fever, for example, was shown in volunteer studies by Hornick and colleagues [2], who demonstrated that with an inoculum of 10^3 S. typhosa, no clinical disease developed in normal volunteers. However, when the inoculum was increased to 10^7 salmonellae, there was a 50% attack rate among the volunteers and, with an inoculum of 10^9 organisms, there was a 95% attack rate.

Specificity

Microorganisms may be specific with respect to their range of hosts. St. Louis encephalitis virus, for example, has a broad range of hosts, including many avian species, mammals, and mosquitoes. On the other hand, Rickettsia prowazekii, the species that causes typhus, has a very narrow host range, involving body lice and humans. Brucella abortus is highly communicable in cattle but not in humans. Some Salmonella species, such as S. typhimurium, are common to both animals and humans, but others have a narrow range of specificity; for example, S. dublin primarily infects bovines, and S. typhosa is known to infect only humans.

Other Agent Factors

Other characteristics of the organism, such as the production of enzymes, are directed toward overcoming the defense mechanisms of the host. Streptococci, for example, produce leukocidin, hemolysin, and proteinase, all of which are directed toward overcoming humoral and tissue defense mechanisms of the host. Some agents produce polysaccharide capsules and others, toxins, that may give an advantage to the organism.

Certain antigenic variations within species of microorganisms influence the disease-producing potential of the organism. Of the 83 different pneumococcal serotypes, for instance, 14 cause >80% of human pneumococcal pneumonia infections. Among streptococci, group A organisms are associated with infections of the pharynx, whereas group B organisms are primarily associated with infections of the genitourinary tract.

The antigenic makeup of an organism may change, allowing a new variant to spread through a population because of the lack of host resistance to the new variant. This is seen with influenza A; every 2 to 3 years, a modified variant becomes prevalent and spreads throughout the country. This phenomenon is known as antigenic drift. More significant changes in influenza A may occur irregularly; these changes are known as major antigenic shifts.

Resistance-transfer plasmids also influence the occurrence of nosocomial disease (see Chapters 16). The transfer of R plasmids from one enteric organism to another has occurred in hospital outbreaks and may account for a change in the antibiotic sensitivity of a strain. The antibiotic sensitivity of hospital organisms is also influenced by the use of antibiotics in the hospital (see Chapter 14); more resistant strains are selected as a result of the increased use of a particular antibiotic (or antibiotics) against which specific resistance plasmids are commonly carried by prevalent nosocomial strains. If a common R plasmid-mediated resistance pattern of E. coli in a hospital is ampicillin, tetracycline, and sulfonamide, for example, then the pressures deriving from the use of any one of these drugs will concurrently select for strains with the other two resistances as well. This change in antibiotic sensitivity may make therapy difficult; it can result in an increasing prevalence of the resistant strain, reduce the necessary infecting or colonizing doses of the organism in those receiving drugs to which these strains are resistant, increase the numbers of organisms disseminated from persons colonized with these strains, and potentially increase the frequency of nosocomial infections due to this more resistant strain.

Other organism factors, some plasmid-mediated, include the ability to adhere to intestinal mucosa, resist gastric acid and disinfectants, and produce bacteriocins active against endogenous flora.

Reservoir and Source

All organisms have a reservoir and a source; these may be the same or different, and it is important to distinguish between these potentially different sites if control and/or prevention measures are to be directed at this aspect of the chain of infection. The reservoir is the place where the organism maintains its presence, metabolizes, and replicates. Viruses generally survive better in human reservoirs; the reservoir of gram-positive bacteria is usually a human, whereas gram-negative bacteria may have either a human or animal reservoir (e.g., Salmonella) or an inanimate reservoir (e.g., Pseudomonas in water). The reservoir may be highly specific: For poliomyelitis virus, for example, the reservoir is always human. On the other hand, Pseudomonas species may be found in either an animate or an inanimate reservoir.

The source is the place from which the infectious agent passes to the host, either by direct or indirect contact, air, or a vector as the means of transmission. Sources also may be animate or inanimate. The source may become contaminated from the reservoir. For example, a reservoir for Pseudomonas organisms may be the tap water in a hospital; however, the source from which it is transmitted to the patient may be a humidifier that has been filled directly with the contaminated tap water. In a common-source outbreak of measles, the reservoir and source may be the same—a person.

The source may be mobile or fixed. A susceptible patient may be brought to a fixed source (e.g., a patient who comes to use a contaminated whirlpool bath), or the source may be mobile and brought to the patient (e.g., contaminated food brought from the kitchen to the patient's bedside).

Period of Infectivity

Infectivity refers to the ability of an organism to spread from a source to a host. An infected human may be infective during the incubation period, the clinical disease state, or convalescence. Additionally, an asymptomatic carrier (or colonized person), who does not show evidence of clinical disease, may be infective. An example of a disease that is primarily infectious during the incubation period is hepatitis A: The infected individual is infective during the latter half of the incubation period and during the first several days of clinical disease. In measles, the patient is infective during the prodromal stage to ~ 4 days after the onset of the rash. In chickenpox, the individual is infective from ~ 5 days before the skin eruption to ≤ 6 days after the appearance of the eruption. A disease in which the individual is infective primarily during the initial clinical disease phase is exemplified by influenza, in which the individual is infective for a period of several days after the onset of symptoms. In cases of tuberculosis and typhoid fever, the individual may be infective for essentially the entire pretreatment clinical phase, with infectivity usually significantly decreasing when there is clinical evidence of successful chemotherapy. Examples of diseases that are infectious into the convalescent period are salmonellosis, shigellosis, and diphtheria. In some diseases, such as typhoid fever and hepatitis B, a chronic carrier state may develop in which the individual may be infective for a long time, possibly years, while showing no symptoms of illness. However, the microorganisms that most commonly cause nosocomial infections such as E. coli, Klebsiella, Enterobacter, and Pseudomonas do not demonstrate the same patterns of infectivity or evoke the protective immune responses that typhoid fever and hepatitis B do.

Asymptomatic or subclinical carriers may be the more important source of infection than the clincally infected individual. This is seen, for example, in poliomyelitis and hepatitis A. In poliomyelitis, the ratio is ~ 100 carriers to 1 clinical case, and in hepatitis A, 10:1. In spite of not showing clinical evidence of infection, the person with a subclinical infection may be an active transmitter of infection, and clinical disease may result from such transmission. Dissemination from an asymptomatic carrier may be related to a specific event, such as the occurrence of a second disease process (see previous discussion). However, dissemination may also occur that is unrelated to any definable event. The staphylococcus carrier provides a classic example of the asymptomatic dissemination of infectious organisms; in this case, the site of dissemination may be the anterior nares or, at times, the skin. Similarly, the site of asymptomatic streptococcal carriage may be in the pharynx, perianal area, or vagina.

The source of an infection may be an atypical case of a specific disease whose clinical course has been modified by therapy, vaccine (as in measles), or prophylaxis (such as the use of immune serum globulin in hepatitis A). Also, the source may be an abortive case of disease in which the typical expression of the disease has been modified by treatment with antibiotics.

Animals may also provide a source of infection, although this is of less concern in the hospital setting.

Exit

The portal of exit for organisms from humans is usually single, although it may be multiple. It may not always be the obvious portal of exit; in bubonic plague, for example, in which the skin lesions are the most visible concern, exit by the airborne route from unrecognized secondary pneumonia is also of great importance in transmission. In general, the major portals of exit are the respiratory and gastrointestinal tracts as well as the skin and wounds. Blood may also be the portal of exit, as in hepatitis B or human immunodeficiency virus (HIV) infections. However, depending on the organism, any bodily secretion or excretion can be infectious.

Transmission

Transmission, the second link in the chain of infection, describes the movement of organisms from the source to the host. Spread may occur through one or more of four different routes: contact, common-vehicle, airborne, or vectorborne. An organism may have a single route of transmission, or it may be transmissible by two or more routes. Tuberculosis, for example, is almost always transmitted by the airborne route; measles is primarily a contact-spread disease but may also be transmitted through the air; salmonellae may be transmitted by contact or by the common-vehicle, airborne, or vectorborne routes. Thus in defining the route of transmission, although one route may be the obvious one involved in a nosocomial infection problem, another route may also be operative. Knowledge regarding the route of transmission for a specific disease can be very helpful in the investigation of a nosocomial infection problem. Such information can point to the source and may allow control measures to be introduced more rapidly.

Contact Spread

In contact-spread disease, the victim has contact with the source, and that contact is direct, indirect, or by droplets. Direct contact, of which person-to-person spread is an example, occurs when there is actual physical contact between the source and the victim, such as in the oral-oral spread of infectious mononucleosis virus. Infections resulting from organisms within the patient may be referred to as autogenous infections; that is, the mode of acquisition is autogenous, even though acquisition or transmission may have occurred earlier, namely, at the time the host became colonized with the organism.

Indirect-contact transmission is distinguished from direct-contact transmission by the participation of an intermediate object (usually inanimate) that is passively involved in the transmission of the infectious agent from the source to the susceptible host. The intermediate object may become contaminated from an animate or inanimate source. An example is the transfer to susceptible hosts of enteric organisms on an endoscope that initially became contaminated when brought in contact with an infected patient (the index patient).

Droplet spread refers to the brief passage of the infectious agent through the air when the source and the victim are relatively near each other, usually within several feet, such as when there is transmission by talking or sneezing. Droplets are large particles (~ 5 μm or larger) that rapidly settle out on horizontal surfaces; thus they are not transmitted beyond a radius of several feet from the source. Examples of droplet-spread infections include measles and streptococcal pharyngitis.

Common-Vehicle Spread

In common-vehicle-spread infection, a contaminated inanimate vehicle, such as food, water and other liquids, and drugs, serves as the vector for transmission of the agent to multiple persons. The victims become infected after contact with the common vehicle. This transmission may be active if the organisms replicate while in the vehicle, such as salmonellae in food, or passive if the organisms are passively carried by the vehicle, such as hepatitis A in food. Other types of common vehicles include blood and blood products (hepatitis B and HIV), intravenous fluids (gram-negative septicemia), and drugs (salmonellosis), in which units or batches of a product become contaminated from a common source and serve as a common vehicle for multiple infections. Thus multiple vehicles may all become contaminated from a single common source. Even though there are multiple vehicles involved, these infections may be considered to be transmitted by a common vehicle because the epidemiologic principles are the same. It should be noted that common source and common vehicle are not interchangeable terms. A common source is just that: a source common to multiple vehicles from which the vehicles become infected. A common vehicle, on the other hand, is a vehicle of infection associated with two or more cases of a disease. If only a single infection results, the designation of direct-contact or indirect-contact spread, whichever is appropriate for the circumstances, should be used.

Airborne Spread

Airborne transmission describes organisms that have a true airborne phase in their route of dissemination, which usually involves a distance of more than several feet between the source and the victim. The organisms are contained within droplet nuclei or dust particles or on skin squames; the droplet nuclei are airborne particles that result from the evaporation of droplets, that originate from the oral cavity, typically by coughing or sneezing. Droplet nuclei are commonly 1 to 5 μm in size, though some particles ≤ 10 mm in size may also be transmitted by the airborne route and they may remain suspended in air for prolonged periods of time. Dust particles that have settled on surfaces may become resuspended by physical action and may also remain airborne for a prolonged period. Skin squamae may become airborne and provide a mechanism for the airborne transmission of organisms such as staphylococci. Airborne particles may remain suspended for hours or possibly days, depending on environmental factors. Movement may be within a room, or—again depending on environmental factors, especially air currents—transmission may be over a longer distance. The size and density of the airborne particle will also influence the distance it moves.

Airborne spread by means of droplet nuclei is exemplified in the transmission of tuberculosis and, in some instances, staphylococcal infections. The classic experiments of Riley and co-workers [3] demonstrated the airborne route of infection for tubercle bacilli, in which the source of the organisms was disseminating patients with active, sputum-positive, cavitary disease. Some nosocomial staphylococcal disease has been shown to be transmitted by the airborne route. In one report, several postoperative wound infections were said to have resulted from the airborne spread of staphylococci from a staff member who remained at the periphery of the operating room throughout the surgical procedure; the only route for transmission of the organisms was through the air, there being no opportunity in this case for contact or common-vehicle spread [4].

Organisms may be transmitted in dust, as was seen, for example, in an outbreak of salmonellosis, in which transmission occurred by means of contaminated dust contained in a vacuum cleaner bag; the dust became resuspended each time the vacuum cleaner was used [5].

Skin squamae are the superficial cells of skin that become airborne by the rubbing of the skin such as by clothing that moves across the skin under normal conditions. The squamae may carry organisms such as staphylococci that can be infectious if deposited on a susceptible host. Several outbreaks of streptococcal wound infections have been reported in which the reservoir and source was a hospital staff person with skin squamae being the hypothesized means of transmission.

The airborne route of transmission is more frequently assumed to be the route of an infection than is the case. Creation of an infectious aerosol is more difficult than is usually recognized.

Vectorborne Spread

Vectorborne-spread nosocomial disease, although unreported in the United States, could occur; it includes external and internal vector transmission. External vectorborne transmission refers to the mechanical transfer of microorganisms on the body or appendages of the vector; shigellae and salmonellae are reported to be transferred in this way by flies, for example. Internal vectorborne transmission includes harborage and biologic transmission. In transmission by harborage, there is no biologic action between the vector and the agent; this is seen with Y. pestis organisms in the gastrointestinal tract of the flea. Biologic transmission occurs when the agent (e.g., a parasite) goes through a biologic change within the vector, as malaria parasites do within the mosquito.

Host

The third link in the chain of infection is the host or victim. Disease does not always follow the transmission of infectious agents to a host. As previously discussed, various agent factors play a part; similarly, a variety of host factors must also be surmounted before infection occurs and disease develops. Host factors that influence the development of infections are the site of deposition of the agent and the host's defense mechanisms, referred to as immunity, either specific or nonspecific.

Entrance

Sites of deposition include the skin, mucous membranes, and respiratory, gastrointestinal, and urinary tracts. Organisms such as leptospires can gain entrance through normal skin. Other organisms, such as staphylococci, need a minute breach in the integrity of the skin to gain entrance to the body. There may be mechanical transmission through the normal skin, as with hepatitis B or HIV viruses on a contaminated needle or in contaminated blood. Abnormal skin, such as a preexisting wound, may be the site of deposition of organisms such as Pseudomonas aeruginosa. Mucous membranes may be the site of entrance, as the conjunctiva is for adenovirus type 8.

Another site of deposition is the respiratory tract. The exact area of deposition will depend on the size of the airborne particle and the aerodynamics at the time of transmission. Generally, particles 5 μm or larger in diameter will be deposited in the upper respiratory tract, whereas those < 5 μm in diameter will be deposited in the lower respiratory tract.

Infectious agents may gain entrance to the body through the intestinal tract by means of ingestion of contaminated foods or liquids, contaminated supplemental feedings, contaminated medications, or through contaminated equipment, such as endoscopes inserted into the intestinal tract. Within the gastrointestinal tract, some organisms cause disease by secreting a toxin that is absorbed through the mucosa (enterotoxigenic E. coli), whereas others invade the wall of the intestinal tract (Shigella). Some microorganisms involve primarily the upper part of the gastrointestinal tract (Staphylococcus), and others, the lower part of the tract (Shigella). The urinary tract may become infected from contaminated foreign objects such as catheters or cystoscopes inserted into the uretha, or by the retrograde movement of organisms on the external surface of a catheter inserted into the bladder.

Organisms may gain entrance into the host via the placenta, as occurs in rubella and toxoplasmosis. Transplantation is another method by which microorganisms enter the host; infection may follow renal transplantation if the donated kidney is infected with cytomegalovirus.

An organism may colonize one site and cause no disease, but the same organism at another site may result in clinical disease. E. coli, for example, routinely colonizes the gastrointestinal tract and under normal circumstances does not cause disease; however, the same organism in the urinary tract may cause infection. S. aureus may colonize the external nares without any evidence of disease but, when the same organism colonizes a fresh surgical wound, a postoperative wound infection may develop.

Nonspecific Defense Mechanisms

Nonspecific defense mechanisms include the skin, mucous membranes, certain bodily secretions, and certain other factors. The skin forms the first barrier against infection; it is a mechanical barrier and contains secretions that have an antibacterial action. Tears, a form of epithelial secretion, have an antibacterial action (due to lysozyme), and they also mechanically remove entrapped organisms. The gastrointestinal tract secretes acid that acts as a barrier against enteric organisms. Other secretions, such as mucus and enzymes, bolster the defense mechanisms. The muscular contractions of the intestinal tract act to move the contents through the tract and thus reduce the available time for organisms to invade the mucosa. Within the nose and upper respiratory tract, the cilia act to remove organisms that impinge on them. The blanket of mucus serves to entrap and remove infectious agents. The lower respiratory tract is protected by secretions and macrophages that ingest microorganisms and carry them to regional lymph nodes.

The local inflammatory response provides another nonspecific host defense mechanism. Other nonspecific protective mechanisms include genetic, hormonal, and nutritional factors, as well as behavioral patterns and personal hygiene. Age, as influenced by these nonspecific factors, is associated with decreased resistance at either end of the spectrum; the very young and the very old frequently are more susceptible to infection. Surgery and the presence of chronic diseases-such as diabetes, blood disorders, certain lymphomas, and collagen diseases-alter host resistance, which again reflects the influence of the nonspecific factors just cited.

Specific Defense Mechanisms

Specific immunity results from either natural or artificially induced events. Natural immunity may be either active or passive. Active natural immunity results from having had certain diseases-such as rubella and poliomyelitis (type-specific)-and usually persists for the life of the host. Immunity may also develop after inapparent infection, such as in hepatitis A or poliomyelitis. With some other diseases, there is a latent stage following clinical illness in which immunity is imperfect; the agent will remain in the latent stage until some triggering mechanism initiates disease. Such latency is shown in infection with herpes simplex virus and cytomegalovirus.

Transplacental antibodies, such as measles antibodies from the mother to the new born child represents active immunity. These antibodies reflect the maternal immunity status and will protect the newborn for several months, often for six months or more.

Artificial immunity can be either active or passive. Active artificial immunity follows the use of vaccines. There are attenuated vaccines, such as those used against poliomyelitis (Sabin vaccine), yellow fever, and tuberculosis; killed vaccines, used against such diseases as typhoid fever and poliomyclitis (Salk vaccine); and toxoids, which are used against diphtheria and tetanus. For some vaccines, booster inoculations are recommended. The duration of artificial immunity is variable, depending on the disease.

Passive artificial immunity results from the use of immune serum globulin (i.e., serum that contains antibody); this is employed, for example, in prophylaxis against hepatitis A infections. Passive protection is of relatively short duration, usually several months at most.

Host Response

The spectrum of the host's response to a microorganism may range from a subclinical (or inapparent) infection to a clinically apparent illness, the extreme being death. The host may become a carrier of the organism. The clinical spectrum of disease varies from mild, to a typical course (although a disease may typically be mild), to severe disease and possible death. There may be atypical or modified forms of the disease. The degree of host response is determined by both agent and host factors and includes the dose of the infecting organism, its organ specificity, the pathogenicity of the infecting organism, its virulence and invasiveness, and its portal of entry. Host factors include the quantitative and qualitative level of the specific and nonspecific immunologic factors previously discussed.

The same organism infecting different hosts can result in a clinical spectrum of disease that is the same, similar, or different in various individuals. In an epidemic, for example, many cases of what appears to be the epidemic disease may meet the clinical case definition, whereas other cases that epidemiologically are related to the same epidemic may not meet the same case definition. They may, in fact, be cases of the epidemic disease but with a different clinical spectrum (as can occasionally be demonstrated by serologic tests). They may also be cases of other diseases occurring concurrently with the epidemic.

Environment

The environment significantly influences the multiple factors in the chain of infection. The transmission of the agent from its source to the host occurs in an environment that represents the summation of many individual factors; changes in any of these can have an impact on any link in the chain of infection. Some environmental factors are under strict control, such as the air in an operating room, whereas others are not.

At times, too much emphasis is placed on the role of the environment; for example, it is inappropriate to take environmental cultures routinely throughout a hospital (see Chapters 9, 20). However, in investigating nosocomial infections, it may be appropriate to obtain environmental cultures as suggested by the circumstances of the specific problem under investigation (see Chapter 6). In other instances, not enough attention is paid to the environment. There needs to be a healthy respect for the environment, with maintenance that does not deliberately promote the transmission of disease-causing agents to hosts but without excessive control measures that impose unnecessary and ineffective actions on the hospital staff and a consequent loss of efficiency and effectiveness, and a wasting of resources such as personnel time and money. Knowledge of environmental factors and their influence on the chain of infection as well as an awareness of adverse changes in the environment should be sufficient to alert one to the need to investigate these environmental factors to ascertain their role in a nosocomial infection problem.

Some environmental factors can influence all the links in the chain of infection, whereas others are more limited in their range of action. Humidity, for example, can influence a multiplicity of factors; it can affect the persistence of an agent at its source, its transmission through the air, and the effectiveness of a host's mucous membranes in resisting infection. Other environmental factors, however, have a more limited effect on the occurrence of infection; for example, the temperature-pressure relation in a specific autoclave affects sterilization within that autoclave, but it has no direct effect on the host.

Certain environmental factors directly affect the agent. Replication of the agent at its reservoir may depend on certain substances in the environment. The agent's survival is influenced by the temperature, humidity, pH, and radiation at its reservoir or source; its survival is even influenced by such factors during its transmission. There may also be toxic substances in the environment that are lethal for the agent.

The transmission of agents will be affected by environmental factors such as temperature and humidity, as mentioned earlier. Airborne transmission is influenced by air velocity and the direction of its movement. The stability and concentration of an aerosol are directly related to environmental factors. In winter, people tend to be indoors with closed windows and reduced air circulation, and this increases the risk of airborne disease compared with summer, when room air is air-conditioned or diluted with outside air. In epidemics associated with common-vehicle transmission, the temperature of the environment will influence the level of contamination in the vehicle. The spread of vectorborne disease also reflects favorable conditions in the environment for the survival and movement of the vector.

The host's resistance mechanisms are affected by environmental factors; for example, in an excessively dry atmosphere, mucous membranes become dry and are less able to protect against microbial invasion. Also, the host's behavioral patterns are influenced by temperature.

Only after each link in the chain of infection has been carefully described can the most appropriate methods of control and prevention be determined. There may be similarities among cases of disease in different epidemics; until all the factors involved in the chain of infection are determined for each epidemic, however, it is not possible to be certain that extrapolation of control and preventive measures from one epidemic will be appropriate to another epidemic.

REFERENCES

1. Gregg MB. *Field epidemiology*. New York: Oxford University Press, 1996: 65–70.
2. Hornick RB, Greisman SE, Woodward TE. Typhoid fever: pathogenesis and immunologic control. *N Engl J Med* 1970;283:739–746.
3. Riley RL, et al. Aerial dissemination of pulmonary tuberculosis: A two-year study of contagion in a tuberculosis ward. *Am J Hyg* 1959;70:185.
4. Walter CW, Kuntsin RB, Brubaker MM. The incidence of airborne wound infections during operation. *JAMA* 1963;186:908–913.
5. Bate J, James U. *Salmonella typhimurium* infection dust-borne in a children's ward. *Lancet* 1958;2:713.

Hospital Infections, Fourth Edition,
edited by John V. Bennett and Philip S. Brachman.
Lippincott–Raven Publishers, Philadelphia © 1998

CHAPTER 2

The Hospital Epidemiologist

Bryan P. Simmons

HISTORY

Hospital epidemiology has been practiced since the mid-1800s; Nightingale, Semmelweis, Lister, and Holmes all made significant contributions to the field. The term "hospital epidemiologist" was first used in an article published in 1940 that described measures to prevent outbreaks of diarrhea [1]. When used in this chapter, "hospital epidemiologist" will refer to anyone who concerns themselves with the determinants of hospital-acquired diseases or injuries; such efforts are usually undertaken with prevention in mind. Hospital epidemiology traditionally has referred to infection control but is increasingly being applied to clinical performance and quality management. Usually the hospital epidemiologist is a physician, and the infection control practitioner is a nurse, although there are important exceptions to this rule.

Modern hospital epidemiology began in the 1950s in Great Britain, when infection control sisters were used to address hospital outbreaks of staphylococcal infections. Such staphylococcal outbreaks also swept hospitals in the United States. In the 1960s, the American Hospital Association (AHA) formed the Committee on Infections Within Hospitals, and the Communicable Disease Center (CDC, now the Centers for Disease Control and Prevention) formed the Hospital Infections Unit. These two organizations supported an organized approach to nosocomial infections, including use of an infection control practitioner. The AHA also published a manual on prevention of hospital infections that was extensively used for almost two decades [2].

In 1970 the Joint Commission on Accreditation of Hospitals (now the Joint Commission on Accreditation of Healthcare Organizations, or JCAHO) had a relatively meager set of infection control standards requiring an infection control committee, surveillance, a sanitary environment, facilities for isolation of infected patients, microbiology services, and measures to protect against contamination of food [3]. As time went on, JCAHO standards became increasingly more demanding such that an infection control practitioner was needed to comply with them. By 1970, however, < 10% of hospitals had an infection control practitioner [4].

In 1970 there was a need to organize and promote the scientific basis of hospital infection control programs and to encourage expansion of such programs. The CDC addressed this need by convening the first International Conference on Nosocomial Infections in 1970 [5]. The proceedings of this conference represented the state of the art about the various aspects of hospital-acquired infections [6]. However, it was clear that there was much more work to be done. In closing the conference Sir Robert E. O. Williams said that "convincing evidence" was still needed to make the changes necessary to prevent nosocomial infections [7].

Since this historic conference, there have been two more international conferences sponsored by the CDC, in 1980 and 1990, and a fourth is planned for the year 2000. These conferences have demonstrated that hospital epidemiology is a science full of information not generally known by any other specialty. Even though there is a unique body of knowledge encompassed by hospital epidemiology, there was no proof that the hospital epidemiologist could use this knowledge to prevent infections until the CDC concluded its SENIC (Study on the Efficacy of Nosocomial Infection Control) project (see Chapter 4). The SENIC project showed that a physician specially trained in infection control could reduce the rate of nosocomial infections [8]. These findings added momentum to the movement to train physicians to become hospital epidemiologists.

The first hospital epidemiologists concentrated their efforts on preventing nosocomial infections. Yet in 1975 only 9% of hospital epidemiologists were infectious diseases physicians; ~40% were pathologists [9]. Infectious

B.P. Simmons: Department of Preventive Medicine, Division of Biostatistic and Epidemiology, University of Tennessee School of Medicine, Memphis, Tennessee 38104.

diseases physicians have increasingly filled the role of hospital epidemiologist. The epidemic of AIDS stimulated enormous interest in hospital epidemiology in the mid-1980s and gave advantages to the epidemiologist trained in infectious diseases. The boundaries of hospital epidemiology have expanded well beyond infection control into clinical performance and quality management. It remains to be seen whether the association between the field of hospital epidemiology and physicians specializing in infectious diseases will persist if infection control no longer dominates the practice of hospital epidemiology.

In 1980 a group of physicians practicing hospital epidemiology formed the Society for Hospital Epidemiology of America (SHEA), now called the Society for Healthcare Epidemiology of America (see Chapter 11). Similar organizations were formed overseas, for example, in Great Britain. Most SHEA members are infectious diseases specialists, but most infectious diseases physicians do not believe that their specialty training adequately prepares them for hospital epidemiology [10]. The discipline of infection control has more and more incorporated epidemiologic principles and statistical analyses that are generally not learned in clinical training. Thus, formal training in hospital epidemiology has become important. Many of the early hospital epidemiologists learned their skills as Epidemic Intelligence Service officers or by attending training courses at the CDC. Recently the SHEA, CDC, and AHA together have offered a course on hospital epidemiology. Additional courses are being developed to address issues not related specifically to infection control, such as clinical performance and quality management. Other courses are offered by universities as summer programs or special courses.

THE ROLE OF THE HOSPITAL EPIDEMIOLOGIST

Infection Control

The hospital epidemiologist can provide many services to a hospital (Table 2-1), but the most important is administering an infection control program together with the infection control practitioner. The functions of the infection control program can be divided into the following areas: surveillance, control of endemic infections, outbreak investigation and control, education, employee health, antibiotic use as it effects the infection control program, development of policies and procedures, and new product evaluation (see Chapters 3, 5, 6, 14, 30). For each of these areas the hospital epidemiologist should develop a practical hospital-specific plan of improvement. Such a plan needs to consider hospital priorities and address questions concerning which patient or procedure categories are high risk, high volume, or problem prone in terms of nosocomial infections; which strategies are most cost effective; which solutions are most politically palatable; and what resources are available or needed to solve problems.

TABLE 2-1. *Hospital epidemiology services*

- Infection control
- Performance assessment and quality
- Employee health
- Risk management
- Microbiology consultation
- Pharmacy consultation

Surveillance is an integral component of any quality improvement process. Good surveillance data allow the hospital epidemiologist to detect problems and determine endemic and epidemic rates (see Chapter 5). These data should be used to help set priorities, develop policy, and monitor the results of interventions to ensure ongoing improvement. Surveillance encompasses more than just collecting data and calculating rates. In the process of surveillance, the infection control/quality management practitioner's presence in clinical areas serves as a reminder to other personnel that infection control/improvement activities are ongoing and important. It also provides an opportunity for consultation, feedback, and networking.

Surveillance alone has been shown to lower rates of nosocomial infections [7]; perhaps the impact of the "Hawthorne effect" (a phenomenon of improved performance associated solely with monitoring activities) will be seen, at least in part, when surveillance is applied to other quality problems. The hospital epidemiologist who is also a clinician can use clinical rounds as an opportunity to verify that policy is being implemented, to look for evidence of cross-infection, to discover new devices introduced (often without input from the infection control committee), and to interact with other physicians and personnel. The clinician/epidemiologist can also see problems as a "customer" of the hospital rather than as an administrator. Quality problems that can be detected during clinical rounds include failure of reports to arrive on the chart in a timely manner, excess waiting times, antibiotic administration errors, evidence of microbiology laboratory derived cross-contamination, and so on.

Policies are generally developed by the infection control department and then submitted to the Infection Control Committee for approval. Such policies should be designed to minimize the risk of nosocomial infections. Once these policies are approved by the hospital, educating the staff in their implementation becomes very important. The infection control practitioner usually takes responsibility for educating hospital personnel, and the hospital epidemiologist is responsible for educating the medical staff.

Product evaluation is another important role for both the infection control practitioner and hospital epidemiologist. Many products are marketed with the claim of reducing the rate of nosocomial infections. Purchasing personnel need assistance in determining which products are useful and cost effective. The hospital epidemiologist needs to maintain interest in this seemingly mundane area, at least for those products with infection control implications.

The hospital epidemiologist should develop a strategy, in partnership with infection control practitioners, about what they want to accomplish in the foreseeable future. Trying to do too much at once can result in unnecessary stress for everyone and policies that aren't adopted because of inadequate preparation. Obviously, epidemics or other important problems require immediate attention. However, most improvement projects should be prioritized and subject to strategic planning. One author feels that one long-term (annual) goal and two short-term (3 to 6 months) goals are a reasonable objective [11]. Such a strategy allows time for monitoring the implementation of the new policy, education, follow-up surveillance, and so forth.

Performance Assessment and Quality Management

Many hospital epidemiologists have become involved in quality management because epidemiology is as useful to quality assessment as it is to infection control [12–14]. Continuous quality improvement (CQI) programs have become the most popular method of quality management and are strongly encouraged by JCAHO [15]. Data management and statistical analysis are the backbone of CQI programs [16,17]. The hospital epidemiologist can also expand into other areas of quality management, such as clinical practice guideline development [18]. Use of such guidelines can minimize unwanted practice variation, length of stay, and hospital costs. The tools of CQI can also be applied to infection control programs to reduce the rate of endemic infections, which constitute the majority of nosocomial infections [19] (see Chapter 30).

Employee Health

The head of employee health often needs to collaborate with the hospital epidemiologist (see Chapter 3). Opportunities to collaborate lie in determining vaccination strategies (hepatitis B, hepatitis A, influenza, varicella, rubella, measles, mumps, and BCG), managing needle sticks and infection exposures (human immunodeficiency virus, meningococcus, tuberculosis, hepatitis, varicella, measles, rubella, scabies, etc.), and determining hiring and return-to-work practices related to infection control. The mandates of the U.S. Occupational Safety and Health Administration (OSHA) have created many opportunities for the hospital epidemiologist to assist the hospital.

Risk Management

The hospital's risk management department can also use the services of the hospital epidemiologist. Preventing adverse outcomes can be done most efficiently if the tools of epidemiology are used, whether these outcomes are infections or another undesirable event [17]. The hospital epidemiologist also can evaluate infection control issues related to litigation and help develop litigation defense strategies.

Microbiology Consultant

The hospital epidemiologist can assist the microbiology laboratory by selecting the antibiotics to report on sensitivity testing, including use of an antibiotic sensitivity "cascade" (see Chapter 9). An antibiotic cascade is a microbiology reporting system in which sensitivity to broad-spectrum antibiotics is not mentioned unless resistance to more narrow spectrum agents is found. These efforts can help control the prescribing practices of physicians, which, in turn, can affect the development of antibiotic-resistant microorganisms. The hospital epidemiologist can also help develop policies to prevent the spread of microorganisms to the microbiologists who are handling them in the lab (see Chapter 23).

Consultant to the Pharmacy

The pharmacy and therapeutic committee can also use the services of the hospital epidemiologist. Opportunities to help include use of surveillance to monitor medication use and adverse effects (pharmacoepidemiology [20]), selection of an antibiotic formulary, restriction of certain antibiotics as needed for infection control, and determination of proper antibiotic prophylaxis regimens. All of these activities can help prevent infections, lessen the number of side effects of antibiotics, and save money.

Inspecting/Regulating Agencies

The OSHA, JCAHO, and state regulatory bodies all inspect hospitals and can have a major impact on hospital functions if quality problems are discovered. The hospital epidemiologist plays an important role in preparing for such inspections and in ensuring compliance with pertinent regulations, standards, and recommendations. During JCAHO accreditation surveys, the epidemiologist should be available to answer questions about the epidemiology program and be prepared to defend the program's priorities and policies. Careful preparation is necessary, starting ≥ 6 months before the JCAHO survey.

HEALTHCARE EPIDEMIOLOGY

Managed care and health maintenance organizations are increasingly prevalent in providing healthcare. These organizations manage patients both in and out of the hospital. To control costs, hospital admissions are discouraged. Thus, there is an emphasis on prevention, an area of expertise familiar to most epidemiologists. When epidemiologists apply their skills outside the hospital, they are best called "healthcare" rather than "hospital" epidemiologists. Healthcare epidemiologists can assist with the following activities aimed at care out of the hospital: developing guidelines for efficient use of hospitals, quality management, employee health, home health, long-term care, product evaluation, risk management, pharmacoepidemiology, and prevention.

SKILLS AND SUPPORT NEEDED FOR THE HOSPITAL EPIDEMIOLOGIST

Knowledge

The hospital epidemiologist needs many skills to succeed (Table 2-2) but the most important one is a thorough knowledge of the science of epidemiology and its associated statistical tools. Those who treat hospital epidemiology as a hobby are unlikely to make the impact necessary for their healthcare systems to compete in the future. Scientific skills will allow the epidemiologist to prevent infections and other complications and to seek out and eliminate costly but ineffective infection control traditions (ritual) and quality management busywork. These skills should also help in product evaluation and selection. Most new products cost more than the products that they are designed to replace, but few are worth the extra cost. Good epidemiology skills also are needed to present accurate data to the administration and the medical committees in a concise and forceful format. Such data are difficult to ignore and can drive necessary change and improvement.

TABLE 2-2. *What you need to succeed as a hospital epidemiologist*

- Epidemiology/statistical skills
- Management skills
- Computer/software support
- Partnership with epidemiology nurses
- Committee participation
- Administrative support
- "People" skills
- A contract

Management Skills

The hospital epidemiologist needs to learn management skills to be effective. Management activities that are important include setting priorities, budgeting, planning, using time efficiently, and making polices. Making sound policy is only part of the solution to most problems. Someone must be able to effect change and implement policy, sometimes over the objections of many other physicians and hospital employees. The tools of CQI are very helpful in promoting necessary change; these tools should become familiar to the hospital epidemiologist [13]. In addition, the hospital epidemiologist should consider special training in management, for example, as provided by the American Management Association in Chicago or the American College of Physician Executives. One of the first management decisions a hospital epidemiologist should make is to determine what support is needed to do a good job.

Computer Support

Computers and software are very important to the modern hospital epidemiology program [21] (see Chapter 8). Computers will allow storage of surveillance data and efficient and rapid retrieval of it to assess trends and find solutions to problems. Computers can eliminate the need for retrospective chart review for all but the most complex problem. In addition, computers can be programmed to actually prevent problems rather than just count them. The hospital epidemiologist, in partnership with the infection control practitioner, needs to select the best software for the hospital's needs. Thus, the hospital epidemiologist must be familiar with the advantages and disadvantages of various software programs.

Partnership with Epidemiology Nurses

The infection control/quality management practitioners will be the greatest asset to your department. These nurses should be well trained or the epidemiologist will be constantly dealing with day-to-day department management rather than issues that require his/ or her input. The best-trained infection control nurses are those that are certified in infection control by Certification Board of Infection Control. It is best that infection control and quality management nurses report to the epidemiologist's department rather than to nursing because of conflicts that can arise when nursing personnel fail to follow established policy or resist important changes.

Committee Participation

The hospital epidemiologist should be a member of the most important committees dealing with issues strongly linked to hospital epidemiology. Certainly, the hospital epidemiologist should be a member of the Infection Control Committee. Some hospital epidemiologists prefer to chair this committee. Being the chair has its advantages but can be seen as putting too much power in the hands of one individual. If a major controversy evolves out of an infection control decision, the hospital epidemiologist who is not chair can depend on the chair for support. This is especially helpful if the chair is an influential member of the medical staff.

Infection Control Committee meetings can be the place to develop important policy and address politically unpopular issues, such as dealing with certain physicians who fail to follow policy, departments that won't cooperate with implementing committee policy, or a surgeon with an unacceptable infection rate. However, it is usually best to contact the departments or individuals first, and even resolve the issue if possible, before presenting it to the committee. Such issues can be addressed, at least initially, without mentioning names or identifying individuals. The committee acts to insulate the hospital epidemiologist from such thankless work, but ultimately the hospital epidemiologist must see that committee policy is implemented and followed. Often one-on-one discussions are needed to ensure that policy is communicated to those who ignore it. The hospital epidemiologist should not trivialize Infection Control Committee meetings or consider them a waste of time [11].

"People" Skills

It is useful to know how to interact with people in order to get things done. The hospital epidemiologist should be friendly, visible, approachable, and known. The hospital epidemiologist must have the confidence of the medical staff in order to persuade physicians to change their ways when necessary. Often this requires appearances before several committees and individual discussions with key physicians. Change must often be negotiated rather than mandated. The hospital epidemiologist must also have the confidence of the administration and be able to negotiate with them. Often monetary and other support is necessary to get things done and make improvements. It is important that the administration be kept informed of the activities, successes, and needs of the hospital epidemiology department.

GETTING PAID

Many administrators are unwilling to pay for hospital epidemiology services and consider them part of the duties that the medical staff provides to the hospital through committee activities. However, in the current environment of capitation and fixed reimbursement for care, complications such as nosocomial infections are a source of monetary loss for the hospital [22,23]. Thus, there is a premium on preventing infections and other complications. Dr. Robert Haley used SENIC data to devise a formula for calculating cost savings by instituting various components of a well-run infection control program [24]. In addition to money saved by preventing infections, the knowledgeable hospital epidemiologist can save the hospital money by eliminating unnecessary ritual, by controlling excess use of prophylactic antibiotics, and by rejecting expensive new products that are not cost effective. These savings can be presented to the administration when seeking reimbursement. In addition, the administrator should keep in mind that the infectious diseases physician, who is also a hospital epidemiologist, is likely to experience a decline in private practice income when nosocomial infections are prevented.

EMPORIATRICS

Infections that affect international travelers are occasionally introduced into hospitals. "In the context of infectious diseases, there is nowhere in the world from which we are remote and no one from whom we are disconnected" [25]. This is especially true for hospitals. Thus, the hospital epidemiologist needs to keep current on important international epidemics, especially if the pathogens causing these epidemics are transmissible in hospitals. A classic example of a worrisome group of such pathogens are the hemorrhagic fever viruses [26]. The hospital epidemiologist can stay current on such topics by reading the CDC's *Morbidity Mortality Weekly Report*.

CONSORTIUMS

Consortiums are useful for hospitals that do not have access to a well-trained hospital epidemiologist, e.g., most rural hospitals (see Chapter 10). Policies, surveillance techniques, data analysis, instructional material, outbreak investigation, and new product evaluations are some aspects of the infection control program that can be provided efficiently by a consortium [27]. The opportunities for such consortiums may increase as hospitals form managed care networks.

TABLE 2-3. *Future opportunities for the health care epidemiologist*

- Multi-drug-resistant bacteria control
- Increased computer support
- Increased outpatient focus
- Clinical performance management and assessment
- New product/new technology assessment
- Quality service despite reduced resources

THE FUTURE

There will be many opportunities for hospital epidemiologists to apply their skills in the future (Table 2-3), provided they are willing to adapt to meet the needs created by a changing healthcare delivery system [28]. This may be especially true for infectious diseases physicians [29]. Perhaps the most pressing of these needs will be controlling the spread of multi-drug-resistant microorganisms, but improving quality in the face of declining resources represents a major challenge. In any case, it is clear that the well-trained and experienced epidemiologist will have many challenges and opportunities ahead.

REFERENCES

1. Felson J, Wolarsky W. The hospital epidemiologist. *Hospitals* 1940; 14:41.
2. Weinstein RA, Pugliese G. The American Hospital Association. *Infect Control Hosp Epidemiol* 1994;15:269–273.
3. *Standards for Accreditation of Hospitals, Plus Provisional Interpretations*. Chicago: Joint Commission on Accreditation of Hospitals, 1969.
4. Haley RW, Shachtman RS. The emergence of infection surveillance and control programs in U.S. hospitals: an assessment, 1976. *Am J Epidemiol* 1980;111:574–591.
5. Eickhoff TC. Historical perspective: the landmark conference in 1970. *Am J Med* 1991;91(suppl 3B):S3–S5.
6. Brachman PS, Eickhoff TC, eds. *Proceedings of the International Conference on Nosocomial Infections*. Chicago: American Hospital Association, 1971.
7. Williams REO. Summary of conference. In: Brachman PS, Eickhoff TC, eds. *Proceedings of the International Conference on Nosocomial Infections*. Chicago: American Hospital Association, 1971:318–381.
8. Haley RW, Culver DH, White JW, et al. The efficacy of infection surveillance and control programs in preventing nosocomial infections in U.S. hospitals. *Am J Epidemiol* 1985;121:182–205.
9. Haley RW. The "hospital epidemiologist" in U.S. hospitals, 1976–1977: a description of the head of the infection surveillance and control program. *Infect Control Hosp Epidemiol* 1980;1:21–32.
10. Hamory BH, Hecks LL, and the Manpower and Training Committee, Infectious Diseases Society of America. Infectious diseases manpower in the United States—1986 (changes in practice patterns over time and training needs). *J Infect Dis* 1992;165:218–223.
11. Wenzel RP. The hospital epidemiologist: practical ideas. *Infect Control Hosp Epidemiol* 1995;16:166–169.
12. Simmons BP, Kritchevsky SB. Epidemiologic approaches to quality assessment. *Infect Control Hosp Epidemiol* 1995;16:101–104.
13. Kritchevsky SB, Simmons BP. The tools of quality improvement: CQI versus epidemiology (editorial). *Infect Control Hosp Epidemiol* 1995; 16:101–104.
14. Wenzel RP. Infection control: the premier quality assessment program in United States hospitals. *Am J Med* 1991;91:27S–31S.
15. *1995 Comprehensive Accreditation Manual for Hospitals*. Oakbrook Terrace, Ill.: Joint Commission on Accreditation of Healthcare Organizations 1984:30–33.
16. Kritchevsky SB, Simmons BP. Continuous quality improvement: concepts and applications for physician care. *JAMA* 1991;266: 1817–1823.
17. Kritchevsky SB, Simmons BP. The tools of quality improvement: CQI versus epidemiology [Editorial]. *Infect Control Hosp Epidemiol* 1995; 16:499–502.
18. Epstein PE. Clinical practice guidelines. *Ann Intern Med* 1990;113: 645–647.
19. Haley RW, Tenney JH, Lindsey II JO, Garner JS, Bennett JV. How frequent are outbreaks of nosocomial infection in community hospitals? *Infect Control Hosp Epidemiol* 1985;6:233–236.
20. Burke JP, Tilson HH, Platt R. Expanding roles of hospital epidemiology: pharmacoepidemiology. *Infect Control Hosp Epidemiol* 1989;10:253.
21. Classen DC. Information management in infectious diseases: survival of fittest. *Clin Infect Dis* 1994;19:902–909.
22. Haley RW, White JW, Culver DH, Hughes JM. The financial incentive for hospitals to prevent nosocomial infections under the prospective payment system: an empirical determination from a nationally representative sample. *JAMA* 1987;257:1611–1614.
23. Miller PJ, Farr BM, Gwaltney JM. Economic benefits of an effective infection control program: case study and proposal. *Rev Infect Dis* 1989;11:284–288.
24. Haley RW. *Managing hospital infection control for cost-effectiveness: a strategy for reducing infectious complications*. Chicago: American Hospital Association Publications, 1986.
25. Institute of Medicine. *Emerging infections: microbial threats to health in the United States*. Washington, D.C.: National Academy Press, 1992.
26. Centers for Disease Control and Prevention. Update: managing patients with suspected viral hemorrhagic fever—United States. *MMWR* 1995; 44:475–479.
27. Ehrenkranz NJ. Starting an infection control network. *Infect Dis Clin Pract* 1995;4:194–198.
28. Wenzel RP. Instituting healthcare reform and preserving quality: role of the hospital epidemiologist. *Clin Infect Dis* 1993;17:831–834.
29. Sande ME. Health care reform: implications for professions related to infectious diseases. *J Infect Dis* 1994;169:1197–1200.

Hospital Infections, Fourth Edition,
edited by John V. Bennett and Philip S. Brachman.
Published by Lippincott–Raven Publishers, Philadelphia, 1998

CHAPTER 3

Personnel Health Services

Ofelia C. Tablan, Elizabeth A. Bolyard, Craig N. Shapiro, and Walter W. Williams

Healthcare workers (HCWs)[1] are at risk of exposure to communicable diseases in both the workplace and the community. If disease develops in them, they may in turn pose a risk for transmission of that disease to patients, other HCWs, members of their households, or other community contacts. Health care workers or others who have frequent and prolonged direct contact with patients may be at great risk of exposure to infectious agents.

This chapter outlines infection control objectives of an HCW health service and discusses important aspects of selected transmissible diseases excluding HIV infection, which is discussed in Chapter 43. General objectives and control measures are set forth, which may need to be broadened for certain HCW groups, depending on the needs of the institution, local and state regulations, and local disease risks.

INFECTION CONTROL OBJECTIVES OF A PERSONNEL HEALTH SERVICE

As part of the general program for infection control, hospitals should establish policies to minimize the risk of transmission of infections between HCWs and patients. The personnel health service should coordinate its activities with the infection control program and other hospital departments to ensure prompt implementation of prevention and control measures. The support of the administration, medical staff, and other HCWs is essential for goals to be met.

In collaboration with infection control staff, the personnel health service can contribute to infection control activities by establishing such policies and procedures as placement evaluations, health and safety education, immunization programs, monitoring potentially harmful infectious exposures and instituting appropriate preventive measures, coordinating plans for managing outbreaks among HCWs, providing care to HCWs for work-related illnesses or exposures, providing information regarding infection risks related to employment or special conditions, developing guidelines for restricting work because of infectious disease, and maintaining health records on all HCWs.

Placement Evaluations

Placement evaluations should be done before or at the time HCWs are hired or allowed to work. A placement evaluation can be used to assist in ensuring that persons are able to perform job tasks safely and efficiently and that they are not placed in jobs that would pose unusual risk of infection to themselves, other HCWs, patients, or visitors. Determining the existence of, or susceptibility to, certain infectious diseases may be an important part of this evaluation and should include determining an HCW's immunization status and history of previous medical conditions, such as chicken pox or tuberculosis, or immunodeficient conditions that may predispose the HCW to acquiring or transmitting infectious diseases. In addition, the preplacement evaluation can be used to educate HCWs about their role in the prevention of nosocomial infections.

Physical examinations for job placement may help detect unusual susceptibility to infection, conditions that may increase the likelihood of transmitting disease to patients, and the presence of communicable diseases or conditions, and they may serve as a baseline for future evaluation of conditions that may be related to work.

O. C. Tablan, E. A. Bolyard: Hospital Infections Program
C. N. Shapiro: Division of Viral and Rickettsial Diseases
W. W. Williams: Adult Vaccine Preventable Diseases Branch, National Immunization Program, Centers for Disease Control and Prevention, Atlanta, Georgia 30333.

[1]For purposes of this chapter, personnel who work directly with, or in close proximity to, patients are referred to as *healthcare workers*. They include not only the hospital staff but also emergency or first-responders and trainees and volunteers who work in the same capacity or under the same circumstances as the hospital staff members.

There are no data, however, to suggest that routine complete physical examinations are needed for infection control. Neither are there data to suggest that routine laboratory testing (such as complete blood cell counts, serologic tests for syphilis, urinalysis, or chest roentgenograms) or preemployment screening for enteric or other pathogens are beneficial in terms of cost. In some areas, however, local public health ordinances may mandate that certain screening procedures be employed.

Because of the resurgence of tuberculosis in the United States in recent years, tuberculosis screening should be part of the HCW's initial evaluation and should be completed before the HCW has any direct contact with patients (see Tuberculosis in this chapter and Chapter 33) [1].

Personnel Health and Safety Education

Health care workers' education, including an initial job orientation and ongoing in-service education, should be a central focus of the personnel health program. In the initial and ongoing educational program, it is important to stress that HCWs can lower their risk of acquiring or transmitting infection by rigorous adherence to infection control practices when caring for patients and, in particular, careful hand washing after touching patients or materials that are likely to be contaminated [2]. Ongoing educational activities may include the use of lectures, discussion groups, display materials, newsletters, in-service training directly on the unit, or any other innovative technique that will assist in maintaining HCW awareness of infection control issues.

A mechanism should be in place for HCWs to obtain advice in a timely manner about infections they may acquire or transmit to patients. In addition, this mechanism should address the policy for immediate evaluation of the HCW after occupational exposure to infectious agents.

Immunization Programs

Because of their contact with patients or infective material from patients with infections, many HCWs are at risk of exposure to and transmission of certain vaccine-preventable diseases [3]. Using immunizing agents to maintain immunity is therefore an essential part of prevention and infection control programs for HCWs. Optimal use of immunizing agents will not only safeguard the health of HCWs but will also protect patients from becoming infected through exposure to HCWs, lower the risk for transmission of preventable infections from HCWs to others in the hospital, and avoid unnecessary work restrictions. Preventing illness by developing and implementing comprehensive staff immunization policies is far more cost-effective than case management and outbreak control. Mandatory programs are more effective than voluntary programs in ensuring that susceptible persons are vaccinated, and programs for which the hospital bears the cost have had higher vaccination rates. In addition, hospital-based immunization programs for patients can potentially be a vehicle through which to immunize susceptible persons in the community.

Comprehensive immunization programs should be an essential part of a personnel health and infection control program. The following considerations should be included in selecting the vaccines for HCW immunization programs: the likelihood of HCW exposure to the agents included in the vaccine; the nature of employment (i.e., type of contact with patients); and the potential consequences of not vaccinating HCWs.

The Advisory Committee on Immunization Practices (ACIP) of the U.S. Public Health Service develops vaccination guidelines for HCWs and the general population in the United States (Table 3-1). Persons administering

TABLE 3-1. *Recommendations of the Advisory Committee on Immunization Practices on HCW immunizations*[a]

Subject	*MMWR* publication
General recommendations on immunizations	1994;43(RR-1):1–39
Adult immunization	1991;40(RR-12):1–94
Altered immunocompetence	1993;42(RR-4):1–18
Bacille Calmette-Guérin vaccine	1996;45(RR-4):1–18
Diphtheria, tetanus, and pertussis	1991;40(RR-10):1–28, 1997 (in press)
Hepatitis B	1991;40(RR-13):1–25, 1997 (in press)
Hepatitis A	1996;45(RR-15):1–30
Influenza[b]	1997;46(RR-9):1–25
Japanese encephalitis	1993;42(RR-1):1–15
Measles	1989;38(S9):1–18
Measles, mumps, rubella (MMR)	1997 (in press)
Meningococcal disease and outbreaks	1997;46(RR-5):1–21
Mumps	1989;38:388–400
Pertussis, acellular (see also Diphtheria);	1992;41(RR-1):1–10 1997;46(RR-7):1–25
supplementary statements:	1992;41(RR-15):1–5
Pneumococcal pneumonia	1989;38:64–76, 1997; 46(RR-8):1–24
Poliomyelitis	1997;46(RR-3):1–25
Rabies	1991;40(RR-3):1–19
Rubella	1990;39(RR-15):1–18
Typhoid	1994;43(RR-14):1–7
Vaccine adverse reactions, contraindications, and precautions	1996;45(RR-12):1–8
Vaccinia (smallpox)	1991;40(RR-14):1–10
Varicella	1996;45(RR-11):1–36

[a](Published in the *Morbidity and Mortality Weekly Review* as of August 1, 1997.)

[b]Each year influenza vaccine recommendations are reviewed and amended to reflect updated information on influenza activity in the United States for the preceding influenza season and to provide information on the vaccine available for the upcoming influenza season. These recommendations are published in the *MMWR* annually, usually during May or June.

TABLE 3-2. *Immunizing agents and vaccination schedules for HCWs*

Generic name	Primary schedule and booster(s)	Indications	Major precautions and contraindications	Special considerations
		Immunizing agents strongly recommended		
Hepatitis B (HB) recombinant vaccine	Two doses i.m. 4 wk apart, third dose 5 mo after second, booster doses not necessary	For pre-exposure vaccination of HCWs at risk of exposure to blood or body fluids For postexposure vaccination	On the basis of limited experience, there is no apparent risk of adverse effects to developing fetuses. Pregnancy should not be considered a contraindication to vaccination of women. Previous anaphylactic reaction to common baker's yeast is a contraindication to vaccination	The vaccine produces neither therapeutic nor adverse effects in HBV-infected persons. Prevaccination serologic screening for susceptibility before vaccination may or may not be cost effective depending on costs of vaccination and testing and on the prevalence of immune individuals in the group. HCWs who have contact with patients or blood should be tested 1–2 mo after vaccination to determine serologic response
Hepatitis B immune globulin (HBIG)	A dose of 0.06 ml/kg i.m. should be administered as soon as possible after exposure. A second dose of HBIG should be given 1 mo later if the HB vaccine series has not been started	For postexposure prophylaxis, 0.06 ml/kg i.m.should be given as soon as possible to persons exposed to HBsAg-containing blood or body fluids and who are not immune to HBV infection		
Influenza vaccine (inactivated whole- and split-virus)	Annual vaccination with current vaccine; either whole- or split-virus vaccine may be used	For HCWs with contact with high-risk patients or working in chronic care and workers with high-risk medical conditions and/or > 65 yr of age	History of anaphylactic hypersensitivity to egg ingestion	No existing evidence of maternal or fetal risk when vaccine is given during pregnancy because of an underlying high-risk condition in a pregnant woman. Influenza vaccination should be considered for all pregnant women because of their increased risk of hospitalization during influenza season
Measles live-virus vaccine	One dose s.c., second dose ≥ 1 mo later	For HCWs born in or after 1957 who have not had two doses of live vaccine on or after their first birthday, physician-diagnosed measles, or laboratory evidence of immunity. Vaccine should be considered for all workers, including those born before 1957, who have no proof of immunity	Contraindicated in pregnant women; immunocompromised state, including HIV-infected persons with severe immunosuppression; persons with history of anaphylaxis after gelatin ingestion or receipt of neomycin; and anyone who has recently received immune globulin	MMR is the vaccine of choice if recipients are likely to be susceptible to rubella and/or mumps as well as to measles. Persons vaccinated between 1963 and 1967 with a killed measles vaccine alone, killed vaccine followed by live vaccine, or a vaccine of unknown type should be revaccinated with two doses of live measles virus vaccine
Mumps live-virus vaccine	One dose s.c., no booster	For HCWs believed to be susceptible Adults born before 1957 can be considered immune	Contraindicated in pregnant women, immunocompromised patients[a], persons with a history of anaphylaxis after gelatin ingestion or receipt of neomycin	MMR is the vaccine of choice if recipients are likely to be susceptible to measles and rubella as well as to mumps

HCWs; healthcare workers.

TABLE 3-2. *Continued.*

Generic name	Primary schedule and booster(s)	Indications	Major precautions and contraindications	Special considerations
Rubella live-virus vaccine	One dose s.c., no booster	For HCWs, both male and female, who lack documentation of receipt of live vaccine on or after their first birthday or laboratory evidence of immunity. Adults, except women of childbearing age, can be considered immune	Contraindicated for pregnant women; immunocompromised patients[a]; patients with a history of anaphylactic reaction after receipt of neomycin	Women who are pregnant when vaccinated or who become pregnant within 3 mo of vaccination should be counseled on the theoretical risks to the fetus. (The risk of rubella vaccine–associated malformations in these women is so small as to be negligible.) MMR is the vaccine of choice if recipients are likely to be susceptible to measles or mumps as well as to rubella.
Varicella zoster live-virus vaccine	Two 0.5-ml doses s.c. 4–8 wk apart if >13 years of age	For HCWs who do not have a reliable history of varicella or evidence of immunity	Contraindicated during pregnancy, in immunocompromised patients[a], with history of anaphylactic reaction after receipt of neomycin or gelatin. Use of salicylate should be avoided for 6 wk after vaccination	Vaccine is available from the manufacturer for certain patients with acute lymphocytic leukemia in remission. Because 71%–93% of persons without a history of varicella are immune, serologic testing before vaccination is likely to be cost effective
Varicella zoster immune globulin (VZIG)	Persons > 50 kg: 125 u/10 kg i.m.; persons > 50kg: 625 u[b]	For persons (particularly those at high risk of complications, e.g., pregnant women) who are known or likely to be susceptible to VZ and have close and prolonged exposure to an infectious patient or HCW		Serologic testing may help in assessing whether or not to administer VZIG. If varicella is prevented by using VZIG, vaccination should later be offered to the person
		Immunizing agents that may be indicated in particular situations		
Immune globulin (hepatitis A)	Postexposure: one i.m. dose of 0.02 ml/kg given within 2 wk of exposure	For HCWs exposed to feces of infected persons during outbreaks; household and sexual contacts of persons with hepatitis A; staff, attendees, and parents of diapered children in day-care-center outbreaks	Administer into large muscle mass (deltoid, gluteus); contraindicated in persons with IgA deficiency. Do not administer within 2 wk after MMR vaccination or within 3 wk after varicella	
Hepatitis A vaccine	Two doses of vaccine either 6–12 mo apart (HAVRIX) or 6 mo apart (VAQTA)	Not routinely indicated for HCWs in the United States. Persons who work with HAV-infected primates or with HAV in a research laboratory should be vaccinated.	Contraindicated during pregnancy or in those with a history of anaphylactic hypersensitivity to alum or in the case of HAVRIX, to the preservative 2-phenoxyethanol	HCWs who travel to endemic areas should be evaluated for vaccination
Meningococcal polysaccharide vaccine (tetravalent A, C, W135, and Y)	One dose (volume and route specified by manufacturer; need for boosters unknown)	Not routinely indicated for HCWs in the United States	The safety of the vaccine in pregnant women has not been evaluated; it should not be given during pregnancy unless the risk of infection is high	

TABLE 3-2. *Continued.*

Generic name	Primary schedule and booster(s)	Indications	Major precautions and contraindications	Special considerations
Typhoid vaccine, i.m., s.c., and oral	One 0.5-ml dose i.m.,booster of 0.5ml every 2 yr, two 0.5-ml doses s.c. ≥ 4 wk apart, booster of 0.5 ml s.c. or 0.1 ml ID every 3 yr if exposure continues; or 4 oral doses on alternate days. The manufacturer recommends revaccination with the entire four-dose series every 5 yr	For workers in microbiology laboratories who frequently work with *S. typhi*	Severe local or systemic reaction to a previous dose	Vaccination should not be considered as an alternative to the use of proper procedures when handling specimens and cultures in the laboratory
Vaccinia vaccine (smallpox)	One dose administered with a bifurcated needle, boosters to be administered every 10 yr	For laboratory workers who directly handle cultures or animals contaminated with recombinant vaccinia viruses or orthopox viruses that infect humans	The vaccine is contraindicated in pregnancy, and in persons with eczema, a history of eczema, or immunodeficiency in themselves or in their household contacts	Vaccination may be considered for health care personnel who have direct contact with contaminated dressings or other infectious material from volunteers in clinical studies involving recombinant vaccinia virus
BCG vaccine (tuberculosis)	One percutaneous dose of 0.3 ml, no booster dose recommended	Should be considered only for HCWs in areas where multidrug-resistant tuberculosis is prevalent, a strong likelihood of infection exists, and comprehensive infection control precautions have failed	Should not be given to immunocompromised persons or pregnant women[a]	In the United States, tuberculosis-control efforts are directed toward early identification, treatment of patients, and preventive therapy with isoniazid
Immunizing agents for other vaccine-preventable diseases				
Tetanus and diphtheria (toxoids Td)	Two doses i.m. 4 wk apart, third dose 6–12 mo after second dose, booster every 10 yr	All adults	Not contraindicated in pregnancy except during the first trimester Contraindicated in persons with a history of a neurologic, immediate hypersensitivity, or severe local (Arthus type) reaction after a previous dose. Such individuals should not be given further routine or emergency doses of Td for 10 yr	Tetanus prophylaxis in wound management
Pneumococcal polysaccharide vaccine (23 valent)	One dose, revaccination recommended for those at highest risk 75 yr after the first dose	Adults who are at increased risk of pneumococcal disease and its complications because of underlying health conditions;- older adults, especially those age > 65 who are healthy	The safety of the vaccine in pregnant women has not been evaluated; it should not be given during pregnancy unless the risk of infection is high	Previous recipients of any type of pneumococcal polysaccharide vaccine who are at highest risk of fatal infection or antibody loss may be revaccinated > 6 yr after the first dose.

ID; intradermal.

[a]Persons who are immunocompromised because of immune deficiency diseases, HIV infection (who should primarily not receive BCG, OPV, and yellow fever vaccines), leukemia, lymphoma, or generalized malignancy or who are immunosuppressed as a result of therapy with corticosteroids, alkylating drugs, antimetabolites, or radiation.

[b]Some researchers have recommended 125 u/10 kg body weight for all persons.

immunizing agents should be familiar with the recommendations of the ACIP and other professional organizations as well as the regulations of individual states or localities and should be well informed about indications, storage, dosage, preparation, and contraindications for each of the vaccines, toxoids, and immune globulins (Table 3-1). Product information should be available at all times, and a pertinent health history should be obtained from each HCW before an agent is given. Table 3-2 summarizes information on the major indications, regimens, and major contraindications of the vaccines and immunizing agents generally recommended for HCWs.

Immunization of Immunocompromised HCWs

Immunization of immunocompromised HCWs is discussed in the ACIP recommendations on "the use of vaccines and immune globulins in persons with altered immunocompetence" (Table 3-1); specific recommendations by vaccine and type of immunocompromising conditions are listed in Table 3-3.

A physician must assess the degree to which an individual HCW is immunocompromised. Severe immunosuppression can be the result of congenital immunodeficiency, human immunodeficiency virus (HIV) infection, leukemia, lymphoma, generalized malignancy, or therapy with alkylating agents, antimetabolites, radiation, or large amounts of corticosteroids. For some of these conditions, all affected persons will be severely immunocompromised; for others, such as those with HIV infection, there will be a spectrum of severity owing to the particular disease or treatment stage that will determine the degree of immunosuppression. The determination of whether a HCW is severely immunocompromised ultimately must be made by a physician. In addition, the risk of exposure to a vaccine-preventable disease should be weighed against the risks and benefits of vaccination for an immunocompromised HCW.

The exact amount of systemically absorbed corticosteroids and the duration of administration needed to suppress the immune system of an otherwise healthy individual are not well defined. Most experts agree that steroid therapy usually does not contraindicate administration of live-virus vaccines, such as MMR and its component vaccines, when the therapy is short term (i.e., < 14 days) at a low to moderate dose; given daily or on alternate days at low to moderate dose, given as a long-term alternate-day treatment with short-acting preparations, used as replacement therapy (at maintenance physiologic

TABLE 3-3. *Summary of ACIP recommendations on immunization of HCWs with special conditions*

Vaccine	Pregnancy	HIV infection	Severe immunosuppression[a]	Asplenia	Renal failure	Diabetes	Alcoholism and alcoholic cirrhosis
BCG	UI	C	C	UI	UI	UI	UI
Hepatitis A	UI	UI	UI	UI	UI	UI	R[b]
Hepatitis B	R	R	R	R	R	R	R
Influenza	R[c]	R	R	R	R	R	R
Measles, Mumps, Rubella	C	R[d]	C	R	R	R	R
Meningococcus	UI	UI	UI	R[b]	UI	UI	UI
Polio, inactivated[e]	UI	UI	UI	UI	UI	UI	UI
Polio, oral[e]	UI	C	C	UI	UI	UI	UI
Pneumococcus[b]	UI	R	R	R	R	R	R
Rabies	UI	UI	UI	UI	UI	UI	UI
Tetanus/diphtheria[b]	R	R	R	R	R	R	R
Typhoid, inactivated & V_i	UI	UI	UI	UI	UI	UI	UI
Typhoid, Ty21a	UI	C	C	UI	UI	UI	UI
Varicella	C	C	C	R	R	R	R
Vaccinia	UI	C	C	UI	UI	UI	UI

R, recommended; C, contraindicated; UI, use if indicated; V_i, V_i antigen.

[a]Severe immunosuppression can be the result of congenital immunodeficiency, leukemia, lymphoma, generalized malignancy, or therapy with alkylating agents, antimetabolites, radiation, or large amounts of corticosteroids.

[b]For women who will be in the second or third trimester of pregnancy during influenza season.

[c]Recommendation is based on the person's underlying condition rather than occupation.

[d]Contraindicated in persons with HIV infection and severe immunosuppression; see text.

[e]Vaccination is recommended for vaccinated HCWs who may have close contact with patients who may be excreting wild polioviruses. IPV is recommended for primary vaccination of adults because vaccine-associated paralysis after OPV administration is higher in adults than in children. A single-dose booster vaccination with either IPV or OPV may be administered to HCWs who have had a primary series of OPV or IPV (who are directly involved with providing care to patients who may be excreting poliovirus).

doses), or administered topically (to skin or eyes), by aerosol, or by intraarticular, bursal, or tendon injection. The immunosuppressive effects of steroid therapy vary, but many clinicians consider a dose equivalent to 2 mg/kg/day of prednisone (or ≤ 20 mg of prednisone per day to persons who weigh ≥ 10 kg) sufficiently immunosuppressive to raise concern about the safety of vaccination with live-virus vaccines.

Although persons receiving high doses of corticosteroids daily or on alternate days for < 14 days generally can receive MMR or its component vaccines immediately after cessation of treatment, some experts prefer waiting until 2 weeks after completion of therapy. MMR and its component vaccines and varicella vaccine should be avoided for ≥ 1 month after cessation of therapy if high doses (i.e., > 2 mg/kg per day or > 20 mg per day) of systemic steroids are given daily or on alternate days for a period of ≥ 14 days or if clinical or laboratory evidence of systemic immunosuppression results from prolonged or extensive topical, aerosol, or other local therapy. Persons with a disease that, in itself, suppresses the immune response and who are receiving either systemic or topically administered corticosteroids should generally not be given MMR, its component vaccines, or varicella vaccine.

Killed or inactivated vaccines do not represent a danger to immunocompromised HCWs and generally should be given as recommended for healthy workers. Frequently, the immune response of immunocompromised persons to these vaccines is not as good as that of nonimmunocompromised persons; higher doses or more frequent boosters may be required. Even with these modifications, the immune response may be suboptimal.

Persons with immunosuppression due to specific conditions may be at higher risk of certain diseases; additional vaccines may be recommended for them. For example, persons with asplenia should receive bacterial polysaccharide vaccines, such as *Haemophilus influenzae* type b, pneumococcal, and meningococcal vaccines.

Immunization of HIV-infected HCWs

In general, live-virus or live bacterial vaccines should not be administered to persons known to be HIV infected. However, the evaluation and testing for HIV infection of symptomatic HCWs is not necessary before decisions concerning immunization with live-virus vaccines are made. Specific recommendations by vaccine are listed in Table 3-3.

Symptomatic HIV-infected children and adults usually have suboptimal immunologic responses to vaccines [4–6]. The response to both live and killed antigens may decline as the disease progresses [6]. However, the response to higher doses of vaccine and persistence of antibody in HIV-infected patients has not been systematically evaluated. Although higher doses or more frequent boosters may be considered in these patients, firm recommendations cannot be made at this time.

Limited studies of MMR immunization in both asymptomatic and symptomatic HIV-infected patients who had no evidence of severe immunosuppression have not documented serious or unusual adverse events after vaccination [7]. Because of the increased risk for severe complications associated with measles infection and the absence of serious adverse events after measles vaccination among HIV-infected persons without evidence of severe immunosuppression, MMR vaccine is recommended for all asymptomatic HIV-infected HCWs and should be considered for all symptomatic HIV-infected HCWs who have no evidence of severe immunosuppression. However, measles vaccine is not recommended for HIV-infected persons with evidence of severe immunosuppression because of (a) the report of a case of progressive measles pneumonia following receipt of MMR vaccine by a person with acquired immunodeficiency syndrome (AIDS) and severe immunosuppression [8], (b) the very low incidence of measles in the United States [9], (c) reports of vaccination-related morbidity in persons with severe immunosuppression unrelated to HIV infection [10], and (d) evidence of a diminished antibody response to measles vaccine among severely immunocompromised HIV-infected persons [11]. The only polio vaccine recommended for those who have HIV infection is the enhanced inactivated polio vaccine. Pneumonococcal vaccine is indicated for all HIV-infected persons ≥ 2 years of age.

Immunization Records

An immunization record should be maintained for all HCWs. The record should reflect both documented histories of vaccine-preventable illnesses and immunizing agents administered at the provider site. At each immunization encounter, the record should be updated and the HCW should be encouraged to maintain the record, as appropriate.

Catch-up Vaccination Programs

In addition to the implementation of existing immunization policies for new HCWs, health facility managers should consider catch-up programs for HCWs already employed. This strategy will help prevent outbreaks of vaccine-preventable diseases. To help ensure acceptance of the program goals, it may be necessary to conduct educational workshops or seminars several weeks before the initiation of the program. In addition, reference materials should be available to assist in answering questions regarding the diseases, vaccines, and toxoids and the program or policy being implemented.

Outbreak Control

Outbreaks of vaccine-preventable diseases are costly and disruptive and may require different control strategies. The best approach is to prevent outbreaks by ensuring full immunity of all HCWs who have direct contact with patients. Hospitals should develop comprehensive policies and protocols for management and control of outbreaks should they occur. More information on outbreak control for specific diseases can be found in published ACIP recommendations for prevention of each disease (Table 3-1).

Work Restrictions and Management of HCW Illnesses and Exposures

A major function of the personnel health service may be to arrange for prompt diagnosis and management of potentially transmissible illnesses or exposures and provide prophylaxis, when appropriate, to HCWs who have experienced an occupational exposure. Hospitals should have well-defined policies for employees who have transmissible infections. Such policies should address the responsibility of the HCW in using the health service and reporting illness, exclusion from direct contact with patients, and clearance for return to work after recovery from an infectious disease or condition. For any exclusion policy to be enforceable and effective, all personnel, especially department heads, area supervisors, and head nurses, should know when and where an illness is to be reported. Any policy for work restriction should be designed to encourage HCWs to report their illnesses or exposures and, as much as possible, not to penalize them with loss of wages, benefits, leave time, or job status.

Table 3-2 briefly lists recommendations for prophylaxis of HCWs after certain exposures; Table 3-4 summarizes the recommendations for hepatitis B postexposure prophylaxis. However, issues regarding HCW exposure to HIV are not discussed in this chapter; they are taken up in Chapter 43. Tables 3-5 and 3-6 briefly summarize recommendations and suggested work restrictions for staff with selected infectious diseases. More detail on selected infectious diseases or conditions that may be transmitted nosocomially and thus require consideration in placement or work restrictions is discussed in the remainder of the chapter.

Epidemiology and Control of Selected Infections Transmitted Among Hospital Personnel and Patients

Cytomegalovirus

Healthcare workers may be exposed to patients with cytomegalovirus (CMV) infection. The principal reservoirs of CMV in the hospital are infants infected with CMV and immunocompromised patients, such as oncology patients, patients with AIDS, and those undergoing solid-organ transplantation (see Chapters 42, 45). In contrast to reports from day-care centers, however [12,13], conclusive evidence of an increased risk of transmission of CMV to HCWs working in hospitals with a high prevalence of CMV infection, when compared with HCWs with no contact with patients, is lacking [14,15], probably because of observance of appropriate infection control measures by hospital personnel.

Primary infection with CMV during pregnancy may damage the fetus [16]; however, pregnancy per se does not increase a woman's susceptibility to CMV infection. Nosocomially, CMV is transmitted mainly through infected body fluids that come into contact with the hands and are inoculated into the nose or mouth of a susceptible person. Virus can be shed in the urine, saliva, respiratory secretions, tears, feces, breast milk, semen, and cervical secretions.

TABLE 3-4. *Recommendations for postexposure prophylaxis for percutaneous or permucosal exposure to hepatitis B virus, United States*

	Treatment when source is found to be		
Exposed person	HBsAg positive	HBsAg negative	Source not tested or unknown
Unvaccinated	HBIG × 1 and initiate HB vaccine[a]	Initiate HB vaccine	Initiate HB vaccine
Previously vaccinated			
Known responder[b]	No treatment	No treatment	No treatment
Known nonresponder	HBIG × 2, or HBIG × 1 and initiate revaccination	No treatment	If known high-risk source, treat as if source is HBsAg positive
Response unknown	Test exposed for anti-HBs 1. If response is adequate, no treatment 2. If response is inadequate, HBIG × 1 and vaccine booster[b]	No treatment	Test exposed for anti-HBs 1. If adequate, no treatment 2. If inadequate, initiate revaccination

[a]HBIG dose, 0.06 ml/kg i.m.
[b]Response to vaccine is considered adequate if anti-HBs level is ≥ 10 mIu/ml.

TABLE 3-5. *Work restrictions for HCWs exposed to or infected with certain vaccine-preventable diseases*

Disease/problem	Work restriction	Duration
Hepatitis A	Relieve from contact with patients	Until 7 days after onset of jaundice
Hepatitis B		
Acute or chronic infection in personnel who do not perform exposure-prone invasive procedures	Universal precautions should be observed	Standard precautions should always be observed
Acute or chronic antigenemia in personnel who perform exposure-prone invasive procedures	If hepatitis Be antigen (HBeAg) positive, these HCWs should not perform exposure-prone invasive procedures until they have sought counsel from an expert review panel, which should review and recommend the procedures the worker can perform, taking into account the specific procedure as well as the skill and technique of the worker [21]	Until HBeAg is negative
Influenza	During winter, when influenza is prevalent, consider excluding personnel with symptoms of acute febrile upper-respiratory infection from providing care to high-risk patients[a]	Until acute symptoms resolve
Measles		
Active	Exclude from duty	Until 7 days after the rash appears
Postexposure (susceptible personnel)	Exclude from duty	From the 5th day after the first exposure through the 21st day after the last exposure and/or 7 days after the rash appears
Mumps		
Active	Exclude from duty	Until 9 days after onset of parotitis
Postexposure (susceptible personnel)	Exclude from duty	From the 12th day after the first exposure through the 26th day after the last exposure or until 9 days after onset of parotitis
Pertussis		
Active	Exclude from duty	From the beginning of the catarrhal stage through the 3rd wk after onset of paroxysms or until 5 days after start of effective antimicrobial therapy
Postexposure (asymptomatic personnel)	Need not relieve from contact with patients; prophylaxis recommended	
Postexposure (symptomatic personnel	Relieve from direct contact with patients	
Rubella		
Active	Exclude from duty	Until 5 days after the rash appears
Postexposure (susceptible personnel)	Exclude from duty	From the 7th day after the first exposure through the 21st day after the last exposure and/or 5 days after rash appears
Varicella		
Active	Exclude from duty	Until all lesions dry and crust
Postexposure (susceptible personnel)	Exclude from duty	From the 10th day after the first exposure through the 21st day (28th day if VZIG given) after the last exposure or, if varicella occurs, until all lesions dry and crust
Zoster (localized in normal person)	Cover lesions; relieve from care of high-risk patients	
Generalized or localized in immunocompromised person	Relieve from direct contact with patients[b]	
Postexposure (susceptible personnel)	Restrict from patient contact	
Same as varicella		

[a]High-risk patients are defined by the ACIP—see Table 3-1).
[b]High-risk patients are those susceptible to varicella and who are at increased risk of complications of varicella, such as neonates and immunocompromised persons of any age.

TABLE 3-6. *Work restrictions for HCWs exposed to or infected with non-vaccine-preventable infectious diseases of importance in health care settings*

Disease/problem	Work restriction	Duration
Conjunctivitis	Relieve from contact with patients	Until discharge ceases
Cytomegalovirus infections	No restriction	
Diarrheal diseases		
Acute stage (diarrhea with other symptoms)	Relieve from contact with patients or food handlers	Until symptoms resolve and infection with *Salmonella* is ruled out
Convalescent stage		
Salmonella spp	Relieve from care of high-risk patients	Until symptoms resolve. Consult with local health authorities regarding the need for negative stool cultures
Other enteric pathogens	No restriction	
Enteroviral infections	Relieve from care of infants, newborns, and immunocompromised patients	Until symptoms resolve
Herpes simplex		
Genital	No restriction	
Hands (herpetic whitlow)	Relieve from contact with patients, patient	Until lesions heal
Orofacial	Relieve from care of high-risk patients	Until lesions heal
Scabies	Relieve from direct contact with patients	Until treated
Staphylococcus aureus		
Active, draining skin lesions	Relieve from contact with patients, patient materials and food handlers	Until lesions have resolved
Carrier state	No restriction, unless personnel is shown epidemiologically to be disseminating the organism	
Streptococcal disease, Group A	Relieve from patient care or food handling	Until 24 hr after adequate treatment is completed
Tuberculosis		
Active pulmonary or laryngeal tuberculosis	Exclude from duty	Until proven noninfectious, i.e., until adequate treatment is instituted, cough is resolved, and sputum is free of bacilli on three consecutive smears
Asymptomatic, PPD-positive	No restriction	
Upper respiratory tract infections	Relieve from care of high-risk patients[a]	Until acute symptoms resolve

[a]High-risk patients as defined by the ACIP for complications of influenza.

Screening Programs for CMV Infection

Screening programs to detect CMV-infected patients are not practical because the tests are costly and would entail screening all high-risk patients, including newborns. In addition, because CMV shedders can excrete the virus intermittently, screening tests to identify shedders may have to be performed repeatedly. Likewise, the drawbacks of mass screening of workers include its expense, the absence of assurance for those found to be seropositive that if they become pregnant they will not transmit CMV to their offspring [17,18], and the possibility that HCWs found to be seronegative may feel undue fear of acquiring the infection. Moreover, since there are no studies to indicate clearly that seronegative personnel may be protected by transfer to areas of less contact with infants, children, or other high-risk patients, identifying women without antibodies to institute such measures may not reduce the number of primary infections.

Preventing Transmission of CMV

When hygienic practices are used, the risk of acquiring infection through contact with patients is low [19,20]. Therefore, a practical approach to reducing the risk of infection with CMV is to stress standard precautions, including gloving for contact with secretions and excretions of all patients, careful hand washing after all contacts with patients or materials that are potentially infective and after removing gloves, and using other protective barriers (gown, mask, eye protection) when performing procedures likely to generate splashes or sprays of body fluids [2]. Pregnant employees should be informed of the potential risk to the fetus of primary CMV infection and should practice appropriate precautions (as outlined) to minimize the risk of acquiring primary CMV infection.

Personnel who contract illnesses believed to be due to CMV need not be restricted from work. They can lower the risk of transmitting CMV to patients or other staff members by careful hand washing and by preventing their body fluids from coming into contact with other persons.

Gastrointestinal Illness

Various agents may cause acute gastrointestinal infections in patients and hospital personnel. *Salmonella*, *Shigella*, *Campylobacter*, *Escherichia coli*, and *Clostridium difficile* are among the bacterial pathogens [21–28]. Viruses such as rotavirus, calicivirus (e.g., Norwalk and Norwalk-like viruses), and adenovirus [24,29] and such parasites as *Giardia lamblia*, *Cyclospora*, and *Cryptosporidium* [30,31] may also cause gastroenteritis (see Chapters 22,34).

If employees experience acute diarrheal illness accompanied by fever, cramps, or bloody stools, they are likely to be excreting potentially infective organisms at high titers in their feces. Usually, the specific cause of acute diarrhea cannot be determined solely on the basis of clinical symptoms; thus, some laboratory tests may be necessary. Evaluation of personnel may include any one or more of the following studies, as appropriate: serologic tests or cultures for bacterial or viral pathogens or stool examination for intestinal protozoa.

Nosocomial transmission from workers infected with any of the agents named may take place via the hands of those infected. Thus, employees with acute symptoms of diarrheal illness should not provide direct care to patients or handle food or items that may go into the patient's mouth.

Carriage of Enteric Pathogens by Personnel

Carriage of enteric pathogens may persist after resolution of the acute illness. In general, however, the risk to patients of personnel who have recovered from clinical manifestations of illness and are having formed stools appears to be minimal, provided standard infection control precautions (including meticulous hand washing after toileting activities and before handling food or items that may go into the patient's mouth) are observed by the staff [2]. Personnel infected by enteric pathogens can normally safely return to care of patients after symptoms resolve.

Carriage of *Salmonella* pathogens by personnel, however, calls for special precautions because it may be prolonged [32] and because the clinical effects of acute salmonellosis are often severe in high-risk patients (i.e., newborns, the elderly, immunocompromised patients, and the severely ill, such as those in intensive care units [33]). In some U.S. states and localities, personnel with *Salmonella* enteric infections are excluded from direct care of patients until their stool cultures are *Salmonella*-free on two consecutive specimens collected not less than 24 hours apart.

Hepatitis

Viral hepatitis has long been recognized as a nosocomial hazard (see Chapter 42). In the United States, the agents that most commonly cause viral hepatitis are hepatitis A virus (HAV), hepatitis B virus (HBV), and hepatitis C virus (HCV). Each of these viruses has the potential for transmission within the healthcare setting. For the HCW, the risks and consequences of HBV and HCV infections are greater than those of HAV infection.

Hepatitis A Virus

Hepatitis A virus is the etiologic agent of hepatitis A. Because HAV is excreted in high concentrations in the stool of infected persons [34], the most common mode of HAV transmission is the fecal-oral route between close contacts. Because viremia is a component of infection, bloodborne transmission can occur (e.g., via blood transfusion from an asymptomatic blood donor incubating HAV infection); however, it has been infrequently reported [35,36]. Transmission of HAV through accidental or other needle sticks has not been reported.

The incubation period for hepatitis A is 15 to 50 days, with an average of 28 days. In general, fecal excretion of HAV and infectivity are greatest during the 2-week period immediately before the onset of symptoms [34,37]. However, fecal shedding of HAV, especially in infants and children, may continue after onset of clinical symptoms. In neonates, viral shedding has been documented by using the polymerase chain reaction (PCR) for as long as 6 months after onset of infection [36]. Because immunoglobulin M anti-HAV (the serologic marker used for the diagnosis of acute HAV infection) can persist for months after onset of illness and because PCR to detect the presence of HAV in feces is not routinely available, it is often difficult to assess infectivity. For practical purposes, adults with acute hepatitis A can be assumed to be noninfectious 1 week after onset of symptoms.

Nosocomial HAV infection is usually associated with two unique circumstances: first, the source of infection is typically a patient hospitalized for other reasons whose hepatitis has not been diagnosed or become clinically apparent and, second, the patient is incontinent or has diarrhea [34]. However, because HAV does not cause chronic infection and the incidence of asymptomatic HAV infection among hospitalized patients is relatively low, nosocomial hepatitis A is relatively uncommon. In addition, viral titers in stool decline substantially after the onset of symptoms in patients with symptomatic hepatitis A.

Outbreaks of HAV transmission in healthcare settings have been reported in neonatal intensive care units and on pediatric and adult patient wards [36,38–40]. The outbreaks generally involved HAV transmission from patient to patient indirectly via HCWs and from infected patients to HCWs. Risk factors for acquisition of hepatitis A by HCWs during outbreaks include practices that contribute to fecal contamination of hands (not washing hands routinely, not wearing gloves for procedures) and practices that increase hand-to-mouth contact (smoking, eating, and drinking beverages on the unit) [40]. Transmission from infected HCWs to patients has been extremely rare [41–43].

Prevention of HAV Transmission in Health Care Settings. Routine measures for preventing hepatitis A transmission consist of maintenance of standard precautions, including good personal hygiene, attention to hand washing, and use of barriers (e.g., gloves, gowns) when there is a potential for contact with feces or material contaminated with the feces of any patient [2].

There are two types of agents available for preventing hepatitis A, immune globulin (IG) and hepatitis A vaccine. However, neither one is recommended for *routine* use in HCWs (see later discussion). The first immunizing agent, IG, is > 85% effective in preventing hepatitis A when it is administered intramuscularly before a person's exposure or within 2 weeks after exposure to HAV. However, routine IG prophylaxis of HCWs providing care to patients with hepatitis is not indicated; instead, HCWs should follow standard precautions [2]. On the other hand, because IG has been effective in limiting transmission of hepatitis A during outbreaks in healthcare settings, it is recommended that when an outbreak appears at a healthcare facility, a single dose of IG (0.02 ml/kg) should be given as soon as possible, and no later than 2 weeks after exposure, to each HCW or patient exposed to feces of infected patients.

The second product, inactivated hepatitis A vaccine, has been developed to provide long-term protection against hepatitis A. The vaccine preparations have been shown to be safe, highly immunogenic, and very efficacious. Two vaccines are commercially available in the United States, HAVRIX, manufactured by SmithKline Beecham Pharmaceuticals, and VAQTA, manufactured by Merck & Co.; both are licensed for administration to persons ≥ 2 years of age. For adults, the recommended dosing schedules are as follows: for HAVRIX, two doses (1,440 ELISA u), 6 to 12 months apart, and for VAQTA, two doses (25 u) 6 to 12 months apart. Because seroprevalence studies do not show a higher risk of HAV infection in HCWs compared with control populations [41–43], the routine use of hepatitis A vaccine in HCWs is not indicated. The role of hepatitis A vaccine in helping control outbreaks of hepatitis A in the healthcare setting is not known.

To prevent HAV transmission from HCWs to patients, personnel who become infected with HAV are advised not to provide care to patients until 7 days after the onset of jaundice, which is the usual time when viral shedding and infectivity (in adults) decline to minimal levels.

Hepatitis B Virus

HBV infection (see Chapter 42) is one of the major infectious occupational hazards to HCWs [44]. Transmission may happen after parenteral or mucosal exposure to blood or serum-derived body fluids from persons who are HBV carriers or who have acute HBV infection. The risk of HBV transmission depends on the viral titer in the source blood as well as the inoculum volume and route of inoculation. Because the presence of hepatitis B e antigen (HBeAg) in blood correlates with high titers of circulating HBV particles [45], infection rates are higher after exposure to blood with detectable HBeAg compared with blood with detectable hepatits B surface antigen (HBsAg) alone [46–49].

The average incubation period of HBV infection is 4 months (range 2 to 6 months). Symptoms associated with acute infection are more common in adults (33% to 50%) than in children (< 10%) [50]. The risk of acquiring chronic HBV infection after acute infection is inversely proportional to the age of infection. In adults, most infections (90% to 95%) are self-limited, with clearance of the virus and the development of lifelong immunity to reinfection. Between 5% and 10% of persons, however, experience chronic infection with the virus and are at risk of chronic hepatitis, cirrhosis, and liver cancer [50].

In infected persons, the highest concentrations of virus are found in serum, serum-derived body fluids, semen, vaginal fluid, and saliva. Thus, the principal modes of HBV transmission are parenteral, sexual, and vertical (from mother to infant) at the time of birth. Transmission can also ensue from injection of saliva through a bite that breaks the skin and indirectly from person to person through contamination of environmental surfaces. In the healthcare setting, the principal modes of HBV transmission in order of decreasing efficiency appear to be of two kinds—overt parenteral transmission and inapparent parenteral transmission.

In the first case, there is direct percutaneous inoculation by a needle or instrument contaminated with serum or plasma (e.g., accidental needle sticks) [47,49]. In the second case [51,52], transmission may result from (a) percutaneous inoculation without overt needle puncture (e.g., contamination of open skin lesions with infective serum or plasma), (b) contamination of mucosal surfaces with infective serum or plasma (e.g., accidental eye splash or other direct contact with mucous membranes of the eyes or mouth, such as touching the hand to mouth or eye when contaminated with infective blood or serum), (c) transfer of infective material to skin lesions or mucous membranes via inanimate environmental surfaces or contaminated medical devices, or (d) contamination of mucosal surfaces with infective secretions other than serum or plasma (e.g., contact involving bloody saliva).

Within the hospital, persons working in certain locations and occupational categories may have a higher risk of acquiring HBV infection. Generally, the highest risk of HBV infection is among employees working in locations and occupations in which contact with blood or sharps is frequent [53,54]. Examples include emergency room nurses, intensive care unit nurses, and laboratory staff. Health care workers who are not directly exposed to blood are at no greater risk of HBV infection than the general population [55].

Prevention of HBV Infection in HCWs. Measures to prevent HBV infection in HCWs include preexposure immunization with hepatitis B vaccine; postexposure use of hepatitis B vaccine and/or hepatitis B immune globulin (HBIG), when appropriate; and implementation of infection control practices to prevent exposure to blood and blood-derived body fluids.

Hepatitis B Vaccine. Two recombinant vaccines are available in the United States, Recombivax HB, manufactured by Merck & Co., and Engerix B, manufactured by SmithKline Beecham Pharmaceuticals. Numerous studies have shown both vaccines to be safe and highly effective in preventing HBV infection: in > 90% of vaccine recipients protective antibody levels develop, and adults who respond are completely protected from clinical disease and chronic infection [56]. Studies of cohorts vaccinated in the early 1980s indicate that the duration of protection from the vaccine is ≥ 13 years, even though antibody levels may decline to low or undetectable levels. Therefore, administration of vaccine booster doses or testing to determine antibody persistence in vaccine recipients is not routinely recommended.

Hepatitis B vaccine is recommended for HCWs with reasonably anticipated exposure to blood or blood-contaminated body fluids. Ideally, vaccination should be done during training, before working in clinical or laboratory settings. In 1991, the Occupational Safety and Health Administration issued the bloodborne standard that required employers to offer hepatitis B vaccine, at no cost to the employee, to all employees who anticipate contact with blood or other potentially infectious materials [57]. Since then, a progressive increase in hepatitis B vaccine use among HCWs has taken place: in 1991, 72% and 58% of surveyed surgeons in South Carolina and nationwide, respectively, had received the hepatitis B vaccine [58,59]; by 1992, in several East Coast urban areas, 90% of hospital-based surgeons aged 20 to 29 years had received the vaccine [60]. A 1994 survey indicated that 98% of graduating medical students had received hepatitis B vaccine [F. Hall, Association of American Medical Colleges, personal communication].

The decision to screen potential vaccine recipients for susceptibility to HBV, in order to identify previously infected persons and prevent unnecessary vaccination, is primarily an economic one. The cost-effectiveness of screening is determined by balancing the prevalence of previous infection in any targeted group, the cost of screening, and the cost of immunizing personnel without screening. Prevaccination screening in groups with the highest risk of previous HBV infection (HBV marker prevalence > 30%) may be cost beneficial. The most appropriate screening test is total antibody to hepatitis B core antigen (total anti-HBc), which will detect both immune persons and persons who are chronically infected with HBV. For HCWs, prevaccination testing is generally not indicated unless they are at high risk of HBV infection for another reason (e.g. they are from a country with a high endemic rate of HBV infection).

Postvaccination testing of HCWs who receive hepatitis B vaccine is useful because the results can help determine appropriate prophylaxis if they should have exposure to HBV. Postvaccination antibody testing is recommended for HCWs who are at risk of occupational exposure to blood or body fluids. Testing is not indicated for persons who are at low risk of exposure (e.g., HCWs without direct contact with patients or laboratory specimens). When indicated, postvaccination anti-HBs testing should be performed with an appropriate quantitative method. Testing should be done within 1 to 2 months after completion of the vaccine series. Persons who do not respond to three doses of hepatitis B vaccine should be revaccinated with one or more additional doses of vaccine.

Postexposure Prophylaxis. Any HCW who sustains occupational exposure (percutaneous or permucosal) to blood or other body fluid should undergo a thorough postexposure evaluation that includes an assessment of the exposed HCW's preexposure immunity to HBV and determination, if possible, of the source patient's HBV infection status. Since available data indicate that persons who respond to hepatitis B vaccine are protected even if antibody levels become undetectable, known vaccine responders do not need additional prophylaxis after an HBV exposure. Persons who are nonresponders require HBIG. Table 3-4 summarizes the approach to the treatment of exposed HCWs.

Other Infection Control Precautions. To further prevent HBV transmission, hospital personnel should be aware of the modes of HBV transmission and adopt appropriate precautions (i.e., standard precautions; see Chapter 13) for contact with or handling of blood and certain body fluids of all patients [2]. Standard precautions apply to blood, all body fluids, secretions, and excretions except sweat, regardless of whether they contain visible blood, nonintact skin, and mucous membranes, and are designed to cut down the risk of transmission of microorganisms from both recognized and unrecognized sources of infection in hospitals. Standard precautions include the use of barriers (e.g., gloves, gowns or aprons, masks, and goggles) for appropriate circumstances. For example, when performing certain dental procedures, dentists should protect their eyes, nose, and mouth from exposure to the patient's oral secretions and blood by using masks and protective eyewear; they can minimize the likelihood of direct contact with infective material in the patient's mouth by routinely wearing gloves [61,62].

Recommendations for HCWs with HBV Infection. Since the introduction of serologic testing for HBV infection in the early 1970s, at least 42 HBV-infected HCWs have been reported to have transmitted HBV to at least 375 patients worldwide [63]. Most reports were linked to surgeons (including obstetricians/gynecologists and cardiac and general surgeons), oral surgeons, or dentists; others were linked to workers in other healthcare fields, among them, cardiopulmonary bypass pump technician, general practitioner, and inhalation therapist.

Several risk factors for HBV transmission were identified from these reports. First, of the HCWs whose HBeAg status was determined, all were HBeAg-positive, except for several, whose virus was genetically unable to produce HBeAg. Second, most of the procedures implicated in transmission were relatively invasive. Finally, in most of the reported clusters or occurrences of transmission, the potential existed for contamination of surgical wounds or traumatized tissue, either from a major break in standard infection control practices (such as not wearing gloves during invasive procedures) or from unintentional injury to the HCW during the procedures (such as needle sticks incurred while palpating needles blindly during suturing). In one reported cluster, there were no major breaks in infection control practices or history of needle sticks; one postulated mechanism of HBV transmission was the surgeon's acquisition, after prolonged suture tying, of "paper-cut-like" finger lesions which, in combination with the presence of nonintact gloves, might have allowed exposure of patients to HBV [64].

The overall experience with HBV transmission from HCWs to patients indicates that when HCWs adhere to recommended infection control procedures, the risk of HBV transmission from HCW to patient is low. Most reported U.S. clusters occurred before awareness of the risks of transmission of bloodborne pathogens in healthcare settings was heightened and before emphasis on the use of universal precautions and hepatitis B vaccination among HCWs.

Recommendations published by Centers for Disease Control and Prevention (CDC) for prevention of HBV transmission from infected HCWs during invasive procedures are similar to recommendations to prevent HIV transmission from infected HCWs (see Chapter 43) [65]. These recommendations indicate that HCWs who perform exposure-prone invasive procedures should be vaccinated against hepatitis B. In addition, they should know their HBeAg status. Those HCWs who are HBeAg-positive should not perform exposure-prone, invasive procedures unless they have sought counsel and received advice from an expert review panel as to the circumstances, if any, under which they may continue to perform exposure-prone, invasive procedures. Such circumstances would include notifying prospective patients of the HCW's seropositivity before they undergo exposure-prone, invasive procedures. There is no scientific basis to restrict the activities of HCWs who are not HBeAg-positive or who do not perform exposure-prone, invasive procedures.

In a subsequent publication, the CDC issued additional information indicating that determination of whether a procedure is exposure-prone should be done on a case-by-case basis, taking into consideration the specific procedure as well as the skill, technique, and possible impairment of the healthcare worker [63]. Subsequently, states have developed guidelines implementing these recommendations. Many state-specific guidelines do not include the stipulation that patients undergoing exposure-prone, invasive procedures performed by infected HCWs should be notified of the HCW's status.

Hepatitis C Virus

Epidemiology of HCV Infection. Hepatitis C virus was identified in 1989 and has been determined to be the primary etiologic agent of parenterally transmitted non-A, non-B (NANB) hepatitis and a major cause of chronic liver disease. The average incubation period for hepatitis C following a blood transfusion or needle stick is ~7 weeks [66]. Of persons with acute HCV infection, ≤ 25% have symptoms of acute hepatitis. However, it is believed that nearly all persons with acute HCV infection will experience chronic HCV infection with persistent viremia. Follow-up studies after HCV infection show that an average of 67% of patients have persistently elevated liver enzymes, 26% to 50% will show signs of chronic active hepatitis, and 3% to 26% will develop cirrhosis within several years [66].

Tests to detect antibody to HCV (anti-HCV) have been developed. However, the anti-HCV test has limitations in detecting HCV infection. Only ~90% of patients with HCV infection (determined by using more sensitive tests, including the PCR for HCV genetic material) are anti-HCV positive. In addition, there may be a delay in the appearance of anti-HCV after onset of acute HCV infection [66].

HCV transmission occurs mainly after exposure to contaminated blood. The risk of HCV transmission after a needle stick contaminated with blood from an anti-HCV-positive source has been estimated to be ~10%, based on results from second-generation tests and PCR used to detect infection among needle stick recipients [67]. The role of the environment in the transmission of HCV is believed to be unimportant because compared with HBV, HCV is relatively fragile and rapidly degraded in serum at room temperature [68].

Because the major mode of HCV transmission is via blood, HCWs who have occupational exposure to blood or body fluids are at risk of HCV infection, although the epidemiology of HCV infection in the occupational setting is not well defined. Documented cases of HCV transmission from anti-HCV-positive patients to HCWs as a result of accidental needle sticks or cuts with sharp instruments [67,69–72] and one case of HCV transmission from a blood splash to the conjunctiva [73] have been reported. In two studies, the anti-HCV seroprevalence in HCWs ranged from 0% to 1.7% [60, 74–79]; however, few of these studies have used comparison groups. In two studies, dentists were shown to have a 12-fold higher anti-HCV prevalence compared with age-matched blood donors [76] and HCWs who reported a history of frequent needle sticks had a significantly higher prevalence than HCWs who did not [79].

Prevention of HCV Infection in HCWs. General measures for the prevention of HCV infection in HCWs are similar to those for other bloodborne diseases; they include the use of barrier precautions and personal protective devices (see section on hepatitis B). Unfortunately, there is no effective postexposure prophylaxis against HCV transmission. Studies of blood transfusion recipients in the 1970s showed equivocal efficacy of IG in preventing the transmission of parenteral NANB hepatitis, and before 1994 the ACIP recommended that IG be considered for recipients of blood from patients with NANB hepatitis [65]. However, since the discovery of HCV, several lines of evidence have indicated that IG is not effective in preventing HCV infection. These sources include animal experiments in which previous administration of either standard IG or high-titer anti-HCV IG failed to prevent HCV infection in animals later challenged with HCV [80]. Consequently, in 1994, the ACIP concluded that there was no evidence to support the use of IG for hepatitis C postexposure prophylaxis.

Testing and follow-up of HCWs who have percutaneous or permucosal exposure to blood or body fluids from anti-HCV-positive persons is the subject of controversy. Screening of source patients and persons exposed percutaneously will enable persons who may become infected to take precautions to prevent further transmission to others (e.g., sexual partners) and allow persons who acquire infection to receive counseling regarding possible treatment, for example, with interferon [81]. However, the risks of sexual, household, and perinatal transmission are not well defined, and interferon is effective in only a relatively modest percentage (< 20%) of patients. Nevertheless, because of the potential benefits of follow-up to HCWs who manifest HCV infection, the CDC recommends that institutions consider implementation of policies and procedures for such follow-up of HCWs who have percutaneous or permucosal exposure to anti-HCV-positive blood. Such policies might include baseline testing of the source for anti-HCV antibody and baseline and 6-month follow-up testing of the exposed person for anti-HCV and alanine aminotransferase activity. All anti-HCV test results reported as repeatedly reactive by Enzyme Immunoassay (EIA) should be confirmed by supplemental anti-HCV testing.

HCWs with HCV Infection. There are only a few reports of HCV transmission from infected surgeons to patients during invasive procedures. In a report from Spain, five patients acquired acute HCV infection after open heart surgery performed by an HCV-infected surgeon; the sequence of viral isolates from the surgeon and the patients showed a high degree of homology [82]. The factors responsible for transmission were not identified.

The relative infrequency of reports of surgeon-to-patient HCV transmission suggests that the risk of such transmission is low. Management of surgeons who are anti-HCV positive is somewhat difficult, primarily because there is no serologic assay that can definitively determine infectivity. While it is possible that PCR-detected HCV RNA is better than anti-HCV as an indicator of infectivity, PCR tests are not standardized. In addition, it is not known if there is a threshold viral concentration that determines infectivity, and since HCV RNA detection by PCR may be intermittent, the meaning of a single negative PCR test is not conclusive. Thus, to date, the CDC and other advisory groups have not made recommendations regarding the restriction of HCWs who are anti-HCV positive and instead suggest that such HCWs should follow strict aseptic techniques when performing invasive procedures.

Herpes Simplex Virus

Herpes simplex virus (HSV) can be transmitted among personnel and patients through direct contact with the vesicle fluid or from secretions containing the virus (e.g., saliva, vaginal secretions, and infected amniotic fluid) (see Chapter 42). Exposed areas of the skin, such as the fingers or hands, are the sites of infection that are of most concern in the healthcare setting.

Transmission of HSV from Patients to HCWs

Health care workers may acquire an HSV infection of the fingers (herpetic whitlow or paronychia) from exposure to contaminated secretions. Such exposure is a distinct hazard for nurses, anesthesiologists, dentists, respiratory care personnel, and other HCWs who have direct contact with oral lesions, saliva, or respiratory secretions. Less frequently, HCWs may be exposed to HSV lesions on the skin, genitals, or mucous membranes of patients. To prevent such exposure, HCWs should avoid direct contact with any lesion, wear gloves when anticipating contact with lesion fluid or patients' secretions, and always wash hands thoroughly after contact with patients [2].

Transmission of HSV from HCWs to Patients

An HCW with active HSV infection should take extreme care to ensure that there is no possibility that patients could have contact with his or her lesion fluid. If lesions are localized and covered, and the infected HCW uses recommended infection control practices (e.g., thorough hand washing), it is unlikely that the HCW poses any risk of transmission of HSV to the patient. The risk posed to patients by HCWs with uncovered orofacial lesions is believed to be low, but it has not been quantified. However, that risk can be reduced by covering the lesion to prevent hand contact, careful hand washing before all contact with patients, not kissing or nuzzling newborn infants or children with dermatitis, and restricting HCWs with active lesions from providing care to high-risk patients.

Personnel with herpetic whitlow should not have direct contact with patients until the lesions have completely crusted. Although some have suggested that HCWs with herpetic whitlow should be allowed to perform direct care while wearing gloves, the efficacy of wearing gloves to prevent HSV transmission is unknown [83].

Measles

Measles is transmitted both by large droplets during close contact between infected and susceptible persons and by airborne spread [84,85]. Nosocomial measles transmission has been documented in private doctors' offices, emergency rooms, and on hospital wards [86–88]. Although only 3.5% of all cases of measles reported between 1985 and 1989 occurred in a medical setting, the risk of infection among medical personnel is estimated to be up to 13 times greater than in the general population [86,87,89]. During 1990 to 1991, 1,788 (4.8%) of 37,429 cases of measles in the U.S. were reported to have been acquired in medical settings. Of these, 668 (37.4%) were diagnosed in HCWs, 561 (84%) of whom were unvaccinated. Three of the HCWs died, and 187 (28%) were hospitalized with measles [CDC, unpublished data]. From 1992 to 1995, there were 3,659 cases of measles. For 2,765 of these cases there was a known site of transmission; 385 (13.9%) were transmitted in a medical setting [CDC, unpublished data].

Because measles is highly transmissible and frequently misdiagnosed during the prodromal stage, prevention of nosocomial measles entails ensuring that hospital personnel are immune to measles, promptly identifying and isolating persons with fever and rash, continuing the use of appropriate isolation precautions once the diagnosis of measles is established [2], and providing measles vaccine to patients in medical settings, especially emergency rooms.

Documenting measles immunity is essential for all hospital personnel regardless of their involvement with care of patients. A person is considered immune to measles if he or she has had physician-diagnosed measles, serologic evidence of measles immunity, or adequate vaccination. (Health care workers born during or after 1957 are considered adequately vaccinated if they have received two doses of live measles-containing vaccine. Health care workers needing a second dose of measles-containing vaccine should be revaccinated ≥ 28 days after receipt of their first dose.) Most persons born before 1957 were once believed to have been infected naturally with measles and were therefore considered immune. However, recent studies indicate that ≤ 9.3% of hospital personnel born before 1957 may not be immune to measles [90,91]. In addition, from 1985 to 1992, 27% of all measles cases among HCWs in the U.S. were diagnosed in those born before 1957 [86; CDC, unpublished data]. Although birth before 1957 is still generally considered an acceptable indication of measles immunity, administration of a dose of MMR vaccine to unvaccinated workers born before 1957 who do not have a history of measles disease or laboratory evidence of measles immunity should be considered.

Health care workers exposed to measles may be infectious during the incubation period of 5 to 21 days after their exposure. In addition, persons with measles continue to be infectious for several days after the rash appears because the virus is shed from the nasopharynx of infected, immunocompetent persons beginning with the prodrome until 3 to 4 days after the onset of rash [92]; immunocompromised persons with measles may shed virus for extended periods of time.

Screening for Susceptibility to Measles

The cost-effectiveness of prevaccination screening for susceptibility to measles in hospital personnel depends on the costs of the screening tests and of the vaccine and on the expected prevalence of immunity to the virus. Both the expected prevalence of immunity to measles acquired from previous vaccination or disease (90% to 95%) and the vaccine cost are relatively constant throughout the U.S.; therefore, the key variable for a hospital is the cost of screening. The targeted, screen-and-vaccinate approach to measles vaccination (i.e., serologic screening of personnel for immunity to measles and vaccination of those found to be seronegative) has been shown to be cost effective when the serologic test is performed in-house (Table 3-1) [93–96]. However, when serum samples are sent for testing to reference laboratories outside the hospital, the cost of screening may offset the potential savings from not administering vaccine to those immune to measles.

A screen-and-vaccinate approach to measles alone does not take into consideration rubella and mumps. Although hospital outbreaks of rubella and mumps are reported less frequently than those of measles, a recent study among U.S. Army recruits suggests that as many as 16% to 18% of young adults may be susceptible to these infections [97]. In addition, because of the potential impact of these diseases, particularly the devastating effect of rubella infection in a pregnant woman, the opportunity to ensure the immunity of HCWs to these viruses cannot be overlooked. The additional cost of screening for immunity to rubella and mumps eliminates the cost savings from the screen-and-vaccinate approach to measles prevention and favors the administration of MMR vaccine to employees who do not have documentation of previous MMR vaccination (see sections on mumps and rubella herein).

Serologic screening to determine immunity before vaccination can be a barrier to timely immunization. In general, routine serologic screening to determine immunity to measles, rubella, or mumps is not recommended. Serologic screening is appropriate only in situations in which tracking systems are used to ensure that persons identified as susceptible are subsequently vaccinated in a timely manner, as when hiring new HCWs. However, during an outbreak, serologic screening before vaccination is generally not recommended because arresting disease transmission requires rapid vaccination.

Meningococcal Disease

Nosocomial transmission of *Neisseria meningitidis* either to hospital personnel taking care of patients with meningococcemia, meningococcal meningitis, or lower respiratory infections or to laboratory personnel processing specimens containing *N. meningitidis* is uncommon (see Chapter 36). In rare instances, transmission in these settings has occurred through intensive direct contact with respiratory secretions or cultures of *N. meningitidis* [98–100].

In the clinical setting, the most likely mode of spread from a person with respiratory or systemic infections is by large droplets from the respiratory tract. Thus, meningococcal lower-respiratory infections may present a greater risk of transmission than meningococcemia or meningitis alone, especially if the patient has an active, productive cough [99,100]. Airborne transmission and patient-to-patient spread via hands of personnel have been suggested but not well documented [101]. The risk to personnel from casual contact with an infected patient (e.g., as usually occurs with housekeepers) appears to be negligible. To lessen the risk of infection in the clinical setting, staff taking care of patients with known or suspected *N. meningitidis* infection should, in addition to observing standard infection control precautions, wear a mask when close contact with the patient is anticipated [2].

In the laboratory, workers may be exposed to *N. meningitidis* by inoculation, ingestion, and droplet or aerosol exposure of the mucous membranes. It has been recommended that for their protection, laboratory employees who handle meningococci should wear gloves and gowns, decontaminate all infectious wastes, and, when performing procedures that may aerosolize meningococci, use a class II biologic safety cabinet [98].

Prophylaxis After Unprotected Exposure

Antimicrobial prophylaxis can prevent *N. meningitidis* infections in personnel who have unprotected exposure to the microorganism. Prophylaxis is indicated for persons who, without using appropriate precautions, have intensive direct contact with patients with known or unrecognized meningococcal infection or whose cultures are positive for *N. meningitidis*.

When prophylaxis is deemed necessary, it is important to begin treatment immediately, before the results of antimicrobial susceptibility testing are available. The ACIP recommends that personnel with mucosal exposure to meningococci receive rifampicin (600 mg orally twice daily for 2 days) for chemoprophylaxis [102]. However, rifampicin should not be given to pregnant employees. Ceftriaxone, has been found to be effective in eradicating pharyngeal carriage of *N. meningitidis*, and should be considered for exposed personnel who are pregnant or cannot take rifampicin for other reasons [102–105]. In addition, single-dose (500 mg) ciprofloxacin is also recommended for prophylaxis [106]; however, ciprofloxacin is contraindicated for pregnant women. Because of sulfonamide-resistance in meningococci, sulfonamides are no longer recommended for prophylactic use [102,107,108].

Carriage of N. Meningitidis *by Staff*

Carriage of *N. meningitidis* in the nasopharynx of healthy persons has been recognized for many years, but the prevalence is variable [108–110]. Carriage may be transient, intermittent, or chronic [110]. In non-outbreak situations, asymptomatic carriers among personnel need not be identified, treated, or removed from the care of patients.

Mumps

In recent years, the overall incidence of mumps in the United States has fluctuated only minimally, but an increasing proportion of cases has been reported in persons ≥ 15 years of age [111]. Outbreaks have arisen among unvaccinated adolescents and young adults on college campuses and in the workplace. Outbreaks have also taken place in vaccinated populations; these have been attributed to primary vaccine failure [112]. Mumps transmission in medical settings has been reported in many locations nationwide [113; CDC, unpublished data].

Mumps is transmitted by direct contact with virus-containing respiratory secretions or saliva; the portals of entry are the nose and mouth (see Chapter 42). The incubation period varies from 14 to 25 days and is usually 16 to 18 days. The virus may be present in saliva for 6 to 10 days before parotitis and persists for ≤ 9 days after onset of disease. Because mumps virus is shed by infected persons long before any clinical symptom is manifested and because many infected persons remain asymptomatic, an effective vaccination program is the best approach to preventing mumps transmission (Table 3-1).

Vaccination with the live, attenuated Jeryl Lynn strain mumps vaccine is recommended, unless otherwise contraindicated, for all those who are susceptible to mumps (Table 3-1) [3]. Because of its favorable cost-benefit ratio, the combined MMR vaccine is the vaccine of choice for routine mumps vaccination [114], especially if the recipient is likely to be susceptible also to measles and rubella.

Persons are considered susceptible to mumps unless they have documentation of physician-diagnosed mumps or adequate immunization with live mumps vaccine on or after the first birthday or laboratory evidence of immunity or were born before 1957 (Table 3-1). This latter arbitrary cutoff date, however, does not preclude vaccinating possibly susceptible persons born before 1957 who may be exposed in an outbreak. Revaccination with MMR is recommended under certain circumstances for measles (see section on measles) and may also be important for mumps because recent studies have shown that mumps can break out among vaccinated populations [115]. Isolation precautions to prevent droplet transmission are recommended for patients with mumps; these precautions are maintained for 9 days after the onset of parotitis [2].

Parvovirus Infection

Human parvovirus B19 is the causative agent of erythema infectiosum (EI), or fifth disease, which manifests as a rash illness in children or acute arthropathy in adults [116–118]. Although most B19 infections are mild and self-limited, certain groups of persons are at risk of more serious manifestations or complications of B19 infection [118]. Among these groups are patients with chronic hemolytic anemia, who may manifest a pure red-cell aplasia, also known as transient aplastic crisis (TAC) [119]; immunodeficient patients, who may show signs of chronic anemia [120]; and pregnant women, who may experience spontaneous abortions and stillbirths [121] (see Chapter 42).

Transmission of B19 has been confirmed after close-contact exposure (e.g., to susceptible household contacts of patients with EI or TAC [122] or, rarely, to HCWs giving care to patients with B19-associated sickle cell aplastic crisis [117]). It is hypothesized that B19 may be transmitted via direct person-to-person contact, fomites, and droplets [116].

Transmission of Parvovirus B19 from Patients to Personnel

Isolation precautions are not indicated for most patients with EI because they are already past the period of infectiousness at the time of clinically evident illness [118,123]. However, patients in aplastic crisis due to B19 or patients with chronic B19 infection may transmit the virus to susceptible HCWs or other patients; therefore, patients with chronic hemolytic anemia who are admitted to the hospital with febrile illness and TAC or patients known or suspected to be chronically infected with B19 are placed on droplet precautions on admission until the infection resolves [2,117].

Pregnant Employees

Pregnant employees do not have a greater risk of acquiring B19 infection compared with nonpregnant personnel; however, if a pregnant woman acquires B19 infection during the first half of pregnancy, the risk of fetal death (spontaneous abortion and stillbirth) is increased [123]. Because of this increased risk, and until a B19 vaccine becomes available, workers who are pregnant or who might be pregnant should know the potential risks to the fetus that are associated with B19 infection and the dangers of working with high-risk patients and should practice appropriate infection control precautions when performing their duties [2,123].

Pertussis

Pertussis is highly contagious; secondary attack rates exceed 80% in susceptible household contacts [124,125]. Transmission occurs by direct contact with respiratory secretions or large droplets from the respiratory tract of infected persons. The incubation period is 7 to 10 days. The period of communicability starts at the onset of the catarrhal stage and extends into the paroxysmal stage. Vaccinated adolescents and adults, whose immunity wanes 5 to 10 years after the last vaccine dose (usually given at 4 to 6 years of age), play an important role in transmitting pertussis to susceptible infants. Pertussis can be transmitted from adult patients to close contacts, especially nonimmunized children. Such transmission may occur in the household or in hospitals, where chains of transmission have been known to involve both patients and personnel [126–129]. These outbreaks have been costly and disruptive; although the numbers of persons with clinical pertussis were relatively small (2 to 17 patients and 5 to 13 HCWs), many more HCWs who were evaluated for cough required nasopharyngeal cultures, serologic tests, prophylactic antibiotics, and exclusion from work.

Preventing secondary transmission of pertussis is especially difficult during the early stages of the disease because pertussis is highly communicable in the catarrhal stage, when the symptoms are nonspecific and the diagnosis is uncertain. Because of the lack of a good definition of what constitutes exposure to pertussis, a patient's or HCW's risk of contracting the disease during a pertussis outbreak in a hospital is often difficult to quantify. Serologic studies conducted in HCWs during two outbreaks indicate that exposure to pertussis is much more frequent than is suggested by the attack rates of clinically manifest disease [126,129]. However, the level of serum agglutination antibodies to pertussis were found to correlate with the degree of contact with patients. Seroprevalence was highest among pediatric house staff (82%) and ward nurses (71%) and lowest among nurses with administrative responsibilities (35%) [127].

Prevention of pertussis transmission in healthcare settings calls for early diagnosis and treatment of clinically evident cases, placement of hospitalized infectious patients on appropriate isolation precautions, exclusion of infectious HCWs from work, and postexposure prophylaxis. Early diagnosis of pertussis, before secondary transmission occurs, is difficult because the disease is highly communicable during the catarrhal stage, when symptoms are still nonspecific. Pertussis should be considered in the differential diagnosis of any patient with illness manifesting with an acute cough lasting ≥ 7 days without a clear cause, particularly if the symptoms include paroxysms of cough or post-tussis vomiting, whoop, or apnea. Nasopharyngeal cultures should be obtained whenever possible.

Patients admitted to the hospital with suspected or confirmed pertussis should be placed on precautions to prevent large-droplet transmission or spread by direct contact [2]. Precautions should remain in effect until patients' clinical symptoms have improved and they have completed ≥ 5 days of appropriate antimicrobial therapy. Health care workers who have symptoms (e.g., unexplained rhinitis or acute cough) following known pertussis exposure may be at risk of transmitting pertussis and require exclusion from work (Table 3-5).

Postexposure Prophylaxis

Erythromycin has been given to personnel following exposure to pertussis [130]; however, the efficacy of this treatment has not been determined [131]. In persons with hypersensitivity or intolerance to erythromycin, sulfa-containing animicrobials have been used as substitutes.

Rubella

Nosocomial rubella can affect both hospital personnel and patients [132–139]. Rubella can pass from both male and female personnel (including medical and dental students) to susceptible co-workers and patients and from patients to personnel and other patients [134,135]. Rubella in adults is usually a mild disease, lasting only a few days (see Chapter 42). From 30% to 50% of cases may be subclinical or inapparent. The incubation period is variable, but it may range from 12 to 23 days; most persons show signs of rash 14 to 16 days after exposure. The disease is most contagious when the rash is erupting, but virus may be shed from one week before to 5 to 7 days after the onset of the rash.

To minimize introduction and transmission of rubella at medical facilities, all HCWs, both male and female, who might transmit rubella to pregnant patients or other HCWs, should be immune to rubella (Table 3-1) [4,113, 140]. Persons should be considered susceptible to rubella unless they have documentation of vaccination on or after their first birthday or laboratory evidence of immunity. Although birth before 1957 is generally accepted as an indication of rubella immunity, a dose of MMR vaccine should be considered for unvaccinated HCWs born before 1957 who do not have serologic evidence of rubella immunity. Rubella vaccination or laboratory evidence of rubella immunity is particularly important for HCWs born before 1957 who might become pregnant.

Serologic screening need not be done before vaccinating HCWs against rubella unless the medical facility considers it cost effective or the potential vaccinee requests it. Serologic screening is appropriate only if tracking systems are used to ensure that tested persons identified as susceptible are subsequently vaccinated in a timely manner. The ACIP states that administering rubella vaccine to women not known to be pregnant and to men is justifiable without prevaccination screening (Table 3-1); the risk of adverse events following rubella vaccination of persons already immune to rubella is not increased [141]. MMR trivalent vaccine is the vaccine of choice (see sections on measles and mumps).

Ideally, all personnel should be immune, but priority in terms of vaccination should be given to employees who are at increased risk of exposure to rubella or who are in direct contact with pregnant patients. To maximize compliance, mandatory programs may need to be considered; voluntary programs are usually inadequate [142,143]. Many local and state health departments mandate rubella immunity for HCWs; thus, staff in charge of personnel health programs should consult with their local or state health departments.

On the basis of the periods of incubation and communicability of rubella, susceptible personnel who are exposed to or show signs of rubella are relieved from direct contact with patients from the 7th day after the first exposure through the 21st day after the last exposure or until 5 days after rash appears (Table 3-5).

Scabies

Scabies is caused by infestation with the mite *Sarcoptes scabiei*. It is transmitted in hospitals primarily through skin-to-skin contact with an infested person [144]. Health care workers should observe contact precautions when taking care of infested patients, to prevent acquiring the disease [2].

In most cases of typical scabies, including scabies in hospital personnel, treatment with a single correct application of agents (e.g., permethrin cream, crotamiton 10%, or a 1% lindane lotion) used to treat scabies is curative and lowers substantially the risk of transmission immediately after the first treatment [145–151]. Repeating the treatment 7 to 10 days after the initial therapy usually kills mites that are newly hatched from eggs that remain viable after the first treatment. Between treatments, the risk of transmission from these persons is negligible.

Because most infested HCWs have low mite loads (exceptions are those with Norwegian [crusted] scabies or those who are old and/or immunocompromised) [152, 153], the risk of transmission from them is low after they receive the first treatment, even if they may later require a second treatment for complete cure. Thus, personnel infested with scabies are excluded from work until after they receive initial treatment, and they are advised to report for further evaluation if symptoms do not subside. It may be prudent to exclude HCWs with confirmed scabies from providing care to immunosuppressed patients until the second treatment is completed, unless they wear gloves and gowns for any such contact. Postexposure prophylaxis of HCWs is not warranted if the HCWs do not have signs of infestation.

Staphylococcus Aureus

Staphylococcal carriage or infection is common among humans. In the case of nosocomial transmission, there are two sources: a person with a lesion or an asymptomatic carrier (see Chapter 41). Persons with skin lesions due to *Staphylococcus aureus* are most likely to disseminate these organisms. Direct contact is the major route of transmission. Even minor or entirely inapparent skin infections in employees may represent a hazard to patients. One way to lessen the possibility of dissemination is to not allow HCWs to work until skin infection caused by this organism resolves.

The anterior nares are among the most commonly colonized sites, but *S. aureus* may be found at other sites, such as any draining or crusted lesion, the nasopharynx and oropharynx, and the skin of the axilla, fingers, and perineum [154] (see Chapter 41). Methicillin-susceptible (but penicillin-resistant) *S. aureus* (MSSA) used to account for most staphylococcal infections. However, methicillin-resistant *S. aureus* (MRSA) has become a prevalent nosocomial pathogen [154,155]. The epidemiology of MRSA does not appear to differ much from that of MSSA, except that outbreaks due to MRSA tend to happen more frequently in intensive care and burn units [156].

The most important source of *S. aureus* in hospitals are infected or colonized patients. Hospital personnel who are infected or colonized with *S. aureus* can also serve as reservoirs and disseminators of the microorganism and have been identified as a link for transmission between patients [156]. The main mode of transmission of *S. aureus* is via employees' hands, which can become contaminated by contact with colonized or infected sites on patients or on personnel themselves. In patients on burn units or in patients with pneumonia or draining skin lesions, droplet transmission of *S. aureus* may occur. In addition, when fomites are heavily contaminated with *S. aureus*, contact transmission is facilitated.

Culture surveys of staff members can detect carriers of *S. aureus* [157] but do not indicate whether carriers are likely to disseminate the organism. For most hospitals, routine culture survey data are difficult to interpret. A more reasonable approach is to emphasize effective surveillance that permits prompt recognition of *S. aureus* infections in both personnel and patients. If workers are linked epidemiologically to an increased or unusual cluster of infections, cultures should be done on those persons and, if they are positive for the same strain(s) of *S. aureus* cultured from patients, such employees should be removed from contact with patients until the organism is eradicated (see Chapter 41).

Streptococcus Groups A and B

Groups A and B streptococci (*S. pyogenes* and *S. agalactiae*) are important nosocomial pathogens (see Chapter 42).

Group A Streptococci

Patient-to-Personnel Transmission. Although pharyngeal and skin infections are the most common group A streptococcal infections, clusters of invasive group A streptococcal infections, including the toxic shock–like syndrome (TSLS), have been recognized [158–160]. Secondary spread and illness (including TSLS, cellulitis, lymphangitis, and pharyngitis) in hospital staff can occur after direct contact by them with secretions from infected patients. To prevent patient-to-personnel transmission of group A streptococci, personnel should wash their hands thoroughly after each contact with patients, wear gloves when contact with potentially contaminated secretions is anticipated, and wear gowns when soiling with infective material is likely [2].

Personnel-to-patient transmission. Sporadic outbreaks of surgical wound infections or postpartum infections caused by group A streptococci have been associated with carriers among operating room or delivery room personnel [161–164]. The main reservoirs of group A streptococci in implicated carriers are the pharynx, the skin, the rectum, and the female genital tract. Direct contact and airborne spread are the major modes of transmission of this organism in these settings [161–164].

Since surgical wound infections or postpartum infections due to group A streptococci are rare, any isolate from cases should be saved for possible typing should an outbreak ensue. The occurrence of two or more cases should prompt an epidemiologic investigation and a search for a carrier-disseminator. Isolates obtained from personnel and patients should be typed to determine strain relatedness. Ideally, only personnel who are epidemiologically linked to cases should have cultures of skin lesions, pharynx, rectum, and vagina and, if they are positive for the same strain(s) of streptococci isolated from patients, the infected staff should be removed from contact with patients until treatment is completed and follow-up cultures show negative results. However, in situations in which epidemiologic studies cannot establish any links between cases and personnel, the identification of a carrier-disseminator may be facilitated by taking cultures of all personnel associated with cases and the operating room environment [162]. Routine screening of personnel for group A streptococcal carriage in the absence of cases of nosocomial infection is not recommended.

Because experience is limited regarding the treatment and follow-up of personnel carriers implicated in outbreaks of surgical wound infections due to group A streptococci, and because carriage of the organism by an HCW may recur over long periods of time [161,164], treatment and follow-up of these personnel carriers should be individualized.

Group B Streptococci

Personnel who are carriers of group B streptococci may play a role in its nosocomial transmission. However, the epidemiology of early-onset group B streptococcal infections in neonates suggests that maternal colonization with group B streptococci, followed by the infant's acquisition of the organism during passage through the birth canal, accounts for most infections. In late-onset neonatal infections, spread of the organism occurs from colonized to uncolonized infants via the hands of staff members or by direct contact from colonized hospital personnel. In both types of infections, careful observance of standard precautions will minimize the risk of spread from colonized infants or personnel to uncolonized infants [2].

Tuberculosis and Bacille Calmette-Guérin Vaccination

Mycobacterium tuberculosis (TB) continues to pose a serious problem for HCWs. In the hospital, exposure is most likely to occur when a patient has unsuspected pulmonary or laryngeal TB, has bacilli-laden sputum or respiratory secretions, and is coughing or sneezing into air that remains in general circulation (also see Chapter 33). The best ways to protect others from a patient with TB in a healthcare facility is to develop and implement a comprehensive TB infection control plan that includes maintaining vigilance about the possibility of TB, instituting appropriate engineering controls and isolation precautions with all known or suspected TB patients, and administering appropriate chemotherapy promptly [1]. Episodes of nosocomial transmission of multidrug-resistant TB to patients and HCWs further emphasize the importance of complying with current guidelines [1].

Approaches to the treatment of infected HCWs or those with active TB disease include the recommendations for surveillance and control in the general population issued jointly by the American Thoracic Society, the CDC, and the Infectious Diseases Society of America [165]; those of the CDC Guideline for Preventing the Transmission of *Myobacterium tuberculosis* in Healthcare Facilities, [1] the CDC Guideline for Isolation Precautions in Hospitals [2]; and the recommendation of the American Thoracic Society for the Treatment of Tuberculosis and Tuberculous Infection in Adults and Children [166].

Screening Programs

Healthcare facilities providing care to patients at risk of TB should maintain active surveillance for TB among patients and healthcare facility personnel and for skin-test conversions among HCWs. When TB is suspected or diagnosed, public health authorities should be notified so that appropriate contact investigation can be performed. The TB screening program should be based on the facility-specific risk assessment [1].

At the time of employment, all healthcare facility personnel, including those with a history of bacille Calmette-Guérin (BCG) vaccination, should receive a Mantoux tuberculin skin test (purified protein derivative of tuberculin (PPD)) unless a previously positive reaction can be documented or completion of adequate preventive therapy or adequate therapy for active disease can be confirmed. A two-step procedure should be used for baseline testing of HCWs who have not had a negative PPD test during the preceding 12 months. This is done to minimize the likelihood of misinterpreting a boosted reaction as a true conversion due to recent infection. Initial and follow-up tuberculin skin tests should be administered and interpreted according to current guidelines [1,165–166].

Healthcare workers with a documented history of a positive tuberculin test or adequate treatment for disease or preventive therapy for infection should be exempt from further screening unless they develop symptoms suggestive of TB. Periodic retesting of PPD-negative HCWs should be conducted to identify persons whose skin tests convert to positive [1]. The frequency of conducting these repeated tests after the initial screening can be established on the basis of the facility's periodic risk assessment [1].

Persons with tuberculous infection can be identified by a significant reaction to a Mantoux method skin test after the administration of 5 tuberculin units (TU) of PPD standard (see Chapter 33 for interpretation of PPD test results). The Mantoux technique (intracutaneous injection of 0.1 ml PPD-tuberculin containing 5 TU) is the preferred method for screening persons for TB infection [1] because it is the most accurate test available.

Recommendations for Treatment of Infected HCWs

Healthcare workers with positive tuberculin skin tests or with skin-test conversions on repeated testing or after exposure should be clinically evaluated for active TB [1]. Persons with symptoms suggestive of TB should be evaluated regardless of skin-test results. If TB is diagnosed, appropriate therapy should be instituted according to published guidelines [1,166,167]. Personnel diagnosed with active TB should be offered counseling [1].

Personnel who have positive tuberculin skin tests or skin-test conversions but who do not have clinical evidence of TB should be evaluated for preventive therapy according to published guidelines [1]. Staff members with positive skin tests should be evaluated for risk of HIV infection. If HIV infection is considered a possibility, counseling and HIV antibody testing should be strongly encouraged [1]. All persons with a history of TB or positive tuberculin tests are at risk of future manifestations of TB. These persons should be reminded periodically that they should promptly report any pulmonary symptoms. If symptoms of TB should develop, the person should be evaluated immediately [1].

Routine chest films are not recommended for asymptomatic, tuberculin-negative HCWs. After the initial chest radiograph is taken, personnel with positive skin-test reactions do not need any more chest radiographs unless symptoms develop that may be related to TB [1,168]. Chest radiographs cannot take the place of tuberculin skin tests, because they will not identify persons who are infected but who do not have radiographic evidence of current or past disease.

Healthcare workers with ongoing pulmonary or laryngeal tuberculosis pose a risk to patients and other personnel while they are infectious. They should be excluded from work until adequate treatment is instituted, cough is resolved, and sputum is free of bacilli on three consecutive smears. Employees with active TB at sites other than the lung or larynx usually do not need to be excluded from work if concurrent pulmonary TB has been ruled out. Personnel who discontinue treatment before the recommended course of therapy has been completed should not be allowed to work until treatment is resumed and they have negative sputum smears on 3 consecutive days.

Staff members who are otherwise healthy and receiving preventive treatment for tuberculous infection should be allowed to continue usual work activities. Health care workers who cannot take or do not accept or complete a full course of preventive therapy should not be excluded from the workplace. They should be counseled about the risk of active TB and should be instructed to seek evaluation promptly if symptoms that may be due to TB manifest [1]. Consultation on TB surveillance, screening, and other methods to reduce TB transmission should be available from state health department TB control programs. Facilities are encouraged to use the services of health departments in planning and implementing their surveillance and screening programs.

Tuberculosis and BCG Vaccination of HCWs in High-Risk Settings

Because the overall risk of TB infection is low for the total U.S. population, routine vaccination with BCG vaccine is not indicated. Instead, TB prevention and control efforts are focused on interrupting transmission from patients who have active infectious TB, skin testing those at high risk of TB infection, and preventive therapy whenever appropriate. In certain situations, BCG vaccination contributes to the prevention and control of TB when other strategies are inadequate. In the United States, BCG vaccination has not been recommended for general use because of the uneven distribution of TB risk in the population, uncertainty regarding the protective efficacy of BCG, and its interference with detection of *M. tuberculosis* infection.

Vaccination of HCWs should be considered on an individual basis in healthcare settings where a high percentage of TB patients are infected with *M. tuberculosis* strains resistant to both isoniazid and rifampin, transmission of such drug-resistant *M. tuberculosis* strains to HCWs is likely, and comprehensive TB infection-control precautions have been implemented and have not been successful. Vaccination with BCG should not be required for employment or for assignment in specific work areas.

Vaccination with BCG is not recommended for HIV-infected persons or other persons who are immunocompromised. In settings where there is a high risk of transmission of *M. tuberculosis* strains resistant to both isoniazid and rifampin, employees and volunteers who are infected with HIV or are otherwise immunocompromised should be fully informed about the risk of acquiring TB infection and active disease.

Healthcare workers considered for BCG vaccination should be counseled regarding the risks and benefits of both BCG vaccination and preventive therapy. They should be informed about the variable data regarding the efficacy of BCG vaccination, the interference with diagnosing a newly acquired *M. tuberculosis* infection, and the possible serious complications of BCG vaccination of immunocompromised persons, especially those infected with HIV. They also should be informed of the lack of data regarding the efficacy of preventive therapy for *M. tuberculosis* infections caused by strains resistant to isoniazid and rifampin and the risks of drug toxicity associated with multidrug preventive therapy.

At the request of an immunocompromised HCW, employers should offer, but not compel, a work assignment in which the HCW would have the lowest possible risk of infection with *M. tuberculosis*. Health care workers who contract TB are a source of infection for other HCWs and patients. Immunocompromised persons are at higher risk of manifesting active disease after exposure to TB; therefore, managers of healthcare facilities should develop written policies to limit activities that might result in exposure of immunocompromised HCWs to active TB.

Vaccination with BCG is not recommended for HCWs in low-risk settings. In most areas of the United States, most *M. tuberculosis* isolates are fully susceptible to isoniazid or rifampin or both, and the risk of TB transmission in healthcare facilities is very low if adequate infection control practices are maintained.

Varicella Zoster Virus

Nosocomial transmission of varicella zoster virus (VZV) is well recognized [169–179]. Sources for nosocomial exposure of patients and HCWs have included patients, HCWs, and visitors who are infected with either varicella or zoster. Airborne VZV transmission in hospitals—from people with varicella or zoster—has been verified: nosocomial varicella infection arose in susceptible persons who had no direct contact with the index case patient [180–184] (see Chapter 42).

Although all susceptible hospitalized persons are at risk of severe varicella and its complications, certain patients are at particularly high risk. They include premature infants born to varicella-susceptible mothers; infants born at < 28 weeks' gestation or weighing ≤ 1,000 g, regardless of maternal immune status; and immunocompromised patients of all ages, including persons undergoing immunosuppressive therapy and those with malignant disease and/or immunodeficiency.

Although only a few HCWs are susceptible to varicella, it is useful to identify them when they begin employment in the hospital. It is advisable to allow only HCWs who are immune to varicella to take care of patients with known or suspected varicella or zoster. Adults with a history of varicella can be assumed to be immune. Those without a history or with uncertain history of varicella may either be considered susceptible or be tested serologically to determine their immune status.

In March 1995, a live attenuated varicella vaccine prepared from a cell-free preparation of the Oka strain of VZV was licensed for use in the U.S. Administration of varicella vaccine is recommended for susceptible persons who will have close contact with persons at high risk of serious complications (Table 3-1)]. In hospitals, prevaccination serologic screening of HCWs who have a negative or equivocal history of varicella may be cost effective depending on the relative costs of the test and vaccine.

Varicella vaccination should help control, but not eliminate, the spread of VZV to and from HCWs [187]. Varicella vaccination programs may not be as simple as those for measles, mumps, and rubella. Two doses of the vaccine are required to achieve high seroconversion rates in adults [185]. The need for and response to booster doses of vaccine are unknown. Some experience with the vaccine will be required to optimize varicella prevention and control strategies.

Varicella Antibody Testing

A reliable history of chicken pox has been found to be a valid measure of immunity [179,186–188]; in adults, a positive history of varicella is highly predictive of serologic immunity (97% to 99% seropositive). In addition, the majority (71% to 93%) of adults with negative or uncertain histories are seropositive. Numerous methods have been used to detect antibodies to VZV; they include complement fixation, the indirect fluorescent antibody test, the fluorescent antibody to membrane antigen test, neutralization, indirect hemagglutination, immune adherence hemagglutination, radioimmunoassay, latex agglutination, and the enzyme-linked immunosorbent assay [189–201].

Varicella virus vaccine provides 70% to 90% protection against infection and 95% protection against severe disease for ≥ 7 to 10 years after vaccination. Breakthrough infections have occurred among vaccinees after exposure to natural varicella virus. In studies of vaccinees of all ages who were followed for ≤ 9 years, 1% to 4% per year developed chicken pox, depending on the vaccine lot and interval from vaccination [Merck, unpublished data]. The disease in vaccinated persons is markedly less severe (skin lesions number ≤ 50 [median] and are less apt to be vesicular; most patients are afebrile, and the illness is shorter in duration) than in unvaccinated persons, who generally manifest fever and several hundred vesicular lesions [202,203].

The rate of transmission of disease from vaccinees who contract varicella is low for vaccinated children, but it has not been studied in adults. Active surveillance for 1 to 8 years after vaccination of 2,141 children between 1981 and 1989 in 10 different trials resulted in reports of secondary cases in 11 (12.2%) of 90 vaccinated siblings of 78 vaccinated children who showed signs of varicella [204]. Illness was mild in both index and secondary cases. There also has been a report of transmission from a vaccinated child (in whom breakthrough disease occurred) to a susceptible mother.

Current data concerning vaccine efficacy and persistence of antibody in vaccinees are based on research conducted when natural VZV infection has been prevalent and has not been affected by the wide use of vaccine. Thus, the extent to which boosting from exposure to natural virus increases the protection provided by vaccination remains unclear. Whether longer term immunity may wane as the circulation of natural VZV declines is also unknown.

Transmission of Vaccine Virus to Contacts

The risk of transmission of vaccine virus was assessed in placebo recipients who were siblings of vaccinated healthy children [205] and among healthy siblings of vaccinated children with leukemia [206]. The results suggest that healthy children have a minimal risk of transmitting vaccine virus to susceptible contacts; the risk may be higher in vaccinees in whom a varicella-like rash develops after vaccination; in contrast, immunocompromised vaccinees have a high risk of transmitting the virus, probably because they usually manifest a rash after vaccination.

More information is needed on the risk of transmission of vaccine virus from vaccinees with and without varicella-like rash after vaccination. The risk, if any, appears to be very low, and the benefits of vaccinating susceptible HCWs clearly outweigh this potential risk. (In clinical trials, 3.8% of children and 5.5% of adolescents and adults showed signs of nonlocalized rash [median, five lesions] after the first injection, and 0.9% of adolescents and adults had nonlocalized rashes after the second injection.) As a safeguard, infection-control precautions may be considered for personnel who manifest rashes after vaccination and for other vaccinated staff members who will have contact with susceptible persons at high risk of serious complications from varicella.

Varicella Control Strategies

Strategies for managing clusters of VZV infection in hospitals generally have included isolation of patients with varicella and of exposed susceptible patients; control of air flow; rapid serologic testing of patients and HCWs to determine susceptibility; furlough or daily screening of exposed susceptible HCWs for skin lesions, fever, or constitutional symptoms; and temporary reassignment of susceptible personnel to locations remote from areas dedicated to care of patients [186,187,207–212]. Implementation of appropriate isolation precautions for hospitalized patients with known or suspected VZV infection can minimize the risk of transmission to HCWs [2]. It is generally advisable to allow only HCWs who are immune to varicella to take care of these patients. Adults with a history of varicella can be assumed to be immune. Those without a history or with uncertain history of varicella may be considered susceptible or may be tested serologically to determine susceptibility or immunity.

Until all their lesions dry and crust, HCWs with localized zoster should not take care of high-risk patients because of the possibility of transmission to and development of severe illness in these patients. HCWs with localized zoster may not pose a special risk to other patients if the lesions can be covered; however, some institutions may wish to institute more strict precautions for all patients, including placing HCWs with zoster on furlough until all lesions dry and crust [178].

Treatment of Exposed HCWs

Susceptible HCWs who are exposed to varicella are potentially infectious 10 to 21 days after exposure and should be relieved from direct contact with patients from the 10th day after the first exposure through the 21st day after the last exposure or, if varicella occurs, until all lesions dry and crust [2].

The use of VZIG after exposure of potential susceptibles to varicella can be costly, does not necessarily prevent varicella, and may prolong the incubation period by a week or more, thus extending the time during which personnel should not work with patients. Thus, VZIG is not recommended for routine use in immunocompetent HCWs. Instead, it is reserved for use in immunocompromised (e.g., HIV-infected) HCWs. Immunologically competent workers are placed under observation for clinical signs and symptoms of varicella, which can be treated with acyclovir.

Several options for the treatment of vaccinated HCWs who may be exposed to varicella are available. One approach is to not test vaccine recipients for varicella immunity after two doses of vaccine have been administered, since 99% of persons are seropositive after the second dose and seroconversion does not always result in full protection against disease. A second approach potentially offers an effective strategy to identify people who remain at risk: to test vaccinees for seropositivity immediately after their exposure to VZV. Prompt serologic results at reasonable cost may be obtained using the latex agglutination test.

Persons with detectable antibody are unlikely to manifest varicella. Those without antibody can be retested in 5 to 6 days to determine if an anamnestic response is present, in which case it is unlikely that they will show signs of disease; those who remain susceptible should be furloughed at once or observed further for development of signs and symptoms of varicella, at which time they would be furloughed. Institutional guidelines will be needed for treatment of exposed vaccinees without detectable antibody as well as for those who show clinical symptoms of varicella.

Vaccination should be considered for unvaccinated HCWs without documented immunity who are exposed to varicella. However, because the protective effects of postexposure vaccination are unknown, persons vaccinated after exposure should be treated as previously recommended for unvaccinated persons.

Viral Respiratory Infections

Viral respiratory infections are common problems for infection control programs (see Chapters 32,42). Respiratory viruses are mainly transmitted via airborne small-particle aerosols or droplet nuclei and via droplets (large particles) [2] (see Chapter 1). Different respiratory viruses may vary in the way in which they are transmitted.

Aerosols are produced by talking, sneezing, or coughing and may transmit infection over a considerable distance (> 3 feet). Large particles (droplets) are produced by sneezing and coughing and require close person-to-person contact for transmission. In addition, however, person-to-person transmission can also take place through contaminating the hands by direct contact with infective areas or materials, then transferal of infective virus to mucous membranes of a susceptible person [213–215]. Self-inoculation can also occur in this way. The nose and eyes appear to be important portals of entry [215].

Pediatric patients seem to be at particular risk of complications from nosocomial respiratory tract infections. Infection in the elderly, patients with chronic underlying illness, and immunocompromised patients may also be associated with significant morbidity. Thus, it may be prudent to exclude HCWs with viral respiratory infections from the care of these high-risk patients. Because large numbers of HCWs may have viral respiratory illnesses during the winter, it may not be possible to restrict all such HCWs from taking care of patients who are not in high-risk groups. In all instances, implementation of transmission-based (airborne and/or droplet) isolation precautions when appropriate, in addition to standard precautions (which include careful hand washing and appropriate gloving), is essential in preventing transmission [2].

Respiratory Syncytial Virus Infection

Respiratory syncytial virus (RSV) is the most important cause of lower respiratory tract disease in infants and young children (see Chapter 42). The disease outbreaks are usually seen during winter. Infants with congenital diseases of the heart or lung, those who are premature, or those with immunosuppression are at particular risk of severe or fatal RSV infection. Respiratory syncytial virus infection in adults is usually mild [216]; however, HCWs are not spared from illness and usually play a major role in transmitting the virus during nosocomial outbreaks [213]. The virus enters a susceptible host via the conjunctiva or nasal mucosa [215] and appears to be transmitted mainly by hand inoculation of virus into one's own eye or nose, after the hand has touched RSV-laden secretions or fomites, or by large-droplet deposition, as occurs during close contact with an infected individual who sneezes, coughs, or talks [214–217].

Transmission from Patients to HCWs

Healthcare workers acquire RSV infection mainly by self-inoculation with hands that have been contaminated with the virus from infected patients [213–215]. Direct large-droplet deposition onto the worker's conjunctiva or nasal mucosa during close contact with infected patients may also play a role but probably happens less frequently [213–215]. Therefore, measures that deter self-inoculation of the virus by hand, combined with precautions against virus inoculation of the eye and nose, should adequately prevent RSV transmission from patients to HCWs. In theory, meticulous hand washing by HCWs after each contact with a patient and after touching potentially contaminated articles should lessen RSV transmission. However, lapses in routine hand-washing practices are common [218,219], and hand-to-eye or hand-to-nose contact occurs frequently [220]. The additional use of eye-nose barriers (e.g., eye-nose goggles) was found to be beneficial in lowering the incidence of RSV infection in HCWs at one institution [221]. At another center, the use of gloves and gowns halted transmission of RSV [222]. The use of private rooms and/or patient cohorting, cohorting of HCWs, and pre-admission screening of patients for RSV have been helpful in containing nosocomial RSV outbreaks [223,224].

Transmission from HCWs to Patients

Healthcare workers infected with RSV may directly transmit the virus to patients during close contact with them. Ideally, HCWs with active RSV infection should not have direct contact with infants. Personnel also may transfer the virus passively by hand, from contaminated fomites or infected patients to other patients [217]. As in patient-to-worker transmission, gloving and careful hand washing by staff between contacts with patients and after contact with RSV-contaminated fomites should significantly diminish transmission of RSV between patients via the hands of personnel. Gowns may further decrease the potential for indirect RSV transmission via the hands of HCWs by minimizing the likelihood of fomite soiling with infectious secretions that may contaminate the hands [225].

Influenza

Influenza epidemics may require other measures. Nosocomial spread of influenza can be reduced by immunizing HCWs and high-risk patients several weeks or longer before the influenza season. Antiviral drugs, such as amantadine and rimantadine, may be useful in limiting the spread to and from patients and nonimmunized HCWs during an epidemic of influenza A [226,227].

Influenza is associated with significant morbidity and mortality in the elderly, patients with chronic underlying disease, and immunocompromised patients [228] (see Chapters 32, 42). Unlike RSV, influenza is spread mainly by small-particle aerosol (i.e., airborne transmission) [229]. Consequently, nosocomial outbreaks of influenza can be explosive once susceptible persons in an institution are exposed to an infected individual. Prevention of nosocomial outbreaks of influenza necessitates prospective immunization of both susceptible HCWs and high-risk patients before the influenza season each year [226]. Ideally, efforts to vaccinate high-risk people should be directed not only at hospital inpatients and long-term care facilities but also at high-risk individuals in the community (who may introduce the virus into the hospital if they are admitted with influenza infection) [226].

Once an outbreak takes hold within a hospital or long-term care facility, the most effective control measure (against influenza A) is chemoprophylaxis with amantadine or rimantadine [226]. Other measures have been advocated, but their exact roles in controlling influenza outbreaks have not been fully elucidated. These measures include early identification, isolation, or cohorting of infected patients, preferably in rooms with negative air pressure; cohorting of staff; strict hand washing; gowning when soiling with respiratory secretions is likely; limiting visitors; and avoiding elective admissions and surgery during an influenza outbreak [230] (see Chapter 13).

REFERENCES

1. Centers for Disease Control and Prevention. Guidelines for preventing the transmission of *Mycobacterium tuberculosis* in health-care facilities, 1994. *MMWR* 1994;43(RR-13):1–132.
2. Garner JS, Hospital Infection Control Practices Advisory Committee. Guideline for isolation precautions in hospitals. *Infect Control Hosp Epidemiol* 1996;17:53–80.
3. Williams WW, Preblud SR, Reichelderfer PS, Hadler SE. Vaccines of importance in the hospital setting: problems and developments. *Infect Dis Clin North Am* 1989;3:701–722.
4. Opravil M, Fierz W, Matter L, et al. Poor antibody response after tetanus and pneumococcal vaccination in immunocompromised, HIV-infected patients. *Clin Exp Immunol* 1991;84(2):185–189.
5. Huang KL, Ruben FL, Rinaldo CR Jr., et al. Antibody responses after influenza and pneumonococcal immunization in HIV-infected homosexual men. *JAMA* 1987;257:2047–2050.
6. Vardinon N, Handsher R, Burke M, et al. Poliovirus vaccination responses in HIV-infected patients: correlation with T4 cell counts. *J Infect Dis* 1990;162:238–241.
7. Onorato IM, Markowitz LE. Immunizations, vaccine-preventable diseases, and HIV infection. In: Wormser GP, ed. *AIDS and other manifestations of HIV infection*. New York: Raven Press, 1992: 671–681.
8. Centers for Disease Control and Prevention. Measles pneumonitis following measles-mumps-rubella vaccination of a patient with HIV infection, 1993. *MMWR* 1996;45:603–606.
9. Centers for Disease Control and Prevention. Measles—United States, 1995. *MMWR* 1996;45:305–307.
10. Mitus A, Holloway A, Evans AE, Enders JF. *Am J Dis Child* 1962;103: 413–418.
11. Bellini WJ, Rota JS, Greer PW, Zaki SR. Measles vaccination death in a child with severe combined immunodeficiency: report of a case. Annual Meeting of United States and Canadian Academy of Pathology, Atlanta, GA, 1992. *Lab Invest* 1992;66:91A.
12. Pass RF, Hutto C, Lyon MD, Cloud MT, Cloud G. Increased rate of cytomegalovirus infection among daycare center workers. *Pediatr Infect Dis J* 1990;9:465–470.
13. Murph JR. Day care associated cytomegalovirus: risk for working women. *J Am Med Wom Assoc* 1993;48:79–82.
14. Adler SP. Hospital transmission of cytomegalovirus. *Infect Agents Dis* 1992;1:43–49.
15. Adler SP, Bagget J, Wilson M. Molecular epidemiology of cytomegalovirus in a nursery: lack of evidence for nosocomial transmission. *J Pediatr* 1986;108:117–123.
16. Adler SP. Cytomegalovirus and pregnancy. *Curr Opin Obstet Gynecol* 1992;4:670–675.
17. Ahlfors K, Harris S, Ivarsson S, Svanberg L. Secondary maternal cytomegalovirus infection causing symptomatic congenital infection. *N Engl J Med* 1981;305:284.
18. Yeager AS. Longitudinal, serological study of cytomegalovirus infections in nurses and in personnel without patient contact. *J Clin Microbiol* 1975;2:448–452.
19. Gerberding KL, Bryant-LeBlanc CE, Nelson K, et al. Risk of transmitting the human immunodeficiency virus, cytomegalovirus, and hepatitis B virus to healthcare workers exposed to patients with AIDS and AIDS-related conditions. *J Infect Dis* 1987;156:1–8.
20. Finney JW, Miller KM, Adler SP. Changing protective and risky behaviors to prevent child-to-parent transmission of cytomegalovirus. *J Appl Behav Anal* 1993;26:471–472.
21. Standaert SM, Hutcheson RH, Schaffner W. Nosocomial transmission of *Salmonella* gastroenteritis to laundry workers in a nursing home. *Infect Control Hosp Epidemiol* 1994;15:22–26.
22. Centers for Disease Control and Prevention. Outbreaks of *Salmonella enteritidis* gastroenteritis—California, 1993. *MMWR* 1993;42: 793–797.
23. Watier L, Richardson S, Hubert B. *Salmonella enteritidis* infections in France and the United States: characterization by a deterministic model. *Am J Public Health* 1993;83:1694–1700.
24. Cohen MB. Etiology and mechanisms of acute infectious diarrhea in infants in the United States. *J Pediatr* 1991;118:S34–S39.
25. Lee LA, Shapiro CN, Hargrett-Bean N, Tauxe RV. Hyperendemic shigellosis in the United States: a review of surveillance data for 1967–1988. *J Infect Dis* 1991;164:894–900.
26. Allos BM, Blaser MJ. *Campylobacter jejuni* and the expanding spectrum of related infections. *Clin Infect Dis* 1995;20:1092–1099.
27. MacDonald KL, Osterholm MT. The emergence of *Escherichia coli* O157:H7 infection in the United States: the changing epidemiology of foodborne disease. *JAMA* 1993;269:2264–2266.
28. Wust J, Sullivan NM, Hardegger U, Wilkins TD. Investigation of an outbreak of antibiotic-associated colitis by various typing methods. *J Clin Microbiol* 1982;16:1096–1101.
29. Centers for Disease Control and Prevention. Viral agents of gastroenteritis. *MMWR* 1990;39(RR-5):1–24.
30. Lengerich EJ, Addiss DG, Juranek DD. Severe giardiasis in the United States. *Clin Infect Dis* 1994;18:760–763.
31. Baxby D, Hart CA, Taylor C. Human cryptosporidiosis: a possible cause of hospital cross-infection. *Br Med J* 1983;287:1760–1761.
32. Buchwald DS, Blaser MJ. A review of human salmonellosis. II. Duration of excretion following infection with nontyphi *Salmonella*. *Rev Infect Dis* 1984;6:345–356.
33. Miller SI, Hohmann EL, Pegues DA. *Salmonella* (including *Salmonella typhi*). In: Mandell GL, Bennett JE, Dolin R, eds. *Principles and practice of infectious diseases*, 4th ed. New York: Churcill Livingstone, 1995:2013–2033.
34. Carl M, Kantor RJ, Webster HM, Fields HA, Maynard JR. Excretion of hepatitis A virus in the stools of hospitalized patients. *J Med Virol* 1982;9:125–129.
35. Noble RC, Kane MA, Reeves SA, Roeckel I. Posttransfusion hepatitis A in a neonatal intensive care unit. *JAMA* 1984;252:2711–2715.
36. Rosenblum LS, Villarino ME, Naiman OV, et al. Hepatitis A outbreak

in a neonatal intensive care unit: risk factors for transmission and evidence of prolonged viral excretion among preterm infants. *J Infect Dis* 1991;164:476–482.
37. Coulepis AG, Locarnini SA, Lehman NI, Gust ID. Detection of hepatitis A virus in the feces of patients with naturally acquired infections. *J Infect Dis* 1980;141:151–156.
38. Goodman RA. Nosocomial hepatitis A. *Ann Intern Med* 1985;103: 452–454.
39. Klein BS, Michaels JA, Ryter MW, Berg KG, Davis JP. Nosocomial hepatitis A: a multi-nursery outbreak in Wisconsin. *JAMA* 1984;252: 2716–2721.
40. Doebbeling BN, Li N, Wenzel RP. An outbreak of hepatitis A among healthcare workers: risk factors for transmission. *Am J Public Health* 1993;83:1679–1684.
41. Szmuness W, Purcell RH, Dienstag JL, Stevens CE. Antibody to hepatitis antigen in institutionalized mentally retarded patients. *JAMA* 1977;237:1702–1705.
42. Gibas A, Blewett DR, Schoenfield DA, Dienstag JL. Prevalence and incidence of viral hepatitis in healthcare workers in the prehepatitis B vaccination era. *Am J Epidemiol* 1992;136:603–610.
43. Kashigawi S, Hayashi J, Ikematsu H, et al. Prevalence of immunologic markers of hepatitis A and B infection in hospital personnel in Miyazaki Prefecture, Japan. *Am J Epidemiol* 1985;122:960–969.
44. Shapiro CN. Occupational risk of infection with hepatitis B and hepatitis C virus. *Surg Clin North Am* 1995;75:1047–1056.
45. Shikata T, Karasawa T, Abe K, et al. Hepatitis B antigen and infectivity of hepatitis B virus. *J Infect Dis* 1977;136:571.
46. Alter HJ, Seeff LB, Kaplan PM, et al. Type B hepatitis: the infectivity of blood positive for e antigen and DNA polymerase after accidental needlestick exposure. *N Engl J Med* 1976;295:909.
47. Seeff LB, Wright EC, Zimmerman HJ, et al. Type B hepatitis after needlestick exposure: prevention with hepatitis B immunoglobulin. Final report of the Veterans Administration Cooperative Study. *Ann Intern Med* 1978;88:285–293.
48. Werner B, Grady GF. Accidental hepatitis-B-surface-antigen-positive inoculations. *Ann Intern Med* 1982;97:367–369.
49. Grady GF, Lee VA, Prince AM, et al. Hepatitis B immune globulin for accidental exposures among medical personnel: final report of a multicenter controlled trial. *J Infect Dis* 1978;138:625–638.
50. McMahon BJ, Alward WLM, Hall DB, et al. Acute hepatitis B virus infection: relation of age to the clinical expression of disease and subsequent development of the carrier state. *J Infect Dis* 1985;151: 599.
51. Francis DP, Favero MS, Maynard JE. Transmission of hepatitis B virus. *Semin Liver Dis* 1981;1:27–32.
52. Petersen NJ, Barrett DA, Bond WW, et al. Hepatitis B surface antigen in saliva, impetiginous lesions, and the environment in two remote Alaskan villages. *Appl Environ Microbiol* 1976;32:572.
53. West DJ. The risk of hepatitis B infection among health professionals in the United States: a review. *Am J Med Sci* 1984;287:26.
54. Hadler SC, Doto IL, Maynard JE, et al. Occupational risk of hepatitis B infection in hospital workers. *Infect Control Hosp Epidemiol* 1985; 6:24.
55. Lewis TL, Alter HJ, Chalmers TC, et al. A comparison of the frequency of hepatitis-B antigen and antibody in hospital and nonhospital personnel. *N Engl J Med* 1973;289:647–651.
56. Hadler SC, Margolis HS. Hepatitis B immunization: vaccine types, efficacy, and indications for immunization. In: Remington JS, Swartz MN, eds. *Current topics in infectious diseases*. Boston: Blackwell Scientific Publications, 1992:282.
57. Department of Labor. Occupational Safety and Health Administration. Occupational exposure to bloodborne pathogens: final rule. *Fed Reg* 1991;56:64004–64182.
58. Barie PS, Dellinger EP, Dougherty SH, et al. Assessment of hepatitis B virus immunization status among North American surgeons. *Arch Surg* 1994;129:27.
59. Lettau LA, Smith JD, Williams D, et al. Transmission of hepatitis B with resultant restriction of surgical practice. *JAMA* 1986;255: 934–937.
60. Panlilio AL, Shapiro CN, Schable CA, et al. Serosurvey of human immunodeficiency virus, hepatitis B virus, and hepatitis C virus infection among hospital-based surgeons. *J Am Coll Surg* 1995;180: 16–24.
61. Centers for Disease Control and Prevention. Recommendations for prevention of HIV transmission in health-care settings. *MMWR* 1987;36(S-2):1S–18S.
62. Centers for Disease Control and Prevention. Update: universal precautions for prevention of transmission of human immunodeficiency virus, hepatitis B virus, and other bloodborne pathogens in health-care settings. *MMWR* 1988;37:377–388.
63. Bell DM, Shapiro CN, Ciesielski CA, et al. Bloodborne pathogen transmission from health-care workers to patients: the CDC perspective. *Surg Clin North Am* 1995;75:1189–1203.
64. Harpaz R, Seidlein LV, Averhoff FM, et al. Transmission of hepatitis B virus from a surgeon without evidence of inadequate infection control. *N Engl J Med* 1996;334:549–554.
65. Centers for Disease Control and Prevention. Recommendations for preventing transmission of human immunodeficiency virus and hepatitis B virus to patients during exposure-prone invasive procedures. *MMWR* 1991;40(8):1–9.
66. Alter MJ. The detection, transmission, and outcome of hepatitis C virus infection. *Infect Agents Dis* 1993;2:155.
67. Mitsui T, Iwano K, Masuko K, et al. Hepatitis C virus infection in medical personnel after needlestick accident. *Hepatology* 1992;16: 1109–1114.
68. Cuypers HTM, Bresters D, Winkel IN, et al. Storage conditions of blood samples and primer selection affect yield of cDNA polymerase chain reaction products of hepatitis C virus. *J Clin Microbiol* 1992;30: 3320–3324.
69. Seeff LB. Hepatitis C from a needlestick injury. *Ann Intern Med* 1991; 115:411.
70. Kiyosawa K, Sodeyama T, Tanaka E, et al. Hepatitis C in hospital employees with needlestick injuries. *Ann Intern Med* 1991;115:367–369.
71. Nakano Y, Kiyosawa K, Sodeyama T, et al. Acute hepatitis C transmitted by needlestick accident despite short duration interferon treatment. *J Gastroenterol Hepatol* 1995;1095:609–611.
72. Cariani E, Zonaro A, Primi D, et al. Detection of HCV RNA and antibodies after needlestick injury. *Lancet* 1991;337:850.
73. Sartori M, La Terra G, Aglietta M, et al. Transmission of hepatitis C via blood splash into conjunctiva. *Scand J Infect Dis* 1993;25:270–271.
74. Herbert AM, Walker DM, Kavies KJ, et al. Occupationally acquired hepatitis C virus infection. *Lancet* 1992;339:305.
75. Jochen ABB. Occupationally acquired hepatitis C infection. *Lancet* 1992;339:305.
76. Klein RS, Freeman K, Taylor PE, et al. Occupational risk for hepatitis C virus infection among New York City dentists. *Lancet* 1991;338: 1539–1542.
77. Cooper BW, Krusell A, Tilton RC, et al. Seroprevalence of antibodies to hepatitis C virus in high-risk hospital personnel. *Infect Control Hosp Epidemiol* 1992;13:82.
78. Shapiro CN, Tokars JI, Chamberland M, et al. Hepatitis B vaccine use and infection with hepatitis B and hepatitis C virus infection among orthopedic surgeons. *J Bone Joint Surg* 1996;78:1791–1800.
79. Polish LB, Tong MJ, Co RL, et al. Risk factors for hepatitis C virus infection among healthcare personnel in a community hospital. *Am J Infect Control Hosp Epidemiol* 1993;21:196–200.
80. Krawczynski K, Alter MJ, Tankersley DL, et al. Effect of immune globulin on the prevention of experimental hepatitis C virus infection. *J Infect Dis* 1996;173:822–828.
81. Fried M, Hoofnagle JH. Therapy of hepatitis C. *Semin Liver Dis* 1995; 15:82–91.
82. Esteban JI, Gomez J, Martell M, et al. Transmission of hepatitis C virus by a cardiac surgeon. *N Engl J Med* 1996;334:555–560.
83. American Academy of Pediatrics. Summaries of infectious diseases: herpes simplex. In: Peter G, ed. *1994 Red book: report of the Committee on Infectious Diseases*, 23rd ed. Elk Grove Village, IL: American Academy of Pediatrics, 1994:251–252.
84. Bloch AB, Orenstein WA, Ewing WM. Measles outbreak in a pediatric practice: airborne transmission in an office setting. *Pediatrics* 1985;75:676–683.
85. Remington PL, Hall WN, Davis IH, Herald A, Gunn RA. Airborne transmission of measles in a physician's office. *JAMA* 1985;253: 1574–1577.
86. Atkinson WL, Markowitz LE, Adams NC, Seastrom GR. Transmission of measles in medical settings—United States, 1985–1989. *Am J Med* 1991;91(suppl 3B):320S–324S.
87. Davis RM, Orenstein WA, Frank JA Jr, et al. Transmission of measles in medical settings, 1980 through 1984. *JAMA* 1986;255:1295–1298.

88. Sienko DG, Friedman C, McGee HB, et al. A measles outbreak at university medical settings involving healthcare providers. *Am J Public Health* 1987;77:1222–1224.
89. Centers for Disease Control and Prevention. Measles—United States, 1985. *MMWR* 1986;35:366–370.
90. Braunstein H, Thomas S, Ito R. Immunity to measles in a large population of varying age. *Am J Dis Child* 1990;144:296–298.
91. Smith E, Welch W, Berhow M, Wong VK. Measles susceptibility of hospital employees as determined by ELISA. *Clin Res* 1990;38:183A.
92. Kempe CH, Fulginiti VA. The pathogenesis of measles virus infection. *Arch Ges Virusforsch* 1967;16:103.
93. Sellick J, Longbine D, Schiffeling R, Mylotte J. Screening hospital employees for measles is more cost-effective than blind immunization. *Ann Intern Med* 1992;116:982–984.
94. Subbarao EK, Amin S, Kumar ML. Prevaccination serologic screening for measles in healthcare workers. *J Infect Dis* 1991;163:876–878.
95. Grabowsky M, Markowitz LE. Serologic screening, mass immunization, and implications for immunization programs. *J Infect Dis* 1991; 164:1237–1238.
96. Stover BH, Kuebler CA, Cost KM, Adams HG. Measles-mumps-rubella immunization of susceptible hospital employees during a community measles outbreak: cost-effectiveness and protective efficacy. *Infect Control Hosp Epidemiol* 1994;15:20–23.
97. Kelly PW, Petrucelli BP, Stehr-Green P. The susceptibility of young adult Americans to vaccine-preventable infections. *JAMA* 1991;266: 2724–2729.
98. Centers for Disease Control and Prevention. Laboratory-acquired menigococcemia—California and Massachusetts. *MMWR* 1991;40:46.
99. Centers for Disease Control and Prevention. Nosocomial meningococcemia—Wisconsin. *MMWR* 1978;27:358.
100. Riewerts-Eriksen NH, Espersen F, Laursen L, et al. Nosocomial outbreak of group C meningococcal disease. *Br Med J* 1989;289: 568–569.
101. Rose HD, Lenz IE, Sheth NK. Meningococcal pneumonia: a source of nosocomial infection. *Arch Intern Med* 1981;141:575.
102. Immunization Practices Advisory Committee. Meningococcal vaccines. *MMWR* 1997;46(RR-5):1–21.
103. Schwartz B. Chemoprophylaxis for bacterial infections: principles of and application to meningococcal infections. *Rev Infect Dis* 1991;13 (suppl 2):S170–S173.
104. Schwartz B, Al-Tobaiqi A, Al-Ruwais A, et al. Comparative efficacy of ceftriaxone and rifampicin in eradicating pharyngeal carriage of group A *Neisseria meningitidis*. *Lancet* 1988;2:1239–1242.
105. Judson FN, Ehret JM. Single-dose ceftriaxone to eradicate pharyngeal *Neisseria meningitidis*. *Lancet* 1984;2:1462–1463.
106. Euceres CW, Lambert BE, Gaunt PN. A description of the outbreak of meningitis in HMS Raleigh in February 1987. *J Roy Naval Med Service* 1988;74:187–193.
107. Leedom JM, Ivler D, Mathies AW. Importance of sulfadiazine resistance in menigococcal disease in civilians. *N Engl J Med* 1963;273: 1395–1401.
108. Caugant DA, Hoiby EA, Magnus P, et al. Asymptomatic carriage of *Neisseria menigitidis* in a randomly sampled population. *J Clin Microbiol* 1994;32:323–330.
109. Caugant DA, Hoiby EA, Rosenqvist LO, Froholm LO, Selander RK. Transmission of *Neisseria meningitidis* from a population of asymptomatic carriers. *Epidemiol Infect* 1992;109:241–253.
110. Broome CV. The carrier state: *Neisseria meningitidis*. *J Antimicrob Chemiother* 1986;18:25–34.
111. Van Loon RPL, Holmes SJ, Sirotkin BI, Williams WW, et al. Mumps surveillance—United States, 1988–1993. In: CDC Surveillance Summaries, Aug. 11, 1995. *MMWR* 1995;44:1–14.
112. Briss PA, Fehrs LJ, Parker RA, et al. Sustained transmission of mumps in a highly vaccinated population: assessment of primary vaccine failure and waning vaccine-induced immunity. *J Infect Dis* 1994;169:77.
113. Wharton M, Cochi SL, Hutcheson RH, Schaffner W. Mumps transmission in hospitals. *Arch Intern Med* 1990;150:47–49.
114. Koplan JP, Preblud SR. A benefit-cost analysis of mumps vaccine. *Am J Dis Child* 1982;136:362–364.
115. Hersh BS, Fine PEM, Kent WK, et al. Mumps outbreak in a highly vaccinated population. *J Pediatr* 1991;119:187–193.
116. Anderson MJ, Lewis E, Kidd IM, et al. An outbreak of erythema infectiosum associated with human parvovirus infection. *J Hyg* 1984; 93:85.
117. Bell LM, Noides SJ, Stoffman P, Hodinka RL, Plotkin SA. Human parvovirus B19 infection among hospital staff members after contact with infected patients. *N Engl J Med* 1989;321:485–491.
118. Anderson LJ, Gillespie SM, Torok TJ, Hurtwitz ES, Tsou CJ, Gary GW. Risk of infection following exposures to human parvovirus B19. *Behring Mitt* 1990;85:60–63.
119. LaFrere JJ, Courouce AM, Bertrand Y, et al. Human parvovirus and aplastic crisis in chronic hemolytic anemias: a study of 24 observations. *Am J Hematol* 1986;23:271–275.
120. Kurtzman GJ, Cohen B, Meyers P, et al. Persistent B19 parvovirus infection as a cause of severe chronic anaemia in children with acute lymphocytic leukemia. *Lancet* 1988;2:1159–1162.
121. Anand A, Gray ES, Brown T, et al. Human parvovirus infection in pregnancy and hydrops fetalis. *N Engl J Med* 1987;316:183–186.
122. Chorba T, Coccia P, Holman RC, et al. The role of parvovirus B19 in aplastic crisis and erythema infectiosum. *J Infect Dis* 1986;154:183–193.
123. Centers for Disease Control and Prevention. Risks associated with human parvovirus B19 infection. *MMWR* 1989;38:81.
124. Mortimer EA Jr. Pertussis vaccine. In: Plotkin SA, Mortimer EA, eds. *Vaccines*. Philadelphia: WB Saunders, 1995:94–137.
125. Mortimer EA Jr. Pertussis and its prevention: a family affair. *J Infect Dis* 1990;161:473–479.
126. Kurt TL, Yeager AS, Guennette S, Dunlop S. Spread of pertussis by hospital staff. *JAMA* 1972;221:264–267.
127. Linneman CC, Ramundo M, Perlstein PH, et al. Use of pertussis vaccine in an epidemic involving hospital staff. *Lancet* 1975;2:540–543.
128. Valenti WM, Pincus PH, Messner MK. Nosocomial pertussis: possible spread by a hospital visitor. *Am J Dis Child* 1980;134:520–521.
129. Christie C, Glover AM, Willke MJ, Marx ML, Reising SF, Hutchinson NM. Containment of pertussis in the regional pediatric hospital during the greater Cincinnati epidemic of 1993. *Infect Control Hosp Epidemiol* 1995;16:556–563.
130. Weber DJ, Rutala WA. Management of healthcare workers exposed to pertussis. *Infect Control Hosp Epidemiol* 1994;15:411–415.
131. Halsey NA, Welling MA, Lehman RM. Nosocomial pertussis: a failure of erythromycin treatment and prophylaxis. *Am J Dis Child* 1980; 134:521–522.
132. Greaves WL, Orenstein WA, Stetler HC, Preblud SR, Hinman AR, Bart KJ. Prevention of rubella transmission in medical facilities. *JAMA* 1982;248:861–864.
133. Centers for Disease Control and Prevention. Rubella in hospitals—California. *MMWR* 1983;32:37–39.
134. Poland GA, Nichol KL. Medical students as sources of rubella and measles outbreaks. *Arch Intern Med* 1990;150:44–46.
135. Storch GA, Gruber C, Benz B, Beaudoin J, Hayes J. A rubella outbreak among dental students: description of the outbreak and analysis of control measures. *Infect Control Hosp Epidemiol* 1985;6:150–156.
136. Strassburg MA, Stephenson TG, Habel LA, Fannin SL. Rubella in hospital employees. *Infect Control* 1984;5:123–126.
137. Fliegel PE, Weinstein WM. Rubella outbreak in a prenatal clinic: management and prevention. *Am J Infect Control* 1982;10:29–33.
138. Strassburg MA, Imagawa DT, Fannin SL, et al. Rubella outbreak among hospital personnel. *Obstet Gynecol* 1981;57:283–288.
139. Gladstone JL, Millian SJ. Rubella exposure in an obstetric clinic. *Obstet Gynecol* 1981;57:182–186.
140. Polk FB, White JA, DeGirolami PC, Modlin JF. An outbreak of rubella among hospital personnel. *N Engl J Med* 1980;303:541–545.
141. Preblud SR. Some current issues related to the rubella vaccine. *JAMA* 1985;254:253–256.
142. Sachs JJ, Olson B, Soter J, et al. Employee rubella screening programs in Arizona hospitals. *JAMA* 1983;249:2675–2678.
143. Heseltine PNR, Ripper M, Wohlford P. Nosocomial rubella: consequences of an outbreak and efficacy of a mandatory immunization program. *Infect Control Hosp Epidemiol* 1985;6:371–374.
144. Centers for Disease Control and Prevention. Scabies in health-care facilities—Iowa. *MMWR* 1988;37:178–179.
145. Taplin D, Arrue C, Walker JG, Roth WI, Rivera A. Eradication of scabies with a single treatment schedule. *J Am Acad Dermatol* 1983;9: 546–550.
146. Taplin D, Rivera A, Walker JG, Roth WI, Reno D, Meinking T. A comparative trial of three treatment schedules for the eradication of scabies. *J Am Acad Dermatol* 1983;9:550–554.
147. Gooch JJ, Strasius SR, Beamer B, Reiter MD, Correll GW. Nosocomial outbreak of scabies. *Arch Dermatol* 1978;114:897–898.

148. Belle EA, D'Souza TJ, Zarzour JY, Lemieux M, Wong CC. Hospital epidemic of scabies: diagnosis and control. *Can J Public Health* 1979; 70:133–135.
149. Yonosky D, Ladia L, Gackenheimer L, Schultz MW. Scabies in nursing homes: an eradication program with permethrin 5% cream. *J Am Acad Dermatol* 1990;23:1133–1136.
150. Schultz MW, Gomez M, Hansen RC, et al. Comparative study of 5% permethrin cream and 1% lindane lotion for the treatment of scabies. *Arch Dermatol* 1990;126:167–170.
151. Marty P, Gari-Toussaint M, LeFichoux Y. Efficacy of ivermectin in treatment of an epidemic of sarcoptic scabies. *Ann Trop Med Parasitol* 1994;88:453.
152. Hopper AH, Salisbury J, Jegadeva AN, Scott S, Bennett GCJ. Epidemic Norwegian scabies in a geriatric unit. *Age Aging* 1990;19:125–127.
153. Clark J, Friesen DL, Williams WA. Management of an outbreak of Norwegian scabies. *Am J Infect Control* 1992;20:217–222.
154. Mulligan ME, Murray-Leisure KA, Ribner BS, et al. Methicillin-resistant *Staphylococcus aureus*: a consensus review of the microbiology, pathogenesis, and epidemiology with implications for prevention and management. *Am J Med* 1993;94:313–328.
155. Boyce JM. Methicillin-resistant *Staphylococcus aureus*: detection, epidemiology and control measures. *Infect Dis Clin North Am* 1989; 3:901.
156. Boyce JM, Opal SM, Byone-Potter G, Medeiros AA. Spread of methicillin-resistant *Staphylococcus aureus* in a hospital after exposure to a healthcare worker with chronic sinusitis. *Clin Infect Dis* 1993;17: 496–504.
157. Opal SM, Mayer KH, Stenberg MJ, et al. Frequent acquisition of multiple strains of methicillin-resistant *Staphylococcus aureus* by healthcare workers in an endemic hospital environment. *Infect Control Hosp Epidemiol* 1990;11:479–485.
158. Schwartz B, Schuchat A, Oxtoby MJ, Cochi SL, Hightower A, Broome CV. Invasive group B streptococcal disease in adults: a population-based study in metropolitan Atlanta. *JAMA* 1991;266: 1112–1114.
159. Butler JC, Schwartz B, Kimball J, Davis JP. Severe illness associated with group A-hemolytic streptococcal infections. *Wis Med J* 1991;90: 525–529.
160. Schwartz B, Facklam RR, Breiman RF. Changing epidemiology of group A streptococcal infection in the USA. *Lancet* 1990;336: 1167–1171.
161. Berkelman RL, Martin D, Graham DR, et al. Streptococcal wound infections caused by a vaginal carrier. *JAMA* 1982;247:2680–2682.
162. Mastro TD, Farley TA, Elliott JA, et al. An outbreak of surgical-wound infections due to group A streptococcus carried on the scalp. *N Engl J Med* 1990;323:968–972.
163. Schaffner W, Lefkowitz LB, Jr., Goodman JS, Koenig KC. Hospital outbreak of infections with group A streptococci traced to an asymptomatic anal carrier. *N Engl J Med* 1969;280:1224.
164. Viglionese A, Nottebart VF, Bodman HA, Platt R. Recurrent group A streptococcal carriage in a healthcare worker associated with widely separated nosocomial outbreaks. *Am J Med* 1991;91:329S–333S.
165. American Thoracic Society, Centers for Disease Control and Prevention, Infectious Diseases Society of America. Control of tuberculosis in the United States. *Am Rev Respir Dis* 1992;146:1623–1633.
166. American Thoracic Society, CDC. Treatment of tuberculosis and tuberculosis infection in adults and children. *Am J Respir Crit Care Med* 1994;149:1359–1374.
167. Centers for Disease Control and Prevention, Initial therapy for tuberculosis in the era of multidrug resistance: recommendations of the Advisory Council for the Elimination of Tuberculosis. *MMWR* 1993; 42:(RR-7):1–8.
168. Barrett-Connor E. The periodic chest roentgenogram for the control of tuberculosis in healthcare personnel. *Am Rev Respir Dis* 1980;122:153.
169. Morens DM, Bregman DJ, West CM, et al. An outbreak of varicella-zoster virus infection among cancer patients. *Ann Intern Med* 1980; 93:414–419.
170. Baltimore RS. Infections in the pediatric intensive care unit. *Yale J Biol Med* 1984;57:185–197.
171. Gustafson TL, Shebab A, Brunell PA. Outbreak of varicella in a newborn intensive care nursery. *Am J Dis Child* 1984;138:548–550.
172. Hyams PJ, Stuewe MCS, Heitzer V. Herpes zoster causing varicella (chicken pox) in hospital employees: cost of a casual attitude. *Infect Control* 1984;12:2–5.
173. Shehab ZM, Brunell PA. Susceptibility of hospital personnel to varicella-zoster virus. *J Infect Dis* 1984;150:786.
174. Weitekamp MR, Schan P, Aber RC. An algorithm for the control of varicella-zoster virus. *Am J Infect Control* 1985;13:193–198.
175. Alter SJ, Hammond JA, McVey CJ, Myers MG. Susceptibility to varicella-zoster virus among adults at high risk for exposure. *Infect Control* 1986;7:448–451.
176. Krasinski K, Holzman RS, LaCouture R, Florman A. Hospital experience with varicella-zoster virus. *Infect Control* 1986;7:312–316.
177. Haiduven-Griffiths D, Fecko H. Varicella in hospital personnel: a challenge for the infection control practitioner. *Am J Infect Control* 1987;15:207–211.
178. Weber DJ, Rutala AW, Parham C. Impact and costs of varicella prevention in a university hospital. *Am J Public Health* 1988;78:19–23.
179. McKinney WP, Horowitz MM, Battiola RJ. Susceptibility of hospital-based healthcare personnel to varicella-zoster virus infections. *Am J Infect Control* 1989;17:26–30.
180. Asano Y, Iwayama S, Miyata T, et al. Spread of varicella in hospitalized children having no direct contact with an indicator zoster case and its prevention by a live vaccine. *Biken J* 1980;23:157–161.
181. Sawyer MH, Chamberlin CJ, Wu YN, Aintablian N, Wallace MR. Detection of varicella-zoster virus DNA in air samples from hospital room. *J Infect Dis* 1994;169:91–94.
182. LeClair JM, Zaia JA, Levin MJ, Congdon RG, Goldmann DA. Airborne transmission of chickenpox in a hospital. *N Engl J Med* 1980; 302:450–453.
183. Gustafson TL, Lavely GB, Brawner ER Jr, Hutcheson RH, Wright PF, Schaffner W. An outbreak of airborne nosocomial varicella. *Pediatrics* 1982;70:550–556.
184. Josephson A, Gombert M. Airborne transmission of nosocomial varicella from localized zoster. *J Infect Dis* 1988;158:238–241.
185. Gershon AA, Steinberg SP, LaRussa P, et al. Immunization of healthy adults with live attenuated varicella vaccine. *J Infect Dis* 1988;158: 132–137.
186. Ferson MJ, Bell SM, Robertson PW. Determination and importance of varicella immune status of nursing staff in a children's hospital. *J Hosp Infect* 1990;15:347–351.
187. Kelly PW, Petruccelli BP, Stehr-Green P, Erickson RL, Mason CJ. The susceptibility of young adult Americans to vaccine- preventable infections. *JAMA* 1991;266:2724–2729.
188. Struewing JP, Hyams KC, Tueller JE, Gray GC. The risk of measles, mumps, and varicella among young adults: a serosurvey of US Navy and Marine Corps recruits. *Am J Public Health* 1993;83:1717–1720.
189. Weller TH. *Varicella and herpes zoster*, 5th ed. Washington, D.C.: American Public Health Association, 1979:375–398.
190. Williams V, Gershon A, Brunell PA. Serologic response to varicella-zoster antigens measured by direct immunofluorescence. *J Infect Dis* 1974;130:669.
191. Zaia JA, Oxman MN. Antibody to varicella-zoster virus induced membrane antigen: immunofluorescence assay using monodisperse glutaraldehyde-fixed target cells. *J Infect Dis* 1977;136:519–530.
192. Schmidt NJ, Lennette EH, Woodie JD, Ho HH. Immunofluorescence staining in the laboratory diagnosis of varicella-zoster infections. *J Lab Clin Med* 1965;66:403–412.
193. Asano Y, Albrechy P, Vujcic LK, Quinnan GV Jr., Takahashi M. Evaluation of humoral immunity to varicella-zoster virus by an enhanced neutralization test and by the fluorescent antibody to membrane antigen test. *Arch Virol* 1983;75:225–228.
194. Furukawa T, Plotkin SA. Indirect hemagglutination test for varicella-zoster infection. *Infect Immun* 1972;5:835–839.
195. Wreghitt TG, Tedder RS, Naginton J, Ferns RB. Antibody assays for varicella virus: comparison of competitive enzyme-linked immunosorbent assay (ELISA), competitive radioimmunoassay (RIA), complement fixation, and indirect fluorescence assays. *J Med Virol* 1984;13:361–370.
196. Demmler GJ, Steinberg SP, Blum G, Gershon AA. Rapid enzyme-linked immunosorbent assay for detecting antibody to varicella-zoster virus. *J Infect Dis* 1988;157:211–212.
197. LaRussa P, Steinberg S, Waite E, Hanna B, Holzman P. Comparison of five assays for antibody to varicella-zoster virus and the fluorescence-antibody-to-membrane-antigen test. *J Clin Microbiol* 1987;25: 2059–2062.
198. Bogger-Goren S, Baba K, Hurley P, Yabuuchi H, Takahashi M, Ogra OL. Antibody response to varicella-zoster virus after natural or vaccine-induced infection. *J Infect Dis* 1982;146:260–265.

199. Provost PJ, Krah DL, Kuter BJ, et al. Antibody assays suitable for assessing immune responses to live varicella virus vaccine. *Vaccine* 1991;9:111–116.
200. Steinberg SP, Gershon AA. Measurement of antibodies to varicella-zoster virus by using a latex agglutination test. *J Clin Microbiol* 1991; 29:1527–1529.
201. Gershon AA, Steinberg SP, LaRussa PS. Detection of antibody to varicella-zoster virus using the latex agglutination assay. *Clin Diagn Virol* 1994;2:271–278.
202. White CJ, Kuter BJ, Ngai A, et al. Modified cases of chicken pox after varicella vaccination: correlation of protection with antibody response. *Pediatr Infect Dis J* 1992;11:19–23.
203. Bernstein HH, Rothstein EP, Pennridge Pediatric Associates, et al. Clinical survey of natural varicella compared with breakthrough varicella after immunization with live attenuated Oka/Merck varicella vaccine. *Pediatrics* 1993;92:833–837.
204. Watson BM, Piercy SA, Plotkin SA, Starr SE. Modified chicken pox in children immunized with the Oka/Merck varicella vaccine. *Pediatrics* 1993;91:17–22.
205. Weibel RE, Neff BJ, Kuter BJ, et al. Live attenuated varicella vaccine: efficacy trial in healthy children. *N Engl J Med* 1984;310: 1409–1415.
206. Tsolia M, Gershon AA, Steinberg SP, Gelb L, The National Institute of Allergy and Infectious Diseases Varicella Vaccine Collaborative Study Group. Live attenuated varicella vaccine: evidence that the vaccine virus is attenuated and the importance of skin lesions in transmission of varicella-zoster virus. *J Pediatr* 1990;116:185–189.
207. Preblud SR. Nosocomial varicella: worth preventing but how? *Am J Public Health* 1988;78:13–15.
208. Myers MG, Rasley DA, Hierholzer WJ. Hospital infection control for varicella zoster virus infection. *Pediatrics* 1982;70:199–202.
209. Steele RW, Coleman MA, Fiser M, Bradsher RW. Varicella zoster in hospital personnel: skin test reactivity to monitor susceptibility. *Pediatrics* 1982;70:604–608.
210. Anderson JD, Bonner M, Scheifele DW, Schneider BC. Lack of nosocomial spread of varicella in a pediatric hospital with negative pressure ventilated patient rooms. *Infect Control Hosp Epidemiol* 1985;6: 120–121.
211. Stover BH, Cost KM, Hamm C, Adams G, Cook LN. Varicella exposure in a neonatal intensive care unit: case report and control measures. *Infect Control Hosp Epidemiol* 1988;16:167–172.
212. Lipton SV, Brunell PA. Management of varicella exposure in a neonatal intensive care unit. *JAMA* 1989;261:1782–1784.
213. Hall CB. The nosocomial spread of respiratory syncytial viral infections. *Ann Rev Med* 1983;34:311.
214. Hall CB, Douglas RG. Modes of transmission of respiratory syncytial virus. *J Pediatr* 1981;99:100.
215. Hall CB, Douglas G, Schnabel KC, Geiman JM. Infectivity of respiratory syncytial virus by various routes of inoculation. *Infect Immun* 1981;33:779.
216. Hall WJ, Hall CB, Speers DM, et al. Respiratory syncytial virus infection in adults: clinical, virologic, and serial pulmonary function studies. *Ann Intern Med* 1978;88:203–205.
217. Hall CB, Douglas RG, Geiman JM. Possible transmission by fomites of respiratory syncytial virus. *J Infect Dis* 1980;141:98.
218. Albert RK, Condie F. Hand-washing patterns in medical intensive-care units. *N Engl J Med* 1981;304:1465.
219. Doebbeling BN, Stanley GL, Sheetz CT, et al. Comparative efficacy of alternative hand-washing agents in reducing nosocomial infections in intensive care units. *N Engl J Med* 1992;327:88–93.
220. Gwaltney JM Jr., Mowkalsky PB, Hendley JO. Hand-to-hand transmission of rhinovirus colds. *Ann Intern Med* 1978;88:463.
221. Gala CL, Hall CB, Schabel KA, et al. The use of eye-nose goggles to control nosocomial respiratory syncytial virus infection. *JAMA* 1986; 256:2706–2708.
222. LeClair JM, Freeman J, Sullivan BC, et al. Prevention of nosocomial respiratory syncytial virus infections through compliance with glove and gown isolation precautions. *N Engl J Med* 1987;317:329–334.
223. Madge P, Paton JY, McColl JH, Mackie PLK. Prospective controlled study of four infection control procedures to prevent nosocomial infection with respiratory syncytial virus. *Lancet* 1992;340:1079–1083.
224. Krasinski K, LaCouture R, Holzman RS, Waithe E, Bank S, Hanna B. Screening for respiratory syncytial virus and assignment to a cohort at admission to reduce nosocomial transmission. *J Pediatr* 1990;116: 894–898.
225. Carbary L. Volunteers help nurses tend boarder babies. *RN* 1991;54 (8):12.
226. Centers for Disease Control and Prevention. Prevention and control of influenza: recommendations of the Advisory Committee on Immunization Practices (ACIP). *MMWR* 1996;46(RR-9):1–25.
227. Arden NH, Patriarca PA, Fasana MB, et al. The roles of vaccination and amantadine prophylaxis in controlling an outbreak of influenza A (H3N2) in a nursing home. *Arch Intern Med* 1988;148:865–868.
228. Eickhoff TC, Sherman IL, Serfling RE. Observations on excess mortality associated with epidemic influenza. *JAMA* 1961;176:104–110.
229. Alford RH, Kasel JA, Gerone PJ, Knight V. Human influenza resulting from aerosol inhalation. *Proc Soc Exp Biol Med* 1966;122: 800–804.
230. Tablan OC, Anderson LJ, Arden NH, et al. Guideline for prevention of nosocomial pneumonia. *Respir Care* 1994;39:1191–1236.

Hospital Infections, Fourth Edition,
edited by John V. Bennett and Philip S. Brachman.
Lippincott–Raven Publishers, Philadelphia © 1998

CHAPTER 4

The Development of Infection Surveillance and Control Programs

Robert W. Haley

HISTORICAL PERSPECTIVE

Nosocomial infections have been a serious problem ever since sick patients were first congregated in hospitals. The explosiveness of spread of the classic epidemic diseases led to the concept of quarantine, from which evolved modern techniques of isolation. The ubiquitous threat of wound infections after surgery stimulated the stringent aseptic tradition of the operating room, including meticulous aseptic surgical technique, environmental cleanliness, and disinfection and sterilization processes. The observations of Semmelweis and Holmes, later bolstered by the popularization of the germ theory of infectious diseases, established the importance of hand washing for reducing the spread of infection among patients. The unique observations and management abilities of Florence Nightingale established the modern basis for the design of hospitals and the strategies for patients' care that minimize infection risks. And, finally, the advent and widespread availability of antimicrobial agents in the 1940s revolutionized the treatment of infectious diseases and promised virtually to eliminate infections as a threat to hospitalized patients. Thus by the postwar period of the late 1940s, most of the concepts and tools for preventing nosocomial infections were in the hands of individual physicians and nurses who were to apply them, but no organized group at the hospital level was considered necessary to oversee the activity of infection control.

In the mid-1950s, hospitals in the United States and abroad were struck by a pandemic of staphylococci infections that were increasingly resistant to available antibiotics and more virulent than previous strains. In response to this widespread problem, hospitals organized infection control committees to develop new strategies for controlling the epidemic and for coordinating the infection control efforts of the diverse groups and departments of the hospital. In addition, the Centers for Disease Control and Prevention (CDC), then called the Communicable Disease Center, designated a new investigations unit, one purpose of which was to assist infection control committees in investigating hospital epidemics.

This nationwide effort was summarized and discussed at two national conferences on the control of staphylococcal disease in 1958. The proceedings of the conferences indicated the leading approaches to be stringent disinfection and monitoring of the inanimate environment, detection and treatment of staphylococcal carriers among the hospital staff, more vigorous encouragement of aseptic technique, and the reporting of staphylococcal infections to an infection control committee [1,2].

By the mid-1960s, the pandemic began to subside for reasons that are still unclear. It left in its wake, however, a new awareness of nosocomial infections and committees of hospital personnel interested in controlling the problem. At the same time, hospitals were experiencing another strong current of change—the use of increasingly complex technology bequeathed by the World War II technological explosion and the burgeoning space race. As staphylococcal infection epidemics declined, new types of infections were noticed; they were caused by opportunistic pathogens, such as gram-negative rods, fungi, and parasites, and infected an increasing number of patients undergoing invasive and immunocompromising medical treatments.

These developments were described in 1963 at the National Conference on Institutionally Acquired Infections, the name of the conference well illustrating the awareness that a broader problem was emerging [3]. The

R. W. Haley: Department of Internal Medicine, Division of Epidemiology, University of Texas Southwestern Medical Center at Dallas, Dallas, Texas 75235-8874.

proceedings of the conference indicated the development of a much wider range of approaches to control of the problem, including the application of epidemiologic methods, the recommendation of organized systems for surveillance of nosocomial infections, and the importance of personnel education [3].

Through the middle and late 1960s, a few hospitals developed organized infection control programs to conduct surveillance, develop control measures, and monitor the control process for the infection control committee, although most hospitals continued to depend on the individual efforts of doctors and nurses. These programs were focused somewhat and encouraged by an infection control manual published and distributed widely by the Committee on Infections Within Hospitals, under the American Hospital Association (AHA) [4]. Meanwhile researchers at the CDC were engaged in pilot studies in several community hospitals to develop and test technology for conducting more effective surveillance of nosocomial infections [5].

After demonstrating the futility of depending on voluntary reporting of infections by doctors or nurses, these pilot studies first relied on a physician infection control officer to identify infections. Later, borrowing from the British the concept of the infection control sister [6], which was being tried in two other U.S. hospitals [7,8], the CDC researchers thoroughly tested the feasibility of surveillance by trained infection control nurses and found that one full-time nurse was needed to perform surveillance and control for approximately every 250 beds [9]. On the basis of these findings, the CDC set up a training course for infection control nurses, and the first classes were held in 1968. These developments were summarized and discussed in the First International Conference on Nosocomial Infections held at the CDC in 1970 [10]. The proceedings focused on a debate between the proponents of surveillance of infections by infection control nurses and their critics, who considered the approach infeasible, unnecessary, or too costly.

Following the First International Conference, the CDC developed a strong recommendation for the surveillance approach, which was also supported and promoted by the AHA [11,12]. Popularized by scientific articles, presentations at scientific meetings and regional and local conferences, practical manuals, training courses, and individual consultations with hospital staffs by medical and nurse epidemiologists from the CDC, the approach was adopted to varying degrees by virtually all U.S. hospitals in the early to middle 1970s. For example, although infection control committees had emerged earlier, in 1970 few hospitals had infection control nurses, practiced active surveillance of infections, or had formal policies prescribing aseptic practices; by 1976, however, the majority of hospitals had adopted these measures and had begun reducing their levels of wasteful routine environmental culturing [13]. Since there were virtually no government or private regulations or standards of much force during those years, this revolution in infection control was entirely a voluntary movement by hospitals to address an emerging problem.

Noteworthy signs of the vitality of the movement were the demand for the CDC training course for infection control nurses, the huge circulation of the various books and manuals on infection control, and the formation of a professional society for infection control nurses (the Association for Practitioners in Infection Control [APIC], established in 1972). During the 1970s, the CDC operated a network of ~ 70 voluntary hospitals, the National Nosocomial Infections Surveillance System, to maintain nationwide surveillance of the problem [14].

In 1974, the CDC began a nationwide study to evaluate the effectiveness of the approach that had been adopted throughout the country. Termed the Study of the Efficacy of Nosocomial Infection Control (the SENIC Project), the multiphased project had two objectives: first, to measure the extent to which these new programs, labeled infection surveillance and control programs (ISCPs), had been adopted by U.S. hospitals, and, second, to determine whether these programs led to reduced nosocomial infection rates in the country and, if so, to what extent [15]. The study was stimulated by the prediction that future financial pressures on hospitals would cause them to discontinue costly preventive programs of unproved value. If the programs were truly effective, their efficacy should be documented scientifically to perpetuate their support; if not, a demonstration of the lack of efficacy should help redirect the efforts of the nation's hospitals toward more effective approaches.

During the ten years (1974 to 1983) that the SENIC Project was conducted, the infection control movement in U.S. hospitals was going through a maturation phase. In this period, > 5,000 infection control nurses received training in the CDC training courses, and diverse organizations began sponsoring their own courses for nurses, physicians, and microbiologists. A professional society for physician epidemiologists, the Society of Hospital Epidemiologists of America (SHEA), was formed in 1980. More efficient methods of detecting infections through surveillance were developed. Extensive environmental culturing programs virtually disappeared. National conferences on infection control, including the Second International Conference on Nosocomial Infections in 1980, disseminated new information and provided a forum for infection control personnel to exchange experiences. Finally, a host of new risk factors that predispose patients to infection and cause epidemics were identified and studied. Despite much continued debate over the cost-effectiveness of routine infection surveillance, the hospitals that increased the intensity of their surveillance efforts outnumbered those that limited or discontinued the activity [16].

The early 1980s saw a consolidation of the experiences of the previous decade. Of particular importance was the CDC project to record the increasingly complex set of findings and recommendations into a series of guidelines for hospitals. The physician and nurse epidemiologists of the CDC Hospital Infections Program had been providing consultation to hospital personnel on diverse technical issues ranging from questions on disinfection techniques to the management of outbreak investigations. By 1980, they were responding to > 10,000 inquiries per year. The philosophy behind the effort to write guidelines was to provide to all U.S. hospitals simultaneously the answers to the most important and frequently asked questions [17].

In the end, the effort produced a valuable checklist of the issues that should be addressed by the policies of all hospitals [18]. To make the guidelines most useful, each recommendation was classified according to the strength of its backing by scientific evidence or the consensus of experts [17]. This system was to allow hospitals to discriminate between approaches very likely to prevent infections and those with a good rationale but of untested value. The intent of the process was to provide a body of useful information and to avoid the aura of governmental regulatory pressures.

Since their initial release from 1981 through 1983, the CDC guidelines have generated widespread interest and discussion. A 1985 nationwide survey to evaluate the dissemination and adoption of the guidelines found that although 84% of infection control personnel across the country were familiar with them, actual adoption varied widely for the specific recommendations [19]. For example, 78% of hospitals reported having adopted the recommendation for changing intravenous tubing every 48 hours, whereas only 23% reported having taken up the recommendation for computing procedure-specific clean wound infection rates for each surgeon, with feedback of results to the surgeons. Small hospitals were found to have been significantly less likely both to have heard of the guidelines and to have adopted them. It is probable that the guidelines have achieved even wider adoption with the passage of time since the survey.

The late 1980s promised to be a period of innovation in infection control. With the release of the results of the SENIC Project [20] and the financial incentives for hospitals to support infection control created by the national Prospective Payment System [21–23], it appeared that hospitals would rapidly adopt the new outcome-oriented approaches to surveillance and feedback of epidemiologic data and make major reductions in nosocomial infection risks [24]. The onslaught of the acquired immunodeficiency syndrome (AIDS) epidemic [25,26] (see Chapter 43) followed by the resurgence of tuberculosis [27] (see Chapter 33), however, monopolized the time of infection control personnel in most hospitals, and progress slowed. In addition, the parallel quality assurance movement, based on the review of individual patients' medical records for sentinel events, pervaded U.S. hospitals and threatened to co-opt the epidemiologic orientation of infection control programs. Epidemiologists involved in infection control struggled to interject epidemiologic methods into quality assurance programs [28–32].

Nonetheless, by the early 1990s, new developments in infection control revitalized the epidemiologic movement. After establishing systems for dealing with AIDS, tuberculosis, and the resulting personnel health problems (see Chapter 3), infection control personnel proceeded rapidly to computerize the data collection, analysis, and reporting of their surveillance programs [33,34], capitalizing on the emergence of commercial infection control software [35,36] (see Chapter 8). By 1993, > 80% of U.S. hospitals were using computers to process infection surveillance data [37].

Computers also came into use in hospitals in Europe [38–41]. The wide availability of computers made possible the increase in sophistication of epidemiologic rate measures, typified by the introduction of device-day rates for measuring the risk of infection associated with indwelling catheters or ventilators [42]. The greater control over confounding factors afforded by device-day rates and increasingly sophisticated multivariate risk indexes [43–46] made interhospital comparisons of nosocomial infection rates valid and feasible [47–49]. These technological advances bred new enthusiasm for surveillance in many countries of the world where it had not been previously practiced [50,51].

In the early 1990s, the public process of formulating guidelines for infection surveillance and control were transferred to a new, formal federal advisory committee, the Hospital Infection Control Practices Advisory Committee. This committee revised old guidelines and formulated new ones [52–56]. Private professional organizations also developed guidelines [57,58] (see Chapter 11).

Finally, by mid-decade, the threat to the survival of the epidemiologic infection control movement from the parallel quality assurance movement had ended with the widespread abandonment of traditional individual-patient review approaches. In its place, however, arose a new force in the form of "quality management" and "continuous quality improvement" [59]. This movement stressed the techniques of industrial quality control, such as statistical control charts, training programs to change hospital culture, and systematic problem solving [60–62]. Whether these statistical techniques, such as control charts and "fish-bone diagrams," which were developed in manufacturing environments [60], will prove useful for lowering infection risks in hospitals remains to be seen.

STRATEGIES FOR SURVEILLANCE AND CONTROL

The main lesson derived from the past 2 decades of research and experience is that preventing nosocomial infections and controlling infection outbreaks in hospitals require an organized management system staffed by dedicated personnel to influence the behavior of practicing doctors, nurses, and paramedical workers [20]. In this respect, the system is similar to an office or department of quality control on the management staff of an industrial corporation [63]. Many nosocomial infections are analogous to product defects resulting from the human errors of workers on the assembly line. Without careful management to ensure quality and without statistical feedback of the product defect rates, quality tends to decline, whereas a system for managing quality usually improves the products. This is the general rationale behind the need for an organized ISCP.

The basic model for an effective ISCP is portrayed in Figure 4-1 [15]. The nosocomial infections that are preventable, perhaps between 30% and 50%, are primarily caused by problems in *patient care practices*, such as the use and care of urinary catheters, intravenous and central venous monitoring catheters, and respiratory therapy equipment, as well as in hand-washing practices and surgical skill. As in most work situations, in the absence of a system for managing these practices, they are generally determined by the inertia of ward routine—that is, the apprentice system, in which practices are passed on from generation to generation of doctors and other hospital workers.

Since old practices become strongly ingrained, changing behavior in the hospital environment meets stiff resistance and, if pursued persistently, generates interpersonal conflict. To change old methods to preventive practices requires an infection control program, consisting of an organized intervention system with specific goals for changing behavior. For this program to be successful, it must be guided by sound principles and current information; consequently, the infection control personnel must learn correct preventive techniques from studying the published literature, including articles in scientific journals, textbooks, and technical manuals, and they must conduct regular surveillance over the occurrence of nosocomial infections and the patient care practices in their hospital. The information obtained from surveillance not only allows infection control personnel to direct their efforts toward the most serious problems but also arms them with information with which to obtain the support of hospital workers and provide feedback on the results of preventive changes. Information is power, and the more immediately relevant the information is to the individual hospital's situation, the more powerful it is.

A more detailed model of the infection control process is pictured in Figure 4-2 [15,64]. There are basically two routes by which the infection control staff can influence patient care practices and reduce infection risks: taking direct action to change behavior without having to rely on the voluntary compliance of hospital personnel (the direct approach) and working with hospital personnel through training or other activities to motivate them to practice correct techniques (the indirect approach). Taking the direct approach—for example, having the purchasing department switch to a new type of phlebotomy needle that lowers the risk of a needle-stick injury to personnel—generally requires a less personnel-intensive effort and is more certain to be effective, but, unfortunately, only a minority of infection risks are susceptible to this approach.

In contrast, the majority of infection risks require changing behavior, a more difficult and less certain endeavor [65–69]. To change behavior successfully requires a complex management process involving the following steps. First, the preventive practice must be correctly defined; all too frequently medical, nursing, or support service departments use written or informal policies that run counter to proven preventive approaches. Given correct policies, the infection control staff must achieve a unity of purpose among the power brokers of the hospital (e.g., the hospital administrator, nursing service director, chiefs of involved medical departments, or directors of support service departments). A dissenting department head will ensure the failure of any attempt to influence the care of patients in his or her domain.

Achieving unity of purpose requires a skillful and diplomatic approach, involving a realistic effort to balance infection control needs against practical constraints. The importance of peer relations must be recognized by having a knowledgeable infection control physician to deal with the medical staff and an influential nurse or other practitioner as the infection control coordinator to work with the nursing and support service staffs.

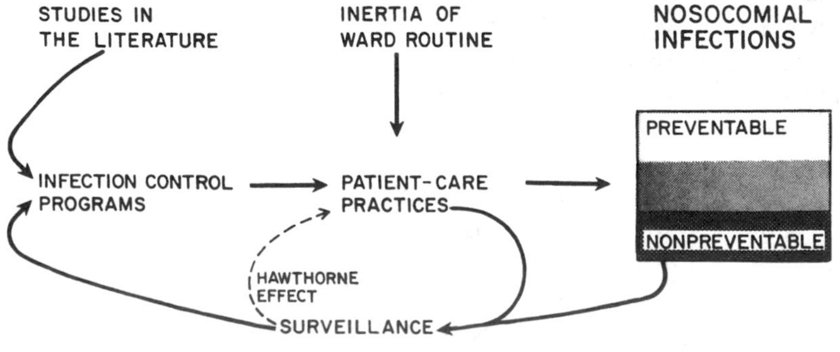

FIGURE 4-1. Simplified theoretical model of an infection surveillance and control program. (Reproduced from Haley RW, Quade D, Freeman HE, et al. Study on the Efficacy of Nosocomial Infection Control (SENIC Project): summary of study design. *Am J Epidemiol* 1980;111:474, with permission.)

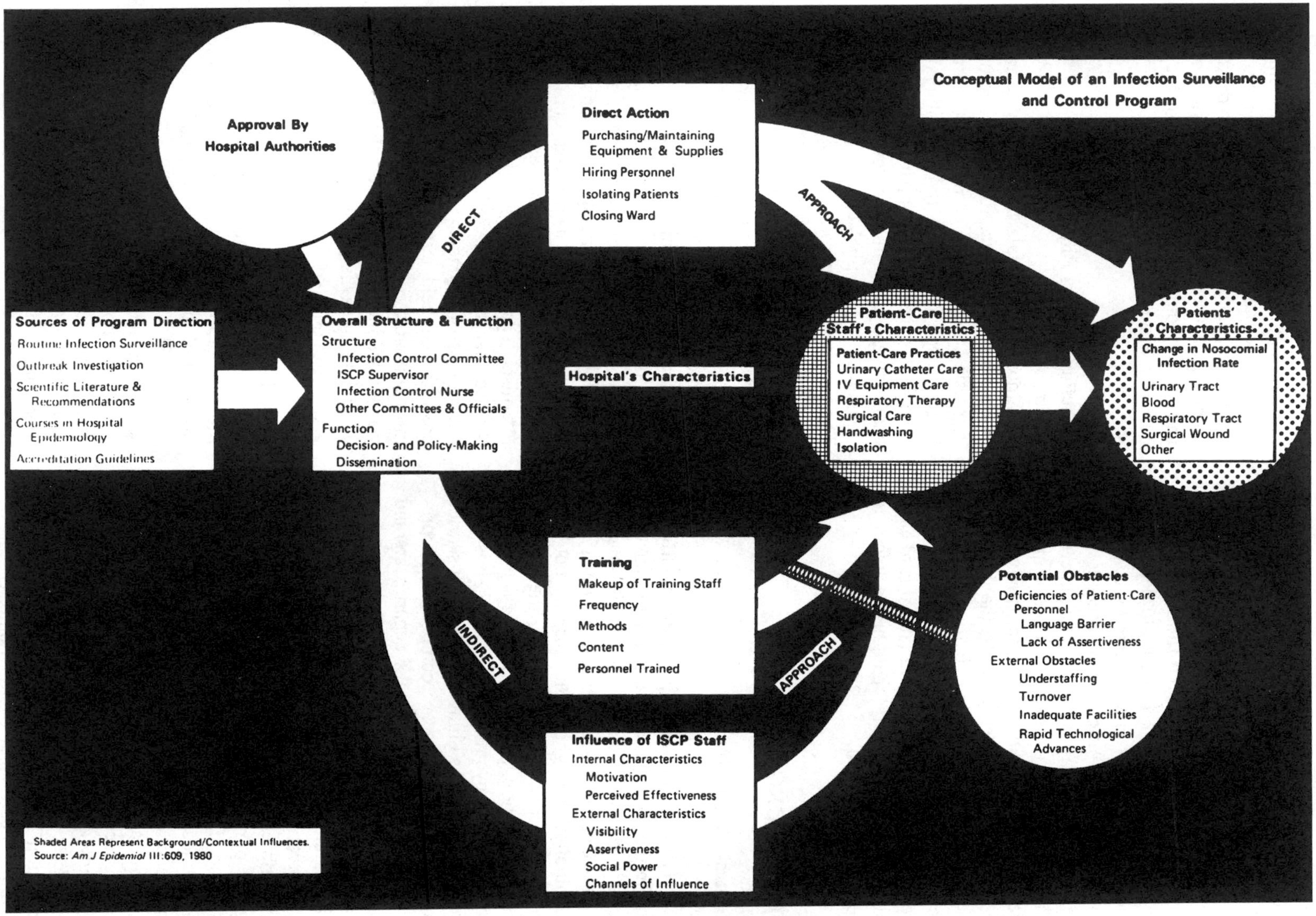

FIGURE 4-2. Detailed conceptual model of an infection surveillance and control program. Shaded areas represent background/contextual influences. (Reproduced from *Am J Epidemiol* 1980;111: 608–612, with permission.)

With unity of purpose established, training efforts must be designed to provide all relevant personnel with the skills and knowledge required to carry out the new preventive practice according to the agreed-on standard. Various motivational techniques can be used to increase compliance; potential obstacles to correct performance, such as understaffing or inadequate hand-washing facilities, must be removed. Once these prerequisite steps are taken, the practice must be monitored to measure compliance, and the results must be reported to department heads and particularly to first-line workers to reward the desired behaviors and focus attention on breakdowns in performance. With unity of purpose among supervisors and department heads and quantitative data on performance, correct practice can be maximized. If any of the steps in the process is neglected or fails, the degree of prevention will be diminished. Since halfway programs are often ineffective, a well-organized system to manage the process of infection control is essential if it is to have a substantial effect in the rapidly changing technologic milieu of the modern hospital.

PERSONNEL AND ORGANIZATION

Infection Control Committee

An Infection Control Committee is present in virtually every hospital in the United States and usually functions as the hospital's central decision- and policy-making body [70,71] (see Chapter 2). Its decisions are often independent and binding throughout the hospital but may require review and approval by higher authorities, such as the hospital administration. Since its purpose is to be the hospital's advocate for prevention of infections, it is usually placed above the various clinical and support service departments. Most committees are composed of representatives from most of the hospital's departments and meet regularly, usually monthly, to deal with current developments and problems. Its multidisciplinary representation is important for at least three reasons.

First, since infection problems and control measures often cross departmental lines, effective decision making requires regular participation of members from most departments. Second, to carry out the committee's decisions, it is often most effective to have committee members exert influence in their respective departments to ensure agreement and compliance. Third, the multidepartmental representation of the committee bolsters its authority as an advocate for the hospital that transcends the special interests of any single department. When a committee decision is opposed—as, for example, by a strong department head—this overall authority can be very important in ensuring that the final compromise position is in the best interests of patients' care in all departments.

The activities of the infection control staff members, such as the infection control practitioner and the hospital epidemiologist or infection control physician (see next section), are generally performed, at least in principle, at the direction of the infection control committee. The job of executive staff of the committee is to provide technical information and surveillance data, to draft policies for the committee's use in the final decision-making process, and to carry out or promote many of the prevention and control measures that are adopted.

Infection Control Physician

Almost all hospitals have a physician acting as the chairperson of the infection control committee [72]. An increasing number of committees, particularly in the larger hospitals and in those affiliated with medical schools, also have a full- or part-time position for a physician with special training in hospital epidemiology functioning as the hospital epidemiologist (see Chapter 2). The hospital epidemiologist may be the chairperson of the committee or may occupy a separate position as either a technical adviser or a member of the executive staff of the committee. The former seems preferable in smaller hospitals, whereas the latter creates a separation of the epidemiologic and decision-making roles that could strengthen both activities, particularly in the more complex situations present in larger hospitals.

Most persons occupying the position of hospital epidemiologist are practicing physicians who serve on a part-time basis, often as a 2-year committee assignment [72]. In the mid-1970s, 40% were pathologists, 18% were internists (approximately half of these were infectious disease specialists), 12% were surgeons, and 20% were other types of physicians; in 10% of U.S. hospitals, the position was held by someone other than a physician, most commonly a microbiologist. By 1983, the tendency was toward increased representation of internists, particularly infectious disease specialists, with a commensurate decrease of non-physicians and pathologists [unpublished SENIC data]. Infectious disease specialists are increasingly filling the position of epidemiologist in teaching hospitals, but not in nonteaching hospitals, and they are more likely to be receiving remuneration for their infection control duties and to have had specific training for the job [73].

The average tenure in this position tends to be 2 to 3 years, and most appointees tend to spend < 4 hours per week on the job, although pathologists and infectious disease specialists tend to remain much longer and devote more time. More and more hospitals, particularly those that are large and affiliated with medical schools, are creating full-time positions for hospital epidemiologists, some of whom provide the same service for groups of smaller hospitals in the surrounding locale (see Chapter 10).

The degree of knowledge and interest of these infection control physicians appears to vary widely. In the mid-1970s, only ~60% of U.S. hospitals had an infection control physician who indicated special interest in the problem, and by 1983 the percentage had not risen [16]. In both periods, only one third or so of the physicians had taken a training course in infection control. Without a training course, physicians are generally unprepared to manage infection control activities, since little, if any, time has been devoted to the subject in the curricula of medical schools, medical residencies, or even infectious disease fellowships.

Following the publication of the results of the SENIC Project in 1985 [16,20,24], in which the deficiencies in the number and training of infection control physicians were stressed, there appears to have been an growth in the percentage of U.S. hospitals with a trained physician in this position. A survey of U.S. hospitals in 1988 found that 46% had a physician with training in infection control [74]. To expand this percentage, in 1990 the AHA, SHEA, and CDC began conducting training courses for physicians across the United States. (see Chapters 2,11).

Infection Control Practitioner

The infection control practitioner (ICP), or infection control nurse, occupies the key position in the ISCP (see Chapter 2). Without a qualified, energetic person in this post, the efforts of the infection control committee will be largely ineffective. This fact has become so apparent that by 1983 virtually 100% of U.S. hospitals had established such a position on at least a part-time basis [16], and this remained true into the late 1980s [74].

These positions have been filled predominantly by nurses. In the mid-1970s, 96% of ICPs were nurses, the rest being mostly trained in microbiology and laboratory technology [75]. This predominance held true through 1983, when 85% of ICPs were nurses, and the rest were medical technologists, microbiologists, and personnel from other backgrounds [unpublished data from the 1983 SENIC survey]. The national survey in 1987 conducted by Turner and colleagues [76] found that 75% were nurses, but a response rate of only 58% leaves the possibility of a large error in the results. The most common job titles for the position are infection control nurse (34% of U.S. hospitals in 1983), infection control coordinator (18%), nurse epidemiologist (12%), and infection control practitioner (5%) [unpublished data from the 1983 SENIC survey].

In U.S. hospitals, only approximately one fourth of ICPs work on infection control full-time. A much higher percentage (> 70%) work full-time in larger hospitals (more than 300 beds) in contrast to a much lower percentage (14%) in smaller hospitals [77]. In 1976 only about one half of U.S. hospitals met the recommendation for one full-time-equivalent ICP per 250 hospital beds [77]. Since most hospitals tended to have either one half-time or one full-time ICP position, smaller hospitals were more likely to have met this recommendation than large hospitals, even though some larger hospitals have more than one position. By 1983, however, two thirds of hospitals had established enough ICP positions to meet the recommendation [16].

In small hospitals in which ICPs work less than full-time on infection control, the appointee often has one or more other titles, including director or assistant director of nursing service, in-service education coordinator, operating room supervisor, utilization review nurse or, more recently, risk management coordinator [77]. In an increasing number of large medical school–affiliated hospitals, infection control is combined with risk management or utilization review in a single department. Although this situation offers advantages in efficient use of personnel and in bringing epidemiologic techniques to the risk management or utilization review activities, it runs the risk of seriously impairing the personnel's commitment to infection control if sufficient staff are not provided to cover all of the added responsibilities.

The advent of the AIDS epidemic in the mid-1980s added new responsibilities to the jobs of most ICPs, who were already overworked. These additional responsibilities varied widely from such duties as monitoring and minimizing employee exposures to patients' blood to writing policies for implementing new isolation precautions. In the early 1990s, the impact of AIDS on the ICP's job diminished somewhat as the epidemic became better understood (see Chapter 43).

The ICP position is most often located organizationally in the quality assurance or the nursing service department, although the ICP usually obtains advice and supervision from the infection control physician, if one is present in the hospital [77]. The majority of ICPs hold a nursing position equivalent to nursing supervisor or higher. Choosing more experienced nurses for the job is important, to give the ICP greater insight into the patient care practices that are to be influenced and more experience in the clinical milieu, which facilitates the detection of infections for surveillance and increases rapport with clinical nurses and doctors. In contrast to the levels of training of infection control physicians, almost all ICPs have taken at least one training course in infection control; two thirds of them were trained in the CDC training course, but more and more are taking courses offered by local and national APIC organizations, academic institutions, and private firms [77]. In 1983, as an indication of the growing training opportunities available for ICPs, the CDC, in cooperation with the Association of Schools of Public Health, consulted with a group of infection control training experts and recommended that the CDC cut back or discontinue its direct training efforts and turn these resources toward developing training materials and guidelines for others to use in training [78]. Subsequently, the CDC discontinued training in infection control, and courses were developed by private and professional groups.

ICPs across the country have tended to spend their time in similar ways. Regardless of the number of hours per week worked or the size of the hospital, they spend, on the average, approximately half their time on surveillance of infections, one fourth on policy development, and the rest about equally divided among training, consulting, and investigating potential outbreaks [77] (although it is important to note that time usage of ICPs has not been resurveyed in recent years). Recent task analyses performed by APIC have further specified what the infection control job entails [79–82].

In the early 1970s, it appeared that there would be a high turnover rate of nurses in the ICP position; however, by the mid-1970s the turnover rate had fallen significantly below that of hospital nurses in general, suggesting that the earlier trend was a temporary feature of the position's formative period [77]. In a 1985 national survey, the rate of turnover of ICPs was found to be 50% over 5 years, with a much lower turnover rate (28%) in large hospitals (> 500 beds) than that (54%) in small hospitals (< 50 beds) [19].

EFFICACY OF SURVEILLANCE AND CONTROL PROGRAMS

The question of the efficacy of ISCPs has been posed almost from the beginning of the movement in the 1960s but has been of increasing interest since the First International Conference in 1970. This debate has centered on several issues, including the efficacy and cost-effectiveness of routine infection surveillance over and above vigorous control measures, the need for ICPs, the best ratio of ICPs to hospital beds, the need for interested and trained infection control physicians, and the effectiveness of reporting surgical wound infection rates to surgeons. Although several studies in individual hospitals have verified dramatic reductions of their nosocomial infection rates after the establishment of various combinations of these features [7,33,38,62,83–102], they have not been influential in settling the efficacy questions because of the lack of simultaneous control observations, the possibility of selective reporting of positive results in the literature, and other methodological problems.

In the early 1970s, CDC investigators designed the protocol for a large historical prospective study, building in numerous design features to avoid or control for the many potential biases that might be encountered. After clearance through internal scientific peer review at the CDC, presentations at scientific meetings, and formal review through government channels, the project was undertaken by the CDC staff with technical assistance from the Department of Biostatistics of the University of North Carolina School of Public Health, the UCLA Institute for Social Science Research, and the National Center for Health Statistics, with financial support from the CDC, the National Institute of Allergy and Infectious Diseases, the Health Care Financing Administration (HCFA), and the office of the Assistant Secretary for Health, HHS.

After the initial design phase spanning 1974 to 1976, pilot studies were completed to validate the various data collection methods developed specifically for the project [15]. The study was then performed in three phases. First, a questionnaire was mailed to all U.S. hospitals to measure specific surveillance and control characteristics needed to construct indexes of these activities and other measures of the ICP and the other components under study. After stratifying all acute-care U.S. hospitals with these two indexes, 338 hospitals were selected randomly from the strata [15]. The sample provided a representative group of hospitals that had established different levels of surveillance and control efforts, including hospitals that had established no programs at all. Second, each of the 338 sample hospitals was visited by trained CDC interviewers to validate the surveillance and control indexes and collect more detailed descriptive information about the programs.

The third phase involved a review by trained CDC medical records analysts of random samples of the medical records of patients admitted in 1970 and in 1975 to 1976 to the 338 sample hospitals. In each hospital, 500 patients were selected randomly from each of the 2 years, and their records were reviewed to diagnose all nosocomial urinary tract infections, surgical wound infections, pneumonia, and bacteremia from the clinical data found in all parts of the record. These four sites account for > 80% of nosocomial infections. From these data on approximately 339,000 patients, the change of the nosocomial infection rates from 1970 (before any of the hospitals had programs) to 1975 to 1976 (after the program activities measured in the first two phases had been established) were estimated. In addition, measurements were made of other hospital and patients' characteristics, changes in which could have confounded the evaluation. Following the data collection phase (1976 to 1978), the large computerized database was extensively edited and made ready for analysis (1978 to 1980), and the statistical analysis of the influence of the programs on the change in infection rates, controlling for changes in other characteristics, was performed (1980 to 1983).

The results, published in early 1985 [20], are summarized in Table 4-1. In comparison with hospitals that started no program activities, those that established ISCPs with one full-time-equivalent ICP per 250 occupied beds, an effectual infection control physician with special interest in infection control, and a program for reporting wound infection rates to surgeons reduced their nosocomial infection rates by ~32%, a result that was highly statistically significant for all four types of infections studied. Separate analyses for cohorts of high- and low-risk patients showed similar results for each type of infection, although programs to prevent infection among low-risk patients had to be somewhat more intensive than those needed for high-risk patients. The importance of these results was emphasized by the finding that among hospitals that started no programs, the nosocomial infection rate rose at a rate of 18% over 5 years, presumably reflecting the increasing infection risks accompanying the continual introduction of invasive and immunocompromising medical technology.

Whereas approximately one third of nosocomial infections could be prevented if all U.S. hospitals established the programs found to be the most effective, the fact that relatively few hospitals actually had all of the required components meant that in the mid-1970s only 6% of nosocomial infections were actually being prevented nationwide [20]. The widespread adoption of the most effective programs might therefore be expected to prevent an additional one fourth of the infections. A second survey of a random sample of U.S. hospitals in 1983 found that hospitals had substantially strengthened the intensity of their surveillance and control activities, but the failure to implement certain specific critical components, such as an adequate staffing ratio for ICPs, training of hospital epidemiologists, or reporting wound infection rates to surgeons, had muted the degree of improvement in prevention to the extent that still only 9% of infections were being prevented [16].

POTENTIAL IMPACTS OF THE SENIC PROJECT

As the first controlled study of the effectiveness of ISCPs, the SENIC Project provided "a powerful justification for the American infection control strategy" [103]. Sufficient time has now passed since the release of the results of the SENIC Project to begin to assess its impact on the practice of infection control in the United States. Evidence to date suggests that the results have favorably influenced at least five areas: preservation of the role of infection control, a rekindling of interest in surveillance, a fundamental reorientation of surveillance from process to outcome, an enhanced emphasis on training for infection control physicians, and the use of multivariate analytic methods in the development of infection risk indexes.

Preservation of the Role of Infection Control

When the SENIC results were published in the mid-1980s, the roles of infection control, quality assurance, risk management, utilization review, and other oversight functions of the hospital were undergoing a restructuring under the changing priorities of the Joint Commission on Accreditation of Healthcare Organizations (JCAHO) and the HCFA. In an effort to make these activities more efficient, it was recommended that they be merged, preferably under the supervision of the directors of quality assurance. This was an unfortunate choice in many hospitals because most quality assurance programs were strongly oriented toward detecting individual cases of clinical errors and had little involvement with epidemiologic methods. This nationwide change threatened to extinguish the epidemiologic approach from hospitals. The release of the SENIC results, which constituted the first evidence of the efficacy of any of these patient care review functions, gave ICPs ammunition in persuading their quality assurance supervisors and hospital administrators of the need to preserve their epidemiologic orientation. With its survival now more assured, the epidemiologic approach appears to be gaining advocates among the other patient care review departments as well.

Rekindling of Interest in Surveillance

In the 1970s, when most hospitals started their organized ISCPs, surveillance of nosocomial infections and calculation of infection rates was a central focus of the programs. In the late 1970s and the early 1980s, however, many hospitals began lessening the intensity of surveillance, some discontinuing it altogether [16]. Since the release of the SENIC findings in early 1985, this trend appears to have reversed. For example, the practice of feeding back surgeon-specific wound infection rates to individual surgeons—the surveillance activity found to have had the greatest effect in SENIC [20]—was reportedly performed regularly in 19% of U.S. hospitals in 1976 [13], in 13% of hospitals in 1983 [16], and in only 6% in early 1985. But by the end of 1986, almost 2 years after publication of the SENIC findings, Landry [104] reported that this figure had risen to 28% of hospitals in Virginia, and, in 1987, an independent nationwide survey by the General Accounting Office found a similar prevalence [74]. There may have been further increases since 1987 as a result of policy recommendations for this practice by the Surgical Infection Society [105] and the JCAHO [71], based on the SENIC findings.

Change to Outcome Orientation

Perhaps the most important finding from SENIC, one that was not immediately recognized, was a strong dissociation of infection control program effectiveness for different types of infections. Programs that were effective in reducing the numbers of surgical wound infections were usually not the same as those that were effective in lowering the rate of urinary tract infections, bacteremias, and pneumonias, and vice versa. Only 0.2% of U.S. hospitals had programs that were effective in reducing all four of the main types of infection [20]. This finding led to the startling and controversial proposal that hospitals should stop doing routine surveillance of all nosocomial infections playing into the overall hospital infection rate and instead develop specific outcome objectives for which separate, targeted surveillance systems ought to be developed [24,106]. Initially opposed by proponents of routine hospital-wide surveillance, the new concept has been adopted increasingly by U.S. hospitals and has been incorporated as a recommended model in the 1990 standards for accreditation of hospitals by the JCAHO [71].

Increase in Physician Training

As discussed earlier, the percentage of U.S. hospitals with a physician trained in infection control remained at ~25% from 1976 to 1983 [16]. Following the release of the SENIC findings, the percentage appears to have risen substantially [74] and should continue to grow as a result of the training initiative for physicians launched by the AHA, SHEA, and CDC.

Multivariate Risk Indexes

The idea of controlling infection rate comparisons for intrinsic infection risk is an old concept, dating back to the late nineteenth century, when surgeons confined analysis to "clean" surgical wounds. Before the SENIC Project, analyses were being stratified by wound classification based on the likely level of bacterial contamination of the wound [105]. Using as a model the multivariate analyses of risk factors for wound infection done by previous investigators, SENIC investigators applied multivariate analysis to construct a simple, practical risk index combining the traditional wound classification with measures of intrinsic patient susceptibility to infection and predicted wound infection far more powerfully [43]. Whereas this particular multivariate index will undoubtedly be improved in the future [44–46], the concept of employing multivariate risk indexes rather than unidimensional risk measures will make nosocomial infection surveillance data far more useful for informing personnel involved in the care of patients of infection risks in their patients (see Chapters 7,8).

REFERENCES

1. U.S. Public Health Service Communicable Diseases Center and the National Academy of Sciences National Research Council. *Proceedings of the National Conference on Hospital-Acquired Staphylococcal Disease*, Atlanta, September 15–17, 1958. Atlanta: Centers for Disease Control, 1958.
2. U.S. Public Health Service Communicable Diseases Center and the National Academy of Sciences National Research Council. *Proceedings of the Conference on Relation of the Environment to Hospital-Acquired Staphylococcal Disease*, Atlanta, December 1–2, 1958. Atlanta: Centers for Disease Control, 1958.
3. University of Michigan School of Public Health, Mayo Foundation, Communicable Disease Center. *Proceedings of the National Conference on Institutionally Acquired Infections*, Minneapolis, September 4–6, 1963. Atlanta: Centers for Disease Control, 1963.
4. American Hospital Association. *Infection control in the hospital*. Chicago: American Hospital Association, 1968.
5. Eickhoff TC, Brachman PW, Bennett JV, et al. Surveillance of nosocomial infections in community hospitals. I. Surveillance methods, effectiveness, and initial results. *J Infect Dis* 1969;120:305–317.
6. Gardner AMN, Stamp M, Bowgen JA, et al. The infection control sister. *Lancet* 1962;2:710.
7. Streeter S, Dunn H, Lepper M. Hospital infection: a necessary risk? *Am J Nurs* 1967;67:526–533.
8. Wenzel K. The role of the infection control nurse. *Nurs Clin North Am* 1970;5:89–98.
9. Centers for Disease Control and Prevention. *Outline for surveillance and control of nosocomial infections*. Atlanta: Centers for Disease Control, 1972.
10. Centers for Disease Control and Prevention. *Proceedings of the First International Conference on Noscocomial Infections*, Atlanta, August 5–8, 1970. Chicago: American Hospital Association, 1970.
11. American Hospital Association. *Infection control in the hospital*. Chicago: American Hospital Association, 1970.
12. Stamm WE. Elements of an active, effective infection control program. *Hospitals* 1976;50:60.
13. Haley RW, Shachtman RH. The emergence of infection surveillance and control programs in U.S. hospitals: an assessment, 1976. *Am J Epidemiol* 1980;111:574–591.
14. Centers for Disease Control and Prevention. *National Nosocomial Infections Study: quarterly reports*. Atlanta: Centers for Disease Control, 1970–1983.
15. Haley RW, Quade D, Freeman HE, et al. Study on the Efficacy of Nosocomial Infection Control (SENIC Project): summary of study design. *Am J Epidemiol* 1980;111:472–485.
16. Haley RW, Morgan WM, Culver DH, et al. Hospital infection control: recent progress and opportunities under prospective payment. *Am J Infect Control* 1985;13:97–108.
17. Haley RW. CDC guidelines on infection control. *Infect Control Hosp Epidemiol* 1981;2:117–118.
18. Centers for Disease Control and Prevention. *Guidelines for the prevention and control of nosocomial infections*. Springfield, Va.: National Technical Information Service, U.S. Department of Commerce, 1982.
19. Celentano DD, Morlock LL, Malitz FE. Diffusion and adoption of CDC guidelines for the prevention and control of nosocomial infections in U.S. hospitals. *Infect Control* 1987;8:415–423.
20. Haley RW, Culver DH, White JW, et al. The efficacy of infection surveillance and control programs in preventing nosocomial infections in U.S. hospitals. *Am J Epidemiol* 1984;121:282.
21. Haley RW, White JW, Culver DH, et al. The financial incentive for hospitals to prevent nosocomial infections under the prospective payment system: an empirical determination from a nationally representative sample. *JAMA* 1987;257:1611–1614.
22. Inglehart JK. The new era of prospective payment for hospitals. *N Engl J Med* 1982;307:1288.
23. Wenzel RP. Nosocomial infections, diagnosis-related groups, and study on the efficacy of nosocomial infection control: economic implications for hospitals under the prospective payment system. *Am J Med* 1985;78:3–7.
24. Haley RW. *Managing hospital infection control for cost-effectiveness*. Chicago: American Hospital Publishing, Inc., 1986.
25. Decker MD, Schaffner W. Changing trends in infection control and hospital epidemiology. *Infect Dis Clin North Am* 1989;3:671–682.
26. Hughes JM. Universal precautions: CDC perspective. *Occup Med* 1989;suppl 4:13–20.
27. Fridkin SK, Manangan L, Bolyard E, et al. SHEA-CDC TB survey. I. Status of TB infection control programs at member hospitals, 1989–1992. Society for Healthcare Epidemiology of America. *Infect Control Hosp Epidemiol* 1995;16:129–134.
28. Crede W, Hierholzer WJ Jr. Linking hospital epidemiology and quality assurance: seasoned concepts in a new role. *Infect Control Hosp Epidemiol* 1988;9:42–44.

29. Massanari RM. Risk management: an epidemiologic approach. *Infect Control Hosp Epidemiol* 1987;8:3–6.
30. Crede W, Hierholzer WJ Jr. Surveillance for quality assessment. I. Surveillance in infection control success reviewed. *Infect Control Hosp Epidemiol* 1989;10:470–474.
31. McGeer A, Crede W, Hierholzer WJ Jr. Surveillance for quality assessment. II. Surveillance for noninfectious processes: back to basics. *Infect Control Hosp Epidemiol* 1990;11:36–41.
32. Crede WB, Hierholzer WJ Jr. Surveillance for quality assessment. III. The critical assessment of quality indicators. *Infect Control Hosp Epidemiol* 1990;11:197–201.
33. Collier C, Miller DP, Borst M. Community hospital surgeon-specific infection rates. *Infect Control* 1987;8:249–254.
34. Gaunt PN. Audit in infection control: data analysis and infections in the intensive care unit. *J Hosp Infect* 1993;24:291–300.
35. LaHaise S. A comparison of infection control software for use by hospital epidemiologists in meeting the new JCAHO standards. *Infect Control Hosp Epidemiol* 1990;11:185–190.
36. Evans RS, Burke JP, Classen DC, et al. Computerized identification of patients at high risk for hospital-acquired infection. *Am J Infect Control* 1992;20:4–10.
37. Schifman RB, Howanitz PJ. Nosocomial infections: a College of American Pathologists Q-probes study in 512 North American institutions. *Arch Pathol Lab Med* 1994;118:115–119.
38. Gil-Egea MJ, Pi-Sunyer MT, Verdaguer A, et al. Surgical wound infections: prospective study of 4,468 clean wounds. *Infect Control Hosp Epidemiol* 1987;8:277–280.
39. Ziesing S, Weber S, Will S, et al. Introduction of an infection registration program for surgical wound infection based on the WHOCARE software of WHO. *Zentralbl Hyg Umweltmed* 1994;195:288–298.
40. Melcher GA. Computer-assisted prospective wound infection monitoring. II. Experiences and practical application. *Swiss Surg I* 1995;45–47.
41. Ryf C. Computer-assisted prospective wound infection monitoring. I. Ideas and principles. *Swiss Surg I* 1995;40–44.
42. Anonymous. Nosocomial infection rates for interhospital comparison: limitations and possible solutions. A report from the National Nosocomial Infections Surveillance (NNIS) System. *Infect Control Hosp Epidemiol* 1991;12:609–621.
43. Haley RW, Culver DH, White JW, et al. Identifying patients at high risk of surgical wound infection: a simple multivariate index of patient susceptibility and wound contamination. *Am J Epidemiol* 1984;121:206.
44. Culver DH, Horan TC, Gaynes RP, et al. Surgical wound infection rates by wound class, operation, and risk index in U.S. hospitals, 1986–90. *Am J Med* 1991;91(suppl 3B):152S–157S.
45. Haley RW. Nosocomial infections in surgical patients: developing valid measures of intrinsic patient risk. *Am J Med* 1991;91(suppl 3B): 145S–151S.
46. Haley RW. Measuring the intrinsic risk of wound infection in surgical patients. In: Nichols RL, ed. *Problems in general surgery*. Philadelphia: JB Lippincott, 1992.
47. Gaynes RP, Martone WJ, Culver DH, et al. Comparison of rates of nosocomial infections in neonatal intensive care units in the United States: National Nosocomial Infections Surveillance System. *Am J Med* 1991;91:192S–196S.
48. Gaynes RP, Culver DH, Martone WJ, et al. Comparison of rates of nosocomial infections in neonatal intensive care units in the United States. *Am J Med* 1991;91(suppl 3B):192S–196S.
49. Haley RW. JCAHO infection control indicators, parts I and II. *Infect Control Hosp Epidemiol* 1990:11:545–546.
50. Cookson BD. Progress with establishing and implementing standards for infection control in the U.K. *J Hosp Infect* 1995;suppl 30:69–75.
51. Jepsen OB. Towards European Union standards in hospital infection control. *J Hosp Infect* 1995;suppl 30:64–68.
52. O'Rourke EJ. The first HICPAC guideline: well done, CDC Hospital Infection Control Practices Advisory Committee. *Am J Infect Control* 1995;23:50–52.
53. Tablan OC, Anderson LJ, Arden NH, et al. Guideline for prevention of nosocomial pneumonia. The Hospital Infection Control Practices Advisory Committee, Centers for Disease Control and Prevention. *Infect Control Hosp Epidemiol* 1994;15:587–627.
54. Anonymous. Recommendations for preventing the spread of vancomycin resistance. Hospital Infection Control Practices Advisory Committee (HICPAC). *Infect Control Hosp Epidemiol* 1995;16: 105–113.
55. Anonymous. Guideline for isolation precautions in hospitals. II. Recommendations for isolation precautions in hospitals. Hospital Infection Control Practices Advisory Committee. *Am J Infect Control* 1996;24:32–52.
56. Goldmann DA, Weinstein RA, Wenzel RP, et al. Strategies to prevent and control the emergence and spread of antimicrobial-resistant microorganisms in hospitals: a challenge to hospital leadership. *JAMA* 1996;275:234–240.
57. Dellinger EP, Gross PA, Barrett TL, et al. Quality standard for antimicrobial prophylaxis in surgical procedures: the Infectious Diseases Society of America. *Infect Control Hosp Epidemiol* 1994;15:182–188.
58. Larson EL. APIC guideline for handwashing and hand antisepsis in healthcare settings. *Am J Infect Control* 1995;23:251–269.
59. French GL, Wong SL, Cheng AFB, et al. Repeated prevalence surveys for monitoring effectiveness of hospital infection control. *Lancet* 1989;2:1021–1023.
60. Sellick JA Jr. The use of statistical process control charts in hospital epidemiology. *Infect Control Hosp Epidemiol* 1993;14:649–656.
61. Scheckler WE. Continuous quality improvement in a hospital system: implications for hospital epidemiology. *Infect Control Hosp Epidemiol* 1992;13:288–292.
62. Kelleghan SI, Salemi C, Padilla S, et al. An effective continuous quality improvement approach to the prevention of ventilator-associated pneumonia. *Am J Infect Control* 1993;21:322–330.
63. Deming WE. The statistical procedure in the SENIC Project. *Am J Epidemiol* 1980;111:470–471.
64. Haley RW. The usefulness of a conceptual model in the Study on the Efficacy of Infection Surveillance and Control Programs. *Rev Infect Dis* 1981;3:775–780.
65. Raven BH, Freeman HE, Haley RW. Social science perspectives in hospital infection control. In: Johnson AW, Grusky O, Raven BH, eds. *Contemporary health services: social science perspectives*. Boston: Auburn House, 1981:137–176.
66. Raven BH, Haley RW. Social influence in a medical context. *Appl Soc Sci Annu* 1980;1:255–277.
67. Raven BH, Haley RW. Social influence and compliance of hospital nurses with infection control policies. In: Eiser JR, ed. *Social psychology and behavioral medicine*. New York: Wiley, 1982.
68. Raven BH. The bases of power: origins and recent developments. *J Soc Sci Issu* 1993;49:227–251.
69. Seto WH, Ong SG, Ching TY, et al. The utilization of influencing tactics for the implementation of infection control policies [Brief Report]. *Infect Control Hosp Epidemiol* 1990;11:144–150.
70. Joint Commission on Accreditation of Healthcare Organizations. Standards: Infection Control. In: *JCAHO: Accreditation manual for hospitals*. Chicago: Joint Commission on Accreditation of Healthcare Organizations, 1990.
71. Joint Commission on Accreditation of Hospitals. *Accreditation manual for hospitals*, 1976. Chicago: Joint Commission on Accreditation of Hospitals, 1976.
72. Haley RW. The "hospital epidemiologist" in U.S. hospitals, 1976–1977: a description of the head of the infection surveillance and control program. Report from the SENIC project. *Infect Control* 1980;1:21–32.
73. Haley RW. The role of infectious disease physicians in hospital infection control. *Bull N Y Acad Med* 1987;63:597–604.
74. U.S. General Accounting Office. *Infection control: military programs are comparable to VA and nonfederal programs but can be enhanced*. Washington, D.C.: U.S. General Accounting Office, 1990. Report to Congressional Requestors no. GA0/HRD-90-74.
75. Emori TG, Haley RW, Garner JS, et al. Comparison of surveillance and control activities of infection control nurses and infection control laboratorians in United States hospitals, 1976–1977. *Am J Infect Control* 1982;10:3–16.
76. Turner JG, Booth WC, Brown KC, et al. National survey of infection control practitioners' educational needs. *Am J Infect Control* 1990;18: 86–92.
77. Emori TG, Haley RW, Stanley RC. The infection control nurse in U.S. hospitals, 1976–1977: characteristics of the position and its occupant. *Am J Epidemiol* 1980;111:592–607.
78. Centers for Disease Control Association of Schools of Public Health. *A Report of the Meeting of the CDC/ASPH Working Group on Nosocomial Infection Control Training*, April 12–13, 1983. Atlanta: Centers for Disease Control, 1983.
79. Larson E, Eisenberg R, Soule BM. Validating the certification

process for infection control practice. *Am J Infect Control* 1988;16: 198–205.
80. McArthur BJ, Pugliese G, Weinstein S, et al. A national task analysis of infection control practitioners, 1982. I. Methodology and demography. *Am J Infect Control* 1984;12:88–95.
81. Pugliese G, McArthur BJ, Weinstein S, et al. A national task analysis of infection control practitioners, 1982. III. The relationship between hospital size and tasks performed. *Am J Infect Control* 1984;12: 221–227.
82. Shannon R, McArthur BJ, Weinstein S, et al. A national task analysis of infection control practitioners, 1982. II. Tasks, knowledge, and abilities for practice. *Am J Infect Control* 1984;12:187–196.
83. Moore WL Jr. Nosocomial infections: an overview. *Am J Hosp Pharm* 1974;31:832–838.
84. Shoji KT, Axnick K, Rytel MW. Infections and antibiotic use in a large municipal hospital 1970–1972: a prospective analysis of the effectiveness of a continuous surveillance program. *Health Lab Sci* 1974;11: 283–292.
85. Edwards LD. The epidemiology of 2,056 remote site infections and 1,966 surgical wound infections occurring in 1,865 patients: a four year study of 40,923 operations at Rush-Presbyterian–St. Luke's Hospital, Chicago. *Ann Surg* 1976;184:758–766.
86. Fuchs PC. *Epidemiology of hospital-associated infections*. Chicago, American Society of Clinical Pathologists, 1979:74–78.
87. Cruse PJE, Foord R. The epidemiology of wound infection: a 10-year prospective study of 62,939 wounds. *Surg Clin North Am* 1980;60:27.
88. Kaiser AB. Effective and creative surveillance and reporting of surgical wound infections. *Infect Control Hosp Epidemiol* 1982;3:41–43.
89. Condon RE, Schulte WJ, Malangoni MA, et al. Effectiveness of a surgical wound surveillance program. *Arch Surg* 1983;118:303–307.
90. Lennard ES, Hargiss CO, Schoenknecht FD. Postoperative wound infection surveillance by use of bacterial contamination categories. *Am J Infect Control* 1985;13:147–153.
91. Mead PB, Pories SE, Hall P, et al. Decreasing the incidence of surgical wound infections: validation of a surveillance-notification program. *Arch Surg* 1896;121:458–461.
92. Borst M, Collier C, Miller D. Operating room surveillance: a new approach in reducing hip and knee prosthetic wound infections. *Am J Infect Control* 1986;14:161–166.
93. Onesko KM, Wienke EC. The analysis of the impact of a mild, low-iodine, lotion soap on the reduction of nosocomial methicillin-resistant *Staphylococcus aureus*: a new opportunity for surveillance by objectives. *Infect Control Hosp Epidemiol* 1987;8:284–288.
94. Nystrom B. Hospital infection control in Sweden. *Infect Control Hosp Epidemiol* 1987;8:337–338.
95. Braun M. Five years' infection statistics of an orthopedic clinic: pathogen spectrum, resistance status, therapeutic consequences. *Z Orthop Ihre Grenzgeb* 1989;127:471–473.
96. Kjaersgaard E, Jepsen OB, Andersen S, et al. Registration of postoperative wound infections by ADB: a trial of the DANOP program. *Ugeskr Laeger* 1989;151:994–996.
97. Larsen RA, Evans RS, Burke JP, et al. Improved perioperative antibiotic use and reduced surgical wound infections through use of computer decision analysis. *Infect Control Hosp Epidemiol* 1989;10:316–320.
98. Bremmelgaard A, Raahave D, Beier-Holgersen R, et al. Computer-aided surveillance of surgical infections and identification of risk factors. *J Hosp Infect* 1989;13:1–18.
99. Sejberg D, Cordtz T, Kjaeldgaard P, et al. Postoperative wound infections at a mixed surgical department: 1 year's registration employing a PC-based system. *Ugeskr Laeger* 1989;151:991–994.
100. Manian FA, Meyer L. Comprehensive surveillance of surgical wound infections in outpatient and inpatient surgery. *Infect Control Hosp Epidemiol* 1990;11:515–520.
101. Kirk SJ, Cooper GC, Moorehead RJ, et al. Wound sepsis in 10,000 surgical patients. *Ulster Med J* 1990;59:36–40.
102. Olson MM, Lee JT Jr. Continuous, 10-year wound infection surveillance: results, advantages, and unanswered questions. *Arch Surg* 1990; 125:794–803.
103. Goldmann DA. Nosocomial infection control in the United States of America. *J Hosp Infect* 1986;8:116–128.
104. Landry S. Survey of infection control practices in Virginia [Abstract]. *Proceedings of the International Conference on Practit Infection Control*, May 1–8, 1988.
105. Condon RE, Haley RW, Lee JT Jr, et al. Does infection control control infection? *Arch Surg* 1988;123:250–256.
106. Haley RW. Surveillance by objectives: a priority-directed approach to the surveillance of nosocomial infection. *Am J Infect Control* 1985; 13:78.

Hospital Infections, Fourth Edition,
edited by John V. Bennett and Philip S. Brachman.
Published by Lippincott–Raven Publishers, Philadelphia, 1998

CHAPTER 5

Surveillance of Nosocomial Infections

Robert P. Gaynes

DEFINITION OF SURVEILLANCE

Surveillance is defined as "the ongoing, systematic collection, analysis, and interpretation of health data essential to the planning, implementation, and evaluation of public health practice, closely integrated with the timely dissemination of these data to those who need to know" [1]. A nosocomial infection surveillance system may be based on a sentinel event or on a population, or both. A sentinel infection is one that clearly indicates a failure in the hospital's efforts to prevent infections and, in theory, requires individual investigation [2,3]. For example, blood transfusion from a source patient already identified as a hepatitis carrier should always prompt investigation, since it clearly indicates a failure of a hospital's efforts. Denominator data are usually not collected in sentinel event–based surveillance. Such surveillance will find only the most serious problems and should not be the only surveillance system in the hospital. Population-based surveillance, that is, surveillance of patients with similar risks, requires both a numerator (the infection) and a denominator (the number of patients or days of exposure to the risk).

HISTORICAL PERSPECTIVE

In the time since the first edition of this book was published, a great deal of discussion and debate has concerned the desirability of continuing routine surveillance, argued by some to be too personnel-intensive in a milieu of constrained hospital budgets. As this discussion continues, an account of how the modern concepts and techniques of surveillance came to be—how we got where we are now—should be considered. Many of these practices were developed to meet emerging problems, and the basic idea of surveillance has been found to reduce infection risks. Knowledge of the historical reasons for these developments may help improve the efficiency and effectiveness of our current surveillance activities without discarding well-conceived approaches that remain effective.

The use of surveillance methods to control nosocomial infections dates back at least to the classic work of Ignaz Semmelweis in Vienna in the 1840s [4]. Although the Semmelweis story is best remembered as the first demonstration of person-to-person spread of puerperal sepsis and of the effectiveness of washing the hands with an antiseptic solution, an equally important achievement was Semmelweis's rigorous approach to the collection, analysis, and use of surveillance data. In contrast, the concurrent work of Oliver Wendell Holmes on the same subject in the United States was based primarily on the traditional anecdotal case-study approach of clinical medicine.

Semmelweis's investigation constitutes an amazingly contemporary example of the effective use of surveillance in addressing a widespread infection problem. When he assumed the directorship of the obstetric service at the Vienna Lying In Hospital in 1847, the apparent risk of maternal mortality had been at high levels for > 20 years, so long that the eminent clinicians of the day considered the risks to be no more than the expected endemic occurrence that could not be influenced. Semmelweis first undertook a retrospective investigation of maternal mortality and set up a prospective surveillance system to monitor the problem and the effects of later control measures. The initial results of his retrospective study of annual hospital mortality lists showed clearly that the maternal mortality level, which he measured by simply calculating annual mortality rates, had indeed increased tenfold after the introduction in the 1820s of the new anatomic school of pathology, which used the autopsy as its primary teaching tool.

His second discovery, based on the use of ward-specific mortality, was that the risk of death in the ward used

R. P. Gaynes: Hospital Infections Program, National Center for Infectious Diseases, Centers for Disease Control and Prevention, Atlanta, Georgia 30333.

by the obstetricians for teaching medical students was at least four times higher than that in the ward used by midwifery students. After the septic death of his mentor suggested the presence of a transmissible agent, Semmelweis used the findings from his retrospective surveillance study to implicate the practices of the obstetricians and medical students. After observing their daily routines, he surmised that professors and students might be transferring the infection from their cadavers to the parturient women and that washing hands with a chlorine solution might prevent transmission. Subsequently, his prospective surveillance data documented a dramatic reduction in maternal mortality immediately after the institution of the policy of mandatory hand washing before entering the labor room.

Here the great insights of Semmelweis ended, as often happens to infection control efforts today. Apparently owing to his abrasive manner and lack of diplomacy as well as an inability to organize his statistical data into a concise and convincing report, Semmelweis failed to win over his clinical colleagues to his discovery. Within 2 years, he was dismissed from the staff of the hospital, and his successor gradually allowed the strict hand-washing measures to lapse. In the absence of hand washing and continuing surveillance, the epidemic promptly resumed and lasted well into the early part of the twentieth century, its severity and means of prevention apparently unrecognized by several more generations of clinicians.

This story well illustrates one of the main impediments to infection control today, namely, that in the absence of careful epidemiologic data and a diplomatic presentation, clinicians, who are oriented almost entirely toward the treatment of their individual patients, often fail to note the severity of the infection transmission problem and sometimes even resist control measures. It also points out the utility of surveillance in identifying problems and developing and applying control measures. From a methodologic viewpoint, Semmelweis's efforts encompassed almost all aspects of the modern surveillance approach: retrospective collection of data to confirm the presence of a problem; analysis of the data to localize the risks in time, place, and person; controlled comparisons of high- and low-risk groups to identify risk factors; formulation and application of control measures; and prospective surveillance to monitor the problem, evaluate the control measures, and detect future recurrences. The main shortcoming of his approach was not diplomatically educating his powerful colleagues with a careful report of his findings.

As good a model as Semmelweis's work was, the modern era of nosocomial infection surveillance grew as much out of different currents of the mid-twentieth century as from the Semmelweis tradition. The importance of surveillance for disease control in general was demonstrated in the late 1940s by the Communicable Diseases Center, now called the Centers for Disease Control and Prevention (CDC). Since a large number of reports of malaria indicated the disease to be widespread in the United States, a surveillance system was immediately set up to define the problem. As investigators examined each reported case, however, they found virtually all the reports to be errors in diagnosis. Thus, the mere activity of surveillance "eradicated" the malaria epidemic in the United States.

With this and similar successes fresh in memory, when the pandemic of staphylococcal infections swept the nation's hospitals in the mid-1950s, CDC staff members were quick to apply the concepts of surveillance to the problem [5]. Once asked to assist in investigating a staphylococcal epidemic in a particular hospital, those early investigators often met with strong resistance from clinicians and hospital administrators convinced that no unusual infection problems were present in their hospitals. In instances where CDC staff members were able to continue their investigations, the collection and reporting of surveillance data regularly changed those attitudes to strong concern over the documented problems and eagerness to apply control measures. These initial inquiries thus confirmed a nationwide staphylococcal epidemic and led the CDC to sponsor several national conferences to discuss the problem.

As the epidemic subsided in the early 1960s, the CDC's Hospital Infections Unit continued to develop more effective surveillance methods specifically geared to the hospital environment. By 1970, on the basis of pilot studies, the CDC began recommending that surveillance be practiced routinely in all hospitals. The results were that by the late 1970s almost all U.S. hospitals had adopted the approach of routine surveillance of nosocomial infections. Surveillance that consisted of culturing the inanimate environment had been virtually abandoned (see Chapters 4, 20). In 1976, the Joint Commission on Accreditation of Hospitals (JCAH) incorporated a detailed surveillance system into their standards for accreditation.

By the early 1970s, some critics questioned the effectiveness and cost benefit of routine infection surveillance, although more hospitals were expanding their surveillance efforts than were curtailing them [6]. Surveillance was (and is) a very time-consuming activity, requiring ~40% to 50% of an infection control practitioner's time. The inability of some hospitals to establish an adequate number of positions for infection control practitioners (at least one full-time-equivalent practitioner per 250 beds) was a major contributor to their disenchantment with routine infection surveillance.

Several factors have influenced the contemporary practices favoring a strong surveillance component in infection control programs. First, the results of the Study on the Efficacy of Nosocomial Infection Control (SENIC) substantiated the importance of surveillance along with control measures to cut down infection rates and provided the scientific basis for surveillance of nosocomial infections [7–9]. The strong conclusion was that hospitals that are effective in lowering their nosocomial infection rates have an organized, routine, hospital-wide surveillance system. Second, the requirements of the Joint Commission on Accreditation of Healthcare Organizations (JCAHO, formerly JCAH) have legitimized the need for personnel to perform surveillance [10,11]. Third, the surveillance practices developed within the context of infection control have begun to influence other aspects of hospitals' patient care review activities.

At the same time that the strategy of targeting surveillance to reduce specific endemic problems and monitoring to assess the effectiveness of intervention measures was incorporated into the JCAHO's 1994 infection control standards for accreditation, the strategy was also applied to hospital quality assurance programs to lower rates of noninfectious complications [12,13]. The increasing pressure to continually improve quality is certain to broaden the use of surveillance to aid in the prevention of nosocomial infections.

THE PURPOSE OF SURVEILLANCE

A hospital should have clear goals for surveillance. These goals must be reviewed and updated frequently to address new infection risks in changing populations of patients, such as the introduction of high-risk medical interventions and changing pathogens and their resistance to antibiotics. The collection and analysis of surveillance data must be performed in conjunction with a prevention strategy. It is vital to identify and state objectives of surveillance before designing and starting surveillance.

Reducing Infection Rates Within a Hospital

The most important goal of surveillance is to lower the risks of acquiring nosocomial infections. In order to attain this goal, specific objectives for surveillance must be defined based on how the data are to be used and the availability of financial and personnel resources for surveillance [7,8]. Objectives for surveillance can be either outcome- or process-oriented. Outcome objectives, such as comparative rate analysis and feedback to patient care personnel, are aimed at reducing infection risks and costs. Process objectives, on the other hand, are activities necessary to achieve outcome objectives. Examples of process objectives are defining and identifying infections, analyzing and interpreting data, observing and evaluating patient care practices, monitoring equipment and the environment, and providing education. Much of the time spent performing surveillance is devoted to process objectives. However, these activities are of limited value without clearly stated outcome objectives. While there are other legitimate purposes for surveillance of nosocomial infections, the ultimate goal is to use the process objectives to achieve outcome objectives—decreases in infection rates, morbidity, mortality, and cost.

Establishing Endemic Baseline Rates

Surveillance data can be used to quantify baseline rates of endemic nosocomial infections. This measurement provides hospitals with knowledge about the ongoing infection risks in hospitalized patients. Most nosocomial infections, perhaps 90% to 95%, are endemic, that is, not part of recognized outbreaks [14]. Thus, the main purpose for surveillance activities should be to lower the endemic rate rather than identify outbreaks. Many hospitals' infection control practitioners (ICPs) have stated that their presence on the wards may be sufficient to influence infection rates, and 91% of hospitals have reported using surveillance data simply to establish endemic baseline rates [15]. However, the mere act of collecting data does not usually influence infection risks appreciably unless it is linked with a prevention strategy. Otherwise, surveillance is no more than bean counting, an expensive exercise without focus that today's hospitals can ill afford and that ICPs will ultimately find dissatisfying.

Identifying Outbreaks

Once endemic rates are established, one may be able to recognize deviations from the baseline that sometimes represent outbreaks of infection. This benefit must be balanced with the relatively time-consuming task of ongoing collection of surveillance data, since only a small proportion of nosocomial infections, perhaps 5% to 10%, manifest as outbreaks [14]. Moreover, outbreaks of nosocomial infections are often brought to the attention of infection control personnel by astute clinicians or laboratory personnel much more quickly than by the analysis of routine surveillance data. This lack of timeliness often limits the use of routine surveillance in identifying outbreaks in a hospital.

Persuading Medical Personnel

One of the most difficult tasks of an infection control program is persuading hospital personnel to adopt recommended preventive practices. Familiarity with the scientific literature on hospital epidemiology and infection control is effective in influencing behavior only if the hospital personnel believe the information is relevant to the specific situation in question. Often, studies in the literature do not address the varied situations encountered in a particular hospital. Using information on one's own hospital to influence personnel is one of the most effective means to address a problem and apply the recommended techniques to prevent infection. If surveillance data are analyzed appropriately and routinely presented in a skillful manner, medical personnel usually come to rely on them for guidance. The feedback of such information is often quite effective in influencing healthcare workers to adopt recommended preventive practices [9]. A team approach, using ICPs working with clinicians from a variety of disciplines, is particularly effective.

Evaluating Control Measures

After a problem has been identified through surveillance data and control measures have been instituted, continued surveillance is needed to ensure that the problem has come under control. By continual monitoring, some control measures that seemed rational can be shown to be ineffective. In one example, the use of daily meatal care to prevent nosocomial urinary tract infections seemed appropriate but did not control infection [16]. Even after the initial success of control measures, there can be lapses in applying them that require ongoing vigilance (including the continued collection of surveillance data).

Satisfying Regulators

Satisfying the requirements of regulators, such as the JCAHO, is a very commonly reported application of surveillance data, but one of the least justifiable if used only for that purpose. The collection of surveillance data merely to appease a surveyor who visits a hospital once every three years (or occasionally more often) is an extraordinary waste of resources. The JCAHO also viewed this process-oriented task of collecting data as unproductive when it altered its standards in 1990. Hospitals are now required to apply surveillance in a directed manner to bring about change in the risk of infection to patients [10]. The JCAHO's Agenda for Change has impelled hospitals to use surveillance for its originally intended purpose—to change the outcome of care of patients by reducing infection risks.

Defending Malpractice Claims

One concern about collection of surveillance data has been that it would create a record that could be used against the hospital in a malpractice claim related to a nosocomial infection. It is now the opinion of most legal experts that a strong surveillance component in an infection control program demonstrates that a hospital is attempting to detect problems rather than conceal them (see Chapter 18). This has proved to be an important defense against unwarranted claims. Additionally, the records of infection control committees are considered privileged in most states and are not available in the context of the process of discovery in civil court proceedings. Therefore, surveillance is often helpful in defending against malpractice claims; it is rarely, if ever, a hindrance.

Comparing Hospitals' Nosocomial Infection Rates

Traditionally, surveillance has been recommended solely for gaining understanding of and cutting down nosocomial infection rates within individual hospitals. The idea of comparing infection rates among hospitals, though it is often suggested by administrators and quality assurance supervisors, has generally been discouraged by infection control physicians and practitioners because the large differences in the mix of intrinsic infection risks of the patients in different hospitals render differences among the rates virtually uninterpretable.

Recent studies performed by the CDC, however, have suggested that interhospital comparisons can be useful in lowering infection risks [17–20] if the rates are specific to a particular site of infection (e.g., urinary tract) and control for variations in the distributions of the major risk factor(s) for that type of infection (e.g., duration of indwelling urinary catheterization). Conversely, it must be emphasized that a single number expressing the hospital's overall nosocomial infection rate is not a valid measure of the efficacy of the hospital's infection control programs, largely because of the lack of suitable overall risk adjusters for infections of all types [20–23]. Therefore, a hospital's overall nosocomial infection rate, as presently derived, should not be used for interhospital comparisons.

The importance of interhospital comparison of infection rates has captured the interest of the JCAHO. The JCAHO Board of Commissioners selected three infection control indicators for inclusion in the Indicator Measurement System (IM System) beginning in 1996. An infection control task force of 17 field experts considered findings from 2 years of beta-testing of eight indicators. The final indicators endorsed by the task force include (a) patients undergoing selected surgical procedures complicated by surgical site infections, (b) ventilated patients who get pneumonia, and (c) inpatients with a central intravascular line who show signs of a primary bloodstream infection.

The JCAHO expects hospitals to analyze the data that they collect for the indicators to make improvements in care and then transmit the data for analyses comparing hospitals [24]. The distributions of hospitals on the indicator rates, stratified by intrinsic risk indexes, will be reported to hospitals for their use in identifying potential problems in care that could be addressed by further surveillance and control efforts in the hospital. Accreditation decisions will not be made on the basis of the interhospital comparisons but instead on the basis of how hospitals respond to the findings of the comparisons. In January 1995 the board of directors of the JCAHO elected not to require hospitals to participate in the IM System. Rather, hospitals may use the IM System but can implement other performance measurement systems in their attempts to compare rates. The Council on Performance Measurements convened by the JCAHO in 1996 devised criteria to evaluate a performance measurement system in order to recommend its use in place of participation in the JCAHO's IM System.

METHODS OF SURVEILLANCE

Collecting the Data

Defining Events to Be Surveyed

In developing a surveillance system, it is of utmost importance to define carefully those events to be surveyed and then to apply the accepted definitions systematically in the data-collecting process. In attempting to understand the relationship between urinary tract infection and urinary catheterization, for example, it is necessary first to define or establish criteria to decide what will be called a urinary tract infection and what will be considered urinary catheterization. Once the event to be surveyed has been defined as concisely and precisely as possible and the criteria for determining its presence or absence have been established, then it is imperative that these definitions and criteria be applied systematically and uniformly henceforth. Ideally, all members of the population judged at risk of the adverse event would be systematically and continuously assessed for the presence or absence of the properties specified by the criteria that define the event or the infection being sought.

The CDC has published guidelines for determining the presence and classification of nosocomial infections [25, 26]. These guidelines are not rigorous definitions of disease but instead serve as practical, operational definitions for most hospitals, regardless of their size or medical sophistication. The exact definitions to be used in surveillance in individual hospitals are not as critical as having the infection control committee obtain the concurrence of key hospital staff members. Such widespread advance agreement is necessary to avoid later disqualification of the results of surveillance as a result of disagreements over the definitions.

Role of the ICP

A number of methods of collecting infection data have been described in the literature [27–30]. In general, the most satisfactory and practical method at present employs a person (or persons), often called the ICP, whose job description includes collecting and analyzing surveillance data. Details of the qualifications, functions, and responsibilities of the ICP were given previously (see Chapter 4). The ICP is responsible to the infection control committee and should be under the immediate supervision of the committee chairperson or the hospital epidemiologist, if the hospital has one. The traditional choice of a nurse to fill this position has been primarily based on his or her professional training and ability to interact with other nursing personnel in the data collection process, but experience has shown that persons other than nurses can also function well in this position, particularly in the surveillance process.

The original studies of surveillance conducted by the CDC in the 1970s indicated that one full-time-equivalent ICP could conduct surveillance for ~250 acute-care hospital beds and have sufficient remaining time for other infection control duties and responsibilities [9]. As the average length of a patient's hospital stay has shortened and the patients' severity of illness has increased with changes in medical care (e.g., managed care), the ICP's job has become more demanding. Therefore, ICPs have had to set priorities for the use of their time in ways that will maximize their impact on infection risks.

Minimal Data to Collect About Infections

The precise information collected in conjunction with each infection depends upon the surveillance objective and may vary according to the institution, service, site of infection, or causative agent. Certain essential identifying data, however, can be recommended: the patient's name, age, sex, hospital identification number, ward or location within the hospital, service, and date of admission; the date of onset of the infection; the site of infection; the organism(s) isolated in culture studies; and the antimicrobial susceptibility pattern of the organisms isolated. Most hospitals collect too much data that is never analyzed. This excessive data collection often interferes with or delays the surveillance process. Additional information should be collected only if it will be analyzed and used by the hospital.

Some institutions may wish to include the primary diagnoses of the infected patients, an assessment of the severity of underlying illness(es), the name(s) of the attending physician(s) or other staff who cared for the patient, whether the patient was exposed (before the onset of infection) to therapies that can predispose to infection (e.g., surgery; antibiotic, steroid, or immunosuppressive therapy; or instrumentation), what antimicrobial agents were used to treat the infection, and some assessment of mortality related to the infection. Hospitals may also want to record the presence or absence of particular exposure factors, for example, the use of invasive devices such as urinary catheters for urinary tract infections, respiratory therapy equipment for respiratory infections, and intravascular catheters for primary bacteremia.

Denominators

The methods for obtaining the denominators for infection rates have always been the most controversial and have sometimes been the most labor-intensive aspect of generating nosocomial infection rates. The most common method was to use the number of patients admitted to or discharged from the hospital, or from a particular ward or service, as a crude estimate of the number of patients at risk of infection. Another denominator used was patient-days rather than admissions or discharges. Patient-day denominators are derived by summing the number of days that all patients stayed in the hospital during the surveillance period.

Since the patient-day denominator includes length of stay, the resulting infection rates are at least partly adjusted for differences among patients' lengths of stay. Admissions, discharges, and patient-days can be acquired for the hospital as a whole and by each service, usually from the hospital medical records department or business office. However, these denominators fail to consider differences in patients' risks for nosocomial infection, such as exposures to certain invasive devices. Accordingly, calculation of overall rates using these denominators is not recommended [20].

Another method is to compile a record on every patient at risk, rather than on only infected patients, and using summary denominator data for rate calculation. As hospitals rely more and more on computers, this will become easier and more common. Using this method, the record contains the risk factors for individual patients (e.g., each patient undergoing a surgical operation), and the information about nosocomial infections is added to an affected patient's record when infections are detected. A computer system is usually necessary for compiling such detailed records. From this type of complete patient database, the computer simply calculates infection rates for whatever time period and population the ICP selects, and the denominators are generated automatically for the calculations.

While entering data on all patients at risk might seem more time-consuming than the traditional method, it is preferable for targeted surveillance projects, such as generating for surgeon-specific rates by class or for intensive care unit (ICU) surveillance, because ICPs have far more flexibility in the types of rates that they can generate. With a full database, they can calculate rates by any risk factor, or combination of risk factors, contained in the database. This alternative is made even more attractive by the ability to download the denominator records from other hospital computers. For example, the records of all operations can be downloaded daily from the operating room computer. As surveillance becomes increasingly targeted toward specific prevention objectives, detailed denominators on individual patients at risk are expected to be employed more often (see Chapters 7, 8).

Sources of Infection Data

To ensure the most complete enumeration of infections, ICPs must use a wide variety of sources of infection information, from within and outside the hospital [15]. The main methods used for detecting cases of infection and the frequency of use of each in U.S. hospitals in the mid-1970s are shown in Figure 5-1. The active techniques of case finding, which are used in almost all hospitals, are strongly preferred to the passive techniques. The active techniques allow more complete detection of cases and also provide for the ICP to visit the areas of patient care regularly, to interact with and provide consultation to the medical and nursing staffs and to gain firsthand awareness of infection problems. The passive techniques, particularly the practice of asking physicians or staff nurses to fill out infection report forms, have been extremely inaccurate for the routine detection of infections. Hospitals relying on passive techniques typically find extremely low nosocomial infection rates, but they are usually due to underreporting rather than good practice [30].

The Microbiology Laboratory

Of the case-finding methods listed in Figure 5-1, one of the most useful is the periodic (usually daily) review of microbiology laboratory reports. This may be done each morning before making ward rounds, so that any new or potential infections can be inspected during ward rounds. Such review requires that the ICP understand the infectious and epidemiologic potential of various microorganisms; this knowledge can be gained in a laboratory training period at the time of employment and should be reinforced by periodic in-service review sessions. It must be stressed that a review of microbiology laboratory reports alone is not sufficient for the identification of nosocomial infections for several reasons. First, cultures are not obtained for all infections or may be handled incorrectly. Second, some infectious agents (e.g., viruses) will not be identified in many hospital laboratories. And, last, for some types of infections (e.g., surgical site infections and pneumonia), the identification of a potentially pathogenic organism from a culture specimen does not mean that infection is present; such infections require clinical detection and verification (see Chapter 9).

Ward Rounds

Periodic (preferably daily) ward rounds conducted by the ICP should be an integral part of an effective surveillance program. The purposes of such rounds are to identify new infections and to follow up previously identified infections. New infections may be identified outright by

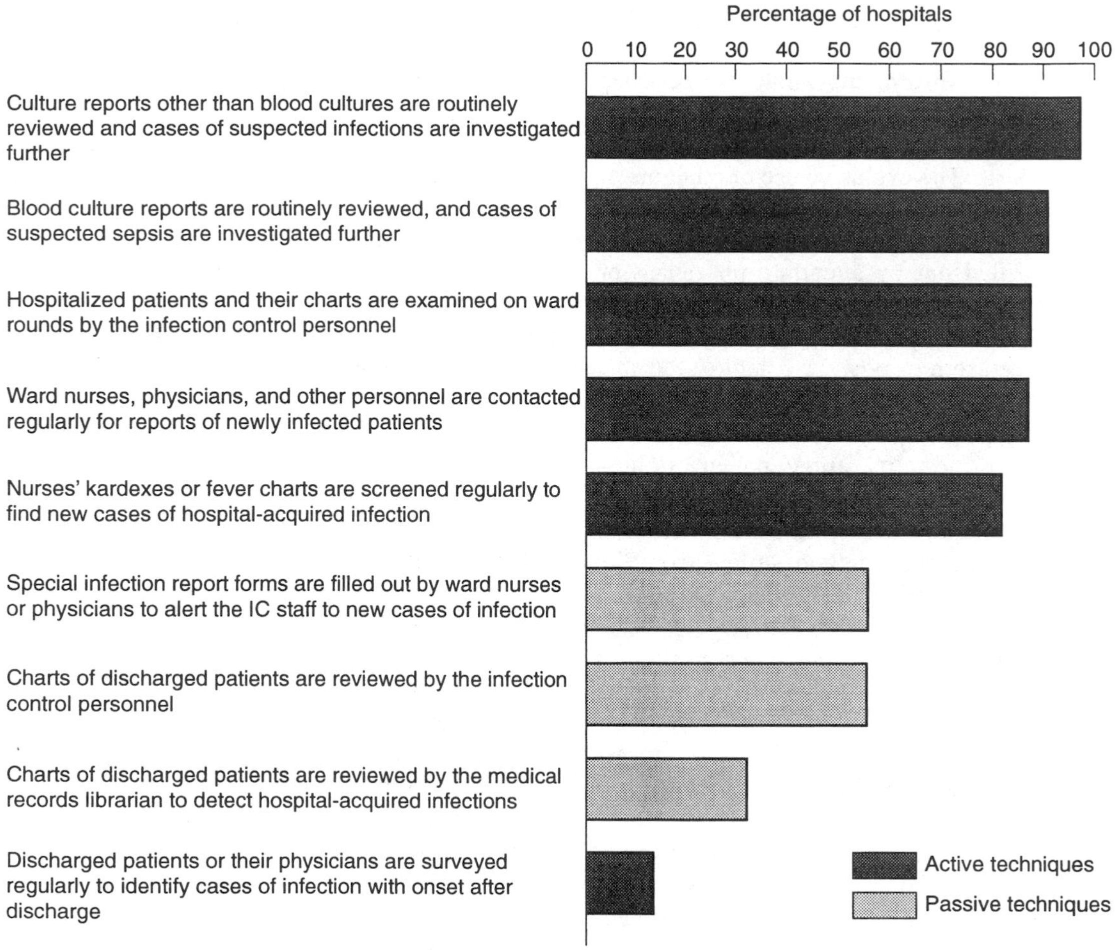

FIGURE 5-1. Active and passive case-finding methods used in surveillance. IC, intensive care.

physicians or nurses working in the area visited and by review of patients' records, temperature records, patients undergoing high-risk procedures (such as surgery, urinary tract instrumentation, or maintenance on indwelling urinary or intravenous catheters), and patients in isolation or receiving antimicrobial therapy. Ward visitation also allows direct inspection and documentation of visible infections, which bolster the validity of the data collected.

Postdischarge Follow-up

With the progressive reduction in the average length of stay of patients in U.S. hospitals, the percentage of certain nosocomial infections that manifest after patients' discharge from the hospital has grown. This appears to be particularly true for surgical site infections (SSIs). In various studies, the percentage of SSIs that become apparent after discharge has ranged from 20% to 60% [31–37], and at least one study has shown the presence of a strong selection bias in rates based only on in-hospital surveillance [37]. Since the average postoperative length of stay of surgical patients will influence the probability that wound infections will be recognized while the patient is still in the hospital, this variable must be taken into account when analyzing and evaluating a hospital's wound infection rate.

Multi-hospital analyses of wound infection rates in the SENIC Project used length of stay as a covariate in multiple regression analyses [9]; others have suggested using the incidence density (i.e., patient-days as the denominator of the wound infection rates) [38]. The method of postdischarge surveillance is the subject of controversy. Some surgeons recommend that surgical patients be followed up by postcard or telephone call to the patients or surgeons at 21 to 30 days after the date of the operation, to determine whether the wound has become infected [34–38]. Although this plan creates additional work for the surveillance staff, the amount of work may offset the gain in completeness and accuracy of the rates. Others suggest that postdischarge antibiotic exposure may be a resource-efficient adjunct for surveillance of SSIs after discharge [39].

Other Sources

Additional infection information may be obtained through a periodic review of radiologic, pharmacy, and laboratory reports; records of personnel health clinic visits; and autopsy reports. The exclusive use of other methods of infection data collection, such as reviewing patients' medical records after discharge or using infection report forms filled out by attending physicians or floor nurses, is less satisfactory from the standpoint of infection control. Reviewing patients' medical records after discharge suffers from its post facto nature. Valuable time may be lost between the onset of the infection and its discovery by this method, and such delay may result in excessive morbidity or mortality among patients or hospital personnel. Infection report forms filled out by attending physicians or floor nurses have been used in a number of hospitals, but this method suffers from the lack of systematic application of standard definitions and criteria for detecting infection as well as from great variation from person to person in the completeness of reporting infection.

Consolidating and Tabulating Data

Since it is difficult to recognize potentially important relationships or patterns of infection from the raw data on the file cards, worksheets, or line-listing forms, it is necessary to consolidate the data in ways that make the information more understandable. The most effective analyses of surveillance data may take many forms, depending on the objective being addressed by the surveillance system. When doing routine, total hospital surveillance, ICPs often simply analyze infection data in single-variable frequency tables (e.g., number of infections by service, site, or pathogen) and two-way cross-tabulations (e.g., a line listing with the number of infections by site for each hospital service, by pathogen for each hospital service, and by pathogen for each site) and tally antimicrobial susceptibility patterns for each pathogen by site of infection. In recent years, however, more imaginative analyses have been done using three-way rate tables (e.g., pathogen by site by service), four-way rate tables (e.g., susceptibility patterns by pathogen by site by service) and more complex cross-tabulations. Usually these tabulations are performed for subsets of patients, such as those on a particular unit or those of a specific surgeon. To do these tabulations adequately requires a computer to analyze the database information.

Although infection control personnel just starting out should first master the standard frequency and cross-tabulation routines mentioned previously, more experienced personnel should begin to try more creative ways of organizing the infection data. The basic purpose of tabulating the infections is to gain a new understanding of when, where, and in whom the infections are occurring. One of the most common mistakes at this stage is to make the initial tabulations hastily and proceed with calculating rates without pausing to examine the data and think about them. It is often very useful just to read over the original listings and the initial simple tabulations to let the mind synthesize the data and suggest additional tabulations, graphs, listings, and so on. For example, finding an increased rate of bacteremias among surgery patients might call for a tabulation of bacteremias for each surgical subspecialty or for each surgical ward and the surgical ICU and for comparisons with similar rates from previous months or for the same months the previous year. This process of freewheeling exploration of the data has no rigid rules; if it works, it's right!

Calculating Rates

Definition of Rate

After the initial tabulations of the infections are complete, the infection control staff should have strong suspicions of where infection problems might be taking place. Since these hunches are based solely on examination of the overall number of infections (numerator data), further analysis involving the calculation of rates is necessary to develop stronger evidence. A practical way of doing this is to write in the denominator data, obtained in the data collection stage, below the appropriate numerator figures in the frequency and cross-tables of infections tabulated earlier. From these numerators (indicating the numbers of infections) and their denominators (indicating the numbers of patients, or patient-days, at risk of infections), infection rates can be calculated. Alternatively, currently available computer software can display the numerator and denominator and calculate the rate automatically from a database containing all patients at risk and the nosocomial infections that were documented in them.

A rate is an expression of the probability of occurrence of a particular event, and it has the form $k(x/y)$, where x, the numerator, equals the number of times an event has occurred during a specific time interval; y, the denominator, equals a population from which those experiencing the event were derived during the same time interval; and k equals a round number (100, 1,000, 10,000, 100,000, and so on) called a base. The base that is used depends on the magnitude of x/y, and it is selected to permit the rate to be expressed as a convenient whole number.

For example, if five infections were found among 100 patients in a given month, the value of x/y would be 0.05 infections per patient per month; to express the rate as a convenient whole number, x/y would be multiplied by the base number 100, giving five infections per 100 patients per month. If 50 infections were found among 10,000 patients in a month, the base number 1,000 would be used to express the rate as five infections per 1,000 patients per month. It is important to emphasize that in determining a rate, both the time interval and the population must be specified, and they must apply to both the numerator *(x)* and the denominator *(y)* of the rate expression.

Types of Rates

Three specific kinds of rates—prevalence, incidence, and attack rates—are fundamental tools of epidemiology and, as such, must be familiar to infection control personnel. Prevalence is the number of cases of the disease found to be active within a defined population either during a specified period of time (period prevalence) or at a specified point in time (point prevalence); these concepts are discussed in a later section of this chapter. Incidence is the number of new cases of disease that appear in a defined population during a specified period of time. The incidence rate is obtained by dividing the number of new cases by the number of people in the population at risk during the specified time period. In Figure 5-2, which portrays the infection status of 10 hospitalized patients, the incidence of infection during time period A or B, for example, would be three, since three new infections began among the 10 patients in each time period. Assuming that period A was 1 month and period B was 3 months, the incidence rates would be three infections per 10 patients at risk, or 30%, per month in period A and 10% per month in period B (i.e., exactly equivalent to 30% per 3 months).

An attack rate is a special kind of incidence rate. It is usually expressed as a percentage (i.e., $k=100$ in the rate expression), and it is used almost exclusively for describing epidemics where particular populations are exposed for limited periods of time (e.g., in common-source outbreaks). Since the duration of an epidemic is reasonably short, the period of time to which the rate refers is not stated explicitly but is assumed. This is what distinguishes an attack rate from an incidence rate, where the period of time is always stated. If 100 infants in a newborn nursery, for example, were exposed to a contaminated lot of infant formula over a 3-week period, and if 14 of the infants developed a characteristic illness believed to be caused by the contaminated formula, then the attack rate for those infants exposed to the formula would be 14%. Notice that the incidence rate would be 14 cases per 100 infants per 3 weeks, preferably expressed as 4.67 cases per 100 infants per week.

Choice of Numerator and Denominator

The fact that several infections occasionally appear in individual patients somewhat complicates the calculation of rates. Basically two types of incidence rates can be calculated. The infection ratio is the number of infections divided by the number of patients at risk during the specified period, and the infection proportion is the number of patients with one or more infections divided by the number of patients at risk during the time period. Since ~18% of patients with nosocomial infections have more than one infection, the infection ratio is usually nearly 1.27 times larger than the infection proportion [30]. In practice, most researchers have found the infection ratio to be far easier to obtain than the infection proportion (and equally useful), and consequently the commonly used term infection rate has come to refer specifically to the infection ratio. In either case, however, when presenting the results it is important to specify which method has been used for calculating the rate.

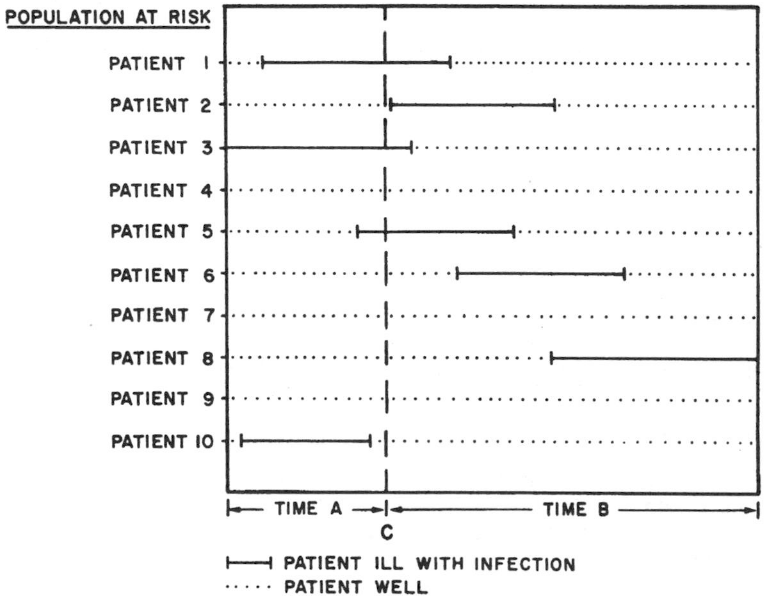

FIGURE 5-2. Infection status of 10 hospitalized patients. The incidence of infection is three during either time period A or B (3 new cases were added during each time period). The prevalence rate of infection during time period A is 40% and during time period B is 60% (4 cases and 6 cases, respectively, in each period). The point prevalence rate of infection at time C is 30% (at that point, 3 cases exist).

Another approach is to use for the denominator the number of patient-days at risk during the period of surveillance (i.e., the sum of all of the days spent by all patients in the specified area during the time period covered). This rate is referred to as the incidence density. To get an idea of how the two types of rates compare, rates based on the number of patient-days *(R)* are usually smaller than those based on admissions or discharges *(r)* by a factor approximately equal to the average length of stay of the patients *(k)*, that is, $R=k \times r$. For example, if the infection rate was five infections per 100 admissions per month and the patients' average length of stay was 10 days, one would expect to find a rate of approximately five infections per 1,000 patient-days.

The incidence density is useful primarily in two situations: when the infection rate is a linear function of the length of time a patient is exposed to a risk factor (e.g., in-dwelling urinary or intravenous catheter) and when the duration of follow-up will influence the measured infection rate (e.g., SSI rates when no postdischarge surveillance is done). The relative merits of the alternative ways of controlling for differences of stay, including using incidence density, performing postdischarge follow-up of surgical patients, and applying multivariate analytic methods, are yet to be clearly defined.

It is especially important that the denominator reflect the appropriate population at risk as precisely as possible. In determining the attack rate of SSIs among patients on the urology service, for example, only those urology patients who actually undergo a surgical procedure that results in a wound capable of becoming infected would ideally be included in the denominator. Practical difficulties in obtaining such refined denominators, however, often dictate the use of a less precise, summary denominator, such as the total number of admissions or discharges from the urology service during the appropriate period of time.

In the National Nosocomial Infections Surveillance System, hospitals conducting surveillance in ICUs are

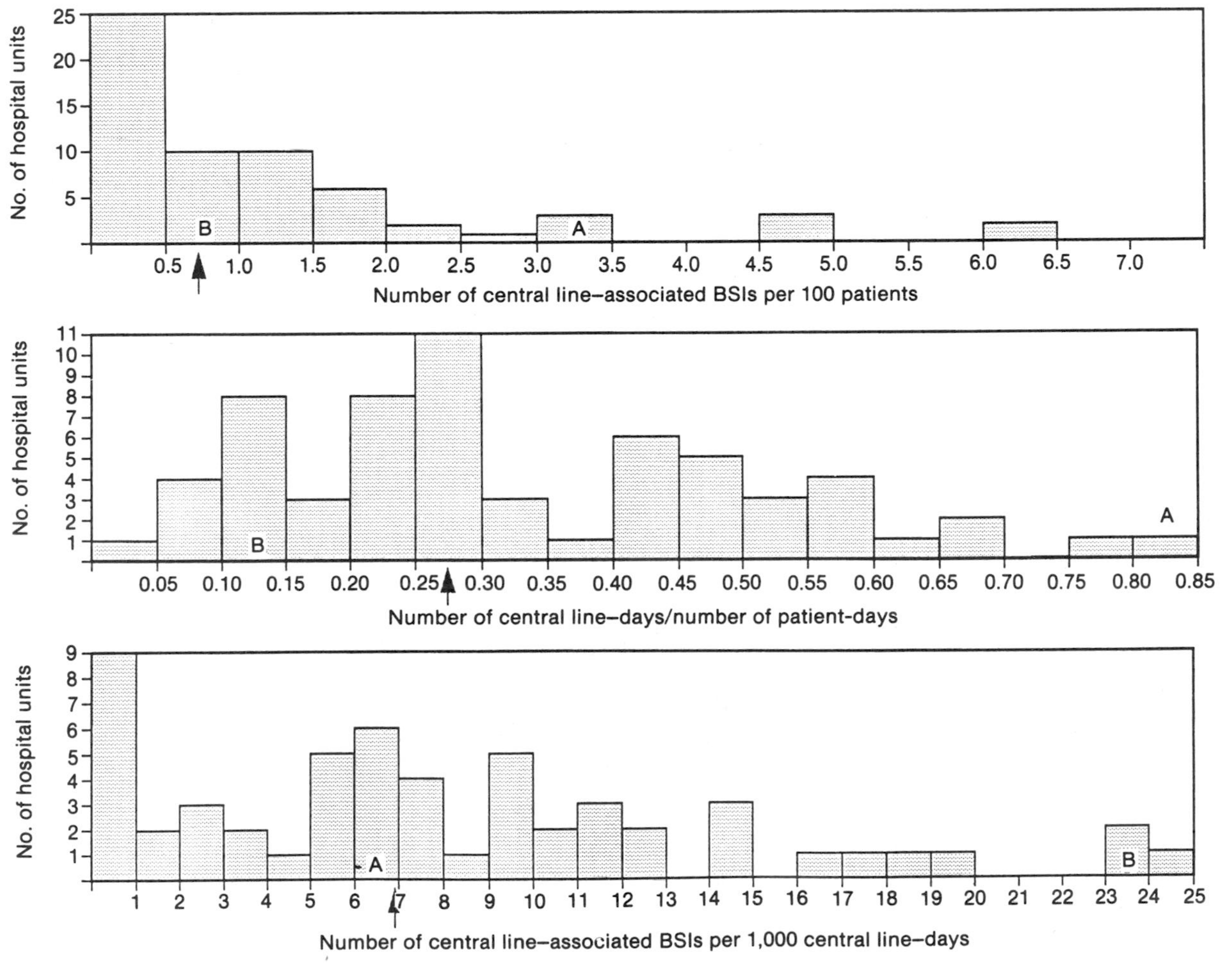

FIGURE 5-3. Comparison of the distribution of bloodstream infection (BSI) rates (patient-based and based on central line days) and central line use in combined coronary and medical intensive care units, National Nosocomial Infection Surveillance (NNIS) System, Intensive Care Unit Component, October 1986–December 1990. A and B indicate the specific location of individual hospital unit rates. Arrows indicate the median.

using device-days (e.g., ventilator-days or central line days) as the denominator data. The use of device-days may seem like a subtle change from patients, but the choice of denominator was critical for purposes of inter-hospital comparison. This is more fully illustrated by the distribution of several rates for hospital ICUs (Figure 5-3). The top histogram of Figure 5-3 shows the number of central line–associated bloodstream infections per 100 patients, the middle histogram shows the number of central line days divided by patient-days (i.e., central line use), and the bottom histogram shows central line–associated bloodstream infections per 1,000 central line days. For Hospital Unit A, the rate on the top histogram, which uses the number of patients as the denominator, was nearly five times higher than the median. However, the middle histogram shows that Hospital Unit A had the highest central line use rate; that is, > 80% of patient-days were also central line days. Using central line days as the denominator helps take into account this high rate of use of central lines.

Hospital Unit A's device-associated, device-day bloodstream infection rate was slightly lower than the median (bottom histogram). Although Hospital Unit A was no longer an outlier, its high level of central line use may need to be reviewed for appropriateness. On the other hand, for Hospital Unit B, the central line–associated bloodstream infection rate (top histogram) was near the median, and its central line use (middle histogram) was low. When its rate was calculated using central line days as the denominator, it was quite high, suggesting the need to review central line placement and maintenance practices.

Analysis

Comparing Groups of Patients

Analysis implies careful examination of the body of tabulated data in an attempt to determine the nature and relationship of its component parts. This includes comparison of current infection rates to determine whether significant differences exist among different groups of patients. Suppose, for instance, that both the gynecology and general surgery services have had eight catheter-associated urinary tract infections during a given month; however, during the same month 20 patients with in-dwelling catheters were discharged from the gynecology service, and 100 such patients were discharged from the general surgery service. Thus, the rates for gynecology and general surgery patients are 40% and 8%, respectively. Determination of whether the difference observed between these infection rates is significant (i.e., greater than what we would expect by random or chance occurrence alone, if indeed no real difference exists) requires the use of a statistical process known as significance testing [16].

Several tests of significance, such as the chi-square test and Fisher's Exact Test for cross-tables, and the Student's *t* test for comparison of sample means should be familiar to epidemiologists and ICPs (see Chapter 7). Currently available software packages for microcomputers make even the most sophisticated statistical testing procedures very accessible to all infection control departments [23, 40] (see Chapter 8). In the preceding example, the difference between the observed infection rates (40% versus 8%) is highly significant at a p value < 0.001 according to Fisher's Exact Test. This means that a difference as large as or larger than that observed would be expected to occur by chance alone less than one time in 1,000. Thus it is very likely that there is a real difference between the infection rates on the two services, and further investigation is indicated to explain why such a difference exists.

Comparing Rates over Time

Another type of analysis involves the comparison of current infection rates with previous rates to determine whether significant changes have taken place over time. Tables of current rates and those of each of several preceding time periods can simply be visually inspected, or the rates can be plotted on graph paper to detect changes of possible importance. Potentially important deviations from baseline rates should then be tested for statistical significance (see Chapter 7), and further investigation should be undertaken if indicated (see Chapter 6). Although it is convenient to compare rates each month, one should exercise caution when the denominator of a rate is small. This is more often the case when examining SSI rates. Tests of significance must often be performed when the estimate of a surgeon's SSI rate is poor owing to the small number of procedures performed.

Clusters

Screening to identify clusters of similar strains or specific patterns of antimicrobial susceptibility of organisms is another potentially valuable analytic tool for detecting outbreaks, especially when it is applied to particular pathogens on specific wards or in particular geographic areas. Epidemiologic typing can be useful in identifying clusters (see Chapter 9).

Appropriateness of Medical Care

Analysis of surveillance data must not be limited to infection rates. Most ICPs are familiar with analyzing the numerator data, specifically the numbers and types of infections and their associated pathogens, but an analysis of the denominator data alone can be extremely revealing. For example, if an ICP determines that a hospital's use of central lines in ICUs is high compared with that in other hospital ICUs (see Hospital A in the middle panel of Figure 5-3), a review of appropriateness of device use may be needed. Also, after SSI rates have been assessed, useful information can be obtained by further exploring the distribution of risk factors in each of the risk index categories. For example, while a surgeon with more than the expected number of herniorrhaphies in the higher SSI index categories may be operating on more high-risk patients, he or she may also be consistently exceeding the seventy-fifth percentile for the duration of surgery for the procedure and thus raising the patients' risk of SSIs. The question must be asked, "Are patients unnecessarily being placed at risk of a nosocomial infection?" Because examination of appropriateness of medical care and device use is of major interest to quality assurance personnel in U.S. hospitals [21,40–43], ICPs may find areas for collaboration with their quality assurance colleagues.

Interpretation

Interpretation of the data is considered by many to be the final step in analysis; it is simply an intellectual process by which meaning is ascribed to the tabulated and analyzed body of information. The interpretation may vary from no significant change in the infection rates to the detection of a serious endemic problem or epidemic in the hospital. Often, however, more information—particularly that obtained through further investigation directed at problem areas identified by the analysis of the surveillance data—will be necessary for final interpretation of the data. Additional uses of other information collected through surveillance, such as the time of onset of infection, are described in Chapters 4 and 6.

Reporting the Data

It is essential that the tabulated data, or at least the analyses and interpretations of the data, come to the attention of those people in the hospital who are interested and who can take appropriate actions. A periodic report containing the tabulated data and the analytic results and their interpretations should routinely be submitted to the infection control committee and maintained on record in the hospital. Of course, weekly, or even daily, reports may be necessary during epidemics or unusual situations. It is not necessary—in fact, it is often very inefficient—to include a line listing of infections in this report. When the analysis yields tables that contain insufficient data to justify inclusion in the report, the tables should be retained and a summary table released whenever sufficient data have accumulated.

The data should be displayed in graphic form to provide nurses, clinicians, administrators, and others with visual evidence of the existence of a problem and the need for preventive action. Simple, creative, and neatly drawn graphics are particularly effective. The ICP must not assume that those persons have the time or epidemiologic expertise to interpret the data without clearly presented graphics and narratives. The availability of computer software for infection control allows graphic analyses to be performed far more efficiently and accurately than by hand.

In the reporting phase, as well as throughout the surveillance process, measures should be taken to ensure the privacy of the information collected on patients and hospital staff members. For example, the ICP should keep all surveillance forms that list patients by name under tight security, using a locked filing cabinet or other secure storage. Reports should not mention patients or staff members by name unless there is a good reason and the distribution of the reports should be limited to those who need to know. The infection control committee should establish a policy on privacy of information, prescribing the procedures for handling records or reports that identify patients or staff members (e.g., surgeon-specific wound infection rates or laboratory data implicating an employee as a disseminator of an epidemic organism).

PREVALENCE

Definition

Prevalence measures the number of all current cases of active disease (new and old) within a specified population at risk during a specific period of time, and the prevalence rate is the prevalence divided by the number of patients at risk during the period. When the period of time used for the calculation is relatively long, say a month or longer, the measurement is called period prevalence. In Figure 5-2, the period prevalence rate of infection during period A would be 4/10, or 40%, and during time period B, it would be 6/10, or 60%. When the period of time used for the calculation is relatively short, say a day or less, the measurement is called point prevalence (i.e., the number of all currently active cases of disease, old and new, at a given instant in time). For example, the point prevalence rate of infection at point C in Figure 5-2 would be 3/10, or 30%. The difference between point and period prevalence is arbitrary; an interval that is considered a point on one time scale may become a period on a different time scale.

The Prevalence Survey

The prevalence survey, as it is applied to nosocomial infections, consists of a systematic study of a defined population for evidence of infection at a given point in time; such a survey derives the point prevalence rate for the population. Typically, after a short period of training to standardize definitions and methods, a team of surveyors visits every patient in the hospital on a single day and detects all active infections from studying the patients' medical records and examining each patient or discussing the case with the clinical staff when necessary. When there are more patients than the survey team can visit in one day, the prevalence study is conducted over several days, with care taken to ensure that each patient is visited only once.

If the object is to obtain the prevalence rate of infections (the usual procedure), then those infections that have resolved before the day of the visit are not counted, and the point prevalence rate is calculated by dividing the number of infections active on the day of the visit by the number of beds visited and multiplying by an appropriate base number (usually 100). If, on the other hand, the object is to obtain the point prevalence rate of infected patients, then all patients with active or resolved infections contracted during the current hospitalization are counted, and the point prevalence rate is calculated by dividing the number of infected patients by the number of beds visited and multiplying by the appropriate base number. To be consistent with the usual way of defining the incidence rate (i.e., the infection ratio), prevalence surveys should be designed to measure the point prevalence rate of infections.

The relative magnitudes of these various measures are complicated, but they can be deduced from the fundamental relationship between prevalence and incidence [44]: Prevalence ≈ Incidence × Duration. From this general relationship it is apparent that prevalence rates (both point and period) are always higher than the comparable incidence rates, and the longer the duration of the infections, the greater the difference will become. As explained in the earlier discussion of the two types of incidence rates, the infection ratio is always higher than the infection proportion measured on the same population as long as some patients have more than one infection. In contrast, the prevalence rate of infections is always lower than the prevalence rate of infected patients, because the duration of an infected patient's hospitalization is almost always longer than the duration of the active infection. It is interesting to note that point and period prevalence rates measured on the same population are usually approximately the same, although estimates of period prevalence are usually more precise than those of point prevalence owing to the larger number of patients studied in a period prevalence survey.

In general, the most useful measure to derive from surveillance is the incidence rate, because it provides an estimate of the risk of infection uncluttered by differences in the durations of various infections. The main reason that prevalence rates were used in the past was simply that a point prevalence survey requires much less effort and can be completed much more rapidly than the ongoing, daily surveillance needed to obtain incidence rates. There are two main disadvantages of point prevalence surveys. First, because of the complex influence of the duration of infections, the prevalence rate overestimates patients' risk of acquiring infection. Second, except in the largest hospitals, the number of patients included in a point prevalence survey (i.e., the number of beds) is usually too small to obtain precise enough estimates of rates to detect important differences (e.g., a difference between the bacteremia rates on medicine and surgery wards) with statistical significance. Because of these limitations, prevalence surveys are useful primarily when a "quick and dirty" estimate is needed and there is insufficient time or resources to obtain a more useful measure of the incidence [45]. Since prevalence rates do not provide data that is true surveillance data, as determined from the definition of surveillance, incidence rates are more useful in the long run for an institution.

Uses of Prevalence Surveys

Secular Trends

Repeated prevalence surveys in the same institution have been used to document secular trends in the epidemiology of nosocomial infections. Prevalence studies in large hospitals have demonstrated shifts in the predominant pathogens associated with nosocomial infections and in the patterns of antimicrobial use for hospitalized patients [46]. However, limitations in the numbers of patients studied and variations in the types of prevalence rates determined in the various surveys have complicated the interpretation of these results. In general, incidence rates derived from ongoing surveillance, although it is more time-consuming, are much better for detecting and examining secular trends.

Estimating Surveillance Accuracy

Prevalence surveys have been used to evaluate a hospital's ongoing surveillance system. Typically, a survey team, using the same standard definitions as are used for routine surveillance by the ICP, visits all patients in the hospital to detect all active infections. By comparing the infections identified in the course of the prevalence survey with those detected by the routine surveillance system, and under the assumption that the survey team correctly detected all active infections, an estimate is derived of the percentage of true infections detected by the routine surveillance system. Although this percentage approximates the sensitivity of routine surveillance (i.e., the probability that the routine surveillance system will detect all true infections), the statistic has been referred to as an efficiency factor, since the difficulty of determining reliably whether infections are active at the time of the prevalence survey introduces error into the assessment [47]. Because the efficiency factor approximates the sensitivity, it can be used to correct the monthly routine estimates of the incidence rates for the degree of underassessment.

One of the weaknesses of this application in past studies has been the failure to estimate the specificity of routine surveillance in addition to its sensitivity (efficiency). Specificity is the probability of correctly classifying a patient as uninfected, and it reflects how often the ICP records an infection when one was not really present. Unfortunately, the ICP's specificity in estimating incidence rates in routine surveillance has not been thoroughly studied [48,49]. The process of correcting incidence rates with the efficiency factor assumes that specificity is perfect at 1.0. Corrections for lower levels of specificity would give lower estimates of the incidence rates.

Estimating Incidence from Prevalence

Modified prevalence surveys can be used to derive a crude approximation of the incidence rates that would have been obtained from continuous surveillance [50]. In this use, surveys are performed at regular intervals (e.g., weekly) that must be considerably shorter than the average duration of stay of infected patients. Only infections that began since the preceding survey are tabulated. The denominator of the rates should include the number of admissions during the interval plus the census at the start of the period. Obviously, the shorter the interval between prevalence surveys, the more closely the final estimate approximates the true incidence rate. Some loss in completeness, accuracy, and timeliness in detecting infections, compared with the results of surveillance studies, must be weighed against the potential benefit from a smaller time commitment to case finding.

Other Uses

Perhaps the best uses of prevalence studies are to make valuable estimates of antimicrobial usage patterns, to evaluate the adherence to proper isolation practices, and to monitor practices related to high-risk procedures, such as prevalence of intravenous or urinary catheter use [51,52]. In one study, the investigators used sequential prevalence surveys to estimate the impact of their infection control program on the risks of nosocomial infection [45].

Finally, the use of the prevalence survey to establish a single infection prevalence (or incidence) rate for comparison with those of other hospitals is controversial. Since a single overall rate ignores differences in risk in each hospital (i.e., case mix and frequency of exposure to high-risk procedures) and differences in surveillance methodology, it may engender a false sense of complacency or alarm. It is impossible to assess the quality of care of patients or the effectiveness of intervention measures using a single, overall rate. Last, prevalence rates should not be compared with incidence rates.

TARGETED SURVEILLANCE

A recent trend has been to find creative ways of targeting surveillance more directly toward potential infection problems. The purpose of these efforts is to focus on surveillance strategies that will lead to prevention measures. Although these new approaches were initially motivated by the need to cut down the amount of personnel time devoted to surveillance in hospitals with inadequately staffed programs, they actually increase the efficiency of surveillance in hospitals. Indeed, these approaches fit well into current concepts of continuous quality improvement [53].

Unit-Directed Surveillance

Some large hospitals have sought to maximize the use of personnel time by directing surveillance toward infections in areas of patient care with the highest infection risks, such as ICUs, oncology units, or the like [20,54]. For example, in one hospital, the infection rate in the ICU was found to be three times higher than among medical-surgical patients in general [54]. Intensive care units tend to house patients who are most susceptible to infection, that is, the patients most likely to have suppressed immunologic systems, to be undergoing invasive diagnostic and therapeutic procedures, and to be receiving intensive nursing and medical care with the attendant risk of person-to-person spread of infection.

Focusing scarce resources on a few relatively small units has the advantages of greatly simplifying the surveillance effort and of preventing infections in the patients with the highest risks and greatest likelihood of suffering severe and life-threatening infections. In these units the focus could be further narrowed by monitoring only patients being treated with devices that are associated with high infection risks. For example, in the ICU component of the National Nosocomial Infections Surveillance System, the incidence density is calculated as the number of ventilator-associated pneumonias per 1,000 ventilator-days [20]. Despite the limitations of surveillance of ventilator-associated pneumonia, device-related infection rates have proved more useful for interhospital comparison than have overall infection rates [18,19].

Another unit worth considering for unit-directed surveillance is the high-risk nursery. Neonates in the high-risk nursery are highly susceptible to nosocomial infection. Host and environmental factors unique to patients in this unit contribute to the high infection risk (e.g., low birth weight). Bloodstream infections are among the most common nosocomial infections in all birth-weight groups; this rate differs dramatically from that found in adult patients with nosocomial infections and should be a major focus of prevention measures [55].

Priority-Directed Surveillance

While unit-directed surveillance is efficient and effective for high-risk areas such as ICUs, this approach is less practical when dealing with the remaining areas of the hospital. An alternative approach, referred to as surveillance by objectives, matches the level of surveillance effort to the seriousness of the infection problem [7,8]. Instead of focusing on geographic areas, as the previous two types of surveillance do, this priority-directed approach targets the types of infections to be prevented and assigns levels of effort commensurate to the relative seriousness of the problems.

The first prerequisite of this approach is to establish priority rankings based on the relative seriousness of the different types of infections. Several possible parameters for setting these priorities are compared in Table 5-1, based on further analysis of data collected in three hospitals in the SENIC pilot studies [56]. In the past, the main parameter has been simply the relative frequency of different types of infections. If this measure were to be used, urinary tract infections would be given the highest priority, followed by SSIs and pneumonia, with primary bloodstream infections receiving a lower priority just ahead of a large number of relatively rare infections at other sites.

An alternative parameter that appears to be a better measure of the relative seriousness of various types of infections is the total extra-hospital costs attributable to each of the infections [7,8,57]. This measure reflects both the relative frequency of the infections and the relative degree of morbidity as expressed by the costs of the extra days and extra ancillary services necessary to treat the infections. By this criterion, SSIs would constitute the most serious problem, followed by pneumonias, with urinary tract infections and bacteremias in third and fourth place, respectively (Table 5-1).

Surgical Site Infections

Surveillance of SSIs should be heavily emphasized. Unit-directed surveillance is ineffective for this site, since SSIs may not occur while the patient is on a particular unit. For priority-directed SSI surveillance, all patients undergoing operations would be enrolled into a surveillance registry at the time of the operation, and information on several key risk factors would be recorded at that time. The risk factors most likely to be useful in the analysis (see Chapter 37) are wound classification, type and duration of the operation, and a measure of the severity of the patient's underlying disease, such as the number of underlying conditions or the physical status classification of the American Society of Anesthesiologists [17,58–60]. All of these patients would be visited regularly during hospitalization by the ICP to detect all SSIs. Attempts should be made to follow up all, or a subset, of the patients for infection that appears after discharge [31,37].

The tabulation process should be conducted monthly and should involve three steps. First, each patient would be assigned to an intrinsic infection risk category, using a multivariate risk factor scale. Second, the SSI rate would be calculated for the patients in each subcategory of the intrinsic infection risk category—not just clean wound or low-risk groups. Third, two reports would be compiled, one displaying each surgeon's category-specific monthly rates over time (e.g., over 1 or 2 years) and a second comparing the category-specific rates of each surgeon with those of his or her colleagues, with the rate of the service overall, and, possibly, with an SSI rate aggregated from other hospitals [20]. Finally, the reports would be given to the chief of the surgical service to distribute among and

TABLE 5-1. *Comparison of the relative frequency of the major types of nosocomial infections and alternative measures of their relative importance*

Type of infection	Percent of all nosocomial infections	Total extra days[a] (%)	Total extra charges[a] (%)	Percent preventable[b]
Surgical wound infection	24	889 (57)	$102,286 (42)	35
Pneumonia	10	370 (24)	95,229 (39)	22
Urinary tract infection	42	175 (11)	32,081 (13)	33
Bacteremia	5	59 (4)	7,478 (3)	35
Other	19	69 (4)	8,680 (3)	32
Total (all sites)	100	1,562 (100)	245,754 (100)	32

Note that charges are in 1975 dollars.

[a](Data are drawn from SENIC pilot studies: R. W. Haley et al. Extra days and prolongation of stay attributable to nosocomial infections: a prospective interhospital comparison. *Am J Med* 1981;70:51.)

[b](Data are drawn from SENIC analysis of efficacy: R. W. Haley et al. The efficacy of infection surveillance and control programs in preventing nosocomial infections in U.S. hospitals. *Am J Epidemiol* 1984;121:282.)

discuss with the practicing surgeons. With this plan, the surveillance time devoted to SSIs would be directed toward the surveillance effort shown to be the most effective in solving the problem [9,31,61].

Pneumonia

A surveillance plan targeted outside ICUs and toward specific prevention objectives for nosocomial pneumonia should be used. The development of nosocomial pneumonia in ventilated patients has been the subject of great scrutiny. Although clinical criteria together with cultures of sputum or tracheal specimens may be sensitive for bacterial pathogens, they are nonspecific in patients on mechanically assisted ventilation [62,63]. Consensus recommendations for standardization methods to diagnose pneumonia in clinical research studies of ventilator-associated pneumonia have been proposed [64–66]. However, these approaches are generally not applicable to surveillance. Further studies are needed to help in the diagnosis of this common clinical entity in the nonresearch context.

For nosocomial pneumonia in patients who are not on ventilators, the first consideration is to distinguish the generically different problems of pneumonia among surgical and medical patients. The vast majority of preventable cases of pneumonia among surgical patients are postoperative pulmonary infections representing progression of the usual atelectasis syndrome most commonly seen after operations of the chest and upper abdomen. In contrast, most preventable pneumonias among adult medical patients are hypostatic infections related to the failure to turn frequently enough those patients with diminished levels of consciousness.

On pediatric and newborn services, the most serious preventable pneumonias follow person-to-person spread of nosocomial infections with viruses such as respiratory syncytial virus (see Chapters 26, 42). Postoperative pneumonias can be detected with little additional effort if surgical patients are already being followed for SSIs. Analysis of these rates can be performed for each nursing unit or for the patients of each surgeon. Reports of these analyses should then be discussed just as the SSI rates are (see preceding section).

The ICP should also identify nursing units where patients with strokes, drug overdoses, and other conditions that carry high risks of hypostatic pneumonia are congregated. In only these areas, all patients at high risk should be followed regularly to detect all cases of pneumonia, the pneumonia rates among these patients should be regularly reported to the charge nurses of the specified nursing units, and continuing in-service education should be provided on the importance of frequently turning these patients and providing pulmonary assistance to prevent pneumonia.

In addition, the ICP should regularly visit units caring for infants or children at high risk of pneumonia from respiratory syncytial virus and similar agents, to monitor informally the frequency of upper-respiratory infections among patients and employees, especially in the fall and winter months [67]. When these infections become evident, virologic studies (if available) should be done immediately to detect the presence of virulent viruses. When they are found, the staff members should be warned of the imminent danger and instructed in meticulous contact precautions for infected patients and employees [25]. Approaches to other types of nosocomial pneumonia, such as legionnaires' disease and influenza, have been described in the revised CDC *Guideline for the Prevention of Nosocomial Pneumonia.*

Bloodstream Infections

While bloodstream infections make up only ~10% to 15% of nosocomial infections, the associated morbidity and mortality and the increasing frequency with which they arise demand a concerted surveillance effort [7,69]. However, one must control for a single major risk factor before rate calculation becomes meaningful—exposure to an intravascular device. Any device-associated bloodstream infection should be examined for correctable errors in the care of patients, such as failure to change the site of intravenous catheters frequently enough or improper sterilization of an arterial pressure–monitoring device. Such errors must be rectified. Calculation of a central line–associated bloodstream infection rate using central line days is useful for monitoring endemic problems that may be remedied by changes in policies, practices, or selection of equipment [20].

Urinary Tract Infections

Many ICPs invest little time in the surveillance of urinary tract infections, since they are generally of less consequence to the patient than are other infections. This relative inattention remains controversial because, overall, these infections remain the most common of all nosocomial infections [9]. Surveillance efforts should be directed toward identifying areas where personnel engaged in the care of patients are not properly managing urinary catheters or other urinary instrumentation. The most efficient way of achieving this goal would be to periodically calculate catheter-associated urinary tract infection rates (stratified or adjusted by categories of the duration of urinary catheterization) on different wards or nursing units and to assess the indications for inserting and discontinuing catheters and the techniques of aseptically caring for them. By periodically reporting how the urinary tract infection rates of the different units compare, practices can be improved in units with consistently higher rates. Alternatively, the infection control staff could annually conduct a 1-month prevalence study of urinary tract infections and catheter care practices. This amount of effort would be commensurate with the magnitude of the problem and would reinforce prevention at least on a yearly basis.

Other Infections

Since nosocomial infections at sites other than those mentioned are comparatively rare, little time should be spent on their surveillance. Instead, the ICP should depend on other hospital departments to recognize the rare outbreaks of unusual infections and to distinguish common factors that might tie the cases together, such as a single unusual organism, spatial clustering, or a relationship with some diagnostic or therapeutic device. For example, the employee health service should maintain surveillance to detect problems of tuberculosis transmission to employees; the director of the newborn nursery should notify the ICP of clusters of staphylococcal pyoderma; and someone in the microbiology laboratory should be alert to clusters of unusual pathogens. Only when a suspicious cluster or relationship is found would a more detailed investigation involving the calculation of rates be undertaken. The level of effort is proportional to the magnitude of the problems, but the efforts are likely to detect problems if they occur. Infection control practitioners must remain alert to such problems regardless of which targeted surveillance approach is employed.

Site-Directed Surveillance

Site-directed surveillance focuses on detecting one or more specific sites of infection (e.g., bloodstream infections) occurring among all hospitalized patients. This method may easily be combined with other strategies. Two potential disadvantages, however, are that clearly defined prevention objectives may not have been established and adequate denominator data may not be readily available across the entire hospital (such as the number of device-specific days).

Another method of this type of targeted surveillance is rotating surveillance. Using this approach, each area of patient care is surveyed for all types of infection for 1 month each year. The disadvantage of this type of surveillance is that the limited period of time that one monitors such an area may be insufficient to accurately estimate the rate of infection. And risk-adjusted denominator data may not be readily available for the whole hospital.

THE ROLE OF COMPUTERS IN SURVEILLANCE

Computers are uniquely suited to handling epidemiologic data and use of them can reduce the drudgery and time expenditure of keeping lists of patients, counting and recording denominators, and repeating standard tabulations of routine data (see Chapter 8). Using computers can solve the chronic problem of underanalyzed surveillance data. However, computers are merely tools and are not capable of setting surveillance strategies or analytic approaches. In addition, they are limited by the ability and willingness of infection control personnel to learn how to operate them efficiently and use them effectively.

Most computers in hospitals are designed for business and accounting purposes rather than for scientific functions and, until recently, the only computer available to the infection control staff was the large mainframe machine owned by and operated for the hospital's business office. Infection control personnel generally do not have sufficient expertise to design their own surveillance systems into mainframe computers. Programming staff are also rarely made available to develop specialized applications that are not directly related to producing revenue. Recently, however, two developments have improved the prospects of using computers for surveillance purposes: integrated database management systems on the mainframe and surveillance software programs designed for the personal computer.

Mainframe Computers

Hospitals have increasingly adopted integrated database management systems for efficiently organizing most information on all hospitalized patients on their mainframe computers. Although administrative efficiency, not infection control, was the objective of these systems, they offer, particularly in large hospitals, a wonderful opportunity to the infection control staff for greatly cutting down the work of surveillance. With the demographic, business, pharmacy, laboratory, and other records of all patients residing in one file or a system of integrated computerized files, two things are needed to generate surveillance reports directly from the mainframe: first, a mechanism for entering the information on nosocomial infections obtained through surveillance into a file in the database management system and, second, a way to merge the infection information into the patient database by the patient's identification number. The computer software must then be capable of performing the required tabulations and rate calculations and constructing the various tables and figures for the printed reports.

Although several such systems are commercially available for hospital mainframe computers, the initial investment is usually high, and operating costs may be prohibitive if the infection control program is charged for computer time and programming. Also, infection data input by infection control staff can itself be time-consuming, although it is often less burdensome if it is kept current on a daily basis (see Chapter 8). To find out whether such a system is available for the computer at a particular hospital, the marketing representative of the company that manufactured the hospital's business computer should be consulted with the assistance of the hospital's data-processing manager.

Personal Computers

The recent introduction of the personal computer (PC) at relatively low prices has suddenly put potentially powerful computers literally on the desks of the infection control staff. Initially, the usefulness of PCs was severely limited by the lack of availability of software designed to accomplish the unique tasks required in infection control. But newly introduced commercial software products have made the PC a very useful tool for infection surveillance and control activity [70–72].

Functions of PC Software

A properly designed software package for infection control serves an important function as a workhorse for entering, analyzing, and reporting surveillance data. It must be designed by infection control experts who structure the computer functions and the user's manual to teach the approaches that have proved effective. In this way, the software product becomes a powerful vehicle for broadening the sophistication of infection control staff members in conducting surveillance.

The software must have the versatility to create special surveillance files and user-defined codes that allow the infection control staff to design new surveillance systems aimed at achieving specific prevention objectives. The user's manual should take the infection control staff step by step through the process of planning a new surveillance system and have the adaptability to support most foreseeable surveillance functions. The infection control staff should be particularly skeptical of software that is oriented mainly toward microbiologic information or that has objectives that are too broad (e.g., infection control plus risk management, quality assurance, and employee health), unless the software's usefulness and efficiency for infection control per se are evident. Also, the infection control staff must be prepared to devote considerable time and effort to becoming familiar with a software package (see Chapter 8).

To serve as a workhorse for surveillance, the software must be designed to handle the required data quickly while minimizing the time required to enter data, edit files, and produce reports. To run efficiently, it should use an efficient language (e.g., assembly language or the C language), and the choice of data items to be collected and processed should be limited to those essential for preventing infections, with only a few nonspecific fields that can be defined by the user for special purposes. For practicality of entering data, it should have a menu-driven format with appropriate help screens, and the data entry fields should fit on as few screens as possible to shorten time consumed in page-turning.

All fields, except perhaps a comments field, should have structured codes with internal edit checks to prevent entry of invalid responses. Since open-ended (noncoded) responses cannot be analyzed easily, such data are rarely used and only impair the efficiency of storage and processing. Codes should be user-designed wherever possible. The package should allow for the creation of separate files for special surveillance projects, such as surgical site, ICU, or procedure surveillance, and, ideally, infections entered into any special file should automatically be added to an infection master file to facilitate overall hospital analysis if needed.

Efficient file structures should be provided for entering, storing, and retrieving large denominator files (e.g., a record for each surgical operation) and later adding infection information to those cases where infections occurred (e.g., wound infection data). Likewise, it should be possible to enter only numerator data (e.g., infections) and supply numerical denominators at the analysis stage. An effective report generator should be able to select records based on a string of search criteria, sort the resulting file, and print line listings of cases, two- and three-way cross-tabulations, and selected rates for virtually all variables in the database. The software should also have the ability to display graphics, including epidemic curves, line graphs, and bar charts, on the computer screen as well as in printed form and to output data files to other computers or software packages. Infection control practitioners should invest extra time in learning how to analyze data with the software package, since surveillance data are often underanalyzed. Extensive analysis will not only lead to increased use (and, it is hoped, prevention of infections) but also spot errors in data collection as ICPs and clinicians come to rely upon the data.

Developing the compact and highly efficient software needed for routine use in community hospitals is made difficult by the need to limit the amount of information collected to maximize efficiency of computer usage and staff time. To limit the amount of information appropriately, software designers must make very difficult judgment calls about what is the minimum of information essential for effective infection control. They must then be ruthless about excluding extra data fields that might have research or other appeals but have only marginal or no actual infection control impact. Since this procedure requires astute epidemiologic insights into the priorities and functioning of infection control programs rather than statistical or computer-programming judgments, one can expect slower progress and fewer good products to emerge in this class of software packages. This fact will necessitate great care in choosing an infection surveillance software package.

Selecting the Best Software Package

As discussed earlier, the most important decisions that must be made before selecting a software system concern the objectives to be achieved by the surveillance activity. In view of the substantial differences among the packages available for testing at the time of this writing, a system selected before one's objectives are formulated and agreed on may not meet one's needs when put into use. For example, if the surveillance objectives include research, the best software package might be one of the general-purpose database management packages that allow considerable flexibility but require broad-based and sophisticated computer skills. On the other hand, if the objectives are limited to routine aspects of controlling and preventing infections, one of the software packages designed specifically for infection control would probably be a better choice. Furthermore, a significant change in the infection control program's objectives may require the acquisition of a new software package. Various methods have been used for comparing computer software packages for use in infection surveillance and control programs [71–73]. These methods have highlighted broad differences in speed of computation, time required for the ICP to complete analyses, and accuracy of numerical computations.

Starting a Computerized Surveillance System

Perhaps the greatest impediment to the effective use of microcomputers in infection control is the lack of computer literacy among infection control personnel. Not uncommonly, microcomputers and powerful software systems have been purchased and placed in the infection control office only to sit idle amid growing disillusionment with computers. Often this stems from the inability of the staff to master the basic workings of the computer rather than the deficiencies in the hardware or software. (See Chapter 8 for additional problems in implementing surveillance by computer.) To avoid this common pitfall, the infection control staff must invest the time to learn how to operate the computer and the software program.

After mastering the basics, one should schedule at least a month to read the infection control software manual thoroughly, become familiar with its functions, and design the surveillance system, including the types of surveillance studies to perform, the user-defined variables and codes, and the types of reports that will be needed. All of this planning should be based on the objectives to be accomplished and should be approved by the infection control committee before the system is put into operation. If introduced in this carefully planned manner, the microcomputer can indeed become a useful and indispensable tool for infection surveillance in the hospital.

REFERENCES

1. Centers for Disease Control and Prevention. *CDC surveillance update*. Atlanta: Centers for Disease Control, 1988.
2. Scheckler WE. Continuous quality improvement in a hospital system: implications for hospital epidemiology. *Infect Control Hosp Epidemiol* 1992;13:288–292.
3. Seligman PJ, Frazier TM. Surveillance: the sentinel health event approach. In: Halperin W, Baker EL, eds. *Public Health Surveillance.* New York: Van Nostrand Reinhold, 1992:16–25.
4. Semmelweis IP. *The etiology, the concept and the prophylaxis of childbed fever*. Leipzig: C. A. Harleben, 1861.
5. Hughes JM. Nosocomial infection surveillance in the United States: historical perspective. *Infect Control Hosp Epidemiol* 1987;8(11):450.
6. Haley RW, Morgan WM, Culver DH, et al. Hospital infection control: recent progress and opportunities under prospective payment. *Am J Infect Control* 1985;13:97–103.
7. Haley RW. Surveillance by objectives: a priority-directed approach to the surveillance of nosocomial infection. *Am J Infect Control* 1985;13: 78–85.
8. Haley RW. *Managing hospital nosocomial control for cost-effectiveness*. Chicago: American Hospital Publishing, 1986.
9. Haley RW, Culver DH, Morgan WM, et al. The efficacy of infection surveillance and control programs in preventing nosocomial infections in U.S. hospitals. *Am J Epidemiol* 1984;121:282–287.
10. Joint Commission on Accreditation of Healthcare Organizations. Standards: infection control. In: *JCAHO accreditation manual for hospitals*. Chicago: Joint Commission on Accreditation of Healthcare Organizations, 1994.
11. Joint Commission on Accreditation of Hospitals. *Accreditation manual for hospitals, 1976*. Chicago: Joint Commission on Accreditation of Hospitals, 1976.
12. Lynch P, Jackson M. Monitoring: surveillance for nosocomial infections and uses for assessing quality of care. *Am J Infect Control* 1985; 13(4):161–165.
13. Massanari RM, Wilkerson K, Swartzendruber S. Designing surveillance for noninfectious outcomes of medical care. *Infect Control Hosp Epidemiol* 1995;16:419–426.
14. Stamm WE, Weinstein RA, Dixon RE. Comparison of endemic and epidemic nosocomial infections. *Am J Med* 1981;70:393–397.
15. Emori TG, Haley RW, Garner JS. Technique and uses of nosocomial infection surveillance in U.S. hospitals, 1976–1977. *Am J Med* 1981; 70:933–940.
16. Stamm WE. Catheter-associated urinary tract infections: epidemiology, pathogenesis, and prevention. *Am J Med* 1991;91(3B):65S–71S.
17. Culver DH, Horan TC, Gaynes RP, et al. Surgical wound infection rates by wound class, operation, and risk index in U.S. hospitals, 1986–90. *Am J Med* 1991;1(suppl 3B):152S–158S.
18. Gaynes RP, Martone W, Culver DH, et al. Comparison of rates of nosocomial infections in neonatal intensive care units in the United States. *Am J Med* 1991;91(suppl 3B):192S–197S.
19. Jarvis WR, Edwards JR, and the National Nosocomial Infectious Surveillance Sustem. Nosocomial infections in adult and pediatric intensive care units in the United States, 1986–90. *Am J Med* 1991;91(suppl 3B):185S–189S.
20. National Nosocomial Infections Surveillance System. Nosocomial infection rates for interhospital comparison: limitations and possible solutions. *Infect Control Hosp Epidemiol* 1991;12:609–621.
21. Chassin MR, Kosecoff J, Park RE, et al. Does inappropriate use explain geographic variations in the use of healthcare services? A study of three procedures. *JAMA* 1987;258:2533–2539.
22. Haley RW. JCAHO infection control indicators, parts 1 and 2. *Infect Control Hosp Epidemiol* 1990;11:545–548.
23. Larson E. A comparison of methods for surveillance of nosocomial infections. *Infect Control Hosp Epidemiol* 1980;1:377–381.
24. (no author) Framework for evaluating performance measurement systems established. *Joint commission perspectives*. 1996;16(1):1–8.

25. Garner JS, Simmons BP, eds. CDC guideline for isolation precautions in hospitals. *Infect Control Hosp Epidemiol* 1983;4:245–280.
26. Horan TC, Gaynes RP, Martone WJ, et al. CDC definitions of nosocomial surgical site infections, 1992: a modification of CDC definitions of surgical wound infections. *Infect Control Hosp Epidemiol* 1992;13: 606–608.
27. Centers for Disease Control and Prevention. *Outline for surveillance and control of nosocomial infections*. Atlanta: Centers for Disease Control, 1972.
28. Abrutyn E, Talbot GH. Surveillance strategies: a primer. *Infect Control* 1987;8(11)459–464.
29. Altemeir WA. *Manual on the control of infection in surgical patients*. Philadelphia: Lippincott, 1976:29–30.
30. Emori TG, Culver DH, Horan TC, et al. National Nosocomial Infections Surveillance System (NNIS): description of surveillance methodology. *Am J Infect Control* 1991;19:19–35.
31. Condon RE, Haley RW, Lee JT, Meakins JL, Does infection control control infection? *Arch Surg* 1988;123:250–254.
32. Manian FA, Meyer L. Comprehensive surveillance of surgical wound infections in outpatient and inpatient surgery. *Infect Control Hosp Epidemiol* 1990;11(10):515–520.
33. Reimer K, Gleed C, Nicolle LE. Impact of postdischarge infection in surgical wound infection rates. *Infect Control Hosp Epidemiol* 1987; 8(6):237–240.
34. Weigelt JA, Dryer D, Haley RW. The necessity and efficiency of wound surveillance after discharge. *Arch Surg* 1992;152:77–82.
35. Zoutman D. Surgical wound infections occurring in day surgery patients. *Am J Infect Control* 1990;18(4):277–281.
36. Holtz TH, Wenzel RP. Postdischarge surveillance for nosocomial wound infection: a brief review and commentary. *Infect Control Hosp Epidemiol* 1992;20:206–213.
37. Sheretz RJ, Garabaldi RA, Kaiser AB, et al. Consensus paper on the surveillance of surgical wound infections. *Infect Control Hosp Epidemiol* 1992;13:599–605.
38. Mertans R, Jans B, Kurz X. A computerized nationwide network for nosocomial infection surveillance in Belgium. *Infect Control Hosp Epidemiol* 1994;171–179.
39. Yokoe DS, Platt R. Surveillance for surgical site infections: the uses of antibiotic exposure. *Infect Control Hosp Epidemiol* 1994;15:717–723.
40. Donabedian A. Contributions of epidemiology to quality assessment and monitoring. *Infect Control Hosp Epidemiol* 1990;11:117–121.
41. McGeer A, Crede W, Hierholzer WJ Jr. Surveillance for quality assessment. II. Surveillance for noninfectious processes: back to basics. *Infect Control Hosp Epidemiol* 1990;11:36–41.
42. Myers SA, Gleicher N. A successful program to lower caesarean section rates. *N Engl J Med* 1988;319:1511–1516.
43. Massanari RM, Wilkerson K, Swartzendruber S. Designing surveillance for noninfectious outcomes of medical care. *Infect Control Hosp Epidemiol* 1995;16:419–426.
44. Rhame FS, Sudderth WD. Incidence and prevalence as used in the analysis of the occurrence of nosocomial infections. *Am J Epidemiol* 1981;113:1–10.
45. French GL. Repeated prevalence surveys for monitoring effectiveness of hospital infection control. *Lancet* 1989;2:1021–1023.
46. McGowan JE Jr., Finland M. Infection and usage of antibiotics at Boston City Hospital: changes in prevalence during the decade 1964–1973. *J Infect Dis* 1974;129:421–424.
47. Bennett JV, Scheckler WE, Maki DG, Brachman PS. Current national patterns: United States. In: Brachman PS, Eickhoff TC, eds. *Proceedings of the International Conference on Nosocomial Infections*. Chicago: American Hospital Association, 1971.
48. Haley RW, Culver DH, Emori TG, et al. The accuracy of retrospective chart review in measuring nosocomial infection rates: results of validation studies in pilot hospitals. *Am J Epidemiol* 1980;111:534–540.
49. Wenzel RP, Osterman CA, Hunting KJ, Gwaltney JM Jr. Hospital-acquired infections. I. Surveillance in a university hospital. *Am J Epidemiol* 1976;103:251–256.
50. Wenzel RP. Hospital-acquired infections in intensive care unit patients: an overview with emphasis on epidemics. *Infect Control Hosp Epidemiol* 1983;4:371–375.
51. Scheckler WE, Garner JS, Kaiser AB, Bennett JV. Prevalence of infections and antibiotic usage in eight community hosptitals. In: Brachman PS, Eickhoff TC, eds. *Proceedings of the International Conference on Nosocomial Infections*. Chicago: American Hospital Association, 1971.
52. Quality Indicator Study Group. An approach to the evaluation of quality indicators of the outcome of care in hospitalized patients, with a focus on nosocomial infections. *Infect Control Hosp Epidemiol* 1995; 16:308–316.
53. Donowitz LG, Wenzel RP, Hoyt JW. High risk of hospital-acquired infection in the ICU patient. *Crit Care Med* 1982;10:355–359.
54. Gaynes RP, Edwards JR, Jarvis WR, Culver DH, Tolson JS, Martone WJ, and the National Nosocomial Infections Surveillance System. Nosocomial infections among neonates in high-risk nurseries in the United States. *Pediatrics* 1996;98:357–361.
55. Haley RW, Morgan WM, White JW, et al. Extra days and prolongation of stay attributable to nosocomial infections: a prospective interhospital comparison. *Am J Med* 1981;70:51–54.
56. Emori TG, Gaynes RP. An overview of nosocomial infections including the role for the microbiology laboratory. *Clin Microbiol Rev* 1993;6: 428–442.
57. Haley RW. Nosocomial infections in surgical patients: developing valid measures of intrinsic patient risk. *Am J Med* 1991;91(suppl 3B): 145S–149S.
58. Haley RW, Culver DH, White JW, et al. Identifying patients at high risk of surgical wound infections: a simple multivariate index of patient susceptibility and wound contamination. *Am J Epidemiol* 1984;121: 206–216.
59. Keats AS. The ASA classification of physical status: a recapitulation. *J Anesthesiol* 1978:49:233–238.
60. Cruse PJE, Foord R. The epidemiology of wound infection: a 10-year prospective study of 62,939 wounds. *Surg Clin North Am* 1980;60Z: 27–32.
61. Fagon JY, Chastre J. Hance AJ, et al. Evaluation of clinical judgment in the identification and treatment of nosocomial pneumonia in ventilated patients. *Chest* 1993;103:547–553.
62. Torres A, De La Bellacasa JP, Xaubet A, et al. Diagnostic value of quantitative cultures of bronchoalveolar lavage and telescoping plugged catheter in mechanically ventilated patients with bacterial pneumonia. *Am Rev Respir Dis* 1989;140:306–310.
63. Meduri GU, Chastre J. The standardization of bronchoscopic techniques for ventilator-associated pneumonia. *Chest* 1992;102(suppl): 557S–563S.
64. Baselshi V, El-Torky M, Coalson S, Griffen J. The standardization of criteria for processing and interpreting laboratory specimens. *Chest* 1992;102(suppl 1):571S–579S.
65. Wunderink RG, Mayhall G, Gilbert C. Methodology for clinical investigation of ventilator-assisted pneumonia: epidemiology and therapeutic intervention. *Chest* 1992;102(suppl 1):580S–588S.
66. Goldwater PN, Martin AJ, Ryan B, et al. A survey of nosocomial respiratory syncytial viral infections in a children's hospital: occult respiratory infection in patients admitted during an epidemic season. *Infect Control Hosp Epidemiol* 1991;12:231–238.
67. Tablon OC, Anderson LJ, Arden NH, et al. Guideline for the prevention of nosocomial pneumonia. *Infect Control Hosp Epidemiol* 1994;15: 587–627.
68. Banerjee S, Emori G, Culver DH, et al. Trends in nosocomial bloodstream infections in the United States, 1980–89. *Am J Med* 1991;91 (suppl 3B):86S–89S.
69. Berg R. Reviews: software. *Am J Infect Control* 1986;14:139–143.
70. Gaynes RP, Friedman C, Copeland TA, Mauck-Thiele GA. Methodology to evaluate a computer-based system for surveillance of hospital-acquired infections. *Am J Infect Control* 1990;18:40–45.
71. LaHaise S. A comparison of infection control software for use by hospital epidemiologists in meeting the new JCAHO standards. *Infect Control Hosp Epidemiol* 1990;11:185–190.

Hospital Infections, Fourth Edition,
edited by John V. Bennett and Philip S. Brachman.
Published by Lippincott–Raven Publishers, Philadelphia, 1998

CHAPTER 6

Investigating Endemic and Epidemic Nosocomial Infections

William R. Jarvis

Although healthcare facility infection control programs have been shown to be effective in reducing the rate of nosocomial infections, endemic and/or epidemic infections associated with the delivery of healthcare continue to occur [1]. It has been estimated that only approximately one third of all nosocomial infections are preventable [2]. However, infection control programs at U.S. hospitals prevent only ~ 6% of these nosocomial infections because of incomplete implementation of recommended control measures [2,3]. The goals of any healthcare facility infection control program should be to educate healthcare workers on the recommended measures to prevent and control nosocomial infections; conduct active, prospective surveillance to detect nosocomial infections; analyze surveillance data to identify endemic or epidemic nosocomial infection problems warranting further investigation; conduct epidemiologic investigations to identify the source of these problems; and implement control measures and assess their efficacy in preventing and controlling these problems. The purpose of this chapter is to describe the epidemiology of endemic or epidemic nosocomial infections, discuss criteria for determining whether to investigate endemic or epidemic nosocomial infections, and outline the systematic approach to such investigations.

DEFINING ENDEMIC OR EPIDEMIC NOSOCOMIAL INFECTIONS

Endemic infections are defined as sporadic infections that constitute the background rate of infection at the healthcare facility; the rate of such infections usually fluctuates from month to month but overall is not statistically significantly different from the background rate of these infections (see Chapters 6, 30). Of all nosocomial infections, endemic infections account for the majority of infections and are the focus of most infection control activities. The predominant pathogens and sites of endemic infection are somewhat similar at different types of healthcare facilities but do differ based on the mix of patients (including underlying diseases and severity of illness) and types of procedures performed and devices used (Tables 6-1 and 6-2) [4,5]. Endemic infections can change in type (pathogen, site, or both) and/or rate as the result of a variety of factors, including opening or moving to a new facility, introducing a new or expanding existing clinical services or specialties (e.g., bone marrow or organ transplant, neonatal intensive care unit, surgical or medical subspecialty), introducing new diagnostic methods (e.g., laboratory or radiology), and so on.

Most endemic nosocomial infections result from breaks in aseptic technique, most commonly from person-to-person transmission via transient healthcare worker hand carriage of the colonizing or infecting pathogen. Numerous studies have documented that healthcare workers often fail to wash their hands before and between contacts with patients [6]. Nevertheless, investigating endemic problems transmitted in this way focuses attention on the importance of general infection control recommendations (including identifying and isolating infectious patients, healthcare worker hand washing, environmental cleaning, and existing guidelines to prevent these infections) and can be associated with a reduction (often transient) in the rate of these infections. Since many endemic infections are preventable, investigation of such problems by the hospital epidemiologist or other infection control personnel may be warranted if the

W. R. Jarvis: Hospital Infections Program, National Center for Infectious Diseases, Centers for Disease Control and Prevention, Atlanta, Georgia 30333.

TABLE 6-1. *Most common nosocomial pathogens by site and unit, National Nosocomial Infections Surveillance, October 1986–December 1990*

Site	Pathogen	Component (%) Hospital-wide	Component (%) Intensive care unit
Blood	Coagulase-negative staphylococci	27.9	28.2
	S. aureus	16.5	16.1
	Enterococci	8.3	12.0
	Candida spp	7.8	10.2
	E. coli	5.6	—
	Enterobacter spp	—	5.3
Surgical wound	*S. aureus*	17.1	11.7
	Enterococci	13.3	15.8
	Coagulase-negative staphylococci	12.6	13.8
	E. coli	9.4	—
	P. aeruginosa	8.2	9.5
	Enterobacter spp	—	10.3
Respiratory tract	*P. aeruginosa*	16.9	20.8
	S. aureus	16.1	17.1
	Enterobacter spp	10.5	11.1
	S. pneumoniae	6.5	—
	H. influenzae	6.3	—
	Acinetobacter spp	—	6.4
	K. pneumoniae	—	5.6
Urinary tract	*E. coli*	25.8	17.5
	Enterococci	15.9	13.0
	P. aeruginosa	12.0	11.3
	Candida spp	9.4	25.0
	K. pneumoniae	6.4	—
	Enterobacter spp	—	6.1

E. coli, Escherichia coli; P. aeruginosa, Pseudomonas aeruginosa; S. pneumoniae, Streptococcus pneumoniae; H. influenzae, Haemophilus influenzae; K. pneumoniae, Klebsiella pneumoniae.

(Adapted from Jarvis WR, Martone WJ. Predominant pathogens in hospital infections. *J Antimicrob Chemother* 1991; 28:15–19.)

rate of endemic infection is gradually increasing at the institution or the rate of these infections is higher than expected, than reported in the literature, or than reported from other similar institutions.

Epidemic infections are defined as the occurrence of infection at a rate statistically significantly higher than the background rate of such infections; recognized infection clusters often are unexpected and involve either an unusual organism or an organism with an unusual antimicrobial susceptibility pattern (see Chapter 9). Recognition of clusters of common organisms with common antimicrobial susceptibility patterns may be difficult because they merge with the existing endemic infections. Often infection control personnel attempt to determine whether a cluster represents an outbreak based on numerator data only. In such a situation, it is difficult if not impossible to determine whether a detected cluster represents an outbreak, unless it involves either a very rare organism (e.g., *Vibrio cholera* diarrhea) or a common organism with an unusual antimicrobial susceptibility pattern (e.g., vancomycin-resistant *Staphylococcus aureus*).

TABLE 6-2. *Distribution of nosocomial infections by date, National Nosocomial Infections Surveillance, January 1993–April 1995*

Major site	No. of infections	Percentage
Urinary tract	7,376	27.2
Surgical site	5,058	18.7
Pneumonic lungs	4,673	17.3
Primary bloodstream	4,287	15.8
Other	5,700	21.0

(Adapted from National Nosocomial Infections Surveillance (NNIS) Semiannual Report, May 1995. *Am J Infect Control* 1995;23:377–385.)

Determination of an outbreak should not be based on numerator data alone. Although one episode of nosocomial malaria or cholera in a U.S. hospital represents an epidemic, one cannot determine whether a cluster of nosocomial *S. aureus* bloodstream infections represents an outbreak unless one can calculate and compare the *S. aureus* bloodstream infection rates in the time periods during and before the cluster. Because of the abrupt nature of epidemics and the feeling that most such outbreaks are preventable, in most situations epidemics warrant investigation.

RECOGNITION OF ENDEMIC OR EPIDEMIC NOSOCOMIAL INFECTIONS

Surveillance is the cornerstone for rapid recognition of endemic or epidemic nosocomial infections (see Chapter 5). In order to detect either endemic or epidemic nosocomial infections, one must have a surveillance method in place to detect such infections. Since the majority of nosocomial infections arise in severely ill patients exposed to invasive devices (e.g., patients in intensive care units) or those undergoing surgical procedures, surveillance for infections in these populations is most important. If no systematic surveillance system is in place, many clusters may not be recognized and if they are recognized, it is impossible to determine whether the cluster identified is endemic or epidemic unless appropriate denominator data are obtained and rates are calculated and compared.

If active prospective surveillance using standard definitions and methodologies is not conducted, it may be necessary to carry out a specific retrospective study to determine the background rate of infection before one can determine whether the infection problem detected or recognized is endemic or epidemic [7–12]. In institutions in which active prospective surveillance is not being conducted in the area, when a cluster is detected, a retrospective study must be undertaken to attempt to reconstruct the current and past rates of such infection in the area. Only then can one differentiate between an endemic and epidemic problem.

The early detection of infection clusters and the determination of whether the cluster identified is endemic or epidemic are most readily done if active surveillance for such infections and calculation of infection rates in the area are part of an ongoing, validated process. Once the cluster is identified, the investigator next determines whether the problem is endemic or epidemic in nature.

Differentiating endemic from epidemic infections requires review of how the numerator and denominator are collected, validation of the accuracy of these data, and assessment of whether factors exist that might influence either the numerator or denominator data (i.e., surveillance artifact) (Table 6-3). Care must be taken to ensure that surveillance artifact is not leading to an erroneous conclusion that either the number of infections or the infection rate is increasing. A wide variety of factors that can inflate or deflate the numerator or denominator data can lead to surveillance artifact; they include changes in the definitions used to ascertain infections, infection detection methods—including surveillance or laboratory methods—changes in the populations of patients served, devices used, or procedures performed.

Since surveillance artifact influencing either the numerator or the denominator data can prejudice infection rate comparisons, it is important that the accuracy of these data be determined before rate comparisons are made. Although it is tempting to quickly begin comparative epidemiologic studies to ascertain the source and risk factors for infection, it is imperative that sufficient time be taken, before embarking on such analyses, to ensure the accuracy of the numerator and denominator data used to demonstrate that the infection rate is increasing. Otherwise, one will be misled and devote precious personnel resources to conducting an investigation of a less urgent, nonemerging or now important problem.

Numerator data often are the first finding that leads to a belief that there is an epidemic. Thus, confirmation of the validity and accuracy of the numerator data is an important first step. To be consistent, the numerator data should be obtained using the same definition over the time periods being compared. For instance, if the infection control practitioner has changed the nosocomial infection definitions used, it may appear that the rate of infection also changed when it did not; case ascertainment has altered, and reclassification of the infections using the "old" surveillance definitions may show no change in the number of infections or the infection rate. Even if the same surveillance definitions are used, for some sites of infection it may still be necessary to validate the accuracy of the surveillance data.

TABLE 6-3. *Selected conditions that can result in surveillance artifact*

- Introduction of new infection definitions
- New infection control practitioner(s)
- Initiation of surveillance in new area or population of patients
- Introduction of new laboratory tests
- Introduction of new population of patients
- Increased or decreased frequency of culturing/testing of patients
- Introduction of new medical procedure (e.g., endoscopy, cardiac surgery)

For instance, if bloodstream infections are being classified by infection control personnel as primary or secondary bloodstream infections based on microbiology data, but data concerning the presence of a catheter in the patients with bloodstream infections are not being collected, there may be misclassification of bloodstream infections. If a review of the surveillance definitions used for case ascertainment suggests that the sensitivity and/or specificity of the definitions used is low or allows for considerable subjectivity, it may be necessary to validate the accuracy of the case ascertainment method by having several members of the infection control team review each "case" independently and ensure its accuracy.

Since the existence of an outbreak usually cannot be determined by evaluation of the numerator data alone, one needs to be equally precise in assuring the validity and accuracy of the denominator data that will be used to calculate the rates of infections in the epidemic and pre-epidemic periods. Selection of the denominator to use in calculating infection rates is critically important. Previous studies have shown that for intensive care unit patients, the duration of a patient's intensive care unit stay, device (e.g., central venous or urinary catheters or mechanical ventilation) exposure and the duration of that exposure, and severity of illness all contribute to the patient's infection risk [10,11].

Thus, these important confounding variables must be controlled for by using intensive care unit–specific, device-specific denominator data (e.g., the number of urinary catheter days for the surgical intensive care unit) if valid infection rate comparisons are to be made [8]. Similarly, use of a surgical patient risk index that attempts to control for some of the most important factors determining a surgical patient's infection risk, such as the type and duration of the surgical procedure, severity of illness, and wound class, is essential if valid infection rate comparisons are to be made in surgical patients [12,13].

In most instances, one can determine whether a perceived problem is an endemic or epidemic problem only by comparison of infection rates during the suspected epidemic and pre-epidemic periods. Care should be taken when comparing the rate of infection at one's own institution with that reported either in the literature or from other institutions. Unless the surveillance methods used (including nosocomial infection definitions and case ascertainment methods), the populations served, the invasive device used, and types and number of procedures performed are similar, and the type of denominator data used for rate calculations are the same, it may be misleading to compare one's rate with that of another institution. Thus, because of the large number of confounding variables that can influence the numerator, denominator, or infection rate, one often is safest comparing rates over time at one's own institution. However, even within one's own institution, one must be cautious in making such comparisons, ensuring that the comparisons include both similar numerator and similar denominator data.

For example, comparison of nosocomial bloodstream infection rates in an intensive care unit to which only medical patients are admitted with rates in another unit at that same institution to which both medical and surgical patients are admitted or comparison of nosocomial bloodstream, urinary tract, surgical site, or pneumonia infection rates among patients in a medical intensive care unit to rates in patients in surgical intensive care units may be misleading. Since both the mix of patients and the devices used can influence infection rates, controlling for these factors by making comparisons with similar populations and controlling for the duration of patients' stays and devices used is necessary if valid rate comparisons are to be made. These factors are most easily controlled for by making infection rate comparisons in a particular unit or population within an institution over time.

Differentiating Endemic from Epidemic Infections

No one definition can be used in all situations to differentiate endemic from epidemic infections or define epidemic infections. Depending upon the severity of the problem and the administrative and other pressures present, one may be able to precisely and accurately define the numerator and denominator data or perform a "quick and dirty" analysis to determine whether an epidemic is present and an investigation must be initiated. Once one is confident of the validity and accuracy of these data, one is in a position to compare the rate of the infections or other adverse events recognized in the cluster to the background rate of such events and determine whether the cluster is an epidemic or endemic occurrence. If one can confirm the accuracy of the numerator data but not the denominator data, one may be forced to use a less accurate denominator (e.g., the number of patients or the number of patient-days) to calculate the "rate."

It must be realized that depending on the variation in the possible confounding variables, the findings of the comparison of the "epidemic" to "pre-epidemic" rates (i.e., statistically significantly higher, lower, or unchanged) may be misleading. Furthermore, it may sometimes be difficult, even given the appropriate numerator and denominator data, to determine whether a cluster of infections is endemic or epidemic. For instance, if an endemic rate of infection continues to rise, at some point it may be considered epidemic in nature if recent experience is compared with suitable remote baseline data. In other situations, the lack of background rate data (e.g., no surveillance conducted, new patient population or new diagnostic test introduced at the facility) may preclude the possibility of making rate comparisons. However, in most situations, it is possible to either determine or estimate the background rate and to decide whether the detected cluster of infections represents an epidemic or endemic problem. The recent development of a variety of computer statistical software packages has simplified the calculation and comparison of infection rates; however, the ease with which it is possible to make such comparisons has further highlighted the importance of ensuring the accuracy and validity of the numerator and denominator data used.

Some researchers have suggested conducting prospective surveillance and using threshold programs to determine when the rate of infection increases above a certain level that warrants further investigation. Such programs were used in the 1970s in the National Nosocomial Infections Surveillance system and were found to be unreliable because of normal variations in the rate of infections at most institutions. Although it may be easy to establish a high rate of infection above which further investigation is indicated, the sensitivity of such a system would be low. To date it has been impossible to design a sensitive and specific threshold program that would identify all epidemics when they occur and yet not also highlight other nonoutbreaks as clusters requiring investigation. It has been equally difficult to develop a sufficiently sensitive and specific threshold program for the detection of clusters requiring further investigation.

More recently, data have been published from national surveillance and other studies providing rate distributions for a variety of groups of patients [10–12]. These data can be used to compare the rate of infection at one's own institution and assist in determining whether the endemic rate of infection is too high and should be investigated or whether the rate of infection documented at the institution is significantly higher than at your institution in the past and significantly higher than national averages. These national benchmark data are most useful for evaluating one's endemic infection rate rather than for determining whether an epidemic is in progress. Despite these data, there are many populations for which there are no published benchmark infection rates. Furthermore, some of the published benchmark rates have not carefully controlled for intrinsic or extrinsic risk factors. Thus, one is often forced to decide whether to further investigate an epidemic or endemic problem based upon the limited data one has at the institutional level.

DECIDING WHEN TO CONDUCT AN INVESTIGATION

Making the decision to conduct an epidemiologic investigation and determining the extent of that investigation are dependent upon a number of factors. These factors differ at the institutional, local health departmental, state health departmental, federal governmental (Centers for Disease Control and Prevention (CDC)), and private consultant levels. In all situations, factors that influence the decision to initiate the investigation include whether the cluster is endemic or epidemic in nature, the morbidity and mortality associated with the cluster of infections, and staff availability and expertise.

If a decision is made within the hospital that an investigation is warranted, the necessary staff will be mobilized and the investigation initiated. If the staff's availability or expertise is insufficient to conduct the investigation, hospital personnel can call in a private consultant, the local or state health departments, or the CDC for assistance. Regardless of the outside source, the exact nature and scope of the investigation desired by hospital personnel and what the outside consultant or organization is offering to do should be well defined and outlined before a request for assistance is extended. In addition, because of the changing epidemiology of nosocomial infections and the possible complexity of an investigation, combined epidemiologic and laboratory investigations may be indicated and the capability to perform these investigations should be documented before an invitation is initiated or as soon as the need for such expertise is realized.

At the federal level (Hospital Infections Program, CDC), the decision to initiate an epidemiologic investigation at a healthcare facility is based on the public health importance of the problem, whether the cluster may represent a nationwide problem (e.g., intrinsic product contamination or a serious problem related to a newly introduced medical device), the morbidity and mortality associated with the cluster, the extent to which the investigation may further our knowledge of healthcare epidemiology and infection control, and staff availability [14]. Moreover, since combined epidemiologic and laboratory investigations are frequently most useful, the ability to obtain and genetically type the colonizing or infecting isolates associated with the cluster may influence the decision to collaborate in the investigation. Since the CDC is a nonregulatory agency, for the CDC to collaborate in the investigation, requires the approval of and invitation from both the healthcare facility's infection control department and administration and the local and/or state health department. Each year, the CDC is consulted about 70 to 100 nosocomial epidemics and actively assists in conducting 10 to 20 on-site investigations.

Clusters of infection caused by very unusual organisms, those associated with great morbidity or mortality, and those of epidemiologic importance (introduction of a new multidrug-resistant pathogen) may warrant initiating an investigation without carefully comparing infection rates in the epidemic and pre-epidemic periods. These clusters include infections caused by very unusual or never previously reported pathogens (i.e., vancomycin-resistant *S. aureus*, *Rhodococcus* or *Nocardia* sp infections in surgery patients), two or more infections caused by organisms usually indicative of a carrier (e.g., Group A streptococcus), isolated infections caused by a multidrug-resistant nosocomial pathogen (e.g., vancomycin-resistant enterococcus, multidrug-resistant *Mycobacterium tuberculosis*) that, if not controlled, could become endemic, or dissemination of a clonal organism, which often suggests an eradicable common source [15–18].

Once a cluster is identified and the decision is made to conduct an investigation, the extent of the investigation must be determined. If the cluster is associated with little morbidity and mortality and involves only colonization or infection of a small number of patients, a brief investigation may be performed. In such circumstances, the possible case patients' medical records are reviewed, a hypothetical mode of transmission is identified, and interventions are implemented. If a full-scale investigation is to be initiated, a systematic approach should be taken (discussed later herein). In general, it is recommended that cultures of personnel, products, solutions, or environmental sources be directed by the epidemiologic data.

Documentation of an epidemiologic association between the outbreak and a product, device, or healthcare worker, with subsequent culture confirmation, is preferred to widespread culturing of personnel, solutions, or equipment with the hope that the source will be identified. Widespread culturing of animate or inanimate objects with the object of serendipitously identifying the source is wasteful of the time of both infection control and laboratory personnel (see Chapter 20). On the other hand, if one cannot preserve the area in which the outbreak is taking place and the inanimate environment is going to be cleaned or the product reprocessed, selected cultures should be obtained before the scene of the outbreak is altered. In addition, it may be important to immediately interview healthcare workers in the area where the outbreak has occurred, since practices may change or recall bias be introduced if these persons are interviewed days or weeks later.

Last, careful consideration should be given to whether the unit/ward/area should be closed or surgery or other procedures discontinued. If a large number of deaths is associated with the outbreak in one area, closing the area may be warranted. However, if such a decision is made, infection control personnel should realize the seriousness of the message being sent. Before closing the area, there should be discussion, and a consensus should be developed concerning what criteria must be met before reopening the area. The decisions to close and reopen an area can be made only at the institutional level. Regardless of whether the unit is closed, infection control and administrative personnel should ensure that all potentially relevant materials (devices, medications, solutions, etc.), are saved and quarantined for future evaluation)

If there is serious morbidity or a large number of deaths or if many patients are affected, serious consideration should be given to identifying a spokesperson, best coordinated through infection control and public relations staff, who will regularly update both appropriate institutional (e.g., staff and patients) and external (e.g., regulatory, governmental, or media) personnel. The spokesperson should present enough information to assure others that an appropriate institutional investigation is being conducted but should not prematurely reveal preliminary information. All public inquiries should be directed to the identified spokesperson to ensure that one voice is being heard and conflicting stories do not emerge. Open and honest communication with the local or national media is preferable to dessiminating misinformation or refusing to speak to them.

It should be remembered that state and federal laws require that healthcare facilities notify public health authorities of selected adverse events (see Chapter 18). Since laws differ in each state, infection control personnel should consult the law in the state where their healthcare facility is located. Any outbreaks that may have a public health impact at the county, state, or national level should be reported to local, state, or federal health officials. Any outbreaks associated with intrinsically contaminated or defective products (including solutions, blood or blood products, or devices) should be reported to the Food and Drug Administration (FDA) through the MedWatch Program (1-800-FDA-1088) and the CDC (404-639-6413). If such an outbreak involves many healthcare facilities in more than one state, federal public health agencies are responsible for the investigations.

CONDUCTING AN EPIDEMIOLOGIC INVESTIGATION

Saving Critical Materials

The first step in any investigation is to ensure that critically important isolates and/or materials that may be associated with the outbreak are saved. At the first sign of an outbreak, the infection control staff should get in touch with the director of the microbiology laboratory and request that any of the infecting organisms from current and past possible "cases" be saved. Laboratory personnel also should be alerted to keep any subsequent isolates of the outbreak strain that may be recovered during the investigation. If this is not done, laboratory confirmation of the subsequent epidemiologic findings in the form of isolate typing will be impossible. In addition, if there is the possibility that an intrinsically or extrinsically contaminated product device may be the source of the outbreak, such solution or devices should be immediately quarantined.

For example, if there is an unusual cluster of bloodstream infections with the same organism(s) in one unit over a short period of time (1 to 5 days), a contaminated product should be seriously considered; it may be prudent to collect all medications, multidose vials, or solutions from the involved area and immediately move them to an area where they can be preserved and protected. If extrinsic contamination of a product or solution is suspected, it may be useful to have personnel save products or solutions used in the area as the epidemiologic investigation is being conducted so that these solutions/products can be cultured or studied if epidemiologic studies establish an association between them and the adverse outcome.

The Source, the Pathogen, the Host, and the Mode of Transmission

Epidemiologic investigations have similarities and differences. The approach is similar, although the risk factors assessed may be different. For this reason, we do not have standardized forms to use in our investigations; instead the data collected during each epidemiologic investigation is individualized depending upon the data available on the pathogen, host, and known or suspected modes of transmission. Although the approach may differ slightly for each investigation initiated, in general, epidemiologists use a fairly standard system (Table 6-4). Four major areas assessed in any epidemiologic investigation include the source(s), the pathogen(s), the host, and the mode of transmission. Factors in these four areas contribute to the the outbreak, and modification of one or more of these elements usually can terminate the outbreak. In order for infection to occur, sufficient organisms must be present, the host must be susceptible to the organism, and opportunity must exist for the host to have contact with the organism. The goal of the epidemiologic investigation is to determine which one or more of these factors is the most important in causing the outbreak and which can most easily be modified to interrupt transmission.

It is important to understand the pathogen and the ecologic niche the organism prefers. For instance, *Sternotrophomonas maltophilia* or *Burkholderia cepacia* are increasingly common nosocomial pathogens that often can be traced to water sources [19,20]. *Malassezia* sp are lipid-loving organisms that usually infect patients receiving intralipid. A nosocomial *Malassezia pachydermitis* outbreak among neonates in a neonatal intensive care unit was traced via colonization of the hands of healthcare workers via colonization of the ears of their dogs [22,23]. *Aspergillus* sp usually infect immunocompromised patients and can be found in soil and air [24,25]. *Acinetobacter* or *Serratia* sp emerge in situations of high antimicrobial pressure, and the latter organisms have been traced to intrinsic or extrinsic contamination of antiseptics [26,27]. *Legionella* sp are typically associated with water sources and primarily infect immunocompromised hosts [28]. Some salmonella and most Group A streptococcus infections are traced to personnel carriers [29,30].

In general, molecular typing of the infecting pathogen can provide valuable information [31] (see Chapter 9). If the infecting organisms are identical (i.e., clonal), the chances are great that there is a common source (e.g., a solution, device, or healthcare worker) and that an epidemiologic investigation can identify the source, the source can be removed, and the outbreak can be terminated. On the other hand, if molecular typing of the infecting organisms shows that they are not identical (i.e., nonclonal), most likely the organism is being introduced from multiple sources and/or transmitted from person to person via the hands of healthcare workers. An epidemiologic investigation may pinpoint factors increasing the risk of infection (failure to rapidly identify colonized/infected patients and isolate them, failure of healthcare workers to wash their hands, etc.), but the empiric reinforcement of such practices as isolation of patients and handwashing may terminate the outbreak without a more complete investigation. Thus, reviewing the microbiology of the infecting pathogen can provide valuable clues to the likely source of an infection and facilitate generation of hypotheses about that source.

Next, host factors need to be evaluated. In order for the host to become infected, there must be sufficient numbers of organisms and the patient must be susceptible to infection. In some instances, host susceptibility is related to age or immunosuppression that is condition specific (e.g., low birthweight neonates), disease specific (e.g., human immunodeficiency virus–infected patients) or condition or medication induced (patients with hematologic malignancy or bone marrow or organ transplant patients). In other instances, the host has become susceptible to colonization or infection because of exposure to medical devices or other surgical or invasive procedures.

The next factor to be considered is the mode of transmission. Infection may be transmitted by contact (direct, indirect, droplet) or a common source, or it may be airborne (droplet nuclei, skin squamae) or vectorborne (see Chapter 1). Although nosocomial pathogens can be transmitted by the airborne route (e.g., *Aspergillus* spp, influenza organisms, *M. tuberculosis*, measles or varicella-zoster viruses), the majority are passed by contact, usually necessitating transfer of the organisms from an infected or colonized patient to a susceptible patient via transient hand colonization of the healthcare worker [23,32] or by droplet (< 3 feet) spread (e.g., respiratory syncytial viruses or adenoviruses). In the case of most organisms transmitted by contact, the infected or colo-

TABLE 6-4. *General approach to an outbreak investigation*

- The preliminary investigation: quick and dirty
  - Review existing information
    - Surveillance records
    - Interviews with clinical/laboratory staff
    - Microbiology records
    - Patients' records
  - Verify the diagnosis
  - Develop tentative case definition (may be broad, i.e., fairly sensitive but not too specific)
    - Microbiologic
    - Other clinical laboratory
      - Hematology
      - Chemistry
      - Other (e.g., toxicology)
    - Radiologic
    - Pathologic
    - Clinical signs/symptoms
    - Other (e.g., skin testing)
    - Combinations of these areas
  - Ascertain cases
  - Descriptive epidemiology
    - Establish the nature of the problem (e.g., SWI), population at risk, location, severity of illness, and timeframe
    - Construct the epidemic curve
      - Time
      - Place
      - Person
  - Establish existence of an outbreak
    - Compare rates
    - Exclude surveillance artifact or pseudo-epidemic
  - Assess adequacy of control measures
    - Enforce existing control measures
    - Supplement with additional control measures
  - Decide on a course of observation vs. definitive investigation, taking into account
    - Severity of illness
      - Colonization vs. disease
      - Morbidity vs. mortality
    - Effectiveness of control measures
- The comprehensive investigation
  - Refine the case definition (e.g., increasing specificity)
  - Ascertain additional cases
    - Record reviews
    - Surveys
      - Microbiologic
      - Other (e.g., skin testing, antibody testing)
  - Refine descriptive epidemiology
  - Refine evaluation establishing the existence of an outbreak
  - Develop hypotheses
  - Test hypotheses—analytical epidemiology
    - Case control vs. cohort studies
    - Retrospective vs. prospective studies
    - Control selection
  - Reevaluate control measures
    - Implement additional measures if warranted
    - Ask whether additional epidemiologic/laboratory studies are needed
- Draw conclusions and formalize recommendations for control
- Continue surveillance for new cases
- Evaluate the effectiveness of implemented control measures
- Write and distribute a comprehensive report

SWI, surgical wound infection.

nized patient is the source; for some organisms, such as vancomycin-resistant enterococci, multidrug-resistant *S. aureus*, and respiratory syncytial viruses and rotavirus, the environment may play a role in infection transmission by fomites.

The predominant site of infection also can help the epidemiologist focus the investigation on the most likely route of transmission. For instance, a cluster of bloodstream infections is most likely related to an intrinsically contaminated common vehicle or extrinsically contaminated solution or device (including transducers) or to lapses in aseptic technique on the part of healthcare workers during intravascular catheter device manipulation [33]. Nosocomial pneumonia is often traced to contamination of respiratory therapy equipment or person-to-person transmission of infecting pathogens via the hands of healthcare workers [34]. Nosocomial urinary tract infections are typically attributed to contamination during urinary tract manipulation, of open urinary drainage systems, or in the insertion or maintenance of a urinary catheter [35]. Surgical site infections are often traced to sources in the operating room [15,24,29,32,36,37] or, more rarely, to the postoperative intensive care unit [38] or the preoperative ward.

When initiating an investigation, a review of the source, pathogen, the host, and the mode of transmission can help guide the direction of the epidemiologic investigation. The more that is known about these areas, the more focused the investigation can be. In contrast, the less that is known about these areas (for instance, the first nosocomial outbreak of *Rhodococcus bronchialis* among surgery patients), the broader the scope of the investigation must be at the beginning (15).

Initial "Case" Review

Regardless of whether a brief or detailed epidemiologic study is being carried out, one of the first steps in the investigation of a possible epidemic or outbreak is to review some or all of the medical records of possible case patients. The purpose of this review is to characterize the population at risk by time, place, and person so that a "case" definition can be developed. If possible, this review should encompass all known possible case patients. If the number of possible case patients is large, one may select a sample of them; if either a random or convenience sample is chosen, the reviewer should be aware that bias may thus be introduced and lead to erroneous conclusions.

For infections that have a long incubation period, meaning that the majority of patients experience onset of symptoms after hospital discharge, review of the medical records of only those who are still hospitalized may lead to an underestimation of the extent of the outbreak and may not describe the affected population accurately. Examples of such outbreaks include many insidious postoperative surgical site infections (caused by, e.g., nontuberculous mycobacteria, *Nocardia* spp *Rhodococcus* spp), *S. aureus* infections among newborns, and infections with long incubation periods [15,24,39,40]. In outbreaks with long incubation periods, after the case definition is developed, extensive case ascertainment is necessary.

Line Listing

During the initial case review, a detailed line listing should be developed for each patient (Table 6-5). Data collected should include demographic and clinical data, the date of hospital admission, wards/units admitted to and the dates of admission to and discharge from each ward/unit, underlying diseases, date of onset of infection and/or colonization, and, if the outbreak involves infection, whether colonization with the infecting pathogen preceded the onset of infection and at what site infection was noted. Additional information is collected specific to the site of the infection/colonization. For example, in the case of surgical site infections, information is collected on the pre-, intra-, and postoperative courses of the case patients; these data should include whether a patient was admitted to an intensive care unit before the surgery, the date and type of each surgical procedure, the personnel who took part in the surgery, and exposures specific to the surgical procedure, including the type and timing of administration of prophylactic antimicrobials.

For bloodstream infection outbreaks, the types of catheters, their dates of insertion, and the duration of intravascular catheterization and the types of intravenous fluids, medications, and monitors should be documented. The epidemiologist or infection control personnel should collect adequate information to characterize the population at risk sufficiently so that the type of outbreak (i.e., colonization or disease), population (i.e., patients affected), place (i.e., specific wards, intensive care units, or surgical areas), and estimated outbreak period can be defined. Sufficient detail should be collected to establish a case definition, taking care to avoid generating an enormous amount of useless information. The primary purpose of this review is to try to identify common characteristics among the patients so that one can describe the time period of the outbreak, the group of patients at greatest risk, and the affected area(s) of the healthcare facility. In the course of this review, investigators should ensure that the infections are real and that neither surveillance nor diagnostic artifact has resulted in the "appearance" of an outbreak.

Case Definition

The next step in the investigation of an outbreak is the development of a case definition. Initially, unless the disease is known or the time or place of exposure is well defined, the case definition should be broad. This tentative case definition can be further refined as more infor-

TABLE 6-5. *Example of line listing*

Case	Age	Sex	Ward	Type of surgery	Date of surgery	Operating room	Parenteral antibiotic prophylaxis	Duration of surgery (min)	Wound drain	Fever after surgery (hr)[a]	Date of wound inflammation	Culture	
												Date	Site
1	46	F	5NW	TAH, BSO	4/23	A	No	100	No	17	4/29	4/30	Wound
2	77	M	3C	Cholecystectomy choledocholith-ectomy	5/02	F	No	150	Yes	32	5/04	5/06	Wound
3	47	M	5SW	Laminectomy	5/06	G	No	120	Yes	24	5/09	5/09	Wound
—	—	—	—	—	—	—	—	—	—	—	—	5/08	Blood
—	—	—	—	—	—	—	—	—	—	—	—	5/10	Blood
4	33	F	3C	Lobar resection & pleural stripping	5/08	D	No	120	Yes	17	5/12	5/16	Wound
5	84	F	2SE	Pyelolithotomy	5/14	C	No	60	Yes	36	5/19	5/21	Wound
—	—	—	—	—	—	—	—	—	—	—	—	5/21	Blood
—	—	—	—	—	—	—	—	—	—	—	—	5/24	Blood
6	55	M	3C	Sigmoid resection	5/20	F	No	105	Yes	48	5/23	5/23	Wound
7	22	F	5SW	ORIF ankle	7/06	A	No	150	No	20	7/07	7/08	Wound
8	65	F	5SW	Bunionectomy	7/21	F	No	45	No	18	7/23	7/23	Wound
9	40	F	4SW	Melanoma resection with skin graft	7/21	A	No	145	Yes	99	7/25	7/25	Wound
10	37	F	5NW	TAH, BSO	7/30	A	No	105	No	32	8/01	8/04	Wound

TAH, total abdominal hysterectomy; BSO, bilateral salpingo-oophorectomy; ORIF, open reduction, internal fixation.

[a]Temperature $\geq 101°F$.

mation is obtained during the conduct of the investigation. Each case definition should specify the estimated *time period* of the outbreak, the *place or places* in the healthcare facility where the outbreak is taking place, and the types of *persons* who are becoming case patients. In outbreaks of a pathogen-specific disease, development of the case definition may be relatively simple, for instance, all neonatal intensive care unit patients from June 2 to August 30, 1997, with blood cultures testing positive for *M. pachydermitis* [22]. For syndromes for which a direct association with a specific infectious agent cannot be established from the information available (e.g., initial investigations of toxic shock, legionnaires' disease, or toxic exposures), development of the case definition can be more challenging. In these instances, the case definition should include all the signs and symptoms common to all the "tentative cases" reviewed.

In addition, the case definition may include combinations of signs and/or symptoms common to the majority of the cases reviewed. One such case definition might be any patient in the surgical intensive care unit from January 5 to March 19, 1997, who had a temperature > 102°F and a > 20 mm drop in systolic blood pressure together with any one or more of the following signs: a white blood cell count > 25,000 cells/mm^3, a platelet count < 20,000/mm^3, a bilirubin level of >5 mg/dL, or splenomegaly. When formulating a case definition, a balance must be drawn between sensitivity and specificity. It may be preferable to have a case definition that is very specific rather than overly sensitive; in this way, you can be more certain that each "case" identified is a true case. Furthermore, in subsequent analytic epidemiologic studies missed "case patients" may be included in the control or noncase group and create bias toward not finding differences between the case and control or noncase patients; thus, any significant differences identified are probably even more significant. Alternatively, one may wish to identify "definite," "probable," or "possible" case patients; this approach helps ensure that controls do not include possible or probable case patients and that case patients are only those patients most likely to be cases for case-control comparisons.

Case Ascertainment

Having established a case definition, the next step is to conduct extensive case ascertainment. In this process, the infection control staff try to identify all the cases that may have arisen. All potential sources of information should be examined for possible case-identifying information. If the case definition is microorganism based, usually a careful review of the existing microbiology records is all that is needed to identify case patients. A review of microbiology methods may be necessary, to exclude the possibility that the organism might not be identified or that specimens are referred to an outside laboratory.

Thus, case ascertainment in organism-based outbreaks of bloodstream, urinary tract, or most surgical site infections is simplified. Nevertheless, one must be aware of the possibility of changes in culturing frequency on case detection [41]. However, depending upon the site of infection, outbreaks where culturing bias (i.e., clinicians are less likely to document the infection by culture) may exist, for example, nosocomial pneumonia (where a review of radiology reports in addition to microbiology records may be necessary) or surgical site infections caused by multiple pathogens (where it may be necessary to review the records of all patients undergoing the procedure to identify those with signs or symptoms of surgical site infections from whom cultures were not taken), may require more extensive and rigorous case ascertainment. During the case ascertainment process, all computerized and noncomputerized data sources (including microbiology, radiology, infection control, pharmacy, operating room, surgery, hemodialysis, other invasive procedures, nursing, or patients' medical records) that may facilitate case ascertainment should be considered.

At the same time that case ascertainment is being conducted, one should review an arbitrarily defined pre-outbreak period (usually 6 months to 2 years) for the occurrence of the outbreak adverse event. In this way, one can define the background number of such events. This information will be used to calculate the pre-epidemic rate of the adverse event which will be compared to the epidemic period rate to determine whether an outbreak has or is occurring.

The Epidemic Curve (Time)

Using the information obtained from case definition and case ascertainment, an epidemiologic curve (epi curve) should be drawn. This curve depicts the number of case patients on the vertical axis, or y-axis, and time on the horizontal axis, or x-axis (Figure 6-1). The line-listing information and epi curve can provide data to facilitate generation of hypotheses about the mode of transmission. The time scale used should be shorter than the presumed incubation period of the adverse event, since otherwise person-to-person transmission may appear to be common-source transmission. By plotting the time course of the adverse event during the epidemic and pre-epidemic periods, one can compare the occurrence of the adverse event during the epidemic and background periods, identify clusters of the event, and, based on the shape of the epi curve, generate hypotheses about the mode of transmission.

The shape of the epi curve can suggest the possible mode of transmission. If there is an abrupt increase in the number of adverse events over a short time period, it suggests a single exposure to a point source of contamination, such as a contaminated product (Figure 6-1a). In

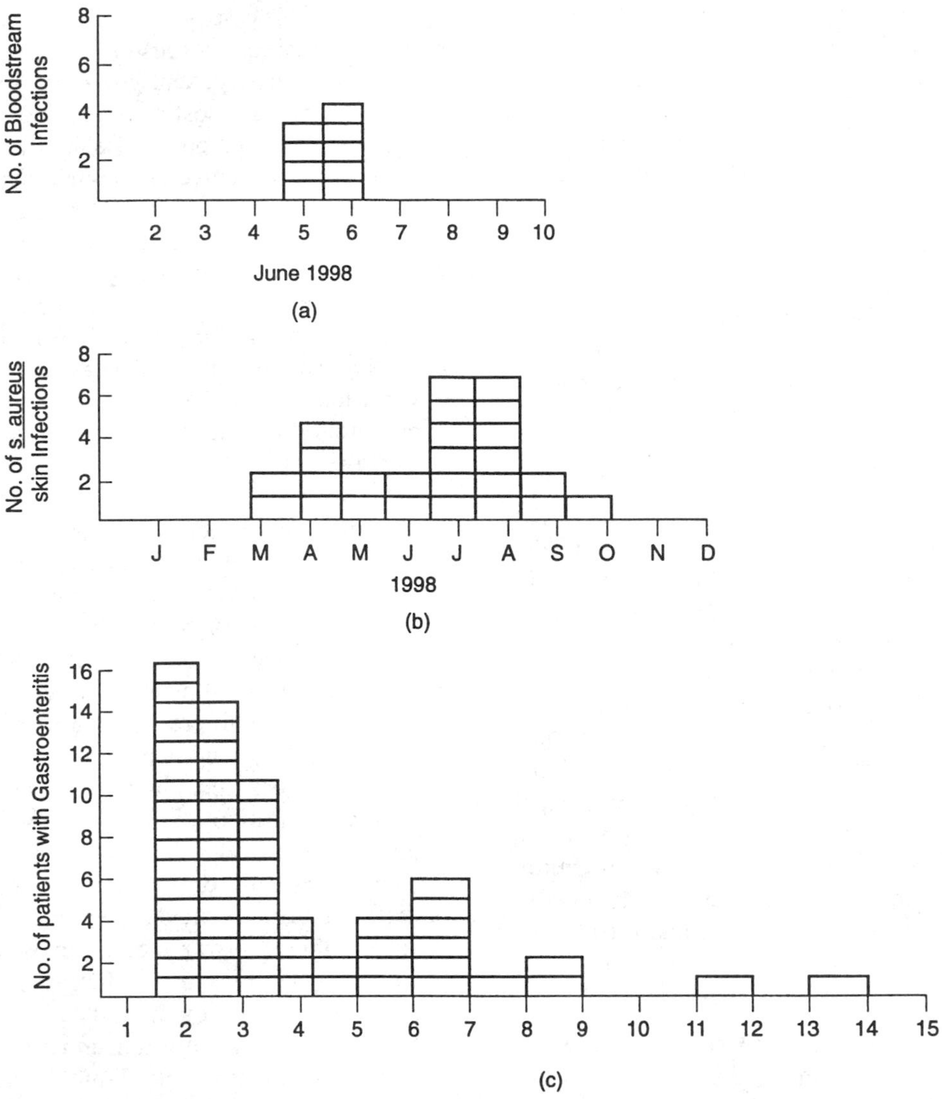

FIGURE 6-1. Example of epidemic curves. **a:** Distribution of patients with bloodstream infections associated with a contaminated common source medication. **b:** Distribution of patients with *S. aureus* skin infections associated with person-to-person transmissions. **c:** Distribution of patients with gastroenteritis associated with a common contaminated food source followed by patient-to-patient transmission.

contrast, when the epi curve depicts patients over a more prolonged time course, it is most suggestive of person-to-person transmission (Figure 6-1b). In some situations, there may be more than one mode of transmission operating either sequentially or simultaneously (Figure 6-1c). Additional epi curves depicting the dates of culture or possible exposure also may be informative—particularly when the incubation period is long. It also may be useful to draw epi curves with different time intervals (i.e., day, week, month) on the horizontal axis.

Geographic Assessment (Place)

It is useful to closely examine the place of the outbreak to determine whether there is geographic clustering. Use of spot maps may facilitate recognition of clustering of case patients that is not otherwise obvious. Do all of the case patients come from one ward or unit? If all the case patients are from one ward/unit, one can plot graphically the dates of admission and discharge from that unit (or multiple units) for each case patient and ask if there is continuous overlap among the patients. If so, this finding would suggest person-to-person transmission from one colonized or infected patient to the next. If all case patients have an infection that can be transmitted via the airborne route, is plotting of the patients by room location consistent with the ventilation system airflow diagrams or direction of airflow demonstrated by smoke tube? If the case patients are located on several different wards or units, have they all had common exposure to medications, solutions, devices, procedures, or rooms where a procedure may have been performed? If the outbreak is at one surgical site, have all the procedures been performed in one operating room or outpatient surgical suite? Geographically plotting the case patients by a variety of dates, including those of the time of culture, onset of illness, possible exposures, and so forth, may all be useful.

Host Factors (Person)

Further review of the characteristics of the case patients is then undertaken to try to define the most likely risk factors of infection. What role are specific underlying host factors playing in the outbreak? For instance, are all neonatal intensive care unit patients at risk or only those < 1,500 g? Are all surgical patients at risk or only those undergoing cardiac surgery? Are all hematology-oncology patients at risk or only those who have prolonged neutropenia? Each of the case patients' host characteristics should be reviewed to determine if there are common features among these patients.

Factors to assess include those intrinsic to the host (i.e., age, sex, race, underlying diseases, and nutritional status) and those extrinsic to the host (e.g., receipt of medications or solutions or environmental exposures—admission to an intensive care unit or procedure room; personnel exposures; exposure to therapeutic measures that might alter host susceptibility, such as receipt of antimicrobials; or exposure to invasive procedures or to invasive devices, such as central venous or urinary catheters, mechanical ventilation, or arterial pressure monitoring).

Refining the Case Definition and Reassessing the Need for Further Investigation

At this point, the basic elements of the simple epidemiologic investigation are complete. Infection control personnel should refine the case definition based upon the data accumulated. Only the essential elements reflecting the time, place, and persons who have experienced the adverse event should be included. For example, if the line listing shows that all (or nearly all) the case patients are < 1,500 g and have stayed in the neonatal intensive care unit for a median of 5 days, the case definition might be modified from that of all neonatal intensive care unit patients to those < 1,500 g who stayed in the unit for ≥ 5 days. Careful addition or deletion of patients initially thought to be case patients who do not fit the case definition should take place. It is imperative that the refined case definition be as precise and accurate as possible, since the results of subsequent epidemiologic studies are contingent upon this case definition.

If the case definition is in error, it may lead to erroneous conclusions. As mentioned previously, an overly restrictive case definition will exclude true case patients and diminish the likelihood of finding an association between an exposure and the case patients. In contrast, an overly inclusive case definition will result in the inclusion of noncase patients in the case patient group and may obscure possible associations. In most circumstances, it is preferable to begin the investigation by being overly inclusive and become more restrictive as the investigation proceeds. In some investigations, it may not be possible to divide all patients into case patient and noncase patient or control populations. If it has not already been done, one may at this point need to define possible and/or probable case patients and then perform further analyses including and then excluding these patients in the case patient group.

Occasionally, the review of the case patient's medical and microbiology records suggests that there is a cluster of positive cultures but that the patients do not have clinical illness [14]. Such findings should alert one to the possibility of a pseudo-epidemic, that is, an apparent cluster of positive cultures that may be false-positives or contaminants. In the 1960s and 1970s, such outbreaks were most often associated with cross-contamination in the laboratory during manual processing of cultures. In the 1980s and 1990s, clusters of positive cultures increasingly have been associated with cross-contamination via automated systems [14,36]. Pseudo-epidemics have been traced to a variety of sources, including intrinsically or extrinsically contaminated antiseptics or culture media, cross-contamination of cultures during manual or automated processing, or intrinsically or extrinsically contaminated blood collection tubes. Whenever there is an unusual cluster of positive cultures, particularly if it is an uncommon or environmental organism, and the case patients do not have clinical signs or symptoms indicating infection, evaluation of the specimen collection and processing methods to exclude a pseudo-epidemic should be initiated.

At this point in the investigation, infection control personnel may have arrived at the most likely source and mode of transmission of the outbreak. Because of personnel, time, or other constraints, it may be decided to introduce a number of infection control interventions thought likely to reduce or interrupt transmission and then discontinue the investigation. If the outbreak is similar to others previously reported, it may be possible to simply implement the previously documented successful infection control measures. If this is done, it is imperative that surveillance be maintained for the adverse event so that one can document the effectiveness of the implemented interventions. If the interventions do not reduce (to acceptable levels) or interrupt transmission, it may be necessary to initiate a more comprehensive comparative investigation.

Is Outside Assistance Needed?

If it is decided that a more comprehensive epidemiologic investigation is warranted because the outbreak (a) has not been terminated by the introduced control measures; (b) is unusual, complex, or associated with substantial morbidity or mortality; (c) is of major public health importance; or (d) represents an opportunity to advance our knowledge and/or understanding of healthcare epidemiology, one should reevaluate whether the personnel, time, and/or expertise are sufficient to conduct the required comprehensive studies. Such investigations may demand a substantial investment in infection control, laboratory, and statistical/computer resources. The comprehensive investigation may involve exhaustive evaluation of potential risk factors; a series of several case-control and/or cohort studies; complex analytic techniques, including multivariate analyses and modeling to control for confounding variables; healthcare worker questionnaires, interviews, or observational studies; epidemiologically directed environmental, product, device, and/or healthcare worker cultures; and implementation of interventions and evaluation of the effectiveness of these interventions.

If the adverse event is serious enough to consider a comprehensive investigation, then sufficient resources should be dedicated to the investigation to permit the rapid initiation of the study, identification of the source, and introduction of control measures. If healthcare facility infection control personnel add the conduct of such an investigation to their ongoing responsibilities, it may mean that the comparative studies will be conducted over several months. By the time the probable source of the outbreak is identified, it is possible either that the device, solution, or source will have been reprocessed or discarded or that the epidemiologically implicated healthcare worker will no longer be colonized with the infecting strain.

If outside advice or assistance is desired, a variety of experts are available. They include personnel at the local or state health departments, colleagues at other healthcare facilities in the same area, experts at nearby academic centers with an interest in healthcare epidemiology, private consultant epidemiologists, or the CDC. State and local health departments may be able to assist in arranging epidemiologic and/or laboratory support. Health care facility administrative and infection control personnel or personnel at the state health department can request CDC assistance. In CDC-conducted on-site investigations, both epidemiologic and laboratory support is provided at no cost to the healthcare facility.

Regardless of the outside source of assistance, the investigation should be considered and conducted as a collaborative effort with the healthcare facility personnel. Without the assistance of healthcare facility personnel, a comprehensive investigation cannot be efficiently conducted, and it will be these personnel who will need to implement the recommended control measures. Furthermore, local personnel are likely to be much more knowledgeable about available data sources, local infection control and other policies and practices, personnel changes, and the particular control measures that can realistically be successfully implemented at their institution.

The Comprehensive Investigation

The first step in conducting the comprehensive investigation is to review the basic investigation's line listing, case definition, and case ascertainment methods to ensure that no shortcuts were taken that may influence the comparative studies. Was the case definition based on a review of all the possible cases or just a sample? If sampling was used, was it random sampling, which may be representative of all case patients, or convenience sampling (i.e., those medical records that were readily available)? Could the case review sampling have biased the case definition? Except in very large outbreaks, it is preferable to review the medical records of all potential case patients.

Occasionally, it is the small number (often one or two) of patients who are otherwise very similar to the case patients but who did not have the adverse condition who provide insight into the possible cause of the outbreak. Was the case ascertainment complete? If not, it should be extended and repeated. Does the case ascertainment need to be broadened to a review (and/or contacting) of patients who have been discharged from the hospital or to communicating with infection control personnel at nearby hospitals or home care? Was the line listing extensive enough, or is further review of the case patient medical records necessary to obtain information on additional exposures or clinical findings? Was the denominator used to calculate the rate of the adverse event and to compare the rates of these events in the epidemic and pre-epidemic periods the correct denominator to use? If the denominator was not correct, is there a way to obtain the correct denominator or must one estimate the denominator?

For example, if the outbreak involves bloodstream infections in the medical intensive care unit but in the initial investigation one had to use either the number of medical intensive care unit patients or the number of patient-days as the denominator, can one obtain the more appropriate denominator, that is, the number of days medical intensive care unit patients spent on central venous catheters? If these data are not available or have not been collected, it may be unrealistic to try to derive them by reviewing the medical records of all medical intensive care unit patients (assuming that the central venous catheter insertion, presence, and removal dates are well documented in the medical records).

However, it would be possible to estimate these denominator data. One could randomly sample time periods during the pre-epidemic and epidemic time periods and, for several days or a week in the pre-epidemic and epidemic periods, determine for all patients in the medical intensive care unit how many had central venous catheters and what proportion of the intensive care unit days those patients were on such catheters. Then one can determine a "central venous catheter use factor" (i.e., the proportion of patient-days spent on central venous catheters times the number of patients in the unit) for each time period. In this way, one can estimate the numbers of central venous catheter days in the unit during the epidemic and pre-epidemic periods. Such estimation may be necessary when either the necessary data are not available or review of records containing the needed data would be excessively laborious and/or time-consuming.

Comparative Epidemiologic Studies

Once one has defined the case, performed comprehensive case ascertainment, developed an extensive line listing, and drafted epidemic curves, one is ready to develop and test hypothesized risk factors and modes of transmission. This can be done through either a case-control or a cohort study (see Chapter 1,7). In a case-control study, all or some of the case patients are compared with a group of patients who did not experience the adverse event (controls) for exposure to the potential risk factors. In contrast, in a cohort study, such exposures are compared among all the patients in the involved area during the specified period.

Numerous factors influence the decision to conduct a case-control or cohort study, including statistical and practical considerations. In a cohort study, one can calculate the relative risk, or a quantitative measure of the strength of the association between the exposure and the risk of developing the adverse condition. In contrast, in a case-control study, one can estimate the strength of the association between the exposure and the adverse condition only by calculating an odds ratio; all one can determine is that case patients were more likely to be exposed to the factor than were controls. Adverse conditions with a high attack rate lend themselves to cohort studies, whereas conditions with low attack rates are better evaluated through a case-control study. If the duration of the outbreak is short and the number of patients in the unit during the outbreak is small, it may be feasible to conduct a cohort study. On the other hand, if the duration of the outbreak is long (months or years) and the number of patients in the involved unit(s) is large (e.g., > 100), it may be impractical to conduct a cohort study, and a case-control study may be more realistic. Depending upon the duration of the outbreak, the size of the population at risk, and the extent of the data being obtained from the medical records, a case-control study may take days to weeks, whereas a cohort study may require weeks to months.

Cohort Study

In a cohort study, all patients in the unit or units of interest or undergoing the particular procedure of interest are evaluated for exposures to the variable(s) of interest. Such a study can be conducted either prospectively or retrospectively. Since case-control studies are easier to perform, take less time, and tend to be more powerful, retrospective cohort studies are less frequently undertaken to evaluate nosocomial endemic or epidemic problems. However, if the case-control study data are insufficient to determine the cause of the outbreak and/or the case-control study has narrowed the population at risk, carrying out a prospective cohort study may be useful.

Case-Control Study

In contrast, in a case-control study, the case patients are compared with a similar population without the adverse condition. In a case-control study, selection of the controls is critical. Unless it cannot be avoided, historical controls (i.e., patients present in the unit but in the time period before the outbreak) should not be used. Such patients may not have had the same opportunity for exposure and may not be similar to the population affected. Random selection of patients in the same unit at the same time as the case patients is preferred. If one is concerned that there could be differences in one or more factors influencing the types of exposures of case patients and controls, a small, focused case-control study focusing on these factors can be done before the comprehensive case-control study. For instance, if by examination of the line listing, one becomes concerned that birthweight (e.g., < 1,500 g) and duration of neonatal intensive care unit stay (i.e., > 5 days) influenced the types of exposure of the patients, one can first evaluate these two factors. If they are found to be significantly different between case and control patients, selection of controls could be limited to only those neonates who weighed < 1,500 g and who stayed in the neonatal intensive care unit > 5 days.

There are several other methods to control for such confounding variables—matching, stratification, or multivariate analyses. In matching, one selects controls by matching one or more factors (e.g., birthweight, duration of stay, severity of illness, underlying disease, etc.) with the case patients. It must be realized that such matching factors cannot be evaluated as potential risk factors. Furthermore, the more factors one wishes to match between case and control patients, the more difficult it is to identify controls without reviewing all of their records looking for these factors. It is preferable to randomly select the controls and evaluate the factors under consideration for their strength of association with the adverse condition. Then, if they are found to be statistically significant, they can be controlled for through stratified or multivariate analyses. In contrast, in matched analyses, it is assumed that these factors are significant without assessing whether the assumption is true.

Several important decisions must be made when conducting a case-control study. The first is whether to include all or a sample of the case patients. In general, it is best to include all case patients in order to increase the power of the study and to avoid introduction of bias. Second, one must decide how to select the controls. To enhance the likelihood of determining the source of the outbreak, controls should have similar opportunity for exposure to the potential risk factors as the case patients. In other words, they should be selected from the same population (same ward or unit or undergoing the same procedure) as the case patients and be hospitalized during the same period as the case patients. Third, once the population of potential controls is identified, one must decide how many controls to select for each case patient.

The number of controls selected is based upon statistical power and practical considerations. If the attack rate is high and the number of case patients is large, one control per case patient may be sufficient. If the number of case patients is small (e.g., < 20), one should select two to three controls per case patient. The proportional increase in power associated with selection of more than three controls per case declines markedly, and the proportional increase in power by selecting more than four or five controls usually does not justify the increased volume of work. Last, one must decide how the controls are going to be selected. There are at least two selection methods: random and stratified, or proportional, sampling.

The random selection of controls is the easiest and most widely used method. With this method, all potential controls are listed and then selected using a random numbers table. Random numbers tables can be found in most statistics books and may be generated by numerous statistical software packages. If one has 500 potential controls and wishes to select 50, one just lists the controls in numerical order from 0 to 500 and then generates 50 random numbers between 1 and 500. Alternative random selection methods include choosing every "nth" control from the list of controls or selecting the patient who came before and/or after the admission or surgery of the case patient. The random numbers method is preferred because the other methods may introduce bias—all patients are not admitted to a unit randomly, and in outbreaks associated with surgery, patients at risk may not undergo surgery at night or on weekends.

If one is concerned about the distribution of some factor among the case patients, such as admission to one of several intensive care units or a surgical site infection that affects patients who have undergone a variety of surgical procedures, one may wish to select controls using the proportional, or stratified, method. The more factors one is concerned about, the more difficult and tedious it will be to match these factors. To identify a match, one needs to review the characteristics in the control patients' medical records; this process requires review and discarding of large numbers of controls until the desired factors are identified. In contrast, using the stratified, or proportional, method, controls are placed into categories based upon the variables of concern (e.g., type of surgery, admission into intensive care unit, etc.), and then the proportion of controls desired is randomly selected from each category. For example, if in a surgical site outbreak, 10% of case patients had cardiac surgery, 20% had neurosurgery, 30% had orthopedic surgery, and 40% had general surgery, the controls would be distributed into categories by the type of surgery they had undergone, and then they would be selected from each surgical category in the same proportion as the case patients.

Once the case and control patients are selected, one can compare the exposures of interest. These exposures should be compared statistically using one of the available statistical software packages. If only one risk factor is statistically significantly different between case and control patients, no further epidemiologic analytic studies are necessary. If there are significant differences in two or three risk factors, further analysis using stratification may demonstrate which of these factors is the most important. In addition, if case and control patients differ significantly in two or more factors, multivariate analyses can be performed to identify the independent importance of these factors. For many nosocomial outbreak investigations, numerous risk factors are identified as significant. Because some of these variables are confounding factors, they are highly correlated with the causative risk factors. Multivariate techniques can be used to try to identify the independent importance of the factors found to have significance in univariate analyses. Multivariate techniques require the close cooperation of the epidemiologist and the statistician for appropriate conduct and interpretation.

Observational Studies

Often outbreaks associated with healthcare facilities are the result of failure by healthcare workers to fully comply with current recommendations or policies. Therefore, infection control personnel should observe healthcare workers performing the procedures in question to document the adequacy of their understanding and compliance with infection control recommendations. Observational studies can help generate hypotheses about the cause of the outbreak or they can confirm the findings of the epidemiologic studies. For instance, if the comparative analyses have linked transmission of the etiologic agent to a particular product healthcare worker, observation of this person preparing or manipulating the product may identify how the product was contaminated.

Infection control personnel should review all written policies associated with the practices in question, interview supervisory staff, and identify any changes in the procedures in question before, during, and after the outbreak. Infection control personnel should observe the implicated procedures and/or personnel and directly question the personnel who are performing the implicated procedures. It may be useful to observe staff on all shifts and to distribute a questionnaire asking the healthcare workers about their particular practices. For instance, in questionnaires distributed to healthcare workers, they often claim to wash their hands before and between contacts with patients, but observational studies usually document that such handwashing occurs ~30% of the time [6].

Culture Surveys

Cultures of the environment and personnel should not be performed before the comparative epidemiologic studies are completed. Cultures of the environment may identify the causative agent, but this may represent secondary contamination rather than the source of contamination. Many common nosocomial pathogens, such as gram-negative organisms and fungi, can be isolated from the environment even in the absence of an outbreak. Similarly, a positive culture from a healthcare worker can represent the source of the outbreak but also may represent secondary contamination from the environment, colonized or infected patients, transient carriage, or carriage of the organism independent of the outbreak. Since identification of a healthcare worker carrier may require removal from work, conclusive epidemiologic data identifying a person as associated with transmission in the outbreak is needed to warrant such action. Random culture surveys of products, the environment, or personnel are costly both in materials and time.

Once the comparative epidemiologic studies are completed, cultures should be obtained from the epidemiologically implicated sources (products or personnel). At the same time, several other cultures should be carried out on personnel or products representing controls, to avoid the risk of identifying the product or person before the investigation is completed and appropriate recommendations can be made. The performance of cultures of only those products or personnel who are epidemiologically implicated reduces the number of cultures to be obtained, the personnel resources needed to conduct the cultures (they should not be performed by the implicated person or persons), and the burden on the laboratory. Cultures of nonsterile areas (e.g., floors, sinks, walls) and other animate or inanimate objects that do not have plausible connections to the outbreak, are a waste of valuable resources and may generate uninterpretable data.

If the epidemiologic data identify a source and yet the cultures of the person or product do not disclose the causative agent, one should not abandon the hypothesis. When low-level contamination of a product occurs, it may require cultures of large numbers of the product to pinpoint the contamination. Furthermore, the cultures of the implicated healthcare worker may give negative results if the colonized site is not cultured or if the employee shows positive results only intermittently or has treated him/herself and is no longer culture positive. Infection control personnel should never vindicate a source that has been identified by a well-designed epidemiologic study even in the absence of culture confirmation.

Since the appropriate method of culturing inanimate and animate objects varies, infection control personnel should consult with the microbiologist before such culturing is initiated. For cultures of healthcare workers' hands, the broth hand-wash method is preferred [42]. For water or dialysate used in hemodialysis, the pour-plate or milepore filter method is preferred [43]. For cultures of the environment, where low numbers of organisms are anticipated, use of premoistened swabs and inoculation into nutrient broth may facilitate recovery of the organism. When investigating outbreaks associated with possible airborne transmission, use of settle plates, or air samplers may expedite recovery of the implicated pathogen [15,24,28,29,36].

Typing of the Outbreak Strain

When the outbreak strains are available from the case patients and the environment or implicated personnel or products, it is essential that they be saved for potential future studies. Although outbreaks can be clonal (caused by one strain) or nonclonal (caused by multiple strains of one species), typing of the outbreak strains can be a vital addition to the epidemiologic study. A wide variety of nonmolecular and molecular typing methods is available for many of the pathogens associated with outbreaks in healthcare facilities [31]. The finding of a clonal outbreak increases the likelihood that the outbreak is caused by a contaminated product or colonized healthcare worker, whereas the finding of a nonclonal outbreak increases the likelihood that the pathogen is being transmitted on the hands of healthcare workers from one source (patient or environment) to another patient. For this reason, it may be useful to type some outbreak strains, particularly those that are common to the environment, water, or healthcare worker. Such typing may influence the direction of the comparative studies.

Typing methods include biotyping, antimicrobial susceptibility testing, multilocus enzyme electrophoresis, serotyping, phage typing, and a variety of molecular methods, such as plasmid analysis, restriction endonuclease analysis, chromosomal analysis, ribotyping, restriction fragment length polymorphism, or pulsed-field gel electrophoresis. In general, the molecular methods, in particular, pulsed-field gel electrophoresis, have become the most useful for epidemiologic typing [31]. However, the field of molecular typing is evolving rapidly, and polymerase chain reaction–based pulsed-field gel electrophoresis typing and other methods are proving useful for organisms for which previous nonmolecular or molecular typing methods have been deemed inadequate.

Making Recommendations and Evaluating the Efficacy of the Recommendations

Once the epidemiologic and laboratory studies are completed, one can assess the results and make appropriate recommendations to terminate the outbreak and prevent further transmission. Often, these recommendations are based on existing guidelines. Several outbreak investigations have documented that often transmission stems from failure to fully implement guideline recommendations, not that the guideline recommendations are inadequate [44–49]. Occasionally, the outbreak investigation identifies a practice needing revision or a contaminated product that can be removed. More often, the investigation finds lapses in aseptic technique that require further education of healthcare workers. Thus, it is imperative that once the recommendations are made, follow-up studies be initiated to ensure that there is compliance with the recommendations and that transmission is terminated.

Furthermore, during the investigation one has the opportunity to improve general infection control measures throughout the hospital (even if the outbreak is taking place in only one unit) and to improve methods of documentation of information that would have made the investigation easier. For instance, if, during an investigation of bloodstream infections in intensive care unit patients, it is impossible to determine the dates of central venous catheter insertion and removal, the prospective collection of such data in a standardized manner by intensive care unit staff should be included in the recommendations.

To assure that the outbreak investigation is conducted efficiently and that hospital personnel fully implement the recommendations, hospital administrative personnel should be actively involved in the investigation and follow-up. Infection control personnel should alert hospital administrative staff as soon as the outbreak is detected. Infection control personnel should update administrative staff during the course of the investigation and then review with them the investigation findings and recommendations. Follow-up meetings with administrative staff should review the adequacy of implementation of the recommendations and determine whether the outbreak has been terminated.

For complex outbreaks that involve a variety of services or are causing significant morbidity or mortality, a task force, which should include administrative staff, should be formed at the beginning of the investigation, and this group should be responsible for monitoring the adequacy of implementation of the recommendations and evaluation of their efficacy. The successful conclusion of any investigation of an endemic or epidemic problem is the documentation through follow-up data that the endemic or epidemic problem has been controlled or terminated by the implemented control measures. Any successful investigation requires the close cooperation of a wide variety of people from many hospital departments. It becomes the responsibility of these people to translate the recommendations into action.

If the investigation is conducted in close collaboration with staff members of other departments, they will in turn help with the implementation and monitoring of the recommendations in their departments. To educate and inform those associated with the outbreak or the investigation, it is important that a report be written at the conclusion of the investigation, summarizing the methods used, the results, and the recommendations. This report should be circulated to all those assisting with the study, all the service chiefs or heads of departments where the outbreak took place, and the administrative, risk management, and hospital public relations departments. In this way, all the necessary personnel are informed about the findings and recommendations of the investigative team. Feedback of follow-up data to these departmental staff members will help them improve conditions and practices in their departments. Investigations of endemic or epidemic problems should be viewed as collaborative efforts between the infection control personnel and other departments. With the cooperation of other departments, a successful outcome is enhanced; without it, success is unlikely.

REFERENCES

1. Haley RW, Culver DH, White JW, Morgan WM, Emori TG. The nationwide nosocomial infection rate: a new need for vital statistics. *Am J Epidemiol* 1985;121:159–167.
2. Haley RW, Culver DH, White JW, et al. The efficacy of infection surveillance and control programs in preventing nosocomial infections in U.S. hospitals. *Am J Epidemiol* 1985;121:182–205.
3. Haley RW, White JW, Culver DH, Hughes JM. The financial incentive for hospitals to prevent nosocomial infections under the prospective payment system: an empirical determination from a nationally representative sample. *JAMA* 1987;257:1611–1614.
4. Jarvis WR, Martone WJ. Predominant pathogens in hospital infections. *J Antimicrob Chemother* 1991;28:15–19.
5. National Nosocomial Infections Surveillance (NNIS) Semiannual Report, May 1995: a report from the National Nosocomial Infections Surveillance (NNIS) System. *Am J Infect Control* 1995;23:377–385.
6. Jarvis WR. Handwashing: the Semmelweis lesson forgotten? [Editorial]. *Lancet* 1994;344:1311–1312.
7. Garner J, Jarvis WR, Emori G, Horan TC, Hughes JM. The Centers for Disease Control definitions for nosocomial infections, 1988. *Am J Infect Control* 1988;16:128–140.
8. National Nosocomial Infections Surveillance (NNIS) System. Nosocomial infection rates for interhospital comparison: limitations and possible solutions. *Infect Control Hosp Epidemiol* 1991;12:609–621.
9. Emori TG, Culver DH, Horan TC, et al. National Nosocomial Infections Surveillance System (NNIS): description of methodology and surveillance components. *Am J Infect Control* 1991;19:19–36.

10. Jarvis WR, et al., and the National Nosocomial Infections Surveillance System. Nosocomial infection rates in adult and pediatric intensive care units. *Am J Med* 1991;91:185S–191S.
11. Gaynes RP, et al., and the National Nosocomial Infections Surveillance System. Comparison of rates of nosocomial infections in neonatal intensive care units in the United States. *Am J Med* 1991;91:192S–197S.
12. Culver DH, et al., and the National Nosocomial Infections Surveillance System. Surgical wound infection rates by wound class, operative procedure, and patient risk index. *Am J Med* 1991;91:152S–157S.
13. Haley RW, Culver DH, Morgan WM, et al. Identifying patients at high risk of surgical wound infection: a simple multivariate index of patient susceptibility and wound contamination. *Am J Epidemiol* 1985;121: 206–215.
14. Jarvis WR, and the Epidemiology Branch, Hospital Infections Program. Nosocomial outbreaks: the Centers for Disease Control's Hospital Infections Program experience, 1980–1990. *Am J Med* 1991;9: 3B101S–106S.
15. Richet HM, Craven PC, Brown JM, et al. *Rhodococcus (Gordona) bronchialis* sternal wound infections following coronary artery bypass graft surgery. *N Engl J Med* 1991;324:104–109.
16. Edlin BR, Tokars JI, Grieco MH, et al. An outbreak of multidrug-resistant tuberculosis among hospitalized patients with the acquired immunodeficiency syndrome: epidemiologic studies and restriction fragment length polymorphism analysis. *N Engl J Med* 1992;326:1514–1522.
17. Jarvis WR. Nosocomial transmission of multidrug-resistant *Mycobacterium tuberculosis*. *Res Microbiol* 1993;144:117–122.
18. Shay DK, Maloney SM, Montecalvo M, et al. Epidemiology and mortality of vancomycin-resistant enterococcal bloodstream infections. *J Infect Dis* 1995;172:993–1000.
19. Villarino ME, Stevens L, Schable B, et al. Epidemic *Xanthamonas maltophilia* infections and colonization in an intensive care unit. *Infect Control Hosp Epidemiol* 1992;13:201–206.
20. Tablan OC, Martone WJ, Doershuk CF, et al. Colonization of the respiratory tract with *Pseudomonas cepacia* of patients with cystic fibrosis: risk factors and outcomes. *Chest* 1987;91:527–533.
21. Mangram A, Jarvis WJ. Nosocomial *Burkholderia cepacia* outbreaks and pseudo-outbreaks. *Infect Control Hosp Epidemiol* 1996;17:718–720.
22. Welbel SF, McNeil M. Pramanik A, et al. Nosocomial *Malassezia pachydermitis* bloodstream infections in a neonatal intensive care unit. *Pediatr Infect Dis J* 1994;13:104–109.
23. Chang H, Miller H, Watkins N, et al. *Malassezia pachydermitis* fungemia in neonatal intensive care unit (NICU) patients. *Infect Control Hosp Epidemiol* 1996;17:47 (suppl part 2).
24. Richet HM, McNeil MM, Davis BJ, et al. *Aspergillus fumigatis* sternal wound infection in patients undergoing open-heart surgery. *Am J Epidemiol* 1992;135:48–58.
25. Buffington J, Reporter R, McNeil MM, et al. An outbreak of invasive aspergillosis among hematology and bone marrow transplant patients at a Los Angeles hospital. *J Pediatr Infect Dis* 1994;13:386–393.
26. Beck-Sague CM, Jarvis WR, Brook JP, et al. Epidemic bacteremia due to *Acinetobacter baumanni* in five intensive care units. *Am J Epidemiol* 1990;132:723–733.
27. Archibald LK, Manning ML, Bell LM, et al. Evaluation of the role of the nurse-to-patient ratio in nosocomial infection transmission in pediatric cardiac intensive care unit patients. In: *Abstracts of the 36th Interscience Conference on Antimicrobial Agents and Chemotherapy*, New Orleans, September 15–18, 1996:243.
28. Breiman RD, Fields BS, Sanden G, et al. An outbreak of Legionnaire's disease associated with shower use: possible role of amoebae. *JAMA* 1990;263:924.
29. Mastro TD, Farley TA, Elliot JA, et al. An outbreak of surgical wound infections due to group A *Streptococcus* carried on the scalp. *N Engl J Med* 1990;323:968–972.
30. Cookson ST, Jarvis WR. Nosocomial gastrointestinal infections. In: RP Wenzel, ed. *Prevention and control of nosocomial infections*, 3rd ed. Baltimore, MD: Williams and Wilkins, 1997.
31. Jarvis WR. Usefulness of molecular epidemiology for outbreak investigations. *Infect Control Hosp Epidemiol* 1994;15:500–503.
32. Pertowski CA, Baron RC, Lasker B, Werner SB, Jarvis WR. Nosocomial outbreak of *Candida albicans* sternal wound infection following cardiac surgery. *J Infect Dis* 1995;172:817–823.
33. Jarvis WR, Cookson ST, Robles B. Prevention of nosocomial bloodstream infections: a national and international priority. *Infect Control Hosp Epidemiol* 1996;17:272–275.
34. Tablan OC, Anderson LJ, Arden NH, et al. Guideline for prevention of nosocomial pneumonia. *Respir Care* 1994;39(12):1191–1236.
35. Wong ED, Hooton TM. *Guideline for prevention of catheter-associated urinary tract infections*. Atlanta: Centers for Disease Control and Prevention, 1981.
36. Berkelman RL, Martin D, Graham DR, et al. Streptococcal wound infections caused by a vaginal carrier. *JAMA* 1982;247(19):2680–2682.
37. Garner JS. *Guideline for prevention of surgical wound infections*. Atlanta: Centers for Disease Control and Prevention, 1985.
38. Lowry PW, Blankenship RJ, Gridley W, Troup JN, Tomkins LS. A cluster of legionella sternal-wound infections due to postoperative topical exposure to contaminated tap water. *N Engl J Med* 1991;324:109.
39. Safranek TJ, Jarvis WR, Carson LA, et al. *Mycobacteria chelonae* wound infections after plastic surgery employing contaminated gentian violet skin marking solution. *N Engl J Med* 1987;317:197–201.
40. Nakashima AK, Allen JR, Martone WJ, et al. Epidemic bullous impetigo in a nursery due to a nasal carrier of *Staphylococcus aureus*: role of epidemiology and control measures. *Infect Control* 1984;5(7): 326–331.
41. Haley RW, Culver DH, Morgan WM, White JW, Emori TG, Hooton TM. Increased recognition of infectious diseases in U.S. hospitals through increased use of diagnostic tests, 1970–76. *Am J Epidemiol* 1985;121(2):168–181.
42. Petersen NJ, Collins DE, Marshall JH. A microbiological assay technique for hands. *Health Lab Sci* 1973;10:18–22.
43. Franson MAH, ed. *Standard methods for examination of water and wastewater*, 16th ed. Washington, D.C.: American Public Health Association, 1985.
44. Beck-Sague CM, Dooley SW, Hutton MD, et al. Outbreak of multidrug-resistant tuberculosis among persons with HIV infection in an urban hospital: transmission to staff and patients and control measures. *Am J Med* 1992;268:1280–1286.
45. Edlin BR, Tokars JI, Grieco MH, et al. An outbreak of multidrug-resistant tuberculosis among hospitalized patients with the acquired immunodeficiency syndrome: epidemiologic studies and restriction fragment length polymorphism analysis. *N Engl J Med* 1992;326: 1514–1522.
46. Pearson ML, Jereb JA, Frieden TR, et al. Nosocomial transmission of multidrug-resistant *Mycobacterium tuberculosis*: a risk to hospitalized patients and health-care workers. *Ann Intern Med* 1992;117:191–196.
47. Maloney SM, Pearson M, Gordon M, Del Castillo R, Boyle J, Jarvis WR. Efficacy of control measures in preventing transmission of multidrug-resistant tuberculosis to patients and healthcare workers. *Ann Intern Med* 1995;122:90–95.
48. Wenger P, Otten J, Breeden A, Orfas D, Beck-Sague CM, Jarvis WR. Control of nosocomial transmission of multidrug-resistant *Mycobacterium tuberculosis* among healthcare workers and HIV-infected patients. *Lancet* 1995;345:235–240.
49. Stroud LA, Tokars JI, Grieco MH, et al. Evaluation of infection control measures in preventing the nosocomial transmission of multidrug-resistant *Mycobacterium tuberculosis* in a New York City hospital. *Infect Control Hosp Epidemiol* 1995;16:141–147.

Hospital Infections, Fourth Edition,
edited by John V. Bennett and Philip S. Brachman.
Published by Lippincott–Raven Publishers, Philadelphia, 1998

CHAPTER 7

Statistical Considerations for Analysis of Nosocomial Infection Data

Stanley M. Martin, Brian D. Plikaytis, and Nancy H. Bean

Data that have been collected in a study of nosocomial infections must be reduced from observations on every included patient to summary statistics describing particular groups of patients. While culture results or other information about one or two patients can be important in understanding the cause of infection, information from more patients is needed to determine which of several potentially important factors contributed to the infection. A transition must be made from clinical diagnosis of illness in a single patient to understanding illness in populations of patients in the study of nosocomial infections; the physician's diagnosis of illness in single patients must give way to the "statistical diagnosis" of illness in the group of patients.

This chapter describes basic statistical considerations for understanding nosocomial infection data from the collection phase through interpretation. Several study design considerations are presented as reminders of necessary precursors of a good study. Among them, control group selection by either an independent or matched procedure influences which statistical test should be used in the analysis. Emphasis is placed on data collection procedures because of the need for careful definition of data to be gathered and as much standardization of the collection process as possible. Finally, a scheme for choosing appropriate significance tests is presented.

S.M. Martin, B.D. Plikaytis: Biostatistics and Information Management Branch, Division of Bacterial and Mycotic Diseases, National Center for Infectious Diseases

N.H. Bean: Surveillance and Epidemic Investigations Section, Division of Bacterial and Mycotic Diseases, Centers for Disease Control and Prevention, Atlanta, Georgia 30333.

DATA COLLECTION

In many epidemiologic studies, the inability of investigators to reach conclusions can be attributed to the collection of data with little or no previous planning of the objectives of the study, the failure to gather data relevant to the objectives, the lack of a defined population for study, failure to identify the best locations in the hospital in which to find the data, the absence of understanding about who will record the data, and improper selection of the period to be covered. In the investigation of possible outbreaks of a particular infection type, the investigator should also consider whether it is necessary to extend the scope of investigation beyond the inpatient population of the hospital to the outpatient department, beyond the primary hospital of interest to other hospitals of a similar type or in the same location, or beyond hospitals to the community.

Studies of nosocomial infections previously have involved the collection of data from personal interviews, examinations of patients, patients' chart reviews, laboratory records, personnel health clinic records, or autopsy reports. These sources of data, singly or in combination, continue to provide reliable information for many hospitals. However, the proliferation of computing equipment in the management of patient-related data in hospitals offers a source of more easily obtainable data for investigating nosocomial infections. The investigator of nosocomial infections should learn about the administrative processes within the hospital that can generate useful "machine readable" records of patients. For example, admissions office personnel may enter demographic data and admitting diagnoses on all patients via a computer terminal or keypunched record. Other hospital locations, such as the pharmacy and various laboratories, may generate additional records that arrive in the central computer area for the same patients. Medical procedures, operations, diagnoses, and costs may be entered into the computer system from still other sources, possibly for billing purposes; discharge diagnoses and other information may be recorded as well.

These records can be a valuable resource in hospitals with well-planned computer systems and local area networks. They can be made available with relatively little work beyond determining from administrative personnel, the accounting office, laboratories, and pharmacy which data are part of the hospital computer system and from the computer center how to gain access to the needed data. Preliminary inquiries of this kind can offer the potential for larger and better-controlled studies because of less cost and time spent in the data collection phase.

CONTROL GROUPS

Little information about the association of any factor that may predispose a patient to infection can be gained by studying only a group of patients who have been exposed to the factor. Similarly, studying only cases is descriptive but may not lead to assessment of risks associated with a factor. For example, an attempt to study the association of excisional surgical wound infections caused by *Staphylococcus aureus* with operations by a particular surgeon will be of limited benefit unless a suitable comparison group is also studied. The surgeon performing the operation may be only one of several factors that can potentially influence the risk of incisional infections. Therefore, a suitable control group should include patients receiving the same operation from another surgeon or patients receiving the operation from any of the entire surgical staff performing operations in the hospital other than the suspect surgeon. The control group should include patients expected to be like the infected group with respect to all known possible risk factors except for the surgeon performing the operation. Differences in infection rates between the control group and the group receiving the operation from the suspect surgeon could then be associated with this surgeon.

Studies of this kind can be successfully controlled within a hospital because both exposed and nonexposed patients are present. However, the study of association of infection with the use of a particular, possibly contaminated, product or apparatus may require a multi-hospital study or an intervention study within a single hospital. It would be impossible to study the association of pneumonia with cleaning techniques of respiratory therapy equipment within a single hospital if the hospital's policy dictates one particular cleaning technique for all such apparatus. No control group would be available in this situation, unless, for purposes of the study, the policy could be changed for at least a portion of the equipment. Intervention in the hospital policy regarding the cleaning of respiratory therapy equipment would allow the investigator to design a study to compare pneumonia rates between a group of patients using respiratory therapy equipment cleaned in the usual way and a group of patients using the same type of equipment during the same period but cleaned by a different technique. Of course, intervention studies of this kind must be preceded by careful attention to ethical concerns for the welfare of the patient.

Even though patients can be stratified into groups according to exposure or nonexposure to the factor under consideration, comparability of the patients included in each group must be ensured. The underlying risks of patients of acquiring the infection under study can differ drastically even without considering exposure to a single factor. For example, patients with a particular condition may be immunosuppressed and more susceptible to infection. Other factors, such as catheterization and exposure to respiratory therapy equipment, prophylactic or therapeutic antibiotics, and intravenous fluids, can predispose patients to a greater risk of infection. A well-designed study will attempt to balance the patients in the control and study groups with respect to such known factors, which may require that control patients be matched to the study patients on these factors. The objective, whether control patients are selected by an independent selection process or matched to the study patients, is to remove the effect of underlying factors that might mask or exaggerate the effect of a particular factor under study.

Multi-hospital studies require more than a single study hospital and a single control hospital. Generally, it is not reasonable to expect many of the same potentially important, but not necessarily obvious, factors to exist in any two hospitals. Studies involving more than one hospital must include adequate numbers of hospitals in both the study group and the control group. Factors such as number of beds, hospital policies, ratio of staff to patients, patients' characteristics, numbers of discharges, and hospital type must be considered in selecting suitable study and control groups of hospitals. The scope of this chapter is limited to studies within a single hospital to avoid lengthy discussions of the sampling problems and other statistical concerns accompanying multi-hospital studies.

SUMMARY STATISTICS

When confronted with pages of written observations on infected and noninfected patients, little can be learned about the association between infection and a factor under study until an appropriate summary statistic is found to describe a "typical" value of the factor for the whole group. For example, the proportion of patients who became infected shortly after urinary catheterization can be compared with the proportion of a similar group of patients who were not catheterized and became infected. The proportion summarizes the infection experience in each of the two groups, catheterized and noncatheterized patients. It relates the number of infected patients to the total number at risk of becoming infected in the two groups. The at-risk population usually includes all patients exposed to a factor or combination of factors. It can encompass all patients admitted or discharged (e.g., exposed to the hospital or a particular service) during a particular period, only patients with a particular condition, or only patients who underwent a particular procedure or received a specific drug.

The actual number of patients at risk may be the best available denominator; however, some investigators can measure the at-risk portion of the summary statistic in terms of the duration of each patient's exposure to risk. This can be the number of days hospitalized, number of hours with inserted catheter, or other time of exposure. If the numerator represents the number of patients with a particular infection, the investigator should subtract from the at-risk period in the denominator the total time patients were exposed after they were infected, since, for purposes of the study, exposure while a patient is infected contributes no additional risk. However, this additional exposure should be included in the denominator if the numerator represents the number of episodes of infection for each patient.

The numerator of the summary statistic also can be formed in different ways. A single patient may experience more than one infection episode due to the same organism. In this case, one must decide whether these patients have had a recurrence of infection from the initial organism or a reinfection with the same organism. If several infections occur, the summary statistic can be a count of the total number of infections relative to the total number of patients for whom the numerator was counted. This statistic would be the average number of infections per patient. Decisions about the association of a particular factor with infection can usually be made using the number of infected patients for the numerator and the number of patients at risk (or patient-time exposure) for the denominator.

STUDY DESIGN

Proportions or other summary statistics are obtained to decide whether hospitalized patients exposed to the factor under consideration are at higher risk of infection than patients who are not exposed to the factor. A significance test is used to determine the probability that a difference as large as the observed difference between the two proportions could have occurred by chance. A small probability of chance occurrence of a difference as large as the observed difference leads the observer to conclude that patients exposed to the factor are likely to be at higher risk of infection. The question then becomes, How small should the probability be so that a conclusion associating infection with the factor is correct? In fact there are two probabilities of primary concern in significance testing [1], which can be stated as questions for the investigator of nosocomial infections.

Type 1: Given that there actually is no difference between the proportion of patients infected among those exposed to the factor and the proportion of patients infected among those not exposed to the factor, what is the probability that the particular samples of patients observed in this study would indicate a difference by chance?

Type 2: Given that there actually is a difference between the proportion of patients infected among those exposed to the factor and the proportion of patients infected among those not exposed to the factor, what is the probability that the particular samples of patients observed in this study would indicate no difference by chance?

These two probabilities of error form the basis for decisions made from significance tests and are determined by the investigator in the planning stage of the study. A summary of the major steps leading to significance testing for the difference between proportions is presented. All these should be considered in planning studies of nosocomial infections.

State Hypothesis to Be Tested and Alternative Hypothesis

As an example, the hypothesis (H) that there is no difference between the proportions versus the hypothesis that there is a difference between the proportions (the alternative hypothesis [AH]) can be written as H_0: $P_E = P_{NE}$ and AH: $P_E \neq P_{NE}$, where P_E and P_{NE} are the proportions infected in the exposed and nonexposed groups, respectively. H_0, the null hypothesis, states that the proportion infected in the exposed group is the same as the proportion infected in the nonexposed group. The alternative hypothesis states that the proportion infected in the exposed group is not the same as the proportion infected in the nonexposed group. Because the alternative hypothesis does not state the direction of the difference (and would be favored whether P_E were significantly greater than or significantly less than P_{NE}), significance tests used to test these hypotheses must consider differences in both directions.

These are called two-tailed tests and are generally useful when the investigator does not know before the data are collected whether to expect exposure to the factor to increase or diminish the patients' risk of infection. When the investigator has reason to believe that exposure to the factor would raise (or lower) the patients' risk of infection, a one-tailed test should be used. The hypotheses may be stated as H0: $P_E \leq P_{NE}$ and AH: $P_E > P_{NE}$.

In this case, the null hypothesis states that P_E is less than or equal to P_{NE}, whereas the alternative hypothesis states that P_E is > P_{NE}. This is a directional difference because the investigator expects exposure to increase the patients' risk of infection, if a difference exists at all. Considering the purpose of studies of infection outbreaks within the hospital, one must conclude that one-tailed tests of significance are generally appropriate.

State Desired Probability Levels for Type 1 and Type 2 Errors

These probabilities are not based on statistical computations but on the investigator's willingness to chance an error of either kind. Stating the type 2 error indirectly expresses another probability that is also important in determining how likely the study is to succeed. This probability, defined by $p = (1 - \text{type 2 error})$, is called the power of the test and p is the probability that if a difference actually exists (i.e., the alternative hypothesis is true), the significance test will reject the null hypothesis in favor of the alternative hypothesis. The power of the test is used in initial planning of the study to ensure an adequate study size to achieve the objectives.

Determine Study Design to Achieve Desired Objective

A primary consideration in study design is that of deciding whether the study and control groups should be selected independently or patients selected for the control group should be matched on certain variables to patients in the study group. That is, for each study patient, one or more control patients could be selected to match the study patient on factors determined ahead of time. Many studies of nosocomial infections have required that patients be matched for validity on factors such as age, sex, underlying conditions, and predisposing therapeutic factors. In outbreak investigations, it may not be possible to know the specific factors that should be studied; therefore, the study population may consist of all patients who were infected, and the control population may include patients who were like the infected patients but were not infected. The proportion exposed to particular factors would then be determined from samples of each of these two populations. Whether patients are matched or unmatched, most studies of nosocomial infection outbreaks use comparisons of these proportions. The single-direction hypotheses would be written as H_0: $P_I \leq P_{NI}$ and AH: $P_I > P_{NI}$, where P_I and P_{NI} are the proportions exposed to the factor under study in the infected and noninfected groups of patients, respectively.

Study design must include consideration of study size, which should be based on the requirements to test certain hypotheses or estimate certain parameters and to achieve predetermined error probability levels. Sometimes the size of the study is limited by the time or resources available. In this case, it should be understood that a low-power or large type 2 error may be associated with the study because inadequate sample sizes are used, and a decision must be made about the value of doing the study under these circumstances. Approaches to determining sample size requirements for testing the difference between two proportions often call for approximation formulas that can be programmed relatively easily [2].

Plan Data Collection Procedures and Train Data Collectors

A main consideration in planning the study is the choice of personnel to collect the data. Deciding whether a patient is infected requires a level of medical knowledge that may be beyond that of a secretary or clerical person. Regardless of who the data collectors are, they must be given standard procedures for deciding about each data item, such as the case definition. Some verification of the data collection process should be planned to avoid such problems as drifting away from established procedures, misunderstanding procedures, inability to follow procedures, and random errors.

Too often inadequate attention is given to quality of data collection because data checking and editing require extra effort for the investigator. Often it is tempting to assume good data quality when the data are collected as computer records. Without close scrutiny, computer summary tables and statistics based on incorrect data entries can appear as if they were valid because the formatting of computer output is often independent of the data quality. When this happens, the study can become the victim of poor or misleading data instead of contributing valuable information for control of nosocomial infections. Decisions about data handling must be planned in advance to avoid delays. If computer records are used, coordination with a programmer or other computer personnel is necessary before the study begins.

Collect Data and Begin Data Processing

One early consideration in study design is the data collection instrument. Designing the form with the intention to use present computer technology requires knowledge of computer input and coding schemes. A common tendency is to ask for too much data on a form, but a well-planned study will pare down the questionnaire to include only the important questions. Simplicity for understanding, recording, and tabulating data is the key to a successful data collection document. Data processing may involve no more than hand tabulation, but it can require detailed computer programs for sophisticated analyses. Realizing beforehand that a substantial amount of the time of nursing staff or other personnel may be needed in both the collection and processing phases, and planning ahead, can avoid overburdening these people at what may be an inopportune time.

Perform Analysis and Report Results

A common error made by an investigator heading a study is to spend unlimited effort collecting data but to allow only a very short time for the analysis. However, analyses must take into account all the design considerations, hypotheses to be tested, and level of measurement of the data. Enough analysis time should be allocated to understanding thoroughly what the data indicate. Simply summarizing findings with p values is usually an indication that the data have not been thoroughly analyzed. Studies planned to meet some types of objectives can begin with examination of the stated hypotheses, followed by determination of other features of the data that support the conclusions. However, the analysis of data from nosocomial infection outbreaks might require a different approach.

Usually there is not a single hypothesis to be tested, and the study objective for infection outbreak data is to determine which factors increase the patients' risk of infection. One approach is to test several factors, looking for an association of any factor with infection. When this procedure is used and the seemingly important factors tested, attention must be paid to the effect of multiple significance testing on the overall type 1 error. One way to compensate for several significance tests is to set the type 1 error probability for each test low enough to yield a specified type 1 error over all tests. For example, if it is desired to perform k tests with an overall type 1 error of α, then the type 1 error for each test could be set approximately to $A = \alpha/k$, where A is the approximate significance level for each test [3].

Significance Testing

Before presenting directions for choosing a significance test for a particular study, it is necessary to mention briefly two statistical terms. Significance tests can be separated into two categories—*parametric* and *nonparametric*. Use of parametric statistics calls for making assumptions about the parent population from which the study samples were drawn. For example, observations of urine output volume on a sample of infected patients could be assumed to have come from a population of urine output volumes that were normally distributed around a mean, μ, and variance, σ^2. Because the assumption is made that these values are normally distributed, the significance testing procedure involves a parametric test. On the other hand, if one is not willing to make assumptions about the parameters of the parent distribution, one may choose a nonparametric test.

The parametric test is usually preferred as long as it is reasonable to make the assumptions for it, because there is an associated gain in power. Although the loss of power accompanying the use of a nonparametric test can be substantial, some of the nonparametric tests actually offer power comparable to parametric tests. When both parametric and nonparametric tests are presented in this chapter, the power of the nonparametric test is reasonably close to that of the corresponding parametric test; the tests mentioned here are commonly used in the analysis of nosocomial infection data.

In addition to consideration of the hypotheses and study design, the decision about which of the many statistical tests to use requires consideration of the level of measurement of the observations. For the sake of simplicity, the discussion in this chapter of level of measurement will be limited to two classifications, attributes and measurements. Usually, data collected on nosocomial infections comprise answers to the following questions. Was the patient infected or not infected? Was the patient exposed or not exposed? Was the change in a measurement positive or negative? The attribute responses yes or no, plus or minus, and zero or one simply give the direction of differences, whereas the measurement data height, weight, and blood sugar level give the direction and magnitude of the differences. The scheme shown in Figure 7-1 for selecting an appropriate test takes into account the issues just mentioned and should help the investigator choose a significance test by making three simple choices [4]. This scheme uses a partial list of tests and is not intended to limit broader choices that are available [5].

Two sets of data are used to illustrate the test procedures listed in Figure 7-1. First, assuming that the samples were selected independently, the tests listed for independent samples are illustrated. Next the tests listed for matched samples are depicted, using the assumption that the same samples were selected with control (noninfected) patients matched to study (infected) patients.

Example 1: Attribute Data

Suppose 100 patients on the general medicine service acquired *Escherichia coli* urinary tract infections during a 6-month period. A sample of 30 of these patients is randomly selected to determine whether the infection is associated with urinary catheterization. A control group of 30 noninfected patients is selected from among all other patients on the general medicine service during the same 6-month period. The status of patients in each group with respect to catheterization is presented in Table 7-1.

Example 2: Measurement Data

Suppose times from admission to onset of *E. coli* urinary tract infection for the 30 infected patients and times from admission to discharge of the 30 noninfected patients from example 1 are studied, to determine whether infection occurred at about the time the patients who were infected would have been discharged if they had not been infected. The time in hours for each patient is given in Table 7-2.

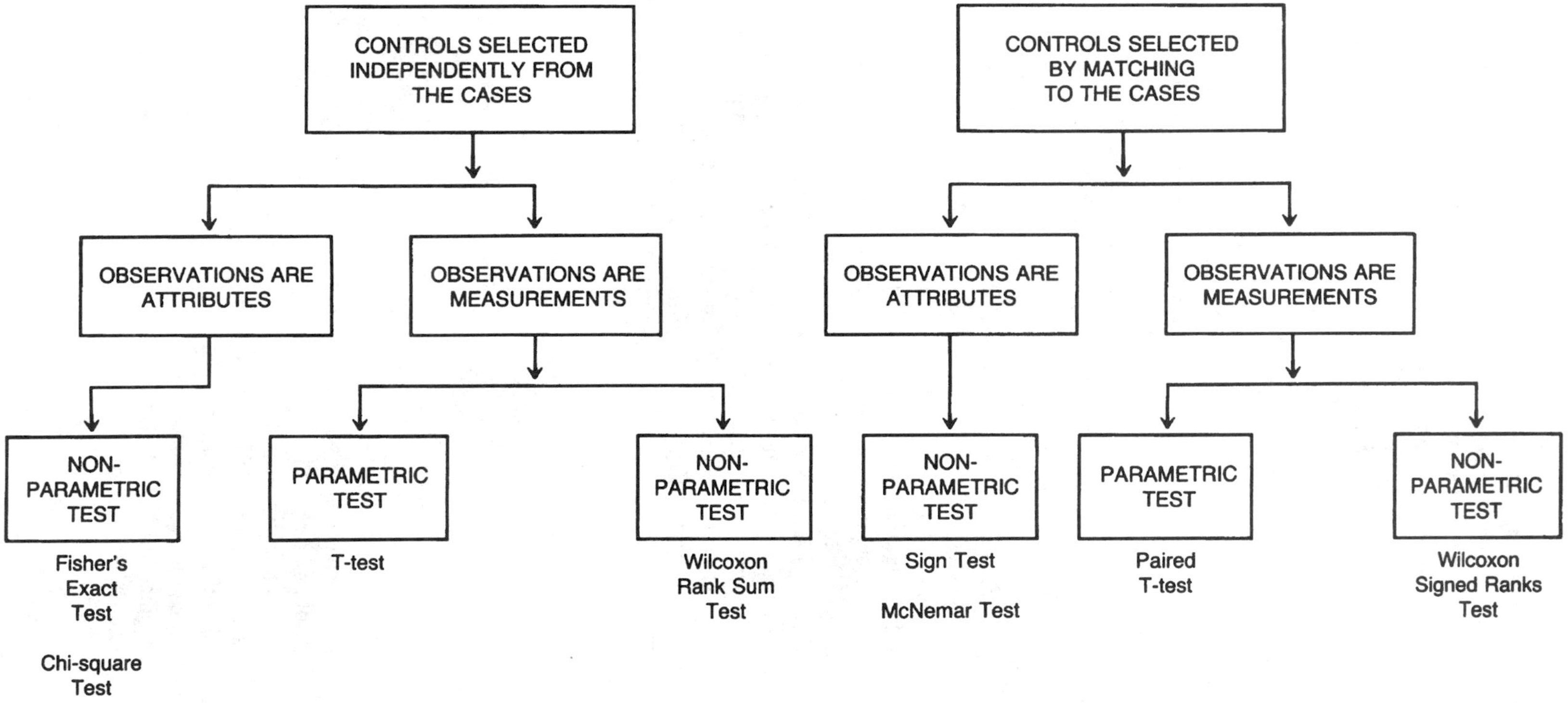

FIGURE 7-1. Scheme for selecting an appropriate significance test. (Reprinted with permission from Martin SM. Choosing the correct statistical tests. In: Wenzel RP, ed. *Handbook of hospital-acquired infections.* Boca Raton, FL: CRC Press, 1981.)

TABLE 7-1. *Catheterization status of patients on general medicine service (example 1)*

Infected patients						Noninfected patients					
Pt. #	Cath.	No cath.	Pt. #	Cath.	No cath.	Pt. #	Cath.	No cath.	Pt. #	Cath.	No cath.
1	X		16	X		1		X	16		X
2	X		17	X		2		X	17		X
3	X		18	X		3		X	18		X
4		X	19	X		4	X		19		X
5	X		20	X		5		X	20	X	
6		X	21	X		6		X	21		X
7		X	22	X		7		X	22		X
8		X	23		X	8		X	23		X
9	X		24	X		9		X	24		X
10	X		25		X	10		X	25	X	
11	X		26	X		11		X	26		X
12		X	27	X		12	X		27		X
13	X		28	X		13		X	28		X
14		X	29	X		14		X	29		X
15	X		30	X		15	X		30		X

Pt. #, patient number; Cath., catheterization.

These examples are used first to illustrate the tests employed when the samples of infected and noninfected persons are independently selected. Since studies of nosocomial infection outbreaks usually use one-tailed tests, the tests illustrated here, except for the chi-square tests, are one-tailed. The observations from example 1 can be summarized into a 2 × 2 table to determine whether there is an association of catheters with infection. A high proportion (22/30) of infected patients and a low proportion (5/30) of noninfected patients were catheterized (Table 7-3). The purpose of the significance test of these data is to determine whether the proportion catheterized was significantly larger among infected patients (P_I) than among noninfected patients (P_{NI}). The single-direction hypotheses can be stated as $H_0 = P_I \leq P_{NI}$ and AH: $P_I > P_{NI}$.

Fisher's Exact Test

Fisher's Exact Test [6] computes the probability of occurrence of the observed arrangement of the data in Table 7-3 plus the probability of occurrence of all other arrangements more divergent than the observed data in the direction of the alternative hypothesis, subject to the condition that all marginal totals of the tables remain fixed. The formula for computing the test probability for each derived table can be stated in terms of the cell val-

TABLE 7-2. *Intervals of exposure to the hospital for infected and noninfected patients (example 2)*

Time (in hours) from admission to onset of infection (infected patients)				Time (in hours) from admission to discharge (noninfected patients)			
Pt. #	Hr	Pt. #	Hr	Pt. #	Hr	Pt. #	Hr
1	216	16	234	1	253	16	242
2	187	17	205	2	82	17	233
3	88	18	136	3	125	18	133
4	280	19	253	4	138	19	342
5	310	20	165	5	137	20	102
6	239	21	340	6	116	21	93
7	344	22	325	7	232	22	82
8	315	23	178	8	327	23	248
9	280	24	153	9	171	24	113
10.	293	25	355	10	338	25	294
11	200	26	338	11	335	26	304
12	229	27	77	12	109	27	211
13	208	28	335	13	126	28	104
14	233	29	261	14	182	29	261
15	190	30	93	15	247	30	269

Pt. #, patient number.

TABLE 7-3. *Catheterization status of infected and noninfected patients (example 1)*

	Infected	Noninfected	Total
Catheter	22	5	27
No catheter	8	25	33
Total	30	30	60

TABLE 7-4. *General table for summarizing the association of a factor with infection*

	Infected	Noninfected	Total
Catheter	a	b	$a + b$
No catheter	c	d	$c + d$
Total	$a + c$	$b + d$	n

ues given in Table 7-4. The probability of the observed arrangement for each table is computed by the following equation:

$$p_k = \frac{(a+b)!\ (c+d)!\ (a+c)!\ (b+d)!}{a!\ b!\ c!\ d!\ n!}$$

where $p_k = 0$ is the probability computed for the observed table, $p_k = 1$ is the probability computed for the next most divergent table, and so on, until the probabilities for all such tables are computed. The next most divergent tables can be generated easily by successively adding 1 to the a and d cells while subtracting 1 from the b and c cells, when the data are arranged as shown in Table 7-4. Note that this procedure leaves the marginal totals unchanged, a requirement for this test. The probability is computed for each successive table, and the final probability is determined by summing them.

$$p_0 = \frac{27!\ 33!\ 30!\ 30!}{22!\ 5!\ 8!\ 25!\ 60!} = 0.0000094776297$$

$$p_1 = \frac{27!\ 33!\ 30!\ 30!}{23!\ 4!\ 7!\ 26!\ 60!} = 0.0000006339551$$

$$p_2 = \frac{27!\ 33!\ 30!\ 30!}{24!\ 3!\ 6!\ 27!\ 60!} = 0.0000000273931$$

$$p_3 = \frac{27!\ 33!\ 30!\ 30!}{25!\ 2!\ 5!\ 28!\ 60!} = 0.0000000007044$$

$$p_4 = \frac{27!\ 33!\ 30!\ 30!}{26!\ 1!\ 4!\ 29!\ 60!} = 0.0000000000093$$

$$p_5 = \frac{27!\ 33!\ 30!\ 30!}{27!\ 0!\ 3!\ 30!\ 60!} = 0.0000000000013$$

$$p_{\text{Tot}} = 0.00001014.$$

Because the total probability ($p_{\text{Tot}} = 0.00001014$) is small ($< 0.05$), the conclusion is that there is an increased risk of *E. coli* infection among catheterized patients in this hospital.

It is important to note that the two-tailed probability for testing the hypothesis—H_0: $P_I = P_{NI}$ and AH: $P_I \neq P_{NI}$—can be computed by repeating the computations for the opposite direction, thus determining the appropriate tables for the other tail of the test. This is accomplished by determining the probabilities for tables for which the proportion of catheterized patients is lower in the infected group than in the noninfected group subject to the condition that the marginal totals remain fixed (i.e., the total numbers of infected and noninfected patients is kept constant). Then the second tail of the test is computed by summing the probabilities for all tables in the second direction that have probabilities less than or equal to the probability for the observed table. The probability for the two-tailed test would then be found by summing the probabilities for each of the two tails. When the number of infected patients sampled, n_I, is equal to the number of noninfected patients sampled, n_{NI}, simply doubling the probability for one tail will produce the two-tailed probability [7].

Chi-Square Test for Independent Samples

Computations for the Fisher's Exact Test are tedious without the assistance of a programmable calculator or computer. The chi-square test is a suitable approximation when the expected cell frequencies of the 2×2 table are sufficiently large. Some authors [2] have recommended that the approximation is inadequate if the total sample size, $n = n_I - n_{NI}$, is < 20 or if the total sample size is between 20 and 40 with one or more expected cell frequencies as small as 5. Chi-square is a test of independence of the factor and infection or, equivalently, a test of the hypotheses H_0: $P_I = P_{NI}$ and AH: $P_I \neq P_{NI}$. A simple computational formula makes this test easy to compute:

$$\chi^2 = \frac{(n) \times \left(|ad - bc| - \frac{n_I + n_{NI}}{2} \right)^2}{(a+b)\ (c+d)\ (a+c)\ (b+d)}$$

$$= \frac{(60) \times \left(|22 \times 25 - 8 \times 5| - \frac{60}{2} \right)^2}{27 \times 33 \times 30 \times 30}$$

$$= \frac{13{,}824{,}000}{801{,}900}$$

$$= 17.239.$$

This value is greater than the tabulated value of the chi-square distribution (readily available in standard statistical tables), corresponding to a significance level (type 1 error) of 0.05 ($\chi^2 = 3.84$). Therefore, the test leads to the conclusion that $P_I \neq P_{NI}$, or that infection is not independent of catheterization.

Student's t *Test*

Example 2 will be used to illustrate two tests for measurement data. The assumption that time intervals were sampled from a normal distribution of time intervals permits use of the Student's t test. This is a parametric test of the difference between two means from independent samples. The hypotheses can be written as follows: H_0: $\mu_I \leq \mu_{NI}$ and AH: $\mu_I > \mu_{NI}$, where μ_I and μ_{NI} are the means of time intervals for the infected and noninfected populations, respectively, from which the samples were drawn. The definitions of symbols used in the formula for the t test are given here and are more completely discussed elsewhere [8]. x_{I_i} equals one time interval measured for the ith selected infected patient, x_{NI_i} equals one time interval measured for the ith selected noninfected patient, n_I equals the number of infected patients selected, and n_{NI} equals the number of noninfected patients selected.

The mean interval from the sample of infected patients is calculated as

$$\bar{x}_I = \frac{\sum_{i=1}^{n_I} x_{I_i}}{n_I}.$$

The mean interval from the sample of noninfected patients is calculated as

$$\bar{x}_{NI} = \frac{\sum_{i=1}^{n_{NI}} x_{NI_i}}{n_{NI}}.$$

The variance estimate from the sample of infected patients is calculated as

$$s^2_I = \frac{\sum_{i=1}^{n_I} (x_{I_i} - \bar{x}_I)^2}{n_I - 1} = \frac{\sum_{i=1}^{n_I} x^2_{I_i} - \frac{\left(\sum_{i=1}^{n_I} x_{I_i}\right)^2}{n_I}}{n_I - 1}.$$

The variance estimate from the sample of noninfected patients is calculated as

$$s^2_{NI} = \frac{\sum_{i=1}^{n_{NI}} (x_{NI_i} - \bar{x}_{NI})^2}{n_{NI} - 1} = \frac{\sum_{i=1}^{n_{NI}} x^2_{NI_i} - \frac{\left(\sum_{i=1}^{n_{NI}} x_{NI_i}\right)^2}{n_{NI}}}{n_{NI} - 1}.$$

The variance of the difference between sample means is calculated as

$$s^2_{(\bar{x}_I - \bar{x}_{NI})} = \frac{(n_I - 1)\, s^2_I + (n_{NI} - 1)\, s^2_{NI}}{(n_I + n_{NI} - 2)} \times \left(\frac{1}{n_I} + \frac{1}{n_{NI}}\right).$$

The t statistic is calculated as

$$t = \frac{\bar{x}_I - \bar{x}_{NI}}{s_{(\bar{x}_I - \bar{x}_{NI})}}.$$

These values for the data of example 2 (Table 7-2) are

$$\bar{x}_I = \frac{7{,}060}{30} = 235.33$$

$$\bar{x}_{NI} = \frac{5{,}949}{30} = 198.30$$

$$s^2_I = \frac{1{,}846{,}916 - \frac{7{,}060^2}{30}}{30 - 1} = 6{,}395.2644$$

$$s^2_{NI} = \frac{1{,}398{,}207 - \frac{5{,}949^2}{30}}{30 - 1} = 7{,}535.1828$$

$$s^2_{(\bar{x}_I - \bar{x}_{NI})} = \frac{(29)\,(6{,}395.2644) + (29)\,(7{,}535.1828)}{58} \times \frac{1}{30} + \frac{1}{30}$$

$$= 464.3482$$

$$t = \frac{235.33 - 198.30}{21.5487} = 1.718.$$

A comparison of this computed value of t with tabulated values of the t distribution ($n_I + n_{NI} - 2$ degrees of freedom) reveals that the probability of a chance occurrence of the observed data is < 0.05, the value often used as a criterion for judging significance. Therefore, the null hypothesis is rejected, and the mean time from admission to onset of infection in the infected group is considered significantly greater than the mean time from admission to discharge in the noninfected group.

If, on the other hand, the investigator decides it is unreasonable to assume that the samples were drawn from normally distributed populations, a nonparametric test can be chosen to test the difference between the means. In the following section, the data from example 2 are used without the normality assumption, to demonstrate a nonparametric test for comparing two sample means, again assuming that the samples were independently selected.

Wilcoxon Rank Sum Test

This test procedure begins by ranking the individual observations of numbers of hours from 1 to n ($n = n_I + n_{NI}$), with the least number of hours receiving a rank of 1. The ranks are assigned without regard for the sample from which the observations are drawn. When the original values are tied, equal ranks are assigned as the average of the ranks that would have been assigned to the tied observations if they had not been tied. One of several ties in the example occurred between the time intervals for infected patient 19 and noninfected patient 1 (Tables 7-2 and 7-5). Each of these patients was assigned a rank of 39.5, the average of the next two ranks that would have been assigned if they had not been tied. The ranking (Table 7-5) begins with the assignment of rank 1 to infected patient 27 and ends with the assignment of rank 60 to infected patient 25.

After the ranking is completed, the ranks are separated into two groups corresponding to the original samples (Table 7-5). The sum of ranks for the sample having the fewer number of observations is obtained. Since, in this example, the number of observations is the same for both the infected and noninfected groups, the sum of the ranks of either can be used.

The sums of ranks for the infected and noninfected groups are 1,070 and 812, respectively. Referring to the tables for the Wilcoxon Rank Sum Test [9,10] for a one-tailed probability at $p = 0.05$, the upper boundary is 1,027. Since the sum of ranks for this example is > 1,027, the investigator would conclude that the average time from admission to onset for infected patients is significantly longer than the time from admission to discharge of noninfected patients.

In the design of a study of nosocomial infections, it is usually necessary to match the controls (noninfected patients) to the infected patients. It is difficult to interpret conclusions about the association of factors with nosocomial infection when controls and study groups are selected independently. If the groups are independent, as in the previous examples, no information is available to allow the investigator to determine whether infected patients really had onset of infection at approximately the same time as noninfected patients were being discharged.

If the noninfected patients generally were admitted with more serious underlying illnesses than the infected patients, their lengths of stay in the hospital could have been prolonged, on average, longer than their lengths of stay had they been admitted with illnesses comparable to those of the infected patients. The time from admission to onset of infection could have appeared, from the data, to be nearly the same as the interval from admission to discharge of noninfected patients, yet in truth the time could have exceeded the admission-to-discharge interval. In this case, the investigator might overlook an important feature of the observations under study, that is, that infections were occurring after prolonged stay beyond the usual length of stay for patients with underlying illnesses like those of the infected group. Matching the noninfected patients to the infected patients on such important variables can avoid this problem.

If we discard the assumption that the samples from examples 1 and 2 were independent and assume that patients in the noninfected group were matched to patients in the infected group on the basis of day of admission, underlying condition, age, and sex, then a new group of tests can be introduced (Figure 7-1). Although these examples illustrate the situation for one-to-one matching of controls to cases only, testing procedures are available for situations in which a variable number of controls is matched to cases [11].

First, two tests for attribute data from matched samples are illustrated using example 1. The data from example 1 must be summarized and tested differently if the patients are matched [12]; the arrangements of Tables 7-3 and 7-4 are for the unmatched situation. Infected-noninfected pairs rather than individual patients are counted in the 2 × 2 table for matched studies (Table 7-6).

TABLE 7-5. *Intervals and ranks for infected and noninfected patients (example 2)*

Ranks and time (in hours) from admission to onset of infection (infected patients)						Ranks and time (in hours) from admission to discharge (noninfected patients)					
Pt. #	Hr	Rank	Pt. #	Hr	Rank	Pt. #	Hr	Rank	Pt. #	Hr	Rank
1	216	29	16	234	34	1	253	39.5	16	242	36
2	187	23	17	205	26	2	82	2.5	17	233	32.5
3	88	4	18	136	15	3	125	12	18	133	14
4	280	44.5	19	253	39.5	4	138	19	19	342	58
5	310	49	20	165	19	5	137	16	20	102	7
6	239	35	21	340	57	6	116	11	21	93	5.5
7	344	59	22	325	51	7	232	31	22	82	2.5
8	315	50	23	178	21	8	327	52	23	248	38
9	280	44.5	24	153	18	9	171	20	24	113	10
10	293	46	25	355	60	10	338	55.5	25	294	47
11	200	25	26	338	55.5	11	335	53.5	26	304	48
12	229	30	27	77	1	12	109	9	27	211	28
13	208	27	28	335	53.5	13	126	13	28	104	8
14	233	32.5	29	261	41.5	14	182	22	29	261	41.5
15	190	24	30	93	55.5	15	247	37	30	269	43

Pt. #, patient number.

TABLE 7-6. *General table for summarizing the association of a factor with infection-matched data*

		Infected		
		Catheter	No Catheter	Total
Noninfected	Catheter	*a*	*b*	*a* + *b*
	No catheter	*c*	*d*	*c* + *d*
	Total	*a* + *c*	*b* + *d*	*n*

There were 20 pairs in which the infected patient was catheterized but the matched, noninfected patient was not catheterized. There were only three pairs in which infected patients were not catheterized while their noninfected matches were catheterized. The two cells (Table 7-7) that count the number of pairs having both patients catheterized or neither of the patients catheterized (two and five pairs, respectively) contribute no information about whether infected or noninfected patients were catheterized more often. Therefore, these two cells are not used in the significance tests for attributes. Only the cells counting discordant pairs add information about the association of infection and catheterization. The effective sample size for this example, therefore, is 23 pairs.

Sign Test

The sign test takes into account only the direction of differences between members of each pair and has a relatively low power. If there were no difference in the frequency of catheterization among infected and noninfected patients, there would be as many pairs in which the infected patient was catheterized and the matched, noninfected patient not catheterized as there would be pairs with the infected patient not catheterized and the matched, noninfected patient catheterized. For this example of 23 untied pairs, it is expected that, if no difference in the frequency of catheterization exists between infected and noninfected patients, there should be 11.5 pairs with a catheterized, infected patient and a noncatheterized, noninfected patient, and 11.5 pairs with a noncatheterized, infected patient and a catheterized, noninfected patient. The probability of observing a given number of pairs or fewer having a noncatheterized, infected patient and a catheterized, noninfected patient is given by the sum of binomial probabilities:

$$p_{\text{Tot}} = \sum_{x=0}^{c} \frac{n!}{x!\,(n-x)!}\,(0.5)^x\,(1-0.5)^{n-x}$$

where n is the number of untied pairs [1] and c is the smaller of the two cells (b and c) in Table 7-6. The formula sums the probabilities of obtaining 0, 1, . . . , c noncatheterized, infected patients paired with a catheterized, noninfected patient when half the total untied pairs, 11.5, are expected to be in this cell. The probabilities for example 1 are

$$p_x = \frac{23!}{x!\,(23-x)!}\,(0.5)^x\,(1-0.5)^{23-x}$$

$$p_0 = \frac{23!}{0!\,(23-0)!}\,(0.5)^x\,(1-0.5)^{23-0}$$
$$= 1.19209290 \times 10^{-7}$$

$$p_1 = \frac{23!}{1!\,(23-1)!}\,(0.5)^x\,(1-0.5)^{23-1}$$
$$= 2.74181366 \times 10^{-6}$$

$$p_2 = \frac{23!}{2!\,(23-2)!}\,(0.5)^x\,(1-0.5)^{23-2}$$
$$= 3.01599503 \times 10^{-5}$$

$$p_3 = \frac{23!}{3!\,(23-3)!}\,(0.5)^x\,(1-0.5)^{23-3}$$
$$= 2.11119652 \times 10^{-4}$$

$$p_{\text{Tot}} = 2.44140625 \times 10^{-4}.$$

This low probability leads to a rejection of the null hypothesis, H_0: $P_I \le P_{NI}$, in favor of the alternative hypothesis, AH: $P_I > P_{NI}$. The conclusion is that catheterized patients were at higher risk of infection.

TABLE 7-7. *Pairs of patients by catheterization status (example 1)*

		Infected		
		Catheter	No Catheter	Total
Noninfected	Catheter	2	3	5
	No catheter	20	5	25
	Total	22	8	30

McNemar Test

The McNemar Test [13] is a chi-square test that uses pairs of patients rather than single patients; therefore, it differs from the ordinary chi-square test presented earlier. As in the sign test, the McNemar Test uses only those pairs with untied observations for the infected and noninfected patients. The formula presented next and the previous formula for chi-square for independent observations both include a correction for continuity. Many elementary statistics textbooks present discussions of appropriate use of the continuity correction [2,8].

$$\chi^2 = \frac{(|b-c|-1)^2}{b+c} = \frac{(|3-20|-1)^2}{23} = \frac{(|-17|-1)^2}{23} = \frac{16^2}{23} = 11.1.$$

Again, this is a two-tailed test for an association between infection and catheterization in either direction (i.e., more risk associated with catheterization or less risk associated with catheterization). Although computed from matched samples, the value of chi-square from the McNemar Test should be compared with the same tabulated values of the chi-square distribution that were used for the chi-square test computed from independent samples. The inference about the populations from which the samples from example 1 were drawn, if they were matched, would be that catheterization is associated with infection, since the probability associated with a chi-square of 11.13 is only 0.00085.

Next, tests for measurement data from matched samples are presented, using example 2 and assuming that the noninfected patients were selected by matching to the infected patients. These tests use the differences between observations for members of the pairs instead of the two observations separately. The hypotheses to be tested are H0: $\mu_I \leq \mu_{NI}$ and AH: $\mu_I > \mu_{NI}$. The hypothesis that the mean of the intervals from admission to onset of infection for infected patients is less than or equal to the mean of the intervals from admission to discharge for noninfected patients is tested against the alternative hypothesis that the mean interval from admission to onset of infection for the infected patients exceeds the mean interval from admission to discharge of noninfected patients.

The investigator wishes to decide whether the risk of infection is increased because hospital stay is longer than it would have been if the patients had not acquired infections or, instead, if the length of stay for infected patients is increased because of infection. If the mean time from admission to onset of infection is approximately the same as the mean time from admission to discharge of noninfected patients, the investigator could conclude that prolonged stay in the hospital is not the underlying cause of infection. Additional study, such as examining the distribution of intervals from onset of infection to discharge, would then be necessary to understand to what extent infections actually lengthened the stay. The assumption that the sample observations were selected from a population of normally distributed time intervals must be made for the parametric test presented next.

Paired t *Test*

The paired t test uses the statistical theorem that the distribution of differences between two normally distributed, random variables (the sample time intervals) is also normal. Once these differences (Table 7-8) between the time intervals of the two members of each pair are determined, the t test can be used to decide whether the mean difference is greater than zero. The formula for this t test is

$$t = \frac{\bar{d}}{s_{\bar{d}}}$$

$$\text{where } \bar{d} = \frac{\sum_{i=1}^{n} d_i}{n} = \frac{1{,}111}{30} = 37.0333$$

TABLE 7-8. *Summary of differences for the paired* t-test *(example 2)*

Pair #	Infected patient	Noninfected patient	Difference	Pair #	Infected patient	Noninfected patient	Difference
1	216	253	−37	16	234	242	−8
2	187	82	105	17	205	233	−28
3	88	125	−37	18	136	133	3
4	280	138	142	19	253	342	−89
5	310	137	173	20	165	102	63
6	239	116	123	21	340	93	247
7	344	232	112	22	325	82	243
8	315	327	−12	23	178	248	−70
9	280	171	109	24	153	113	40
10	293	338	−45	25	355	294	61
11	200	335	−135	26	338	304	34
12	229	109	120	27	77	211	−134
13	208	126	82	28	335	104	231
14	233	182	51	29	261	261	0
15	190	247	−57	30	93	269	−176

d_i being the difference between time intervals for the members of the ith pair,

$$\text{and } s^2 = \frac{\sum_{i=1}^{n}(d_i - \bar{d})^2}{n(n-1)} = \frac{\sum_{i=1}^{n} d_i^2 - \frac{\left(\sum_{i=1}^{n} d_i\right)^2}{n}}{n(n-1)}$$

$$= \frac{397{,}253 - \frac{(1{,}111)^2}{30}}{30\,(30-1)}$$

$$= 409.3206$$

$\bar{d}$ and s^2 being the mean and standard error of the mean of differences in the time intervals and n being the number of pairs. Then

$$t = \frac{37.0333}{20.2317} = 1.83$$

is > 1.699, the tabulated value of t, with $n - 1 = 29$ degrees of freedom, corresponding to a one-tailed probability of 0.05. The null hypothesis that the interval from admission to onset of infection is less than or equal to the interval from admission to discharge of noninfected patients is rejected in favor of the alternative hypothesis, that $\mu_I > \mu_{NI}$. These data would support the hypothesis that infections occurred after a prolonged stay in the hospital rather than that prolonged stay resulted from infection.

Wilcoxon Signed Ranks Test

If the assumption of normality is not acceptable, the hypothesis can be tested from the matched data using a nonparametric test. The Wilcoxon Signed Ranks Test [10] is easy to apply in this case. The results of each step in the test procedure are given in Table 7-9. First, the differences are determined (column 4) for all pairs without considering the sign of the difference. Then these unsigned differences are ranked from lowest to highest (column 5), with the smallest difference receiving rank 1 (pair number 18). Differences of 0 (e.g., pair number 29) are omitted from the test procedure. Tied differences are assigned the average value of the ranks that would have been assigned if the differences had not been tied (e.g., pair number 1 and pair number 3). Finally, the signs of differences are assigned to the ranks (column 6), and the sums of absolute values of positive and negative ranks are obtained separately. The value of the smaller of the two sums is compared with the critical value [9] for a one-

TABLE 7-9. *Summary of the ranking procedure for Wilcoxon Signed Ranks test (example 2)*

Pair #	Infected patient	Noninfected patient	Difference (unsigned)	Rank (unsigned)	Rank (signed)[a]
1	216	253	37	6.5	−6.5
2	187	82	105	17	17
3	88	125	37	6.5	−6.5
4	280	138	142	24	24
5	310	137	173	25	25
6	239	116	123	21	21
7	344	232	112	19	19
8	315	327	12	3	−3
9	280	171	109	18	18
10	293	338	45	9	−9
11	200	335	135	23	−23
12	229	109	120	20	20
13	208	126	82	15	15
14	233	182	51	10	10
15	190	247	57	11	−11
16	234	242	8	2	−2
17	205	233	28	4	−4
18	136	133	3	1	1
19	253	342	89	16	−16
20	165	102	63	13	13
21	340	93	247	29	29
22	325	82	243	28	28
23	178	248	70	14	−14
24	153	113	40	8	8
25	355	294	61	12	12
26	338	304	34	5	5
27	77	211	134	22	−22
28	335	104	231	27	27
29	261	261	0	Omit	Omit
30	93	269	176	26	−26

[a]Sum of positive = 292; sum of negative ranks = 143.

tailed test at the 0.05 level. This value, 140, is exceeded by the sum of negative ranks in this example, supporting the hypothesis that the mean interval from admission to onset was greater than the mean interval from admission to discharge of the noninfected patients.

Relative Risk and Odds Ratios

Another approach to analyzing hospital-acquired infection data uses estimates of relative risk and odds ratios. These two quantities measure the association between the infection status and exposure histories of two groups of patients. Referring to Table 7-4, the infection rate or risk of infection in the exposed (catheterized) group is

$$I_E = \frac{a}{(a+b)}$$

and this rate in the unexposed (noncatheterized) group is

$$I_{NE} = \frac{c}{(c+d)} .$$

The relative risk measures the strength of the exposure effect and is defined as

$$R = \frac{\text{Risk of disease, exposed group}}{\text{Risk of disease, unexposed group}} = \frac{I_E}{I_{NE}}$$

$$= \frac{\dfrac{a}{(a+b)}}{\dfrac{c}{(c+d)}} .$$

Prospective Cohort Versus Case-Control Studies

If the data in Table 7-1 had been collected by identifying two groups of patients—one group of catheterized patients and the other group not catheterized—these two groups could have been observed prospectively to determine which ones would develop a urinary tract infection. Using the data summarized in Table 7-3, the risk of acquiring a urinary tract infection would be 22/27 = 0.8148 for catheterized patients and 8/33 = 0.2424 for noncatheterized patients. The ratio of these two risks, or the relative risk of acquiring a urinary tract infection for those patients who were catheterized, is 0.8148/0.2424 = 3.36. Thus, in this example, catheterized patients were 3.36 times more likely to have developed a urinary tract infection than those who were not catheterized.

Relative risks greater than 1 imply an association of the exposure factors with infection. If there is no increased risk of acquiring an infection associated with a particular exposure, then

$$\frac{a}{(a+b)} = \frac{c}{(c+d)}$$

and the relative risk is 1.0. If there is a decreased risk in acquiring an infection for a particular exposure, then

$$\frac{a}{(a+b)} < \frac{c}{(c+d)}$$

and the relative risk is between 0.0 and 1.0. This implies a potentially protective effect of the exposure because the exposed group has proportionally fewer infected persons than the unexposed group. In general, relative risk can be interpreted according to the summary provided in Table 7-10.

The second measure for describing the relationship between infection status and exposure is the odds ratio. If an infection occurs with probability p, the odds of that infection occurring is defined as $p/(1-p)$. For example, if a particular infection occurs with 3:1 odds, this means it occurs with a 0.75 probability and that the odds are

$$\frac{0.75}{(1.0-0.75)} = \frac{0.75}{0.25} = \frac{3}{1} .$$

This is expressed as 3:1 odds.

Referring to Table 7-4, the odds of acquiring an infection for the exposed group of patients are expressed as

$$\frac{\dfrac{a}{(a+b)}}{\dfrac{b}{(a+b)}} = \frac{a}{b} .$$

The odds of acquiring an infection for patients in the unexposed group are

$$\frac{\dfrac{c}{(c+d)}}{\dfrac{d}{(c+d)}} = \frac{c}{d} .$$

The ratio of the odds of acquiring an infection for the exposed group to the odds for the unexposed group is the infection-odds ratio:

$$\frac{\dfrac{a}{b}}{\dfrac{c}{d}} = \frac{ad}{bc} .$$

TABLE 7-10. *Interpretation of relative risk (R)*

R	<1	risk factor potentially protective
	=1	no association between risk factor and acquiring an infection
	>1	risk factor associated with acquiring an infection

Using Table 7-3, the odds ratio for acquiring an infection for catheterized patients is

$$\frac{(22 \times 25)}{(8 \times 5)} = 13.75.$$

Therefore, the odds of acquiring an infection are 13.75 times greater for the catheterized patients than for the noncatheterized patients.

If the infection in question is rare, then $a + b$ can be estimated by b, and $c + d$ can be estimated by d. This provides a simple estimate of the relative risk using the odds ratio:

$$\hat{R} = \frac{\frac{a}{(a+b)}}{\frac{c}{(c+d)}} \simeq \frac{\frac{a}{b}}{\frac{c}{d}} = \frac{ad}{bc}.$$

The numbers in Table 7-3 indicate that a urinary tract infection is common in the two groups of patients. For this reason, the odds ratio is not a good approximation of the relative risk for these data.

In a prospective cohort study, cohorts are defined as the two exposure groups, patients are assigned to each group according to their catheterization status, and the patients' infection outcomes are recorded. Relative risks can then be calculated. Typically, these studies are difficult to perform for both economic and logistic reasons. If the incidence of the particular infection is low, the groups must be large to ensure the inclusion of infected patients in the study. These large groups of patients must be followed for extended periods to acquire reliable estimates for risk of disease. Often the number of required patients can exceed the population at hand in the hospital. Also, in the hospital setting, ethical and practical considerations often make it impossible to assign patients randomly to two different treatment or exposure groups.

One way to circumvent these problems is to use the concepts outlined previously and identify all patients with a particular infection and then select a suitable group of noninfected patients for a comparison group. Each patient in these two groups is then classified as exposed or unexposed to the factor in question. This design is known as a retrospective case-control study, in that infected (case) and noninfected (control) patients are identified and their exposure histories are tabulated retrospectively.

In this situation, the numbers of infected and noninfected patients may be determined by the resources available to do the study and may not reflect the actual frequencies in the hospital population. For this reason, it is not possible to calculate the risk of disease in the two exposure categories. In fact, in this context,

$$\frac{a}{(a+b)} \quad \text{and} \quad \frac{c}{(c+d)}$$

are meaningless, and relative risk cannot be calculated.

Odds ratios, however, can be determined by calculating the odds of exposure among the infected group as

$$\frac{\frac{a}{(a+c)}}{\frac{c}{(a+c)}} = \frac{a}{c}.$$

and the odds of exposure among the noninfected group as

$$\frac{\frac{b}{(b+d)}}{\frac{d}{(b+d)}} = \frac{b}{d}.$$

This leads to the summary exposure-odds ratio, which expresses the exposure in the infected group relative to the exposure in the noninfected group, as

$$\frac{\frac{a}{c}}{\frac{b}{d}} = \frac{ad}{bc}.$$

Summarizing these results, the odds ratio is the same for both the prospective cohort study and the retrospective case-control study. For rare diseases, it closely approximates the relative risk, which can be calculated only in the prospective cohort study. In the case-control study, the relative risk can be approximated only using the odds ratio.

Testing the Significance of Odds Ratios

A variety of methods are available [15,16] to determine whether the infection-odds ratio is statistically greater than unity. The Fisher's Exact Test described earlier can be used to make this determination. The hypotheses can be stated as H_0: odds ≤ 1 and AH: odds > 1. From the earlier analysis of these data, the chi-square value was 17.239, indicating that the proportion of infected patients who were catheterized was not equal to the proportion of noninfected, catheterized patients. Likewise, the hypothesis that the odds ratio is less than or equal to unity would be rejected by Fisher's Exact Test in favor of the alternative hypothesis that the odds ratio is greater than unity. The resulting conclusion would be that the odds of infected patients being catheterized are greater than the odds of noninfected patients being catheterized.

In addition to investigating exposure factors or underlying predisposing factors that increase the risk of infection, infection control personnel may wish to examine the possibility that a factor decreased the risk of acquiring the infection. Since these "protective" factors have odds ratios of < 1, the hypotheses to be tested are H_0: odds ≥ 1 and AH: odds < 1. Fisher's Exact Test, discussed earlier, is appropriate to evaluate these hypotheses.

Confidence Intervals for Odds Ratios

The odds ratio calculated from a sample of patients from the hospital provides a single number that is an estimate of the true odds ratio, the ratio that would be observed if all patients in the hospital population were used in the calculations. Since only a sample of patients was used, the odds ratio is a point estimate of the true odds for that setting. In addition to the point estimate, the investigator can calculate an interval of values that will include, with a particular level of confidence (often 99% or 95%), the true odds ratio. This interval is known as a confidence interval for the odds ratio and can be interpreted in the following way. If the investigator could take many samples—100, for example—from this population and compute the confidence interval (e.g., 95% confidence interval) from each sample, then 95 of the intervals would be expected to include the true odds ratio. Loosely stated, the investigator would be 95% confident that the true odds ratio would be included in the interval calculated from the sample.

One method of estimating the confidence interval is based on the ln(odds) [14]. In large samples, the $\ln$(odds) has a normal distribution and the variance of the $\ln$(odds) is defined as

$$\text{var}\,[\ln(\text{odds})] = \left[\frac{1}{a} + \frac{1}{b} + \frac{1}{c} + \frac{1}{d}\right].$$

This procedure provides a reasonable estimate of the variance when all cell frequencies are relatively large; when cell sizes are small, other procedures are more appropriate [15,17]. The upper and lower confidence limits of an approximate $1 - \alpha$ confidence interval for $\ln$(odds) are

$$\text{Lower} = \text{Odds} \times \exp\,\{-Z_\alpha \sqrt{\text{var}[\ln(\text{odds})]}\}$$

$$\text{Upper} = \text{Odds} \times \exp\,\{+Z_\alpha \sqrt{\text{var}[\ln(\text{odds})]}\}$$

where α is the type 1 error described earlier and Z_α is the point corresponding to the standard normal distribution that is exceeded with $\alpha/2$ probability. These values may be readily found in statistical tables that present the cumulative normal frequency distribution. In most applications, α is set at 0.01, corresponding to $Z_\alpha = 2.58$, or 0.05, corresponding to $Z_\alpha = 1.96$, and would provide a 99% or 95% confidence interval, respectively.

The odds ratio for the data in Table 7-1 was 13.75, and the variance of the odds was determined by

$$\text{var}\,[\ln(\text{odds})] = \frac{1}{22} + \frac{1}{5} + \frac{1}{8} + \frac{1}{25} = 0.4105.$$

The lower and upper limits of the 95% confidence interval are

$$\text{Lower limit} = 13.75 \times \exp\,[-1.96\sqrt{0.4105}] = 3.92$$

$$\text{Upper limit} = 13.75 \times \exp\,[1.96\sqrt{0.4105}] = 48.27.$$

The investigator would be 95% confident that the population odds ratio estimated from the sample is included in the interval 3.92 to 48.27. Other methods for calculating these confidence intervals are available [15,17].

Confounding Factors

Although the odds ratio is easy to compute, it can give misleading results if other factors are present that are related to both the risk of infection and the exposure. These other associated factors are called confounding factors. For example, patients may be catheterized for the same reasons that they are treated with antibiotics, and their treatment with antibiotics can affect their infection status. To evaluate confounding, the investigator could stratify the patients into two groups—those receiving antibiotic treatment and those not receiving antibiotic treatment—and then compute the odds ratios for each stratum separately.

If the odds ratios obtained in the two strata are different from the odds ratio obtained in the nonstratified analysis (both antibiotic treatment groups combined), the investigator would conclude that antibiotic treatment status modified the relationship between catheterization and infection. The statistical procedures to evaluate the effects of stratification on odds ratio estimates are described by Mantel and Haenszel [18]. This technique tests the hypothesis of association of a single variable with infection while keeping a second variable fixed, which allows the second variable to be tested in the presence of the first variable.

These so-called classical or stratified data analysis techniques for case-control studies have been a mainstay of epidemiologic analysis for years. Most of the calculations can be carried out using a variety of available computer programs. Working closely with the data, deriving tables, observing the configuration of the cell counts, and calculating odds ratios or relative risks, researchers may gain a good deal of insight into the associations and trends among the different variables included in the analysis.

These techniques, however, are limited and lack statistical power when used to analyze hypotheses composed of several variables, which would occur when several variables are identified as potentially confounding factors. If the factors are controlled simultaneously, the resultant strata may be so large in number and small in cell frequencies that the classic techniques would not be useful. As an example, if an exposure variable of interest and three variables thought to be confounders are each composed of two levels (yes/no), the classic techniques would involve analyzing $2 \times 2 \times 2 \times 2 = 16$ data strata or 2×2 tables. If the study consists of 100 people, there would be, on average, 100/16 or 6.25 persons per strata, which is quite small for robust Mantel-Haenszel estimates. Additionally, stratified techniques are not well suited for handling continuous variables or for investigating patterns of interactions among variables. Even if interactions are detected, the stratified techniques do not offer a way to include them into estimates of odds ratios or relative risks. Modeling procedures using nonlinear regression functions have been developed to deal with these circumstances.

Logistic Regression

Regression techniques offer another powerful method for examining more than one variable and the joint effects of several variables in a case-control study of nosocomial infections. Multiple linear logistic regression has been applied to a variety of situations, including matched study designs [19–23]. These procedures allow the investigator to develop models that incorporate important variables and interaction terms for determining possible joint effects among these variables. One can also use regression techniques to construct models with continuous, dichotomous, and categorical variables. This is a particularly helpful development for studying nosocomial infection outbreaks when the causative factors are unknown, because one can explore the data for associations of several potential factors with infection. However, the computations are beyond those that can be done practically with a small calculator. Computer programs that require access to desktop computers have been published for this procedure [24], and versions of them have been included in several statistical programming packages [25,26].

A high level of statistical expertise is required to fully appreciate the use of logistic regression because this technique is more advanced than the classic stratified procedures. While the available software to construct complicated multivariate models can be easily mastered, extreme care must be exercised in model formation and the subsequent interpretation of results.

Regression techniques directly address the problems encountered by using classical techniques when data stratification leads to many tables containing sparse data. While it may be possible to compute odds ratios for a few levels of a particular variable, stratified analysis usually cannot provide meaningful estimates for most of the categories owing to the lack of data in each of the stratified tables. Regression techniques are able to borrow information from neighboring categories (those that have the same levels for some of the risk factors and similar levels for the remaining factors) and create smoothed estimates for the odds ratios.

This smoothing is accomplished via the use of a model composed of a series of risk factors and confounders that define or describe an outcome measure through the use of a mathematical function (the logistic function). The logistic model possesses several attributes that make it a powerful tool in case-control studies of nosocomial infections. In unmatched studies, the coefficients of the risk factors are the natural logarithms of the odds ratios obtained from stratified analysis. In matched studies, these coefficients are smoothed estimates using information gathered from bordering categories. The models also generate variances for the parameter estimates, which simplifies statistical hypothesis testing. With this information, it is easy to determine the significance of factors in a case-control investigation.

Regression techniques offer several advantages over stratified analysis in case-control studies. The primary benefit is the ability to derive odds ratios and variance estimates for models composed of several variables. Multivariable models may be constructed with the goal of determining which are the key or most important confounders and risk factors. It would be difficult or impossible to conduct this type of analysis using stratified techniques alone. It is important to recognize, however, that the modeling procedures operate under a stricter set of criteria or assumptions than do the stratified techniques. To derive Mantel-Haenszel estimates, one need assume only that the factors under study are independent and that the odds ratio for each factor is constant over all levels of the other factors. The regression procedures also require the assumption that the odds ratios combine multiplicatively. That is, the odds ratio associated with exposure to factors A and B (OR_{AB}) is equal to $OR_A \times OR_B$. While it is not possible to compute valid Mantel-Haenszel estimates for odds ratios if interactions are present between factors, it is a simple matter to include interaction terms in logistic regression models as a means of further adjustment.

OTHER CONSIDERATIONS IN RETROSPECTIVE STUDIES

Several things must be considered before extrapolating the results of a retrospective study to the entire hospital population or to patients from a group of hospitals. One major concern is the degree to which the infected and noninfected patients in the study represent infected and noninfected patients in the target population with respect to the exposure factors being evaluated. Commonly, in a case-control study, all infected patients are included, and a suitable sample of noninfected patients is then selected as controls. Since the infected patients are not randomly chosen and the noninfected patients are often chosen to match certain characteristics of the selected infected patients, the degree to which these groups in the study represent the population in the hospital will determine the appropriateness of inferences about that hospital population. If a study were conducted in a hospital serving a limited portion of the population (e.g., a Veterans Administration hospital or a municipal hospital serving a crowded urban area), any inferences made from the study subjects might not be applicable to other hospital populations (e.g., those patients treated at university-affiliated hospitals) [27].

Another concern about using odds ratios or relative risk estimates in a retrospective study is ascertainment bias when recording exposure histories for infected and noninfected patients. In a prospective cohort study, where the exposures are predetermined, if the infection control nurse, hospital epidemiologist, or other investigator is not aware of the exposure status of a study subject, the determination of infection status can more likely be made in an unbiased fashion. However, in a retrospective case-control study, if the infection status is known to the data collector, determination of risk factors can be more prone to bias. Also, infected patients may more easily recall exposure histories than will noninfected patients, hospital charts may be incomplete or unavailable, and the time required to review charts or other documents may add stress to overworked staff and result in a less thorough review. Investigators should take care to avoid these sources of bias.

Another important consideration in ensuring a successful retrospective study is that data related to the infected group should be obtained in the same manner as data for the noninfected group. If exposure histories are collected through questionnaires, the interviewers should not question the infected patients more vigorously than the noninfected patients. Indeed, to the extent possible, data collectors should be kept unaware of the infection status of the patient to guarantee impartiality in this regard. Interviewers and chart reviewers should each collect data on infected and noninfected patients so that the same techniques and interpretations are used for both groups.

Finally, the data source should be the same for both groups. If hospital records are used for data collection on the infected patients, then hospital records should also be used for the noninfected patients. If relatives or other surrogate respondents answer questions for the infected patients, they should provide the same information for the noninfected patients [27].

INTERPRETATION OF STATISTICALLY SIGNIFICANT DIFFERENCES

The practical implications of a statistical result on hospital policies call for the judgment of the investigator in conjunction with hospital staff. Strictly setting policies contingent on the result of a statistical test or the size of the odds ratio is not a prudent strategy, since many factors discussed earlier can affect statistical results (e.g., sample size, confounding factors, study design, and measurement error).

For example, if the odds ratio from a particular study is determined to be not significant when the size of the odds ratio is large enough to indicate a possible association between exposure and infection, several questions should be addressed. First, what was the power of the study? Was the sample size large enough to detect a statistically significant result if a real association was present? If not, the investigator may wish to conduct another study with a larger sample. If an increase in sample size is not possible but another study with the same sample size could be performed, then results from both studies would help in deciding about an association. If results from the second study are similar to those of the first study, there would be more reason to believe the earlier study results. If the second study results do not support the findings from the first study, the results of the two studies would be difficult to interpret, and the first study's results would be questionable.

Second, what was the level of significance in the study? Were the significance test probabilities close to 0.05, hinting at an association, or were they remarkably greater, indicating that no association existed? The investigator may not wish to use the 0.05 level of significance as the only determining factor because other events may have influenced the study's outcome. Third, what was the width of the confidence interval? If the odds ratio confidence interval was narrow, the investigator could be more confident about the value of the true odds ratio. Otherwise, the true value would be difficult to ascertain.

DISCUSSION

Several principles of study design have been presented to remind those responsible for studying nosocomial infections of ways to improve their studies and potentially gain access to computer records for selecting study and control patients. Simple testing procedures and a scheme for deciding when each is appropriate have been outlined. The investigator must be careful to avoid oversimplification of the problems associated with data on nosocomial infections. Using a simple significance test without understanding the underlying assumptions, without considering the study design, and without giving attention to possible confounding variables can lead to meaningless interpretation of the data.

The significance tests presented in this chapter are in no way intended as a complete list of available tests. They were chosen as commonly used examples that are available in each of the situations presented. The objective has been to show the readers, presumably hospital personnel, how the approach to analyzing nosocomial infection data is affected by assumptions, study design, and level of measurement of data. There is no intention to limit analyses to a single factor in any study. Although the scope of this chapter is limited to the single-factor (univariate) case, help for analyses of multiple factors (multivariate) can be found in the references cited.

The selection scheme (Figure 7-1) is intended to assist with correct application of common test procedures, but even the correct choice of test for a single variable (univariate test) may not produce an accurate conclusion about the association of the factor and infection. There are two reasons for this inaccuracy. First, conclusions from hypothesis testing are based on error probabilities that the investigator sets before the data are collected. Second, the investigator must understand the complete data set, possibly including interrelations among several factors (e.g., confounding and interactions). For the data of example 1, inquiring into the possible increased risk of infection caused by catheterization would include examination of underlying illnesses and other elements that might be considered confounding factors. A factor that may itself be associated with exposure to the factor under study and with the risk to infection should be considered as a potential confounding factor.

One might ask whether the catheterized patients were infected as a result of catheterization or whether their infections occurred as a result of serious underlying illness that not only predisposed the patients to infection but also required that the patients be catheterized. Questions like these can sometimes be answered on the basis of a scan of cross-tabulations of the data. Some of these possible confounding variables can be handled in the study design by matching [28]. However, multivariate statistical tools are also available to help in understanding the effects of several variables at the same time.

The study of nosocomial infections can be simplified, as previously suggested, by taking advantage of data that may be routinely collected in machine-readable form. Rarely do such data contain judgments of the infected or noninfected status of patients; therefore, many data items, such as culture results, pharmaceuticals, or other indicators, must be used to signal that a particular record may be for an infected patient. Usually the infection control practitioner, the hospital epidemiologist, or the infection control committee must solicit the hospital computer center to make provision for entry of the infection status and data about the infection. Of course, this requires active infection surveillance or comprehensive record review by the infection control practitioner. The return in simplified selection of study and control groups from computer files and the potential for computer-assisted analysis can, in many instances, easily offset the cost of additional data collection to obtain machine-readable records.

REFERENCES

1. Ostle B. *Statistics in research.* Ames: Iowa State University Press, 1954.
2. Snedecor GW, Cochran WG. *Statistical methods.* Ames: Iowa State University Press, 1968.
3. Miller RB Jr. *Simultaneous statistical inferences*, 2nd ed. New York: Springer-Verlag, 1981:67.
4. Martin SM. Choosing the correct statistical tests. In: Wenzel RP, ed. *Handbook of hospital-acquired infections.* Boca Raton: CRC Press, 1981.
5. Siegel S. *Nonparametric statistics for the behavioral sciences.* New York: McGraw-Hill, 1956.
6. Fisher RA. *Statistical methods for research workers.* Darien, Conn.: Hafner, 1970:96–97.
7. Maxwell AE. *Analysing qualitative data.* London: Methuen, 1971:23.
8. Steel GD, Torrie JH. *Principles and procedures of statistics.* New York: McGraw-Hill, 1960.
9. Wilcoxon F, Kattie SK, Wilcox RA. *Critical values and probability levels for the Wilcoxon Rank Sum Test and the Wilcoxon Signed Rank Test.* Pearl River, N.Y.: American Cyanamid Co. and Florida State University, 1963.
10. Wilcoxon F, Wilcox RA. *Some rapid approximate statistical procedures.* Pearl River, N.Y.: American Cyanamid Co., 1964.
11. Pike MC, Morrow RH. Statistical analysis of patient-control studies in epidemiology, factor under investigation an all-or-none variable. *Br J Prev Soc Med* 1970;24:42.
12. Cochran WG. The comparison of percentages in matched samples. *Biometrika* 1971;37:256.
13. McNemar Q. *Psychological statistics.* New York: Wiley, 1955.
14. Woolf B. On estimating the relation between blood group and disease. *Ann Hum Genet* 1955;19:251.
15. Cornfield J. A statistical problem arising from retrospective studies. In: Neyman J, ed. *Proceedings of the Third Berkeley Symposium*, vol. 4. Berkeley: University of California Press, 1956:135–148.
16. Gart JJ. The comparison of proportions: a review of significance tests, confidence intervals and adjustments for stratification. *Rev Int Stat Inst* 1971;39:148.
17. Fisher RA. Confidence limits for a cross-product ratio. *Aust J Stat* 1962;4:41.
18. Mantel N, Haenszel W. Statistical aspects of the analysis of data from retrospective studies of disease. *J Natl Cancer Inst* 1959;22:719.
19. Breslow NE, Day NE. The analysis of case-control studies. Lyon, France: International Agency for Research on Cancer, 1980:192–279. (*Statistical Methods in Cancer Research*, vol. 1.; International Agency for Research on Cancer, Scientific Publications, No. 32).
20. Gail MH, Lubin JH, Rubenstein LV. Likelihood calculations for matched case-control studies and survival studies with tied death times. *Biometrika* 1981;68:703.
21. Schlesselman JJ. *Case-control studies.* New York: Oxford University Press, 1982:227–280.
22. Hosmer DW, Lemeshow S. *Applied logistic regression.* New York: John Wiley & Sons, 1989.
23. Kleinbaum DG. *Logistic regression: a self-learning text.* New York: Springer-Verlag, 1994.
24. Lubin JH. A computer program for the analysis of matched case-control studies. *Comput Biomed Res* 1981;14:138.
25. *BMDP statistical software manual.* Berkeley: University of California Press, 1990.
26. *SAS/STAT user's guide*, version 6. Cary, N.C.: SAS Institute, Inc., 1990.
27. Kahn HA, Sempos CT. *Statistical methods in epidemiology.* New York: Oxford University Press, 1989.
28. Cornfield J, Haenszel W. Some aspects of retrospective studies. *J Chron Dis* 1960;11:523.

Hospital Infections, Fourth Edition,
edited by John V. Bennett and Philip S. Brachman.
Lippincott–Raven Publishers, Philadelphia © 1998

CHAPTER 8

The Use of Computerized Systems in Hospital Epidemiology

Jonathan Freeman

When properly designed, computerized systems can be tireless servants that do error-free fetching, sorting, ordering, copying, and calculating. On the other hand, poorly planned computerized systems can be voracious consumers of resources that never justify their cost [1,2]. The informed epidemiologist-consumer must be able to determine in what contexts computerized systems will be helpful and when computerization will result in a net loss of time, money, and efficiency [1]. The computerized system, and not the computer itself, is the functional unit. In most situations, the cost of the software and the personnel resources required to computerize some function far exceed the cost of the computer hardware. Merely buying computer hardware without effective planning for the continuing financial support of personnel and critical scrutiny of the software is worse than useless.

The computer software and hardware industry is one of the most rapidly developing in the world. A complete generation of computer hardware and software tends to evolve over about two years, so that approximately two generations matured between editions of this book. While most of the general comments and guidelines in this chapter will remain applicable for decades, specific comments and advice can relate to the computer world only as it was when this chapter was being written. Competition has been so fierce in the computer industry that new products are often released before they have been properly tested. As a result, readers should be aware that it is usually better to delay purchasing a brand new product, either hardware or software, until it has been available for months or years and the bugs have been corrected, or at least well defined.

J. Freeman: Department of Epidemiology, Harvard School of Public Health, Boston, Massachusetts 02115.

It is the purpose of this chapter to describe which functions in hospital epidemiology might reasonably be addressed with a computerized system, the advantages that might accrue, and the additional resources that will be required. Many erstwhile computer users will be surprised to find that computerization of a task generally calls for increases in cost, so the potential gain in usefulness of information that can be manipulated by an electronic servant must be compared with the substantially added cost of creating and maintaining the system in which it can function effectively. In most cases, hospital epidemiology units will find that the paper- or card-based data systems they are currently using are relatively inexpensive. The cost of computerizing an already functioning paper-based system must be weighed against any potential gains.

Particularly faulty programs, such as some graphic operating systems, are also discussed. On the basis of substantial experience, users have developed strategies to minimize the damage that can be caused by flawed software programs. If potential consumers are aware of the types of defects found in popular commercial software, then users can make informed choices that will not needlessly complicate their lives.

Epidemiology units will find computers to be essential for word processing and for accessing literature databases, such as Medline, because these expensive databases were created and are maintained by other agencies. Universities, hospitals, and other institutions tend to be connected to the Internet, so that communication via E-mail is simple and commonly available. E-mail has largely replaced telephone conversation. Beyond those three functions, the potential usefulness of computers must be weighed objectively for each individual job and setting. For example, with substantial additional investment of resources, it is possible to create an electronic surveillance database from the paper- or card-based system for one's own hospital. In addition, for those few epidemiology units that regularly publish the results of serious epidemiologic research, acquiring one of the statistical packages and teaching someone to apply it might be useful. In each instance, the real needs and abilities of the potential users must be assessed. Working systems in use at other similar institutions or hospitals should be tried and evaluated before making any purchase.

RESEARCH IN COMPUTERIZED SYSTEMS FOR HOSPITAL EPIDEMIOLOGIC USE

Several groups of investigators have pioneered in the investigation of the application of computerized systems to hospital epidemiology [3–12]. These research systems have been developed over decades at a cost of tens of millions of dollars and apply only to the institutions in which they were developed. Each of these systems is based on the incorporation of electronic databases created and maintained by other departments of the hospital, such as microbiology, clinical pathology, pharmacy, radiology, and administration. Data from these different departments within each hospital are maintained in different ways, and the development of functional systems to download, recode, combine, and analyze data from these diverse sources in a timely manner is what has made these systems so expensive.

The resources required to create or acquire such systems are far beyond the scope of most hospital epidemiology units. Rather, we can simply look to these systems as the initial steps in the development of generally applicable systems in the distant future. Accurately differentiating between these costly research systems and what is currently practical for the daily work of an individual hospital epidemiology unit will prevent epidemiologists from making the major errors in judgment that characterized the introduction of computers into the business world.

THE NATURE OF PAST DISAPPOINTMENT ENGENDERED BY THE COMPUTER INDUSTRY

Personification of the Computer

There are many reasons why computers, especially personal computers (PCs), failed to live up to the expectations of eager consumers. A mistaken belief existed that a computer would somehow just reach out and take over large portions of an individual's work. Computers are completely passive, however, and do not imitate human thought patterns. They do exactly what they are programmed to do, including perfoming all the errors written into a program, at great speed and with outstanding accuracy.

Ultimately, a computer can do an extraordinary number of mindless tasks that are regarded by humans as drudgery, but there is a steep price. First, simply learning to use a computerized system takes much longer than inexperienced purchasers might anticipate. Second, computerizing an epidemiologic database, for example, often requires substantial additional resources, especially financial resources, for data entry, editing, and correction.

The Difficulty of Learning to Use Common Software

Essential software, such as some operating systems and elaborate word-processing, database, and spreadsheet programs, took much longer to learn to use than advertisements and computer hobbyists acknowledged. One of the best-kept secrets among the manufacturers of these complex and expensive programs manufactured for business use is that no more than 10% to 15% of the software packages they sell are ever used. Computerized systems can be extremely helpful, for they can augment the writing and editing process, facilitate communications, manipulate large databases, and perform complex calculations with seemingly magical speed and accuracy. However, this magic comes at a much higher price than inexperienced purchasers might imagine.

PITFALLS OF COMPUTERIZATION

Potential Computer Users: Hobbyists Versus Occasional Users

The computer user is the most important element and the most variable aspect of any computerized system. Before making decisions regarding the computerization of any task in hospital epidemiology, it is essential to consider the interests and capabilities of the identified computer operators. There are several choices open to a hospital epidemiology unit that wishes to implement a computerized system. Personnel involved in hospital epidemiology usually have arrived at their calling through their interest and expertise in medical areas and thus are generally only occasional users of computers. Rarely, one may have access to a gifted computer hobbyist or hacker who is willing to undertake the large job of system design and personnel education. Unfortunately, hobbyists may overestimate both their ability and the amount of time they are willing to devote to such an enterprise. In the absence of free services, substantial resources will have to be invested in training casual or occasional computer users if they are to become facile operators of the complex programs that are standard in the business arena of the PC industry. The other alternative is to seek out computerized systems that are specifically designed for simplicity.

The Added Costs of Computerizing Almost Any Function

If the computer user views learning to use software programs as recreation, to be performed in spare time outside working hours, then there is little additional time and cost associated with this phase of instituting a computerized system. On the other hand, when the days or weeks required to become facile with a complex piece of new software are taken from other activities normally performed during the working day, then the salary costs of learning about a new program may reach tens of thousands of dollars, far exceeding the purchase price of the computer hardware and software.

Furthermore, even after one has learned to use new software, there are usually costs associated with continued use of a program. The clearest example is the database that would arise from normal surveillance activities in a hospital. The data are originally recorded on paper forms or cards and are immediately useful as a paper or card system. If the decision is made to enter these data into an electronic database, then there will be the additional ongoing expense of data entry, editing, and correction. These last two functions are especially important, since it must be recognized that errors are introduced at the rate of 3% to 5% per step; after data have been collected, transcribed, and keypunched, the cumulative error rates may be high enough to distort results of analyses substantially. Although surveillance data may be more useful in an electronic format, for many hospitals the cost of computerizing, editing, and correcting surveillance data will far exceed any possible benefit.

Estimating Total Costs of Computerization Beforehand

It is necessary to understand what human, software, and hardware resources are required to set up and maintain a computerized system [6]. The most important are the human resources, followed by suitable software and, least important, the hardware, or the computer itself. Obtaining a realistic estimate of the resources needed to create and maintain computerized systems calls for estimating the resources necessary to perform an activity with a paper or card system and then formulating a realistic estimate of the additional costs of using a computerized system to accomplish the same result. The added cost of computerizing a function includes the cost of acquiring the software and the hardware; installing the system; learning to use the software; entering, editing, and correcting data; repeating these procedures as more data are added periodically; and maintaining the system.

Let us look at a common example—the desire to computerize a hospital surveillance database. Hospital epidemiology units are obligated to conduct some sort of formal surveillance for nosocomial infections. The data are recorded as line lists on paper forms or on individual cards, and monthly or weekly tallies may be made of infections by site, service, procedure, and various patients' characteristics. To use a computer to replace paper shuffling with electronic accounting is possible, but computerization of a database involves a number of extra steps, and a practical decision would depend on where the extra resources could be found.

In most hospitals, the budget for hospital epidemiology is fixed, so the extra resources needed to computerize the surveillance database would have to be taken from some other activities within an epidemiology unit. Specifically, it would be necessary to allocate time every week to enter all of the data from the paper forms into the computerized database, to edit the data that have been entered, and to correct data entry errors. The time saved in sorting and summarizing data in a computerized system at the end of each month may be overshadowed by the even greater amount of time required to enter and correct the data in an electronic database.

If additional clerical resources are made available for data entry, then computerizing a database may be a real advantage. On the other hand, when resources are fixed, and a trained epidemiologist would have to be removed from some clinical activities on wards in order to keypunch data, then computerization of a surveillance database may result in a net loss of clinical functionality for a hospital epidemiology unit. These judgments need to be made individually for every hospital.

APPROPRIATE APPLICATIONS OF A COMPUTERIZED SYSTEM

Tasks for Which Computers Are Always Useful

As was mentioned earlier, there are three sorts of tasks for which computers are almost universally useful: word processing, searching a database (such as Medline, a literature database) that somebody else has created and maintains [5], and communication by E-mail over the Internet. These tasks are computerized functions that any hospital epidemiology unit, no matter how small, will probably use. They require minimal investment in hardware and software. If the hospital is already connected to the Internet, then E-mail will be free and, if there is a medical library nearby, literature searches may also be free. Minimal effective hardware and software requirements for these essential functions are discussed later.

Additional Tasks for Which Computers May Sometimes Be Useful

There are three additional specialized tasks for which computers also can be useful: creating, maintaining, and updating simple statistical reports from an individual hospital database; performing complex or repeated epidemiologic or statistical calculations; and desktop publishing, or producing a newspaper or newsletter at regular intervals. Computerization of these last three functions will be cost effective for hospital epidemiology units only under relatively unusual circumstances.

HISTORY OF DATA MANAGEMENT

Functional Speed and Accuracy of Computers

It is important to recognize the relative speeds with which sorting and calculating have been done during this century. Before the advent of electronic computing devices, some epidemiologists and statisticians kept large data sets in giant tables on the backs of rolls of wallpaper. Various card systems were also developed as more efficient paper-based systems of data storage and manipulation. Analysis is hastened if the index cards are marked in color along the edges. A more sophisticated card system is available in the form of McBee cards, which have holes punched along the edges. Once stacked in trays, McBee cards can be sorted quickly and accurately with a long rod resembling a knitting needle.

When the first mainframe computers were developed, they also incorporated a card system for the storage and sorting of data. The ubiquitous computer punch card, or Hollerith card, was actually developed in the previous century to program patterns for weaving on mechanical looms, and its almost universal adoption as the medium for computers was inevitable. The early mainframes allowed neater card storage of data on attributes and events, which could then be sorted and counted with complete accuracy by mechanical card sorters. However, the early mainframes were not easily accessed, even by professionals.

After the data were sorted by a computerized mechanical card sorter, complex statistical and epidemiologic computations could be carried out. Because of the expense, the threatened devastation of forests, and the very slow speeds at which cards could be sorted mechanically, the punch card and the mechanical card sorter are now a part of computing history, and data entry is carried out on magnetic media. At present, sorting is done electronically, and final calculations are easily accomplished with programmable calculators [13] or statistical packages [6,14–17].

Even the slowest computer is incredibly fast and accurate compared with a human performing the same tasks. In the medical world, data sorting on mainframes generally continues to require professional programmers as intermediaries, an aspect that has not changed appreciably since the early days of the mainframe. Because of the intermediary, the turnaround time from formulation of the request until delivery of the results of a successful mainframe sort might range from hours to weeks. However, one can do other work in the interim, and if the program is correctly written, the accuracy of the sorting procedure is assured. Analyses of these sorted data can then be carried out expeditiously with a programmable calculator or PC.

Shortly after the programmable calculator came into wide use, the original Visicalc spreadsheet was developed for the simplest Apple computer. The early spreadsheets could deal with only relatively small data sets, but after data were entered into the spreadsheet, this combination could perform in a minute or two computations that would have taken an experienced user with a calculator a whole day to complete. This represents a five-hundred-fold increase in speed, and an increase of this magnitude has never been approached since. The fastest and most expensive 32-bit PCs now available are only fifty to one hundred times as fast as the original 8-bit machines available 15 years ago.

An additional benefit that accrued from the use of an electronic spreadsheet was that once the data were entered and checked for accuracy, no further errors in data entry or calculation could occur. Since data had to be reentered for many repeated calculations with early calculators, use of a spreadsheet also led to an enormous reduction in errors in data entry. Shortly after the invention of the spreadsheet, electronic databases were developed for PCs that, given enough time, could faultlessly sort data sets of almost any size but had limited abilities to perform calculations. There is now a series of programs for storing and manipulating surveillance data in hospital epidemiology that is based on electronic databases. These database programs devoted to hospital epidemiology will be discussed in more detail later.

The functional speed and efficiency of a computerized system is determined by myriad variables. In practice, speed differences on the order of four- or fivefold are noticeable to operators, but smaller differences are difficult to detect. Many claims about computer speed involve differences so minor that they would not be apparent to the average user. Most advertisements and technical discussions of computers focus on the clock speed of the processor, which is also frequently misleading. The top speed of a computer chip is discussed in the same manner as the top speed of an automobile and has about as much relevance in daily use. Automobiles almost never reach top speed, and, similarly, computers rarely are limited by chip speed.

The efficiency with which a computer can accomplish a particular task is dependent on a multitude of other factors, primarily the presence of a hard disk and disk speed. After that, the amount of RAM, the scratchpad on which the computer works, is important, as is the size of the bus. Perceived speed also depends on how well different parts of a computer keep up with one another. The speed of operation of some programs is limited by the way in which they use the monitor screen, so functional speed is determined by how rapidly the monitor screen can be renewed. Chip speed is one of the least important practical determinants of computer speed as it is perceived by the user. Mainframe computers and workstations can do many things simultaneously, which greatly increases the speed with which they can accomplish complex tasks.

Functional Computer Speed Primarily Dependent on Mechanical Functions

Computerized systems are an integrated mixture of components, many electronic but some mechanical. Electronic processing generally takes place at high speed on a computer, whereas the mechanical tasks progress much more slowly. Most computer programs make extensive use of secondary data storage by reading from a hard disk and writing to a hard disk. Functions performed slowly on mechanical components can be accomplished at an accelerated level by switching to faster mechanical components. This will bring about notable increases in the functional speed of a computer, and moving this same function to the electronic level will enhance performance further still. In the following paragraphs we look at the use of primary RAM and secondary memory, such as floppy disks, the many tape and disk backup systems, hard disks, and electronic RAM disks.

Floppy disks are inexpensive and convenient storage devices for large amounts of text, data, or programs. Hundreds of pages of text may be stored on a single floppy, and the equivalent of a long paper or 40 pages of text can be written to or read off a floppy disk in a period of a few seconds to a minute or two. In mechanical terms, this seems very fast; however, it is glacially slow compared with the electronic capabilities within even the simplest computer. The evolution of tape and disk backup systems has now made them competitive in speed and convenience with standard floppy disks, and these special large-capacity backup disks and tapes can hold 70 times to hundreds of times more data or information.

A hard disk spins ten or more times as fast as a standard floppy disk or a large-capacity backup disk, and information is transferred on and off a hard disk ten or twenty times as rapidly. Nevertheless, the mechanical hard disk is still most likely to be the rate-limiting component of a computer system while it is actively running a program. To circumvent the speed limits imposed by mechanical disk drives, more primary RAM can be installed on a computer (depending on the ability of the operating system to use the extra RAM), or secondary electronic storage on extra RAM may be used to replace mechanical disks. This can be accomplished in a PC by organizing extra RAM to function as an artificial disk drive called a virtual disk. Data can flow to and from an electronic disk at the top speed available from that electronic device. Switching secondary memory storage from floppy disk drives to a hard disk involves an order of magnitude increase in speed, and switching from a mechanical hard disk to an electronic RAM disk will increase speed by approximately another order of magnitude. Only at the electronic level of operation of a RAM disk will the speed of the computer be limited by chip speed, operating system size, and bus size.

The original command line operating systems for PCs were limited in that they could address only 640 kilobytes of primary RAM, so the functional speed of a computer depended heavily on the type of secondary memory available. As was mentioned, extra RAM formulated as a virtual disk was fastest. A better solution was to write new operating systems that could address much larger amounts of primary RAM. The Apple Macintosh graphic operating system was the first to do this, and the graphic operating systems for IBM compatibles soon followed. Although these new graphic operating systems commonly use from 4 to 32 megabytes of primary RAM memory, they are much more complex to use, and because of the addition of the graphics, the speed increases associated with their use are not as great as was anticipated.

Computer Speed for Various Types of Programs

For word processing, the most common task for PCs, chip speed plays almost no role in how well and easily writing, editing, and printing can be accomplished. Likewise, the speed in using a literature database is not determined by the chip in the PC, because the database is being searched by a time-sharing mainframe computer at the other end of a telephone line. Functional speed in using a literature database is most often limited by the nature of the modem used to connect with the central mainframe and the quality of the telephone line over which the transmissions take place. Likewise, E-mail messages are stored on computer servers operated by a third party that are neither the sender nor the receiver, so the characteristics of the PC system used to send or retrieve E-mail are not of major importance in determining functionality. All of the essential functions of computerized systems for most hospital epidemiology units can be implemented with simple, elderly, and even secondhand PCs.

A database program that might be used to manipulate hospital surveillance information and make simple statistical calculations stores data on a hard disk, and the efficiency of such a database program depends primarily on the speed of data exchange between the processor and the hard disk in the computer. This is usually limited by the mechanical speed with which the hard disk can access stored information but may also be influenced by the design of the database program itself and the size of the operating system and bus.

Spreadsheets do generally calculate at chip speed, and even the slowest computer can produce recalculation results with stunning speed and accuracy compared with the time required to perform the same operations on a programmable calculator. Large spreadsheets are recalculated in a minute or two on even the slowest machine. Investigators in hospital epidemiology generally do not make giant spreadsheets, and even a major difference in speed of recalculation is not likely to save very many minutes in a year.

Academic research for publication in the hospital epidemiology field may involve the use of one of the large statistical packages [6,14–17], and this is the only context in which chip speed and machine architecture will have a visible influence on the practical functionality of a computerized system. Statistical calculations generally are the most difficult type of operation for a computer, because many significant figures have to be carried along in classic analysis of variance, and long iterative processes are involved in performing analyses such as logistic or Cox regression. These academic enterprises are the only situations in which an expensive and fast PC is likely to make a noticeable difference. However, one should never consider the purchase of a machine such as this until the data are already in hand and the immediate need for statistical computation is clear. As was mentioned, computer technology is evolving quickly, and prices continue to fall. Since data collection for most research projects in epidemiology takes a year or more to complete, major gains in computing power may be realized simply by postponing purchase of an expensive machine until the end of a research project rather than acquiring a computer at the outset.

RELIABILITY OF COMPUTERIZED SYSTEMS

From the point of view of the reliability of a computerized system, it is convenient to divide system components into three groups: electrical, mechanical, and software. In general, if the electronic components of a computerized system—the circuit boards and chips—function perfectly in the beginning, they will continue to function that way for a long time. However, the power supply may have a shorter lifetime, especially if it was relatively small to start, and if the user has added a number of extra boards to the computer that have relatively high energy requirements. Also, computer hackers who repeatedly plug and unplug chips and boards from their machines may eventually mechanically disrupt some electrical connections on the circuit boards.

Because the electronic components of computerized systems are so trouble-free, beginning users tend to forget that there are also essential mechanical components in a computerized system, such as disk drives and printers. All mechanical devices need regular service, just like an automobile and, like an automobile, will break down on occasion. Because hard disks work so well and are so fast, beginners tend to depend on them completely and store everything on the hard disk. Modern hard disks are very reliable, and most run for years without trouble, but hard disk drives are also mechanical components. Computer sages report that there are only two kinds of hard disk drives: those that have already failed and those that are about to fail.

Every computer user must be prepared to lose the entire contents of the hard disk periodically. If the hard disk contained months or years of work, and there are no other copies, then a hard disk crash is a major catastrophe. In monetary terms, a hard disk may contain data that are worth tens or even hundreds of thousands of dollars. The obvious safeguard is to make multiple copies of all important files on floppy disks or special backup systems using large-capacity floppy disks or cassette tape and to update them regularly. There are a number of programs for the speedy backup of hard disks and special disk and tape drives that will accomplish the backup of tens of megabytes in a few minutes. Although backup takes time, it is obviously cost effective to back up a hard drive at least weekly.

Current software is by far the most common source of difficulty with the use of computerized systems. Competition in the computer industry has caused a new problem with the premature release of new and incompletely tested software. It can no longer be assumed that software programs will perform as indicated on the box, so a wise beginner will read critical reports and comparisons of new products in computer magazines, consult experienced computer users, and try out an installed version of a new product before purchase. The graphic operating systems for IBM-compatible computers are a major source of difficulty for naive users, as are some of the large and complex programs that are written for them.

GENERAL CONSIDERATIONS IN CHOOSING A COMPUTER SYSTEM

There is no such thing as the best computer; there is only the simplest and least expensive computerized system to be used by a specific operator that will perform the tasks essential for the defined needs. The most important single determinant of success with a computerized system is the inclination and training of the identified computer operator. Proponents of the two major standards for PCs, IBM and Apple, tout their favorite systems with religious fervor. Historically, less expensive IBM compatibles generally have provided more computing power for the hardware dollar but require more in the way of human resources to learn. The expense of training and maintaining the operator can be prohibitive. Apple systems have been more expensive to purchase but are substantially easier for non-experts to use. Apple has brought out new lines of less expensive Macintosh computers to compete more directly with the large array of low-cost IBM compatibles, and both IBM and Microsoft have copied the Macintosh graphic operating system and transported it to the IBM-compatible lines. Apple has finally licensed other computer companies to manufacture less expensive Macintosh clones.

Using Existing Computer Facilities

Most, if not all, computer systems needed by hospital epidemiology units may already be available within the hospital at no extra cost. A number of tasks can be efficiently carried out on existing computer systems. Many hospitals use mainframe computers for accounting and billing and are willing to allow use of them for hospital epidemiology. The availability and scope of these mainframes and programs varies markedly. Most hospital and medical school libraries already have access to literature databases through PCs and modems. For the purposes of hospital epidemiology, it is far more efficient and less expensive to conduct occasional literature searches through these standard facilities. Many institutions are already connected to the Internet, which makes low-cost E-mail accessible.

Minimizing Cost

There are three considerations for minimizing expenses associated with computer hardware acquisition: borrowing time on underused systems, looking for free PCs, and postponing computer purchase until the last possible moment. There tend to be many unused and underused PCs of various ages sitting in offices and laboratories around hospitals, and borrowing time on an already functioning computer is the best way to learn about simple word processing or a spreadsheet program.

Epidemiologists should constantly be on the lookout to salvage free PCs (such as older Macintosh systems) from offices and laboratories within a hospital to use as the initial system in determining what role computers may play in their professional lives. Word processing and connecting to a modem or network to send E-mail or to search literature databases make minimal demands on any computer. The PC needed for 90% to 100% of the functions of most hospital epidemiology units may well be found free or for little additional cost.

Technical advances are being made at a remarkable pace in the PC industry, and the amount of computing power available per dollar has continued to double approximately every 2 years. It makes sense to delay the purchase of a computerized system until the time when the actual needs are most clearly defined. Then, buy just the software programs available that exactly fulfill the needs of the immediate task at hand and acquire the hardware required to run the software. Suggestions concerning such acquisitions are given later.

Interfaces: First Barrier to PC Use

The computer interface is simply the way an operator communicates with a computer. For the mainframes, for the original Apple II, and for the IBM compatibles, the first interface with the computer was text typed in on a command line via the keyboard. With the Macintosh line, Apple went to a graphic interface, in which basic operations are represented by picture symbols termed icons. There are five things a graphic interface can accomplish, in principle: it makes for uniform use of the freehand drawing device, the mouse, for all programs; it can allow common pictorial elements to be in the control of all programs; it gives documents a similar appearance on the monitor and paper; it permits multiple windows containing different programs to be present on the screen simultaneously (multitasking) and quick switching among programs; and it makes quick interconnections between programs.

In spite of the advertising on the box, some of the operating systems with these graphic interfaces cannot in practice accomplish a number of the potential listed activities, but the popularity of graphic interfaces indicates how many potential computer users were put off by the classic command line interface. The world of IBM compatibles raced to catch up with the Apple Macintosh in the area of graphics, but graphic-based systems for IBM compatibles involve substantially more complexity and expense than simple systems based on the command line interface.

Operating Systems: Second Barrier to PC Use

The operating system and utilities are the primary programs that tell the computer how to control all of its components and how to perform basic housekeeping and accounting chores, such as allocating disk space and moving files around. These operations seem so central to computer use that beginners are surprised that a separate program is needed to accomplish these essential functions. The nature and reliability of the operating systems available for the various computer systems is emblematic of the relative ease of use of the system in general.

PC DOS and MS DOS are the functionally equivalent primary operating systems for IBM and IBM-compatible PCs, respectively. There are many sequential versions of these programs extant, and version 6.22 includes substantial valuable improvements. Ironically, IBM has released version 7.0 of DOS, which is less functional than the previous version 6.22. Earlier versions of these operating system programs were difficult for beginners to master and contained many traps for the unwary. With these versions it was relatively easy for an amateur inadvertently to destroy files or even whole disks with a nonspecific use of a FORMAT, COPY, or DELETE command. And these versions delivered insufficient warning when catastrophic changes were about to take place. Such unfortunate tendencies gave rise to a whole industry devoted to the development of programs to protect the user from these early versions of the DOS operating system for IBM compatibles.

By far the easiest way to learn to use the DOS operating system is to take a course for beginners. The same warning concerning how to learn a program holds true for most of the complex word-processing, spreadsheet, or database programs for the IBM compatibles that are popular in the business world. Many of these programs have tried to minimize the difficulties with the DOS operating system by incorporating simplified DOS functions within the other programs. As a result, some beginners have found it easier to move files around on a hard disk with a word-processing program than with the early versions of the DOS operating system.

Apple Macintosh systems have much simpler and more intuitively grounded windowed operating systems that are accessible to most users without taking a course. The high-end Apple Macintosh systems are the functional equivalents of the expensive IBM compatibles, and word-processing, spreadsheet and database programs with similar capabilities are available for both. Apple systems are ahead when it comes to the interface, the operating system, and programs that use graphics, such as desktop publishing. In contrast, the statistical packages moved from mainframes to PCs have been adapted to the IBM systems first and for some years were available only on IBM-compatible computers. However, these statistical packages are becoming available for the powerful machines at the high end of the Macintosh line as well. The variety of operating systems now available for PCs also represent a range of choices in how much primary RAM they can address and whether they are 16-bit systems, 32-bit systems, or a mixture. Beginners should be aware that all of the operating systems have substantial problems, and more details of operating systems are discussed later in this chapter.

Difficulties with Current Graphic Operating Systems and Comparison with DOS

There are five major problems with graphic interfaces: they require a great deal of space on a hard disk (at least 30 megabytes), they need quite a bit of RAM (8 to 16 megabytes) to function well, they can be difficult to install, they may run programs much more slowly, and they are more unstable than their nongraphic predecessors. Lack of stability simply means that while one is using a program on a computer, the computer may crash or freeze. When this happens the only way to regain control of the computer is to reboot and lose all of the work one did from the last time one saved everything. If several programs are running, everything from all of the programs that were active may be lost.

By contrast, the MS DOS operating system version 6.2 or greater does what it is supposed to, is rock-solid stable, takes little space on a hard disk, and runs most programs substantially faster than the graphic operating systems while requiring much less RAM. With version 6.2, DOS finally has all of the features that were available with the old Apple II and should have been included in DOS years ago. At this point the DOS operating system does many things much better than the graphic operating systems and should be considered first for many applications in hospital epidemiology. The only problem for beginners is that it is not a graphic interface.

The Apple Macintosh, the first computer with a graphic interface, is probably the simplest to install and use—and the most stable. At the time of this writing, users have a choice among at least four copies of the Macintosh operating system for IBM compatibles: OS/2 Warp (version 4.0) from IBM; Windows x.x to 3.1, Windows 95, and Windows NT (New Technology) from Microsoft. Windows 97, an upgrade of Windows 95, is being developed for release in 1998.

In the rush to create a graphic operating system for IBM compatibles similar to that available for the Apple Macintosh, Microsoft introduced a series of operating environments named Windows x.x up to 3.1, which appeared to provide similar graphic functionality to IBM compatibles. These Macintosh look-alikes all ran on top of, and required the use of, the DOS operating system, for which they provided a graphic interface. There are two types of problems with these Microsoft programs: they run slowly and poorly on older and smaller machines, and there is a fundamental flaw in the design of all of them that makes them unstable and prevents them from accomplishing some of the five types of tasks listed in the discussion of graphic interfaces.

The fundamental flaw with all of these Microsoft Windows programs has been that they share RAM and hard disk space while multitasking. When two programs run simultaneously under Windows they both run in common or shared spaces in RAM and on the hard disk. In order to run simultaneously in the same spaces the programs must cooperate, which is termed cooperative multitasking. Multiple programs running in the same space under Microsoft Windows are not controlled by the operating system, and their cooperation is strictly voluntary. Making the products from one software company cooperate with those of another has never been a high priority among the software companies that market popular word-processing, database, and spreadsheet programs, with the result that programs running "cooperatively" in the same spaces tend to behave more like feuding siblings and corrupt each other's files and freeze or crash the system. When this happens, the user usually loses all of the work in all of the programs since the last time it was saved. There are ways to minimize the likelihood of crashes with these Microsoft Windows programs, which will be described later, but potential users should be aware that some graphic operating systems are inherently much more unstable than their command line predecessors, such as MS DOS, and under certain circumstance they may make the attempted use of computerized systems very frustrating.

PRACTICAL COMPUTERIZED SYSTEMS IN HOSPITAL EPIDEMIOLOGY

First Programs for Hospital Epidemiology

There are many PCs available, and almost any of them will serve most needs of hospital epidemiology units. The best beginning computer is the computer one already owns or can use for nothing. Make sure there is no other choice before spending money on hardware. If no free equipment is available and some purchases must be made, then one should try an installed version of any system being considered for purchase to determine what level of sophistication is required from the operator. Personnel costs, and not hardware or software, will ultimately represent the major expense involved in the implementation of any computerized system. In the following sections, hardware needs, according to application, are reviewed with each function.

Choice of an Operating System

There used to be no choice—one simply used the operating system that came with a computer. Now there are many alternatives, beginning with MS DOS for IBM compatibles, and the original windowed graphic operating system for the Apple Macintosh. Currently it is the copies of the Macintosh operating system for the IBM compatibles that are in most common use. These include Microsoft Windows x.x to 3.1, IBM's OS/2, and Microsoft Windows 95 and Windows NT. Although the Apple Macintosh operating system is better developed than any of the copies, historically the higher cost of Macintosh computers prevented them from becoming the dominant machines in business use. Macintosh computers available today are much more competitively priced. Now that Motorola, IBM, and Apple have joined forces to produce the PowerPC chip, they may in the future produce machines and operating systems that will run both Apple Macintosh and IBM operating systems and programs.

The selection of an operating system may determine how useful a computerized system will ultimately become and also what programs will be used with that computer. The evolution of operating systems has not followed the path that might have been anticipated, and current selections are complex and involve many unfortunate trade-offs. Unless you are a computer expert, you will need help and advice, so the first consideration in the choice of an operating system should probably be local expertise and what people around you are using. Whatever system comes with the best local support system should probably be at or near the top of your list.

The simplest and most reliable operating system is unquestionably MS DOS version 6.2 or higher. At this point it resides on more PCs than any other operating system. It will run well on old IBM compatibles with 8086 or 286 processor chips and hard disks and makes older computers, discarded by others, into highly functional word processors. On a 386 or later machine, the automatic memory allocation features of DOS 6.2 will relieve the user of the arcane and difficult tasks of memory management, and the compression program included with this operating system will essentially double the functional size of the hard disk and rejuvenate an older machine with a 386 chip.

The word processors, communications programs, databases and spreadsheets made for DOS have been around for a long time and have the bugs worked out of them. The MS DOS operating system and DOS programs are small by current standards and run fast on old machines with limited RAM and hard disk space. Elderly machines with DOS should not be overlooked by hospital epidemiology units. In fact, at the time of this revision, the four dedicated hospital epidemiology database programs, described later, run only on DOS, although a Windows version of at least one of them is in the planning stages.

There are disadvantages to the MS DOS operating system as well. DOS is the only available operating system that is not graphics based, which matters to some beginning users. Beginners and even advanced users still find the official DOS manual opaque. The easiest way to learn DOS is to take a 1-day course. If courses are not available, and even if they are, most DOS beginners will find DOS much easier to use with one of the many books on MS DOS written to replace the manual. An excellent series of books for beginners on many different types of computer programs are the "Dummies" books, of which *DOS for Dummies* was the flagship [18]. DOS is a 16-bit operating system and can use only 16-bit DOS software programs. And DOS still has the limitation that it can address only 640 kilobytes of RAM at once, but additional RAM can be configured as virtual RAM disks to increase the performance of DOS. However, MS DOS is considered old-fashioned by the industry, and it is unlikely that most software companies will continue to develop and support DOS programs into the next century.

Microsoft rushed to create a Macintosh-like graphics interface for IBM compatibles and developed a series of programs called Windows x.x to 3.1 that operated on top of MS DOS and provided a graphic interface for DOS. The performance of these Windows programs provoked substantial criticism in the trade press, but Windows was a huge commercial success and eventually was shipped already installed on many new computers. The older versions of Windows were very unstable and frequently crashed, but version 3.1 was usable, particularly if one installed ≥ 8 megabytes of RAM in the computer, which was twice the minimum amount required according to the advertisements and reference manual for the product. In addition, further stability could be achieved by making sure that one never ran more than one program at a time, so there was minimal opportunity for two programs to compete and corrupt each other while "cooperatively" sharing the same RAM and hard disk space [18–20].

The popularity of Windows 3.1 resulted from the fact that it was very easy to install and provided a graphic interface for IBM compatibles. Since it runs on top of DOS, Windows 3.1 is also a 16-bit operating environment and will run DOS programs as well as those programs specifically written for Windows. It simply requires a much larger and more expensive computer to run the Windows operating environment as well as the DOS and Windows programs. If used with the precautions described, Windows 3.1 will perform acceptably, but one should recognize that DOS programs will run faster and more reliably on an older and less sophisticated computer with only the MS DOS operating system.

OS/2 is a 32-bit operating system capable of running and controlling DOS and Windows programs simultaneously in individual and separate spaces in RAM and on the hard disk, so that programs do not corrupt each other. Since OS/2 can run Windows programs in separate areas of memory, which is something that neither Windows 3.1 nor Windows 95 (discussed later) can do, OS/2 was marketed by IBM as a "better Windows than Windows," which it certainly is from the point of view of stability. It is a stand-alone operating system that does not require the concurrent presence of MS DOS, though it runs DOS programs. Because this refined design allows programs to run in their own separate spaces, if one program running under OS/2 crashes for its own reasons, all the others will not automatically crash at the same time, nor will the operating system. The major problem with OS/2 is that it is more difficult than Windows to install, and a beginner will need installation help from a more advanced user.

Windows 95 is a combination of a 16-bit and a 32-bit operating system. The chip manufacturer Intel has announced that its next generation of CPU chips (code-named P6) will run only 32-bit operating systems, so it does not appear that Windows 95 will become a long-term standard. Windows NT (New Technology) is another separate, but more expensive operating system designed by Microsoft for businesses. It is purely a 32-bit operating system, which is unrelated to the other Microsoft Windows programs mentioned and does not share their design flaws. Windows NT was created expressly for the business market and includes all of the connectivity features intended for servers on large networks. It is an industrial-strength operating system that is stable and incorporates the security features desired by large businesses. Furthermore, it will not run many current DOS programs, and hospital epidemiology units are unlikely to need the other unique features of Windows NT. This operating system would need to be installed on a network server by the systems person who maintains the network.

None of the copies of the Macintosh OS for IBM compatibles is as elegant as the original Apple Macintosh graphic operating system, but they are coming much closer. The Macintosh operating system is a 32-bit system. Until recently an equivalent Macintosh computer would have been more expensive than an IBM compatible, but prices for Macintosh and IBM-compatible computers have become much more comparable.

There is no longer a simple and clear choice among operating systems. All have different disadvantages. How much RAM and how large a hard disk does your machine have? How important is a graphic interface? How crucial is the stability of the operating system? How critical is ease of installation? The answers to these questions are individual and subjective. Personal computers are not as simple as they once were, and the local availability of expert help with computers and their operating systems should be a strong determinant of the choice of an operating system.

Common Integrated Packages of Software Programs

Simple but very effective programs for word processing, spreadsheets, databases, and telecommunications are available for every computer system in combinations called integrated packages or suites. The names of many of these integrated programs end in the suffix works or office or suite. These integrated programs generally are inexpensive simplified versions of more complex programs and offer the beginner an opportunity to try using a word processor, a communications program, a spreadsheet, and a database with a common set of commands. Almost everyone will find a simple word processor to be cost efficient, but if personnel in a hospital epidemiology unit never use the simple spreadsheet or database programs in an integrated package, then there will probably be no need to consider the purchase of more expensive and complex versions of the same programs.

Word Processing

In excess of 90% of all computer use by hospital epidemiology units is for word processing. Memos and letters are written daily, and minutes of meetings and manuals have to be revised repeatedly. All of this is facilitated by the use of a simple word-processing program. At the most, scientific documents require underlining, subscripting, and superscripting, and the simplest available word-processing programs included in integrated packages provide these functions. Furthermore, word processing makes minimal demands on the computing chip, so computer speed considerations are almost irrelevant in this context.

As long as they have sufficient memory to hold a reasonably sized program either in RAM or on a hard disk, the simplest of PCs can serve as highly functional and efficient word processors. An expensive PC that is one hundred times faster than an elementary PC at performing complex statistical calculations will not be notably better for word processing. Furthermore, the added complexity of alleged state-of-the-art programs that beginners tend to purchase along with expensive high-end machines actually interferes with the accessibility and general utility of a computerized system. It is possible for almost anybody to master a simple word-processing program, and hospital epidemiology personnel should not hesitate to acquire simple hardware and software for word processing.

Searching a Literature Database

Because a literature database is searched by the computer at the other end of the telephone line, the power and speed of the PC used to address the distant computer is irrelevant. Connections with computers at distant sites can be accomplished either by direct cable network connection or by modem over telephone lines. Direct cable connections allow faster and clearer transmission than telephone connections. The type of network card necessary for direct cable connections is dictated by the network system. If telephone lines are used, then the quality and speed of the modem used for transmission of messages between computers over telephone lines will determine the functional speed of the system. Modem speeds are rated in baud, which refer to the approximate bits per second. Remember that 8 bits form 1 byte, or one character. Inexpensive modems have the ability to transmit and receive at common speeds $\leq$ 2,400 baud. Somewhat higher-priced modems are available that transmit at 28,800 baud and will transmit a document to a fax machine as well.

Electronic noise on telephone lines is the factor that most often limits the speed at which communication can take place between computers. Modems have built-in electronic circuitry to filter out unwanted noise, and the higher-speed modems have better filter systems. Almost any modem will work at low speeds. Furthermore, the total cost of telecommunication between computers includes the cost of the modem and software plus the cost of using the telephone line. If telephone charges are considered as well, a cheap but really slow modem is not an economically wise choice. A 28,800-baud modem may work at 28,800 baud for good telephone connections, but it will work better than a 2,400-baud modem at 2,400 baud because of its improved filter system. Unlike most areas in computing reviewed in this chapter, the purchase of the more expensive item in this case, a 28,800-baud modem, may prove cost-effective in any situation where a modem is used a substantial amount of time and results in extra measurable monthly telephone charges.

Communication between computers also requires a telecommunications program to connect the modem with the computer. Modems are usually packaged with usable software, and the integrated packages include a telecommunications program as well, so there is little need to buy a separate program for searching a literature database or contacting another computer with a modem.

Communications, the Internet, and E-mail

If you join one of the online services for a monthly subscription fee, you can gain access to the Internet and send and receive E-mail with your modem via the online service. If your institution is connected directly with the Internet you will need a network card instead of a modem to connect your PC with the local area network. Consult your local area network or systems manager before purchasing a network cable card and compatible network software.

Although it is not essential for hospital epidemiology, there is much information available over the Internet on the Worldwide Web. For easy access to the Web you will need a Web browser. The most popular browser is the Netscape Navigator, but Microsoft includes the Internet Explorer with Windows 95, and Windows 97 will incorporate this browser in the graphics interface.

Creating and Managing a Database

An electronic database is simply a program for recording and sorting data. Simple databases such as the ones included with integrated packages can be used effectively to store and sort data from a study or outbreak investigation. Data sets with dozens of variables for every subject can be sorted rapidly according to one or several variables at once with complete accuracy. This is the electronic equivalent of instant shuffling and reshuffling of paper data forms. Using a simple electronic database system for a limited study will acquaint the beginning user with the potential costs and benefits of such a computerized system.

Since surveillance is an integral function of the hospital epidemiology unit, it is also natural to consider the creation of a database for storing and accessing surveillance information [21]. At least four companies market database systems that are designed and customized for hospital epidemiology. These systems are expensive to acquire initially, and substantial time must be invested in order to learn how to use an electronic database. Furthermore, they require additional investment of time daily or weekly to enter all of the surveillance data. Once the program has been mastered and the data are entered, it is relatively easy to generate reports and summaries of the data. The potential usefulness of such a system for keeping records of an intensive care unit or an entire hospital depends on the balance between the time and money costs of entering the data into the electronic database versus the savings that might be realized when the data have to be sorted and summarized. It is substantially more difficult to master and maintain a database than a word processor, and thoughtful reflection is necessary before investing in an expensive database.

THE NEW HOSPITAL ACCREDITATION PROGRAM SCORING GUIDELINES

The new Accreditation Manual for Hospitals issued by the Joint Commission on Accreditation of Healthcare Organizations (JCAHO) includes a specific set of scoring guidelines on which the compliance of a hospital will be judged [22] (see Chapter 11). According to this new manual, to obtain the highest score, an individual hospital must provide evidence of having switched from processes such as surveillance of antibiotic use and nosocomial infections as ends in themselves [17] to the measurement of patients' outcomes as indicators of hospital performance [22]. According to the new manual, use of patients' outcomes requires that the system be performance-based and functionally organized to integrate with hospital-wide quality-improvement programs.

In the future performance will be based on "indicators," which are supposed to be valid and reliable quantitative or outcome process measures related to one or more dimensions of performance, such as appropriateness or effectiveness. There is a system called ORYX that consists of about 70 currently approved indicators for use in hospitals, only a few of which relate specifically to nosocomial infections. Only three of the eight proposed nosocomial infection indicators that underwent beta testing in hospitals survived the process, and these three are part of the ORYX system [22]. The first three infection control indicators are some surgical site infections, ventilator pneumonias, and some central line bacteremias. Because of the very limited and specific nature of the approved infection control indicators, small and even moderately sized hospitals may have very few patients to whom these three indicators apply. By 1998 all hospitals must begin reporting data to JCAHO on two of the 70 indicators from their own populations, and at least one of these two indicators must apply to inpatients. At least initially there is no requirement that anything related to nosocomial infections be included in the two required quality indicators.

What is allegedly new with this version is the requirement that results be linked to a hospital-wide system to assess and improve quality. The JCAHO scoring guidelines require that data trend analyses generated by surveillance activities be reviewed at least annually and the effectiveness of prevention and control intervention strategies in reducing nosocomial infection risk be evaluated at the same time. This calls for consideration of the manner in which hospital epidemiology units collect, sort, analyze, and store surveillance data. Of central importance will be the practical operational functionality of the database.

Attributes Defining the Functionality of a Database System

A user of any database system must be able to enter, store, retrieve, and sort data accurately in order to allow analyses of the data and the timely generation of reports. All of this must take place with minimal expenditure of resources. After data have been collected, all database systems require some form of data entry, data editing, and error correction before data sorting. A number of hospitals have been maintaining paper- or card-based systems for decades that have been used to analyze nosocomial infection data on various subgroups, such as those suggested in the new standard issued by the JCAHO [22]. The manner in which each of these steps is accomplished for paper, card, and electronic database systems and combinations of such systems is outlined here.

Paper-Based Systems

The original and still commonly used paper databases consist of line listing individuals in rows down the side with attributes defined as column headings along the top. Data from microbiology records, Kardexes, temperature sheets, medical records, interviews with nurses and physicians, and examinations of patients are added. Daily updating of line lists can be accomplished. Line lists are still in common use because they are the simplest to create, maintain, and store. Different types of line lists are easily made for various types of patients.

The disadvantages of line lists are that complex analyses may require reentry of data onto another medium because paper forms may not stand up well to repeated handling; moreover, counting and page turning is done by hand and is subject to human error. Furthermore, if substantial additional data concerning patients are taken from other offices in the hospital, these additional data must then be copied by hand onto the line lists. The benefits of line lists are that data entry is immediate and the organization self-evident, so that virtually no training time or user sophistication is required. Paper and pencils are very inexpensive, and updated line lists are immediately useful for simple report generation.

Card-Based Systems

Decks of common index cards are relatively efficient when used for analyzing moderately sized to large data sets. The data for one subject is recorded on each card, and then colored marks can be made in specified locations along the edges of each card to indicate the presence of various exposures, attributes, or events. These color-coded cards can then be sorted and counted quickly by hand and will stand up to repeated hand sortings.

The next level of sophistication involves McBee cards, which have holes punched along the edges. When the cards are stacked in a tray, the holes line up and a long rod can be used to sort cards by passing it through any specified hole location. Thus, sorting of McBee cards is much faster and more accurate than sorting color-coded index cards, and large data sets are conveniently handled using this system.

One disadvantage of a card-based system is similar to the problem with the paper-based system—namely, data from other offices in the hospital must still be transferred onto cards by hand. However, cards retain the inherent organizational simplicity of line lists and have some additional advantages. A card system is particularly efficient when the card is also the primary data collection form and cards rather than line lists are carried onto the wards. No additional steps of data transfer are required, and analyses can be carried out directly on the primary data collection form. Cards hold up well to multiple sortings and can be regrouped and resorted repeatedly. Cards are likewise inexpensive, and sorting and counting cards is faster and more accurate than shuffling papers and counting ticks on line lists. As with the paper-based systems, data on cards remain immediately available for the timely production of reports. Cards are also more resistant than paper forms to physical insults such as coffee spills.

Combining Numerators from Cards with Denominators from the Hospital Administrative Database

An efficient system for small to moderately large hospitals can be created simply by combining nosocomial infection surveillance data from cards with data taken from the administrative or discharge abstract electronic database already maintained by the hospital. If a card is used to record the data related to each patient who acquires a nosocomial infection, then these specific infection numerator data can be used in conjunction with other denominator data generally available from the electronic database maintained by the administrative offices of a hospital.

For example, denominator data for all surgical procedures of a specific type or all procedures performed by an individual surgeon or all patients with a specific diagnosis or a diagnosis-related group in a year are often readily available from an administrative electronic database. Detailed information on the nosocomial infections experienced by these subgroups of patients can be taken from surveillance data recorded on cards to provide incidences of procedure-, surgeon-, diagnosis-, or diagnosis group–specific incidences of nosocomial infection. Experience with such mixed systems suggests that they are relatively inexpensive and practical if the number of dischargees who acquire a nosocomial infection during hospitalization is not more than 500 to 1,000 per year. If ~5% of discharged patients experience a nosocomial infection, then hospitals with as many as 10,000 to 20,000 discharges annually could consider using a mixed system.

Dedicated Infection Control Electronic Databases

Now that nosocomial infection rates for subgroups of patients are of interest, computer enthusiasts have incorrectly suggested that dedicated computerized database systems have become essential in hospital epidemiology [23]. In fact, the actual usefulness of electronic database systems has become the focus of a major controversy, as evidenced by editorials and record numbers of letters to the editor [24]. Nosocomial infection rates according to site, service, physician, geographic location, and risk factors have been produced for decades using the paper- and card-based systems already described.

Dedicated computerized database systems for record keeping and sorting of hospital epidemiologic surveillance data have been tested and reviewed by various groups [23,25–27], and their usefulness will depend on the long-term availability of extra resources to enter, edit, and correct data from original data collection forms and the resources to train and maintain an operator to manipulate the electronic database. In addition, the computer hardware and software must be purchased, the system assembled, and the programs installed.

One exceptional potential advantage to an electronic database is that computerized data from other offices in the hospital may be accessed and downloaded into the system without the necessity of reentry of data by hand. The availability of computerized data from other sources, such as administration and billing, various laboratories, the radiology department, and the pharmacy, will vary among hospitals, and the ease with which such data can be acquired varies among database programs. At the expense of tens of millions of dollars, some research institutions have been able to create systems with interfaces to access virtually all of the information available in tertiary care hospitals as it becomes available and to feed back the information to physicians and epidemiologists in real time, so that it can be put to use immediately in the care of patients [3–5,8–11].

However, the creation of an electronic database that will be useful in the timely analysis of data and production of reports is far from a trivial undertaking. At the Centers for Disease Control and Prevention, the National Nosocomial Infections Surveillance (NNIS) System was created as a standardized electronic database system for recording the data generated from line lists in many individual hospitals nationwide. Although this was a very laudable goal, there were some difficulties in keeping current. The objective of maintaining an electronic database that will be useful in the timely analysis of data and generation of reports has eluded even experienced central authorities with substantial resources. Currently the NNIS system is being revitalized.

Features of an Individual Hospital That Determine the Usefulness of a Dedicated Electronic Database

Each hospital epidemiology unit must judge individually whether it has the additional resources that will be required to create and maintain a large electronic database dedicated to infection control and whether such an investment would result in a reasonable return. Two extreme situations are presented here, and most hospitals will fall somewhere between the two.

A hospital that already maintains administrative, billing, laboratory, radiology, and pharmacy data in computerized format and is willing to supply a programmer who will make these data easily available to downloading into a hospital epidemiology database has an ideal situation in which to switch to an electronic database. In such a setting, large amounts of information will already be available for each patient, and infection control personnel need only add their own data to what already exists. The extra time required to enter data into this system will be more than compensated for by the vast amount of information available from other sources within the hospital. At present, this situation exists in only a few research settings [3–5,8–11], but the potential to create another should not be overlooked. An appropriately maintained and updated electronic database is a joy to use when it is time to generate routine reports and can also facilitate investigations of unusual events.

On the other hand, for many small and moderately sized hospitals and for hospitals with no additional resources for programming and data entry, the use of a dedicated infection control electronic database would require removing personnel from clinical responsibilities to enter, edit, and correct data. Furthermore, if data are not easily accessible electronically from other offices in the hospital, then these additional data would have to be entered manually into the electronic database. The need for additional personnel may negate the advantages of a dedicated electronic database. A compromise used by several hospitals has been to keep data on patients in intensive care units in an electronic database while maintaining data from the remainder of the hospital in a card or paper based system.

Safeguards for Implementing an Electronic Database System

If it is decided that a hospital epidemiology unit will switch, altogether or in part, from a paper or card system to an electronic database for surveillance, there are certain safeguards that should be instituted. For a period, the old paper- or card-based system and the new electronic database must be maintained side by side, until all personnel involved are convinced that the new system can be used to analyze data accurately and produce the desired reports without unreasonable delays.

Several kinds of backup for an electronic system are also essential. Hard disks on PCs are simple to use and thus easy to ignore. Hard disks are precision mechanical devices and will fail eventually, so all data on hard disks must be backed up at least weekly onto conventional floppy diskettes, large-capacity diskettes, or tapes. A convenient large-capacity disk or tape backup system should be considered an integral part of any electronic database used in hospital epidemiology and should be used at least weekly. Additionally, if data are originally collected on cards, then the card-based system can be retained as a precaution in case of computer malfunction or lack of availability of the trained database operator.

Dedicated Hospital Epidemiology Databases

For those who would like to use an electronic database but do not wish to spend the time that would be required to customize one of the commercially available databases for use in their hospital, there are four commercially available dedicated hospital epidemiology databases for general use in hospitals. These are AICE, NNIS-IDEAS, QLOGIC II, and WHOCARE [28–31]. AICE is now in version 5; it is the oldest and the most common, and is thus user friendly, but it is also expensive. It has some graphics capability. NNIS-IDEAS is available from the Centers for Disease Control and Prevention only to those hospitals that participate in CDC's NNIS project. While the program is free, it requires the purchase of the PRODAS database program and continued participation in NNIS. QLOGIC II is a quality management program that includes an infection control module. QLOGIC bought the old NOSO3 program and runs on the Paradox Database. It is complex and expensive but has good graphics and a good query feature. WHOCARE/HAI is a basic program that comes from Europe. It is much less expensive and less comprehensive than the others, and it also has European date formats. Although reviews of available software have been published in the past [23–25], the information in the reviews has been of varying quality, and there is only one up-to-date paper available for those interested in the purchase of a dedicated electronic database. Be sure to try out an installed version of one of these databases before selecting one.

The vast majority of U.S. hospitals do not use dedicated hospital epidemiology electronic databases. Most commonly they use paper- or card-based systems and, occasionally, generic electronic databases, spreadsheets, and graphics programs. Epidemiology units in hospitals that use one of the dedicated electronic databases often apply it only to a small segment of the hospital population, such as patients in intensive care units. Before settling on any one of these programs, be sure to try out a working version in another hospital.

COMPUTERIZED SYSTEMS IN ADVANCED EPIDEMIOLOGIC RESEARCH

The computerized system that is optimal for effective analysis of a complex data set originating from a disease outbreak, or for the analysis of data for research into an endemic problem, is different from the software described earlier. The area in which computers can be most helpful in advanced epidemiologic research is in the removal of distortions from confounding [32–34].

Confounding

For the sake of understanding, we prefer to estimate the magnitude of the effect of one determinant at a time. The bench biologist has control of the environment and can set up experiments to change one variable at a time. To accomplish that same end in observational epidemiology, we must somehow nullify or correct for the effects of many other unwanted determinants or exposures that are actually acting jointly with the exposure under study (see Chapter 7).

Since several factors or determinants acting jointly are almost invariably responsible for a single outcome in hospital epidemiology, confounding can be seen as the distortion of the estimate of the magnitude of the effect of one cause of an outcome when it is mixed with some of the effects of other causes of the same outcome [32–34]. We know that older age, female gender, and instrumentation of the urinary tract are all determinants, or causes, of nosocomial urinary tract infections. In a hospital population, patients with urinary tract infections tend to be older and are more likely to be female than the patients without urinary tract infections. Urinary tract infections would be jointly determined by all three of these exposures, and this is called confounding. If we want to measure the effect of instrumentation alone, then we must somehow nullify the effect of age and gender. If we fail to adjust for the effect of age and gender, then our estimates of the effect of instrumentation of the urinary tract will be distorted, or confounded, by the effects of these other unwanted, extraneous variables.

Variation in the Severity of Underlying Disease

The most overarching problem in the analysis of data from observational studies in hospital epidemiology is confounding by severity of underlying disease [32]. With the change in approach to accreditation by the JCAHO, hospital epidemiology has recently been subsumed into the relatively new area of quality assurance [22,35–37], and difficulties with confounding have been best illustrated by the initial efforts of the Health Care Financing Administration (HCFA) to judge quality of hospital care through monitoring and reporting hospital death rates and rates of nosocomial infections. Both death and infection have many causes, and to measure the effect of one of them, say, the effect of quality (or lack of quality) of hospital care in the analysis, one must adjust successfully for the effects of all of the other determinants of death or infection.

The first attempts of the HCFA demonstrate the hazard of failing to consider the confounding effect of different degrees of severity of underlying illness in the comparison of crude hospital death rates. Despite the fact that the need for adjusting for severity of underlying disease when comparing hospital death rates was clearly established [38], this agency failed to adjust for variations in the severity of underlying illness and so identified a hospice as the hospital with the highest "abnormal" mortality in the country, without consideration of the terminal nature of the illnesses of patients admitted to a hospice [39].

Increasingly sophisticated means for adjusting for severity of illness (case mix) were gradually employed by this agency. However, perhaps because of the errors in the initial effort, the intended consumers of these data—the hospital leaders—generally rejected the results [40]. Further research has indicated that after adjustment for severity of illness, using objective comparisons, it remains extremely difficult to detect differences in hospital care that lead to excess mortality rates [41]. Because of the failure of the HCFA to adjust appropriately for severity of underlying disease, this system of judging the quality of hospital care through hospital mortality fell into disrepute and was eventually discontinued. Sicker patients are more likely to acquire nosocomial infections, and, similarly, these same sicker patients are more likely to have adverse outcomes of hospitalization.

Unfortunately, most studies in hospital epidemiology are observational in nature. In any comparison in an observational study, no matter whether the subjects are neonates [42–44] or adults [32,45,46], separating the effects of severity of illness from the effects of the exposure under study remains the major challenge. Sicker patients have more exposures and more bad outcomes, and the interpretability of almost any study in hospital epidemiology depends on how well adjustment can be made for varying degrees of severity of underlying illness [32].

At the Second International Conference on Nosocomial Infections held in 1980, there was but a single paper on the effects of differential risks of nosocomial infection [47], whereas a large number of such papers were presented at the Third International Conference held a decade later [48]. Despite the clear importance of underlying disease in determining nosocomial infection, the HCFA, the same government agency that failed to adjust for underlying illness when comparing hospital death rates, also concluded that the frequency of occurrence of nosocomial infections reported by hospitals or their epidemiology units should be used as a generic screen for comparing quality of care among hospitals. In their view, every nosocomial infection indicated a problem with quality of care, irrespective of the underlying illness of the patient [49].

This reasoning erroneously suggested that a patient with a terminal underlying illness and compromised host defenses who acquired an infection with his or her own flora suffered a nosocomial infection that was somehow preventable. Before constructing this generic quality screen, the HCFA did not consider the wide range in reported sensitivity (5% to 95%) of available surveillance data from different types of hospitals in different areas of the country [50,51], nor did they consider their own documented inability to adjust for confounding by severity of underlying disease [39,40]. The concerted actions of several national organizations involved with hospital epidemiology were successful in persuading the HCFA to withdraw the quality screen based on unadjusted comparisons of reported occurrences of nosocomial infections. No sooner had the HCFA withdrawn the nosocomial infection screen as a generic quality screen than the Maryland Hospital Association reinvented the concept of nosocomial infections as a quality indicator [52], without noting any of the above-mentioned problems with the epidemiologic interpretation of comparative nosocomial infection rates.

The degree to which the unalterable characteristics of the individual patient determine the inherent susceptibility to infection and probability of death are not yet well defined but clearly are of major importance in modern hospital epidemiology. As recent history, such as that just described, has demonstrated, the frantic search for anything possibly related to the measurement of the quality of hospital care has put a new public focus on several groups within hospitals. Hospital epidemiology personnel have been especially pressured to measure, compare, and make reports public. Insofar as many groups interested in quality have shown little interest in or sophistication with the basic principles of epidemiology, it is incumbent on knowledgeable hospital epidemiology personnel to ensure that reasonable data and comparisons come before the public eye. Adjustment for confounding is clearly a major concern for the future.

There are two general categories of computerized tools for effective adjustment for confounding in comparisons: multiway stratification and the fitting of multivariate models. Stratification is most accessible to the clinically trained individual.

Introduction to Stratification

Stratification is the simplest, most intuitive way to approach this problem, and a simple logical scheme for analyzing complex epidemiologic data sets has been published [32–34,51]. In these references, confounding and a related concept, effect modification, are defined, and several examples of analysis using these concepts are provided. Stratification is easy to understand, makes data visible, and automatically indicates confounding, effect modification, and lack of linear trend. Detailed examples and suggestions are available [51].

Multiway stratification has long been the favorite analytic tool of the epidemiologist, but sophisticated programs for producing adjusted summary estimates of risk ratios and 95% confidence intervals have appeared only relatively recently [6,13,51]; now there are a number of programs for PCs that focus on the epidemiologic analysis of categorical data. These programs are reviewed regularly [6,17]. The dEPID, IDR, MHCHI, and STATCALC (part of EPI INFO) are simple shareware programs for PCs that can be used for sophisticated epidemiologic analyses of categorical data. After data have been sorted into categories, perhaps with one of the database programs, sophisticated stratified analyses can be conducted with these shareware programs. In addition, versions of programs suitable for sophisticated epidemiologic analysis of categorical data are beginning to be included in the standard statistical packages [13–17].

Introduction to Multivariate Modeling Using Statistical Packages

Complex epidemiologic data sets containing data on many variables have commonly been analyzed by multiway stratification, without fitting multivariate models [6,13,32,51]. However, canned statistical programs are available that make the fitting of multivariate models relatively easy for beginners and experts alike [14–17]. All three commonly available statistical packages have versions for both mainframes and PCs. The PC versions are generally available for both Macintosh and IBM compatibles, although versions for Windows 3.1 and the MS DOS operating system are still limited in the amount of RAM that can be used. The limitations in RAM usage for the PC versions using 16-bit operating systems inhibit some of the memory-intensive procedures for analyzing categorical data, such as logistic regression and Cox regression. SAS is available for the IBM OS/2 and Windows 95 operating systems in full 32-bit versions for PCs that provide performance on a PC approaching that available from a workstation.

The programming necessary to use these statistical packages is much more complex than the programming required for the simple shareware programs mentioned earlier and for the other uses of computers described previously in this chapter, so a potential user should experiment with a statistical package before spending any money. The least expensive way to investigate the potential usefulness of one of these statistical packages is to borrow time on a hospital or university mainframe in which one of these packages is already installed. Statistical packages for PC use can be purchased but are very expensive. Most companies make PC versions available through local lease-of-site licenses rather than through purchase [39], which is much less costly.

It requires a substantial formal background to fit multivariate models in an appropriate way. A recent survey of the medical literature has found that investigators with clinical training but little biostatistical or epidemiologic expertise usually misuse these canned statistical programs and report flawed analyses incorporating multivariate models [51,53]. An investigator should be familiar with the concepts in standard epidemiology and biostatistics texts and examples [51–61] before embarking on an analysis that depends on the fitting and interpretation of multivariate models.

Summary of the Epidemiologic Use of Statistical Packages

Many statistical packages contain excellent programs for the analysis of categorical data, especially multiway stratification. These programs are indispensable for the analysis of complex data sets. Additionally, despite this long list of very real problems with the naive application of multivariate models in epidemiology, there are a number of appropriate uses of multivariate analysis.

There are two steps to understanding what is happening in a complex observational data set: elimination of the myriad variables that have no bearing on the outcome under investigation and elucidation of the biologic influence of the few variables that actually are causally related to the outcome [33,34,42,46,47,51,58,60]. Statistical packages on computers are efficient at fitting multivariate models to sort through and discard as unimportant many variables in complex data sets. Although an epidemiologist may be hesitant to render a positive biologic interpretation of the results of a multivariate model, the same model will be very helpful in indicating which variables are of no importance and can be ignored in future analyses of the same data set. In this manner, multivariate models can be used to identify variables that merit further analysis by methods such as stratification, which more easily lend themselves to the causal interpretation of results.

In summary, computerized systems are invaluable for word processing, for searching literature databases, and for communicating via E-mail. The cost-effectiveness of a computerized electronic database system compared with a card-based system or combined system for hospital surveillance data depends on the characteristics of an individual hospital and the resources of the hospital epidemiology unit. Potential users interested in stratified analyses of hospital data to adjust for confounding can experiment with simple but sophisticated available shareware programs. A few hospitals will have use for large and complex canned statistical packages for the analysis of research data.

HARDWARE FOR PERSONAL COMPUTING FOR HOSPITAL EPIDEMIOLOGY

The Minimal Outlay Version Based on Scavenging

A wide range of PCs can be used in hospital epidemiology, and the range from the cheapest to the most expensive is reviewed here. Relatively simple computers and programs needed for most work in hospital epidemiology, word processing and communications often can be obtained free or for little money from other areas or departments in a hospital. What constitutes a minimal but useful PC? Obviously the answer to this question varies, and computer enthusiasts will tell you that old and limited machines of the sort described here are useful only as door stops. Nevertheless, if you can use the MS DOS operating system, then an IBM-compatible computer with a 286 Intel chip, at least 640 kilobytes of RAM, a 40-megabyte hard disk and a 3.5-inch floppy drive will make a highly functional word processor.

The purchase of a larger hard disk is a cheap way to increase the utility of a scavenged machine. If you can find several such cast-off machines, then you have the potential for an economic form of multitasking (running different programs simultaneously on different computers) without worry about complex and unstable operating systems and program crashes. The author uses such a setup to perform quantitative analyses on one simple machine while actually writing the paper on the word processor of a second. In addition, if one has the same programs on more than one machine, then one can move a file from one machine to another by physically transferring it on a floppy disk. This file transfer without a network and a complex operating system has been termed "sneakernet." Sneakernet works faultlessly between departments of a hospital or between home and work offices, requires no additional programming, and produces no telephone bills. With such a setup one needs only a letter-quality printer for one of the computers. Contrast the specifications in this section on cheap secondhand computers with those recommended for new machines to understand the wide range of computers that can be useful in hospital epidemiology.

The Moderate Outlay Version Based on Buying Discontinued Models

When computer companies introduce new models of computers, they frequently offer older but discontinued models at substantial discounts. By keeping an eye on computer magazines, it is often possible to purchase a new but discontinued previously top-of-the-line computer for one half to one fifth of the original list price. Such discounts make the purchase of these new machines very economical. Make sure you obtain a sufficiently large hard disk and enough RAM (see later discussion) if you purchase a new computer this way. When buying a discontinued model, it is wise to choose a computer from a well-known company that has been in business for a number of years so that you will be able to obtain service for your computer. When machines with Intel 486 chips were discontinued in favor of the Pentium chip, real bargains became available. The author has bought all of his new machines as discontinued models.

Buying New Computer Hardware

At the other end of the economic spectrum is the purchase of a new state-of-the-art model of PC. The graphic operating systems use 30 to 60 megabytes of hard disk space, and the programs designed for these systems are proportionally large. At this time it would seem foolhardy to purchase a new computer with less than about 300 megabytes of hard disk space, and 1.2 gigabytes would be better. The graphic operating systems also require at least 8 megabytes of RAM to function, and 16 or 32 megabytes are better. If you want to be able to read the text easily in several open windows at once, then plan on buying a substantially larger monitor (perhaps 15 inch) than was previously necessary. Look at the size of the text in several windows on another machine to decide how big a monitor is big enough for you.

Most new large software programs are being supplied on a single optical CD rather than on dozens of floppies, so if you plan to buy a state-of-the-art PC you will need a CD-ROM drive as well. Also remember that if you buy one of the new graphic operating systems with programs to match, you will probably need expert advice on installation and configuration.

Choosing a Laptop

Laptop PCs are very useful when one travels and when one is at a distant site where, for example, one might be on call. The capabilities of laptops are close to the capabilities of desktop models, but laptops are somewhat more expensive. Two additional features are especially important in determining the functionality of a laptop: visibility of text on the screen and the size and feel of the keyboard. With a laptop it is especially important to try out the screen and keyboard on the exact model you are considering purchasing.

The ease of viewing of the screen on a laptop is a major determinant of its utility. While a cathode ray tube (CRT) of a conventional monitor actually shines light out toward your eyes, the liquid crystal display (LCD) of a laptop screen may or may not be very difficult to see. There are many varieties of LCD screens, and those with an active matrix display are easier to use and can be viewed effectively from wider angles. There are also major differences between similar products made by different manufacturers. As you look at the display on the screen of a computer you are considering buying, see if you can find the cursor easily on the LCD screen. Can you read text on the LCD screen from various angles and in all kinds of light? Will you be able to view the LCD screen with comfort for hours? If you want to use a program with windows, can you read the text inside the windows, and are you comfortable with the laptop mouse equivalent? Try the keyboard on a laptop. One way for manufacturers to miniaturize a computer is to reduce the size and spacing of keys on a keyboard. If you have large hands, you may find a small keyboard to be a real handicap. If you plan to spend even a moderate amount of time with a computer, it makes no sense to purchase a machine that is difficult or unpleasant to use.

Review of Suggestions for Acquiring PC Hardware

As a final reminder, it is useful to remember that 90% to 100% of your work (word processing, searching literature databases, and communicating via the Internet) can be accomplished equally well on a cheap scavenged machine of the sort described earlier.

REFERENCES

1. Landauer TK. *The trouble with computers: usefulness, usability, and productivity.* Cambridge, Mass.: MIT Press, 1995.
2. Barr RL, Gerzoff RB. Controlling urges and infections: computer system design for epidemiology. *Infect Control Hosp Epidemiol* 1985; 6:317–322.
3. Broderick A, Mori M. Nettleman MD, et al. Nosocomial infections: validation of surveillance and computer modeling to identify patients at risk. *Am J Epidemiol* 1990;131:734–742.
4. Classen DC, Burke JP, Pestotnik SL, et al. Surveillance for quality

assessment. IV. Surveillance using a hospital information system. *Infect Control Hosp Epidemiol* 1991;12:239–244.
5. Evans RS, et al. Computer surveillance of hospital-acquired infections and antibiotic use. *JAMA* 1986;256:1007.
6. Foster D, Sullivan K. Software. In: Bernier RH, Mason VM, eds. *Episource: a guide to resources in epidemiology*. Roswell, Ga.: The Epidemiology Monitor, 1991:973–1064.
7. Hierholzer WJ Jr. The practice of hospital epidemiology. *Yale J Biol Med* 1982;55:225.
8. Hierholzer WJ Jr, Miller SP, Streed SA, Wood D. On-line infection control system using PCS/IMS. In: O'Neill JT, ed. *Proceedings of the Fourth Annual Symposium on Computer Applications in Medical Care*. Washington, D.C.: Center for Health Sciences Research, 1980: 540.
9. Evans RS, Burke JP, Classen DC, et al. Computerized identification of patients at high risk for hospital-acquired infection. *Am J Infect Control* 1992;20:4–10.
10. Platt R, Stryker WS, Komaroff AL. Pharmacoepidemiology in hospitals using automated data systems. *Am J Prev Med* 1988;4(suppl 2): 39–47.
11. Miller PL, Paton JA, Roderer NK, et al. Building a cooperative institutional model of IAIMS at the Yale–New Haven Medical Center. In: *Proceedings of the Annual Symposium in Computer Applications in Medical Care* 1994:1002.
12. Birnbaum D. Computers in hospital epidemiology practice. *Infect Control Hosp Epidemiol* 1988;9:81.
13. Rothman KJ, Boice JD Jr. *Epidemiologic analysis with a programmable calculator*. Boston: Epidemiology Resources, Inc., 1982.
14. Dixon WJ, Brown MB, Engleman L, Jennrich RI. *BMDP statistical software manual*. Berkeley: University of California Press, 1990.
15. *SAS/STAT user's guide*, version 6, 4th ed. Cary, N.C.: SAS Institute, 1990.
16. Norusis MJ. *SPSS/PC-base system user's guide*, version 5.0. Chicago: SPSS, 1992.
17. Sullivan K. Epiware. *Epidemiol Monit* 1994;15:5; 1995;16:6; 1996; 17:3.
18. Gookin D. *MS-DOS 6.2 upgrade for dummies*. San Mateo, CA: IDG Books, 1993.
19. Leonard W, Simon B. *The mother of all Windows books*. Reading. Mass.: Addison-Wesley, 1993.
20. Cortese A, Rebello K. Windows 95: Can Microsoft's new software live up to expectations? *Business Week* July 10, 1995:94–104.
21. Proceedings of the International Symposium on Control of Nosocomial Infection, Jerusalem, April 28–May 2, 1980. *Rev Infect Dis* 1981; 3:635.
22. Joint Commission on the Accreditation of Healthcare Organizations. *Hospital accreditation standards*. Oakbrook Terrace, Ill.: Joint Commission on the Accreditation of Healthcare Organizations, 1997.
23. LaHaise S. A comparison of infection control software for use by hospital epidemiologists in meeting the new JCAHCO standards. *Infect Control Hosp Epidemiol* 1990;11:185.
24. Letters to the editor. *Infect Control Hosp Epidemiol* 1990;11:400.
25. Berg R. Reviews: software. *Am J Infect Control* 1986;14:139.
26. Gaynes R, Friedman C, Copeland TA, Thiele GH. Methodology to evaluate a computer-based system for surveillance of hospital-acquired infections. *Am J Infect Control* 1990;18:40.
27. Reagan DR. Microcomputers in hospital epidemiology. *Infect Control Hosp Epidemiol* 1997;18:440–448.
28. Infection Control and Prevention Analysts. *AICE 5.0*. Austin: 1995.
29. Hospital Infections Program, Centers for Disease Control. *NNIS IDEAS*. Atlanta: 1995.
30. Epi-Systematics. *QLOGIC II infection control*. Fort Myers, Fla.: 1995.
31. WHO/EURO Quality of Care Technologies. *WHOCARE/HAI*. Copenhagen: Statens Seruminstitut, 1995.
32. Freeman J, Goldmann DA, McGowan JE Jr. Methodologic issues in hospital epidemiology. IV. Risk ratios, confounding, effect modification, and the analysis of multiple variables. *Rev Infect Dis* 1988;10: 1118.
33. Keinbaum DG, Kupper LL, Morgenstern H. *Epidemiologic research: principles and quantitative methods*. Belmont, Calif.: Lifetime Learning Publications, 1982.
34. Rothman KJ. *Modern epidemiology*. Boston: Little, Brown, 1986.
35. Crede W, Hierholzer WJ. Surveillance for quality assessment. I. Surveillance in infection control success reviewed. *Infect Control Hosp Epidemiol* 1989;10:470.
36. McGeer A, Crede W, Hierholzer WJ. Surveillance for quality assessment. II. Surveillance for noninfectious processes: back to basics. *Infect Control Hosp Epidemiol* 1990;11:36.
37. Crede WB, Hierholzer WJ. Surveillance for quality assessment. III. The critical assessment of quality indicators. *Infect Control Hosp Epidemiol* 1990;11:197.
38. Hebel RJ, Kessler II, Mabuchi K, McCarter RJ. Assessment of hospital performance by use of death rates: a recent case history. JAMA 1982; 248:3131.
39. Brinkley J. U.S. releasing lists of hospitals with abnormal mortality rates. *The New York Times* March 12, 1986:1.
40. Berwick DM, Wald DL. Hospital leaders' opinions of the HCFA mortality data. *JAMA* 1990;264:247.
41. Park RA, et al. Explaining variations in hospital death rates: randomness, severity of illness, quality of care. *JAMA* 1990;264:484.
42. Freeman J, Goodman DA, Smith NE, et al. Association of intravenous lipid emulsion and coagulase-negative staphylococcal bacteremia in neonatal intensive care units. *N Engl J Med* 1990;323:301–308.
43. Goldmann DA, Durbin WA Jr, Freeman J. Nosocomial infections in the neonatal intensive care unit. *J Infect Dis* 1981;144:449.
44. Goldmann DA, Freeman J, Durbin WA Jr. Nosocomial infection and death in a neonatal intensive care unit. *J Infect Dis* 1983;147:635.
45. Freeman J, McGowan JE Jr. Risk factors for nosocomial infection. *J Infect Dis* 1978;138:811.
46. Freeman J, McGowan JE Jr. Methodologic issues in hospital epidemiology. III. Investigating the modifying effects of time and severity of underlying illness on estimates of the cost of nosocomial infection. *Rev Infect Dis* 1984;6:285.
47. Freeman J, McGowan JE Jr. Differential risks of nosocomial infection. *Am J Med* 1981;70:915.
48. Final program and abstracts of the Third International Conference on Nosocomial Infections, Atlanta, July 31–August 3, 1990.
49. Health Care Financing Administration. *Generic quality screens*. Peer Review Organization, Third Scope of Work, Attachment 1. September 1989.
50. Haley RW, Culver DH, Morgan WM, et al. Increased recognition of infectious diseases in U.S. hospitals through increased use of diagnostic tests, 1970–1976. *Am J Epidemiol* 1985;121:168–181.
51. Freeman J. Modern quantitative epidemiology in the hospital. In: Mayhall CG, ed. *Hospital epidemiology and infection control*. Baltimore: Williams and Wilkins, 1995.
52. Scheckler WE. Interim report of the quality indicator study group. *Infect Control Hosp Epidemiol* 1994;15:265–268.
53. Concato J, Feinstein AR, Holford TR. The risk of determining risk with multivariable models. *Ann Intern Med* 1993;118:201–210.
54. Mosteller F, Tukey JW. *Data analysis and regression: a second course in statistics*. Reading, Mass.: Addison-Wesley, 1977.
55. Sall J. *Technical report: A-102. SAS regression applications*. Cary, N.C.: SAS Institute, 1981.
57. Greenland S. Modeling and variable selection in epidemiologic analysis. *Am J Public Health* 1989;79:340–349.
58. Hill AB. *Principles of medical statistics*, 9th ed. New York: Oxford University Press, 1971.
59. Snedecor GW, Cochran WG. *Statistical methods*, 7th ed. Ames: Iowa State University Press, 1980.
60. Rinehart E, et al. Rapid dissemination of β-lactamase-producing, aminoglycoside-resistant *Enterococcus faecalis* among patients and staff on an infant-toddler surgical ward. *N Engl J Med* 1990;323:1814.
61. Pestotnik SL, Classen DC, Evans RS, Burke JP. Implementing antibiotic practice guidelines through computer-assisted decision support: clinical and financial outcomes. *Ann Intern Med* 1996;124:884–890.

Hospital Infections, Fourth Edition,
edited by John V. Bennett and Philip S. Brachman.
Lippincott–Raven Publishers, Philadelphia © 1998

CHAPTER 9

The Role of the Laboratory in Control of Nosocomial Infection

John E. McGowan, Jr. and Robert A. Weinstein

Nosocomial infections continue to present a major problem in hospitals today. Because of the importance of this subject, each hospital laboratory has the responsibility of supporting activities related to surveillance, control, and prevention of nosocomial infections [1,2]. Each laboratory can make major contributions toward infection control, as long as the people responsible for infection control efforts and those in charge of the clinical microbiology laboratory cooperate closely to attack this problem. Often the same people have both of these responsibilities; nearly half of those who chair Infection Control Committees are laboratory personnel [3].

Laboratory personnel attempt to minimize the occurrence of nosocomial infection in the following seven ways: 1) participation in hospital-wide infection control activities, especially those of the hospital Infection Control Committee or Service Team; 2) recovery and accurate identification of responsible organisms; 3) determining antimicrobial susceptibility of selected nosocomial pathogens; 4) reporting in timely fashion of laboratory data relevant to infection control and participation in surveillance of nosocomial infection; 5) provision of additional studies, when necessary, to establish similarity or difference of organisms; 6) provision, on occasion, of microbiologic studies of the hospital environment; and 7) training of infection control personnel.

Since 1990, improvements in laboratory instrumentation and procedures have provided dramatic aid to infection control efforts in several ways [4]. Among these are techniques for more rapid detection and differentiation of organisms and improved systems of reporting for both patient data and trend analysis. Perhaps the most dramatic advances have come in special procedures for examining ("typing") hospital organisms for similarity or difference; here, molecular and other techniques have permitted more definitive examination of a wider range of organisms than was possible before [5,6].

J. E. McGowan, Jr.: Department of Pathology, Emory University, Department of Laboratory Medicine, Grady Memorial Hospital, Atlanta, Georgia 30335.

R. A. Weinstein: Department of Medicine, Rush Medical College, Division of Infectious Diseases, Cook County Hospital, Chicago, Illinois 60612-9985.

PARTICIPATION IN HOSPITAL-WIDE INFECTION CONTROL ACTIVITIES

Relationship of the Laboratory to the Infection Control Committee

A clinically oriented member of the laboratory staff can contribute significantly by serving on the Infection Control Committee, or Service Team, as it may be called today. Such participation is essential in contributing to a harmonious relationship among clinical, infection control, and microbiology personnel [7].

In the typical hospital, most members of the Infection Control Committee do not have a background in microbiology [8]. Thus, it is of great importance for the representative of the laboratory to provide the microbiologic expertise that is critical to many decisions of the group. This knowledge may be required for the assessment of the significance of culture data, for determining the validity of laboratory techniques used to identify cases of nosocomial infection, and in the design and implementation of investigations and survey projects.

The diagnostic microbiology laboratory is engaged primarily in the evaluation of cultures related to infection. Because these are crucial data for successful infection control, the laboratory activities should be closely coordinated with the Infection Control Committee. For example, the adequacy of the basic techniques for primary isolation, speciation, and antimicrobial susceptibility testing should be discussed by the microbiologists and the Infection Control Committee. Laboratory resources often are stretched by patient care requirements, especially in smaller hospitals [9]. Laboratory support for infection control activities must be given with discretion. For example, use of laboratory resources to assess colonization or to sample personnel and the environment for bacterial or other organisms should never be permitted when the epidemiologic indications are unclear [9].

Major changes have occurred in reimbursement methods for hospitals in the United States as managed care has become popular [10]. In view of these changes, there seems to be an added service that the laboratory microbiologist can provide to the Infection Control Committee and other hospital committees concerned with infection control. Under managed care, there will continue to be new and intensive attempts to evaluate the validity and usefulness of hospital programs such as infection control [11]. Techniques for assessment are familiar to clinical microbiology personnel, who have to make similar cost–benefit judgments for laboratory equipment, instruments, and procedures almost daily [12]. The insights and methods used for such laboratory activities should be helpful to the infection control team and the various committees (e.g., infection control, quality assurance, pharmacy and therapeutics) as they review the benefit of their activities and attempt to improve the productivity of the program [13].

Budgetary Considerations

Costs for laboratory procedures that are not related directly to care of patients (e.g., bacteriologic sampling of personnel and the environment) should be borne by a budget separate from that of the laboratory. To facilitate all the microbiologic activities necessitated by an outbreak, the laboratory (or the hospital epidemiologist, or the Infection Control Committee, depending on the organizational structure of the hospital) should have a contingency fund to enable personnel, materials, and space to be temporarily assigned to epidemic aid support [14]. An investigation of an outbreak should not be financed by charging individual patients for cultures taken during the study. This will become less of an issue as capitated care becomes more prominent and direct charges to patients for specific services decline.

ACCURATE IDENTIFICATION OF ORGANISMS INVOLVED IN NOSOCOMIAL INFECTION

Infection control personnel search constantly for evidence that a common organism has spread from patient to patient or from staff to patient. Thus, information permitting the successful tracing of organism movements within the hospital may be of value to the hospital infection control team, whether the positive cultures represent episodes of infection or indicate colonization of the patient [15]. Although some clinical features of illness provide information about etiology, the main sources for this determination usually are the data provided by the clinical laboratory. Hence, the ability of the laboratory staff to isolate and identify responsible microorganisms is crucial to infection control [16].

The spectrum of organisms causing nosocomial infection has changed dramatically since the mid-1980s [17]. Enterobacteriaceae, *Staphylococcus aureus*, *Pseudomonas aeruginosa*, and coagulase-negative staphylococci remain frequently associated with nosocomial infection [2,18]. Among the patterns of special concern are the appearance of fungi and viruses as they become more frequent agents of nosocomial infection [18]. Fortunately, technologic developments in the laboratory over the same period have continued to increase the efficiency with which nosocomial organisms can be recognized and recovered [4]. There are three main aspects to this. First, new instruments and devices have become widely available. These permit easier detection of the presence of organisms in blood cultures, organism identification, and testing of susceptibility to antimicrobials. Some of these devices are automated, permitting the laboratory to provide these improved services with the same or fewer personnel [19]. Many of the instruments can be cost effective for limited numbers of specimens; as a result, smaller laboratories as well as large ones can now include some of these methods in their program. Use of these instruments and devices also has led to a more standard approach throughout the United States to the identification and susceptibility testing of nosocomial pathogens. Thus, most of the organisms causing outbreaks or special endemic problems of nosocomial infection can be identified in the hospital laboratory.

Second, nonculture tests have permitted identification of agents of nosocomial infection that would not have been recognized in earlier years [20]. Immunologic and nucleic acid testing methods have added to our ability to recognize viruses and other organisms that are difficult or impossible to grow in culture; some of these are involved in nosocomial infection. Amplification techniques such as the polymerase chain reaction (PCR) and other gene-based methods are making tests for diagnosis of infection even more sensitive [21,22]. Some of these tests are useful for rapid identification of isolates even if they cannot be characterized by routine biochemical methods [23].

Third, these newer tests and instruments not only permit identification of additional agents but allow more rapid diagnosis of both new and old pathogens. This speedier testing should provide earlier recognition of outbreaks and more efficient handling of organisms in endemic nosocomial and community-acquired infections [24], which should reduce the likelihood for community-acquired organisms to serve as a source for nosocomial infection.

Even with these new technologic developments, certain basic principles of operation remain crucial to producing reliable microbiologic data. Several of these are discussed here.

Collection and Transport of Specimens

Specimen collection, transport, and handling must be of sufficiently high quality to provide valid data [25]. Specimens that are not collected or transported properly may give inaccurate results, even when handled as well as possible once they reach the laboratory. In turn, these inaccurate results may lead to improper clinical decisions by physicians, unnecessary labor by laboratory personnel, and unnecessary patient charges. This is especially true for the newer molecular techniques [26].

The laboratory must monitor specimen handling continually and work closely with both inpatient and ambulatory care units to make sure that the possibility of contaminated specimens is minimized. This is a necessity to ensure that laboratory information presented to the hospital epidemiologist reports organisms actually associated with the patient's site of culture rather than contaminants.

Certain laboratory findings suggest specific handling errors [1]. For example, a frequent failure to isolate organisms from deep wounds or abscesses of patients who are not on antibiotics, or inability to recover pathogens seen on Gram stain in cases of presumed anaerobic infections, suggests inadequate anaerobic transport media, delay or inappropriate refrigeration of specimens in transit, or use of inadequate techniques for isolating anaerobes. The frequent recovery of three or more different organisms in clean-voided, midstream urine specimens suggests unsatisfactory technique in collecting specimens, a delay in transporting specimens to the laboratory, or a delay in culturing the specimens. The finding of negative cultures from a high percentage of patients with positive smears for bacteria suggests unsatisfactory specimen collection or handling, errors in staining, contaminated reagents, or errors in culture techniques [27].

Specimen collection and handling should be assessed regularly to detect and correct such problems; the frequency with which probable contaminants are isolated from clinical specimens can be a measure of the quality of specimen collection in a specific hospital area. For example, determining frequency of urine specimens with characteristics that suggest specimen contamination permits wards with high rates to be singled out for evaluation and, if necessary, for inservice education programs instituted by laboratory or infection control personnel. In addition, identifying people who draw blood cultures that frequently contain diphtheroids, coagulase-negative staphylococci, or other probable skin contaminants may permit reinstruction of these personnel in aseptic technique. Periodic review of the relative incidence of false-positive smears for acid-fast bacilli or of specimens with heavy bacterial contamination may highlight problems in sputum collection and processing [25].

Many hospitals record both the time the specimen was collected and the time the laboratory received it so that transport time can be monitored periodically or continuously and the culturing of old specimens avoided. Evaluation of turnaround time has become an important element of laboratory quality assurance [28].

Initial Evaluation of Specimens

Assessment of specimens at the time they are received in the laboratory is one of the best ways to evaluate their suitability. For example, microscopic review of Gram stain of sputum specimens remains the best way to determine whether these specimens are contaminated [29]; specimens identified as inadequate are not processed further and do not confuse either clinician or epidemiologist. A new specimen should be requested unless the clinician provides notice of special circumstances (e.g., immunosuppression) that might make it worthwhile to proceed with culture [24].

Culture or smear results for other types of specimens may also suggest contamination at the time of collection. For example, urine specimens with three or more different organisms present ordinarily suggest contamination in patients without chronic indwelling urine catheters. Such specimens should be held for 2 to 3 days without further processing. The patient's physician should be notified so that unusual clinical situations requiring further identification of the specimen can be recognized. Scoring systems for use in determining acceptable wound, vaginal, cervical, and other specimens also have been described [30]. Application of such criteria ensures that the information generated from the specimens that are processed completely will more likely correlate with true infecting organisms and will reduce unnecessary laboratory costs. Repeat specimen collection should be requested for these inadequate specimens, and additional processing of organisms isolated from poor specimens (for example, speciation, susceptibility testing) should be delayed or eliminated. The culture report should alert the clinician about the questionable value of the specimen so that results are used cautiously, if at all, for guidance in diagnosis and therapy.

For specimens from sputum and wounds, reporting of the morphologic characteristics of bacteria seen on Gram stain may be misleading if no statement is made regarding the presence or absence of white blood cells. Both sites may be extensively contaminated with skin, oropharyngeal, or intestinal bacterial flora. When organisms are found only in the presence of abundant squamous epithelial cells, it is unlikely that they are the causative agents, and reports of such mixed flora without qualification about the accompanying cells may lead the clinician falsely to assume mixed flora as the cause of the infection. Substantial effort will be conserved and superior information ultimately provided if repeat collection is requested for such specimens.

Microscopy at the time of specimen submission can help other aspects of microbiologic diagnosis. For example, examination on Gram stain for morphology can identify organisms that might be epidemiologically important but not reflected by culture. Thus, presence of a mixed flora on Gram stain of a sputum specimen, when coupled with an aerobic culture yielding only *Hemophilus influenzae*, may indicate possible mixed aerobic–anaerobic infection rather than pneumonia due to *Hemophilus*. Because infection control implications of these two causes may differ, evaluations of this type by the laboratory can be important. Similarly, nonculture methods for identifying the presence of parvovirus B19 (e.g., demonstration by electron microscopy or gene probe) have helped us learn more about this organism as a cause of nosocomial infection [31].

Anaerobic culture of specimens should be limited to 1) those that show leukocytes on Gram stain, 2) those with no evidence of contaminating squamous cells and organisms suggestive of anaerobic species, or 3) specimens from patients whose unusual circumstances suggest a need for anaerobic culture. This limitation results in reporting of isolates that have a much higher probability of association with infection. The application of sensitive techniques for culturing and identifying anaerobes to specimens containing endogenous flora is costly and productive of misleading information [32]. Large numbers of anaerobic organisms are present in the normal flora of skin, oral cavity, and genital and gastrointestinal tracts. Therefore, swabs from superficial portions of skin or mucous membrane lesions, specimens of expectorated sputum, and any materials contaminated with feces should be considered inappropriate for anaerobic culture [32]. Submission for anaerobic culture of such specimens or of specimens from sites that are rarely infected by anaerobes (e.g., urine) suggests the need for inservice education of hospital personnel.

Efforts such as those outlined substantially reduce errors in diagnosis and use of unnecessary antimicrobial therapy. Such an approach also improves the specificity of infection surveillance data, which otherwise might include isolates of questionable etiologic significance.

Identification of Isolates

Once a specimen has been received in the laboratory, it must be processed in a way that maximizes the likelihood of recovering older agents as well as the many newer agents causing hospital cross-infection.

Often it is difficult to determine the causative agents in nosocomial infection. Recovery of an organism does not ensure that it is the causative agent of the nosocomial infection [24], and thus etiologic diagnosis cannot be made with certainty in many cases. Most cases today for which the cause is known involve gram-positive cocci and gram-negative aerobic bacilli [17]. Most frequent among these gram-negative rods are *Klebsiella, Enterobacter, Pseudomonas, Serratia, Proteus*, and *Escherichia coli* (in approximately that order) (see Chapter 30). More recently, organisms such as *Acinetobacter, Flavobacterium, Legionella*, and *Pseudomonas* species other than *P. aeruginosa* have become increasingly prominent.

Anaerobic bacterial organisms (usually found in mixed aerobic–anaerobic infections) have become less frequent in nosocomial infection since the mid-1980s. However, viral agents (e.g., rotavirus) and fungi and parasites such as *Pneumocystis* and *Toxoplasma* have been identified as important causes of nosocomial infection [17]. This expansion of the list of possible microbial pathogens for hospitalized patients has made it more difficult for both microbiologist and clinician to deal effectively with hospital infection. Effective handling of such problems requires the laboratory staff to keep up with the steadily unfolding panorama of organisms important in cross-infection and to implement and maintain culture and other techniques that bring these to light.

Need for Complete Identification

The degree to which organism identification routinely is carried can be important to nosocomial infection control efforts. Infection control personnel constantly are searching for evidence that a common organism has spread from patient to patient [4]. The ability to detect such an event is enhanced by identification of the organism at least to the level of species. Reporting of "biotyping" information (pattern of response to biochemical testing) on occasion can be of value in differentiating organisms that are frequently encountered, but this identification is not needed on a routine basis [16].

In today's environment of cost controls, the value of complete identification of all isolates is questionable [33]. Regardless of the extent to which full identification is conducted, it is important that standard criteria and nomenclature be consistently applied. Otherwise, attack rates for nosocomial infections with various species may identify false problems (e.g., because of previously unreported species or strains) or fail to identify true problems. Furthermore, such surveillance data may not be comparable to data developed in other institutions or in cooperative surveillance programs.

Even more important, incomplete or incorrect identification of organisms may obscure real problems and make retrospective epidemiologic investigation impossible. For example, a report of "*Klebsiella–Enterobacter* group" fails to distinguish between two organisms (*Klebsiella* and *Enterobacter*) that have different epidemiologic patterns of infection within the hospital [34]. Similarly, identifying an isolate as *Burkholderia cepacia* (formerly *Pseudomonas cepacia*), an organism frequently associated with illness or pseudoepidemics caused by contaminated water or other solutions [35], provides more useful epidemiologic information than identifying the organism only as "nonfermenting gram-negative bacillus," in which the strain is lumped with a group of organisms that may not have as characteristic a hospital reservoir.

Because of these considerations, laboratories should maintain the capability to identify gram-negative aerobic bacilli to the genus level. The laboratory should also have the capability of identifying organisms to the species level when special or recurring problems in a given institution make such information useful for dealing with nosocomial infection problems.

Many hospitals find it advantageous to use commercial, multiple test media for biochemical testing that provide this degree of characterization. Acceptable methods for microbiologic identification procedures are described in detail elsewhere [36]; additional assistance in identifying unusual isolates beyond the stated expertise of an individual laboratory is available from state and national reference laboratories.

Sometimes it is the pattern of susceptibility to antimicrobials that discriminates epidemiologically significant organisms from other apparently similar hospital organisms. For example, many U.S. hospitals encounter nosocomial infections due to *Enterococcus* strains resistant to vancomycin [37]. Such organisms can be the subject of infection control activities only if the laboratory maintains effective and efficient means for their identification [38].

Need for Accuracy and Consistency

Many spurious outbreaks have been traced to inaccurate or inconsistent microbiologic procedures. An "outbreak" of *S. aureus* infection, for example, may be caused by delayed reading of coagulase tests, resulting in misidentification of coagulase-negative organisms as coagulase positive. Unfortunately, most of the rapid tests available identify organisms that are not common nosocomial pathogens. The challenge therefore remains to develop rapid testing methods for the organisms closely associated with nosocomial infection (especially staphylococci, enterococci, and gram-negative aerobic bacilli).

Performance characteristics (e.g., sensitivity, specificity, reproducibility) of some of the rapid tests for identification of hospital pathogens are not good [39]. This means that the rapid tests are used only as an adjunct to other testing. Such tests tend to *increase* care costs rather than decrease them, and their utility is not clear. Improving test methodology will be essential if tests such as these are to assume a strong role in infection control [40].

The renaming of organisms that results from more precise knowledge of organism relationships also can cause confusion for nosocomial infection personnel. For example, the renaming as *Xanthomonas maltophilia* of the emerging nosocomial pathogen formerly called *Pseudomonas maltophilia* gave false alarm to institutions not used to seeing or dealing with what appeared to be a new intruder [41]. That organism now has again been renamed as *Stenotrophomonas maltophilia*. This constant effort to be more and more precise in taxonomy is less desirable in the era of managed care, and some now question the practice of slavish adherence to taxonomic and nomenclatural changes in the clinical setting [33].

Introduction of New Procedures

The laboratory must also consider whether additional laboratory techniques can make testing results more relevant. For example, cultures of intravenous catheter tips may become positive because of contamination at the time of catheter removal or from the intravascular device becoming infected. Several semiquantitative and quantitative methods for culture of intravenous catheters [42] have been shown to be useful in distinguishing between these possibilities (see Chapter 44). Similar claims of usefulness have been made for cultures of other fluids, burn wounds (see Chapter 38), and surgical wounds (see Chapter 37). It is not clear that these special techniques generate useful information.

Quality Control

Just as an effective clinical microbiology laboratory is essential to an effective infection control program, adequate quality control is essential to the practice of good clinical microbiology [30]. Such a quality control program begins with a comprehensive procedure manual that establishes standards for performance, including definition of acceptable and unacceptable quality of specimens and specimen containers, permissible delay between collection and receipt of the specimen in the laboratory, and times during which specimens are accepted for processing. The action to be taken by workers when specimens are not in accord with these standards also must be defined. These standards should be communicated to clinicians and nurses as well as to laboratory personnel.

The procedure manual also should cover administrative aspects of laboratory operation related to infection control and employee safety [43]. Minimum standards for identification of isolates should be provided, including a listing of the equipment and reagents to be monitored and the measures to be made to ensure reproducible and accurate performance. The periodic evaluation of skills of all workers, including evening, night, and weekend workers, should be included in the program.

Participating in proficiency testing programs helps the laboratory maintain competence, particularly if proficiency test specimens are submitted to the laboratory in a blinded fashion and are handled by routine procedures [44]. If problems develop with such an evaluation, the identity of the problem specimens should be made known and the personnel challenged to deal with the specimen in as careful a fashion as possible, to ensure that the laboratory actually has within its capability the correct handling and identification procedures for the organisms.

In addition to such outcome-oriented projects, periodic review of selected laboratory materials, media, and other equipment should be performed. On occasion, erroneous microbiologic results related to the inadvertent use of contaminated or faulty materials may occur. For example, an epidemic of pseudomeningitis was traced to contamination of funnels and an automated Gram-staining apparatus [45]. Such "pseudo-outbreaks" must be considered when laboratory culture or stain results do not correlate with clinical or epidemiologic findings.

Hospital-supported continuing education is essential for high-quality work in the microbiology laboratory. It is especially important for personnel in smaller hospital laboratories to stay abreast of technologic advances and trends in nosocomial infection occurrence and diagnosis [9]. Fortunately, a number of organizations, including the American Society for Microbiology, the Association for Practitioners in Infection Control, and the American Society of Clinical Pathologists, provide frequent programs on nosocomial infection topics.

ACCURATE CHARACTERIZATION OF ANTIMICROBIAL SUSCEPTIBILITY OF NOSOCOMIAL PATHOGENS

A standardized method of antimicrobial susceptibility testing subject to quality control evaluation is essential in any clinical microbiology laboratory and is equally critical to infection control studies. Occasionally, the epidemiologist will suspect that a group of nosocomial infections with organisms of the same species have a common origin. To investigate whether strains in this cluster are common or different, the usual practice is to examine results of speciation, biochemical tests, and the pattern of susceptibility to antimicrobial agents [4]. Often, these results answer the question of relationships. Occasionally, additional tests are needed; these are described in a later section of this chapter.

New patterns of antimicrobial resistance have been characteristic of the organisms causing hospital infection in the recent past (see Chapters 14–16). Organisms that had been consistently susceptible to older antimicrobials have developed resistance to these drugs, and some nosocomial organisms have developed resistance to new antimicrobials almost as soon as the drugs have been marketed [46]. Methicillin-resistant *S. aureus* (see Chapter 41) and coagulase-negative strains are involved in hospital infections nationwide [47]. Enterococci have increased in importance as nosocomial pathogens; some of these strains have become resistant to aminoglycoside and β-lactam drugs that used to be the drugs of choice for treatment of serious infection due to this organism. In the 1990s, strains of enterococci resistant to vancomycin (see Chapter 15) also have become widespread [48]. *Enterobacteriaceae*, a common source of nosocomial infection, have developed resistance to some of the newer β-lactam and fluoroquinolone antibiotics. The sequential appearance and persistence of these resistant organisms suggests spread of the resistant organisms within the hospital [34].

Several of these current resistance patterns require new or modified laboratory techniques for detection. For example, detection of vancomycin-resistant *S. aureus* requires several modifications of susceptibility testing techniques and is especially a problem for automated systems of detection [49]. Vancomycin-resistant enterococcal strains also require special means for identifying resistance, and for these organisms as well, automated detection systems are less reliable [48]. Detection of high-level aminoglycoside resistance in enterococci also presents challenges [50]. Detection of resistance to newer cephalosporins, ureidopenicillins, and β-lactamase inhibitor compounds in enterobacteriaceal strains poses special problems as well, although the role of automated testing systems seems more secure [51].

The Kirby-Bauer disk agar-diffusion method or an equivalent test system is used in many laboratories for routine testing of antimicrobial susceptibility of bacteria [52]. However, many other laboratories routinely perform a more quantitative evaluation of sensitivity, using broth-dilution or agar-dilution test methods [52]. In addition, tube dilution, E-test, or other methods of establishing minimum inhibitory concentration or susceptibility to "gate" concentrations of antibiotics must be used for testing organisms that have not been standardized for testing by a disk method. The latter include a number of anaerobic bacteria, fungi, and yeasts. Other sources may be consulted for detailed discussion of the performance and quality control of these procedures [36,53].

Some microorganisms can be additionally differentiated by indicating the relative degree to which susceptibility or resistance to antimicrobials is present [4]. This can be done by noting the absolute value of zone size in agar-diffusion testing or by providing assessment of minimum inhibitory concentration. Situations in which this more quantitative information would be useful should be delineated jointly by the laboratory and infection control team.

Selection of Strains for Susceptibility Testing

Applications of susceptibility tests to bacteria that are doubtfully related to infection must be avoided, and specific guidelines for the selection of isolates for susceptibility determination should be established by the laboratory. For example, the request for testing of susceptibility should be carefully evaluated when the organisms isolated are endogenous flora present at sites in which they are not normally pathogens. Similarly, the testing of organisms from mixed culture should be avoided in most cases because of the unclear role of the various isolates [32]. Direct testing of urine and spinal fluid is not essential in most cases. Potential pathogens with well established susceptibility to antimicrobials (for example, *Streptococcus pyogenes* to penicillin) should not be tested routinely.

Selection of Drugs for Routine and Special Testing

The selection of drugs for routine testing should be undertaken by the laboratory after consultation with the Infection Control Committee and the Pharmacy and Therapeutics Committee; the chosen agents should reflect both common usage practices of physicians in the hospital and the spectrum of pathogens that are frequently encountered [54]. Occasionally, testing of susceptibility to certain drugs is performed for epidemiologic purposes; results of such testing may be omitted from routine clinical reporting. Similarly, certain antimicrobials for which the hospital wishes to control usage may be tested but not reported routinely, or tested only after consultation.

Different groups of antimicrobials often are used for gram-negative and gram-positive aerobic organisms. Drugs included in each panel should be periodically evaluated and updated. The epidemiologic value of susceptibility patterns may be enhanced by inclusion of certain antibiotics that are not in routine clinical use. Such additional information can also provide valuable taxonomic and quality control information, but these benefits must be weighed against the extra time and cost required for testing and recording of the additional studies.

For some of the newer nosocomial pathogens, susceptibility testing methods are not very good. For example, susceptibility testing methods for fungi do not correlate well with clinical outcome [55]. Thus, another challenge is the need to develop susceptibility testing methods for some of the newer organisms closely associated with nosocomial infection, especially gram-negative nonfermentive bacilli, fungi, and viruses.

Quality Control

Consistent and accurate identification of organisms over time is necessary for susceptibility data to be useful for clinical and epidemiologic purposes. In addition, errors in performance of susceptibility tests may result in information that is misleading about therapy. To minimize this possibility, detailed quality control procedures must be maintained for all elements of the susceptibility testing process [52,53]. Special attention must be given to storage of reagents, control of batch-to-batch variation in media, use of control strains for testing, and monitoring of incubation temperatures and atmosphere. When results of these quality control tests exceed acceptable limits, reports on clinical isolates should be withheld until satisfactory control results are obtained. The reproducibility of susceptibility tests can also be assessed by participation in quality control programs of groups such as the College of American Pathologists or the Centers for Disease Control and Prevention, which periodically distribute unknown specimens for evaluation. Such testing programs focus on clinically and epidemiologically important strains; correct identification assures the laboratory and infection control personnel that the laboratory applies proper techniques and skills.

TIMELY REPORTING OF LABORATORY DATA AND PARTICIPATION IN SURVEILLANCE OF NOSOCOMIAL INFECTION

To deal with individual problems of nosocomial infection in the hospital as they arise, control measures must be taken as quickly as possible and must be based on accurate assessment of the problem and its causes [4]. Without rapid identification and reporting of the organisms involved, control measures cannot be efficiently designed and implemented.

Laboratory records are an important tool for infection control practitioners [7]. Development of computerized laboratory information systems has progressed rapidly in the 1990s, and this has led to major improvements in several ways that the laboratory can provide infection control information [56].

Surveillance

Laboratory records are an important tool for surveillance of infections [7]. More than 80% of infections defined by other criteria as nosocomial may be identified by review of positive cultures from the microbiology laboratory. Review of laboratory records is the most common method for surveillance of hospital infection carried out in the United States. Therefore, data gathered by infection control personnel during laboratory visits form an important base to which additional surveillance data from clinical rounds must be added. Both sources must be used to obtain an accurate estimate of the true rate of occurrence of nosocomial infection in a given hospital (see Chapter 5).

For both endemic and epidemic nosocomial infection, microbiologic and immunologic reports may be the starting point for additional epidemiologic investigations. These investigations often require information about attributes of the patient, the personnel involved in care, or the diagnostic and therapeutic procedures provided to the patient. Obtaining these nonlaboratory data usually is easier when the patient is still present in the hospital or at least is fresh in the minds of hospital personnel. Prompt reporting of pertinent laboratory results facilitates information retrieval of this type.

Computer programs have been developed to identify clusters of infections with the same organism and susceptibilities that occur at the same time in the same patient care area (ward or service) [57]. Such programs have permitted identification of outbreaks; whether they provide such information in rapid enough fashion to permit use of control measures remains open to question [58].

The laboratory can indicate only which organisms were present in culture. The epidemiologist must supplement this information with clinical data to determine whether organisms found in culture indicate infection or colonization [15]. If colonization is present, the identification of organisms in the culture may be of little help to the clinician. To the epidemiologist, however, both the organisms involved in episodes of exogenous colonization and those of infection are of interest. Either may be evidence of spread of organisms from one site to another, indicating an area in which control measures may halt transmission. Data used for this purpose must be accurate, which emphasizes the role of continuing quality control studies in the laboratory.

Reporting of Results

To facilitate the surveillance of nosocomial infections and of all infections requiring isolation or notification of public health authorities, a copy of positive culture results should be provided to the infection control personnel. Physicians and nurses sometimes are lax about notifying public health authorities of reportable diseases. Isolation of such organisms is reported to health authorities more efficiently if the responsibility for reporting is delegated to the infection control nurse or some other person designated by the Infection Control Committee (see Chapter 12).

Availability of a computerized laboratory information system can make it possible for the laboratory routinely to produce frequent and tailored reports for the infection control practitioner (see Chapter 5). For example, such a report is generated at the start of each day at Grady Memorial Hospital [7]. The report lists selected positive cultures and immunologic tests from the previous day, sorted by ward in the order in which each practitioner makes daily rounds. The *only* culture results selected and printed on this report are those specified as relevant by the infection control personnel. This maintains a relatively concise report, while ensuring that the infection control officer has access to all information of current interest. The list of results to be selected is changed on a periodic basis to make sure that current needs are addressed (e.g., when the name of an organism has changed or when a new nosocomial pathogen has arisen at the institution).

Prompt reporting by telephone to both clinicians and infection control personnel is essential when presumptive identification is made of isolates of nosocomial significance; this is the only way to ensure proper treatment of the patient and the application of proper control measures [59]. Occasions for reporting include incidents such as the presumptive identification of certain agents in meningitis, isolation of *Salmonellae* or *Shigellae* from stool specimens, positive smears and cultures of tuberculosis bacilli from any patient or employee, and isolation of *S. aureus* from lesions of a newborn or other nursery patient.

Laboratory studies may provide early warning of the emergence within a hospital of highly infectious microorganisms, multiply drug-resistant organisms, and clusters of unusual infections. In some hospitals, laboratory workers may be the first to detect these and other trends of infection. When findings suggest a possible outbreak, notification requires quicker action than a final report, because rapid epidemiologic investigations triggered by the first preliminary data from the laboratory often are profitable. The major elements needed in any early warning are the interest and expertise of the laboratory worker in calling results to the attention of infection control colleagues. This may be done by telephone or page, if urgent; if not, discussion during the daily visit of the infection control staff usually suffices.

Such reporting facilitates the efforts of the infection control personnel. At the same time, early warning must not be requested for so many situations that this becomes an unreasonable burden on the laboratory personnel. The key here is consultation between laboratory and infection control personnel to establish which findings need to be given critical-value status [59].

Laboratory Records

In addition to instituting control measures, infection control workers often need to analyze laboratory data from various periods to try to detect patterns of infection [4]. To assist in this effort, it is helpful if the laboratory can provide an archival summary of organisms on a periodic basis. Data of particular usefulness here might include compiled listings of organisms by culture site, date, patient, and ward; a summary of susceptibility testing results for various species of organisms for given time periods might also be of help. Computer storage and retrieval of all results can aid this process considerably. Some newer laboratory information systems permit downloading of information pertinent to infection control to a desktop computer [58]. These data then can be used both by the laboratory and in infection control, if these departments have a compatible desktop computer. The specific laboratory data that can aid epidemiologic analyses vary from hospital to hospital. The information to be included and the frequency with which such summaries are made should be determined by the people providing and working with the data in each hospital.

Laboratory records should be retained in such a way that they facilitate such retrospective epidemiologic investigations and quality control activities. The source of each specimen, date of collection, patient identification, hospital number, hospital service, ward, and organisms identified in the final report should be recorded. Records also should be kept of results of antimicrobial sensitivity tests and of any special biochemical or typing reactions.

All cultures should be recorded so that results are readily available by date, type of specimen, and pathogens isolated. Culture data on inpatients and outpatients should be maintained separately. Computer storage and retrieval of all results is optimal [58]. These records also can be maintained in simple, inexpensive, and epidemiologically useful fashion by bound log books, which are kept chronologically for each major type of specimen (e.g., blood, wound, skin, cerebrospinal fluid, urine, stool, sputum). Sole reliance on a filing system of loose laboratory slips is not desirable because specific data are difficult to retrieve and easily lost.

The permanent records of the microbiology laboratory should include dates and other details of any major changes in culturing techniques or laboratory procedures. Dates of changes in the criteria for identification and taxonomic designations applied to isolates should be recorded as well.

Retention Period for Records

No analysis of previous data can be made if the records are not available. To this end, it is incumbent on the laboratory staff to maintain the microbiologic records in some accessible format (e.g., final report sheets, disc or tape storage) for a reasonable period. The length of time such records can be maintained depends on hospital size, work volume of the laboratory, and available storage facilities, as well as on infection control needs. Thus, storage time should be determined by laboratory personnel after consultation with the hospital infection control staff. One author considers 18 months to be a reasonable minimum [16].

Summary Reports for Clinical Use

Development of profiles for susceptibility of frequently tested pathogens to drugs commonly in use can be of considerable assistance in guiding therapy for sepsis of unclear cause and other infections. Testing other organisms (e.g., slow-growing bacteria or organisms requiring special test procedures) may be performed at intervals to develop a profile of their susceptibility. As long as susceptibility patterns can be presumed to remain stable, such testing may be a useful substitute for testing each isolate at the time of recovery.

These summaries of susceptibility patterns should be available to the medical staff on at least an annual basis [7]. In addition to the hospital epidemiologist (see Chapter 2), any or all of the Infection Control Committee, medical staff committees, and quality assurance committee may also wish to receive susceptibility summaries to guide their review of antibiotic utilization. The use of a laboratory information system to tabulate the data directly or to download the raw data to a desktop computer for calculation of results has eased the burden of performing this task by hand. The laboratory information system also can be used to provide information about proper use of antimicrobial agents [46].

Tabulations that may be of particular use include frequency of susceptibility to individual drugs by site of infection or ward (which may provide guidance to the clinician for empiric therapy of infection before the causative organism has been identified) and tabulation of frequency of susceptibility to individual antimicrobials by pathogen (which may be used to direct therapy after an organism has been identified but before susceptibility tests have been completed) [57].

A listing of the relative costs of the currently used antimicrobials may be developed with cooperation of the pharmacy; inclusion of this information with susceptibility summaries may increase the incentive to reduce costs of antimicrobial use [57].

ADDITIONAL STUDIES TO ESTABLISH SIMILARITY OR DIFFERENCE OF ORGANISMS

On occasion, the epidemiologist suspects that a group of nosocomial infections with organisms of the same species have a common origin. Determining the features of the epidemiologic problem, or testing certain hypotheses about reservoir or mode of spread, may be helped if the laboratory can define whether the individual strains are related or unrelated to each other [4]. To investigate whether strains in this cluster are common or different, the usual initial practice is to examine results of speciation, biochemical tests, and pattern of susceptibility to antimicrobial agents. However, for organisms commonly encountered in the hospital (e.g., *S. aureus* or *Klebsiella*), the general pattern of these results may be similar on the basis of chance alone. Conversely, for other organisms (e.g., *P. aeruginosa*), the variation in these characteristics from strain to strain is so small that the tests provide little information about similarity or difference of tested strains. Testing of additional antimicrobials not ordinarily included, or of susceptibility to other antibacterial substances (e.g., silver) may differentiate strains in some cases. Many times, however, no differences can be shown by these tests. In these situations, examination ("typing") of additional organism characteristics (markers) can be of great assistance [60].

Although hospital laboratory personnel may not have the facilities to perform specialized typing procedures, they should know which organisms can be typed and which cannot and where specific procedures can be obtained. When epidemiologically important isolates require special typing, it may be necessary to forward them to public health or private reference laboratories. Potentially pathogenic materials should be packaged for air transport in conformance with federal regulations [61].

TABLE 9-1. *Typing systems for organisms causing nosocomial infection: some phenotypic methods and examples of use for specific organisms*

I. Pattern of susceptibility to antimicrobials ("antibiogram")
  - *Klebsiella* [62]
  - *Legionella* [63]
  - MRSA [64]
  - *Pseudomonas aeruginosa* [65]

II. Pattern of susceptibility to heavy metals ("resistotyping")
  - MRSA [66]
  - *Candida albicans* [67]

III. Biotyping
  - *Serratia marcescens* [68]
  - Enterococci [69]
  - *Burkholderia cepacia* [70]

IV. Phage susceptibility ("phage typing")
  - MRSA [64,71]

V. Serotyping
  - *Klebsiella* [72]
  - *Streptococcus agalactiae* [73]
  - *Serratia* [74]
  - *P. aeruginosa* [65]

VI. Bacteriocin production
  - *Enterobacter* [75]
  - *Serratia* [76]

VII. Immunoblotting
  - MRSA—Southern blot hybridization after protein electrophoresis [77]

VIII. Multilocus enzyme electrophoresis
  - *S. agalactiae* [73]
  - Enterococci [78]
  - Coagulase-negative staphylococci [79]

MRSA, methicillin-resistant *Staphylococcus aureus*.

Methods for Typing of Isolates

A variety of techniques have been used for typing isolates [60]. Selected typing systems of special value in investigating nosocomial infection problems are summarized in Tables 9-1 and 9-2. So many typing systems are being used today for so many organisms that only a few examples can be provided in the Tables. Several reviews provide detailed descriptions of the procedures used for each [1,60]. Many are beyond the capabilities of the usual clinical laboratory, but a number can be conducted when circumstances dictate.

Although routine typing of all strains is not cost effective, some laboratories store selected isolates for later typing should it prove desirable.

Some typing systems monitor changes in characteristics expressed by the microorganism (phenotype; see Table 9-1), and others analyze changes from organism to organism in chromosomal or extrachromosomal genetic elements (genotype; see Table 9-2). Each is considered in turn.

Phenotypic Techniques

A number of organisms involved in nosocomial infection have been differentiated successfully by *antimicrobial susceptibility testing*. The pattern of resistance or susceptibility to several different antimicrobials often is referred to as the "antibiogram" of the organism. Test antimicrobials not in routine clinical use can be of assistance here [106]. However, the antibiogram of strains in the same clone can change over time [107]. Susceptibility to various chemicals, especially heavy metals (*resistotyping*), also has proved of value in selected instances [66].

Biotyping is the use of certain characteristic biochemical reactions to identify subgroups of bacteria. Typing schemes using this method have been devised for a variety of bacterial organisms, both anaerobes and aerobes, and found to be useful in infection control investigations. The process can be simplified by automated performance and analysis by use of computerized methods [108]. Unfortunately, the biotype codes generated by many of the commercial identification systems are poorly reproducible [107]. The method is most useful when unusual biotypes characterize the nosocomial pathogen.

Bacteriophages are viruses that can kill certain bacteria by lysis. Susceptibility to bacteriophages (*phage typing*) is a characteristic used for typing a number of organisms of nosocomial importance. The technique has been especially useful for grouping strains of *S. aureus*. However, this procedure usually is available only in reference laboratories, and plasmid transfer of phage characteristics apparently can occur, so it has been replaced by genotypic techniques in most situations [71].

TABLE 9-2. *Typing systems for organisms causing nosocomial infection: some genotypic methods and examples of use for specific organisms*

I. Plasmid profile analysis ("fingerprinting")
Serratia marcescens [74]
Coagulase-negative staphylococci [80]
Burkholderia cepacia [70]
II. Restriction endonuclease analysis
A. Restriction endonuclease analysis of plasmids
MRSA [81]
Streptococcus pyogenes [82]
B. Restriction enzyme analysis of chromosomes
Clostridium difficile [83]
III. Ribotyping
S. marcescens [68]
Legionella pneumophila [84]
MRSA [85]
Escherichia coli [86]
B. cepacia [70]
IV. Pulsed field gel electrophoresis
Enterococci [69,87]
L. pneumophila [88]
MRSA [71,81,89]
Pseudomonas aeruginosa [90]
B. cepacia [70]
Mycobacterium tuberculosis [91]
A. Contour-clamped homogeneous electric field electrophoresis
Enterococci [92]
Candida lusitaniae [93]
V. Analysis of nucleic acid amplification products
A. DNA typing by repeated PCR assay
Streptococcus pneumoniae [94]
Citrobacter [95]
B. Arbitrary primed PCR
Acinetobacter [96]
C. difficile [97]
M. tuberculosis [98]
B. cepacia [71]
L. pneumophila [88]
Stenotrophomonas maltophilia [99]
C. Whole-cell repetitive extragenic PCR
Acinetobacter [100]
D. Random amplification of polymorphic DNA
E. coli [86]
Enterococci [87]
Enterobacter [101]
S. maltophilia [102]
Aspergillus [103]
Candida albicans [104]
VI. Nucleotide sequence analysis
Hepatitis B virus [105]

MRSA, methicillin-resistant *Staphylococcus aureus*; PCR, polymerase chain reaction.

Serotyping is a technique used for typing of many gram-negative aerobic bacilli, especially *Klebsiella pneumoniae* isolates [72]. The technique can be of help for other organisms as well, in both outbreak situations and research investigations. However, when reagents are not readily available, or when typing procedures are complex, the techniques are available only in referral laboratories.

Many bacteria produce products that can kill or inhibit the growth of other organisms. Production of such *bacteriocins* by an organism, or susceptibility of the organism in question to those produced by other bacteria, can be used as a typing tool for a number of organisms. However, the method requires careful use of controls; widespread agreement on standards for reagents and interpretation is unusual. In addition, reproducibility of results is a problem; all strains should be tested at the same time [109]. Thus, the method also has been supplanted in favor of genotypic procedures for most situations.

Electrophoretic typing of proteins results from isolating relevant proteins, separating them by protein agar gel electrophoresis, and staining the gel so that the resulting pattern can be observed. The individual enzymes present in a given organism vary in structure from those present in other organisms; this is reflected in their different mobility when subjected to electrophoresis. Separating these compounds by electrophoresis on a starch gel can provide information on variation in a number of different enzymes at the same time. Such testing is called *multilocus enzyme electrophoresis*. A variant of this is *immunoblotting*, in which a nitrocellulose membrane is used as a site for the application of antisera of various sorts.

Genotypic Techniques

Since the mid-1980s, molecular and other, newer techniques have permitted more definitive typing of a wider range of organisms than ever before [60,110,111]. These methods have helped immeasurably in defining mode of spread, reservoirs, and asymptomatic and unsuspected sources of infection [112]. It is now clear that these techniques can provide an epidemiologic picture different from that of prior methods. In many cases these techniques have supplanted the traditional phenotypic methods [113].

The simplest of these genetic techniques is analysis of the *plasmid profile* of a given organism or group of organisms. Most bacterial species carry plasmids, which are extrachromosomal pieces of DNA that encode a variety of genes. After isolation, plasmids are separated by electrophoresis and the pattern (number and size) of the plasmids from different organisms compared (so-called fingerprinting). Of course, if an organism has few or no plasmids, this technique provides little assistance. In addition, the rapid pace of gain or loss of plasmids by a single organism, as well as the frequent exchange of plasmids between different organisms, makes interpretation of this technique difficult [60,114].

Both plasmids and chromosomal DNA can be subdivided further for typing purposes by using *restriction endonuclease enzymes* that divide the genetic material into smaller fragments. The fragments then can be separated by agar gel electrophoresis and compared as a further fingerprinting step. The bacterial chromosome usually contains some regions that are variable and other regions that are quite similar among different strains of the same species ("conserved"). The regions with different nucleotide sequence result in different patterns in the agarose gel for different organisms. These are known as restriction fragment length polymorphisms. Plasmid evaluation by this method usually is simpler than that for chromosomal DNA. The utility of this technique for analysis of chromosomal elements is subject to confounding by presence of DNA in plasmids and may be difficult to interpret because of the number and variety of patterns produced.

Ribotyping is the use of ribosomal RNA as a probe to detect variations in the DNA sequences associated with ribosomal operons [110]. Although most genes are present in bacteria in single copies, ribosomal operon genes are unique in that they are present in multiple copies. This makes analysis easier. In addition, only a small section of the genome is being examined, so a small number of bands are produced in the analysis. These are easier to analyze than the huge number of fragments that result from analysis of the whole chromosome. However, ribosomal gene patterns are relatively stable within a given species, so the ability to discriminate between epidemiologic isolates may be hindered to a certain degree [60].

Pulsed-field gel electrophoresis also begins with lysis of organisms and digestion of their chromosomal DNA with restriction endonucleases [113]. However, the restriction fragments are resolved into a pattern of discrete bands in the gel by switching the direction of current. The number and size of fragments from different organisms then are compared. This alteration of electric field more readily allows resolution of large DNA molecules. The method is gaining wide use because it allows typing of a broad range of bacteria. A hindrance is that there are no standardized criteria for analyzing the fragment patterns; however, consensus approaches are being proposed [113].

A variant of pulsed-field gel electrophoresis is *contour-clamped homogeneous electric field electrophoresis*. It is used primarily to compare large chromosomal DNA fragments [1]. DNA is separated by subjecting the molecules alternately to perpendicular electric fields. The high–molecular-weight DNA then can be subjected to agarose gel electrophoresis or digested by restriction endonucleases. Bacteria, yeast, and mycobacteria all can be studied using this approach.

Amplification techniques like PCR or the ligase chain reaction are widely used in characterizing nosocomial pathogens [115]. Analysis of the products of such amplification can provide information on organism typing. By enhancing the number of target molecules by several logs of concentration, the study of the variability of the individual targets is enhanced. However, specialized equipment and personnel are needed to conduct this procedure, and this is a major problem for many hospitals [116].

Variations using amplification methods are emerging constantly. One is the use of *repeated PCR assay* aimed at different parts of small sections of a genome. *Arbitrary primed PCR assays* are variations of the amplification technique using short primers whose nucleotide sequence is not directed at a known genetic site [99]. These result in amplification of unpredictable loci, and a set of restriction fragments is generated that can be compared for different isolates. Because the discriminatory power of the assay is not clear, interpretation of these tests depends even more strongly than usual on the correlation with epidemiologic data.

There has been a dramatic recent increase in methods and equipment for analyzing the exact *nucleotide sequence* of microbes. It now is technically possible to compare multiple isolates by sequencing the same genetic site from all [60]. Differences in content and arrangement of nucleotides are being used for epidemiologic typing studies [105]. Further work is needed to define the exact role that such techniques should play in cost-effective epidemiologic analysis.

Choosing Typing Systems

Although the potential benefit of these new techniques for hospital infection control is great, some cautions are needed regarding their use [4,113,117]. Sometimes the new systems for analysis have impeded rather than aided in outbreak investigations. For example, some investigations produce conflicting results from typing studies carried out by different techniques [71]. Incorrect results also may arise from contamination of reagents, a special concern with use of newer techniques such as PCR, with which sensitivity is so great that the chance of contamination is high [118]. Some typing methods provide data of doubtful value or results that are difficult to interpret for a given epidemiologic situation [119]. To improve these, further information is needed to evaluate their validity as a tool for infection control [4]. Some have suggested that in analyzing subgroups of clonal organisms, it is necessary to use at least two typing methods [71,114].

Even if the methods are valid, overinterpretation or underinterpretation of the results is a potential problem. Typing never proves that organisms are the same [60]. On the other hand, the use of too many individual markers in several typing methods can cause problems as well [120]. For example, use of 20 different antibiotics in typing a series of specimens in which organisms are defined as different if their pattern of susceptibility varies by more than one drug almost guarantees that organisms that actually are part of the outbreak will be identified as different and thus considered unrelated [4].

Results from some typing methods may be redundant; if so, this needs to be discovered, so that the cheaper method can be used. An important question for current investigation should be not *whether* new tests provide additional discrimination but *how much* discriminating ability they add to tests that are readily available [121]. For example, in a study of infections with coagulase-negative staphylococci, antibiogram, biotyping, phage typing, and plasmid profiling all were performed. The antibiogram, selected as the first stage of the scheme because it was the simplest and cheapest test, proved to be the most discriminatory stage, providing 66% of the discriminating ability between strains [122].

A related issue is how often most hospitals really need these newer techniques. Most of the newer methods are used for research (detailing routes of transmission or reservoirs of organisms) rather than for acting on outbreaks. For most of the newer molecular testing methods, instruments and reagents are not readily available, and have yet to be widely automated [116]. The expertise to perform and interpret the tests is not widespread, and standards are lacking for most assays [116]. In addition, outbreak organisms rarely are all isolated at once, so typing procedures are performed at separate times; the need for control of batch-to-batch variation in media, reagents, phages, and the like is especially crucial with many of these typing procedures. These considerations explain why many newer typing procedures should not be performed in the routine clinical laboratory [116]. Thus, not every laboratory must be able to perform every, or even most, of these tests. The laboratory director must be aware of the tests that are available, determine which can be performed on site when needed, and identify referral laboratories (e.g., colleague, state, private) where other methods are available on request.

Storage of Strains

For supplemental tests to be performed, such as those described in the preceding section, the organisms must be available. Thus, a related duty of the clinical laboratory staff is to retain strains that may relate to nosocomial infection for a given period while it is determined whether additional testing is needed. In cooperation with infection control personnel, the laboratory staff should subculture and save epidemiologically important isolates, whether such isolates are from outbreaks or from single cases of unusual or potentially epidemic diseases. Isolates may be conveniently and inexpensively stored by placing a small amount of growth on a blank paper disk that is placed in a 2-ml glass screw-cap vial containing a few granules of silica gel. If the vial is kept tightly closed, isolates may be held up to 6 months; they can then be easily retrieved by placing the disk in broth.

A system for reviewing and periodically discarding these isolates also must be established. How long a storage period is required for this purpose varies from hospital to hospital and should be agreed on between epidemiologist and clinical laboratory director. The technique used to ensure the viability of the organisms (e.g., freezing, lyophilization) should be determined by the laboratory staff after considering the equipment and personnel that are available for this task.

OCCASIONAL MICROBIOLOGIC STUDIES OF HOSPITAL PERSONNEL OR ENVIRONMENT

In some situations, nosocomial infection may result from environmental or personnel sources. In evaluating such episodes, the infection control staff may ask the laboratory staff to process specimens from employees, environmental sources, or hospital equipment (e.g., respiratory therapy machines) as part of the investigation [4]. Such environmental culturing, however, should focus on investigation of documented infections in patients (see Chapters 6, 20) [2]. When such culturing is necessary, its costs should be considered part of the hospitals' infection control program, and charges for the cultures should not be billed to the patients involved in the outbreak.

A few procedures of this type should be done routinely (Table 9-3). Others are elective, performed in association with episodes of patient illness or as part of an educational program. A third group is specifically not recommended. Each is dealt with in turn.

Routine Environmental Sampling

Surveillance cultures of the hospital environment and personnel once were advocated on a routine basis. During

TABLE 9-3. *Microbiologic studies of hospital personnel and the hospital environment*

- Recommended for routine performance
  - Monitoring of sterilization
    - Steam sterilizers
    - Ethylene oxide sterilizers
    - Dry heat sterilizers
    - Flash sterilizers (but no standard method)
  - Sampling of infant formula prepared in the hospital and other specific high-risk hospital-prepared products
  - Monitoring of dialysis fluid
- Elective environmental monitoring
  - Surveys to investigate a specific problem of patient infection
  - Surveys for educational purposes
- Procedures not recommended
  - Routine culture surveys of patients or hospital personnel
  - Routine culture of commercial products labeled as sterile
  - Routine testing of antiseptics and disinfectants
  - Routine culture of blood units
  - Routine monitoring of disinfection process for respiratory therapy equipment

the 1970s, studies found these programs to be of minimal value in infection control; by 1980, most institutions took the approach that routine environmental culturing should be severely limited. During the past decade, limiting cultures of the environment has become even more imperative because of changes in the economics of healthcare in the United States. Fortunately, further studies have supported this selective approach [123]. Close communication between epidemiologist and microbiologist about the need for such cultures continues to be essential to keep from wasting valuable resources.

In the absence of an epidemic, sampling should be minimal; microbiology and infection control personnel should be firm in not conducting indiscriminate routine microbiologic sampling and testing (see Chapter 20) [2]. However, routine checks on the adequacy of sterilizer function, culture of dialysis infusates and the water used to prepare them, and culture of infant formula and some other products prepared in the hospital may help prevent infections from these sources (Table 9-3).

Monitoring of Sterilization

All steam sterilizers should be checked at least once each week with a suitable live-spore preparation [124]; if sterilization is performed less often, testing should be done on each day that sterilization is done (see Chapters 20, 21). Ethylene oxide gas sterilizers should be checked with each load of items that come into contact with blood or other tissues. In addition, each load in either type of sterilizer should be monitored with a spore test if it contains implantable objects. These implantable objects should not be used until the spore test is reported as negative, usually at 48 hours of incubation. Dry-heat sterilizers should be monitored at least once each month [124].

The process of flash sterilization is used when contaminated items will be needed again in a short period of time. This time requirement makes use of biologic indicator testing impractical [125]. This means that this method of sterilization is not feasible for items that are to be implanted in patients. Products for monitoring flash sterilization are being evaluated, but no consensus exists for the way they should be used. Likewise, low-temperature sterilization technologies are being developed to replace ethylene oxide use; these include vaporized hydrogen peroxide, gas plasmas, ozone, and chlorine dioxide [126]. Some progress has been made in developing biologic indicators for these newer systems [127], but no consensus yet exists. Developing these standard testing systems should remain a high priority.

All sterilizers should be equipped with time–temperature recorders to provide evidence of adequate exposure for each load. However, evidence that a sterilizing temperature has been held for an adequate time does not prove that sterilization took place; the temperature is measured at the outlet valve and does not reflect whether adequate sterilization occurred within dense volumes of fluid or large, dense, fabric-wrapped packs. The use of chemical monitors (e.g., test tapes or heat-sensitive color indicators) within the autoclave is recommended for the outside of each package sterilized [124]. This provides an indication that a sterilizing temperature may have been reached, although such monitors do not show whether there was an adequate duration of exposure. Therefore, additional monitoring systems are required, which ordinarily involve the laboratory: biologic monitoring with spore strips generally has been accepted as the most effective way to determine successful sterilization (see Chapters 20, 21).

Microorganisms chosen for spore strip tests are more resistant to sterilization than are most naturally occurring pathogens. The test organisms are provided in relatively high concentrations to ensure a margin of safety. The spores may be provided either in impregnated filter paper strips or in solution in glass ampules. For steam sterilization, the thermophile *Bacillus stearothermophilus* is used, and, for ethylene oxide and dry-heat sterilizers, *Bacillus subtilis* (var. *niger*) is used. Both species frequently are incorporated simultaneously in the test strips, and these can be used to test for adequate sterilization with either procedure.

Most spore strip preparations are packaged in envelopes that contain one or two test strips and a control strip. The test strips are packaged in separate envelopes and are removed and sterilized at the time other material is processed. Subsequently, the test strips and control strip are cultured by placing the strips in tubes of tryptic-digest casein-soy (TS) broth that are incubated at 37°C (99°F) for *B. subtilis* and 56°C (133°F) for *B. stearothermophilus*. It is not necessary to culture a positive control strip for each test; if strips are obtained from a single lot, only 10% of the positive control strips need be tested.

Spore solutions are prepared in sealed glass ampules for testing the adequacy of sterilization fluids. These ampules should be incubated at 56°C (133°F) in a water bath. If there is no change in the indicator by 7 days, the test is reported as negative. Alternatively, the fluid may be inoculated with a test culture, which may be subcultured after autoclaving.

Other types of spore preparations are commercially available and require different handling. In each case, the manufacturer's directions should be followed closely.

Test strips or spore solutions should always be placed in the center of the specimen to be tested, never on an open shelf in the autoclave. The center of a pack located near the bottom front exhaust valve will be exposed for the least adequate duration and temperature of sterilization and thus provides the best location for a test measurement. Testing of sterilization of fluids is accomplished by placing an ampule containing a spore solution in the largest vessel.

Use of ampules containing spore solutions is not appropriate for checking sterilization of microbiologic culture media, because these media do not require the duration of exposure that is required for sterilization of material known to contain large populations of bacteria. Heating of bacteriologic culture media to a temperature sufficient to ensure sterilization of a test strip or spore ampule results in damage to the medium through overheating.

The likelihood of cross-contamination can be reduced by minimizing the handling of the strip after sterilization. Test strips can be removed from their envelopes and placed in sterile glass tubes before sterilization. The tube then is sterilized with the screw-cap removed or with other closures permeable to steam in place. After sterilization, the tube is sent to the laboratory, where the nutrient broth is added.

The handling of spore strips in the laboratory requires considerable care to prevent secondary contamination. The transfer should be made in a laminar-flow cabinet if available, using sterile forceps and scissors. The forceps and scissors are common sources of contamination, which may be insufficiently sterilized by flaming or wiping with alcohol. Alcohol may contain viable spores that might not be killed by flaming, and flaming may be insufficient to heat instruments to a temperature that destroys viable spores. Care should be taken not to cross-contaminate the sterilized spore strips with the control strips.

Condensation on the cover of a 56°C (133°F) water bath may cause contamination of the caps and closures of tubes. A heating block may be used to avoid this, or the bath may be left uncovered; the latter makes it necessary to provide a reservoir to maintain the water level because the evaporation rate is high at this temperature. Uninoculated culture media should be incubated at 35°C (95°F) or at 56°C (133°F) to ensure that contamination does not yield false-positive reports.

Gram staining and subculturing should be performed to detect secondary contamination of test cultures. If organisms other than gram-positive bacilli are observed, the test should be repeated and reported as "possible laboratory contamination, test being repeated."

Whenever positive results are obtained, the sterilizers should be checked immediately for proper use and function. Careful examination must be made of thermometer and pressure gauge readings, and recent time and temperature records must be reviewed. If any deficiency is observed or if the repeat sterility test still results in growth, engineering personnel and experts in autoclave maintenance and function should be consulted promptly. Objects other than those used for implants do not need to be recalled at this point unless defects are discovered in the sterilizer or its use; if spore tests remain positive after proper use of the sterilizer is documented, the machine should be removed from service until the defects are corrected (see Chapter 20).

Sampling of Infant Formula and Other Food Products Prepared in the Hospital

Few hospitals still prepare their own infant formula. However, infant formula prepared in the hospital kitchen should be monitored on a weekly basis [128]. A guideline for interpretation of culture suggests that < 25 organisms per milliliter be present and that no virulent bacteria, such as *Salmonella* or *Shigella*, be present [128]. The guideline is an arbitrary one, however, and should be a matter of local preference.

On occasion, other food products prepared in hospitals are considered as potential sources for nosocomial infection. Extensive guidelines for appropriate culture techniques have been developed [129]. These should be consulted as necessary.

Culture of Blood Components

The American Association of Blood Banks [130] does not recommend routine sterility culturing of transfusion components. Likewise, surveillance bacterial cultures are not recommended for specific transfusion practices (e.g., exchange transfusions for neonates) [131].

Culture of Dialysis Fluid

The water used for preparation of dialysis fluid should be tested by colony count at least once per month. Guidelines of the Association for Advancement of Medical Instrumentation [132] specify that the water used to prepare dialysis fluid and water used to rinse and reprocess dialyzers should contain fewer than 200 viable organisms per milliliter, and the dialysate < 2,000 colony-forming units (cfu) per milliliter. Defined methods for such testing vary from one regulatory body to the next; in general, the correlation between the specified levels and occurrence of patient disease is poor. Counts obtained vary markedly with media and conditions of incubation [133] (see Chapter 24).

Periodic Sampling of Disinfected Equipment

Any article that makes direct contact with the vascular system or tissue other than unbroken skin should be sterile. Whenever possible, steam or gas sterilization should be applied. If chemical disinfection or pasteurization rather than sterilization is used on equipment such as cystoscopes and other endoscopes or anesthesia equipment, some authorities recommend (and some require) that periodic microbiologic sampling be done to ensure the absence of pathogens after processing. Methods and equipment for testing have been specified [133].

The frequency of sampling such disinfected devices depends on any evidence that nosocomial infection is associated with their use and an assessment by the Infection Control Committee of the adequacy of standards for control of contamination of such equipment. There is little agreement on which items of this type should be tested, or how often. If such a monitoring program is begun, it may be possible to cut back on the frequency of culturing after a period of time in which cultures are negative, as long as no changes are made in equipment and techniques used.

Infections have resulted from contamination of transplant materials like bone marrow during processing [134]. Thus, on occasion, local or regional regulations require routine culture of transplant organs (e.g., eye, bone, and porcine heart valves), laminar flow hoods, or pharmacy admixture solutions.

Elective Environmental Monitoring

A wide variety of items and substances can be responsible for cross-infection. Thus environmental surveys may be useful during investigation of specific problems within a hospital and should be instituted in response to, and specifically address, epidemiologic findings [4]. For example, microbiologic assessment of foods may be needed during investigation of suspected foodborne illness in the hospital setting [135] (see Chapter 22). Elective culturing programs may also be instituted in association with educational efforts.

Support for Investigation of Specific Problems of Nosocomial Infection

These must be dealt with as rapidly as possible [4] (see Chapter 6). This means that the laboratory may face exceptional demands for service at the beginning of, and throughout, an epidemic period [16]. Advance preparation for such situations makes response easier in the time of need. The laboratory personnel should prepare contingency plans for the types of outbreaks that have occurred most frequently in the past in the hospital so that they are ready to deal with these exceptional requests in a smooth fashion.

Investigation of an outbreak of nosocomial infection may require isolation and identification of isolates in specimens not only from patients but from personnel who might be colonized with the outbreak strain and from environmental objects that might be similarly contaminated [4]. Such activity may require the laboratory staff to process and evaluate large numbers of cultures, and special techniques may be necessary to accomplish such projects. For example, reliable detection of colonization with vancomycin-resistant enterococci requires use of selective media like Enterococcsel broth [136]. The laboratory staff and the infection control team can process this work efficiently by making careful assessment of the sites to be cultured and determining which culture media and techniques will be used.

A detailed description of suitable culture techniques for every possible vehicle of cross-infection is beyond the space allocation and practical scope of this chapter. The interested reader is referred to detailed protocols available for culture survey of hemodialysis equipment, dialysis fluid, intravascular devices, air cultures, and environmental and medical device surfaces, blood bank products, and water for *Legionella* [133]. The development of selective media and techniques for culture of environmental objects has continued since the mid-1980s as new potential reservoirs and vectors of hospital infection have been recognized [16]. Methods for sampling sites relevant to infections caused by specific pathogens are described in the appropriate chapters of Part III of this text. The infection control worker and laboratorian must be familiar with general aspects of culture procedures discussed in the following sections, but they should not obtain or process such cultures unless surveillance of infections in patients specifically implicates these items as potential sources of nosocomial infection.

Because standard methods for the microbiologic evaluation of such culture procedures do not exist or are of doubtful validity, considerable expense may be incurred in the production of information that is worthless or misleading. Requests for such cultures therefore should be approached with caution, and the infection control staff should be clear regarding how the culture results will affect patient care or epidemiologic control measures before undertaking such tasks [4]. Specific areas of support are considered in turn.

Culture of Blood Products After a Transfusion Reaction

Bacteria present in blood components can cause a septic transfusion reaction [137]. Fortunately, this is a very rare occurrence. Such reactions usually are due to endotoxin produced by organisms that can grow in the cold. If transfusion reaction is suspected by clinical signs, the transfusion should be halted immediately and the unit examined. If further evaluation of the signs, symptoms, and clinical course of the patient then suggests bacterial contamination of the blood product, cultures of the suspect component(s) may be indicated, at various temperatures [130,133]. It is desirable as well at this time to collect blood culture specimens by venipuncture from the patient and from all intravenous solutions in use for that patient.

Cultures of Parenteral Fluids and Intravascular Therapy Equipment

The investigation of bacteremia associated with parenteral therapy may require investigation of the needle or catheter, portions of the administration set, the fluid being administered, and portions of the cap or closure provided with the fluid [133,138] (see Chapter 44). Blood culture specimens should be collected simultaneously from the patient. It is especially important to keep careful track of lot numbers, which should be recorded on the patient's chart as well as on all subsequent laboratory records.

Needles and catheters must be submitted separately from the hubs and other portions of the administration set that may have been exposed to superficial contamination. If portions of the administration set are suspected, these must be received properly capped to exclude spurious contamination. The bottle and administration set should remain connected and be placed in a plastic bag to minimize contamination during delivery to the laboratory.

The standard method for culture of catheters and needles has been the semiquantitative method in which the catheter tip is rolled across a plate containing solid media. Some authors suggest flushing the inside with nutrient broth or a quantitative sonication method for culture of the catheter instead of (or in addition to) a semiquantitative culture [139]. Substitution of hub cultures and cultures of the skin around the insertion point has been suggested as an alternative sample not requiring removal of the catheter [140]. Quantitative cultures are time-consuming and are a drain on personnel resources; the need to use them rather than the more efficient semiquantitative methods has not been demonstrated [139]. Options for culture of the catheter are discussed further in Chapter 44.

Culture methods for intravenous fluids in containers or collected from administration lines also are described in Chapter 44. Careful aseptic technique is critical.

Methods for Culturing Hands and Skin

Several methods are suitable for culture of hands [133]. The simplest is to take a sterile swab, moisten it with sterile saline or a culture broth appropriate to skin organisms (brain–heart infusion broth is one), and then swab the palmar surface of the hand or hands. A rapid and simple way to obtain these cultures also is provided by pressing the subject's palm gently on a large culture plate containing a suitable agar medium (or a Rodac plate; see section on culture of floors and other surfaces). When a more quantitative estimate of the organisms present is desired, 50 ml of culture broth can be poured into a sterile container or plastic bag. The person to be cultured is asked to rub hands together in the broth for 30 seconds. An estimate of cfu per milliliter can be obtained [141]. A bag-wash method has been found to enhance recovery of yeasts from hands of healthcare workers [142].

In contrast to these simple methods, sampling of hands associated with testing of antiseptics or disinfectants is a more complicated process and requires special techniques [143].

Monitoring of antibiotic-resistant organisms on occasion has involved investigation of skin of patients or healthcare workers as potential sources of resistant organisms. However, quantitative culturing of skin or gastrointestinal tract seldom is indicated [15]. To quantify skin microflora, several methods have been developed [133].

Methods for Culturing Tubes and Containers

Cultures of external surfaces or internal cavities (e.g., tubes and containers) may be conducted by a swab–rinse technique [133].

Sampling of Respiratory Therapy Equipment

Disinfection of respiratory therapy and anesthesia equipment is discussed in Chapter 33. In situations of high endemic or epidemic levels of occurrence of nosocomial respiratory infections, sampling of respiratory therapy apparatus may be of value [144,145].

Sampling of Air

Airborne spread of nosocomial bacterial or viral infection is known to occur [146] but is probably uncommon; air sampling should be required infrequently [147]. Common recent indications for use of this technique in healthcare settings include monitoring of production areas for pharmaceuticals, in operating suites, and in the investigation of suspected episodes of airborne infection [148]. Air sampling may be performed with either settling plates or more sophisticated equipment [133,149].

Particles suspended in hospital air vary greatly in size and in the number of microorganisms they contain. The average diameter of airborne microbial particles in ward air is approximately 13 μm, but 7% are < 4 μm in size and 30% are > 18 μm. Particles with a mean size of 13 μm settle at a rate of approximately 1 foot/minute. Because the surface of a standard 100-mm Petri dish represents an area of approximately 1/15 square foot, and assuming that the air in the study area contains particles of average size, an open Petri dish in still air will sample microbial particles from nearly 1 cubic foot of air during 15 minutes of exposure [150].

Although this is an inexpensive way to evaluate airborne microbial contamination, quantitative results may correlate poorly with those obtained with mechanical, volumetric air samplers because of variation in particle size and unknown influences of air turbulence. Under low-humidity conditions, droplet nuclei of approximately 3 μm can remain suspended indefinitely and can be collected only with high-velocity, volumetric air samplers.

A slit sampler is suitable for many precise air sampling applications [148]. Brain–heart infusion or tryptic soy agar (TSA) media should be used in the sampling plates. A staged sampler [149] should be needed only when there is some reason to determine the size distribution of the particles, which should be an extremely infrequent event in most U.S. hospitals. Efficient vacuum sources must be used for both samplers, and the rate of flow of air must be properly calibrated to ensure accurate results.

The total number of airborne microbial particles is not measured precisely by observing growth after impaction on an agar plate because an airborne microbial particle may contain more than one viable cell. Air-sampling techniques in which volumetric samples are taken by bubbling air through collection fluid break up airborne particulate matter and better reflect the total number of organisms than air samplers that impinge contaminated particles on agar.

Culture of Floors and Other Surfaces

Methods for sampling of floors and other surfaces have been described in detail [133]. Standards for acceptable levels of contamination of floors and bedside tables as sampled by the Rodac plate technique have been suggested by a committee of the American Public Health Association [151]. There is no evidence, however, that any particular level of contamination is directly correlated with an increased risk of infection, and such standards probably are useful only in assessing the adequacy of housecleaning procedures.

Sampling Water and Ice

Water that meets U.S. Public Health Service standards for drinking water frequently contains up to 1 million or more microorganisms per milliliter, and some of these organisms are potential pathogens. Ice also can contain organisms that can pose a threat of infection, especially in patients with compromised host defenses. However, correlation of levels of microorganisms with occurrence of patient illness has been rare.

Samples of water or melted ice can be obtained by collection in a sterile container. If chlorine is present, it can be inactivated by thiosulfate. The specimen is cultured by passing large quantities through a 0.45-µm (or 0.22-µm) Millipore filter and culturing the filter in broth or directly on agar. More than 4 colonies per 100 ml is considered abnormal by this test [150].

When transmission of *Legionella* infection occurs in the hospital setting, culture of water is recommended (see Chapter 32). Guidelines for such cultures have been proposed [152].

Developing Selective Media for Surveys

To reduce the workload in the laboratory and to expedite the processing of specimens, selective survey media should be used whenever possible for culturing specimens during outbreak investigations. Susceptibility data on known or suspected epidemic strains may be used to identify an appropriate selective medium for use in surveys of the animate and inanimate environment of the hospital. Once the implicated organism is isolated and tested on appropriate media containing one or more antibiotics to which it is resistant, the media can be used to exclude numerous bacteria unrelated to the outbreak. This may accelerate the detection of contaminated equipment or infected patients. Pretesting of the media is essential because of possible synergy or antagonism between the added antimicrobials or between these drugs and the media; such interactions could cause inhibition of growth of the epidemic strain or failure to inhibit growth of nonimplicated organisms.

Other selective media also may be useful. For example, cetrimide medium may be helpful in selectively isolating *P. aeruginosa* from contaminated material or mixed cultures. Similarly, tetrathionate broth is an excellent medium for selective preenrichment of *Salmonella* cultures. Mueller-Hinton agar containing sorbitol, a pH indicator, and antibiotics (vancomycin, colistin, and nystatin) provides selective differentiation of *Serratia* species. Many epidemic strains of *S. aureus* are resistant to mercuric chloride, and the incorporation of small amounts of this compound in tryptic soy agar (TSA) can be helpful in inhibiting nonepidemic strains of *S. aureus, Staphylococcus epidermidis*, and most gram-negative organisms except *Pseudomonas*.

Vancomycin-resistant strains of enterococci have become a problem in many U.S. hospitals; agar containing small concentrations of vancomycin have been of use in investigating hospital problems due to these strains [38,136]. The resistance of epidemic microorganisms to heavy metals, dyes, disinfectants, and other antimicrobial substances also may be used to identify and construct selective media for surveys.

Surveys for Educational Purposes

Sampling techniques that are not directly related to epidemiologic surveys may prove useful in educational programs; visible evidence of contamination of hands, clothing, equipment, and surfaces may serve to teach the need for effective aseptic technique and sanitation.

Sampling That Is Not Recommended

Routine Culture Surveys of Patients and Personnel

Routine culturing of patients or hospital personnel is not recommended (see Chapter 3). Surveys may be useful during investigation of specific problems within a hospital and should be instituted in response to, and specifically address, epidemiologic findings.

Routine Culture of Commercial Products

Although commercial patient care items that are labeled sterile (e.g., intravascular catheters and fluids) occasionally have been contaminated with viable organisms that can cause patient disease, routine sampling of these items is not recommended, because the low frequency of contamination makes it difficult (because of the large number of specimens that would have to be taken) and expensive to perform adequate sterility testing.

Routine Testing of Antiseptics and Disinfectants

In-use testing of antiseptics and disinfectants should not be a routine procedure for hospital microbiology laboratories [133]. No consensus is available about the optimal methods for such testing against many organisms, including viruses [153]. If contamination of commercial products sold as sterile is suspected, infection control personnel should be notified and the nearest office of the U.S. Food and Drug Administration contacted immediately [150]. State regulations may require immediate notification of state health authorities as well.

Random Culture of Blood Units

The American Association of Blood Banks [130] does not recommend random culture of blood units to ensure sterility.

Routine Monitoring of Disinfection Process for Respiratory Therapy Equipment

Guidelines from the Centers for Disease Control and Prevention advise to "not routinely perform surveillance cultures of patients or of equipment or devices used for respiratory therapy, pulmonary function testing, or delivery of inhalation anaesthesia" [145].

TEACHING MICROBIOLOGIC ASPECTS OF NOSOCOMIAL INFECTION TO INFECTION CONTROL PERSONNEL

The people responsible for infection control usually are not trained in clinical laboratory procedures. Because the key to success in infection control efforts is communication, it is necessary that all involved speak the same language. For this purpose, training of epidemiology personnel in the language of the clinical laboratory microbiologist is important. The training of many infection control personnel in microbiology is inadequate or out of date. The goal of such teaching is not necessarily to make the infection control staff accomplished laboratory workers but rather to familiarize them with the procedures and practices of the laboratory, the microorganisms involved in nosocomial infection, the validity of test procedures used in identifying these pathogens, and the strengths and weaknesses of the resulting data.

Similarly, it is important for the microbiologist to learn some of the concepts of the epidemiologist, because few laboratory directors or technologists have adequate grounding in epidemiology. Especially important is exposure to techniques used for measuring frequency of infection and the concept of colonization versus infection.

Such joint efforts permit ready communication between the two groups of colleagues. Teaching of this type can be done in a formal fashion but is also effective when included as part of the day-to-day informal contacts between the infection control staff and laboratory personnel (see Chapter 2).

REFERENCES

1. Mahayni R, Zervos M. The clinical laboratory's role in hospital infection control. *Laboratory Medicine* 1994;25:642–647.
2. Emori TG, Gaynes RP: An overview of nosocomial infections, including the role of the microbiology laboratory. *Clin Microbiol Rev* 1993; 6:428–442.
3. Schifman RB. *ASCP check sample—microbiology: surveillance for nosocomial infections: the laboratory component*. Skokie, IL: American Society of Clinical Pathologists, 1989.
4. McGowan JE Jr, Metchock BG. Basic microbiologic support for hospital epidemiology. *Infect Control Hosp Epidemiol* 1996;17:298–303.
5. Sadler HS, Hollis RJ, Pfaller MA. The use of molecular techniques in the epidemiology and control of infectious diseases. *Clin Lab Med* 1995;15:407–431.
6. Arbeit R. Laboratory procedures for the epidemiologic analysis of microorganisms. In: Murray PR, Baron EJ, Pfaller MA, Tenover FC, Yolken RH, eds. *Manual of clinical microbiology.* 6th ed. Washington, DC: American Society for Microbiology, 1995:190–208.
7. McGowan JE Jr. Communication with hospital staff. In: Balows A, Hausler WJ Jr, Herrmann KL, Isenberg HD, Shadomy HJ, eds. *Manual of clinical microbiology.* 5th ed.. Washington, DC: American Society for Microbiology, 1991:151–158.
8. Wiblin RT, Wenzel RP. The infection control committee. *Infect Control Hosp Epidemiol* 1996;17:44–46.
9. Boyce JM. Hospital epidemiology in smaller hospitals. *Infect Control Hosp Epidemiol* 1995;16:600–606.
10. Swartz K, Brennan TA. Integrated healthcare, capitated payment, and quality: the role of regulation. *Ann Intern Med* 1996;124:224–228.
11. Simmons BP, Parry MF, Williams M, et al. The new era of hospital epidemiology: what you need to succeed. *Clin Infect Dis* 1996;22: 550–553.
12. Scott DR. Influence of managed care and health maintenance organizations on the clinical microbiology laboratory. *Diagn Microbiol Infect Dis* 1995;23:17–21.
13. McGowan JE Jr, MacLowry JD. Addressing regulatory issues in the clinical microbiology laboratory. In: Murray PR, Baron EJ, Pfaller MA, Tenover FC, Yolken RH, eds. *Manual of clinical microbiology.* 6th ed. Washington, DC: American Society for Microbiology, 1995: 67–74.
14. McGowan JE Jr, Metchock B. Infection control epidemiology and clinical microbiology. In: Murray PR, Baron EJ, Pfaller MA, Tenover FC, Yolken RH, eds. *Manual of clinical microbiology.* 6th ed. Washington, DC: American Society for Microbiology, 1995.
15. Greene JN. The microbiology of colonization, including techniques for assessing and measuring colonization. *Infect Control Hosp Epidemiol* 1996;17:114–118.
16. Goldmann DA. New microbiologic techniques for hospital epidemiology. *Eur J Clin Microbiol* 1987;6:344–347.
17. Martone WJ, Gaynes RP, Horan TC, et al. National Nosocomial Infections Surveillance (NNIS) semiannual report, May 1995. *Am J Infect Control* 1995;23:377–385.

18. Vincent J-L, Bihari DJ, Suter PM, et al. The prevalence of nosocomial infection in intensive care units in Europe: results of the European Prevalence of Infection in Intensive Care (EPIC) study. *JAMA* 1995; 274:639–644.
19. Jenkins SG. Evaluation of new technology in the clinical microbiology laboratory. *Diagn Microbiol Infect Dis* 1995;23:53–60.
20. Relman DA. The identification of uncultured microbial pathogens. *J Infect Dis* 1993;168:1–8.
21. Haynes KA, Westerneng TJ. Rapid identification of *Candida albicans, C. glabrata, C. parapsilosis* and *C. krusei* by species-specific PCR of large subunit ribosomal DNA. *J Med Microbiol* 1996;44:390–396.
22. Grundy JE, Ehrnst A, Einsele H, et al. A three-center European external quality control study of PCR for detection of cytomegalovirus DNA in blood. *J Clin Microbiol* 1996;34:1166–1170.
23. Thanos M, Schonian G, Meyer W, et al. Rapid identification of *Candida* species by DNA fingerprinting with PCR. *J Clin Microbiol* 1996; 34:615–621.
24. Kiehn TE, Ellner PD, Budzko D. Role of the microbiology laboratory in care of the immunosuppressed patient. *Rev Infect Dis* 1989; 11(Suppl 7):S1706–S1710.
25. Wilson ML. General principles of specimen collection and transport. *Clin Infect Dis* 1996;22:766–777.
26. Farkas DH, Kaul KL, Wiedbrauk DL, et al. Specimen collection and storage for diagnostic molecular pathology investigation. *Arch Pathol Lab Med* 1996;120:591–596.
27. Morris AJ, Tanner DC, Reller LB. Rejection criteria for endotracheal aspirates from adults. *J Clin Microbiol* 1993;31:1027–1029.
28. Valenstein P. Laboratory turnaround time. *Am J Clin Pathol* 1996;105: 676–688.
29. Flournoy DJ, Beal LM, Smith MD. What constitutes an adequate sputum specimen? *Laboratory Medicine* 1994;25:456–459.
30. Baron EJ. Quality management and the clinical microbiology laboratory. *Diagn Microbiol Infect Dis* 1995;23:23–34.
31. Dowell SF, Torok TJ, Thorp JA, et al. Parvovirus B19 infection in hospital workers: community or hospital acquisition? *J Infect Dis* 1995; 172:1076–1079.
32. Washington JA II. Effective use of the microbiology laboratory. *J Antimicrob Chemother* 1988;22(Suppl A):101–112.
33. Wegner DL. Resolved: that taxonomy should be more medically relevant. *Clinical Microbiology Newsletter* 1996;18:121–128.
34. Weinstein RW. Enterobacteriaceae. In: Mayhall CG, ed. *Infection control and hospital epidemiology.* Baltimore: Williams & Wilkins, 1996.
35. Hamill RJ, Houston ED, Georghiou PR, et al. An outbreak of *Burkholderia* (formerly *Pseudomonas) cepacia* respiratory tract colonization and infection associated with nebulized albuterol therapy. *Ann Intern Med* 1995;122:762–766.
36. Murray PR, Baron EJ, Pfaller MA, Tenover FC, Yolken RH, eds. *Manual of clinical microbiology.* 6th ed. Washington, DC: American Society for Microbiology, 1995.
37. Gordts B, Van Landuyt H, Ieven M, et al. Vancomycin-resistant enterococci colonizing the intestinal tracts of hospitalized patients. *J Clin Microbiol* 1995;33:2842–2846.
38. Barton AL, Doern GV. Selective media for detecting gastrointestinal carriage of vancomycin-resistant enterococci. *Diagn Microbiol Infect Dis* 1995;23:119–122.
39. Perkins MD, Mirrett S, Reller LB. Rapid bacterial antigen detection is not clinically useful. *J Clin Microbiol* 1995;33:1486–1491.
40. Robinson A. Rationale for cost-effective laboratory medicine. *Clin Microbiol Rev* 1994;7:185–199.
41. Marshall WF, Keating MR, Anhalt JP, et al. *Xanthomonas maltophilia*: an emerging nosocomial pathogen. *Mayo Clin Proc* 1989;64: 1097–1104.
42. Schmitt SK, Knapp C, Hall GS, et al. Impact of chlorhexidine-silver sulfadiazine-impregnated central venous catheters on in vitro quantitation of catheter-associated bacteria. *J Clin Microbiol* 1996;34: 508–511.
43. August MJ, Hindler JA, Huber TW, et al. *Cumitech 3A: quality control and quality assurance practices in clinical microbiology.* Washington, DC: American Society for Microbiology, 1990.
44. Richardson H, Wood D, Whitby J, et al. Quality improvement of diagnostic microbiology through a peer-group proficiency testing program. *Arch Pathol Lab Med* 1996;120:445–455.
45. Southern PM Jr, Colvin DD. Pseudomeningitis again: association with cytocentrifuge funnel and Gram-stain reagent contamination. *Arch Pathol Lab Med* 1996;120:456–458.
46. McGowan JE Jr. Antibiotic-resistant bacteria and healthcare systems: four steps for effective response. *Infect Control Hosp Epidemiol* 1995; 18:67–70.
47. Casewell MW. New threats to the control of methicillin-resistant *Staphylococcus aureus. J Hosp Infect* 1995;30(Suppl):465–471.
48. Jett B, Free L, Sahm DF. Factors influencing the Vitek gram-positive susceptibility system's detection of *vanB*-encoded vancomycin resistance among enterococci. *J Clin Microbiol* 1996;34:701–706.
49. Centers for Disease Control and Prevention. *Staphylococcus aureus* with reduced susceptibility to vancomycin—United States, 1997. *MMWR* 1997;46:765–766.
50. Swenson JM, Ferraro MJ, Sahm DF, et al. Multilaboratory evaluation of screening methods for detection of high-level aminoglycoside resistance in enterococci. *J Clin Microbiol* 1995;33:3008–3018.
51. Washington JA II, Knapp CC, Sanders CC. Accuracy of microdilution and the AutoMicrobic system in detection of beta-lactam resistance in gram-negative bacterial mutants with derepressed beta-lactamase. *Rev Infect Dis* 1988;10:824–829.
52. Sahm DF, Neumann MA, Thornsberry C, et al. *Cumitech 25: current concepts and approaches to antimicrobial agent susceptibility testing.* Washington, DC: American Society for Microbiology, 1988.
53. National Committee for Clinical Laboratory Standards. *Performance standards for antimicrobial susceptibility testing.* Sixth informational supplement (M100-S6). Villanova, PA: NCCLS, 1995.
54. Jorgensen JH. Selection of antimicrobial agents for routine testing in a clinical microbiology laboratory. *Diagn Microbiol Infect Dis* 1993; 16:245–249.
55. Ghannoum MA, Rex JH, Galgiani JN. Susceptibility testing of fungi: current status of correlation of in vitro data with clinical outcome. *J Clin Microbiol* 1996;34:489–495.
56. Desseau RB, Steenberg P. Computerized surveillance in clinical microbiology with time series analysis. *J Clin Microbiol* 1993;31: 857–860.
57. Stratton CW VI, Ratner H, Johnston PE, et al. Focused microbiologic surveillance by specific hospital unit: practical application and clinical utility. *Clin Ther* 1993;15(Suppl A):12–20.
58. Wenzel RP, Streed SA. Surveillance and use of computers in hospital infection control. *J Hosp Infect* 1989;13:217–229.
59. Lundberg GD. Critical (panic) value notification: an established laboratory practice policy (parameter). *JAMA* 1990;263:709.
60. Maslow JN, Mulligan ME, Arbeit RD. Molecular epidemiology: application of contemporary techniques to the typing of microorganisms. *Clin Infect Dis* 1993;17:153–164.
61. Shea YR. Specimen collection and transport. In: Isenberg HD, ed. *Volume I: Clinical microbiology procedures handbook.* Washington, DC: American Society for Microbiology, 1992:1.1.1.-30.
62. Venezia RA, Scarano FJ, Preston KE, et al. Molecular epidemiology of an SHV-5 extended-spectrum β-lactamase in Enterobacteriaceae isolated from infants in a neonatal intensive care unit. *Clin Infect Dis* 1995;21:915–923.
63. Vickers RM, Stout JE, Tompkins LS, et al. Cefamandole-susceptible strains of *Legionella pneumophila* serogroup 1: implications for diagnosis and utility as an epidemiologic marker. *J Clin Microbiol* 1992; 30:537–539.
64. Bannatyne RM, Wells BA, MacMillan SA, et al. A cluster of MRSA: the little outbreak that wasn't. *Infect Control Hosp Epidemiol* 1995; 16:380.
65. Holder IA, Volpel K, Ronald G, et al. Studies on multiple *Pseudomonas aeruginosa* isolates from individual burn patients by RFLP, O antigen serotyping, and antibiogram analysis. *Burns* 1995;21: 441–444.
66. Rossney AS, Coleman DC, Keane CT. Evaluation of an antibiogram-resistogram typing scheme for methicillin-resistant *Staphylococcus aureus. J Med Microbiol* 1994;41:441–447.
67. Hunter PR. Discrimination of strains of *Candida albicans* isolated from deep and superficial sites by resistotyping. *Mycoses* 1995;38: 37–40.
68. Chetoui H, Delhalle E, Osterrieth P, et al. Ribotyping for use in studying molecular epidemiology of *Serratia marcescens*: comparison with biotyping. *J Clin Microbiol* 1995;33:2637–2642.
69. Kuhn I, Burman LG, Haeggman S, et al. Biochemical fingerprinting compared with ribotyping and pulsed-field gel electrophoresis of DNA for epidemiological typing of enterococci. *J Clin Microbiol* 1995;33:2812–2817.
70. Ouchi K, Abe M, Karita M, et al. Analysis of strains of *Burkholderia*

(*Pseudomonas*) *cepacia* isolated in a nosocomial outbreak by biochemical and genomic typing. *J Clin Microbiol* 1996;33:2353–2357.
71. Jorgensen M, Givney R, Pegler M, et al. Typing multidrug-resistant *Staphylococcus aureus*: conflicting epidemiological data produced by genotypic and phenotypic means clarified by phylogenetic analysis. *J Clin Microbiol* 1996;34:398–403.
72. Trautmann M, Cross AS, Reich G, et al. Evaluation of a competitive ELISA method for the determination of *Klebsiella* O antigens. *J Med Microbiol* 1996;44:44–51.
73. Quentin R, Huet H, Wang F-S, et al. Characterization of *Streptococcus agalactiae* strains by multilocus enzyme genotype and serotype: identification of multiple virulent clone families that cause invasive neonatal disease. *J Clin Microbiol* 1995;33:2576–2581.
74. Bonten MJM, Gaillard CA, van Tiel FH, et al. A typical case of cross-acquisition? The importance of genotypic characterization of bacterial strains. *Infect Control Hosp Epidemiol* 1995;16:415–416.
75. Gaston MA, Strickland MA, Ayling-Smith BA, et al. Epidemiological typing of *Enterobacter aerogenes*. *J Clin Microbiol* 1989;27:564–565.
76. Larose P, Picard B, Thibault M, et al. Nosocomial *Serratia marcescens* individualized by five typing methods in a regional hospital. *J Hosp Infect* 1990;15:167–172.
77. Kreiswirth BN, Lutwick SM, Chapnick EK, et al. Tracing the spread of methicillin-resistant *Staphylococcus aureus* by Southern blot hybridization using gene-specific probes of *mec* and *Tn554*. *Microbial Drug Resistance* 1995;1:307–313.
78. Tomayko JF, Murray BE. Analysis of *Enterococcus faecalis* isolates from intercontinental sources by multilocus enzyme electrophoresis and pulsed-field gel electrophoresis. *J Clin Microbiol* 1995;33: 2903–2907.
79. Tan TQ, Musser JM, Shulman RJ, et al. Molecular epidemiology of coagulase-negative *Staphylococcus* blood isolates from neonates with persistent bacteremia and children with central venous catheter infections. *J Infect Dis* 1994;169:1393–1397.
80. Camargo LFA, Strabelli TMV, Ribeiro FG, et al. Epidemiologic investigation of an outbreak of coagulase-negative *Staphylococcus* primary bacteremia in a newborn intensive care unit. *Infect Control Hosp Epidemiol* 1995;16:595–596.
81. Liu PY-F, Shi Z-Y, Lau Y-J, et al. Use of restriction endonuclease analysis of plasmids and pulsed-field gel electrophoresis to investigate outbreaks of methicillin-resistant *Staphylococcus aureus* infection. *Clin Infect Dis* 1996;22:86–90.
82. Jamieson FB, Green K, Low DE, et al. A cluster of surgical wound infections due to unrelated strains of group A streptococci. *Infect Control Hosp Epidemiol* 1993;14:265–267.
83. Samore MH, Bettin KM, DeGirolami PC, et al. Wide diversity of *Clostridium difficile* types at a tertiary referral hospital. *J Infect Dis* 1994;170:615–21.
84. Schoonmaker D, Heimberger T, Birkhead G. Comparison of ribotyping and restriction enzyme analysis using pulsed-field gel electrophoresis for distinguishing *Legionella pneumophila* isolates obtained during a nosocomial outbreak. *J Clin Microbiol* 1992;30: 1491–1498.
85. Nath SK, Shea B, Jackson S, et al. Ribotyping of nosocomial methicillin-resistant *Staphylococcus aureus* isolates from a Canadian hospital. *Infect Control Hosp Epidemiol* 1995;16:717–724.
86. Bingen E, Bedu A, Brahimi N, et al. Use of molecular analysis in pathophysiological investigation of late-onset neonatal *Escherichia coli* meningitis. *J Clin Microbiol* 1995;33:3074–3076.
87. Barbier N, Saulnier P, Chachaty E, et al. Random amplified polymorphic DNA typing versus pulsed-field gel electrophoresis for epidemiological typing of vancomycin-resistant enterococci. *J Clin Microbiol* 1996;34:1096–1099.
88. Pruckler JM, Mermel LA, Benson RF, et al. Comparison of *Legionella pneumophila* isolates by arbitrary primed PCR and pulsed-field gel electrophoresis: analysis from seven epidemic investigations. *J Clin Microbiol* 1995;33:2872–2875.
89. Cookson BD, Aparicio P, Deplano A, et al. Inter-centre comparison of pulsed-field gel electrophoresis for the typing of methicillin-resistant *Staphylococcus aureus*. J Med Microbiol 1996;44:179–184.
90. Talon D, Cailleaux V, Thouverez M, et al. Discriminatory power and usefulness of pulsed-field gel electrophoresis in epidemiological studies of *Pseudomonas aeruginosa*. *J Hosp Infect* 1996;32:135–145.
91. Bendall RP, Drobniewski FA, Jayasena SD, et al. Restriction fragment length polymorphism analysis rules out cross-infection among renal patients with tuberculosis. *J Hosp Infect* 1995;30:51–56.
92. Donabedian S, Chow JW, Shlaes DM, et al. DNA hybridization and contour-clamped homogeneous electric field electrophoresis for identification of enterococci to the species level. *J Clin Microbiol* 1995; 33:141–145.
93. King D, Rhine-Chalberg J, Pfaller MA, et al. Comparison of four DNA-based methods for strain delineation of *Candida lusitaniae*. *J Clin Microbiol* 1995;33:1467–1470.
94. van Belkum A, Sluijter M, de Groot R, et al. Novel BOX repeat PCR assay for high-resolution typing of *Streptococcus pneumoniae* strains. *J Clin Microbiol* 1996;34:1176–1179.
95. Harvey BS, Koeuth T, Versalovic J, et al. Vertical transmission of *Citrobacter diversus* documented by DNA fingerprinting. *Infect Control Hosp Epidemiol* 1995;16:564–569.
96. Siau H, Yuen KY, Wong SSY, et al. The epidemiology of *Acinetobacter* infections in Hong Kong. *J Med Microbiol* 1996;44:340–347.
97. Collier MC, Stock F, DeGirolami PC, et al. Comparison of PCR-based approaches to molecular epidemiologic analysis of *Clostridium difficile*. *J Clin Microbiol* 1996;34:1153–1157.
98. Cockerill FR, Williams DE, Eisenach KD, et al. Prospective evaluation of the utility of molecular techniques for diagnosing nosocomial transmission of multidrug-resistant tuberculosis. *Mayo Clin Proc* 1996;71:221–229.
99. van Belkum A, van Leeuwen W, Kluytmans J, et al. Molecular nosocomial epidemiology: high speed typing of microbial pathogens by arbitrary primed polymerase chain reaction assays. *Infect Control Hosp Epidemiol* 1995;16:658–666.
100. Snelling AM, Gerner-Smidt P, Hawkey PM, et al. Validation of use of whole-cell repetitive extragenic palindromic sequence-based PCR (REP-PCR) for typing strains belonging to the *Acinetobacter calcoaceticus–Acinetobacter baumanii* complex and application of the method to the investigation of a hospital outbreak. *J Clin Microbiol* 1996;34:1193–1202.
101. Davin-Regli A, Saux P, Bollet C, et al. Investigation of outbreaks of *Enterobacter aerogenes* colonisation and infection in intensive care units by random amplification of polymorphic DNA. *J Med Microbiol* 1996;44:89–98.
102. Davin-Regli A, Bollet C, Auffray JP, et al. Use of random amplified polymorphic DNA for epidemiological typing of *Stenotrophomonas maltophilia*. *J Hosp Infect* 1996;32:39–50.
103. Leenders A, van Belkum A, Janssen S, et al. Molecular epidemiology of apparent outbreak of invasive aspergillosis in a hematology ward. *J Clin Microbiol* 1996;34:345–351.
104. Robert F, Lebreton F, Bougnoux ME, et al. Use of random amplified polymorphic DNA as a typing method for *Candida albicans* in epidemiological surveillance of a burn unit. *J Clin Microbiol* 1995;33: 2366–2371.
105. Roll M, Norder H, Magnius LO, et al. Nosocomial spread of hepatitis B virus (HBV) in a hemodialysis unit confirmed by HBV DNA sequencing. *J Hosp Infect* 1995;30:57–63.
106. Graham DR, Dixon RE, Hughes JM, et al. Disk diffusion antimicrobial susceptibility testing for clinical and epidemiologic purposes. *Am J Infect Control* 1985;13:241–249.
107. Farmer JJ III. Conventional typing methods. *J Hosp Infect* 1988; 11(Suppl A):309–314.
108. Mollby R, Kuhn I, Katouli M. Computerised biochemical fingerprinting: a new tool for typing of bacteria. *Rev Med Microbiol* 1993;4: 231–234.
109. Pfaller MA. Typing methods for epidemiological investigation. In: Balows A, Hausler WJ Jr, Hermann K, Isenberg HD, Shadomy HJ, eds. *Manual of clinical microbiology.* 5th ed. Washington, DC: American Society for Microbiology, 1991;159–169.
110. Bingen EH, Denamur E, Elion J. Use of ribotyping in epidemiological surveillance of nosocomial outbreaks. *Clin Microbiol Rev* 1994;7: 311–327.
111. Miller JM. Molecular technology for hospital epidemiology. *Diagn Microbiol Infect Dis* 1993;16:153–157.
112. Jarvis WR. Usefulness of molecular epidemiology for outbreak investigations. *Infect Control Hosp Epidemiol* 1994;15:500–3.
113. Tenover FC, Arbett RD, Goering RV, et al. Interpreting chromosomal DNA restriction patterns produced by pulsed-field gel electrophoresis: criteria for bacterial strain typing. *J Clin Microbiol* 1995;33:2233–9.
114. Noble WC, Howell SA. Labile antibiotic resistance in *Staphylococcus aureus*. *J Hosp Infect* 1995;31:135–141.
115. van Belkum A. DNA fingerprinting of medically important microorganisms by use of PCR. *Clin Microbiol Rev* 1994;7:174–184.

116. Holzman D. Progress toward practical DNA-based infectious disease diagnostics. *ASM News* 1995;61:329–330.
117. Leading Article. Acceptability of the "bar code doctor." *Lancet* 1996; 347:555–556.
118. McHugh TD, Ramsay ARC, James EA, et al. Pitfalls of PCR: misdiagnosis of cerebral nocardia infection. *Lancet* 1995;346:1436.
119. Pfaller MA. Epidemiology of fungal infections: the promise of molecular typing. *Clin Infect Dis* 1995;20:1535–1539.
120. Fredricks DN, Relman DA. Sequence-based identification of microbial pathogens: a reconsideration of Koch's postulates. *Clin Microbiol Rev* 1996;9:18–33.
121. Hunter PR. Reproducibility and indices of discriminatory power of microbial typing methods. *J Clin Microbiol* 1990;28:1903–1905.
122. Ludlam HA, Noble WC, Marples RR, et al. The evaluation of a typing scheme for coagulase-negative staphylococci suitable for epidemiological studies. *J Med Microbiol* 1989;30:161–165.
123. Rutala WA, Weber DJ. Environmental interventions to control nosocomial infections. *Infect Control Hosp Epidemiol* 1995;16:442–443.
124. Rutala WA. Antisepsis, disinfection, and sterilization in hospitals and related institutions. In: Murray PR, Baron EJ, Pfaller MA, Tenover FC, Yolken RH, eds. *Manual of clinical microbiology.* 6th ed. Washington, DC: American Society for Microbiology, 1995:227–245.
125. Garner J, Favero M. Guidelines for the prevention and control of nosocomial infections: guideline for handwashing and hospital environmental control. *Am J Infect Control* 1985;14:110–129.
126. Rutala WA, Weber DJ. Low-temperature sterilization technologies: do we need to redefine "sterilization?" *Infect Control Hosp Epidemiol* 1996;17:87–91.
127. Wright AM, Hoxey EV, Soper CJ, et al. Biological indicators for low temperature steam and formaldehyde sterilization: investigation of the effect of change in temperature and formaldehyde concentration on spores of *Bacillus stearothermophilus* NCIMB 8224. *J Appl Bacteriol* 1996;80:259–265.
128. Simmons BP. Centers for Disease Control guidelines for hospital environmental control: Microbiologic surveillance of the environment and of personnel in the hospital. *Infect Control* 1981;2:145.
129. Bryan FL. Procedures to use during outbreaks of food-borne disease. In: Murray PR, Baron EJ, Pfaller MA, Tenover FC, Yolken RH, eds. *Manual of clinical microbiology.* 6th ed. Washington, DC: American Society for Microbiology, 1995:229–236.
130. AABB (American Association of Blood Banks). *Technical manual.* 11th ed. Arlington, VA: AABB; 1993.
131. Pillay T, Pillay DG, Hoosen AA, et al. Utility of surveillance bacterial cultures in neonatal exchange blood transfusions. *J Hosp Infect* 1995; 31:67–71.
132. Association for Advancement of Medical Instrumentation. *American national standard for hemodialysis systems.* ANSI/AAMI standard RD-5-1992. Arlington, VA: AAMI; 1992.
133. Gilchrist MJR. Epidemiologic and infection control microbiology. In: Isenberg HD, ed. *Clinical microbiology procedures handbook: Volume 2.* Washington, DC: American Society for Microbiology, 1992:11.1.1–11.1.3.
134. Smith D, Bradley SJ, Scott GM. Bacterial contamination of autologous bone marrow during processing. *J Hosp Infect* 1996;33:71–76.
135. Barrie D. The provision of food and catering services in hospital. *J Hosp Infect* 1996;33:13–32.
136. Landman D, Quale JM, Oydna E, et al. Comparison of five selective media for identifying fecal carriage of vancomycin-resistant enterococci. *J Clin Microbiol* 1996;34:751–752.
137. Haverly RM, Harrison CR, Dougherty TH. *Yersinia enterocolitica* bacteremia associated with red blood cell transfusion. *Arch Pathol Lab Med* 1996;120:499–500.
138. Goetz AM, Rihs JD, Chow JW, et al. An outbreak of infusion-related *Klebsiella pneumoniae* bacteremia in a liver transplantation unit. *Clin Infect Dis* 1995;21:1501–1503.
139. Reimer LG. Catheter-related infections and blood cultures. *Clin Lab Med* 1994;14:51–58.
140. Whitman ED, Boatman AM, Haun WE, et al. Comparison of diagnostic specimens and methods to evaluate infected venous access ports. *Am J Surg* 1995;170:665–670.
141. Horn WA, Larson EL, McGinley KJ, et al. Microbial flora on the hands of healthcare personnel: differences in composition and antibacterial resistance. *Infect Control Hosp Epidemiol* 1988;9:189–193.
142. Strasbaugh LJ, Sewell DL, Tjoelker RC, et al. Comparison of three methods for recovery of yeasts from hands of health-care workers. *J Clin Microbiol* 1996;34:471–473.
143. Larson E, Rotter ML. Handwashing. are experimental models a substitute for clinical trials? Two viewpoints. *Infect Control Hosp Epidemiol* 1990;11:63–66.
144. Cobben NAM, Drent M, Jonkers M, et al. Outbreak of severe *Pseudomonas aeruginosa* respiratory infections due to contaminated nebulizers. *J Hosp Infect* 1996;33:63–70.
145. Tablan OC, Anderson LJ, Arden NH, et al. Guideline for prevention of nosocomial pneumonia. *Infect Control Hosp Epidemiol* 1994;15: 587–627.
146. Gundermann KD. Spread of microorganisms by air-conditioning systems: especially in hospitals. *Ann NY Acad Sci* 1980;353:209.
147. Humphreys H. Microbes in the air: when to count! (the role of air sampling in hospitals). *J Med Microbiol* 1992;37:81–82.
148. Benbough JE, Bennett AM, Parks SR. Determination of the collection efficiency of a microbial air sampler. *J Appl Bacteriol* 1993;74: 170–173.
149. Groschel DH. Air sampling in hospitals. *Ann NY Acad Sci* 1980; 353:230.
150. McGowan JE Jr. Changing etiology of nosocomial bacteremia and fungemia and other hospital-acquired infections. *Rev Infect Dis* 1985;7(Suppl 3):S357–S370.
151. Committee on Microbial Contamination of Surfaces, Laboratory Section, American Public Health Association. A comparative microbiological evaluation of floor-cleaning procedures in hospital patient rooms. *Health Lab Sci* 1970;7:3.
152. Ta CA, Stout JE, Yu VL, et al. Comparison of culture methods for monitoring Legionella species in hospital potable water systems and recommendations for standardization. *J Clin Microbiol* 1995;33: 2118–2123.
153. Woolwine JD, Gerberding JL. Effect of testing method on apparent activities of antiviral disinfectants and antiseptics. *Antimicrob Agents Chemother* 1995;39:921–923.

Hospital Infections, Fourth Edition,
edited by John V. Bennett and Philip S. Brachman.
Lippincott–Raven Publishers, Philadelphia © 1998

CHAPTER 10

The Practices of Epidemiology in Community Hospitals

N. Joel Ehrenkranz

Community hospitals serve most of the hospitalized patients in the United States. These hospitals vary greatly in key characteristics, reflecting differences in patient populations, professional and support staffs, locations, physical structures, stated missions, academic connections, and ownership. In some community hospitals patients may receive subacute care; in others, patients may be treated at sites remote from the primary hospital structure.

The practices of epidemiology in community hospitals are varied. However, along with many opportunities come many challenges. An important organizational deficiency in a number of community hospitals has been the lack of clearly stated patient care missions. Hospital governing boards have generally failed to provide strong direction and unifying influences to support chiefs of services in establishing cohesive patient care policies. Despite actions of utilization and case management teams, this has frequently led to highly individualized patient care practices. Patient populations with similar characteristics may be readily identified at a number of hospitals. Evaluating outcomes of care in comparable patient populations at different hospitals, especially among hospitals within a common consortium, healthcare system, or corporate group, may demonstrate striking differences, thereby providing direction to promotion of meaningful and measurable change.

This chapter focuses on practical and useful approaches in the practice of hospital epidemiology in community hospitals, based on extensive experience of the author. It supports and extends the discussion of the Hospital Epidemiologist in Chapter 2.

N. J. Ehrenkranz: Florida Consortium for Infection Control, South Miami, Florida 33143-5163.

SURVEILLANCE

In the seminal paper in which Langmuir introduced the concept of a hospital epidemiologist, he also indicated the need for the development of systematic hospital surveillance systems: "By centralizing the pertinent data, forewarnings may often be possible and corrective steps taken before trouble begins" [1]. The scope of surveillance should be defined through the following steps:

1. Define boundaries of patient care activities, including sites physically separate from the primary hospital structure.
2. Determine high-risk and high-volume patient populations within the hospital boundaries, in relation to hospital mission and state licensure or certification.
3. Select meaningful time periods after patient treatments to evaluate outcomes.

Although most emphasis has been on nosocomial infection, a new direction is the assessment of various noninfectious adverse events, as a measure of continuous quality improvement. Methodologic problems need to be addressed early on:

1. Is there a systematic method of surveillance, including regular recording and reporting findings to those who should know?
2. Is there consistent use of objective criteria in surveillance? (If subacute or extended patient care facilities are located within hospital boundaries, infection criteria may differ from those of the acute care population.)
3. Is there representative sampling of populations?
4. Is there use of risk-stratified denominators?
5. Is there a process to estimate observer accuracy?

Clear definitions of numerators and denominators permit risk stratification [2]. On-site inspection is a useful surveillance method for prevalence studies. An important task to aid analysis is to implement a system to distinguish between random variations in frequency of adverse events and significant departures from expected findings [3]. Unfortunately, the more thorough the surveillance system is, the more likely the hospital is to appear to provide a lower quality of patient care.

Surveillance and Educational Intervention

Surveyors rarely have the opportunity in one hospital to evaluate treatment processes for a sufficiently large number of patients prospectively, by inspection, to yield a meaningful sample for outcome evaluation. Usually surveyors' observations are used as descriptive prevalence findings to determine patterns of current practices and promote compliance with well established policies, through focused teaching of healthcare personnel. For example, over a brief period, surveyors may record specific practices in care of central vascular catheters by inspection of all patients with central catheters, on a given unit or throughout the hospital. The following would then be expressed as a prevalence rate: the proportion of administration sets in use whose "hang time" for parenteral fluids is within durations established by hospital policy, and the proportion of catheter site dressings that are clean, dry, and securely attached. Such surveillance findings could then be used to establish goals for improvement through feedback and education.

Because nosocomial infection rates may be quite low even when there have been major violations of aseptic technique [4], it is usually not possible to associate prior violation of process with subsequent adverse outcome in a cause-and-effect relation. In the previous example, it is unlikely that a significantly increased frequency of local site infection or bloodstream infections would have occurred had a high rate of vascular catheter care errors been identified. On the other hand, infection surveillance may identify that specific members of the medical staff appear to have a higher rate of infections complicating central vascular catheters they have placed, compared with their colleagues (see Chapter 5). As a first intervention step, the hospital epidemiologist could remind all physicians of the importance of strict adherence to full aseptic technique during central venous catheter placement. Primary bloodstream infections of central vascular catheters may have origins in microbial contamination at catheter insertion, without regard to when infection ultimately becomes manifest [5,6]. If educational efforts fail to resolve the problem, classic epidemiologic studies and more direct interventions would then be required. Because of resource constraints, community hospital epidemiologists may need to limit case control studies (see Chapter 6) to either egregious problems or problems that continue despite educational intervention.

TABLE 10-1. *Routine environmental surveillance*

Autoclaves: Bacterial spore indicators, in-use temperature records
Dialysis machines: Dialysate fluid cultures
Operating rooms: Daily records of room temperature and humidity
Refrigerators: Temperature records, dedicated storage of patient specimens
Tuberculosis isolation rooms: Negative air pressure indicators, ultraviolet light efficacy measurements
Water supply: Functional assessment of system for conditions permitting growth of *Legionella* species

Immediate feedback of findings and education of personnel are essential to decreasing adverse patient occurrences. In critical care units, use of unsterile tap water or permitting an inappropriately long duration of use of initially sterile irrigation fluids or other fluids that readily support microbial growth [7] and easily become contaminated, has the potential to cause patient infections. Exposure of personnel hands to contaminated fluids or sink aerosols may lead to life-threatening bacterial infections in their patients [8]. Bathing postoperative patients with contaminated tap water, in areas close to surgical wounds, may have similar effects [9].

Inspections of kitchens and dietary areas yield valuable information about food safety. Inspections to determine the availability of personal protective equipment, hand disinfection agents, sharp object disposal boxes, adequate ventilation to minimize employee exposure to formaldehyde and glutaraldehyde, and so forth, provide an objective measure of safety of the working environment for healthcare personnel. Some useful environmental surveillance practices are shown in Table 10-1 (see Chapter 20). When new construction is planned, hospital epidemiologists should participate in a review of plans of the proposed structure and its function from the standpoint of patient and employee risks. During construction they should maintain timely surveillance to prevent adverse effects.

There may be unique problems in some community hospitals resulting from occasional needs for temporary rental of certain types of patient care equipment (e.g., mechanical ventilators, air-fluidized beds). After use in one institution, rental equipment may not be adequately disinfected, and pose a threat for other hospitals as a reservoir of such bacteria as vancomycin-resistant enterococci [10]. Part of the surveillance process of on-site inspection is to determine that current practices are adequate for disinfection of rental equipment immediately before and after patient use.

Postdischarge Surveillance

The increasingly short durations of hospitalization in recent years has served to truncate the opportunity for hospital surveillance of patient care outcome (see Chapter 5). This is particularly true in assessing complications of a number of surgical procedures. Moreover, enrollment of indigent Medicaid-funded patients into some health maintenance organizations has dried up this source of follow-up at some community hospitals. Surgeon reporting of operative complications first manifest after hospital discharge is likely to underreport true infection rates [11]. By contrast, telephone calls made to patients after discharge may provide better information than does a passive physician reporting system [12]. Some community hospitals may fund these efforts because information about patient satisfaction, useful for marketing, may also be obtained. Gold standards and estimates of sensitivity and specificity of telephone call surveillance remain to be defined.

Medical Record Audit

At present, and for the foreseeable future, medical records in most community hospitals are not likely to be adequately computerized for evaluating patient process and care. Medical record computer programs have primarily been constructed to retrieve financial data, and at times to capture limited amounts of clinical information that may not be relevant to planned investigations (see Chapter 8). The medical record audit is a powerful and flexible tool to evaluate events that have occurred during hospitalization, and is well defined in sensitivity and specificity [13]. The audit may explore allocations of hospital resources for various patient conditions. Adverse or unplanned events such as medication errors may be explored. In answering certain questions, retrospective medical record audits may be especially useful when combined with concurrent observations. The medical record audit may also be used as a tool to assess the accuracy of concurrent observations and provide an estimate of surveyor sensitivity and specificity in surveillance [14].

As opportunities are presented for medical records to become more fully computerized, epidemiologists should serve among those selecting software to ensure that information identified as necessary for assessment of various patient outcomes will continue to be captured, and that new data bases may be readily added. Purchasing a computer software system for medical record analyses with no consideration given to future uses in detecting events of potential epidemiologic interest will cripple quality improvement efforts.

Regulatory Surveillance

On occasion, surveillance activities may be conducted primarily to meet a requirement of regulatory or quasi-regulatory agencies, rather than because of concern over potential problems (see Chapter 11). For example, the federal Occupational Safety and Health Agency (OSHA) mandates record-keeping of hospital employee tuberculin skin test conversions and exposures to blood and infectious body fluids in the OSHA 200 log form. In some hospitals this may be only a pro forma activity; once data are collected, little is done to explore whether specific hospital areas, personnel, or practices have a possible association with these occurrences, and whether intervention may lead to diminution of their frequency. Efforts to assess the extent of possible underreporting of blood exposures often are not made. A good practice not only includes regular analysis of data and estimation of possible underreporting, but requires testing of hypotheses to reduce the adverse occurrences, with a long-range goal of virtual elimination.

ENDEMIC INFECTION PROBLEMS: SMALL CLUSTER WORK-UP CONSIDERATIONS

A common concern is assessing the significance of occasional episodes of relatively small numbers of nosocomial infections due to a common bacterial species, when these numbers are significantly higher than expected (see Chapter 6). For example, a case–control study may fail to reveal fruitful leads because of the small numbers of case patients. The next decision is whether to proceed to culture healthcare workers and additional patients to seek asymptomatic carriage of the bacterial species, and then to arrange for molecular epidemiologic studies to determine if one or multiple bacterial clones are being spread, or, alternatively, to explore by "shoe-leather" epidemiology a route of common bacterial transmission without regard to the number of bacterial clones being spread. Because molecular epidemiologic studies of some clusters may reveal multiple isolates of the same microbial species or a mixture of single and multiple isolates [15,16]—all being spread by the same route—I prefer investigation of a route of common transmission.

Some patients who are heavily colonized on skin areas close to mucosal surfaces, percutaneous entry sites of invasive devices, or wound sites may be initial sources of transient hand colonization of their caregivers [17]. Colonized healthcare workers may acquire and transmit bacteria such as *Acinetobacter, Serratia, Stenotrophomonas*, and other species readily amplified in environmental reservoirs, or bacteria such as *Clostridium difficile* and multiantibiotic-resistant enterococci, which may be amplified in patients and then heavily disseminated into the environment (see Chapter 15). These bacteria may persist on hands despite bland soap handwashing [18,19], permitting transfer to patient care devices [20]. The importance of hand antisepsis and use of personal barriers, including gloves, to prevent microbial acquisition from patients and the environment, and thereby prevent microbial transmission, cannot be overstated [21,22]. Hence, a key response to contain a cluster of infections should be emphasis on staff education to ensure that these simple measures are fully in force.

Indeed, both the major prevention and intervention roles of epidemiologists in community hospitals are educational ones: teaching routes of microbial spread and methods for interruption. This includes anticipating seasonal outbreaks of viral infections such as influenza, respiratory syncytial virus, and rotavirus. Early planning for control should include specific educational efforts to promote methods of limiting their nosocomial spread [23] (see Chapter 3). Emphasis on environmental disinfection to prevent spread of certain microbes [24] may pay large dividends. Drills, especially directed to nurse managers in critical care areas and simulating care of patients with such infections, may be useful for inculcating nursing staff leaders in proper infection control principles.

CHALLENGES OF MAJOR OUTBREAK INVESTIGATION AND INTERVENTION

Major outbreaks of clinical disease are relatively uncommon. In 1985, it was estimated that one true outbreak per year occurred in the average community hospital [25]. Details of major outbreak work-up are discussed elsewhere (see Chapter 6). However, certain aspects of large outbreak management in community hospitals merit comment.

At times, unusually strenuous infection control efforts may be necessary to deal with protracted episodes among critical care patients. Although not proved, it appears to be helpful on these occasions to employ knowledgeable persons who function as role models, and ensure adherence to proper infection control conduct of all healthcare workers who enter the critical care area [26,27].

Occasionally, colleagues' behavior complicates the challenges faced in the course of an outbreak investigation. When surveillance activities reveal an apparent major outbreak among patients or hospital staff, community hospital epidemiologists may experience considerable pressure "to do something" immediately. In some hospitals overreactions may occur, almost to the point of hysteria, with demands by medical or administrative staff to consider closing all or part of a hospital to new admissions and stopping elective operations, and the like. Others will urge sweeping microbiologic surveys of the environment ("culture everything"), or broad culture surveys among members of the hospital staff ("culture everybody"). Indeed, under these conditions, a calm and rational approach to problem solving, beginning with careful examination of surveillance findings, may be interpreted as nonfeasance of duties. It may be necessary to reassure colleagues of the primacy of analytic studies to establish priorities for intervention and control, to avoid counterproductive and wasteful efforts. Alternatively, in other community hospitals, there may be an overriding fear on the part of some staff and administrators that reporting a serious outbreak to public health authorities may lead to untoward publicity, which could adversely affect the hospital's reputation and finances. These colleagues may seek to trivialize the episode or strongly counsel delay in necessary reporting, in the hope the problem will be an evanescent one. In this setting, epidemiologists must quickly work to convince those at the top of the chain of authority that denial or delay in formal reporting is not in the best interest of the hospital.

To allay rumor and panic, and also to promote acquisition of information that may otherwise be unavailable, communication issues should be addressed by hospital epidemiologists early in an outbreak investigation, and include the following: Does the episode indicate a possible community public health problem, and if so, have public health authorities been informed? Has a method been established for rumor control among personnel? (A telephone "hotline" staffed by infection control personnel with regular updates of outbreak progress is useful.) Is there a method to obtain information from staff who wish to remain anonymous? (A telephone answering machine may be helpful to elicit anonymous reports.) How are exposed people who may no longer be in the hospital (discharged patients, families of exposed patients, visitors, vacationing physicians and hospital staff) to be contacted without creating undue alarm? Who will be the sole hospital spokesperson to deal with news media?

A checklist in management of these occurrence may prove useful:

1. Is the surveillance system identifying true and important excesses, or do the findings simply reflect random variations?
2. Is there laboratory or other objective confirmation of the outbreak?
3. Who has the authority to initiate necessary broad surveillance and control measures, and to prevent unnecessary activities?
4. Have relatively simple hospital measures been fully instituted, such as eliminating possible bacterial reservoirs and interrupting possible contact transmission?
5. How will improvement be demonstrated and total episode costs be calculated?
6. What changes will be implemented to prevent recurrences?

ANTIBIOTIC CONTROL ISSUES

Hyperendemic frequencies or outbreaks of infections due to methicillin-resistant *Staphylococcus aureus,* ceftazidime-resistant *Enterobacter* species, vancomycin-resistant enterococci, or other multiple antibiotic-resistant bacteria do occur in some community hospitals. At times there may be an external source of colonized patients from one or more referring subacute or chronic patient care facilities, which is beyond hospital control and from which there is reintroduction of these bacteria. On these occasions, hospital investigations may reveal that inappropriate or excessive antimicrobial use has appeared to facilitate spread of the resistant bacteria, once introduced (see Chapter 15). Despite absence of a clear cause-and-effect relation between reducing inappropriate antibiotic use and decreasing selection of antibiotic-resistant bacteria [28], episodes of introduction of antibiotic-resistant bacteria provide opportunities for exploring the possibility of association between dissemination of antibiotic-resistant bacteria and excessive antibiotic-prescribing patterns [29]. These episodes may set the stage for bringing about containment of excesses. Moreover, they also provide opportunities to reinforce and improve infection control techniques to prevent transmission of antibiotic-resistant bacteria [20].

The approach to control of inappropriate antibiotic use in community hospitals may require identification of perpetuating mechanisms. For example, some physicians who appear to agree to comply with recommendations to improve their antimicrobial prescription practices, especially when such recommendations flow from quality improvement studies, may simply fail to alter their prescribing habits. This behavior seemingly results from inertia, or perhaps from counterbalancing influences external to the hospital. Other physicians may feel their prerogatives to prescribe freely are being infringed. In these instances, results of studies of inappropriate antibiotic use, comparing individual physicians within departments and groups, (including listing of medical staff members by code), which are presented at various meetings attended by the medical staff and also posted in physicians' lounges, may help to bring about desired changes. Providing a monthly report of antibiotic-resistant bacteria recovered from patients in critical care units [30], together with records of inappropriate empiric antibiotic administration, to physicians who practice in critical care areas may improve antibiotic use. The advantage of graphic feedback of relevant antibiotic observations is that it is nonconfrontational and objective. In yet other instances, small group meetings with the natural leaders of the medical staff, conducted in a collegial fashion, may resolve specific antibiotic use issues.

Other factors that promote continued problems in antibiotic use may relate to the transmission of orders on a preprinted order sheet, sent by electronic facsimile transmission. In this instance it is necessary to persuade the physician to discard the current preprinted orders, or establish a committee for oversight of such orders. Finally, in some physicians' practices, physician assistants may write virtually all antibiotic orders, which are promptly carried out by the nursing staff, and only later countersigned by attending physicians. To bring about change it is necessary to provide new directions to the physician assistants.

Such piecework measures in changing prescription patterns are highly labor intensive and require frequent repetition. The long-range goal should be to bring enduring change, by changing the hospital culture of antibiotic use [31]. A long-term, comprehensive approach might emanate from the hospital governing board, beginning with a new mission statement such as the following: "A hospital mission is to diminish selection and dissemination of antibiotic-resistant bacteria, within the institution and the community-at-large. The best patient care practices consonant with this goal will be carried out by our medical staff, through their judicious use of antimicrobials." The epidemiologist has an important role in promoting this mission.

HOSPITAL CONSORTIA

There is a growing need in community hospitals for epidemiologists to carry out a number of quality improvement activities, such as evaluating use of specific items in patient care in terms of both cost and outcome, cost effectiveness of competing products, and impact of technical and personnel changes. In addition, the epidemiologist often aids implementation of various new regulations mandated by state and federal agencies, helps to prepare for inspections by regulatory and quasiregulatory groups (see Chapter 11), and promotes preventive measures among employee populations, along with carrying out the traditional patient-oriented infection control tasks. However, the constricted financial climate for most community physicians virtually precludes their volunteering to serve in these capacities. Moreover, the financial limitations experienced by many community hospitals sharply restrict their ability to support a full-time epidemiologist. One effective solution is for qualified physicians to establish a consortium, in which a number of hospitals join together and share these professional services and their financial support [32]. This is becoming an increasingly popular undertaking [33]. Shared epidemiologic services permit an emphasis on providing educational programs to various categories of hospital personnel. The increasing number of temporarily employed healthcare workers in high-risk patient care areas, who have little time to consider their potential for spreading infection, makes this an important activity. In addition, there may be an opportunity to develop or improve hospital information systems with the goal of group standardization. This may facilitate a variety of assessments of patient care outcomes and costs among individual hospital members for interhospital comparisons, thereby providing direction to improve patient care or decrease costs. By comparing both outcomes and costs of patient care and making recommendations for measurable changes, consortia epidemiologists may be able to bring about substantial patient care benefits and diminished risks and cost—all of which justify continuation of the program.

National benchmark standards may be composed of data from a variety of hospitals, including large municipal and teaching hospitals; these standards may not necessarily be comparable with those derived entirely from a community hospital group in one region. Despite the many differences among community hospitals, one overriding commonality is that among those in positions of administrative accountability, there is a strong motivation to acquire knowledge of efficiency and efficacy of their hospital relative to neighboring or regional peers. Thus, even if patient outcomes at one community hospital appear to be satisfactory in terms of a national standard, if outcomes are not comparable with those of neighboring hospitals, this will be a major stimulus for change. Epidemiologists at consortia may seek to develop their own data bases. A useful standardized data collection tool for noninfectious disease outcomes has been published [34]. Such data bases are likely to be especially useful as hospitals join together into a single healthcare system. The consortium approach applied to several hospitals in a common healthcare system may be the next step in practices of epidemiology in community hospitals.

Hartstein has pointed out that "efficient and effective solutions to hospital and healthcare problems should be generated at the local level rather than by national mandates" [35].

PLANNING FOR UNCOMMON AND RARE EVENTS

On infrequent occasions, there may be failure of essential city services such as loss of electrical power or potable water, which can adversely affect hospital function. In most North American areas such failures are usually uncommon, and their full effects may not necessarily be anticipated in all day-to-day hospital operations, especially if new hospital services have been recently developed. For example, if no potable water is immediately available, the question whether to cancel elective surgery needs to be addressed. If city electrical power is lost, another question is whether the hospital emergency power supply is adequate to maintain negative pressure in certain isolation rooms. Ideally, such considerations should be addressed before the emergencies occur, and during development of new hospital services.

On very rare occasions, floods, earthquakes, hurricanes, and the like may lead to actual structural hospital damage. Under these circumstances, continued care of all patients becomes problematic—in particular, care of patients capable of efficient dissemination of tuberculosis, such as people with tuberculosis and acquired immunodeficiency syndrome (AIDS). In areas where these natural disasters have repeatedly occurred over a period of years, some community hospitals have now embarked on special programs for care of patients with AIDS; some of these patients may have coexistent pulmonary tuberculosis. Prudent epidemiologists should make contingency plans for their transfer to hospitals at a distance sufficiently remote to be safe. It may be necessary to plan various modes of transportation in event of emergency. Realistically, an alternative program must also be in place because prior commitments may not be honored during emergencies. Local public health and civil disaster authorities should be included in the planning if possible, and kept informed.

In some instances, community hospital marketing efforts for critical care services to patients coming from outside the United States have failed to consider possibilities of introduction of contagious disease not usually seen in metropolitan regions. For example, some community hospitals have established relations with various overseas hospitals, including ones in developing countries of South America, for transfer and sophisticated medical management of seriously ill patients such as those having multiorgan failure. Epidemiologists might provide a valuable service by evaluating whether there is a risk that patients who are referred from outside the United States could have contagious diseases indigenous to their homelands, such as those caused by a pathogenic arenavirus (e.g., Machupo, Junin), and devise screening programs to assess these risks. In theory, correct application of barrier precautions and other pertinent measures should prevent secondary spread of these viruses [36]. However, the lack of complete application of proper precautions by many personnel in community hospitals [37,38], as well as the general absence of protocols for safe triage of febrile patients at the time of admission, underscore the need to consider the full range of implications of care of patients transferred from outside the country. If there is a hospital program to promote transfer of patients from outside the United States who may be capable of disseminating contagious disease, it is sound planning to arrange for drills in specific hospital areas to monitor application of infection control principles in patient screening, as well as to ensure compliance when these patients arrive for care.

EVALUATION OF NEW PRODUCTS

An important activity in community hospital epidemiology is the evaluation of cost effectiveness of new products designed to diminish the risk of nosocomial infections. Answers should be sought to questions such as: 1) Does the problem the new equipment is supposed to remedy actually exist at the hospital? 2) Were studies done in a way to be generalizable to community hospital patients?

and 3) Will use of the product be cost effective for all patients, or only a clearly defined group?

It has been my experience that products reported at scientific meetings to be highly effective in a limited set of patients in tertiary care centers, are at times aggressively marketed based only on the abstracts of these meetings, for wide use among many patients in community hospitals. In these instances, the costs of patient care are likely to increase with little concomitant advantage, unless use of the product is limited to the population already demonstrated to receive benefit. Indeed, in my view, it usually is wise to defer any decision to support large-scale purchases of new products based only on information offered in abstract form. I recommend to wait until published studies are available before making any substantial purchase commitment.

To what extent a community hospital epidemiologist should freely interact with local salespeople may be viewed as an ethical question.

From time to time, there may be consideration of the cost–benefit relations of resterilizing disposable patient care items that have been opened but not used. This may include certain types of surgical sutures, laparotomy pads, ventilatory tubing, invasive devices, and the like. In general, the manufacturer of these materials advises against such practices. The practice of epidemiology in this instance may include exploring the risk of altering the intrinsic structure or integrity of the object by resterilization, estimating the potential gravity of these risks, and calculating potential cost–benefit relations of the resterilization practice. For devices that do not enter body cavities or remain there, these risks are likely to be minimal. An alternate approach may include returning these items to the manufacturer for a partial credit. The epidemiologist's calculations of comparative costs versus benefits of the different options become useful for decision making by purchasing departments and risk managers.

EMPLOYEE HEALTH

Concerns about employee health (see Chapter 3) in community hospitals are similar to those at other hospitals with regard to on-hire assessments, immunizations, blood and body fluid exposures, tuberculin skin tests, employment of handicapped individuals, and so forth. Certain problems may be exaggerated in smaller community hospitals because of a lack of a dedicated employee health program. As a consequence, part-time and temporary employees (e.g., agency personnel, traveling nurses), in particular, may be employed without proper initial health evaluations or assessments when blood or tuberculosis exposure occur. Thus, review of employee health services is an important component of epidemiologic practices to ensure that standards are maintained. One curious problem that may be encountered relates to issues of tuberculin tests. On occasion, personnel may seek advice from senior physicians who are unfamiliar with current concepts of tuberculin skin tests (see Chapter 33). They may receive misinformation, such as tuberculin testing is not to be done in people who have had prior bacillus Calmette-Guerin treatment, or that preventive therapy is not indicated for people who are recent tuberculin test converters if they are 35 years of age or older. At such times, epidemiologists may find it impolitic to contradict the source of the incorrect information. Instead, they may suggest that employees call the toll-free telephone "hotline" at the A. G. Holley State Hospital (800-4TB-INFO or 800-482-4636), a free-standing tuberculosis hospital in Florida. Knowledgeable physicians will speak directly with individual healthcare workers, and provide accurate recommendations. Moreover, the A. G. Holley physicians will specifically contact misinformed physicians to explain these concepts.

A major problem in many community hospitals is the limited staffing of personnel in certain important areas, all of whom are essential to operations. This may motivate employees to avoid reporting possible communicable disease, and department managers to encourage sick employees to work. Moreover, personnel such as most physicians, physician's assistants, some surgical nurses, and certain contract workers (e.g., workers in dialysis services) who are not paid employees of the hospital may not consider themselves subject to the hospital's employee health program. The practice of epidemiology in this setting includes establishing clear guidelines for all healthcare workers, regardless of pay source, as to when specific clinical conditions preclude working, and providing a protocol as to when they may be cleared by hospital personnel to return to work. On the other hand, there is also a need to define minor, noncontagious conditions of respiratory and similar illness—often of an allergic nature—in nonepidemic periods when work may be permitted, to allow departments with a minimal number of staff to continue to function. In this instance, epidemiologists may establish a daily employee health check system for screening working employees having symptoms of minor illness, to ensure that any progress or change in symptomatology is detected promptly. It would also be necessary to evaluate whether the reliability of self-reporting by individual employees is likely to be adequate to detect early onset of contagious disease in time to prevent secondary spread, and to ascertain whether department managers fully support their employees in this program. This activity would not be permitted in high-risk patient care areas. Regular surveillance reports of outcomes of employees who have been permitted to work with minor illness, and of any effects on people who may have been exposed to them, is also necessary to assess untoward consequences.

An important epidemiologic activity is to explore clusters, outbreaks, or hyperendemic occurrences of adverse reactions among hospital employees. Increasingly, problems identified among personnel in some community hospitals are those of occupational origin, including latex allergy [39], other types of allergy, effects of poor indoor air quality (glutaraldehyde, formaldehyde exposure [40]), and "sick building" syndromes [41]. At times, community hospital epidemiologists may find themselves being thrust into the position of functioning as resident experts in occupational health matters. In the event they have no prior experiences in this field, it may be useful if they have already established connections with knowledgeable consultants.

SUMMARY

There is a broad range of opportunities for practices of epidemiology among patients and healthcare workers in community hospitals. These include establishing surveillance activities that may identify problems unique to the special missions and activities of these hospitals, and that may lead to creative solutions. There is a prime role for the epidemiologist as an educator of hospital personnel and medical staff. Systematic studies done in community hospitals have a potential for directly improving the quality of patient care and employee health practices, as well as diminishing healthcare costs.

REFERENCES

1. Langmiur AD. Significance of epidemiology in medical schools. *Journal of Medical Education* 1964;39:39–48.
2. Scheckler WE, Gaynes R, Gross P, et al. An approach to the evaluation of the quality indicators of the outcome of care in hospitalized patients with a focus on nosocomial infection indicators. *Infect Control Hosp Epidemiol* 1995;16:308–316.
3. Birnbaum D. Analysis of hospital infection surveillance data. *Infect Control* 1984;5:332–338.
4. Altemeier WA, Todd J. Studies on the incidence of infection following open chest cardiac massage for cardiac arrest. *Ann Surg* 1963;158: 596–607.
5. Sampath LA, Chowdhury N, Caraos L, et al. Infection resistance of surface modified catheters with either short-lived or prolonged activity. *J Hosp Infect* 1995;30:201–210.
6. Raad II, Holm DC, Gilbreath BJ, et al. Prevention of central venous catheter-related infections by using maximal sterile barrier precautions during insertion. *Infect Control Hosp Epidemiol* 1994;15:231–238.
7. Brown DG, Skylis TP, Sulisz CA, et al. Sterile water and saline solution: potential reservoirs of nosocomial infection. *Am J Infect Control* 1985;13:35–39.
8. Dandalides PC, Rutala WA, Sarubbi FA. Postoperative infections following cardiac surgery: association with an environmental reservoir in a cardiothoracic intensive care unit. *Infect Control* 1984;5:378–384.
9. Lowry DW, Blankenship RJ, Gudley W, et al. A cluster of *Legionella* sternal wound infections due to postoperative topical exposure to contaminated tap water. *N Engl J Med* 1991;324:109–113.
10. Orr KE, Gould FK, Perry JD, et al. Therapeutic beds: the Trojan horses of the 1990s? *Lancet* 1994;344:65–66.
11. Sands K, Vineyard G, Platt R. Surgical site infections occurring after hospital discharge. *J Infect Dis* 1996;173:963–970.
12. Reimer K, Gleed C, Nicolle LE. The impact of postdischarge infection on surgical wound infection rates. *Infect Control* 1987;8:237–240.
13. Haley RW, Schaberg DR, McClisk DK, et al. The accuracy of retrospective chart review in measuring nosocomial infection rates: results of validation studies in pilot hospitals. *Am J Epidemiol* 1980;111: 516–533.
14. Ehrenkranz NJ, Shultz JM, Richter EI. Recorded criteria as a "gold standard" for sensitivity and specificity estimates of surveillance of nosocomial infection: a novel method to measure job performance. *Infect Control Hosp Epidemiol* 1995;16:697–702.
15. Villarino ME, Stevens LE, Schable B, et al. Risk factors for epidemic *Xanthomonas maltophilia* infection/colonization in intensive care unit patients. *Infect Control Hosp Epidemiol* 1992;13:201–206.
16. Laing FPY, Ramotar K, Read RR, et al. Molecular epidemiology of *Xanthomonas maltophilia* colonization and infection in the hospital environment. *J Clin Microbiol* 1995;33:513–518.
17. Eckert DG, Ehrenkranz NJ, Alfonso BC. Indications for alcohol or bland soap in removal of aerobic gram-negative skin bacteria: assessment by a novel method. *Infect Control Hosp Epidemiol* 1989;10: 306–310.
18. Knittle MA, Eitzman DV, Baer H. Role of hand contamination of personnel in the epidemiology of gram-negative nosocomial infection. *J Pediatr* 1975;86:433–437.
19. Wade JJ, Desai N, Casewell MW. Hygienic hand disinfection for the removal of epidemic vancomycin-resistant *Enterococcus faecium* and gentamicin-resistant *Enterobacter cloacae. J Hosp Infect* 1991;18: 211–216.
20. Ehrenkranz NJ, Alfonso BC. Failure of bland soap handwash to prevent hand transfer of patient bacteria to urethral catheters. *Infect Control Hosp Epidemiol* 1991;12:654–662.
21. Boyce JM, Mermel LA, Zervos MJ, et al. Controlling vancomycin-resistant enterococci. *Infect Control Hosp Epidemiol* 1995;16:634–637.
22. Klein BS, Perloff WH, Maki DG. Reduction of nosocomial infection during pediatric intensive care by protective isolation. *N Engl J Med* 1989;320:1714–1731.
23. Raad II, Sherertz RS, Russell BA, et al. Uncontrolled nosocomial rotavirus transmission during a community outbreak. *Am J Infect Control* 1990;18:24–28.
24. Sattar SA, Jacobson H, Rahmay H, et al. Interruption of rotavirus spread through chemical disinfection. *Infect Control Hosp Epidemiol* 1994;15:751–756.
25. Haley RW, Tenney SH, Lindsey JO, et al. How frequent are outbreaks of nosocomial infection in community hospitals? *Infect Control* 1985; 6:233–236.
26. Ehrenkranz NJ, Pfaff SJ. Mediastinitis complicating cardiac operations: evidence of postoperative causation. *Rev Infect Dis* 1991;13:803–814.
27. Haley RW, Cushion NB, Tenover FC, et al. Eradication of endemic methicillin-resistant *Staphylococcus aureus* from a neonatal intensive care unit. *J Infect Dis* 1995;171:614–624.
28. McGowan JE. Do intensive hospital antibiotic control programs prevent the spread of antibiotic resistance? *Infect Control Hosp Epidemiol* 1994;15:478–483.
29. Burmen DR, Baneyee SN, Gaynes RP, et al. Ceftazidime resistance among selected nosocomial gram-negative bacilli in the United States. *J Infect Dis* 1994;170:1622–1625.
30. Swartz MN. Hospital-acquired infections: diseases with increasingly limited therapies. *Proc Natl Acad Sci USA* 1994;91:2420–2427.
31. Goldmann DA, Weinstein RA, Wenzel RP, et al. Strategies to prevent and control the emergence and spread of antimicrobial-resistant microorganisms in hospitals. *JAMA* 1996;275:234–240.
32. Ehrenkranz NJ. Starting an infection control network. *Infectious Disease in Clinical Practice* 1995;4:194–198.
33. Dahl K, L'Ecuyer PB, Jones M, et al. Follow-up evaluation of respiratory isolation rooms in ten Midwestern hospitals. *Infect Control Hosp Epidemiol* 1996;12:816–818.
34. Massanari RN, Wiekerson K, Swartzendruber S. Designing surveillance for noninfectious outcomes of medical care. *Infect Control Hosp Epidemiol* 1995;16:419–426.
35. Hartstein A. Improved understanding and control of nosocomial methicillin-resistant *Staphylococcus aureus: are we overdoing it?* Infect Control Hosp Epidemiol 1995;16:250–259.
36. Barry M, Russi M, Armstrong L, et al. Brief report: treatment of a laboratory-acquired *Sabia* infection. *N Engl J Med* 1995;333:294–296.

37. Henry K, Campbell S, Collier P, et al. Compliance with universal precautions and needle handling and disposal practices among emergency departments at two community hospitals. *Am J Infect Control* 1994;22:129–137.
38. Lund S, Jackson J, Leggett J, et al. Reality of glove use and handwashing in a community hospital. *Am J Infect Control* 1994;22:352–357.
39. Zaza S, Reeder JM, Charles LE, et al. Latex sensitivity among perioperative nurses. *AORN J* 1994;60:806–812.
40. Chan-Yeung M, Malo JL. Occupational asthma. *N Engl J Med* 1995;333:107–112.
41. Sherin KM. Building-related illnesses and sick building syndrome. *J Fla Med Assoc* 1993;80:472–474.

Hospital Infections, Fourth Edition,
edited by John V. Bennett and Philip S. Brachman.
Lippincott–Raven Publishers, Philadelphia © 1998

CHAPTER 11

The Role of Professional and Regulatory Organizations in Infection Control Programs

William E. Scheckler

As a medical student from 1960 to 1964 and a medical intern and resident from 1964 to 1968, I knew very little about nosocomial infections. As a student in surgery, I was aware of the threat of *Staphylococcus aureus* wound infections occurring in patients. I was impressed at the combination of potent antibiotics given to patients before surgery to prevent such infections. The "Hospital Staph" was well described in the 1960s. In 1960, R. E. O. Williams and his colleagues in Great Britain published *Hospital Infection: Causes and Prevention.* This book included a chapter on staphylococcal infections and an important comment in the preface about hospital infections: "The problem is a universal one, and whoever claims that his hospital is free of such trouble need only be invited to open his eyes a little wider" [1]. As the fourth epidemic intelligence service officer assigned to the Hospital Infection Unit at the Communicable Diseases Center (now called the Centers for Disease Control and Prevention (CDC)) in 1968, I checked at my own university hospital before departing for Atlanta to see how wide our eyes were open. In 1968, my university hospital infection control program consisted entirely of line listings generated by the microbiology laboratory of all patients with *S. aureus* infections. A formal comprehensive system of surveillance, management, and prevention of nosocomial infections was yet to be developed. National professional organizations had not yet been formed in the arena of infection control. Williams and colleagues published a second edition [1] of their book a few years after the first epidemic intelligence service officer was assigned to this problem at the CDC at the behest of the editors of this book. The voluntary and federal agencies had not yet made efforts at defining the elements of a hospital infection control program.

W. E. Scheckler: Department of Family Medicine, University of Wisconsin Medical School, Madison, Wisconsin 53715.

The years since the early 1970s, however, have seen an explosion in the knowledge about nosocomial infections and in the new infection problems each new advance in medical and surgical care has caused. The purpose of this chapter, new in this edition, is to put into a frame of reference the role that has been played since the early 1970s by the professional societies, governmental agencies, and regulatory bodies that have developed an interlocking array of guidelines, requirements, rules, suggestions, and laws in hospital infection control.

Table 11-1 lists representative organizations and the main mechanisms they use to influence hospital infection control and prevention.

This chapter expands on the role of these governmental and professional groups in infection control programs, using examples to illustrate their contributions. Hospital epidemiology and infection control professionals of the 1990s might be better able to sort through the complex array of outputs from these groups if those outputs are placed in a framework and illustrated with appropriate case histories.

TYPES OF REQUIREMENTS USEFUL IN PROVIDING OPTIMAL INFECTION CONTROL

Table 11-1 lists a large array of mechanisms used by professional and governmental groups to improve patient care. The most traditional is the *published study* or investigation in a peer-reviewed scientific medical journal. The peer review process helps the editors of such journals find the most valid and useful papers to publish. Virtually all the other mechanisms for improvement depend on this central repository of the scientific literature. Although abstracts of studies selected for presentations at national meetings may be published in journals and accessible by Medline searches, it is the fully published scientific paper

TABLE 11-1. *Principal organizations that influence hospital infection control and prevention*

Organizations	Mechanisms
Federal: Hospital Infections Program—Centers for Disease Control and Prevention (CDC)	Scientific studies reported in the literature Hospital Infection Control Practices Advisory Committee—(HICPAC) Collaborative Studies—National Nosocomial Infection Surveillance System (NNIS) Development and publication of guidelines Training programs and meetings
Joint Commission on the Accreditation of Health Care Organizations (JCAHO)	Certification requirements for Hospital Infection Control Program Publications about requirements
Society for Healthcare Epidemiology of America (SHEA)	Professional journal publications Annual scientific meetings Guidelines and state-of-the-art reports Training programs
Association for Professionals in Infection Control and Epidemiology (APIC)	Professional journal publications Annual scientific meetings Guidelines Training programs
Federal: Occupational Safety and Health Administration (OSHA)	Blood-borne pathogen standards Tuberculosis in health care settings
Federal: Environmental Protection Agency (EPA)	Certification of safety and efficacy of chemical disinfectants
Federal: Food and Drug Administration (FDA)	Certification of safety and efficacy of drugs and medical devices
State statutes and regulations	Reporting of communicable diseases, especially HIV and AIDS—variable from state to state
Federal statutes	Infectious waste requirements
Other professional organizations	Guidelines, scientific meetings, consensus conferences, scientific journals, training programs

AIDS, acquired immunodeficiency syndrome; HIV, human immunodeficiency virus.

that forms the cornerstone for all the other mechanisms listed in Table 11-1. The CDC's journal, *Morbidity and Mortality Weekly Report*, is also crucial as the place new issues and problems in hospital infections first appear in an authoritative way.

Guidelines are usually a combination of why and how to prevent or control a particular nosocomial infection problem. They may address a process such as surveillance of infections or an investigation of a cluster of specific infections. They may provide detailed recommendations on how to use a new medical device in such a way as to minimize the risk of infection. They may specify optimal use of prophylactic antibiotics. But important characteristics of guidelines include their voluntary nature and the usual recognition that "one size fits all" is rarely true in the diverse acute care hospitals that we have, with different sizes, locations, and patient populations. Guidelines are frequently derived from a comprehensive review of the medical literature—a state-of-the-art publication that may precede or accompany the guideline. The Society for Healthcare Epidemiology of America (SHEA) and the Association for Professionals in Infection Control Epidemiology (APIC) make use of the publications of guidelines and state-of-the-art communications in their journals. The more recently formed Hospital Infections Control Practices Advisory Committee (HICPAC) of the CDC uses "guideline" as its official terminology. In the area of infection control, the CDC has issued guidelines, not rules or regulation.

Certification *requirements or standards* are the hallmarks of accrediting organizations such as the Joint Commission on the Accreditation of Health Care Organizations (JCAHO). Formal accreditation by the JCAHO became crucial to hospitals after the passage of Medicare in 1965 when the federal government accepted JCAHO accreditation or certification of hospitals as sufficient to qualify for Medicare payments. JCAHO standards are periodically revised, and new standards with some very new, patient-oriented approaches are being implemented. The text of standards is accompanied by companion literature that provides explanations of how the standards can be met. In general, the standards are changed based both on the scientific literature and a broad consensus of consultants who review them. Again, there is usually some degree of flexibility built into the accreditation process.

Regulations and rules are usually the implementation of statutes by an administrative arm of government charged with implementing and enforcing the law. A good example of a regulating body is the Occupational Safety and Health Administration (OSHA). Originally designed to protect workers from unsafe working conditions, it is only since the acquired immunodeficiency syndrome (AIDS) epidemic that OSHA has become involved in infection control with the "Blood Borne Pathogen Standard" and the "OSHA Enforcement Guidelines for Occupational Exposure to Tuberculosis." OSHA is empowered to enforce these standards by fines. One way to contrast the approaches of CDC guidelines and OSHA standards is depicted in Table 11-2. By their nature, such standards are inflexible rather than flexible.

Other examples of regulations from government bodies include state statutes that cover the reporting of infectious disease and federal statutes defining medical waste. A myriad of other requirements concerning everything from human immunodeficiency virus (HIV) testing to professional licensure are also potentially relevant to infection control practice and may vary from state to state.

TABLE 11-2. *Contrasting federal approaches in infection control*

OSHA	CDC
Rules and regulations	Guidelines
Everything is black or white	Reality is shades of gray
Police enforcers—adversarial	Epidemiologist and scientist
We'll fine you	We'll help you
One size fits all	Diversity is truth

OSHA, Occupational Safety and Health Administration; CDC, Centers for Disease Control and Prevention.

Consensus conferences may occur across governmental and professional organizations. At one time, when no good scientific data could be found concerning a particular process or issue, a panel of "experts" would develop a consensus based on their best professional judgment.

More rigorous evidence based processes have been in place recently—most particularly in the development of "Practice Guidelines" [2]. The early attempts at guidelines from the CDC did address the certainty of the recommendations in several categories, from scientifically based, to consensus by all experts on the panel, to a "might be useful" status.

More recently, interest in the outcomes of medical care has led to the development of a number of *outcome report cards* designed to allow regulatory and accrediting groups to compare hospitals. Such report cards have both useful and dangerous qualities and have been reviewed and reported on elsewhere [3]. Even the federally funded Peer Review Organizations have changed their scope of work to look at outcomes [4].

Another contemporary interest has been the "total quality management paradigm" applied to healthcare as a way of analyzing processes, and called *continuous quality improvement* [5–7]. This approach assumes that all hospital processes, including those in hospital infection control, can be continuously improved by looking at good data and involving the people who use the process in improving it. Several medical journals now address the "CQI" approach, including *Infection Control and Hospital Epidemiology, Clinical Performance and Quality Health Care* from SHEA, and the *Journal of Quality Improvement* from the JCAHO.

CONTEMPORARY EXAMPLES OF THE ROLE OF THE PROFESSIONAL AND REGULATORY ORGANIZATIONS IN INFECTION CONTROL PROGRAMS

The Centers for Disease Control and Prevention, U.S. Public Health Service

The CDC has several working groups that have had a profound impact on infection control programs since the late 1960s. The major mechanisms used to communicate CDC recommendations have been the weekly *Morbidity and Mortality Weekly Report* (MMWR) and the scientific literature.

One of the major groups located at the CDC is the Hospital Infections Program, which has existed in one form or another since 1966. It has run the National Nosocomial Infections Surveillance System (NNIS) since that program was begun in 1970 and has had a major role in setting the programs for the three decennial International Conferences on Nosocomial Infections [8–10]. An ambitious retrospective "Study of the Efficacy of Nosocomial Infection Control Practices" (SENIC) was developed by the Hospital Infection Program group. The SENIC results validated several years of recommendations and continue to be the scientific base on which many current CDC recommendations and guidelines are based [11].

Examples of guidelines promulgated by the CDC are numerous and have been published in the MMWR and elsewhere over many years. Most recently, the issue of the prevention of dissemination of tuberculosis from patients to staff and to other patients has been an important area of study. The CDC guidelines for this area were published in 1990 and an update was reported in the MMWR in 1995 [12]. From 1993 to 1997, a mechanism was put in place to assist in development of authoritative guidelines: HICPAC. Modeled after the very successful Advisory Committee on Immunization Practices, HICPAC is tackling many important and timely issues in infection control and is in the process of issuing guidelines in several areas [13,14].

Through ongoing projects such as NNIS, and through investigation assistance, "epidemiologic aids" in the review of clusters and epidemics of nosocomial infections, the development of guidelines, and panels such as HICPAC, the CDC has been the single most influential agency in infection control. The major professional organizations in hospital infection control, SHEA and APIC, were originated largely by physicians, nurses, and other professionals who either served at the CDC or attended training programs developed and run by the CDC in this area. The CDC's role has been seminal and central to the evolution of the entire field of hospital epidemiology and infection control in the United States. It still is.

The Joint Commission in the Accreditation of Health Care Organizations

The specification of a hospital infection control program and committee and the development of standards by the JCAHO in the 1960s had a profound impact on the growth of the entire field of infection control. Because hospitals were eager to get and retain JCAHO accreditation, infection control programs blossomed throughout the country. This encouraged the development of training programs for infection control practitioners, mostly nurses, and provided employment opportunities for them.

Inclusion of infection control program requirements in JCAHO accreditation is the single most important factor in allowing the work and recommendations of the CDC to be broadly applied.

It is of interest to note that the current JCAHO standards have been modified and shortened. In the quest for looking at outcomes, infection control programs are no longer required as such, but may be part of a broader quality improvement process at a hospital. It remains to be seen whether hospitals will integrate the older, well established knowledge base and epidemiologic expertise of infection control specialists into quality improvement strategies—or misinterpret the intent and use the new standards to eliminate positions [15].

The Society for Healthcare Epidemiology of America

The Society was founded in 1980 by a group of physicians, mostly specialists in infectious diseases, many of whom had served as epidemic intelligence service officers at the CDC in the 1960s and 1970s. The original name was the Society of Hospital Epidemiologists of America. The name changed as the relevance and value of the use of epidemiologic tools in noninfectious problems in hospitals, then in healthcare in general, became appreciated. Hospital infection control, however, continues to be a core activity of the organization.

The Society is now responsible for two journals: *Infection Control and Hospital Epidemiology*, published since 1980, and *Clinical Performance and Quality Health Care*, published since 1993. SHEA sponsors regular short courses in hospital epidemiology and holds an annual scientific meeting in the spring.

The Society has developed independent position papers on several issues, such as *Clostridium difficile*-associated diarrhea and colitis [16], and has spearheaded several joint reviews and guidelines in collaboration with other professional groups, including:

1. With APIC, the Surgical Infection Society (SIS), and the CDC on defining issues concerning the surveillance of surgical site infections [17]
2. With APIC and SIS on looking at clinical outcomes in the *Final Report of the Outcome Indicator Study Group* [3]
3. With JCAHO to monitor outcome indicators [18]

The Association for Professionals in Infection Control and Epidemiology, Inc.

This organization is made up of infection control professionals, most of whom are nurses, who have managed and staffed infection control programs in U.S. hospitals starting in the 1960s. The concept of the position was developed in Great Britain and promoted by the CDC in the late 1960s and early 1970s. A large nucleus of infection control professionals with significant interest evolved, leading to the formation of a professional organization in 1972 [19]. In 1981, APIC created the Certification Board of Infection Control to certify the knowledge and expertise of infection control practitioners [20]. Like SHEA, this group has its own scientific journal, *The American Journal of Infection Control*, which began in 1980 as a formal journal but was published in an earlier form since 1972. Large annual meetings are held in the spring and a major emphasis has been on educational programs. Because of the substantial membership size, many local, regional, or state chapters of APIC also exist and put on their own educational and scientific programs.

In addition to the collaborative work with SHEA, SIS, the CDC, and other organizations, APIC also develops guidelines in a variety of areas. Some examples are:

1. APIC guideline for infection prevention and control in flexible endoscopy [21]
2. A very useful "Resource List for Standards and Guidelines 1993" [22]. This pamphlet enumerates the dozens of organizations and agencies that have some recommendations about infection control issues.

OTHER FEDERAL AND NATIONAL AGENCIES

The Occupational Safety and Health Administration

This agency was originally developed to protect workers in their workplace. The focus was on manufacturing and other occupations where injury, disease, and even death were seen as problems. Hospitals and health professionals had little contact with OSHA until the HIV/AIDS epidemic occurred in the 1980s. Because of the acquisition of HIV by healthcare workers through needlestick injuries, and the aggressive requests of several healthcare worker unions for intervention by OSHA, the Blood Borne Pathogen Standards were developed and enforced [23]. The old relationships between infection control professionals and the CDC had been one of mutual respect and collaboration. The implementation of fines that could come from a sudden inspection by an OSHA inspector called in by an anonymous request was a major change in the way hospital epidemiologists and infection control professionals were used to doing business. The next major standard still in the process of development by OSHA concerns Occupational Exposure to Tuberculosis [24,25] (see Chapter 33). The proposal that high-efficiency particulate air (HEPA) filter masks, fit-tested to the face of healthcare workers screened for pulmonary or heart disease, and then used whenever in a room with someone suspected of having tuberculosis, caused a firestorm of protest in the infection control community because of a lack of a credible scientific basis for this costly and time-consuming requirement.

The HEPA filter mask requirement has been modified. The apparent failure to use the best available scientific and epidemiologic evidence in making the decision, and the huge difference between being put in an adversarial rather than a collaborative role, has made the infection control community very skeptical of the value of OSHA in hospital infection control.

Table 11-2 highlights the difference in approaches between the CDC and OSHA. It will be interesting to see how these differences are handled for other issues in future years.

The American Hospital Association

For well over 30 years, the American Hospital Association (AHA) sponsored the Committee on Infection Within Hospitals. Many distinguished experts from across the country served on this committee. The guidelines and publications of the committee serve as a compendium of historic milestones in the development of infection control programs in American hospitals [26]. The AHA maintained a professional staff to support the committee. There was excellent communication with the Hospital Infections Program at the CDC and other groups.

In the 1960s, the book developed by the AHA was widely disseminated and used as a supplement to JCAHO standards and CDC guidelines [27]. The opinions and recommendations of the committee helped define a national standard of practice.

With the establishment of the formal CDC HICPAC in the 1990s and the continued work by the CDC in this area, the AHA discontinued its professional staff unit in the area of hospital infection "because of all the changes in healthcare." The demise of the committee occurred in December, 1995.

The Association of Operating Room Nurses, Inc.

The Association of Operating Room Nurses (AORN), working cooperatively with professional groups of surgeons such as the American College of Surgeons and the Surgical Infection Society, has for many years provided position statements and recommendations concerning the best nursing practice in operating rooms, operating suites, and associated areas.

For standards of attire, flow of personnel, use of masks, and many other practical matters of practice in and around operating rooms, the AORN recommendations have become the accepted national standard of practice. Their publications are updated every 1 to 2 years and use the format of "recommended practices," "interpretive statement," and "rationale." Studies to support these practices are cited in the bibliography [28].

OTHER IMPORTANT NATIONAL ORGANIZATIONS

Many other important national groups, such as the 500+ members of the Surgical Infection Society, the Committee on Operating Room Environment (CORE) of the American College of Surgeons, the Infectious Diseases Society of America, and other professional and technical organizations, have provided guidelines, recommendations, and consensus reports relating to infection control in all types of healthcare settings. A comprehensive publication reviewing infection control guidelines from all available sources demonstrates the range of groups involved [29].

INTERNATIONAL ORGANIZATIONS

The Hospital Infections Society (HIS) of Great Britain and the Infection Control Nurses Association of Great Britain are examples of national groups parallel to SHEA and APIC in the United States. Many other countries around the world have developed or are in the process of developing similar professional societies to address infection control in hospitals and other healthcare institutions. In many ways the training programs and expertise of the CDC developed several of the leaders (as it did for APIC and SHEA) and provided the impetus for development of programs around the world. HIS has it's own journal: Hospital Infections. Over the past ten years these national professional groups have developed important international collaborative arrangements.

SUMMARY

Governmental agencies and professional organizations have had a long and mostly useful history in helping physicians and nurses better protect their patients from nosocomial infections. It is not possible in the 1990s to consider infection control and related continuous quality improvement programs without the help and the guidelines provided by both types of groups.

As healthcare grows and changes occur both as an industry and as a profession, it will be very important for all to continue to use good epidemiology—good science—in preventing unwanted outcomes in patients such as nosocomial infections. As Williams said in 1960, it is imperative always to open our eyes wide enough to observe what is really happening around us.

Potential threats to continued high-quality science in this area include rigid laws, rules, and regulations not based on good science and the replacement of sound, epidemiologically based and proven infection control strategies with more generic outcome indicator-driven comparisons and tracking systems purporting to enhance quality. Strong independent professional societies will become even more important in the future. Many new resources have been developed or are being developed in nosocomial infection control around the world. New knowledge will also come from the world literature.

REFERENCES

1. Williams REO, Blowers R, Garrod LP, et al. *Hospital infection causes and prevention.* 2nd ed. London: Lloyd-Luke, 1966.
2. Institute of Medicine, Committee to Advise the Public Health Service on Clinical Practice Guidelines. Field MJ, Lohr KN, eds. *Clinical practice guidelines: directions for a new program.* Washington, DC: National Academy Press, 1990.
3. Quality Indicator Study Group, Scheckler WE (chair), et al. An approach to the evaluation of quality indicators of the outcome of care in hospitalized patients, with a focus on nosocomial infection indicators. *Infect Control Hosp Epidemiol* 1995;16:308–316.
4. Jencks S, Wilensky G. The healthcare quality improvement initiative: a new approach to quality assurance in Medicare. *JAMA* 1992;268: 900–903.
5. Berwick DM. The clinical process and the quality process. *Quality in Management in Health Care* 1992;1:1–8.
6. Scheckler WE. Continuous quality improvement in a hospital system: implications for hospital epidemiology. *Infect Control Hosp Epidemiol* 1992;13:288–292.
7. Kritchevsky S, Simmons B. Continuous quality improvement. Concepts and applications for physician care. *JAMA* 1991;266:1817–1823.
8. Nosocomial Infections International Conference. *Proceedings of the international conference on nosocomial infections: Centers for Disease Control and Prevention, August 3–6, 1970.* Baltimore: Waverly Press, 1971.
9. Nosocomial Infections International Conference. Symposium on nosocomial infections (parts 1, 2, and 3). *Am J Med* 1981;70:379–473; 631–744;899–986.
10. Nosocomial Infections International Conference. Proceedings of the third decennial international conference on nosocomial infections. *Am J Med* 1991;91:1S–329S.
11. Haley R, Culver D, White J, et al. The efficacy of infection surveillance and control programs in preventing nosocomial infections in U.S. hospitals. *Am J Epidemiol* 1985;121:182–205.
12. Simone P. Essential components of a tuberculosis prevention and control program. *MMWR Morb Mortal Wkly Rep* 1995;44(September): 1–16.
13. Garner J. The CDC hospital infection control practices advisory committee. *Am J Infect Control* 1993;21:160–162.
14. Tablan O, Anderson L, Arden N, et al. Special report from the HICPAC: guideline for prevention of nosocomial pneumonia. *Infect Control Hosp Epidemiol* 1994;15:587–627.
15. Joint Commission on Accreditation of Healthcare Organizations. *1995 Comprehensive accreditation manual for hospitals. Surveillance, prevention, and control of infection, section 2.* Oakbrook Terrace, IL: Joint Commission on Accreditation of Healthcare Organizations, 1994: 437–450.
16. Gerding D, Johnson S, Peterson L, et al. Society for Healthcare Epidemiology of America position paper on *Clostridium difficile*-associated diarrhea and colitis. *Infect Control Hosp Epidemiol* 1995;16: 459–477.
17. SHEA, APIC, CDC, SIS. Consensus paper on the surveillance of surgical wound infections. *Infect Control Hosp Epidemiol* 1995;16: 599–608.
18. Kritchevsky S, Simmons B, Braun B. The project to monitor indicators: a collaborative effort between the Joint Commission on Accreditation of Healthcare Organizations and the Society for Healthcare Epidemiology of America. *Infect Control Hosp Epidemiol* 1995;16:33–35.
19. Russell B. The Association for Professionals in Infection Control and Epidemiology, Inc. *Infect Control Hosp Epidemiol* 1995;16:522–525.
20. Pirwitz S. The Certification Board of Infection Control, Inc. *Infect Control Hosp Epidemiol* 1995;16:518–521.
21. Martin M, Reichelderfer M. APIC guidelines for infection prevention and control in flexible endoscopy. *Am J Infect Control* 1994;22:19–38.
22. APIC Guidelines Committee. *Resource list for standards and guidelines 1993.* Washington D.C.: Association for Professionals in Infection Control, Inc., 1993.
23. Occupational Safety and Health Administration. Occupational exposure to blood borne pathogens: final rule. *Federal Register* 1991;56 (235):Dec 6:64004–64182.
24. Decker M. OSHA enforcement policy for occupational exposure to tuberculosis. *Infect Control Hosp Epidemiol* 1993;14:689–693.
25. Gerberding J. Occupational infectious diseases of infectious occupational diseases? Bridging the views on tuberculosis control. *Infect Control Hosp Epidemiol* 1993;14:686–688.
26. Weinstein R, Pugliese G. The American Hospital Association. *Infect Control Hosp Epidemiol* 1994;15:269–273.
27. American Hospital Association. *Infection control in the hospital.* Chicago: American Hospital Association, 1968.
28. Association of Operating Room Nurses, Inc. *1996 Standards and recommended practices.* Denver, CO: AORN, 1996.
29. Abrutyn E, Goldman D, Scheckler W, eds. *Saunders infection control reference service.* Philadelphia: WB Saunders, 1997.

Hospital Infections, Fourth Edition,
edited by John V. Bennett and Philip S. Brachman.
Lippincott–Raven Publishers, Philadelphia © 1998

CHAPTER 12

The Relationship Between the Hospital and the Community

Michael D. Decker and William Schaffner

The hospital has always been, in its essence, an act of community. Hospitals, the structural embodiment of hospitality, originally were established to provide shelter to medieval pilgrims. The hospital's subsequent status as a charitable institution for the housing of the needy, destitute, and infirm in Renaissance times has evolved into its modern role as the institution supported by the community to provide care to the seriously ill. The hospital continues to be a linchpin of the local community—an important social symbol, a focus of community pride, and a major employer, as well as a beneficiary of charitable effort. The hospital touches each one of us: virtually all people are born and most will die in a hospital.

This rich, 600-year relationship between the hospital and the community has become vastly more complex in the past few decades as a result of changes in the scientific, commercial, and governmental determinants of healthcare. Moreover, the ongoing changes in the structure and financing of the healthcare system have produced a turbulence that has buffeted hospitals and healthcare workers alike.

Hospitals are the most visible venue in which new research results are applied to patient care, a subject that has always attracted the attention of the news media. In recent years, however, reporters and regulators have devoted at least as much attention to other characteristics of hospitals. Hospitals are big businesses in an industry undergoing massive restructuring. Hospitals are major employers whose employees are at risk of serious occupational infection or other illness. Hospitals are viewed as important sources of offensive, hazardous, or even infectious waste. Hospitals are considered sentinels for (and occasionally sources of) contagious diseases in the community.

Not only is the community paying more attention to hospitals; hospitals must pay more attention to the community. The community expects the hospital to be more responsive and more accessible. Moreover, the community now expects the hospital to evaluate its own performance in the care of the patients entrusted to it and to provide those data for inspection. The hospital also is an expression of its community in less salubrious ways; for example, the hospital increasingly finds itself an unwilling stage for the acts of crime or violence that plague the community.

Only some of these relationships are germane to specialists in infection control; any might fall within the more extended purview of a Hospital Epidemiology Department (see Chapter 2). For all these relationships, an optimal response by the hospital will (or ought to) call on the talents of hospital epidemiologists and infection control practitioners. Such people are the reservoir of expertise in the hospital regarding the collection and evaluation of surveillance data, whether intended for the analysis of nosocomial infections, quality improvement, resource utilization, or adverse events involving patients, employees, or visitors.

SPREAD OF INFECTIONS BETWEEN THE HOSPITAL AND THE COMMUNITY

The hospital is an organic part of the community and, although the characteristic pattern of infections in each differs, infectious events in either may influence the occurrence of infections in the other. This integrated relationship was not appreciated when nosocomial infections first received serious attention.

M. D. Decker: Department of Preventive Medicine.
W. Schaffner: Department of Preventive Medicine, Department of Medicine (Infectious Diseases) Vanderbilt University School of Medicine, Nashville, Tennessee 37232.

Changing Patterns

Before World War II and for a short period thereafter, hospital-acquired infections were recognized as an occasional problem, but usually they were believed to be caused by microorganisms that originated in the community. During the 1950s, hospitals around the world were struck by the well known nosocomial pandemic of *Staphylococcus aureus* infections (see Chapter 41). Thus, attention shifted to the hospital as a special environment, separate from the community. No matter what was going around in the community, staphylococcal infections were prevalent in the hospital. These dire circumstances stimulated intensive laboratory, clinical, and epidemiologic investigation and resulted in the creation of the discipline of hospital epidemiology.

The nature of nosocomial infections, however, did not remain constant. As the staphylococcal problem receded during the 1960s and other nosocomial infections were recognized, it became clear that infections that occurred in the hospital had consequences for the surrounding populace. Some infections that were acquired in the hospital appeared only after the patient was discharged and now were capable of spreading from former patients to community contacts. As these circumstances became known, hospitals began to fear the adverse publicity and lawsuits that could result from nosocomial infections, and patients expressed concern about their admission to institutions that no longer were perceived as completely benign (see Chapter 18).

It now is evident that the proverbial street runs both ways: the hospital and the community are overlapping environments, either of which can be the source of problematic infections that are spread and perhaps even amplified in the other. An early example occurred at the University of Colorado Medical Center, where two small outbreaks of pertussis that originated among children in the community spread to house officers and nurses, then spread from them to children in the outpatient department and to other adults [1]. Thus, the disease originating in the community was transmitted in the hospital and spread back out into the community.

Similarly, before rubella immunization of hospital personnel became commonplace, there were several reports of physicians and nurses transmitting this viral infection to patients, some of whom were pregnant. Major outbreaks of measles in several large cities involved spread within hospitals, to both staff and susceptible patients. Although measles currently is at an all-time low, experience suggests that hospitals may be epicenters of any new outbreaks. Immunization of susceptible staff remains the mainstay of prevention [2] (see Chapter 3).

Community outbreaks of chickenpox have been an almost annual event; it will be interesting to see how soon that pattern is altered by childhood varicella immunization. Regardless, introductions of varicella into the hospital likely will continue to occur for some time; the ease with which chickenpox can spread on pediatric wards makes it an especially vexing problem. Children who are incubating the infection may be admitted for elective surgery, for example, and move freely about the ward, exposing numerous patients and staff. Nosocomial chickenpox presents a serious threat to immunocompromised children, who constitute a growing proportion of the hospitalized pediatric population. Varicella vaccine should be considered strongly for inclusion in healthcare worker immunization programs [3] (see Chapter 3).

The changing epidemiology of methicillin-resistant *Staphylococcus aureus* (MRSA) provides another example of the interaction between the hospital and community environments. Originally seen only as a nosocomial pathogen, in many hospitals MRSA now more commonly is community acquired [4]. A parallel, and probably related, phenomenon has been the rapid increase in the prevalence of resistance to ciprofloxacin among *S. aureus*, and particularly among MRSA, which is over 100 times more likely than methicillin-sensitive *S. aureus* to be ciprofloxacin resistant [5]. A trend of increasing resistance promptly followed licensure of ciprofloxacin in 1989, such that 80% to 90% of MRSA isolates now are resistant to ciprofloxacin [5]. Ciprofloxacin is widely used in ambulatory medicine, and it seems plausible that the increase in community-acquired MRSA is a direct result of this antibiotic pressure, which by selecting for ciprofloxacin resistance, most often also selects for methicillin resistance (see Chapters 14, 15, 41).

Perhaps the most striking recent example of interaction between the hospital and community environments involves tuberculosis. The long-term decline in tuberculosis case rates had the paradoxic effect of increasing the occupational risk of tuberculosis for hospital staff (see Chapter 3): many hospitals dropped their employee tuberculin skin testing and other tuberculosis control programs; hospital workers were likely to be tuberculin negative, and thus susceptible to acquiring primary infection when exposed to tubercle bacilli; and the old tuberculosis hospitals closed, with the result that people with tuberculosis who needed hospitalization would be admitted to general acute care hospitals. Consequently, when the acquired immunodeficiency syndrome (AIDS) epidemic brought into the hospital a new cohort of patients with a remarkable prevalence of contagious tuberculosis, large outbreaks of nosocomial tuberculosis ensued among exposed healthcare workers and patients, the repercussions of which are still being felt (see Chapters 33, 43).

Recent Trends

Recent trends have exacerbated the potential for transport of infection between the hospital and the community. In particular, the continuing drive to shorten inpatient hospitalizations has meant that nosocomial infections of all types increasingly become clinically manifest only after discharge. Such infections can be problematic for the community physician, who may not immediately recognize their derivation and that their causative bacteria are likely to be resistant to usual first-line antibiotics. In addition, resistant hospital-acquired organisms have been demonstrated to spread from patients to their community contacts. For example, infants colonized by enteric organisms containing antibiotic-resistant plasmids were followed after their discharge from an intensive care nursery. After 12 months, nearly half of the infants continued to carry these multiresistant organisms, and one third of their family members also had acquired the same plasmid-positive strains in their fecal flora. No family members of a control group of infants were colonized with such bacilli [6].

Often, discharge from the hospital, particularly for the debilitated patients most likely colonized with nosocomial pathogens, is to a nursing home. It has become evident that nursing homes all too frequently have their own endemic problems of infection with resistant organisms (see Chapter 29). Inevitably, some such patients are readmitted to an acute care hospital, carrying with them their resistant flora. Although resistant gram-negative bacilli participate in this cycle, it more often has involved MRSA [7] and, more recently, vancomycin-resistant enterococci (see Chapter 15). In some communities, this cycle has led to an adversarial situation, with both hospital and nursing home resisting accepting the patients of the other. This is a battle often won by the nursing home, to the detriment of the economic health of the hospital. The diplomatic skill of the infection control staff can be essential to the hospital in managing these situations. Those working in integrated health systems may be able to minimize these internecine conflicts through the development of coordinated infection control programs.

Increasingly, patients who are stable but require continued intravenous therapy are discharged to home, where catheter and other care is provided by the patient, the family, and perhaps visiting nurses from a home health agency. Even if these caregivers have been thoroughly trained in the infection control principles and practices necessary to perform these tasks safely—a questionable proposition—it is apparent that this new clinical environment has new infection control lessons to teach. For example, we have learned that needleless infusion devices, introduced to reduce the risk of injury to healthcare workers, can lead to bloodstream infections among patients [8]. Although this phenomenon was first noted among home care patients, it has obvious implications for infection control practices within the hospital.

Not only are hospitalized patients discharged ever earlier, to complete their care elsewhere; many patients who formerly would have undergone surgical and other procedures in the acute care hospital instead receive their care in one or another venue along a continuum of cost and sophistication. Serious or complex procedures are performed in the inpatient hospital; more routine, yet still major, procedures are performed in the hospital's ambulatory surgical suite; many procedures formerly reserved for the hospital now occur in free-standing surgical centers; and, reversing a long historical trend, physicians increasingly are performing minor (and not so minor) surgical procedures in their offices.

These national trends toward early discharge of inpatients and performing more elaborate surgical procedures on an outpatient basis further increase the likelihood that substantial numbers of nosocomial infections will become manifest in the community rather than in the hospital. This carries two important consequences. First, the infection control team is much less likely to become aware of the infection, and thus less likely to detect adverse trends and implement corrective actions promptly. Second, those witnessing the clinical manifestations of the infections (e.g., family rather than nursing staff) are less likely to appreciate their implications immediately or to institute appropriate management.

Most procedures for the surveillance and control of nosocomial infections were developed and tested for hospitalized patients, and may not be directly applicable to patients outside the hospital (see Chapter 4). Because the emphases on prompt discharge and outpatient care likely will not abate, infection control staff have been exploring strategies to allow better detection of nosocomial infections in patients who have been discharged or who received their care in another facet of their institution's integrated healthcare system (e.g., satellite clinics, surgical centers, affiliated medical practices) [9]. One stratagem we have used is to send home a simple postage-paid form with every patient undergoing an outpatient procedure, to be returned to the epidemiology department in the event of fever, wound redness or discharge, or symptoms of urinary tract infection or pneumonia. The form also urges the patient to contact his or her physician promptly. Such a patient-based surveillance system complements physician-based reporting of postdischarge nosocomial infections; we have found that neither alone is adequate. Although this two-pronged surveillance system represents an improvement, we are confident that it does not approach the sensitivity or specificity of our inpatient surveillance. Clearly, there is an urgent need for innovative research in surveillance methods for the detection of nosocomial infections in the ambulatory setting.

The Hospital Infections Program of the Centers for Disease Control and Prevention (CDC), and the more recent Hospital Infection Control Practices Advisory Committee, have made enormous contributions to the practice of infection control. We hope that these organizations will expand the scope of their activities in response to the changing patterns of healthcare delivery, and help to develop the studies and guidelines necessary to shape effective infection control practices in these new arenas.

RELATIONSHIP OF THE HOSPITAL WITH EXTERNAL AUTHORITIES

As mentioned previously, it no longer is sufficient for the hospital epidemiology staff to limit their responsibility regarding relations with outside authorities to the traditional contacts with public health agencies. New initiatives in the areas of occupational health, evaluation of the quality and utilization of medical care, and the management of wastes and other environmental impacts compel the involvement of the epidemiology team (many of these issues are also reviewed in Chapter 11). Some of these initiatives relate directly to the classic functions of the infection control unit; others are best managed with strong input from those having epidemiologic expertise. Indeed, these nontraditional regulators or evaluators have occupied an extraordinary measure of the energies of the infection control team in the 1990s, a trend likely to continue. Table 12-1 delineates some of the more important external entities and the focus of their activities.

The Public Health Authorities

The best-developed and most collaborative of these external relationships remain those between the hospital and the public health authorities. The health authorities look to the hospital for the reporting of specified sporadic or epidemic diseases. In turn, the hospital looks to health authorities for assistance in three infection control areas:

TABLE 12-1. *A sample of external accrediting, regulating, licensing, standards-setting, or other evaluating entities that affect hospitals*

Entity	Activity
Federal agencies	
Bureau of Alcohol, Tobacco and Firearms	License for ethanol in pharmacy
Drug Enforcement Administration	Regulate dispensing of controlled drugs
Environmental Protection Agency	Regulate emissions, contaminants, and waste disposal
Food and Drug Administration	Audit of the Institutional Review Board; registration of the Blood Bank
Federal Aviation Administration	License heliport
Federal Communications Commission	License radio communications systems
Health Care Financing Administration	Regulate quality and utilization for Medicare/Medicaid
Occupational Safety and Health Administration	Regulate workers' exposure to bloodborne hazards, tuberculosis, chemicals, and radiation
Public Health Service	Oversee Clinical Laboratory Improvement Act (CLIA) registration and inspection
State agencies	
Various entities, usually included within the state health department	Hospital license; broad regulation of hospital activities; certificates of need for capital expenditures; air resources management (incinerators); solid-waste management; water resources management (liquid effluents and nearby waterways); trauma center designation and coordination; licensure of laboratory and other components; radiologic materials licenses and inspection; elevator inspection and licensure; boiler inspection and licensure
Agriculture department	Pest control inspections
Board of pharmacy	License pharmacy
Corporation commissioner	Annual reports
Fire marshall	Fire code compliance
Insurance commissioner	Self-insurance for workers' compensation
Municipal agencies	
Fire department	Inspect fire pump, local hydrants, codes compliance
Health department	Inspect boilers, incinerators, cafeteria, and the like
Solid waste management department	Regulate solid-waste disposal
Transportation authority	Approve alterations of traffic flow; siting of bus stops
Water and sewer department	Inspect meters and backflow preventers; regulate conduct
Private agencies	
American Association of Blood Banks	Blood bank standards and accreditation
College of American Pathologists	Laboratory standards and accreditation
Joint Commission on Accreditation of Healthcare Organizations	Overall accreditation
National accrediting agencies for in-house training programs	Accredit medical student, house staff, nursing, and technologist training programs
Employer groups, health maintenance organizations, other entities that compile comparative databases	Compile and compare data regarding quality of care and utilization of resources

consultation on the establishment of a useful program, training of personnel to carry out the program, and assistance in the investigation of epidemics.

It has long been recognized that a system of prompt and accurate notification of the occurrence of certain communicable diseases was a requisite to their control. In 1883, the state of Michigan adopted legislation establishing a system of communicable disease reporting, and all other states have since followed suit. These laws have been determined by the courts on numerous occasions not to violate the special nature of the doctor–patient relationship.

These reporting systems are pluralist: Typically, physicians, hospitals, and laboratory directors (even those within hospitals) each have an independent obligation to notify the public health authorities of any patients known or reasonably suspected to have certain illnesses (see Chapter 5). It is important for many reasons that hospitals develop a system of disease notification. First, not only do these reporting requirements have the force of law, but compliance with them is usually reviewed by licensing authorities and remains a component of the streamlined infection control standards of the Joint Commission on Accreditation of Healthcare Organizations (JCAHO). Second, by reporting promptly, hospitals can be of assistance to the public health authorities in the control of communicable disease in their own communities. Third, by educating staff physicians and employees of this responsibility, the hospital becomes an advocate of good preventive medical practice. Fourth, the hospital's unique role enables it to be a major contributor to state and national morbidity data collection mechanisms, which strongly influence funding priorities for research and control activities. Finally, as medicine's capacity to detect, treat, and prevent disease increases, there will be a consequent increasing need for precise information on disease occurrence. The sequential addition to disease reporting systems of Legionnaires' disease, toxic shock syndrome, AIDS, Lyme disease, and hantavirus pulmonary syndrome illustrate these points clearly. Table 12-2 provides a representative list of reportable conditions.

When we reviewed the procedures for disease reporting in our institutions, we found that the traditional mechanisms no longer were sufficiently comprehensive (see Chapter 4). Reporting based on laboratory isolates or serologic results is vital, yet a system solely based on laboratory reports misses all those diseases for which diagnosis does not depend on the laboratory (see Chapter 5). Reports from the emergency room are essential for those reportable diseases that often do not require admission (animal bites and foodborne illnesses, for example). Reports generated from routine infection control surveillance are valuable, but in few institutions would the infection control team be assured of reviewing every pertinent chart. Medical records-based surveillance represents the final opportunity to detect the reportable illness; however, not only is it tardy but it often misses a reportable

TABLE 12-2. *Reportable diseases in Tennessee*

Acquired immunodeficiency syndrome (AIDS)[a]
Anthrax[b]
Botulism (all types)[b]
Brucellosis
Campylobacteriosis (outbreaks only)
Chancroid
Chickenpox (number of cases only)
Chlamydia trachomatis infection
Cholera[b]
Cryptosporidiosis
Diphtheria[b]
Disease outbreaks
Foodborne
Waterborne
Related to industrial substances
All other outbreaks
Drug-resistant *Streptococcus pneumoniae* (invasive only)
Ehrlichiosis
Encephalitis, arboviral[b]
California
Eastern equine
St. Louis
Western equine
Escherichia coli, enteropathogenic
Giardiasis (acute)
Gonorrhea
Group A streptococcal disease (invasive infections)[b]
Hemophilus influenzae disease[b]
Hantavirus disease[b]
Hemolytic–uremic syndrome
Hepatitis, viral (acute, types A, B, C)
Human immunodeficiency virus (HIV)[a]
Influenza (number of cases)
Lead poisoning (blood lead levels $\geq$10 μg/dl for children 0–72 months of age)
Legionellosis
Leprosy (Hansen's disease)
Listeriosis (foodborne)[b]
Lyme disease
Malaria
Measles[b]
Meningococcal disease[b]
Mumps[b]
Pertussis (whooping cough)[b]
Plague[b]
Poliomyelitis[b]
Psittacosis
Rabies
Human[b]
Animal
Rocky Mountain spotted fever
Rubella and congenital rubella syndrome[b]
Salmonellosis
Typhoid fever[b]
Other forms
Shigellosis
Syphilis
Tetanus
Toxic shock syndrome
Staphylococcal
Streptococcal
Trichinosis
Tuberculosis (all forms)
Yellow fever

[a]Confidential report form.
[b]Immediate telephonic reporting required.

diagnosis that is secondary to the principal problem. We have established a surveillance and reporting system that incorporates each of these elements, including reviews of autopsy results. Information from all these units is directed to the epidemiology department, which has sole responsibility for transmitting reports to the public health authorities. This minimizes duplicate reporting, permits the earliest possible reports, generates a comprehensive centralized log of reports for review by relevant agencies, and ensures that those charged with infection control are cognizant of the presence in the hospital of patients with these reportable (and, usually, communicable) diseases.

In addition to the foregoing, we participate in several special surveillance programs, including an influenza surveillance system organized by the state health department, and the CDC's National Nosocomial Infection Surveillance system (see Chapter 30). Through such programs, we enhance our own skills and further our community's ability to coordinate the prevention of illness.

So much for the hospital's assistance to the public health authorities; what of the authorities' assistance to hospitals? The first level of support is the closest—the local, regional, or state public health departments. Although the interest and ability of these entities to provide meaningful help to hospital infection control programs has increased considerably in recent years, it still varies widely from jurisdiction to jurisdiction. Health departments and hospitals largely have gone their separate ways in our society, the first concerned with public health and the second with diagnostics and therapeutics. Therefore, the infection control affairs of the hospital often are not identified as a major concern of the health department. Even when such an interest is acknowledged, implementation may be difficult for several reasons. Health departments have traditional responsibilities of impressive diversity and must work within the constraints of tight budgets. Furthermore, the doctors and nurses in the health department may not be comfortable in the highly technologic milieu of the contemporary hospital. Small wonder, then, that local health authorities have been hesitant to open the Pandora's box of nosocomial infection. Hospitals, in turn, value their independence and frequently are wary of close associations with government agencies.

Nonetheless, some state health departments have invested considerable effort in establishing programs for the control of nosocomial infections. Their program content varies, but most have sponsored training courses that emphasize the basic epidemiologic and laboratory aspects of infection control. Some also employ infection control practitioners who are able to provide advice to individual hospitals about their infection control problems.

One example has demonstrated that imaginative local health department officials can play an important role in the monitoring of nosocomial infections and the coordination of efforts to prevent them. Epidemiologists at the New Jersey Department of Health developed a statewide hospital laboratory isolate-based surveillance system for antimicrobial-resistant bacteria [10]. This surveillance system permits estimation of institutional rates of infection, determination of institutional risk factors, and monitoring of changing patterns of antimicrobial resistance. This example can serve as a model for the synergistic collaboration that can result when health departments and hospitals join resources for a common purpose.

Appropriate laboratory support is essential to the investigation of all but the simplest hospital outbreaks (see Chapter 9). Most health department laboratories are reference laboratories, although they may process clinical specimens in selected specialized areas. The techniques required to perform primary isolation of hospital pathogens from diverse clinical specimens, environmental sampling, and antimicrobial susceptibility testing usually are not in the public health laboratory's repertoire. On the other hand, state laboratories usually can assist in identifying unusual organisms and often can provide specialized assays useful in investigating suspected outbreaks. Furthermore, the pathway to the reference laboratories of the CDC generally lies through the state laboratory.

The CDC, through its Hospital Infections Branch, is an important national resource for infection control programs. In addition to its reference laboratories, it provides assistance to local hospitals and health departments in developing effective programs, generates guidelines that are widely followed, offers training courses for personnel (in collaboration with other agencies), provides sophisticated surveillance of nosocomial infections, and assists in the investigation and control of nosocomial outbreaks.

The Food and Drug Administration has regulatory authority over the pharmaceutical and medical device industries and the responsibility for recalling products suspected of being contaminated, as well as intervening in the marketing of those products associated with undue adverse reactions. The surveillance systems of hospital epidemiology programs may detect either type of event.

The Regulators of Employee Health: Occupational Health and Safety Administration and Others

Every worker in infection control has become aware of the Occupational Safety and Health Administration (OSHA) since it launched its major effort to ensure the safety of employees in the healthcare industry, with particular focus on infectious and toxic hazards (see Chapter 11). Acting under the authority of the General Duty clause of the OSHA Act (29 USC 651(5)(a)(1)), the OSHA Bloodborne Hazard Standard (Fed Reg. 56: 64003-64174. December 6, 1991) [11], the Respiratory Protection Standard (29 CFR 1910.134), the Enforcement Procedures for Occupational Exposure to Tuberculosis (OSHA Instruction CPL 2.106, February 9, 1996)

[12], and other pertinent regulations, OSHA regularly conducts rigorous inspections of hospitals and other healthcare institutions. Failure to meet the applicable standards may result in adverse publicity and substantial fines [13].

An OSHA inspection consists of at least the following components: an evaluation of the infection control plan, the bloodborne hazard and tuberculosis control plans, the employee health program, the employee training program, and the monitoring and management of toxic, radioactive, infectious, sharp, and other wastes; a walkaround inspection of the facility; inspection of employee health charts, immunization records, and injury logs; verification of the availability of personal protective equipment; and private interviews of randomly selected employees to establish that they know the policies, know how to follow them, are able to follow them, and agree that they are followed. Hospitals commonly prepare for periodic JCAHO accreditation visits by conducting their own mock surveys; we recommend similar preparation for an OSHA inspection.

The Evaluators of Quality and Utilization: JCAHO, Health Care Financing Administration, and Others

It may seem that the issues of quality assurance and utilization review are of little pertinence in a textbook on infection control. However, it is clear that the major changes occurring in these areas have profound implications for infection control practitioners and hospital epidemiologists. First, infection control programs increasingly are seen by administrators as components of the overall quality effort. Second, JCAHO and other surveyors of hospitals have been moving toward an essentially epidemiologic approach to the evaluation of healthcare. Spurred by the revolution in industrial quality control initiated in postwar Japan by W. Edwards Deming and others, which now has been adopted widely in U.S. industry, JCAHO and others have embraced the concepts of statistical process control and continuous quality improvement [14]. These new approaches are strongly dependent on those analytic thought processes and skills that have served infection control and hospital epidemiology so successfully. Therefore, it is likely that many engaged in these traditional activities will seek or be sought to broaden their role in the hospital through participation in these new activities as well (see Chapter 2).

The Regulators of Waste: Environmental Protection Agency and Others

All hospitals are subject to both municipal and state regulation of solid-waste disposal; most are subject to special regulations for medical or infectious waste; and the possibility remains that Congress will mandate a national standard for the management of medical waste comparable to the now expired Medical Waste Tracking Act of 1988 (40 CFR 22, 259). Hospital infection control programs have two challenges in this regard: to assist in their institution's compliance with local waste disposal regulations and to involve themselves in their community's planning on these issues.

If sharps and body fluids are appropriately contained and disinfected, the hospital's waste stream presents virtually no infectious hazard to the community. Nevertheless, the public and its elected representatives maintain substantial anxiety about these matters. In addition, the elaborate procedures mandated for the disposal of designated infectious waste are expensive. Thus, although the participation of the infection control unit in these matters may not prevent much infection, it surely may prevent much waste [15].

BROADER INFLUENCE OF THE HOSPITAL EPIDEMIOLOGIST

As a person in the medical community with a heightened interest in preventive medicine, the hospital epidemiologist occasionally is in a position to influence decisions in areas beyond those already described (see Chapter 2). The abolition of tobacco use within the hospital is one example, which has been accomplished at our own and many other institutions. Not only does this present a consistent health message, but it may promote a decrease in tobacco use throughout the community.

Similarly, a number of hospitals that provide pediatric or obstetric services have established programs to promote the use of child passenger safety seats among their clients; indeed, in many instances, the hospitals provide the seats. It is well known that motor vehicle crashes are the principal cause of death for children, and that safety seats are highly successful in preventing such deaths; these programs are in the finest traditions of preventive medicine [16].

Another area in which the epidemiologist can be of assistance is in the immediate management of community contacts of patients with certain infections. A 26-year-old married father of two children, for example, is admitted with meningococcal meningitis. Who is responsible—the attending internist, the pediatrician, or the local health officer—for providing antibiotic prophylaxis to his wife and children? There is no absolute rule, but the hospital epidemiologist can help to coordinate the response and ensure that this essential preventive medical service is not overlooked.

It is paradoxic that hospitals, society's most visible healthcare institutions, have lagged in providing preventive medical services for their employees. Although OSHA regulations compel minimum standards in certain aspects of employee health, hospital epidemiologists have the opportunity to persuade hospitals to provide screening programs for hypertension and other coronary risk factors and cervical and breast cancer, as well as to provide comprehensive immunization programs and even family planning services (see Chapter 3). Our own institution (reflecting, perhaps, enlightened self-interest as the health insurer for its employees) now offers its employees programs for fitness, stress management, and other wellness endeavors.

Many hospital epidemiology programs now apply their expertise to the analysis of patterns of noninfectious adverse events among patients; many contribute to the evaluation of various adverse events among employees. Few if any, however, have yet involved themselves in analyses of one of the most rapidly increasing categories of adverse events among employees: workplace violence and other crime [17]. Although our community's crime rate is far lower than that seen in the country's major urban centers, we, like many others, increasingly have witnessed the intrusion of violence and other crime into environments, such as the hospital, that once were relatively spared. In the past few years, for example, we have experienced the murder of a visitor, an employee, and a student by, respectively, an irate family member, a former boyfriend, and an armed robber; the attempted murder of a department head by a disgruntled former resident; and several on-campus rapes of employees or students by off-campus prowlers. In 1995, our security personnel recorded 3 attempted homicides or suicides, 6 rapes or armed robberies, 29 assaults, and 355 thefts; they arrested 156 suspects in or around our medical center. The officers staffing the metal detector at the Emergency Department door have acquired a substantial collection of guns and knives.

It may seem that this particular intrusion of the community into the hospital, although distressing, is not amenable to intervention by the hospital epidemiologist. Of course, the same was thought regarding patient falls, visitor smoking, newborn child passenger safety, and other nontraditional issues that have seen successful risk reduction efforts guided by epidemiologic analyses.

We believe that there remain many opportunities for hospital epidemiologists to apply their skills in innovative ways within their own institutions and their communities so that hospitals, long admired for their sophisticated care of sick patients, can continue to make more comprehensive contributions to medicine's highest goal, the prevention of disease.

REFERENCES

1. Kurt TL, Yeager AS, Guenette S, Dunlop S. Spread of pertussis by hospital staff. *JAMA* 1972;221:264.
2. Decker MD, Schaffner W. Immunization of hospital personnel and other healthcare workers. *Infect Dis Clin North Am* 1990;4:211.
3. Weber DJ, Rutala WA, Hamilton H. Prevention and control of varicella-zoster infections in healthcare facilities. *Infect Control Hosp Epidemiol* 1996;17:694.
4. Layton MC, Hierholzer WJ Jr, Patterson JE. The evolving epidemiology of methicillin-resistant *Staphylococcus aureus* at a university hospital. *Infect Control Hosp Epidemiol* 1995;16:12.
5. Coronado VG, Edwards JR, Culver DH, Gaynes RP. Ciprofloxacin resistance among nosocomial *Pseudomonas aeruginosa* and *Staphylococcus aureus* in the United States. *Infect Control Hosp Epidemiol* 1995;16:71.
6. Damato JJ, Eitzman DV, Baer H. Persistence and dissemination in the community of R-factors of nosocomial origin. *J Infect Dis* 1974;129: 205.
7. Strausbaugh LJ, Jacobson C, Yost T. Methicillin-resistant *Staphylococcus aureus* in a nursing home and affiliated hospital: a four-year perspective. *Infect Control Hosp Epidemiol* 1993;14:331.
8. Danzig LE, Short LJ, Collins K, et al. Bloodstream infections associated with a needleless intravenous infusion system in patients receiving home infusion therapy. *JAMA* 1995;273:1862.
9. Manian FA, Meyer L. Comprehensive surveillance of surgical wound infections in outpatient and inpatient surgery. *Infect Control Hosp Epidemiol* 1990;11:515.
10. Paul SM, Finelli L, Crane GL, Spitalny KC. A statewide surveillance system for antimicrobial-resistant bacteria: New Jersey. *Infect Control Hosp Epidemiol* 1995;16:385.
11. Decker MD. The OSHA bloodborne hazard standard. *Infect Control Hosp Epidemiol* 1992;13:407.
12. Decker MD. OSHA enforcement policy for occupational exposure to tuberculosis. *Infect Control Hosp Epidemiol* 1993;14:690.
13. Valenti AJ, Decker MD. OSHA inspections. *Infect Control Hosp Epidemiol* 1995;16:478.
14. Decker MD. The application of continuous quality improvement to healthcare. *Infect Control Hosp Epidemiol* 1992;13:226.
15. Rutala WA, Mayhall CG, Society for Hospital Epidemiology of America. Medical waste. *Infect Control Hosp Epidemiol* 1992;13:38.
16. Decker MD, Bolton GA, Dewey MJ, Smith G, Schaffner W. Failure of hospitals to promote the use of child restraint devices. *American Journal of Diseases of Children* 1988;142:656.
17. Goodman RA, Jenkins EL, Mercy JA. Workplace-related homicide among healthcare workers in the United States, 1980 through 1990. *JAMA* 1994;272:1686.

Hospital Infections, Fourth Edition,
edited by John V. Bennett and Philip S. Brachman.
Published by Lippincott–Raven Publishers, Philadelphia, 1998

CHAPTER 13

Isolation Precautions in Hospitals

Jeffrey W. Weinstein, Walter J. Hierholzer, Jr. and Julia S. Garner

RATIONALE FOR ISOLATION PRECAUTIONS IN HOSPITALS

Transmission of infection within a hospital requires three elements: a source of infecting microorganisms, a susceptible host, and a means of transmission for the microorganism. A discussion of these three elements provides the basis for understanding the current isolation precautions that are described in this chapter (see Chapter 1).

Source

Human sources of infecting microorganisms in hospitals may be patients, personnel, or, on occasion, visitors, and may include people with acute disease, people in the incubation period of a disease, those who are colonized by an infectious agent but have no apparent disease, or people who are chronic carriers of an infectious agent. Other sources of infecting microorganisms can be the patient's own endogenous flora, which may be difficult to control, and inanimate environmental objects that have become contaminated, including equipment, medications, water, food, and air.

Host

Resistance among people to pathogenic microorganisms varies greatly. Some people may be immune to infection or may be able to resist colonization by an infectious agent; others exposed to the same agent may establish a commensal relationship with the infecting microorganism and become asymptomatic carriers; in still others, clinical disease may develop. Host factors such as age; underlying diseases; certain treatments with antimicrobials, corticosteroids, or other immunosuppressive agents; irradiation; and breaks in the first line of defense mechanisms caused by such factors as surgical operations, anesthesia, and indwelling catheters may render patients more susceptible to infection.

Transmission

Microorganisms are transmitted in hospitals by several routes, and the same microorganism may be transmitted by more than one route. There are four main routes of transmission—contact, common vehicle, airborne, and vectorborne (see Chapter 1). For the purpose of this chapter, common vehicle and vectorborne transmission are discussed only briefly, because neither plays a significant role in typical nosocomial infections.

1. *Contact transmission*, the most important and frequent mode of transmission of nosocomial infections, is divided into three subgroups: direct contact transmission, indirect contact transmission, and droplet transmission.
   a. Direct contact transmission involves a direct body surface-to-body surface contact and physical transfer of microorganisms between a susceptible host and an infected or colonized person, such as occurs when a person turns a patient, gives a patient a bath, or performs other patient care activities that require direct personal contact. Direct contact transmission also can occur between two patients, with one serving as the source of the infectious microorganisms and the other as a susceptible host.
   b. Indirect contact transmission involves contact of a susceptible host with a contaminated intermediate object, sometimes inanimate, such as contaminated instruments, needles, or dressings, or contaminated

J. W. Weinstein: Department of Internal Medicine, Wright State University School of Medicine, Dayton, Ohio 45401.
W. J. Hierholzer, Jr: Department of Internal Medicine, Division of Infectious Disease, Yale University School of Medicine, Yale-New Haven Hospital, New Haven, Connecticut 06504.
J. S. Garner: National Center for Infectious Diseases, Centers for Diseases Control and Prevention, Atlanta, Georgia 30333.

hands that are not washed and gloves that are not changed between patients.

c. *Droplet transmission* is a form of contact transmission, although the mechanism of transfer of the pathogen to the host is quite distinct from either direct or indirect contact transmission. Droplets are generated from the source person primarily during coughing, sneezing, and talking, and during the performance of certain procedures such as suctioning and bronchoscopy. Transmission occurs when droplets containing microorganisms generated from the infected person are propelled a short distance (usually less than 3 feet) through the air and deposited on the host's conjunctivae, nasal mucosa, or mouth. Because droplets do not remain suspended in the air, special air handling and ventilation are not required to prevent droplet transmission; that is, droplet transmission must not be confused with airborne transmission.

2. *Common vehicle transmission* applies to microorganisms transmitted by contaminated items such as food, water, medications, devices, and equipment.
3. *Airborne transmission* occurs by dissemination of either airborne droplet nuclei (small-particle residue [5 μm or smaller in size] of evaporated droplets containing microorganisms that remain suspended in the air for long periods of time) or dust particles containing the infectious agent. Microorganisms carried in this manner can be dispersed widely by air currents and may be inhaled by a susceptible host in the same room or over a longer distance from the source patient, depending on environmental factors; therefore, special air handling and ventilation are required to prevent airborne transmission. Microorganisms transmitted by airborne transmission include *Mycobacterium tuberculosis* and the rubeola and varicella viruses.
4. *Vectorborne transmission* occurs when vectors such as mosquitoes, flies, rats, and other vermin transmit microorganisms; this route of transmission is of less significance in hospitals in the United States than in several other regions of the world.

Isolation precautions are designed to prevent transmission of microorganisms by these routes in hospitals. Because agent and host factors are more difficult to control, interruption of transfer of microorganisms is directed primarily at transmission. The isolation recommendations described later in this chapter are based on this concept.

Placing a patient on isolation precautions, however, often presents certain disadvantages to the hospital, patients, personnel, and visitors. Isolation precautions may require specialized equipment and environmental modifications that add to the cost of hospitalization. Isolation precautions may make frequent visits by nurses, physicians, and other personnel inconvenient, and they may make it more difficult for personnel to give the prompt and frequent care that sometimes is required. The use of a multipatient room for one patient uses valuable space that otherwise might accommodate several patients. Moreover, forced solitude deprives the patient of normal social relationships and may be psychologically harmful, especially to children. These disadvantages, however, must be weighed against the hospital's mission to prevent the spread of serious and epidemiologically important microorganisms in the hospital.

EARLY ISOLATION PRACTICES

The first published recommendations for isolation precautions in the United States appeared as early as 1877, when a hospital handbook recommended placing patients with infectious diseases in separate facilities [1], which ultimately became known as infectious disease hospitals. Later, personnel in these hospitals began to combat problems of nosocomial transmission by setting aside a floor or ward for patients with similar diseases [2] and by practicing aseptic procedures recommended in nursing textbooks published from 1890 to 1900 [1].

In 1910, isolation practices in U.S. hospitals were altered by the introduction of the cubicle system of isolation, which placed patients in multiple-bed wards [2]. With the cubicle system, hospital personnel used separate gowns, washed their hands with antiseptic solutions after patient contact, and disinfected objects contaminated by the patient. These nursing procedures, designed to prevent transmission of pathogenic organisms to other patients and personnel, became known as "barrier nursing."

During the 1950s, U.S. infectious disease hospitals, except those designated exclusively for tuberculosis, began to close. In the mid-1960s, tuberculosis hospitals also began to close, partly because general hospital or outpatient treatment became preferred for patients with tuberculosis. Thus, by the late 1960s, patients with infectious diseases were housed in wards in general hospitals, either in specially designed, single-patient isolation rooms or in regular single- or multiple-patient rooms.

CENTERS FOR DISEASE CONTROL AND PREVENTION (CDC) ISOLATION SYSTEMS

CDC Isolation Manual

In 1970, the CDC published a detailed manual entitled *Isolation Techniques for Use in Hospitals* to assist general hospitals with isolation precautions [3]. A revised edition appeared in 1975 [4]. The manual could be applied in small community hospitals with limited resources, as well as in large, metropolitan, university-associated medical centers.

The manual introduced the category system of isolation precautions. It recommended that hospitals use one of seven isolation categories (Strict Isolation, Respiratory Isolation, Protective Isolation, Enteric Precautions, Wound and Skin Precautions, Discharge Precautions, and Blood Precautions). The precautions recommended for each category were determined almost entirely by the epidemiologic features of the diseases grouped in the category, primarily their routes of transmission. Certain isolation techniques, believed to be the minimum necessary to prevent transmission of all diseases in the category, were indicated for each isolation category. Because all diseases in a category did not have the same epidemiology (i.e., were not spread by exactly the same combination of modes of transmission), with some requiring fewer precautions than others, more precautions were suggested for some diseases than were necessary. This disadvantage of "overisolation" for some diseases was offset by the convenience of having a small number of categories. By the mid-1970s, 93% of U.S. hospitals had adopted the isolation system recommended in the manual [5]. However, neither the efficacy of the category approach in preventing spread of infections nor the costs of using the system were evaluated by empiric studies.

By 1980, hospitals were experiencing new endemic and epidemic nosocomial infection problems, some caused by multidrug-resistant microorganisms and others caused by newly recognized pathogens, which required different isolation precautions from those specified by any existing isolation category. There was an increasing need for isolation precautions to be directed more specifically at nosocomial transmission in special care units, rather than at the intrahospital spread of infectious diseases acquired in the community [6]. Infection control professionals and nursing directors in hospitals with particularly sophisticated nursing staffs increasingly were calling for new isolation systems that would tailor precautions to the modes of transmission for each infection and avoid the overisolation inherent in the category-specific approach.

CDC Isolation Guideline

In 1983, the *CDC Guideline for Isolation Precautions in Hospitals* [7] (hereafter referred to as the isolation guideline) was published to take the place of the 1975 isolation manual; it contained many important changes. One of the most important was the increased emphasis on decision making on the part of users. Unlike the 1975 manual, which encouraged few decisions on the part of users, the isolation guideline encouraged decision making at several levels [8,9]. First, hospital infection control committees were given a choice of selecting between category-specific or disease-specific isolation precautions or using the guideline to develop a unique isolation system appropriate to their hospitals' circumstances and environments. Second, personnel who placed a patient on isolation precautions were encouraged to make decisions about the individual precautions to be taken (e.g., whether the patient's age, mental status, or condition indicated that a private room was needed to prevent sharing of contaminated articles). Third, personnel taking care of patients on isolation precautions were encouraged to decide whether they needed to wear a mask, gown, or gloves based on the likelihood of exposure to infective material. Such decisions were deemed necessary to isolate the infection, but not the patient, and to reduce the costs associated with unnecessary isolation precautions.

In the category-specific section of the guideline, existing categories were modified, new categories were added, and many infections were reassigned to different categories. The old category of Blood Precautions, primarily directed toward patients with chronic carriage of hepatitis B virus, was renamed Blood and Body Fluid Precautions and was expanded to include patients with acquired immunodeficiency syndrome and body fluids other than blood. The old category of Protective Isolation was deleted because of studies demonstrating its lack of efficacy in general clinical practice in preventing the acquisition of infection by the immunocompromised patient for whom it had been described originally [10,11]. The 1983 guideline contained the following categories of isolation: Strict Isolation, Contact Isolation, Respiratory Isolation, Tuberculosis (acid-fast bacilli [AFB]) Isolation, Enteric Precautions, Drainage/Secretion Precautions, and Blood and Body Fluid Precautions. As with the category approach in the former CDC isolation manuals, these categories tended to overisolate some patients.

In the disease-specific section of the guideline, the epidemiology of each infectious disease was considered individually by advocating only those precautions (e.g., private room, mask, gown, and gloves) needed to interrupt transmission of the infection. Because precautions were individualized for each disease, hospitals using the system were encouraged to provide more initial training and inservice education and to encourage a much higher level of attention from patient care personnel.

Because gaps existed in the knowledge of the epidemiology of some diseases, disagreement was expected, and occurred, regarding the placement of individual diseases in given categories. This was especially the case with diseases such as measles, respiratory syncytial virus, and influenza that have a respiratory component of transmission [12,13]. The lack of empiric studies on the efficacy and costs of implementing the recommendations contributed to the disagreements.

As new epidemiologic data became available, several subsequent CDC reports [14–16] updated portions of the isolation guideline dealing with viral hemorrhagic fevers and human parvovirus B19. Recommendations for Tuberculosis (AFB) Isolation were updated in 1990 [17] and again in 1994 [18] because of heightened concern about nosocomial transmission of multidrug-resistant tuberculosis [19,20], particularly in settings where patients with human immunodeficiency virus (HIV) infection were receiving care.

UNIVERSAL PRECAUTIONS

In 1985, largely because of the HIV epidemic, isolation practices in the United States were altered dramatically by the introduction of a new strategy for isolation precautions, which became known as Universal Precautions (UP). In acknowledgment of the fact that many patients with bloodborne infections are not recognized, the new UP approach for the first time placed emphasis to applying Blood and Body Fluid Precautions universally to all people regardless of their presumed infection status [21].

In addition to emphasizing prevention of needlestick injuries and the use of traditional barriers such as gloves and gowns, UP expanded Blood and Body Fluid Precautions to include use of masks and eye coverings to prevent mucous membrane exposures during certain procedures and the use of individual ventilation devices when the need for resuscitation was predictable. This approach, and particularly the techniques for preventing mucous membrane exposures, was reemphasized in subsequent CDC reports that contained recommendations for prevention of HIV transmission in healthcare settings [22–25]. A 1988 report [25] stated that UP applied to blood, to body fluids that had been implicated in the transmission of bloodborne infections (semen and vaginal secretions), to body fluids from which the risk of transmission was unknown (amniotic, cerebrospinal, pericardial, peritoneal, pleural, and synovial fluids), and to any other body fluid visibly contaminated with blood, but not to feces, nasal secretions, sputum, sweat, tears, urine, or vomitus unless they contained visible blood.

BODY SUBSTANCE ISOLATION

In 1987, a new system of isolation, called Body Substance Isolation (BSI), was proposed after 3 years of study by infection control personnel at the Harborview Medical Center in Seattle, Washington, and the University of California at San Diego, as an alternative to diagnosis-driven isolation systems [26]. BSI focused on the isolation of all moist and potentially infectious body substances (blood, feces, urine, sputum, saliva, wound drainage, and other body fluids) from all patients, regardless of their presumed infection status, primarily through the use of gloves. Personnel were instructed to put on clean gloves just before contact with mucous membranes and nonintact skin, and to wear gloves for anticipated contact with moist body substances. In addition, a "Stop Sign Alert" was used to instruct people wishing to enter the room of some patients with infections transmitted exclusively, or in part, by the airborne route to check with the floor nurse, who would determine whether a mask should be worn.

Among the advantages cited for BSI were that it was a simple, easy-to-learn and -administer system, that it avoided the assumption that individuals without known or suspected diagnoses of transmissible infectious diseases were free of risk to patients and personnel, and that only certain body fluids were associated with transmission of infections. The disadvantages of BSI included the added cost of increased use of barrier equipment, particularly gloves [27]; the difficulty in maintaining routine application of the protocol for all patients; the uncertainty about the precautions to be taken when entering a room with a "Stop Sign Alert"; and the potential for misapplication of the protocol to overprotect personnel at the expense of the patient [28].

Controversial aspects of BSI have been summarized [13,29]. BSI appeared to replace some, but not all, of the isolation precautions necessary to prevent transmission of infection. BSI did not contain adequate provisions to prevent 1) droplet transmission of serious infections in pediatric populations (e.g., invasive *Hemophilus influenza, Neisseria meningitidis* meningitis and pneumonia, and pertussis); 2) direct or indirect contact transmission of epidemiologically important microorganisms from dry skin or environmental sources (e.g., *Clostridium difficile* and vancomycin-resistant enterococci); or 3) true airborne transmission of infections transmitted over long distances by droplet nuclei. The lack of emphasis on special ventilation for patients known or suspected of having pulmonary tuberculosis was of particular concern to the CDC in the early 1990s because of multidrug-resistant tuberculosis [16,19].

Body Substance Isolation and UP shared many similar features designed to prevent the transmission of bloodborne pathogens in hospitals. However, there was an important difference in the recommendation for glove use and handwashing. Under UP, gloves were recommended for anticipated contact with blood and specified body fluids, and hands were to be washed immediately after gloves were removed [24,25]. Under BSI, gloves were recommended for anticipated contact with any moist body substance, but handwashing after glove removal was not required unless the hands visibly were soiled [26]. The lack of emphasis on handwashing after glove removal was cited as one of the theoretic disadvantages of BSI [13,30,31].

THE NEED FOR A NEW ISOLATION GUIDELINE

By the early 1990s, isolation had become an infection control conundrum [32]. Although many hospitals had incorporated all or portions of UP into their category- or disease-specific isolation system and others had adopted all or portions of BSI [33,34], there was much local variation in the interpretation and use of UP and BSI, and a variety of combinations were common. Further, there was considerable confusion about which body fluids or substances required precautions under UP and BSI. Moreover, there was continued lack of agreement about the importance of handwashing when gloves were used and the need for additional precautions beyond BSI to prevent airborne, droplet, and contact transmission [12,13,24–27, 29–31,35–38]. Some hospitals had not implemented appropriate guidelines for preventing transmission of tuberculosis, including multidrug-resistant tuberculosis [39]. As other multidrug-resistant microorganisms [40, 41] were emerging, some hospitals failed to recognize them as new problems and to add appropriate precautions that would contain them.

In view of these problems and concerns, no simple adjustment to any of the existing approaches—UP, BSI, the CDC isolation guideline, or other isolation systems—appeared likely to solve the conundrum. Clearly, what was needed was a new synthesis of the various systems that would provide a guideline with logistically feasible recommendations for preventing the many infections that occur in hospitals through diverse modes of transmission. To achieve this, the new guideline would 1) have to be epidemiologically sound; 2) have to recognize the importance of all body fluids, secretions, and excretions in the transmission of nosocomial pathogens; 3) have to contain adequate precautions for infections transmitted by the airborne, droplet, and contact routes of transmission; 4) have to be as simple and user friendly as possible; and 5) have to use new terms to avoid confusion with existing systems.

The 1996 Hospital Infection Control Practices Advisory Committee (HICPAC) Isolation Guideline [42] contains three important changes from previous recommendations. First, it synthesizes the major features of UP [24,25] and BSI [26,43] into a single set of precautions to be used for the care of all patients in hospitals regardless of their presumed infection status. These precautions, called *Standard Precautions*, are designed to reduce the risk of transmission of bloodborne and other pathogens in hospitals. As a result of this synthesis, a large number of patients with diseases or conditions that previously required category- or disease-specific precautions in the 1983 CDC isolation guideline [7] now are covered under Standard Precautions and do not require additional precautions. Second, it collapses the old categories of isolation precautions (Strict Isolation, Contact Isolation, Respiratory Isolation, Tuberculosis Isolation, Enteric Precautions, and Drainage/Secretion Precautions) and the old disease-specific precautions into three sets of precautions based on routes of transmission for a smaller number of specified patients known or suspected to be infected or colonized with highly transmissible or epidemiologically important pathogens. These Transmission-Based Precautions, designed to reduce the risk of *airborne, droplet*, and *contact* transmission in hospitals, are to be used in addition to Standard Precautions. Third, it lists specific syndromes in both adult and pediatric patients that are highly suspect for infection and identifies appropriate Transmission-Based Precautions to use on an empiric, temporary basis until a diagnosis can be made. These empiric, temporary precautions also are designed to be used in addition to Standard Precautions.

HOSPITAL INFECTION CONTROL PRACTICES ADVISORY COMMITTEE 1996 ISOLATION PRECAUTIONS

There are two tiers of the 1996 HICPAC isolation precautions [42]. In the first and most important tier are those precautions designed for the care of all patients in hospitals, regardless of their diagnosis or presumed infection status. Implementation of these "Standard Precautions" is the primary strategy for successful nosocomial infection control. In the second tier are precautions designed only for the care of specified patients. These additional "Transmission-Based Precautions" are for patients known or suspected to be infected by epidemiologically important pathogens spread by airborne or droplet transmission or by contact with dry skin or contaminated surfaces.

Standard Precautions

Standard Precautions synthesize the major features of UP and BSI and applies them to all patients receiving care in hospitals, regardless of their diagnosis or presumed infection status. Standard Precautions apply to 1) blood; 2) all body fluids, secretions, and excretions except sweat, regardless of whether they contain visible blood; 3) nonintact skin; and 4) mucous membranes. Standard Precautions are designed to reduce the risk of transmission of microorganisms from both recognized and unrecognized sources of infection in hospitals.

Transmission-Based Precautions

Transmission-Based Precautions are designed for patients documented or suspected to be infected with highly transmissible or epidemiologically important pathogens for which additional precautions beyond Standard Precautions are needed to interrupt transmission in hospitals. There are three types of Transmission-Based Precautions: Airborne Precautions, Droplet Precautions, and Contact Precautions. They may be combined for diseases that have multiple routes of transmission. When used either singularly or in combination, they are to be used in addition to Standard Precautions. A synopsis of the types of precautions and the patients requiring these precautions is listed in Table 13-1.

Airborne Precautions are designed to reduce the risk of airborne transmission of infectious agents. Airborne transmission occurs by dissemination of either airborne droplet nuclei (small-particle residue [5 μm or smaller in size] of evaporated droplets that may remain suspended in the air for long periods of time) or dust particles containing the infectious agent. Microorganisms carried in this manner can be dispersed widely by air currents and may become inhaled by or deposited on a susceptible host in the same room or over a longer distance from the source patient, depending on environmental factors; therefore, special air handling and ventilation are required to prevent airborne transmission. Airborne Precautions apply to patients known or suspected to be infected with epidemiologically important pathogens that can be transmitted by the airborne route.

Droplet Precautions are designed to reduce the risk of droplet transmission of infectious agents. Droplet transmission involves contact of the conjunctivae or the mucous membranes of the nose or mouth of a susceptible person with large-particle droplets (> 5 μm in size) containing microorganisms generated from a person who has a clinical disease or who is a carrier of the microorganism. Droplets are generated from the source person primarily during coughing, sneezing, or talking, and during the performance of certain procedures such as suctioning and bronchoscopy. Transmission by large-particle droplets requires close contact between source and recipient people, because droplets do not remain suspended in the air and usually travel only short distances (usually 3 feet or less) through the air. Because droplets do not remain suspended in the air, special air handling and ventilation are not required to prevent droplet transmission. Droplet Precautions apply to any patient known or suspected to be infected with epidemiologically important pathogens that can be transmitted by infectious droplets.

TABLE 13-1. *Synopsis of types of precautions and patients requiring the precautions*[a]

Standard Precautions
- Use Standard Precautions for the care of all patients

Airborne Precautions
- In addition to Standard Precautions, use Airborne Precautions for patients known or suspected to have serious illnesses transmitted by airborne droplet nuclei. Examples of such illnesses include:
  1. Measles
  2. Varicella (including disseminated Zoster)[b]
  3. Tuberculosis[c]

Droplet Precautions
- In addition to Standard Precautions, use Droplet Precautions for patients known or suspected to have serious illnesses transmitted by large particle droplets. Examples of such illnesses include:
  1. Invasive *Haemophilus influenzae* type b disease, including meningitis, pneumonia, epiglottitis, and sepsis
  2. Invasive *Neisseria meningitidis* disease, including meningitis, pneumonia, and sepsis
  3. Other serious bacterial respiratory infections spread by droplet transmission, including:
     (a) Diphtheria (pharyngeal)
     (b) Mycoplasma pneumonia
     (c) Pertussis
     (d) Pneumonic plague
     (e) Streptococcal pharyngitis, pneumonia, or scarlet fever in infants or young children
  4. Serious viral infections spread by droplet transmission, including:
     (a) Adenovirus[b]
     (b) Influenza
     (c) Mumps
     (d) Parvovirus B19
     (e) Rubella

Contact Precautions
- In addition to Standard Precautions, use Contact Precautions for patients known or suspected to have serious illnesses easily transmitted by direct patient contact or by contact with items in the patient's environment. Examples of such illnesses include:
  1. Gastrointestinal, respiratory, skin, or wound infections or colonization with multidrug-resistant bacteria judged by the infection control program, based on current state, regional, or national recommendations, to be of special clinical and epidemiologic significance
  2. Enteric infections with a low infectious dose or prolonged environmental survival, including:
     (a) *Clostridium difficile*
     (b) For diapered or incontinent patients: enterohemorrhagic *Escherichia coli* 0157:H7, *Shigella,* hepatitis A, or rotavirus
  3. Respiratory syncytial virus, parainfluenza virus, or enteroviral infections in infants and young children
  4. Skin infections that are highly contagious or that may occur on dry skin, including:
     (a) Diphtheria (cutaneous)
     (b) Herpes simplex virus (neonatal or mucocutaneous)
     (c) Impetigo
     (d) Major (noncontained) abscesses, cellulitis, or decubiti
     (e) Pediculosis
     (f) Scabies
     (g) Staphylococcal furunculosis in infants and young children
     (h) Zoster (disseminated or in the immunocompromised host)[b]
  5. Viral/hemorrhagic conjunctivitis
  6. Viral hemorrhagic infections (Ebola, Lassa, or Marburg)[a]

[a]See HICPAC Guidelines for a complete listing of infections requiring precautions [42].
[b]Certain infections require more than one type of precaution.
[c]See CDC Tuberculosis Guidelines [18].

Contact Precautions are designed to reduce the risk of transmission of epidemiologically important microorganisms by direct or indirect contact. Direct contact transmission involves skin-to-skin contact and physical transfer of microorganisms to a susceptible host from an infected or colonized person, such as occurs when personnel turn patients, bathe patients, or perform other patient care activities that require physical contact. Direct contact transmission also can occur between two patients (e.g., by hand contact), with one serving as the source of infectious microorganisms and the other as a susceptible host. Indirect contact transmission involves contact of a susceptible host with a contaminated intermediate object, sometimes inanimate, in the patient's environment. Contact Precautions apply to specified patients known or suspected to be infected or colonized (presence of microorganism in or on patient but without clinical signs and symptoms of infection) with epidemiologically important microorganisms than can be transmitted by direct or indirect contact.

A comprehensive list of organisms and the corresponding category of precautions recommended can be found in the published guidelines [42]. Criteria for the safe discontinuation of isolation precautions are also included in this list.

EMPIRIC USE OF AIRBORNE, DROPLET, OR CONTACT PRECAUTIONS

In many instances, the risk of nosocomial transmission of infection may be highest before a definitive diagnosis can be made and before precautions based on that diagnosis can be implemented. The routine use of Standard

TABLE 13-2. *Clinical syndromes or conditions warranting additional empiric precautions to prevent transmission of epidemiologically important pathogens pending confirmation of diagnosis[a]*

Clinical syndrome or condition[b]	Potential pathogens[c]	Empiric precautions [42]
Diarrhea		
Acute diarrhea with a likely infectious cause in an incontinent or diapered patient	Enteric pathogens[d]	Contact
Diarrhea in an adult with a history of recent antibiotic use	*Clostridium difficile*	Contact
Meningitis	*Neisseria meningitidis*	Droplet
Rash or exanthems, generalized, cause unknown		
Petechial/ecchymotic with fever	*Neisseria meningitidis*	Droplet
Vesicular	Varicella	Airborne and Contact
Maculopapular with coryza and fever	Rubeola (measles)	Airborne
Respiratory infections		
Cough/fever/upper lobe pulmonary infiltrate in an HIV-seronegative patient and/or a patient at low risk for HIV infection	*Mycobacterium tuberculosis*	Airborne
Cough/fever/pulmonary infiltrate in any lung location in an HIV-infected patient and/or a patient at high risk for HIV infection	*Mycobacterium tuberculosis*	Airborne
Paroxysmal or severe persistent cough during periods of pertussis activity	*Bordetella pertussis*	Droplet
Respiratory infections, particularly bronchiolitis and croup in infants and young children	Respiratory syncytial or parainfluenza virus	Contact
Risk of multidrug-resistant microorganisms		
History of infection or colonization with multidrug-resistant organisms[e]	Resistant bacteria	Contact
Skin, wound, or urinary tract infection in a patient with a recent hospital or nursing home stay in a facility where multidrug-resistant organisms are prevalent	Resistant bacteria	Contact
Skin or wound infection		
Abscess or draining wound that cannot be covered	*Staphylococcus aureus,* Group A streptococcus	Contact

[a]ICPs are encouraged to modify or adapt this table according to local conditions. To ensure that appropriate empiric precautions are always implemented, hospitals must have systems in place to routinely evaluate patients according to these criteria as part of their preadmission and admission care.

[b]Patients with the syndromes or conditions listed below may have atypical signs or symptoms (e.g., pertussis in neonates and adults may not have paroxysmal or severe cough). The clinician's index of suspicion should be guided by the prevalence of specific conditions in the community, as well as clinical judgment.

[c]The organisms listed under the column "Potential pathogens" are not intended to represent the complete or even most likely diagnoses, but rather possible etiologic agents that require additional precautions beyond Standard Precautions until they can be ruled out.

[d]These pathogens include enterohemorrhagic *Escherichia coli* 0157: H7, *Shigella* hepatitis A, and rotavirus.

[e]Resistant bacteria judged by the infection control program, on the basis of current state, regional, or national recommendations, to be of special clinical or epidemiologic significance.

Precautions for all patients should greatly reduce this risk for conditions other than those requiring Airborne, Droplet, or Contact Precautions. Although it is not possible prospectively to identify all patients needing these enhanced precautions, certain clinical syndromes and conditions carry a sufficiently high risk to warrant the empiric addition of enhanced precautions while a more definitive diagnosis is pursued. A listing of such conditions and the recommended precautions beyond Standard Precautions is presented in Table 13-2.

The organisms listed under the column "Potential Pathogens" are not intended to represent the complete or even most likely diagnoses, but rather possible etiologic agents that require additional precautions beyond Standard Precautions until they can be ruled out. Infection control professionals are encouraged to modify or adapt this table according to local conditions. To ensure that appropriate empiric precautions always are implemented, hospitals must have systems in place to evaluate patients routinely according to these criteria as part of their preadmission and admission care.

IMMUNOCOMPROMISED PATIENTS

Immunocompromised patients vary in their susceptibility to nosocomial infections, depending on the severity and duration of immunosuppression. They usually are at increased risk for bacterial, fungal, parasitic, and viral infections from both endogenous and exogenous sources. The use of Standard Precautions for all patients and Transmission-Based Precautions for specified patients, as recommended by the guideline, should reduce the acquisition by these patients of institutionally acquired bacteria from other patients and environments.

FUNDAMENTALS OF ISOLATION PRECAUTIONS

A variety of infection control measures are used for decreasing the risk of transmission of microorganisms in hospitals. These measures make up the fundamentals of isolation precautions.

Handwashing and Gloving

Handwashing frequently is called the single most important measure to reduce the risks of transmitting organisms from one person to another or from one site to another on the same patient. The scientific rationale, indications, methods, and products for handwashing have been well delineated [44–52]. Washing hands as promptly and thoroughly as possible between patient contacts and after contact with blood, body fluids, secretions, excretions, and equipment or articles contaminated by them is an important component of infection control and isolation precautions. In addition to handwashing, gloves play an important role in reducing the risks of transmission of microorganisms.

Gloves are worn for three important reasons in hospitals. First, gloves are worn to provide a protective barrier and to prevent gross contamination of the hands when touching blood, body fluids, secretions, excretions, mucous membranes, and nonintact skin [24–26]; the wearing of gloves in specified circumstances to reduce the risk of exposures to bloodborne pathogens is mandated by the Occupational Safety and Health Administration (OSHA) Bloodborne Pathogens final rule [53]. Second, gloves are worn to reduce the likelihood that microorganisms present on the hands of personnel will be transmitted to patients during invasive or other patient care procedures that involve touching a patient's mucous membranes and nonintact skin. Third, gloves are worn to reduce the likelihood that hands of personnel contaminated with microorganisms from a patient or a fomite can transmit these microorganisms to another patient. In this situation, gloves must be changed between patient contacts and hands washed after gloves are removed.

Wearing gloves does not replace the need for handwashing, because gloves may have small, inapparent defects or may be torn during use, and hands can become contaminated during removal of gloves [12,52,54,55]. Failure to change gloves between patient contacts is an infection control hazard [28].

Patient Placement

Appropriate patient placement is a significant component of isolation precautions. A private room is important to prevent direct or indirect contact transmission when the source patient has poor hygienic habits, contaminates the environment, or cannot be expected to assist in maintaining infection control precautions to limit transmission of microorganisms (i.e., infants, children, and patients with altered mental status). When possible, a patient with highly transmissible or epidemiologically important microorganisms is placed in a private room with handwashing and toilet facilities, to reduce opportunities for transmission of microorganisms.

When a private room is not available, an infected patient is placed with an appropriate roommate. Patients infected by the same microorganism usually can share a room, provided they are not infected with other potentially transmissible microorganisms and the likelihood of reinfection with the same organism is minimal. Such sharing of rooms, also referred to as "cohorting" patients, is useful especially during outbreaks or when there is a shortage of private rooms. When a private room is not available and cohorting is not achievable or recommended [18], it is very important to consider the epidemiology and mode of transmission of the infecting pathogen and the patient population being served in determining patient placement. Under these circumstances, consultation with infection control professionals is advised before patient placement. Moreover, when an infected patient shares a room with a noninfected patient, it also is important that patients, personnel, and visitors take precautions to prevent the spread of infection and that roommates are selected carefully.

Guidelines for construction, equipment, air handling, and ventilation for isolation rooms have been published [56–58]. A private room with appropriate air handling and ventilation is particularly important for reducing the risk of transmission of microorganisms from a source patient to susceptible patients and other persons in hospitals when the microorganism is spread by airborne transmission. Some hospitals use an isolation room with an anteroom as an extra measure of precaution to prevent airborne transmission. Adequate data regarding the need for an anteroom, however, are not available. Ventilation recommendations for isolation rooms housing patients with pulmonary tuberculosis are detailed in the 1994 CDC tuberculosis guidelines [18].

Transport of Infected Patients

Limiting the movement and transport of patients infected with virulent or epidemiologically important microorganisms and ensuring that such patients leave their rooms only for essential purposes reduces opportunities for transmission of microorganisms in hospitals. When patient transport is necessary, it is important that 1) appropriate barriers (e.g., masks, impervious dressings) are worn or used by the patient to reduce the opportunity for transmission of pertinent microorganisms to other patients, personnel, and visitors and to reduce contamination of the environment; 2) personnel in the area to which the patient is to be taken are notified of the impending arrival of the patient and of the precautions to be used to reduce the risk of transmission of infectious microorganisms; and 3) patients are informed of ways by which they can assist in preventing the transmission of their infectious microorganisms to others.

Masks, Respiratory Protection, Eye Protection, Face Shields

Various types of masks, goggles, and face shields are worn alone or in combination to provide barrier protection. A mask that covers both the nose and the mouth, and goggles or a face shield are worn by hospital personnel during procedures and patient care activities that are likely to generate splashes or sprays of blood, body fluids, secretions, or excretions to provide protection of the mucous membranes of the eyes, nose, and mouth from contact transmission of pathogens. The wearing of masks, eye protection, and face shields in specified circumstances to reduce the risk of exposures to bloodborne pathogens is mandated by the OSHA Bloodborne Pathogens final rule [53]. A surgical mask usually is worn by hospital personnel to provide protection against spread of infectious large-particle droplets that are transmitted by close contact and travel only short distances (≤ 3 feet) from infected patients who are coughing or sneezing.

An area of major concern and controversy since the late 1980s has been the role and selection of respiratory protection equipment and the implications of a respiratory protection program for prevention of transmission of tuberculosis in hospitals. Traditionally, although the efficacy was not proven, a surgical mask was worn for isolation precautions in hospitals when patients were known or suspected to be infected with pathogens spread by the airborne route of transmission. In 1990, however, the CDC tuberculosis guidelines [17] stated that surgical masks may not be effective in preventing the inhalation of droplet nuclei and recommended the use of disposable particulate respirators, despite the fact that the efficacy of particulate respirators in protecting people from the inhalation of *M. tuberculosis* had not been demonstrated and the cost of such units is high.

A National Institute of Occupational Safety and Health (NIOSH) certification process, effective in July, 1995, provides a broader range of certified respirators that meet the performance criteria recommended by the CDC in the updated 1994 tuberculosis guidelines [18]. NIOSH has indicated that the N95 (n category at 95% efficiency) meets the CDC performance criteria for a tuberculosis respirator. Such masks became available in late 1995 at a significantly reduced cost.

Gowns and Protective Apparel

Various types of gowns and protective apparel are worn to provide barrier protection and to reduce opportunities for transmission of microorganisms in hospitals. Gowns are worn to prevent contamination of clothing and to protect the skin of personnel from blood and body fluid exposures. Gowns especially treated to make them impermeable to liquids, leg coverings, boots, or shoe covers provide greater protection to the skin when splashes or large quantities of infective material are present or anticipated. The wearing of gowns and protective apparel under specified circumstances to reduce the risk of exposures to bloodborne pathogens is mandated by the OSHA Bloodborne Pathogens final rule [53].

Gowns are also worn by personnel during the care of patients infected with epidemiologically important microorganisms to reduce the opportunity for transmission of pathogens from patients or items in their environment to other patients or environments; when gowns are worn for this purpose, they are removed before leaving the patient's environment and hands are washed. Adequate data regarding the efficacy of gowns for this purpose, however, are not available.

Routine and Terminal Cleaning

The room, or cubicle, and bedside equipment of patients on Transmission-Based Precautions are cleaned using the same procedures used for patients on Standard Precautions, unless the infecting microorganisms and the amount of environmental contamination indicate special cleaning. In addition to thorough cleaning, adequate disinfection of bedside equipment and environmental surfaces (e.g., bed rails, bedside tables, carts, commodes, doorknobs, faucet handles) is indicated for certain pathogens, especially enterococci, which can survive in the inanimate environment for prolonged periods of time [59]. Patients admitted to hospital rooms that previously were occupied by patients infected or colonized with such pathogens are at increased risk of infection from contaminated environmental surfaces and bedside equipment if they have not been cleaned and disinfected adequately. The methods, thoroughness, and frequency of cleaning and the products used are determined by hospital policy.

REFERENCES

1. Lynch T. *Communicable disease nursing.* St. Louis: CV Mosby; 1949.
2. Gage ND, Landon JF, Sider MT: *Communicable disease.* Philadelphia: FA Davis, 1959.
3. National Communicable Disease Center. *Isolation techniques for use in hospitals.* PHS publication no. 2054. Washington, DC: U.S. Government Printing Office, 1970.
4. Centers for Disease Control and Prevention. *Isolation techniques for use in hospitals.* 2nd ed. HHS publication no. (CDC) 80-8314. Washington, DC: U.S. Government Printing Office, 1975.
5. Haley RW, Shachtman RH. The emergence of infection surveillance and control programs in US hospitals: an assessment, 1976. *Am J Epidemiol* 1980;111:574–591.
6. Schaffner W. Infection control: old myths and new realities. *Infect Control* 1980;1:330–334.
7. Garner JS, Simmons BP. CDC guideline for isolation precautions in hospitals. HHS publication no. (CDC) 83-8314. Atlanta, GA: U.S. Department of Health and Human Services, Public Health Service, Centers for Disease Control and Prevention, 1983. Also: *Infect Control* 1983;4:245–325, and *Am J Infect Control* 1984;12:103–163.
8. Garner JS. Comments on CDC guideline for isolation precautions in hospitals, 1984. *Am J Infect Control* 1984;12:163.
9. Haley RW, Garner JS, Simmons BP. A new approach to the isolation of patients with infectious diseases: alternative systems. *J Hosp Infect* 1985;6:128–139.
10. Nauseef WM, Maki DG. A study of the value of simple protective isolation in patients with granulocytopenia. *N Engl J Med* 1981;304:448–453.
11. Pizzo PA. The value of protective isolation in preventing nosocomial infections in high risk patients. *Am J Med* 1981;70:631–637.
12. Goldmann DA. The role of barrier precautions in infection control. *J Hosp Infect* 1991;18:515–523.
13. Goldmann DA, Platt R, Hopkins C. Control of hospital-acquired infections. In: Gorbach SL, Bartlett JG, Blacklow NR, eds. *Infectious diseases.* Philadelphia: WB Saunders 45:378–390;1992.
14. Centers for Disease Control and Prevention. Management of patients with suspected viral hemorrhagic fever. *MMWR Morb Mortal Wkly Rep* 1988;37(3S):1–16.
15. Centers for Disease Control and Prevention. Risks associated with human parvovirus B19 infection. *MMWR Morb Mortal Wkly Rep* 1989; 38:81–88, 93–97.
16. Centers for Disease Control and Prevention. Update: management of patients with suspected viral hemorrhagic fever: United States. *MMWR Morb Mortal Wkly Rep* 1995;44:475–479.
17. Centers for Disease Control and Prevention. Guidelines for preventing the transmission of tuberculosis in health-care settings, with special focus on HIV-related issues. *MMWR Morb Mortal Wkly Rep* 1990;39 (RR-17):1–29.
18. Centers for Disease Control and Prevention. Guidelines for preventing the transmission of tuberculosis in health-care facilities, 1994. *MMWR Morb Mortal Wkly Rep* 1994;43(RR-13):1–132; *Federal Register* 1994; 59(208):54242–54303.
19. Centers for Disease Control and Prevention. Nosocomial transmission of multidrug-resistant tuberculosis to health-care workers and HIV-infected patients in an urban hospital Florida. *MMWR Morb Mortal Wkly Rep* 1990;39:718–722.
20. Centers for Disease Control and Prevention. Nosocomial transmission of multidrug-resistant tuberculosis among HIV-infected persons Florida and New York, 1988–1991. *MMWR Morb Mortal Wkly Rep* 1991;40: 585–591.
21. Centers for Disease Control and Prevention. Recommendations for preventing transmission of infection with human T-lymphotropic virus type III/lymphadenopathy-associated virus in the workplace. *MMWR Morb Mortal Wkly Rep* 1985;34:681–686, 691–695.
22. Centers for Disease Control and Prevention. Recommendations for preventing transmission of infection with human T-lymphotropic virus type III/lymphadenopathy-associated virus during invasive procedures. *MMWR Morb Mortal Wkly Rep* 1986;35:221–223.
23. Centers for Disease Control and Prevention. Update: human immunodeficiency virus infections in health-care workers exposed to blood of infected patients. *MMWR Morb Mortal Wkly Rep* 1987;36:285–289.
24. Centers for Disease Control and Prevention. Recommendations for prevention of HIV transmission in health-care settings. *MMWR Morb Mortal Wkly Rep* 1987;36(2S):1S–18S.
25. Centers for Disease Control and Prevention. Update: universal precautions for prevention of transmission of human immunodeficiency virus, hepatitis B virus, and other bloodborne pathogens in health-care settings. *MMWR Morb Mortal Wkly Rep* 1988;37:377–388.
26. Lynch P, Jackson MM, Cummings J, Stamm WE. Rethinking the role of isolation practices in the prevention of nosocomial infections. *Ann Intern Med* 1987;107:243–246.
27. McPherson DC, Jackson MM, Rogers JC. Evaluating the cost of the body substance isolation system. *Journal of Healthcare Materials Management* 1988;6:20–28.
28. Patterson JE, Vecchio J, Pantelick EL, et al. Association of contaminated gloves with transmission of *Acinetobacter calcoaceticus* var. *anitratus* in an intensive care unit. *Am J Med* 1991;91:479–483.
29. Garner JS, Hierholzer WJ. Controversies in isolation policies and practices. In: Wenzel RP, ed. *Prevention and control of nosocomial infections.* 2nd ed. Baltimore: Williams & Wilkins, 1993:70–81.
30. Garner JS, Hughes JM. Options for isolation precautions. *Ann Intern Med* 1987;107:248–250.
31. Weinstein RA, Kabins SA. Isolation practices in hospitals. *Ann Intern Med* 1987;107:781–782.
32. Jackson MM, Lynch P. An attempt to make an issue less murky: a comparison of four systems for infection precautions. *Infect Control Hosp Epidemiol* 1991;12:448–450.
33. Pugliese G, Lynch P, Jackson MM. *Universal precautions: policies, procedures, and resources.* Chicago: American Hospital Association; 1991:7–87.
34. Birnbaum D, Schulzer M, Mathias RG, Kelly M, Chow AW. Adoption of guidelines for universal precautions and body substance isolation in Canadian acute-care hospitals. *Infect Control Hosp Epidemiol* 1990;11: 465–472.
35. Lynch P, Cummings MJ, Stamm WE, Jackson MM. Handwashing versus gloving [Letter]. *Infect Control Hosp Epidemiol* 1991;12:139.
36. Birnbaum D, Schulzer M, Mathias RG, Kelly M, Chow AW. Handwashing versus gloving [Letter]. *Infect Control Hosp Epidemiol* 1991; 12:140.
37. Gurevich I. Body substance isolation [Letter]. *Infect Control Hosp Epidemiol* 1992;13:191.
38. Jackson MM, Lynch P. Body substance isolation [Letter]. *Infect Control Hosp Epidemiol* 1992;13:191–192.

39. Rudnick JR, Kroc K, Manangan L, Banerjee S, Pugliese G, Jarvis W. Are US hospitals prepared to control nosocomial transmission of tuberculosis [Abstract]? In: *Epidemic intelligence service annual conference*. 1993:60.
40. Institute of Medicine. *Emerging infections: microbial threats to health in the United States*. Washington, DC: National Academy Press; 1992.
41. Centers for Disease Control and Prevention. Nosocomial enterococci resistant to vancomycin United States, 1989–1983. *MMWR Morb Mortal Wkly Rep* 1993;42:597–599.
42. Hospital Infection Control Practices Advisory Committee Guidelines for isolation precautions in hospitals. *Infect Control Hosp Epidemiol* 1996;17:53–80.
43. Lynch P, Cummings MJ, Roberts PL, Herriott MJ, Yates B, Stamm WE. Implementing and evaluating a system of generic infection precautions: body substance isolation. *Am J Infect Control* 1990;18:1–12.
44. Lowbury EJL, Lilly HA, Bull JP. Disinfection of hands: removal of transient organisms. *Br Med J* 1964;2:230–233.
45. Sprunt K, Redmon W, Leidy G. Antibacterial effectiveness of routine handwashing. *Pediatrics* 1973;52:264–271.
46. Steere AC, Mallison GF. Handwashing practices for the prevention of nosocomial infections. *Ann Intern Med* 1975;83:683–690.
47. United States Food and Drug Administration. The tentative final monograph for over-the-counter topical antimicrobial products. *Federal Register* 1978;43:1210–1249.
48. Garner JS, Favero MS. *Guideline for handwashing and hospital environmental control*. Atlanta, GA: U.S. Department of Health and Human Services, Public Health Service, Centers for Disease Control and Prevention; 1985.
49. Larson E. APIC guideline for use of topical antimicrobial products. *Am J Infect Control* 1988;16:253–266.
50. Ehrenkranz NJ. Bland soap handwash or hand antisepsis? The pressing need for clarity. *Infect Control Hosp Epidemiol* 1992;13:299–301.
51. Larson E. Skin cleansing. In: Wenzel RP, ed. *Prevention and control of nosocomial infections*. 2nd ed. Baltimore: Williams & Wilkins, 1993; 450–459.
52. Larson EL. 1992, 1993, and 1994 Association for Professionals in Infection Control and Epidemiology Guidelines Committee: APIC guideline for handwashing and hand antisepsis in healthcare settings. *Am J Infect Control* 1995;23:251–269.
53. United States Department of Labor, Occupational Safety and Health Administration. Occupational exposure to bloodborne pathogens: final rule. *Federal Register* 1991;56(235):64175–64182.
54. Doebbeling BN, Pfaller MA, Houston AK, Wenzel RP. Removal of nosocomial pathogens from the contaminated glove: implications for glove reuse and handwashing. *Ann Intern Med* 1988;109:394–398.
55. Olsen RJ, Lynch P, Coyle MB, Cummings MJ, Bokete T, Stamm WE. Examination gloves as barriers to hand contamination and clinical practice. *JAMA* 1993:270:350–353.
56. Health Resources and Services Administration. *Guidelines for construction and equipment of hospital and medical facilities*. PHS publication no. (HRSA) 84-14500. Rockville, MD: U.S. Department of Health and Human Services, Public Health Service; 1984.
57. American Institute of Architects, Committee on Architecture for Health. General hospital. In: *Guidelines for construction and equipment of hospital and medical facilities*. Washington, DC: The American Institute of Architects Press; 1993.
58. American Society of Heating, Refrigerating, and Air Conditioning Engineers. Health facilities. In: *1991 Application handbook*. Atlanta, GA: American Society of Heating, Refrigerating, and Air Conditioning Engineers, Inc; 1991.
59. Hospital Infection Control Practices Advisory Committee. Recommendations for preventing the spread of vancomycin resistance. *Am J Infect* Control 1995;23:87–94; *Infect Control Hosp Epidemiol* 1995;16: 105–113; *MMWR Morb Mortal Wkly Rep* 1995;44(No. RR-12):1–13.

Hospital Infections, Fourth Edition,
edited by John V. Bennett and Philip S. Brachman.
Lippincott–Raven Publishers, Philadelphia © 1998

CHAPTER 14

Antibiotics and Nosocomial Infections

Theodore C. Eickhoff

The era of chemotherapy for infectious disease is now over 50 years old. Those years have been marked by the continuous development and introduction of new and potent antimicrobial agents and by the relentless development and spread of significant antibiotic resistances among pathogenic bacteria. Contemporary clinicians have available a broad array of potent antibiotic agents of proven efficacy against susceptible pathogens; growing problems with antimicrobial drug resistance, however, are beginning to erode our antibiotic armamentarium.

Since the introduction of antibiotics, significant changes have also occurred in the character of nosocomial infections. The available data strongly suggest that in the 1940s and 1950s nosocomial infection was generally synonymous with gram-positive coccal infection, most notably with β-hemolytic streptococci and staphylococci. In the 1950s, staphylococci—particularly those resistant to the antimicrobial drugs in common use, such as penicillin G, tetracycline, erythromycin, chloramphenicol, and streptomycin—emerged to cause epidemic infection in hospitals. For reasons that are poorly understood, staphylococci subsided somewhat in importance as the major cause of nosocomial infection in the early 1960s, to be replaced by enteric gram-negative bacilli, enterococci, and fungi [1]. During the 1970s and 1980s, staphylococci again became more prominent. Important nosocomial pathogens in the 1990s include coagulase-positive and -negative staphylococci, enterococci, enteric gram-negative bacilli, gram-negative nonfermenting organisms such as *Pseudomonas*, *Stenotrophomonas* (formerly *Xanthomonas* or *Pseudomonas*), *Achromobacter* and *Acinetobacter*, and *Candida* species [2–4]. It is apparent that successful nosocomial pathogens such as these are either intrinsically highly resistant to antimicrobial drugs, or are capable of acquiring such resistance within the hospital (or patient) environment.

T. C. Eickhoff: Division of Infectious Diseases, University of Colorado Health Sciences Center, Denver, Colorado 80262.

It is tempting to relate the changing character of nosocomial infections, as briefly sketched, to the sequential introduction of new antimicrobial agents and to impute a cause-and-effect relation. No one can seriously doubt that antimicrobial drugs have had a profound effect in shaping the character of nosocomial infections, but such an explanation is greatly oversimplified and fails to take into account the enormous changes in the technology of medicine and patterns of healthcare delivery that have also taken place since the introduction of antibiotics.

This chapter explores more fully the way in which antimicrobial drugs are used in hospitals and considers the epidemiologic effects of such drug use on both the host and the microorganism. The biochemical mechanisms of antimicrobial drug resistance and the spread of such resistances among bacteria are fully discussed in Chapters 15 and 16.

ANTIBIOTIC USE IN HOSPITALS

Data on the overall patterns of antibiotic use in hospitals have appeared in the literature frequently in the last several decades. The general thrust of such data indicates that from 25% to 40% of hospitalized patients receive systemic antibiotics at any given time [5,7]. Furthermore, sequentially obtained data suggest that there is a trend toward increasing, rather than decreasing, antibiotic use in hospitals.

A series of four prevalence surveys carried out at the Boston City Hospital during January or February of the years 1964, 1967, 1970, and 1973 provides interesting comparative data from earlier in the antibiotic era [8]. In 1964, 26% of patients in that hospital were receiving at least one systemic antibacterial agent; in 1967, the figure was 27%; in 1970, it was 34%, and, in 1973, 36%. In the 1973 survey, 76% of patients receiving antibiotics were considered to have an active infection at the time.

Scheckler and Bennett [9] reported on antibiotic use in seven community hospitals scattered throughout the United States; they used a survey technique comparable to that used in the Boston City Hospital surveys. Twenty-four such prevalence studies carried out between November, 1967 and June, 1969 indicated that more than 30% of patients were receiving one or more systemic antibiotics but that only 38% of patients receiving antibiotics surveyed in 1969 had recorded evidence of infection.

Kunin and coworkers [10] reported a study of antibiotic use carried out in 1969 at the University of Virginia Hospital. During a 3-month period, all antibiotic therapy given to patients on the medical and surgical services was reviewed by the infectious disease resident and staff, and the use of antibiotics in any given patient was judged by the group to be appropriate or inappropriate. During the survey period, 27% of patients admitted to the medical service and 29% of patients admitted to the surgical service were given antibiotics. Among patients on the surgical service, 48% of the antibiotic therapy given was for prophylaxis, whereas on the medical service, only 6% of antibiotic therapy was for prophylaxis.

Inappropriate therapy included instances in which a different drug was believed to be preferable, the dose was considered inappropriate, or the administration of any antimicrobial therapy or prophylaxis was considered unjustified. In the reviewers' judgment, 52% of all antimicrobial therapy was inappropriate. On the medical service, 42% of all antimicrobial drug use was judged inappropriate, whereas 62% of all antibiotic therapy on the surgical service was considered inappropriate.

Surveys carried out at the Latter Day Saints Hospital in Salt Lake City from 1971 to 1990 [11] have shown that, although the overall prevalence of hospital-acquired and community-acquired infections remained relatively constant, antibiotic usage increased; there was a trend toward increasing use of broad-spectrum agents. Antibiotics were given to 38% of patients in the 1990 survey.

Long-term trends in antibiotic use were also examined at the University of Iowa during the 15-year period from 1978 to 1992 [7]. Use of penicillin G, antistaphylococcal penicillins, first-generation cephalosporins, and aminoglycosides remained relatively constant, but there were sharp increases in the use of extended-spectrum cephalosporins, vancomycin, metronidazole, and amphotericin B. During the period of the study, the percentage of patients who received at least one parenteral antibiotic increased from 23% to 44%, and the average number of agents used in the patients receiving at least one antibiotic rose from 1.8 to 2.1.

Such massive use of antibacterial drugs in hospitals, whether appropriate or inappropriate, has profound effects on both the hosts who receive these drugs and the bacteria exposed to them. There are enormous economic consequences as well. The global antibiotic market was valued at over 20 billion dollars in 1994 [12], and this could well double by the year 2000. There is enormous pressure on the part of the pharmaceutical industry to increase antibiotic use, both to recoup the cost of new drug development, and to accomplish the very legitimate goal of making a profit.

DRUG RESISTANCE OF BACTERIA IN HOSPITALS

Current problems of resistance of bacteria to antimicrobial drugs become more understandable if one recalls some of the history of the development of antibacterial drug resistance. In Paul Ehrlich's laboratory, trypanosomes became resistant to the drug *p*-rosaniline after repeated exposures [13]. Similarly, it was shown that pneumococci could develop resistance to hydrocupreine derivatives after repeated exposure [14]. In the mid-1940s, shortly after the introduction of penicillin G, it was recognized that certain strains of staphylococci elaborated a potent β-lactamase, an enzymatic inactivator of penicillin, and that penicillin G had no therapeutic activity in patients with infections caused by such staphylococci. This recognition surely came as a major disappointment but not as a total surprise. Since that time, it has become abundantly clear that the major nosocomial pathogens either are naturally resistant to clinically useful antimicrobial drugs or possess the ability to acquire resistance. The best-known examples are the staphylococci and aerobic gram-negative bacilli, which together regularly account for most nosocomial infections. Every major class of bacterial pathogens has thus far demonstrated an ability to develop resistance to one or more commonly used antimicrobial agents [15].

Selective pressures favoring drug-resistant bacteria conferred by antibiotic therapy may indeed be principally focused in the institutional setting, but they extend widely into the community as well. The increasing prevalence of ampicillin-resistant *Hemophilus influenzae*, the increasing frequency of β-lactamase-producing gonococci, the widespread dissemination of methicillin-resistant staphylococci, and the emergence of penicillin-resistant pneumococci are more recent examples. Maxwell Finland [15] wrote in 1978, "Little by little, we are experiencing the erosion of the strongest bulwarks against serious bacterial infection."

Finland's concerns have taken on a new urgency in the 1990s. With the development of extended-spectrum cephalosporins and fluoroquinolones in the 1980s, many individuals, including some in the pharmaceutical industry, considered bacterial infections to be controlled; the problem had been solved, and such infections were no longer a threat. Furthermore, other areas of drug development, such as cardiovascular, metabolic, and psychoactive drugs, were considerably more promising. Consequently, effort and investment in new antibiotic development dwindled. Furthermore, all the easy or obvious targets of antibiotic activity had already been identified; hence, new antibiotic development promised to be very costly.

Our position today is thus precarious at best. We face mounting problems of drug resistance in community-acquired infections, best exemplified by the rapid emergence of penicillin-resistant pneumococci; we also face increasingly resistant nosocomial pathogens, best exemplified by methicillin-resistant *Staphylococcus aureus* (MRSA) and *Staphylococcus epidermidis*, vancomycin-resistant enterococci (VRE), and multidrug-resistant gram-negative bacilli (MDRGNB). Certain nosocomial infections caused by VRE and MDRGNB are already resistant to all available antibiotics and therefore essentially untreatable. The threat of emergence of vancomycin-resistant MRSA is real, and believed by many infectious disease physicians to be merely a matter of time. All this is happening at a time in which new antibiotic drug development has rarely been less promising.

Virulence of Antibiotic-Resistant Bacteria

The occurrence of nosocomial infection due to multidrug-resistant organisms is governed by a number of factors, including antibiotic selection pressure, the nature of the resistance determinant, whether the plasmid is conjugative or nonconjugative or is a transposon, and possible linkage with other antibiotic resistances and genetic determinants governing adhesion and pathogenicity [16]. Evidence is conflicting regarding the altered virulence—whether enhanced or diminished—of drug-resistant bacteria compared with that of drug-susceptible organisms. There may prove to be no single answer to such a question, the answer rather depending on the particular bacterial species involved, the specific genetic determinants present, and what these genetic determinants contribute to the metabolic activities of the cell and the specific antigens located on the bacterial cell surface.

Although it is generally true that serious infection, such as bacteremic infection, caused by drug-resistant bacteria results in higher mortality than would be true of comparably serious infections caused by drug-susceptible bacteria, it is usually not clear whether the increased mortality is a reflection of increased virulence, diminished effectiveness of antibiotic therapy, or both. Jessen and colleagues [17], for example, who studied the occurrence of methicillin-resistant staphylococci and staphylococcal bacteremia in Denmark, showed that the combined effects of lysogenicity, transduction, and selection not only influenced the phage type and antibiotic resistance of staphylococci, but involved properties more directly connected with pathogenicity, such as lipase production, which is believed to facilitate the development of abscesses and adversely affect the prognosis in bacteremia. The authors could not determine, however, whether the poorer prognosis was due to the shortcomings of antibiotic therapy or to correlated bacterial properties that enhanced virulence.

Holmberg and associates [18] at the Centers for Disease Control and Prevention reviewed the health and economic impacts of antimicrobial resistance. Working from a data base of 175 reports of investigations of outbreaks, both community and nosocomial, of selected pathogens, they compared mortality, likelihood of hospitalization, and duration of hospital stay in patients in outbreaks of antibiotic-resistant pathogens to patients involved in outbreaks of antibiotic-susceptible pathogens. Included in the data base were outbreaks of salmonellosis, shigellosis, staphylococcal infection, *Serratia* infection, and other gram-negative bacillary infections. As expected, there were many possible confounding variables in such a retrospective analysis but, nonetheless, mortality, likelihood of hospitalization, and hospital stay were at least twofold higher in patients infected with drug-resistant pathogens compared with patients infected with drug-susceptible pathogens. This was true for both community and hospital outbreaks.

Mortality risk associated with bacteremic infection with VRE is clearly higher than in such infections caused by vancomycin-sensitive enterococci [19]. However, it is difficult to conclude that this increased mortality was due simply to the lack of effective antibiotics, because patients infected with VRE also had more severe underlying illness, had greater antibiotic exposure, and had been in hospital longer. Consequently, a direct comparison of mortality rates with bacteremic infection caused by vancomycin-sensitive enterococci and VRE is invalid; the two sets of patients are not directly comparable.

Occasional examples can be found in the literature of linkage of resistance determinants with virulence factors. One such is the linkage of drug resistances with intestinal adherence factors in a diarrheagenic strain of *Escherichia coli* [20]. Such direct linkages of resistance and virulence determinants in nosocomial pathogens seem to be the exception, rather than the rule.

Thus, at the clinical level, the consequences of antimicrobial drug resistance are profound and measurable, even though there may not be in vitro evidence of enhanced virulence. The adverse consequences of antimicrobial drug resistance were due both to ineffective antibiotic therapy and to the higher risk of drug-resistant infection in patients who had been on previous antibiotic therapy as a result of other underlying conditions.

Parallels in Antibiotic Use and Antibiotic Resistance

Evidence from a number of studies suggests that the proportion of bacteria resistant to a given antibiotic may increase as use of the drug increases or, conversely, may decrease if there is decreased use or cessation of use of the drug.

Lepper and coworkers [21] found that after 5 months of intensive use of erythromycin for the treatment of all susceptible infections, three fourths of the strains were highly resistant to that drug. When all erythromycin therapy was discontinued and penicillin and tetracycline therapy resumed, the proportion of erythromycin-resistant strains decreased, whereas the proportion of penicillin-resistant strains, which had declined while erythromycin was used exclusively, rose again rapidly. Similar results were found for tetracycline, to which resistance had increased sharply while it was used for susceptible infections and subsequently declined as its use decreased. Gibson and Thompson [22] described a similar phenomenon with staphylococci from burn wounds that had become highly resistant to tetracycline while that drug was used. When chloramphenicol was substituted for tetracycline, the proportion of chloramphenicol-resistant staphylococci rose sharply during the succeeding 6 months, whereas the proportion of tetracycline-resistant staphylococci fell. When chloramphenicol therapy was discontinued, the proportion of chloramphenicol-resistant strains dropped sharply. Bauer and colleagues [23] reported an entirely comparable experience and demonstrated a correlation between the extent of resistance and use of antibiotics. In an extensive study of staphylococci and staphylococcal infection in Great Britain, Barber and colleagues [24] documented not only a decline in the incidence of staphylococcal infection per patient when a number of anti–cross-infection measures and a controlled antibiotic policy were put into effect, but also a sharp reversal of penicillin and tetracycline resistance of isolates toward increased susceptibility.

Prevailing drug resistance of gram-negative bacilli is also susceptible to alteration by restriction or cessation of use of a given drug. When kanamycin was replaced by gentamicin in an effort to control an outbreak of nosocomial infections caused by kanamycin-resistant enteric organisms, kanamycin-resistant organisms were virtually eliminated from the nursery within a month, which suggested that the selective pressure provided by the extensive use of kanamycin was a major factor in causing and propagating the outbreak. As gentamicin was increasingly used, a significant increase in gentamicin resistance of the infants' intestinal flora occurred [25].

Sogaard and colleagues [26], in studying antibiotic-resistant gram-negative bacilli in a urologic ward in Denmark, found a progressive decrease in the incidence of antibiotic resistance among enteric bacteria over a 9-year period that was coincident with a decreasing use of antibiotics in response to a restrictive antibiotic use policy. In addition, the number of more resistant organisms, such as *Pseudomonas aeruginosa, Proteus, Providencia, Klebsiella*, and *Enterobacter*, declined during the period of study. Bulger and coworkers [27], in surveying resistance among strains of *E. coli* and *Klebsiella–Enterobacter* over a 10-year period, observed a decline in the frequency of resistance to antibiotics; they attributed their findings in part to conservative and selective use of antibiotics and in part to the development of an overall hospital infection control program.

Working in the Birmingham Accident Hospital Burn Unit, Lowbury and associates [28] studied the emergence of strains of *P. aeruginosa* and Enterobacteriaceae that carried a resistance (R) factor conferring resistance to tetracycline, kanamycin, carbenicillin, ampicillin, and cephaloridine. These strains emerged under the selective pressure of carbenicillin therapy, which was widely used on the burn unit. After discontinuation of all use of carbenicillin and restriction of the use of tetracycline, kanamycin, ampicillin, and cephaloridine, strains of *P. aeruginosa* and Enterobacteriaceae carrying this linked multidrug-resistant pattern disappeared. Price and Sleigh [29] reported an unusually dramatic experience in attempting to control an epidemic *Klebsiella* infection by a neurosurgical unit; the epidemic was not curtailed by radical measures for the prevention of cross-infection, and the epidemic strain disappeared only when the use of all antibiotics, both prophylactic and therapeutic, was discontinued in the unit.

A major feature in the appearance of MDRGNB in hospitals has been the spread of extended-spectrum β-lactamases, first in Europe, and then throughout the world, as reviewed by Gold and Moellering [30]. There are many such β-lactamases, which differ in their substrate specificity and which possess the property of inactivating many β-lactam drugs, particularly many of the extended-spectrum cephalosporins.

As use of the extended-spectrum cephalosporins has increased, so have multidrug resistance problems caused by these drugs. Ballow and Schentag [31] have shown that, in the hospitals they surveyed, there was a significant positive correlation between increasing ceftazidime use, and increasing resistance to ceftazidime among isolates of certain microorganisms, notably *Enterobacter cloacae*.

Based on such data, many believe that a policy of restricting the use of the newest and most broadly active antibiotics would minimize the development of resistance to those drugs and hence prolong their useful life span.

In several excellent reviews, McGowan [32,33] has summarized the evidence linking antimicrobial use in the hospital with antimicrobial resistance in hospital bacteria:

1. Antimicrobial resistance is more prevalent among bacteria causing infection in the nosocomial setting than among bacteria causing community-acquired infection. Although exceptions exist, they have been relatively few, and most of the data support the generalization.
2. In outbreak situations in the nosocomial setting, patients infected with resistant outbreak strains are more likely to have received previous antibiotic ther-

apy than patients colonized or infected with susceptible strains of the same species. This has been particularly illustrated in outbreaks of MRSA.

3. Changes in antimicrobial use may lead to parallel changes in the prevalence of resistance to that antibiotic.
4. Areas of most intense antibiotic use in the hospital usually also have had the highest prevalence of antibiotic-resistant bacteria. These are also usually the areas of the hospital in which the most highly susceptible patients are encountered, and include intensive care units, burn units, oncology units, and other special-care units.
5. In general, increased duration of exposure to antibiotics in the hospital increases the likelihood of colonization or infection with resistant organisms. This factor may, however, also simply act as a marker for more highly susceptible hosts.
6. The higher the dose of antibiotic given, the greater the likelihood of superinfection or colonization with resistant organisms. Evidence in support of this contention is not well controlled and is most convincing in the case of respiratory tract infection.
7. Finally, the notion of a cause–effect relation seems to fit the existing data, in biologic terms. The proposed cause precedes the proposed effect. That is, antibiotic therapy produces marked effects on the host's endogenous flora and exerts selective pressure in favor of resistant organisms. Thus, antibiotic therapy appears to act primarily by selecting a drug-resistant causative organism rather than by increasing the frequency of nosocomial infection.

Pathways of Emergence of Resistance

If a population of uniformly susceptible bacteria is exposed to an antibiotic, resistance will not emerge. There must either be a genetic pathway for resistance development, or the introduction of one or more resistant organisms for resistance to develop.

Tenover and McGowan [34] have outlined six possible pathways for emergence of resistance. These are 1) introduction of a few resistant organisms into a population where resistance had previously not been present; 2) acquisition of resistance by a few previously susceptible strains through genetic mutation; 3) acquisition of resistance by a previously susceptible strain through transfer of genetic material; 4) emergence of inducible resistance that is already present in a few strains in the population, usually in the presence of an inducer antibiotic; 5) selection of a small, resistant subpopulation of organisms; and 6) dissemination of inherently resistant organisms within the local setting.

The sixth pathway is considered the major pathway of nosocomial spread of organisms that become resistant as a result of one of the first five pathways. Such transmission or dissemination may, of course, occur from patient to patient, perhaps by way of the hands of healthcare workers, or in contaminated commercial products and the like. Depending on the microbiologic and epidemiologic circumstances, it may or may not be possible to identify which pathway operated in any given situation. Note, however, that the sixth pathway is the only pathway that is amenable to control by barrier precautions, handwashing, and other infection control procedures.

Antibiotic Resistance in Special Care Units

Because of high rates of nosocomial infection in special care units, especially in intensive care units, drug resistance is a particular problem. Multidrug-resistant nosocomial pathogens often are first detected in such units, and if not eradicated or contained, eventually spread through the rest of the hospital.

Schentag has developed the concept of the "genesis patient" [35], best illustrated by ventilator patients with repeated lower respiratory tract infections. Such patients are treated with a succession of existing antibiotics, and then new antibiotics as their pathogens become resistant to older antibiotics. These patients are often the first to yield pathogens resistant to the newer antibiotics. Thus, genesis patients are the focal point for emergence and possible spread of resistant organisms. As medical technology advances and the number of compromised patients increases, the number of genesis patients will only increase.

Investigators at the Indiana University Medical Center studied possible cross-infection in five intensive care units in 1992 [36], and found that, using molecular methods of strain typing, 13% could have arisen by cross-infection. Thus, as previously described by Weinstein [37], most intensive care unit infections appear to originate from the patient's endogenous flora. This lends further support to Schentag's concerns about genesis patients, and also underscores the importance of barrier techniques and other infection control procedures in special care units to minimize the spread of multidrug-resistant pathogens.

Drug-resistant organisms—whether mutants, transductants containing plasmids, or conjugants containing R factors—selected by the pressure of antibiotic drugs are probably at a disadvantage, however slight, in the absence of the selective pressure. Resistance determinants must represent an energy "load" for the host bacterium. If this were not so, "wild" bacteria in the community would likely be drug resistant or would at least be a mixture of sensitive and resistant cells. Although resistant bacteria acquired in the hospital persist for a time in the community free of the selection pressure of antibiotics, they usually decay in the absence of the selective pressure.

ANTIBIOTICS AND HOST SUSCEPTIBILITY

Antibiotics may affect host susceptibility to infection by either a direct effect on host defense mechanisms or an indirect effect resulting from alteration of the metabolic and immunologic state of the host. Antibiotics also exert a profound influence on the nature of host microflora, and although this selection effect may not directly influence host susceptibility to infection, as previously noted, it very directly influences the nature of the organisms that colonize and subsequently infect hospitalized patients.

Direct Effect of Antibiotics on Host Defense Mechanisms

The most obvious and dramatic examples of a direct effect of antibiotics on host defense mechanisms are instances of granulocytopenia or bone marrow aplasia occasionally encountered with the use of several antibiotics, notably chloramphenicol and the sulfonamides. Adverse reactions to penicillins, cephalosporins, sulfonamides, and, less frequently, other antibiotics may take the form of a severe dermatitis, including exfoliation; such direct immunologic injury to the skin may, of course, enhance host susceptibility to infection. These adverse effects of antibiotic therapy are well known and profoundly influence host susceptibility to infection.

Direct effects of individual antibiotics on the components of host defense—that is, polymorphonuclear leukocyte function, immunoglobulin synthesis and function, and cell-mediated immune mechanisms—have not been systematically studied. There is, however, a gradually increasing body of data from which a few conclusions may be drawn [38–41].

With regard to polymorphonuclear leukocyte function, neither β-lactam nor aminoglycoside drugs appear to have any deleterious effects, although there is evidence that tetracycline hydrochloride, chlortetracycline, and doxycycline may inhibit leukocyte chemotaxis and impair phagocytosis. In addition, several sulfonamide drugs, including sulfadiazine, sulfathiazole, and sulfasoxazole, may inhibit leukocyte microbicidal activity. In the case of the tetracyclines, these effects may be seen in clinically attainable concentrations; whether they are of clinical significance has not been established.

Chloramphenicol, in clinically attainable concentrations, can be shown to diminish the antibody response to antigenic stimulation, but this effect has not been shown to be of general clinical significance. Rifampin can be shown in vitro to inhibit antibody production, but the effects of rifampin on antibody response in humans are variable.

Modulation of the host immune response to an infectious agent by specific chemotherapy—such as occurs in the treatment of rickettsial infections with chloramphenicol or tetracycline, penicillin treatment of group A streptococcal infections, or ampicillin treatment of *H. influenzae* type B infections—may, over long periods of time, alter the susceptibility of a population to a particular infectious agent, but this phenomenon probably is of little, if any, significance in the context of nosocomial infection.

The β-lactam, aminoglycoside, and quinolone antibiotics are not known to have any significant effect on host cell-mediated immune mechanisms. Rifampin, the tetracyclines, and trimethoprim have been shown to suppress lymphocyte blastogenesis at concentrations that might be encountered during clinical use. Several other antibiotics, including clindamycin, erythromycin, and nitrofurantoin, can similarly impair lymphocyte blastogenesis, but only at concentrations rarely achieved during clinical use. Rifampin can also be shown to suppress delayed cutaneous hypersensitivity to purified protein derivative of tuberculin in patients with tuberculosis who are receiving the drug. This effect of rifampin, however, has not been shown to alter host susceptibility to infection in patients being treated for tuberculosis, nor has it been associated with a poor therapeutic result.

Concern is frequently expressed about the possible deleterious effect of release of endotoxin when gram-negative bacteria are killed by antibiotics. In the Jarisch-Herxheimer reaction and the tumor lysis syndrome, there is certainly evidence of initial deterioration after initiation of effective chemotherapy. Evidence that antibiotic-induced release of endotoxin is a significant clinical problem is scant [42,43], and this theoretic concern need not affect the choice of appropriate antibiotic therapy.

Thus, there is little evidence that antibiotic therapy has a major, direct effect on host defense mechanisms except in instances of adverse drug reactions precipitating severe dermatitis, bone marrow depression, or other such events. In general, data suggest that antibiotics that are taken up and concentrated in cells (e.g., erythromycin, tetracyclines, rifampin) or that affect intracellular metabolic processes such as protein synthesis, are more likely than others to alter host defense mechanisms. As noted, however, this area has not been systematically studied, and investigational methods have not been standardized. Interested readers are referred to an excellent review [38].

Indirect Effect of Antibiotics due to Alteration of Host Metabolic State

Many antibiotics cause direct toxic or immunologically mediated injury to target organs regulating the metabolic activity of the host, particularly the liver, kidneys, gastrointestinal tract, and lungs. The resulting dysfunction of these organs may alter host susceptibility to infection. These indirect effects of antibiotics can, in most instances, be minimized or avoided altogether by the rational and careful use of potentially toxic drugs.

Kidneys

Interstitial nephritis has been associated with a number of drugs, notably the penicillins, including the penicillinase-resistant penicillins. Direct toxic injury to renal tubular epithelium is caused by many drugs, notably cephaloridine, all of the aminoglycosides, the polymyxins, and amphotericin B. Also, glomerulonephritis has been noted shortly after rifampin therapy in people with previous exposure to the drug. Renal failure and its resulting metabolic consequences have a direct suppressive effect on host defense mechanisms. Clearly, the therapeutic modalities used in the management of renal failure also represent added infection risk factors.

Liver

Minor alterations of hepatic function are found frequently in the course of antibiotic therapy, but, in most instances, such alterations cannot be shown to influence host susceptibility to infection. Intrahepatic cholestasis, such as may occur during therapy with the sodium lauryl sulfate ester of erythromycin, similarly does not appear to represent a major threat to host defense mechanisms. Overwhelming hepatic injury has been associated with both tetracycline and isoniazid therapy, but the unquestionably reduced host resistance to infection is of lesser importance than the more immediate metabolic threat to the host.

Colon

Necrotizing enterocolitis has been recognized as a complication of therapy with many antibiotic drugs, notably the penicillins, cephalosporins, and clindamycin. Thought to be caused by staphylococci during the 1950s and 1960s, necrotizing enterocolitis is now known to be due to an enterotoxin produced by *Clostridium difficile* [44,45]. This adverse effect appears to be related to the alteration of host gastrointestinal tract flora caused by the administered antibiotic.

Lungs

Immunologically mediated injury to the lungs is an occasional consequence of antibiotic therapy, particularly with penicillins and nitrofurans. It is likely that host susceptibility to infection is only mildly enhanced by such injury.

Influence of Antibiotic Therapy on Host Microflora

Virtually all antibiotics in therapeutic doses produce marked changes in the microflora of the skin, upper respiratory tract, gastrointestinal tract, and genital tract—indeed, any site in the host normally colonized by bacteria. Antibiotic-resistant organisms, if present or acquired, are selected out by pathways previously described and multiply freely to replace the susceptible organisms inhibited by antibiotic therapy. In most patients, these changes in host microflora are of no demonstrable consequence. As is well recognized, however, the antibiotic-resistant microflora may, on occasion, result in serious or fatal infection. It is through this mechanism that antibiotic therapy appears to exert its major influence on nosocomial infection—that is, by determining the character, rather than the frequency, of nosocomial infections.

Historically, perhaps the clearest example of alteration of host microflora that led directly to overgrowth and subsequent infection by antibiotic-resistant bacteria was thought to be staphylococcal enterocolitis associated with or following tetracycline therapy. This appeared to be a direct result of antibiotic therapy, which suppressed the normal gastrointestinal tract flora and permitted rapid and uninhibited overgrowth of drug-resistant staphylococci. Today we know that the toxin-producing strains of *C. difficile* may not necessarily demonstrate in vitro resistance to the precipitating antibiotic, but presumably the antibiotic suppresses the more sensitive gastrointestinal tract flora, allowing the less susceptible clostridia to multiply or produce enterotoxin [44,45].

Colonization of the gastrointestinal tract by MDRGNB, under the influence of antibiotic therapy, has been repeatedly demonstrated [46,47]. Evidence has been presented suggesting that hospital food may frequently be contaminated by MDRGNB and that this may be an important source of nosocomial colonization in patients whose normal gastrointestinal tract flora is suppressed by antibiotic therapy (see Chapter 34). The sources of MDRGNB in hospital food, including, for example, fresh garden salads, have not been clarified.

It has become apparent that some kinds of antibiotics, particularly those active against many components of the anaerobic flora of the gastrointestinal tract, are more likely to be associated with colonization by multidrug-resistant organisms than are antibiotics less broadly active against the anaerobic flora of the gastrointestinal tract [46]. This has led to the concept of so-called colonization resistance, suggesting that an intact colonic anaerobic flora is of major importance in decreasing the chance of colonization by new aerobic gram-negative bacilli.

Hooker and DiPiro [47] have published a comprehensive review of the effects of antibiotics on gastrointestinal tract flora. Although antibiotics are the most obvious class of drugs that affect bowel flora, other drug classes have some effects as well, including antineoplastic drugs, immunosuppressive drugs, and histamine H_2 blockers. In general, the most profound changes in bowel flora are caused by oral antibiotics that are poorly or incompletely absorbed from the gastrointestinal tract or antibiotics given by any route that are secreted or excreted in high concentration into saliva, bile, or intestinal secretions. If the antibiotic in question has intrinsic activity against anaerobic bacteria, the alteration of host bowel microflora is even more profound. This leads directly to selection and overgrowth of antimicrobial-resistant strains.

The most profound effects on bowel flora, and disruption of colonization resistance, have been seen with second- and third-generation cephalosporins and extended-spectrum penicillins. Even within these classes, however, effects are variable among different drugs. Cefoperazone, cefuroxime, cefoxitin, cefotetan, and ceftriaxone profoundly suppress both aerobic and anaerobic bowel flora; ceftazidime and cefotaxime have a lesser effect. Parenterally administered aminoglycosides and monobactams have only minor effects on bowel flora. The quinolones have significant activity against the aerobic gram-negative bacteria in the gut, but only limited activity against anaerobes.

The concept of colonization resistance led, in turn, to selective decontamination of the digestive tract (SDD; see Chapter 15). The theoretic basis for this intervention is the belief that most nosocomial pathogens that cause endogenous infection originate in the host's gastrointestinal tract. The goal of SDD is to reduce colonization, and ultimately infection, by potential nosocomial pathogens, especially gram-negative bacilli and sometimes *Candida*, by using those antibiotics that are active against the pathogens of concern, but that preserve the anaerobic flora of the colon. The antibiotics most commonly used include polymyxins, aminoglycosides, trimethoprim–sulfamethoxazole, quinolones, and aztreonam. These are usually given orally in various combinations, sometimes with amphotericin B if candidal infections are of concern.

Selective decontamination of the digestive tract has been evaluated in intensive care units since the mid-1980s as an intervention to reduce oropharyngeal colonization and ventilator-associated pneumonia caused by gram-negative bacilli [48–50]. Over 25 randomized trials have been reported; many show a reduction in the frequency of respiratory tract infection, but overall there has been no reduction in mortality rates. Furthermore, SDD is costly, and has been associated with antibiotic resistance development. The role of SDD thus remains controversial.

Continuing controversy after over a decade of multiple studies suggests that SDD should be abandoned for routine clinical use, and that further use, if any, be restricted to targeted, focused use to help control specific outbreak problems in such units.

The most promising approaches to minimize or prevent the risks of colonization and spread of antibiotic-resistant organisms in the gastrointestinal tract are simple but, unfortunately, not often given much consideration in antibiotic decision making. These are 1) avoidance of unnecessary antibiotic therapy, 2) use of the shortest possible duration of treatment, 3) avoidance of drugs that have antianaerobic activity except when necessary, and 4) the preferential use of antibiotics that are well absorbed after oral administration or are minimally excreted through the biliary tract.

General Conclusions

Thus, there is abundant evidence that antibiotic therapy is a determinant, and perhaps the *major* determinant, of alterations in host microflora and colonization of the host by drug-resistant organisms. There is also evidence, however, that antibiotic therapy is by no means the only determinant involved and that it may be only one of a number of risk factors commonly encountered by hospitalized patients that facilitate colonization and often subsequent disease by drug-resistant organisms.

Interrelation of Antibiotic Therapy, Resistance to Antibiotics, and Nosocomial Infection

The interrelation of antibiotic therapy, intrinsic or acquired resistance to antibiotics in bacteria, and nosocomial infection in the hospitalized host represents an extraordinarily complex equation. Considering the large numbers of other risk factors that affect patients in hospitals, it is perhaps not surprising that data simply do not exist that would permit satisfactory and valid conclusions concerning the exact role of antibiotic use in determining either the magnitude or the frequency of hospital infection.

The use of antimicrobial agents tends to promote the emergence of organisms with intrinsic or acquired resistance to those agents and predisposes patients to colonization by such organisms. With increasing use of instrumentation, immunosuppressive drugs, and other technologic accompaniments of contemporary medical practice, resistant organisms may emerge to cause infection. Infection resulting from multidrug-resistant bacteria is notoriously more difficult to treat than infection by drug-susceptible pathogens, and the results of therapy in such compromised hosts are clearly less satisfactory.

This section has reviewed the adverse effects of antimicrobial therapy, both on bacteria and on the host. These adverse effects must be kept in perspective to keep in sight the enormous benefits of these drugs in curing infections that were major causes of morbidity and mortality in the preantibiotic era. The challenge is to maintain the beneficial effects while minimizing the risks.

EVALUATION OF ANTIBIOTIC USE

Incidence of Antibiotic Abuse

That antimicrobial agents are both widely misused and widely overused is now established beyond reasonable doubt. From 20% to 40% of patients in U.S. hospitals receive antimicrobial agents during the course of their hospitalization, and this accounts for 30% to 50% of hospital drug costs. In one study, no evidence of infection was found in as many as 70% of patients who received antimicrobial therapy [9]. Kunin [10] has estimated that as many as 50% of hospitalized adults who receive antibiotic therapy 1) do not require antibiotic therapy for their medical condition, 2) do not receive the most effective and least expensive drug, or 3) do not receive the lowest dose and duration of therapy that is considered effective.

It is important, however, as emphasized by Kunin [6], to evaluate the problem of antibiotic use in broader perspective rather than to consider it as an isolated example of inappropriate use of drugs. Included in the causation of the problem, and therefore to be considered in resolving the problem, are the ways in which appropriate use of drugs is taught in medical school, how house staff and practicing physicians receive information and advice about new drugs, the nature of the relationship between the pharmaceutical industry and the medical profession, the steadily increasing reliance of the medical profession on drug and laboratory technology in general, and the apparent lack of significant constraints operating to control the escalating cost of healthcare.

Viewed in such a context, antibiotic abuse is simply another reflection of what has become known as the *technologic imperative* and is comparable to well known problems such as the overuse of psychoactive drugs or excessive use of laboratory testing. Nonetheless, there is one major difference between other such problems and antibiotic abuse that is too often ignored or forgotten—that is, the biologic consequences, or ecologic "fallout," of antibiotic therapy. As previously discussed in this chapter, the widespread use of antimicrobial agents in the hospital setting frequently leads to selection of organisms resistant to those antimicrobial agents and thus creates and maintains a population of drug-resistant nosocomial pathogens in the hospital environment. Physicians have been reluctant to recognize that a decision to use an antimicrobial agent in a given patient has ecologic consequences that extend well beyond the patient at hand.

Types of Antibiotic Misuse or Abuse

There are, of course, several different categories of misuse or abuse of antibiotics. For example, antibiotics are widely misused in prophylaxis. A study by the Inter-Society Committee on Antimicrobial Drug Usage organized by the American College of Physicians [51] showed that > 25% of the total antibiotics used in 20 Pennsylvania hospitals was apparently given for surgical prophylaxis and that almost 80% of such prophylactic use was accounted for by administration of antibiotic prophylaxis beyond the 24- to 48-hour postoperative period when prophylaxis can be anticipated to be effective. There was, in fact, a strong correlation between duration of hospital stay and duration of prophylactic therapy [51]. The duration of therapy in surgical prophylaxis has shortened considerably, however, in response to current recommendations [11].

Antibiotic therapy is often used as a diagnostic procedure. Frequently, antibiotics are given as an empiric test for patients with fever or other presumed evidence of infection; if the patient responds to antibiotic therapy, then infection is presumed to have been the cause. There are, unquestionably, legitimate indications for such use of antibiotics, but most such use is clearly inappropriate.

Antibiotics are often used to treat a disease that does not respond to antibiotics. Contributing to abuse in this area are simple physician ignorance [52] and the common use of antibiotics to treat viral respiratory tract infections on the grounds that it is not likely to harm the patient and might prevent subsequent bacterial infection.

There are mistakes in the use of antibiotics, such as incorrect dosage, incorrect route of administration, inappropriate duration of therapy, or inappropriate choice of drug. In addition, physicians frequently fail to look for or recognize adverse reactions; toxic effects are relatively frequent and particularly prominent in aminoglycoside therapy.

The preferential use of newer and more expensive antibiotics, particularly third-generation cephalosporin drugs and carbepenems, in clinical situations in which older and less expensive drugs have proved effective represents another apparent category of misuse. Kunin [6] has referred to many of the antimicrobial agents introduced during the past decade as "drugs of fear," suggesting that the physician is fearful of not giving the best drug for a presumed infection. Fear that an infection may be due to a highly resistant pathogen is a potent stimulus to physicians to use the broadest-spectrum antibiotics available, at least for initial empiric therapy. This syndrome is particularly common in intensive care units, where the practice has become familiarly known as "antibiotic last rites." The use of second- or third-generation cephalosporins for therapy or surgical prophylaxis in situations in which first-generation cephalosporins have been shown to be effective is a clear example of misuse of "drugs of fear."

Controlling and Improving Antibiotic Use

Kunin was among the first to delineate problems of profligate use of antibiotics and explore the epidemiology of antibiotic use [6]. He outlined a number of approaches to improved use, and relied heavily on the surveillance of antibiotic use within the hospital through some form of audit, educational programs, control of contact between pharmaceutical representatives and staff physicians, and restriction of antibiotics within institutions by the hospital formulary. Also included were controls placed on antibiotic sensitivity testing by the microbiology laboratory, restrictions placed on new or highly expensive antibiotics, and control of some antibiotics by the infectious disease service.

A contemporary view of these methods for controlling antibiotic use was published by Jarvis, and is summarized in Table 14-1. It differs little from the views espoused by Kunin in 1981.

The development of guidelines for appropriate antibiotic use began in 1985, when the Infectious Diseases Society of America appointed an Antimicrobial Agents Committee to assess the extent of the problem and to make recommendations. Interestingly, this was prompted in large part by a challenge to the Society by Kunin. Since that time, the Infectious Diseases Society of America has published a number of guidelines for appropriate antibiotic use [54–56], some of them in association with the Society for Healthcare Epidemiology. Other specialty societies have published such guidelines for infections in their own specialty area. For example, the American Thoracic Society has published guidelines for treatment of community-acquired pneumonia [57]. Publication of guidelines alone, however, is unlikely to change patterns of antibiotic use unless accompanied by a variety of additional steps, especially educational steps.

TABLE 14-1. *Selected methods for improving antimicrobial use*

Guidelines
National
International
Specialty society
Microbiology laboratory testing and reporting
Ensure that accepted standardized methods are used for species identification and antimicrobial susceptibility testing
Careful selection of antimicrobials for antimicrobial susceptibility testing
Selected reporting of antimicrobial testing results
Antimicrobial susceptibility secular trend analyses
Formulary and pharmacy
Selection of formulary agents
Elimination of redundant agents
Provision of comparative cost data (agent, preparation, administration, monitoring, and adverse reaction)
Analysis of secular trends in frequency of agent use by service
Antimicrobial audits
Automatic stop orders
Selection of restricted agents (require approval by infectious diseases service)
Systematic review of antimicrobial use
Antimicrobial use evaluation teams
Implement antimicrobial use policies
Optimize antimicrobial use
Select formulary agents
Educate clinicians on antimicrobial use

(Jarvis WR. Preventing the emergence of multidrug-resistant microorganisms through antimicrobial use controls: the complexity of the problem. *Infect Control Hosp Epidemiol* 1996;17:490–95.)

Microbiology laboratory testing and reporting are important components of improving hospital antibiotic use. The laboratory should ensure that the latest national or international standards are being used. Interpretive guidelines should be provided to clinicians. Use of generic terminology and restrictions on the prescription of new and costly drugs, unless specifically requested or indicated, are also important considerations. Pharmaceutical representatives know only too well that one important way to increase use of their newest product is for the drug sensitivity report to contain a specific listing for that drug. Trends in antibiotic susceptibility by organism should be summarized and sent to all staff physicians at intervals of 3 to 6 months. Consideration should also be given to such analyses that are unit specific. Intensive care units may have extraordinary problems with antibiotic resistance that are simply masked if they are submerged in overall hospital susceptibility data [58,59] (see Chapter 25).

The pharmacy and the formulary selection process also have important roles to play. A number of administrative restraints, both major and minor, have been effectively used in some settings to modulate antibiotic use, especially with new, extended-spectrum, or costly agents [60–64]. These range from automatic stop orders for some or all antibiotics, to a mandate for infectious disease consultation and approval for the use of selected antibiotics. The interposition of such administrative restraints must be carefully individualized to the specific hospital setting. For example, the requirement for infectious disease consultation or approval has worked effectively in many academic settings with full-time infectious disease staff and fellows, whereas in community hospital settings, infectious disease physicians on the medical staff have usually rejected the role of policing antibiotic therapy. More broadly applicable is the requirement for written justification, either in the progress notes or on the order sheet, for the use of selected antibiotics, or even a requirement for infectious disease consultation after a period of 24 to 72 hours of use of such agents.

Even after years of experience with antibiotic control programs and policies, however, questions remain as to just how effective such programs are [65].

An antimicrobial use team, consisting of personnel from pharmacy, infectious disease, infection control, and clinical microbiology, can be extremely helpful in guiding the role of the hospital pharmacy in improving antimicrobial use, and in selecting topics for antimicrobial use audit. A list of possible topics is provided in

Table 14-2; this list is intended only as possible suggestions. Local circumstances and problems should guide the selection of specific topics. Vancomycin use is an important topic in light of the emergence of VRE and the recommendations of the Hospital Infection Control Practices Advisory Committee on improving vancomycin use [66]. As much as half of the total vancomycin use in U.S. hospitals may be inappropriate [67].

Although antibiotic use audits are no longer required by the Joint Commission on Accreditation of Healthcare Organizations, their focused use is still strongly recommended because they can play an important role in modifying antibiotic prescribing practices.

The following suggestions are offered to help maximize the potential benefit of antibiotic auditing. First, the focus should be on several specific clinical issues rather than making an attempt to audit all antimicrobial use. Questions should be constructed specifically, remembering that the primary reason for antibiotic audit is to improve medical care and reduce its cost. The purpose is not to introduce conflict among the medical staff or to identify one or more physicians as being "guilty" of antibiotic abuse.

Second, the audit should concentrate on areas of therapy or prophylaxis in which generally accepted national standards exist. Such national standards should be developed by, explained to, and agreed on by that segment of the medical staff involved in a given area of audit. The standards should be agreed on by all concerned as representing appropriate standards of therapy or prophylaxis. Reasonable and nationally acceptable standards of therapy exist or could be developed for a number of medical conditions such as pneumonia, intraabdominal infections, septicemia, endocarditis, and osteomyelitis. In many areas of antibiotic therapy, however, controversy exists; often there are legitimate differences of opinion as to the best approach to therapy. It is important that such areas be avoided as subjects for audit and that efforts be concentrated on areas for which acceptable and reasonable standards do exist.

Third, audits of the prophylactic use of antibiotics in surgery have been emphasized because this area has been identified as a major contributor to antibiotic cost and misuse. Procedures for which prophylaxis is recommended include, among others, prosthetic valve and open heart procedures; coronary artery bypass surgery; insertion of prosthetic joints; colonic surgery; biliary tract surgery in a patient older than 70 years or with acute cholecystitis, obstructive jaundice, or choledocholithiasis; vaginal hysterectomy; cesarean section; and urologic surgery on bacteriuric patients. It is important to emphasize the appropriate preoperative timing of surgical prophylaxis and that prophylaxis should be terminated within 24 hours after completion of surgery (see Chapter 37).

Fourth, the antibiotic audit should be by peer review rather than review strictly by hospital administration, infection control personnel, or pharmacy personnel. Thus, it should be a medical staff responsibility, with standards defined and agreed on by infectious disease consultants among the staff and by the medical staff being audited. Infection control personnel and pharmacy personnel may be extraordinarily helpful in the conduct of the audit, but should not have a dominant role in identifying the standards to be met. Broader acceptance of the results of an audit will follow if it is seen as a medical staff review rather than an administrative one.

Fifth, few, if any, of the standards to be developed should be so rigid as to prohibit exception. Few absolute standards exist; variation from agreed-on standards should appropriately prompt additional review but should not be automatically construed as indicating error. Reviewers must allow for the variety of clinical circumstances that might dictate some degree of variation from generally accepted standards.

If problems are identified in a given area of audit, the audit should be used to bring about change. This requires feedback of the information derived to that segment of the medical staff being audited, together with recommendations to improve use. Whether improvement results can be evaluated only by ongoing or repeat audit.

Bryan has summarized the advantages and disadvantages of many of the various strategies for improving antibiotic use, and these are shown in Table 14-3. As the antimicrobial drug resistance of nosocomial pathogens increases and as the cost of new antibiotics mounts, implementation of these sound and sensible recommendations will become ever more important.

A major contributor to our current problems of antibiotic abuse has been physician failure to appreciate the effects of antibiotic use on the institutional microbial ecology, effects that go well beyond the patient at hand.

TABLE 14-2. *Selected situations for antimicrobial use audits*

Antimicrobial use without a minimum diagnostic evaluation
Concurrent use of > 2 antimicrobials
Use of > 5 antimicrobials during a single hospitalization
Continuous antimicrobial use for > 21 days
Use of parenteral rather than an oral agent
Prophylaxis > 48 hr
Unaccepted prophylaxis
Lack of monitoring (levels, toxicity)
Use of oral vancomycin
Use of intravenous vancomycin for other than indicated uses
Review of conditions receiving antimicrobial prophylaxis and the agent used
Review of empiric antimicrobial use
Review of selected definitive clinical conditions and the antimicrobials used for these conditions

(Jarvis WR. Preventing the emergence of multidrug-resistant microorganisms through antimicrobial use controls: the complexity of the problem. *Infect Control Hosp Epidemiol* 1996;17:490–95.)

TABLE 14-3. *Strategies for improving antibiotic use*

Strategy	Advantages	Disadvantages
Education	Palatable; does not encroach on the "practice of medicine"	Requires continuous reinforcement; effectiveness is difficult to document
Hospital formulary	Immediate impact; enables generic and therapeutic equivalency substitutions	Requires strong Pharmacy and Therapeutics Committee; perception that patient care is being compromised
Ordering policies	Special order sheets have been shown to be effective; automatic stop orders are also useful	Extra paperwork; physicians may be resentful; automatic stop orders may at times compromise patient care
Drug utilization review	Provides feedback to physicians; ongoing, comprehensive review enables intervention	Labor-intensive; requires contact time between reviewers and physicians
Restriction policies	Enables tight control, especially of the newer, more expensive agents	Limits freedom of physicians; may arouse resentment against the "police officers"
Control of laboratory susceptibility testing	Easily accomplished; can influence prescribing habits	May hinder appropriate use, especially of the newer agents
Limitation of contact time between physicians and pharmaceutical representatives	Probably effective in the teaching setting; minimizes confusion among residents	Probably ineffective in the private practice setting

(Reprinted with permission from Bryan CS. Strategies to improve antibiotic use. *Infect Dis Clin North Am* 3:723,1989.)

Among all the factors that physicians consider in selecting one or more antibiotics with which to treat a patient, the impact on patterns of future antibiotic resistance is usually not among them. Some would argue that it is time to restrict prescription of certain antibiotics to selected physicians with special training and expertise in effective use of antibiotics. Such a proposal would, of course, be vigorously opposed by many physician groups on the local, regional, and national levels. Another negative feature of such a proposal is that pharmaceutical companies would be far more hesitant about investing in new antibiotic development if such new drugs were to be prescribed exclusively by an elite cadre of physicians with the right expertise, but who would likely be very conservative in their use of such drugs. If already serious problems of multidrug resistance deteriorate further, however, such steps may ultimately prove necessary.

The report of a multidisciplinary consensus conference on strategies to prevent and control the emergence and spread of multidrug-resistant pathogens in the hospital environment was published in 1996 [69]. Their strategic goals to accomplish this purpose are shown in Table 14-4. Steps to reach these goals were outlined in detail, and various measurements delineated by which to measure progress toward these goals. Barriers to be expected along the way were identified, as were countermeasures and other strategies to overcome the barriers. Thus, a series of steps were outlined that would guide hospitals that really wanted to do something about their resistance problems. Possibly the most critical requirement in this suggested program is the necessity for full support and commitment from the hospital leadership, including administration, the board of directors, and the medical staff leadership. The report is clearly a challenge to hospital leadership, but it is too early to evaluate any possible impact of this challenge. It is a proposal that should be considered by infection control and pharmacy personnel, as well as the hospital leadership in every hospital in the country.

A report from the Latter Day Saints Hospital in Salt Lake City [70] illustrates what can be accomplished when all the critical ingredients are present. The critical ingredients, in this instance, were committed investigators in infectious disease and clinical epidemiology, administrative commitment in the form of a state-of-the-art computer-based hospital information system, and medical staff input and partnership in the process of developing an antibiotic management program using that hospital's infectious disease data base. Using such a system, during the 7-year period from 1988 to 1994, the overall proportion of patients receiving antibiotics increased from 32% to 53% during the study period, yet the inflation-adjusted acquisition costs actually decreased by almost 50%, and the antibiotic costs per treated patient decreased by > 50%. A standardized method to compare antibiotic use showed that there was a 23% decrease in overall antibiotic use during the study period. The average number of antibiotic doses used in surgical prophylaxis dropped from 19 in the base year to 5.3 doses in 1994! Equally important, resistance patterns among nosocomial pathogens at the Latter Day Saints Hospital appeared to stabilize, and showed little change during the study period. It will be critically important to determine whether these encouraging results can be duplicated in other hospitals using comparable methodology, computer technology, and medical staff participation and feedback.

TABLE 14-4. *Strategic goals*

Strategies to optimize the prophylactic, empiric, and therapeutic use of antimicrobials in the hospital:
1. Optimize antimicrobial prophylaxis for operative procedures.
2. Optimize choice and duration of empiric antimicrobial therapy.
3. Improve antimicrobial prescribing practices by educational and administrative means.
4. Establish a system to monitor and provide feedback on the occurrence and impact of antibiotic resistance.
5. Define and implement institutional or health care delivery system guidelines for important types of antimicrobial use.

Strategies for detecting, reporting, and preventing transmission of antimicrobial-resistant microorganisms:
1. Develop a system to recognize and promptly report significant changes and trends in antimicrobial resistance to hospital and physician leaders; medical, nursing, infection control, and pharmacy staffs; and others who need to know.
2. Develop a system for rapid detection and reporting of resistant microorganisms in individual patients to appropriate personnel (caregivers and infection control staff) and for rapid response by caregivers.
3. Increase adherence to policies and procedures, especially hand hygiene, barrier precautions, and environmental control measures.
4. Incorporate the detection, prevention, and control of antimicrobial resistance into institutional strategic goals and provide required resources (e.g., by providing adequate facilities and resources for hand washing, isolation, and environmental hygiene; funding ongoing monitoring and data collection, including infection control/hospital epidemiology and quality improvement in the planning process; and setting managerial goals and accountability for reductions in colonization and infection with resistant microorganisms).
5. Develop a plan for identifying, transferring, discharging, and readmitting patients colonized with specified antimicrobial-resistant microorganisms.[a]

[a]Each hospital should specify a list of problematic pathogens, such as methicillin-resistant *Staphylococcus aureus,* vancomycin-resistant and high-level penicillin-resistant enterococci, and gram-negative bacilli resistant to third-generation cephalosporins and aminoglycosides.

(Goldmann DA, Weinstein RA, Wenzel RP, et al. Strategies to prevent and control the emergence and spread of antimicrobial-resistant microorganisms in hospitals. *JAMA* 1996; 275:234–40.)

We have already reentered the era of having no effective antimicrobial therapy for several multidrug-resistant nosocomial pathogens, and the threat of vancomycin-resistant MRSA looms large on the horizon. Only a few physicians today recall having no effective therapy available for treating staphylococcal infections, but I can attest that it was both frightening and humbling. Hospitals will likely continue to be breeding grounds for the development of more multidrug-resistant pathogens.

There are, nonetheless, reasons for optimism. Emerging problems of drug resistance and multidrug-resistant pathogens are much more readily appreciated by both physicians and the public than ever before. The topic has been widely publicized in popular media in recent years; numerous authorities and professional organizations have taken note and have made recommendations to address the problem [71–77].

Knowledge of resistance mechanisms should guide the pharmaceutical industry in developing new drugs designed to obviate certain resistance genes or gene products, or to identify new targets in pathogenic bacteria for antibiotic action. Even when such advances are made, however, we must continue all efforts to ensure optimal and wise use of antibiotics in hospitals as well as in the community to minimize the selection and spread of antibiotic-resistant pathogens. Otherwise, we are likely to witness continuing erosion in our existing antibiotic armamentarium.

REFERENCES

1. Finland M. Changing ecology of bacterial infections as related to antibacterial therapy. *J Infect Dis* 1970;122:419–431.
2. National Nosocomial Infections Surveillance (NNIS) System, Centers for Disease Control and Prevention. National Nosocomial Infections Surveillance (NNIS) report, data summary from October 1986–April 1996, issued May 1996. *Am J Infect Control* 1996;24:380–388.
3. Swartz MN. Hospital-acquired infections: diseases with increasingly limited therapies. *Proc Natl Acad Sci USA* 1994;91:2420–2427.
4. Jones RN. Impact of changing pathogens and antimicrobial susceptibility patterns in the treatment of serious infections in hospitalized patients. *Am J Med* 1996;100(Suppl 6A):3S–11S.
5. Buckwold, FJ, Ronald AR. Antimicrobial misuse: effects and suggestions for control. *J Antimicrob Chemother* 1979;5:129–136.
6. Kunin CM. Evaluation of antibiotic usage: a comprehensive look at alternative approaches. *Rev Infect Dis* 1981;3:745–753.
7. Pallares R, Dick R, Wenzel RP, et al. Trends in antimicrobial utilization at a tertiary teaching hospital during a 15-year period (1978–1982). *Infect Control Hosp Epidemiol* 1993;14:376–382.
8. McGowan JE Jr, Finland M. Infection and antibiotic usage at Boston City Hospital: changes in prevalence during the decade 1964 1973. *J Infect Dis* 1974;129:421–428.
9. Scheckler WE, Bennett JV. Antibiotic usage in seven community hospitals. *JAMA* 1970;213:264–267.
10. Kunin CM, Tupasi T, Craig WA. Use of antibiotics: a brief exposition of the problem and some tentative solutions. *Ann Intern Med* 1973;79: 555–560.
11. Huth TS, Burke JP. Infections and antibiotic use in a community hospital, 1971–1990. *Infect Control Hosp Epidemiol* 1991;12:525–534.
12. Fernandes PB. Pharmaceutical perspective on the development of drugs to treat infectious diseases. *ASM News* 1996;62(1):21–24.
13. Mitsuhashi S, ed. *Transferable drug resistance factor R.* Baltimore: University Park Press; 1971.
14. Finland M. Changing patterns of susceptibility of common bacterial pathogens to antimicrobial agents. *Ann Intern Med* 1972;76: 1009–1036.
15. Finland M. And the walls come tumbling down: more antibiotic resistance, and now the pneumococcus. *N Engl J Med* 1978;299:770–771.
16. Davies JE. Resistance to aminoglycosides: mechanisms and frequency. *Rev Infect Dis* 1983;5:S261.
17. Jessen O, Rosendahl K, Bulow P, et al. Changing staphylococci and staphylococcal infections. *N Engl J Med* 1969;281:627–635.
18. Holmberg SD, Solomon SL, Blake PA. Health and economic impacts of antimicrobial resistance. *Rev Infect Dis* 1987;9:1065–1070.
19. Shay DK, Maloney SA, Montecalvo M, et al. Epidemiology and mortality risk of vancomycin-resistant enterococcal bloodstream infections. *J Infect Dis* 1995;172:993–1000.
20. Yamamoto T, Echeverria P, Yokota T. Drug resistance and adherence to

human intestines of enteroaggregative *Escherichia coli*. *J Infect Dis* 1992;165:744–749.
21. Lepper MH, Moulton B, Dowling HF, et al. Epidemiology of erythromycin-resistant staphylococci in a hospital population: effect on therapeutic activity of erythromycin. *Antibiotics Annual* 1954;1953–54: 308–313.
22. Gibson CD Jr, Thompson WC Jr. The response of burn wound staphylococci to alternating programs of antibiotic therapy. *Antibiotics Annual* 1956;1955–56:32–34.
23. Bauer AW, Perry DM, Kirby WMM. Drug usage and antibiotic susceptibility of staphylococci. *JAMA* 1960;173:475–480.
24. Barber M, Dutton AAC, Beard MA, et al. Reversal of antibiotic resistance in hospital staphylococcal infection. *Br Med J* 1960;1:11–17.
25. Franco JA, Eitzman DV, Baer J. Antibiotic usage and microbial resistance in an intensive care nursery. *American Journal of Diseases of Children* 1973;126:318–321.
26. Sogaard H, Zimmerman-Nielson C, Siboni K. Antibiotic-resistant gram-negative bacilli in a urological ward for male patients during a nine-year period: relationship to antibiotic consumption. *J Infect Dis* 1974;130:646–650.
27. Bulger RJ, Larson E, Sherris JC. Decreased incidence of resistance to antimicrobial agents among *Escherichia coli* and *Klebsiella–Enterobacter*: observations in a university hospital over a 10-year period. *Ann Intern Med* 1970;72:65–71.
28. Lowbury EJL, Babb JR, Roe E. Clearance from a hospital of gram-negative bacilli that transfer carbenicillin resistance to *Pseudomonas aeruginosa*. *Lancet* 1972;2:941–945.
29. Price DJE, Sleigh JD. Control of infection due to *Klebsiella aerogenes* in a neurosurgical unit by withdrawal of all antibiotics. *Lancet* 1970;2: 1213–1215.
30. Gold HS, Moellering RC Jr. Antimicrobial-drug resistance. *N Engl J Med* 1996;335:1445–1453.
31. Ballow CH, Schentag JJ. Trends in antibiotic utilization and bacterial resistance: report of the National Nosocomial Resistance Surveillance Group. *Diagn Microbiol Infect Dis* 1992;15(Suppl 2):37S–42S.
32. McGowan JE Jr. Antimicrobial resistance in hospital organisms and its relation to antibiotic use. *Rev Infect Dis* 1983;5:1033–1048.
33. McGowan JE Jr. Is antimicrobial resistance in hospital organisms related to antibiotic use? *Bull N Y Acad Med* 1987;63:253–268.
34. Tenover FC, McGowan JE Jr. Reasons for the emergence of antibiotic resistance. *Am J Med Sci* 1996;311:9–16.
35. Schentag JJ. Understanding and managing microbial resistance in institutional settings. *American Journal of Health-Syst Pharm* 1995;52 (Suppl 2):S9–S14.
36. Chetchotisakd P, Phelps CL, Hartstein AI. Assessment of bacterial cross-transmission as a cause of infection in patients in intensive care units. *Clin Infect Dis* 1994;18:929–937.
37. Weinstein RA. Epidemiology and control of nosocomial infections in adult intensive care units. *Am J Med* 1991;91(Suppl 3B):179S–184S.
38. Korzeniowski OM. Effects of antibiotics on the mammalian immune system. *Infect Dis Clin North Am* 1989;3:469–478.
39. Mandell LA. Effects of antimicrobial and antineoplastic drugs on the phagocytic and microbicidal function of the polymorphonuclear leukocyte. *Rev Infect Dis* 1982;4:683–697.
40. Milatovic D. Antibiotics and phagocytosis. *Eur J Clin Microbiol* 1983; 2:414–425.
41. Thong YH. Immunomodulation by antimicrobial drugs. *Med Hypotheses* 1982;8:361–370.
42. Hurley JC. Antibiotic-induced release of endotoxin: a reappraisal. *Clin Infect Dis* 1992;15:840–854.
43. Hurley JC. Antibiotic-induced release of endotoxin: a therapeutic paradox. *Drug Safety* 1995;12:183–195.
44. Jacobs NF Jr. Antibiotic-induced diarrhea and pseudomembranous colitis. *Postgrad Med* 1994;95:117–120.
45. Bartlett JG. Antibiotic-associated diarrhea. *Clin Infect Dis* 1992;15: 573–581.
46. Van der Waaij D. Colonization resistance of the digestive tract: clinical consequences and implications. *J Antimicrob Chemother* 1982;10: 263–270.
47. Hooker KD, DiPiro JT. Effect of antimicrobial therapy on bowel flora. *Clin Pharm* 1988;7:878–888.
48. Bartlett JG. Selective decontamination of the digestive tract and its effect on antimicrobial resistance. *Crit Care Med* 1995;23:613–615.
49. Kollef MH. Antibiotic use and antibiotic resistance in the intensive care unit: are we curing or creating disease? *Heart Lung* 1994;23:363–367.
50. Selective Decontamination of the Digestive Tract Trialists' Collaborative Group. Meta-analysis of randomized controlled trials of selective decontamination of the digestive tract. *Br Med J* 1993;307:525–532.
51. Shapiro M, Townsend TR, Rosner B, et al. Use of antimicrobial drugs in general hospitals: patterns of prophylaxis. *N Engl J Med* 1979;301: 351–355.
52. Neu HC, Howrey SP. Testing the physician's knowledge of antibiotic use: self-assessment and learning via videotape. *N Engl J Med* 1975; 293:1291–1295.
53. Jarvis WR. Preventing the emergence of multidrug-resistant microorganisms through antimicrobial use controls: the complexity of the problem. *Infect Control Hosp Epidemiol* 1996;17:490–495.
54. Marr JJ, Moffet HL, Kunin CM. Guidelines for improving the use of antimicrobial agents in hospitals: a statement by the Infectious Diseases Society of America. *J Infect Dis* 1988;157:869–876.
55. McGowan JE Jr, Chesney PG, Crossley KB, et al. Guidelines for the use of systemic glucocorticosteroids in the management of selected infections. *J Infect Dis* 1992;165:1–13.
56. Dellinger EP, Gross PA, Barrett TL, et al. Quality standard for antimicrobial prophylaxis in surgical procedures. *Infect Control Hosp Epidemiol* 1994;15:182–188.
57. American Thoracic Society. Guidelines for the initial management of adults with community-acquired pneumonia: diagnosis, assessment of severity, and initial antimicrobial therapy. *Am Rev Respir Dis* 1993;148: 1418–1426.
58. Bryce EA, Smith AJ. Focused microbiological surveillance and gram-negative β-lactamase-mediated resistance in an intensive care unit. *Infect Control Hosp Epidemiol* 1995;16:331–334.
59. Gaynes R. Antibiotic resistance in ICUs: a multifaceted problem requiring a multifaceted solution. *Infect Control Hosp Epidemiol* 1995; 16:328–330.
60. Hirschman SZ, Myers BR, Bradbury K, et al. Use of antimicrobial agents in a university teaching hospital: evolution of a comprehensive control program. *Arch Intern Med* 1988;148:2001–2007.
61. Jackson GG. Antibiotic policies, practices, and pressures. *J Antimicrob Chemother* 1979;5:1–4.
62. McGowan JE Jr, Finland M. Usage of antibiotics in a general hospital: effect of requiring justification. *J Infect Dis* 1974;130:165–168.
63. Noone P, Shafi MS. Controlling infection in a district general hospital. *J Clin Pathol* 1973;26:140–145.
64. Recco RA, Gladstone JL, Friedman SA, et al. Antibiotic control in a municipal hospital. *JAMA* 1979;241:2283–2286.
65. McGowan JE Jr. Do intensive hospital antibiotic control programs prevent the spread of antibiotic resistance? *Infect Control Hosp Epidemiol* 1994;15:478–483.
66. Centers for Disease Control and Prevention. Recommendations for preventing the spread of vancomycin resistance: recommendations of the Hospital Infection Control Practices Advisory Committee (HICPAC). *MMWR Morb Mortal Wkly Rep* 1995;44(RR-12):1–13.
67. Evans ME, Kortas KJ. Vancomycin use in a university medical center: comparison with Hospital Infection Control Practices Advisory Committee guidelines. *Infect Control Hosp Epidemiol* 1996;17:356–359.
68. Bryan CS. Strategies to improve antibiotic use. *Infect Dis Clin North Am* 1989;3:723–734.
69. Goldmann DA, Weinstein RA, Wenzel RP, et al. Strategies to prevent and control the emergence and spread of antimicrobial-resistant microorganisms in hospitals: a challenge to hospital leadership. *JAMA* 1996; 275:234–240.
70. Pestotnik SL, Classen DC, Evans RS, et al. Implementing antibiotic practice guidelines through computer-assisted decision support: clinical and financial outcomes. *Ann Intern Med* 1996;124:884–890.
71. Institute of Medicine. *Emerging infections: microbial threats to health in the United States*. Washington, DC: National Academy Press, 1992.
72. Tomasz A. Multiple-antibiotic-resistant pathogenic bacteria: a report on the Rockefeller University Workshop. *N Engl J Med* 1994;330: 1247–1251.
73. Murray BE. Can antibiotic resistance be controlled? *N Engl J Med* 1994;330:1229–1230.
74. American Society for Microbiology. Report of the ASM Task Force on Antibiotic Resistance. *Antimicrob Agents Chemother* 1995;39(Suppl 5):1–23.
75. Kunin CM. Resistance to antimicrobial drugs: a worldwide calamity. *Ann Intern Med* 1993;118:557–560.
76. Cohen ML. Epidemiology of drug resistance: implications for a post-antimicrobial era. *Science* 1992;257:1050–1055.
77. Neu HC. The crisis in antibiotic resistance. *Science* 1992;257: 1064–1073.

Hospital Infections, Fourth Edition,
edited by John V. Bennett and Philip S. Brachman.
Lippincott–Raven Publishers, Philadelphia © 1998

CHAPTER 15

Multiply Drug-Resistant Pathogens: Epidemiology and Control

Robert A. Weinstein and Mary K. Hayden

Our antimicrobial pharmacopeia and the organisms that colonize and infect our patients are in continual competition. At times, the lag between introduction of a new antibiotic and increasing prevalence of resistant bacteria (and fungi and viruses) has been very long; for example, ampicillin was in use for many years before the widespread emergence of resistant *Hemophilus influenzae*, an organism initially susceptible to it. At other times, resistance has occurred even before the clinical use of a specific antibiotic; for example, sulfonamide and aminoglycoside resistance can be found in gram-negative bacilli isolated long before our use of these compounds. Such disparities have led to a controversy over whether antibiotic use and abuse or other host and environmental factors are most responsible for the increasing prevalence of antibiotic-resistant microorganisms in the community and in hospitals [1] (see Chapter 14). Nevertheless, it appears to be conventional wisdom that our antibiotic choices seldom remain more than a very few drugs ahead of the resistant strains.

Since the 1960s, reports of antibiotic-resistant bacteria in hospitals have appeared with increasing frequency. For example, before 1965 no hospital outbreaks involving multiply resistant gram-negative bacilli were investigated by the Centers for Disease Control and Prevention (CDC). During 1965 to 1975, however, 11 of 15 nosocomial epidemics of Enterobacteriaceae studied involved multiply resistant strains [2]. Among gram-positive bacteria, resistance of *Staphylococcus aureus* to penicillins became epidemic in the early 1960s and ultimately has come to be considered the norm. Since the late 1960s, outbreaks of methicillin-resistant *S. aureus* (MRSA) have been reported, first from Europe and, more recently, from the United States [3] (Figure 15-1) (see Chapters 14, 41).

In the 1980s, large families of β-lactamases that mediate resistance to newer cephalosporin antibiotics emerged in Enterobacteriaceae; vancomycin resistance in gram-positive cocci was described; and aminoglycoside-resistant, β-lactamase-containing enterococci surfaced. The 1990s have begun to witness staphylococcal and pseudomonal resistance to the fluoroquinolone antibiotics, and imipenem resistance in Enterobacteriaceae. Moreover, since the mid-1980s, the incidence of nosocomial infections caused by enteric gram-negative bacilli, such as *Klebsiella pneumoniae* and *Escherichia coli*, has decreased, whereas the incidence of infections due to more resistant gram-negative pathogens, gram-positive bacteria, and fungi have increased [4] (see Figure 15-1). Although the reason for this shift is not entirely clear, it may be explained partially by the widespread use of a variety of antibiotics, such as cephalosporins, which inhibit growth of many gram-negative bacteria, but have little or no activity against enterococci, coagulase-negative staphylococci, or *Candida* species. The selective pressure for survival of the latter group of pathogens is therefore increased. In addition, the availability of a range of treatment options for infections caused by gram-negative bacteria may effectively control this population of bacteria and decrease the likelihood of intense selective pressure by any single agent. Emergence and dissemination of resistant bacterial subpopulations would then be less likely.

Bacterial resistance has become a fact of hospital life and is so common that it often goes unnoted until it is either extreme or epidemic. In this chapter, we review the epidemiology of drug-resistant strains in hospitals and discuss prevention and control strategies.

R. A. Weinstein: Department of Medicine, Rush Medical College, Division of Infectious Diseases, Cook County Hospital, Chicago, Illinois 60612-9985.

M. K. Hayden: Department of Medicine, Section of Infectious Disease, Rush Medical College, Chicago, Illinois 60612.

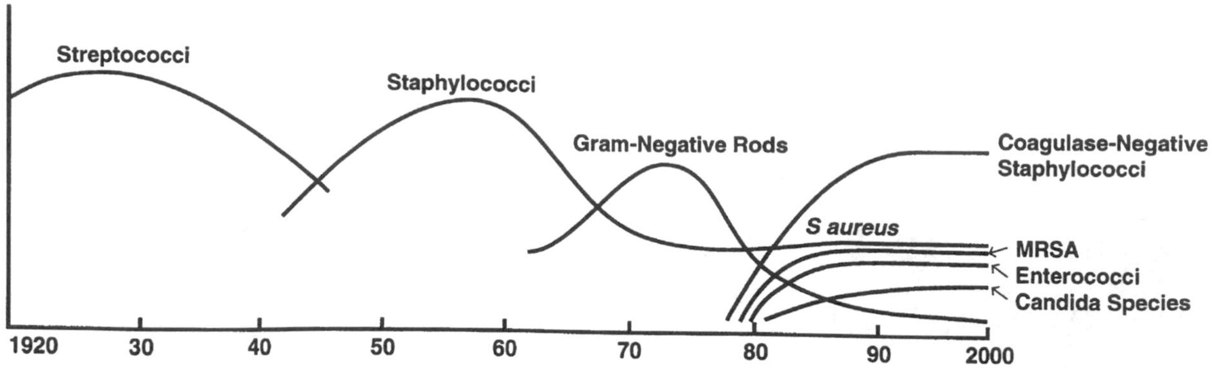

FIGURE 15-1. Schematic representation of the periods during which new pathogens emerged as prominent causes of nosocomial infections. (Reprinted with permission from Herwaldt LA, Wenzel RP. Dynamics of hospital-acquired infections. In: Murray PR, Baron EJ, Pfaller MA, Tenover FC, Yolken RH, eds. *Manual of clinical microbiology.* 6th ed. Washington, DC: American Society of Microbiology Press, 1995:172.)

DEFINITION, MECHANISMS, AND GENETICS OF MULTIPLE RESISTANCE

Although there is no standard definition for multiple resistance in bacteria, one definition commonly used is resistance to two or more unrelated antibiotics to which the bacteria are normally considered susceptible [1,5].

Alternatively, resistance to certain key or first-line drugs may be used as a marker for problems, such as aminoglycoside (gentamicin, tobramycin, amikacin, or netilmicin) or third-generation cephalosporin (e.g., ceftazidime, ceftriaxone) resistance in gram-negative bacilli. Indeed, our level of concern often depends on the nature and availability of other agents. Thus, penicillin-resistant staphylococci were accepted relatively passively once methicillin became available. However, the therapeutic alternative for methicillin-resistant strains, vancomycin, is a relatively toxic agent, which has heightened our concern about resistant staphylococcal strains. More recently, the identification in Japan of a clinical MRSA strain with decreased susceptibility to vancomycin [6] and the transfer of vancomycin resistance from an *Enterococcus faecium* strain to *S. aureus* in vitro [7] raise the concern that vancomycin resistance in MRSA could emerge as a significant clinical problem. While the impact reduced susceptibility to vancomycin on clinical outcome is still uncertain, serious infections due to MRSA with high level vancomycin resistance would potentially be untreatable, making control of vancomycin resistance in enterococci a priority.

The most common mechanisms of resistance include production by bacteria of antibiotic-inactivating enzymes, such as β-lactamases or aminoglycoside-modifying enzymes; changes in cell wall permeability or uptake of antibiotics; alteration in target sites, such as ribosomes; changes in susceptible metabolic pathways; or changes in cell wall binding sites, such as the penicillin-binding proteins [8] (see Chapter 14).

Resistance may be mediated by either the bacterial chromosome or extrachromosomal DNA (plasmids) [8] (see Chapters 14, 16). Chromosomal resistance occurs by spontaneous mutation and darwinian selection of organisms resistant to single (or closely related) agents. In contrast, bacteria may acquire resistance rapidly by the accrual of resistance plasmids (R factors), which often encode multiple resistances to unrelated drugs. Plasmids may spread across species lines and even between genera. An example of extensive spread is the presence of the same plasmid-mediated TEM-1 β-lactamase, an enzyme that confers resistance to ampicillin in a variety of gram-negative bacteria, including Enterobacteriaceae, gonococci, and *H. influenzae*. There has also been a rekindling of interest in the study of environmentally induced or directed mutagenesis [10].

At the molecular level, portions of plasmids called *transposons* may hitchhike from one plasmid to another or between plasmid and bacterial chromosome. Transposons carrying genes for resistance may align with other elements, such as those encoding virulence or colonization factors, creating R factors with an awesome "one-two punch." *Integrons* comprise a related class of mobile genetic elements that allow site-specific integration and efficient expression of multiple different antibiotic resistance genes by a bacterium [11].

PATHOGENS AND INCIDENCE

The problem of resistance occurs in the community and hospital for both gram-positive and gram-negative bacteria. For example, resistance at the community level has affected *Salmonella, Shigella, E. coli, Neisseria gonorrhoeae, H. influenzae* and, most recently, *Streptococcus pneumoniae* and *Neisseria meningitides*. Moreover, resistance problems that traditionally have been considered nosocomial, such as methicillin-resistance in *S. aureus*, are becoming increasingly prevalent outside of acute care settings. Three surveillance studies have reported community acquisition of MRSA in 20% to 62% of cases [12–14]. Resistance in hospitals has appeared in a variety of gram-negative bacilli as well as in common skin flora, such as coagulase-negative staphylococci and corynebacteria. Although the specific "problem bugs" vary from hospital to hospital and depend on the interaction of a number of factors to be described, there are some general correlations between hospital settings and resistant flora (Table 15-1).

One of the greatest concerns in the 1970s and early 1980s was the emergence of aminoglycoside resistance in nosocomial Enterobacteriaceae and *Pseudomonas*. In individual hospitals, the prevalence of aminoglycoside-resistant gram-negative bacilli varies considerably, usually being greatest in large hospitals and teaching institutions [15–19]. Data from the National Nosocomial Infection Surveillance (NNIS) System show that the percentage of *Pseudomonas aeruginosa* resistant to gentamicin increased from 6.6% in 1975 to 13.1% in 1979 [20], but was still 13.4% in 1984 [16] and also in 1990.

More recently, the availability of the second-generation cephalosporins, such as cefamandole, cefoxitin, and cefuroxime, or third-generation agents, such as cefotaxime, cefoperazone, ceftizoxime, ceftriaxone, and ceftazidime, and of combination agents, such as ticarcillin–clavulanate, has called attention to an additional set of potential resistances in nosocomial gram-negative bacilli [21]. For instance, *Enterobacter* species were considered initially susceptible to cefamandole but frequently developed resistance during therapy because of spontaneous derepression of intrinsic chromosomal type I β-lactamase [22, 23]. Now that the second- and third-generation drugs have been available for several years, resistance among *Enterobacter* species is widespread. In a six-hospital study of 136 cases of *Enterobacter* bacteremia, 32% of isolates were resistant to all cephalosporins and penicillins [24]. Similarly, 1987 to 1991 NNIS data revealed that 36.2% of *Enterobacter* species from reporting hospitals were resistant to ceftazidime [25]. In contrast, resistance in *P. aeruginosa* remained stable at ~ 9.7% during this period. Another multicenter survey found a correlation between rising ceftazidime use and increasing ceftazidime resistance among isolates of *Enterobacter cloacae*, but not *P. aeruginosa* [26]. The extent to which the regional differences and increases in resistance correlate with the use of these agents needs to be assessed further.

Families of plasmidborne, extended-spectrum β-lactamases, first identified in 1983 to 1985 in Europe, are also capable of inactivating many of the newer cephalosporins, including ceftazidime, and broad-spectrum penicillins [27]. These enzymes evolved by point mutations from common, older plasmidborne enzymes and are transferable to bacteria that do not have the intrinsic chromosomal genetic material to allow broad-spectrum resistance. These extended-spectrum β-lactamases are now being reported from several centers in the United States [27]. One NNIS hospital reported a rise in ceftazidime-resistant *K. pneumoniae* from 1.0% in 1987 to 1989 to 40% in 1990 to 1991, suggesting that once resistance emerges, it can disseminate rapidly [25].

The broadest-spectrum, commercially available parenteral antimicrobial is the carbapenem, imipenem. Analysis of 1986 to 1989 NNIS data revealed that only 1.3% of 1,282 *Enterobacter* species isolates were resistant to this agent [28]. However, the rate of imipenem resistance in *P. aeruginosa* was already 11.1% in the NNIS hospitals [28]. Imipenem resistance has also been reported in strains of *Serratia marcescens* [29] and *Acinetobacter baumannii* [30]. Interestingly, the *Acinetobacter* outbreak occurred in a hospital that had recently increased its use of imipenem for treatment of increasing numbers of infections due to ceftazidime-resistant *K. pneumoniae* [30].

TABLE 15-1. *Resistance problems in the 1990s*

Setting	Bacteria	Key resistances
General hospitals and intensive care units	Enterobacteriaceae	Newer cephalosporins, aminoglycosides, carbapenems, quinolones
	Pseudomonas aeruginosa	Aminoglycosides, antipseudomonal penicillins, newer cephalosporins, carbapenems, quinolones
	Acinetobacter spp	Aminoglycosides, multiple
	Stenotrophomonas maltophilia	Multiple
	Staphylococcus aureus	Methicillin, quinolones, multiple
	Streptococcus pneumoniae	Penicillin, multiple
	Enterococci	Gentamicin, ampicillin, vancomycin, multiple
Oncology units	Enterobacteriaceae	Trimethoprim-sulfamethoxazole
	JK diphtheroids	Multiple
	Staphylococcus epidermidis	Multiple
	Enterococci	Gentamicin, ampicillin, vancomycin, multiple
Geriatric units	*Proteus, Providencia, Morganella*	Aminoglycosides, newer cephalosporins
	Staphylococcus aureus	Methicillin, quinolones
	Enterococci	Gentamicin, ampicillin, vancomycin, multiple

The prevalence of enteric bacilli resistant to trimethoprim (TMP) and TMP–sulfonamide combinations has been variable [31,32]. For example, TMP has been in use in Finland since 1973; in 1980 to 1981, from 8.6% to 38.3% of nosocomial urinary isolates (*Pseudomonas* excluded) were resistant, depending on the hospital studied [33]. When TMP–sulfamethoxazole has been used in a variety of settings for prophylaxis, prevalence of resistant strains has varied from 0% to 100%. In many U.S. hospitals, however, bacteria resistant to newer cephalosporins are often still susceptible to TMP–sulfamethoxazole [24].

For gram-positive bacteria, methicillin resistance in *S. aureus* and the increasing occurrence of disease caused by multiply resistant coagulase-negative staphylococci have been of concern. In 63 NNIS hospitals during 1974 to 1981, the percentage of *S. aureus* infections resistant to methicillin rose from a low of 2.4% (1975) to a high of only 5% (1981) [3]. This increase was due entirely to four large teaching institutions in which the percentages rose from 0% to 5% to 15% to 50%. By 1992, the pooled percentage of MRSA reported to NNIS had risen to 32.1% [34] (Table 15-2). Hospitals of all sizes were affected, although the rate of increase was greater in larger hospitals. MRSA were reported to be more resistant to non-β-lactam antibiotics than were methicillin-susceptible *S. aureus* (MSSA). In the period 1989 to 1992, gentamicin resistance was reported in 67.2% of MRSA, but only 3.1% of MSSA, whereas resistance to TMP–sulfamethoxazole was 39.2% and 1.4% in MRSA and MSSA, respectively.

The incidence of infection due to coagulase-negative staphylococci and the percentage of these pathogens resistant to methicillin also has been increasing. At one large cancer center, the incidence of infection due to coagulase-negative staphylococci rose from 2 per 1000 days of hospitalization in 1974 to 15 per 1000 days in 1979 [35]. Methicillin resistance occurred in 40% of 87 strains tested. Multiply resistant coagulase-negative staphylococcal strains have also caused symptomatic bacteremia in 3% of newborns in a large referral intensive care unit (ICU) [36] and in increasing numbers of adult patients in some hospitals [37]. Between 1980 and 1989, the incidence of bloodstream infections due to coagulase-negative staphylococci reported to the NNIS System rose between 161% and 754%, depending on the size and teaching status of the hospital [4]. This may have been because of increased recognition of the pathogenic potential of this bacterium, or because of an increase in the use of intravascular devices in seriously ill hospitalized patients. Methicillin resistance among these isolates increased from ~20% to ~60% during this time.

TABLE 15-2. *Percent of nosocomial* Staphylococcal aureus *isolates resistant to methicillin, oxacillin, or nafcillin, in National Nosocomial Infection Surveillance System hospitals*

Hospital size	Hospital's medical school affiliation	Average 1975–1989	1989
≤ 200 Beds	Nonteaching	3.6	3.1
> 200 Beds	Nonteaching	4.9	12.8
≤ 500 Beds	Teaching	5.0	16.0
> 500 Beds	Teaching	8.3	21.6

Prevalence and distribution of methicillin-resistant *Staphylococcus aureus* in the United States. (Adapted from Gaynes R., Culver DH, Horan TC, et al. Trends in methicillin-resistant Staphylococcus aureus in United States Hospitals. *Infectious Diseases in Clinical Practice* 1993;2:452.)

The fluoroquinolone antibiotics, such as norfloxacin and ciprofloxacin, offer a new class of broad-spectrum agents that usually do not show cross-resistance with older classes of antimicrobials. Although in vitro emergence of bacterial resistance appears to be less frequent for fluoroquinolones than for cephalosporins, resistance may be selected rapidly in a patient during treatment [38]. Since the mid-1980s, numerous reports of nosocomial, fluoroquinolone-resistant gram-negative and gram-positive bacteria have been published [39–42]. The prevalence of ciprofloxacin resistance among MRSA is especially striking. Evaluation of NNIS data for 1989 to 1992 revealed that whereas 3.7% of MSSA isolates were ciprofloxacin-resistant, almost 80% of MRSA isolates were also resistant to ciprofloxacin [43], an agent to which all the strains were initially susceptible. Although resistance has been observed primarily in nosocomial infections, the widespread community use of the oral fluoroquinolones may result in selection of resistance among community-acquired bacteria in the future.

CLASSIFICATION AND DIAGNOSTIC CRITERIA

Determining whether resistant bacteria are hospital acquired is often problematic because patients may be colonized asymptomatically when they enter the hospital. For example, in our experience [8,44–47] and others' [48], 15% to 25% of patients colonized or infected with aminoglycoside-resistant gram-negative bacilli and as many as 50% of patients who appear to acquire cefazolin-resistant Enterobacteriaceae after surgery [44, 49] have brought these strains into the hospital. Moreover, the incubation period for many infections caused by resistant bacteria is not clearly delineated.

In addition to the difficulties in defining hospital acquisition, there is often the question of whether the patient is colonized or has clinical disease due to the resistant strain. This is particularly difficult with lower respiratory tract infection (see Chapter 32). Criteria for making this differentiation are discussed in the chapters on site-specific infections; however, we consider colonization an important epidemiologic problem because it increases the reservoir of resistant bacteria and is often a precursor to clinical disease [50].

From a microbiologic standpoint, defining resistance also may have pitfalls (see Chapter 9). In testing by disk diffusion, as a general example, antibiotic-containing disks may be outdated or inadequately stamped onto the agar surface, the bacterial inoculum may be too heavy or too light, the depth or pH of the agar may be incorrect, or the wrong drugs may even be used. Some gram-negative bacilli, such as *Flavobacterium*, are intrinsically resistant to the usual gram-negative panel of antibiotics and, unless the appropriate drugs are tested, such bacteria may appear untreatable. Moreover, some automated systems have difficulty with certain antibiotics against specific bacteria. Problems in testing specific "drug–bug" combinations are cited in the section on Specific Organisms.

Newer DNA-based subtyping methods have been applied to the evaluation of a variety of endemic and epidemic antibiotic resistance problems [51–53]. These techniques, which have been used primarily for the genotypic analysis of bacteria, are often more discriminating, reproducible, and applicable to a larger proportion of strains within a species than are phenotypic methods. Pulsed-field gel electrophoresis appears to be a particularly useful tool; guidelines for interpretation of DNA restriction patterns produced by pulsed-field gel electrophoresis have been published [54]. For most methodologies, however, neither the methodologies nor the interpretation of results have been well standardized and, as with any test, a result should be considered within the overall clinical context. Moreover, discrimination among isolates belonging to a genetically restricted group, such as MRSA, may still be difficult [55,56]. Nevertheless, genotypic analysis of antibiotic-resistant microorganisms in conjunction with conventional epidemiologic techniques should allow more precise delineation of the epidemiology of antibiotic resistance in the future.

SOURCES OF RESISTANT STRAINS

The source of most resistant strains in hospitals appears to be patients who are colonized or infected [5,49]. Because the normal pharyngeal and intestinal flora of hospitalized patients may be displaced by multiply resistant enteric bacteria and *P. aeruginosa* (urine, perineum, and wounds may be similarly affected [57,58]), there are often many colonized patients for each patient with recognized infection, the so-called "iceberg" effect. This shift in flora often occurs within a very few days of admission and affects the older, generally sicker or more debilitated patients. The importance of various risk factors (e.g., specific exposures vs. more hands-on care in general) and the pathophysiology of this shift (e.g., possible changes in membrane receptors or ligands, antibiotic suppression of normal flora) are not well delineated [59]. In our experience, some of this shift in endemic strains may result from emergence of low-count, community-acquired flora in the face of antibiotic exposure rather than from true nosocomial acquisition [49] (Table 15-3).

Personnel have been documented to disseminate resistant gram-positive strains, such as MRSA [60] and even coagulase-negative staphylococci [61]. However, personnel carriage of resistant gram-negative bacilli (other than transient hand carriage described in the following section) appears to be very unusual. Exceptions include outbreaks reportedly traced to carriers of *Acinetobacter, Citrobacter*, and *Proteus*. *Acinetobacter*, one of the few gram-negative bacilli that may be among normal skin flora, was noted in one outbreak to recur periodically despite disinfection of the apparent environmental reservoirs. The outbreak was ultimately traced to the colonized hands of a respiratory therapy technician who had dermatitis and apparently contaminated respiratory therapy equipment while assembling it [62]. There have also been clusters of *Citrobacter* infections of the central nervous system in neonates, traced to hand carriage by nurses [63,64], and an outbreak of *Proteus* infections in newborns traced to a nurse who was a chronic carrier [65].

Foodborne contamination with multiply resistant gram-negative bacilli has been cited in several investigations [3,66] and has been incriminated particularly in oncology units [67]. Despite the potential importance of these observations, however, the overall role of food in

TABLE 15-3. *Characteristics of cardiac surgery patients colonized with cefazolin-resistant gram-negative bacilli*

Species	Number of patients colonized (n=87)	Location at first positive culture (% patients)			Percent of colonization due to horizontal transmission	Percent developing clinical infection
		At admission	48–72 hr into CSICU	>72 hr into CSICU		
Enterobacter spp	58	50	34	16	16	21
Citrobacter spp	37	49	22	29	?	3
Pseudomonas aeruginosa	33	55	12	33	9	27
Serratia marcescens	7	43	57	0	29	29

CSICU, cardiac surgery intensive care unit; ?, unknown (no typing system used).
(Adapted from Flynn DM, Weinstein RA, and Kabins SA. Infections with gram-negative bacilli in a cardiac surgery intensive care unit: the relative role of *Enterobacter*. *J Hosp Infect* 1988;11:367.)

introducing resistant strains into the general hospital remains unclear (see Chapter 22).

Environmental sources and reservoirs of resistant strains have been a recurrent problem, especially when patient care equipment, such as urine measuring devices, become contaminated with enteric bacilli or *Pseudomonas* [5,68]. Extensive outbreaks of urinary tract infections (and respiratory tract, perineal, or intestinal colonization) may result when such contaminated equipment is shared by many patients (see Chapters 31, 34).

Finally, there has been perennial concern about contamination of many areas of the inanimate environment with which patients do not have direct contact, such as flowerpots [68] and sink traps [70–72] (see Chapter 20). Despite heavy contamination, these sites usually have not been implicated epidemiologically in the spread of bacteria in hospitals. However, for high-risk immunocompromised patients, especially those who have the opportunity for environmental exposures (e.g., the debilitated oncology patient who sits at the sink to wash), strains from sink surfaces have been linked to patient colonization and infection [67].

MODES OF TRANSMISSION

The most important way that resistant bacteria are spread in the hospital is from an infected patient to a susceptible patient through transient carriage on hands of personnel. Such spread contributes to the "iceberg" of colonized patients and greatly increases the source and reservoir of resistant strains in the hospital (Figure 15-2). Most of the evidence incriminating hands of personnel is circumstantial [73–75]. However, the weight of experience, dating back to the successful introduction of handwashing as a control measure by Semmelweis, strongly supports this concept. Indexes of hands-on exposure to personnel, used in a few studies to quantitate patients' risk, have provided an additional measure.

Common-source spread of resistant strains has been noted primarily in outbreak settings. The attention of the medical community (and newspaper and journal editors) is often attracted to such epidemics because of striking features, such as large numbers of patients infected with very resistant bacteria, unusual breaks in techniques or protocols, or contaminated commercial products. Perhaps more common than such "extravaganzas" are the ongoing episodes of limited cross-infection due to contamination of shared patient care equipment, such as urine or other measuring containers and other environmental reservoirs, which probably account for a significant portion of seemingly endemic infections [47].

Airborne spread of resistant bacteria has been documented rarely. For MRSA, experience suggests that airborne spread is not a significant problem. For gram-negative bacilli, there was concern in one hospital that contamination in a 16-story chute-hydropulping waste disposal system led to airborne dispersal and transmission of *Pseudomonas* and enteric bacilli [76]. Waste pulp in the chute had 108 colony-forming units (cfu) per

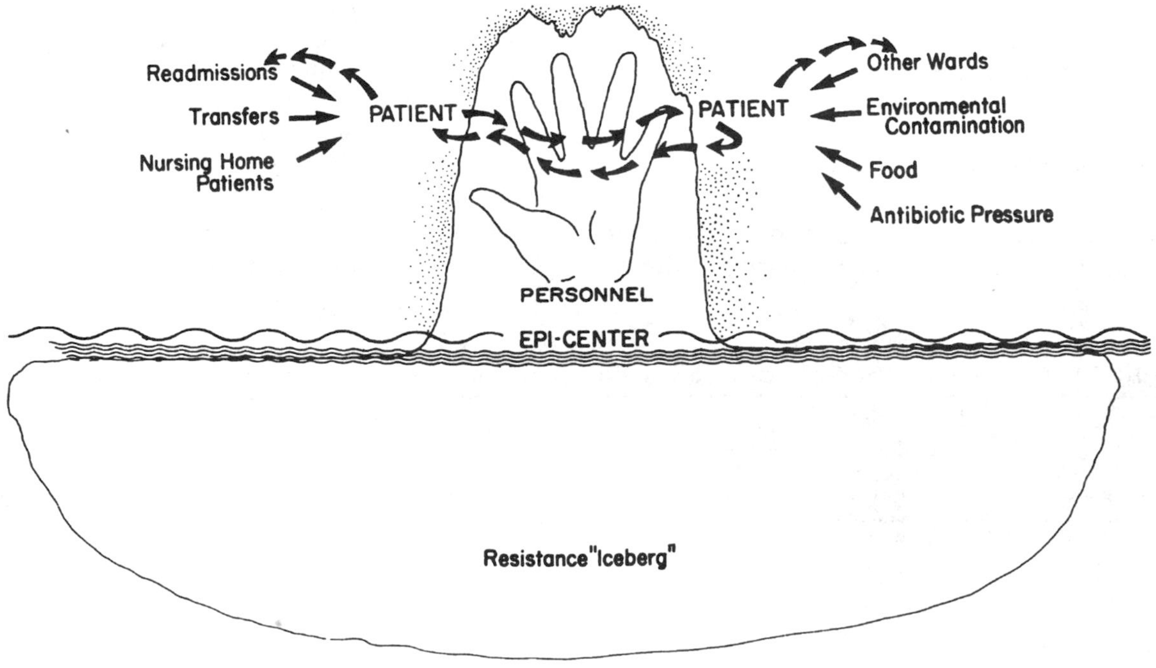

FIGURE 15-2. The dynamics of nosocomial resistance: resistance iceberg. (Reprinted with permission from Weinstein RA, Kabins SA. Strategies for prevention and control of multiple drug-resistant nosocomial infection. *Am J Med* 1981;70:449.)

gram; air samples from hallways connecting the chute and nursing units had greater than 150 cfu per cubic foot of air. After closing the chute, air counts fell by > 75% and the incidence of nosocomial gram-negative bacteremias fell by > 65%. However, this experience appears unique.

Various insect vectors, such as flies and cockroaches, are probably unimportant in the transmission of resistant bacteria in most U.S. hospitals.

PREDISPOSING FACTORS

Patients

A number of host factors have been associated with acquisition of antibiotic-resistant bacteria (Table 15-4). Our epidemiologic understanding of these factors has remained somewhat limited because most work has focused on epidemic and few on endemic situations [19, 47,77,78], most studies have been retrospective and therefore limited in ability to gather complete host profiles, some studies have not included control groups, and, until recently, relatively few of the studies have used multivariate analyses to control for relatedness of host factors [79,80]. Indeed, many of the factors are undoubtedly linked and are serving as indirect markers of frequency of patient–staff contact (i.e., risk of indirect contact spread by hands of personnel).

TABLE 15-4. *Examples of host factors associated with epidemic antimicrobial resistance in selected case-control studies*

Factor	Reference
Antimicrobial drugs Prophylaxis or Therapy	[79,84,35,98,78,59,149,62, 79,140,133,97,99,147,144, 50,157,178,160,172,235]
Apgar score	[79]
Duration of hospital of ICU stay	[61,78,37,149,79,99,50,235]
Decreased WBC	[178]
Elderly age	[59,79]
Endotracheal intubation (or tracheostomy)	[61,79,155,235]
Exchange transfusions	[79]
Gastrointestinal colonization	[78,50]
Gavage feeding	[62]
Genitourinary instrumentation	[144]
Hyperalimentation	[37,79]
Intravenous therapy	[79]
Low birth weight	[79]
Mucocutaneous defects	[178]
Nasogastric suction	[50]
Proximity to other patients	[78,119]
Respiratory therapy	[78,50]
Severity of underlying disease	[29,172]
Sex	[178]
Surgery (or number of operations)	[78,59,160]
Urinary catheter	
Condom	[57]
Indwelling	[15,149,84,147,235]
Urinary irrigation	[145]

ICU, intensive care unit; WBC, white blood cell count.

The studies from which the information is drawn for Table 15-4 include experience with both gram-negative bacilli and gram-positive bacteria. The host factors for both types of epidemics have been generally similar except that gram-negative bacilli more often involve the urinary tract and associated factors, such as indwelling bladder catheters, whereas gram-positive bacteria involve the skin and related factors, such as duration of intravenous catheterization, somewhat more.

Of the many factors, the role of antibiotics has been the most controversial [1,81], and several issues warrant emphasis. Many studies document the emergence of aminoglycoside-resistant strains after use of topical aminoglycoside ointments [80], related to nonabsorbable aminoglycosides in enteral regimens for suppression of gut bacteria in oncology patients [31,82], or after parenteral aminoglycoside therapy [83–86]. In some studies, resistant strains have occurred more frequently in wound and sputum isolates, suggesting emergence of resistance at sites more likely to have poor penetration, and thus subinhibitory levels, of aminoglycosides [47]. The emergence of resistant isolates has also been correlated with inadequate doses of aminoglycosides [47,77,83,87].

There has been some controversy surrounding the relation between amikacin use and resistance [83,88–91]. Some hospitals have used amikacin extensively without noting any increase in resistance [87]. However, the incidence depends to some extent on how prevalent amikacin-inactivating enzymes are in the particular hospital, as well as on the adequacy of dosing. Regardless, cross-resistance to multiple aminoglycosides, including amikacin, occurs in up to 60% of gram-negative bacilli resistant to gentamicin or tobramycin [47,87,91–94].

Use of the newer cephalosporin antibiotics has been associated with emergence of cephalosporin-resistant strains, particularly of *Enterobacter, Serratia, Citrobacter, Klebsiella*, and *Pseudomonas* [21,26,95,96]. For example, as many as 50% of *Enterobacter* species may be resistant by the end of treatment [97].

The use of TMP has been associated with the emergence of TMP-resistant strains in a variety of settings, including treatment of urinary tract infections, prophylaxis of traveler's diarrhea, and gut sterilization in oncology patients. Of particular concern, this resistance is often carried on transferable R factors that confer resistance to multiple antimicrobials, emphasizing the way one agent may affect resistance to many others. In one study, 96% of 165 TMP-resistant *E. coli* were resistant to at least 4 drugs, and 25% were resistant to 7; TMP resistance was transferable in 40 of 100 strains tested [98].

Regarding gram-positive bacteria, studies in the 1960s suggested that patients were at greater risk of being colonized with *S. aureus* after antibiotic treatment [99]. MRSA have been found in hospitalized drug addicts who had self-prescribed oral cephalosporins, emphasizing the potential impact of antibiotic use in the community on hospital flora [100]. The receipt of vancomycin [101–103], ceftazidime [104], metronidazole [105,106], or an antibiotic with significant activity against anaerobic bacteria [106] has been found to be a risk factor for colonization or infection with vancomycin-resistant enterococci in one or more studies.

Epidemics

The events leading to any nosocomial epidemic are probably multifactorial. In most outbreaks of multiply drug-resistant bacteria, precipitating events have not been well elucidated. Factors that could increase person-to-person spread include poor aseptic practices, as in crowded units or when the nurse-to-patient ratio becomes too low. Spread from the environment is facilitated by poor housekeeping practices that lead to reservoirs of resistant organisms within the hospital, as when infected urine is allowed to remain in urine measuring or testing devices. Excessive use of antibiotics may increase the selective pressure for resistant strains [1].

Certain fortuitous events may precipitate outbreaks, such as contamination of a commercial product, admission of a patient who is a heavy shedder of multiply resistant bacteria [82], or acquisition of resistance by a bacterial species that is adept at colonization or unusually resistant to disinfection. Also, advances in medical technology, such as transplantation, dialysis, and new prosthetic devices, create additional epidemic risks.

Particular areas within the hospital, especially intensive care (see Chapter 25), burn (see Chapter 38), neurosurgical, and urology units, are prone to outbreaks. These areas house acutely ill patients who are subjected to many invasive procedures and are often exposed to multiple antibiotics under circumstances in which asepsis may be trampled in the rush of crisis care. We have found that multiply resistant bacteria may breed in such units, which we call *epicenters* (see Figure 15-2) [5]. As colonized patients are transferred to other areas of the hospital, they may leave a trial of resistance.

Plasmid and Transposon Outbreaks

Most reported outbreaks have been due to epidemic spread of single strains. Since the late 1970s, however, several plasmid outbreaks have been described in which a resistance plasmid has caused either simultaneous or sequential resistance to occur in epidemic fashion in different species or genera [107–113] (Table 15-5). City-wide spread of a single–plasmid-mediated ceftazidime, aminoglycoside, and TMP–sulfamethoxazole resistance in multiple strain types of *E. coli* and *K. pneumoniae* has been described in Chicago-area nursing homes [114]. We are also recognizing that transposition of plasmid segments (or other spatial rearrangements of genetic mater-

TABLE 15-5. *Examples of plasmid outbreaks*

Setting [ref.]	Bacteria (no.)	Predominant infections	Appearance of resistance (duration)	Plasmidborne resistances
Neonatal ICU [107]	*Klebsiella* Serotype 30 (21) Serotype 19 (6)	NS	Sequential (9 mo, 5 mo)	Gm, kn, am, cf, cb
Hospitalwide [111]	*Serratia* (71) *Klebsiella* (68) *Citrobacter* (68) *Proteus* (68) *Enterobacter* (68) *Providencia* (68)	UTI	Simultaneous (3 yr)	Gm, tb, kn, am, cf, cb, st, su
Burn unit [105]	*Klebsiella* (NS) *Enterobacter* (NS) Three other genera (NS)	Burn	Simultaneous (11 mo)	Tb, kn, ne
Hospitalwide [110]	*Klebsiella* (69) *Escherichia coli* (16) *Enterobacter* (16) *Proteus* (16)	UTI, wd, resp	Index case admitted with epidemic strain; remainder ~ simultaneous (2 yr)	Gm, tb, kn, am, cf, cb, ch, su
Multiple nursing homes [112]	*K. pneumoniae* (9) *E. coli* (12)	Urine, blood, resp	Simultaneous (2 yr +)	Ceftaz, gm, tb, TMP-SMX

ICU, intensive care unit; NS, not stated; UTI, urinary tract infection; wd, wound infection; resp, respiratory infection; gm, gentamicin; kn, kanamycin; am, ampicillin; cf, cephalothin; cb, carbenicillin; tb, tobramycin; st, streptomycin; su, sulfonamide; ne, neomycin; ch, chloramphenicol; ceftaz, ceftazidime; TMP-SMX, trimethoprim-sulfamethoxazole.

ial) may lead to "transposon outbreaks" involving whole families of related resistance plasmids [110].

The epidemiology of most plasmid outbreaks, specifically the reservoirs for the resistance plasmids, time and place of transfer of plasmids, and pressures involved, has been largely speculative [1,115,116]. Transfer can occur in the gut, on skin, in urine, and in the environment (e.g., in urine containers) and may be facilitated by antimicrobial therapy [116–118]. Moreover, relatively avirulent bacterial strains may serve as reservoirs for resistance. For example, gentamicin resistance in *Staphylococcus epidermidis* or *S. aureus* may be mediated by identical plasmids that can pass between these two species in vitro and on human skin [33].

Plasmid outbreaks may be difficult to detect but should be sought through surveillance for the occurrence of multiple species or genera with identical or very similar multiple drug (or even just key drug) resistance patterns. If available, similar gel electrophoretic patterns of plasmid DNA could facilitate detection (see Chapter 16). Once recognized, plasmid epidemics are controlled much like single-strain outbreaks (see section on Control). Recent technologic refinements may facilitate more extensive epidemiologic investigation of plasmid and transposon resistance and allow more specific control measures.

Other Multiple-Strain Outbreaks

Occasionally, common sources may become contaminated with several bacterial species, leading to outbreaks of otherwise unrelated strains. For example, one multiple-strain outbreak of orthopedic wound infections was traced to a common bucket used to mix cast material. The bucket was not routinely disinfected and contained a variety of contaminants that probably were inoculated into wounds during application of casts. An unusual series of outbreaks of postoperative infection due to multiple organisms at seven different hospitals was linked to exposure to propofol, an anesthetic agent with a lipid-based vehicle that is able to support the rapid growth of a variety of microorganisms at room temperature [119]. Apparently, lapses in aseptic technique by anesthesia personnel at or near the time of surgery resulted in extrinsic contamination of syringes or vials containing this agent. Such outbreaks may go unrecognized unless one strain predominates or the strains or epidemiologic circumstances are very unusual.

CONTROL

Control of Epidemic Resistance

Control of resistant bacteria usually has focused on epidemics (Table 15-6) and traditionally has involved efforts to strengthen aseptic practices while an epidemiologic analysis of cases (and controls) is quickly undertaken to exclude common-source exposures [5] (see Chapter 6). Empiric attempts to decrease transmission usually have also included isolating or cohorting infected or colonized patients. Identifying the colonized patients (see Figure 15-2) often requires culture surveys, which may be facilitated by the use of selective media (see Chapter 9). In some outbreaks, susceptible patients, such as those with indwelling urinary catheters, have been physically separated to decrease the likelihood that personnel would passively carry pathogens from one patient or drainage bag to the next [120]. Use of personnel who act as monitors may be necessary to ensure compliance with isolation precautions [121]. In drastic situations, units have been closed to new admissions.

TABLE 15-6. *Traditional control measures*

Identify reservoirs
Colonized and infected patients
Environmental contamination; common sources
Halt transmission among patients
Improve hand-washing and asepsis
Barrier precautions (gloves, gown) for colonized and infected patients
Eliminate any common source; disinfect environment
Separate susceptible patients
Close unit to new admissions if necessary
Halt progression from colonization to infection
Discontinue compromising factors (Table 15-4) when possible (e.g., extubate, remove nasogastric tube, discontinue bladder catheters, as clinically indicated); rotate intravenous catheter sites; employ proper respirator care (see Chapter 32)
Modify host risk
Treat underlying disease and complications
Control antibiotic use (rotate, restrict, or cease)

In some instances, antibiotic controls may help restrict the spread of resistant bacteria [1,84]. First, in high-density units such as ICUs, restricting antibiotic use may be important [1,31,77,84,85,115]. In rare situations, antibiotic use has been totally suspended [122]. Second, antibiotic restrictions may decrease selective pressures in some plasmid outbreaks. Chemicals that "cure" bacterial plasmids in vitro are currently too toxic for use in humans. Safer agents, such as nalidixic acid, which may prevent transfer of plasmids [123], have yet to be used for this purpose in clinical situations. Third, more careful dosing with aminoglycosides may decrease the chance that subinhibitory levels will select resistant subpopulations (due to spontaneous chromosomal mutations), particularly in sites that have large bacterial populations, such as wounds or the respiratory tract. In a pharmacokinetic model, a peak to minimum inhibitory concentration (MIC) aminoglycoside ratio of greater than 8 : 1 was shown to prevent the in vitro emergence of resistance [124]. Whether aminoglycoside resistance develops less frequently in patients receiving once-daily aminoglycoside dosing, which results in peak antibiotic levels ~ 10 times the MIC of most gram-negative bacteria [125], deserves evaluation. Finally, the control of antibiotics that select for sensitive precursors of resistant organisms (e.g., cephalosporins selecting for *Pseudomonas*) may be necessary.

Experimental Approaches to Epidemic Control

Table 15-7 lists several epidemic control methods that have been tried. Topical and nonabsorbable antimicrobials have been used for prophylaxis in several settings, including epidemics of resistant bacteria. For example, polymyxin spray was used experimentally in one ICU to forestall pharyngeal colonization and pneumonia with *Pseudomonas* (see Chapter 32). In limited studies, this approach appeared to work, but, when applied in the ICU in a continuous fashion, the consequence was a compensatory increase in pneumonias caused by intrinsically polymyxin-resistant bacilli [70]. More recently, use of combinations of topical agents (see later) has been successful in European ICUs in controlling outbreaks of multiply resistant gram-negative bacilli [126,127].

In the 1960s, attempts were made to use avirulent staphylococci to reduce colonization with epidemic strains (see Chapter 41). This form of bacterial interference has been reexplored recently. In one study, pharyngeal implantation of α-hemolytic streptococci successfully displaced resistant enteric organisms in infants in a neonatal ICU [128]. In an outbreak, this approach was used with other measures successfully to control colonization of neonates by amikacin-resistant *Serratia* and *Klebsiella* [129]. However, this work needs to be confirmed and studies extended to adults before any conclusions can be made about its general applicability.

Another control measure from the past that is being reinvestigated is disinfection of urinary catheter drainage bags (see Chapter 31). Earlier use of this method, with formalin in drainage bottles, ended when closed systems were widely adopted. Unfortunately, closed drainage cannot prevent contamination of collection bags indefinitely; in as many as 30% of patients with initially sterile urine, contamination of the bag may precede bladder infection [58]. In one study, disinfection of drainage bags with hydrogen peroxide forestalled urinary infections in a small number of patients with acute spinal injury [130]. Organisms may still ascend from the perineum around the catheter, however, and in a controlled study in a large teaching hospital, bag decontamination did not appear to reduce infection rates [131]. Nevertheless, bag disinfection may reduce reservoirs of contaminated urine in the hospital environment [58] and warrants additional controlled study.

TABLE 15-7. *Experimental approaches for controlling resistance*

Prevention of acquisition by use of topical antimicrobials
Respiratory spray
Oral nonabsorbables
Disinfectants in devices and in environmental reservoirs
Bacterial interference
Treatment of colonized patients
Topical or systemic antimicrobials
Immune enhancement

Attempts to decontaminate relatively remote environmental reservoirs of resistant bacteria, such as sink traps, have been innovative [132]. However, based on the failure of such efforts to decrease infection rates [70] and on the lack of any epidemiologic link between sink traps and patients [71,72], these extraordinary measures do not appear routinely warranted except, perhaps, in units housing oncology patients [67].

Other studies have attempted to alter the host environment to permit the growth of normal commensal flora but discourage colonization with pathogenic bacteria. For example, a randomized, double-blind, placebo-controlled trial investigated whether topically applied intravaginal estriol cream in postmenopausal women with recurrent urinary tract infections would prevent further infections [133]. During 8 months of follow-up, the incidence of urinary tract infection was substantially reduced in women who received estriol, probably because of favorable changes in their vaginal flora. Sixty-one percent of women in the treatment arm of the study became colonized with lactobacilli after 1 month, and colonization with Enterobacteriaceae fell from 67% to 31%. In contrast, lactobacilli were absent from all patients who received placebo, and colonization with Enterobacteriaceae remained stable. Although this study was small (93 patients), the results suggest that further investigation of this type of intervention is warranted.

Finally, in drastic situations, systemic antibiotics have at times been administered to patients who are only colonized with multiply resistant bacteria (e.g., multiply resistant pneumococci) [134].

Control of Endemic Resistance

A variety of epidemic control measures may be applied to endemic situations. For example, we have used antibiotic resistance precautions (Figure 15-3) for all patients who are colonized or infected with resistant gram-negative bacilli [5]. In our experience, such barrier-type precautions have markedly decreased the incidence of aminoglycoside-resistant *E. coli, Klebsiella*, and *Enterobacter*, and probably have limited the extent of recurrent miniepidemics of resistant *Serratia* [47]. In sharp contrast, the incidence of aminoglycoside-resistant *Pseudomonas* infections appears to a greater extent to have paralleled antibiotic use rather than to have been affected appreciably by barrier-type precautions. In fact, we have frequently found that in individual patients, *P. aeruginosa* became resistant in the face of aminoglycoside therapy [46,47,135].

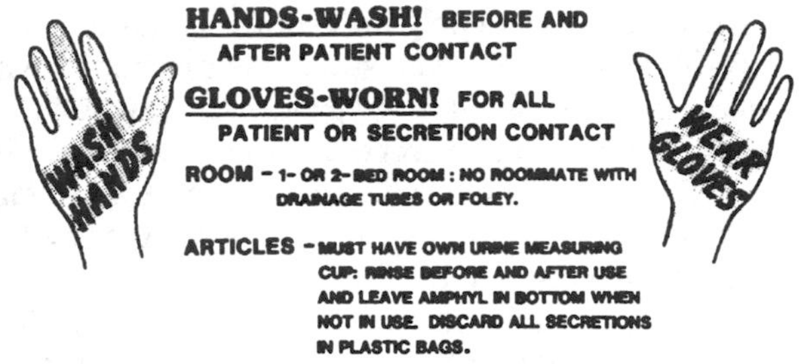

FIGURE 15-3. Placard stating barrier-type antibiotic resistance precautions to be placed on door to patient's room and above bed; stickers with similar precautions may be affixed to urinary drainage bag or other items to alert personnel that patient is colonized or infected with resistant bacteria.

An update of our experience has confirmed these findings [82]. However, we have found that as barrier-type precautions diminished the incidence of plasmid-mediated resistance in Enterobacteriaceae, the remaining resistant isolates followed a pattern like that of *Pseudomonas*, with broad cross-resistant strains emerging from endogenous flora after antibiotic therapy. It is unlikely that the incidence of such strains will be further reduced by barrier-type precautions alone. This emphasizes the need to develop better control strategies. For example, studies of topical antimicrobials for selective decontamination have focused on the use of combinations of agents (e.g., polymyxin with tobramycin [or gentamicin] and amphotericin B [or nystatin]) applied to the oropharyngeal and gastrointestinal reservoir of endogenous gram-negative bacilli [127]. Although such an approach has reduced trauma and cardiac surgery ICU-related infections in several studies by > 50% compared with historical controls [136–138], without emergence of resistant gram-negative bacilli [139], selective decontamination may fail in medical–surgical ICUs and may lead to emergence of resistant enterococci [140].

Based on our studies, we suggest a multifaceted approach to control of endemic, antibiotic-resistant gram-negative bacilli, MRSA, or vancomycin-resistant enterococci in large, acute care hospitals [5]:

1. Antibiotic resistance precautions (see Figure 15-3) should be used for all patients who are colonized or infected with MRSA, vancomycin-resistant enterococci, aminoglycoside-resistant, imipenem-resistant, or broad-spectrum cephalosporin-resistant Enterobacteriaceae. These precautions should be extended to any patient who is a persistent shedder of other multiply resistant bacteria, especially if the patient has draining wounds, receives repeated courses of antibiotics, or requires intensive nursing care. A clean, nonsterile cover gown should be worn for extensive, direct contact with a patient who has heavy colonization or infection of skin, respiratory tract secretions, or uncontrolled wound drainage. Compliance monitoring and feedback to personnel may improve adherence to gloving and gowning recommendations [121].

   The use of universal precautions and body substance isolation should reduce the need for such additional measures (see Chapter 13). However, antibiotic resistance precautions also focus on patients' skin and gut flora and the environment. Moreover, control of epidemics of resistant gram-negative bacilli or staphylococci by increased attention to gloving and cohorting suggests that universal precautions are frequently breached.
2. Such precautions should be used while appropriate cultures are being processed from patients who are admitted (or readmitted) with a history of colonization or infection with resistant organisms.
3. Patients transferred from nursing homes or other hospitals should be evaluated for carriage of resistant bacteria [46,47,82]. Certain patients, such as those who are incontinent, have recently received antibiotics, have indwelling urinary catheters or percutaneous feeding tubes, or come from large nursing homes or hospitals, may warrant precautions while appropriate cultures are processed.
4. Appropriate aminoglycoside usage and dosage should be ensured to decrease selection of spontaneous mutations among *P. aeruginosa* and, to a lesser extent, among Enterobacteriaceae.
5. Surveillance of patients and clinical laboratory results should be maintained to detect miniepidemics (two or more patients with similarly resistant organisms) so that cross-infection or significant environmental reservoirs can be identified and controlled (see Chapter 5). Stratification of clinical isolate antibiotic susceptibility results by hospital unit may detect unit-specific trends in bacterial incidence or antibiotic resistance that would otherwise be masked [141–143]. For example, the emergence of multiply resistant *P. aeruginosa* in the burn and medical ICUs of one hospital was apparent when antibiograms from these areas were analyzed separately, although hospital-wide resistance in *P. aeruginosa* was stable during the same period [143]. These focused microbiologic surveillance reports may be useful in the early detection of outbreaks, or in the evaluation of the impact of infection control measures or changes in antibiotic use, and should be evaluated further.
6. When patients who are colonized or infected with resistant bacteria are transferred to another hospital or nursing home, the receiving institution should be notified of the isolation status.
7. Compromising factors (see Table 15-4) in high-risk patients should be eliminated whenever possible. In certain specialty units, such as ICUs, control of antibiotic usage, as discussed previously, may also help to control endemic resistance. However, several factors may limit the efficacy of this measure. First, use

of one antibiotic may lead to cross-resistance to others, as seen with aminoglycoside cross-resistance as well as with plasmid colinkage of resistance. Next, sequential acquisition of bacterial resistance when antibiotics are rotated has been well described [80]. Finally, when controls are lifted, resistant organisms that have remained in low numbers in colonized patients may reemerge [84].

8. In settings where careful, prospective microbiologic and epidemiologic monitoring is available, selective decontamination, as described earlier, may be considered as an interim epidemic control measure [127].

Threshold for Investigation and Control

In certain situations, ongoing control measures are appropriate. First, some organisms always warrant prompt attention because of key resistances. Such bacteria include MRSA, high-level penicillin-resistant *S. pneumoniae*, aminoglycoside-resistant *P. aeruginosa*, imipenem-resistant gram-negative bacteria, and vancomycin-resistant enterococci. Second, in units such as ICUs, which may serve as epicenters, aggressive containment of multiply resistant strains can be justified. Third, certain types of patients warrant antibiotic resistance precautions. These include patients who are colonized with multiply resistant strains at several sites and whose severity of illness requires frequent physical attention by physicians, nurses, respiratory therapists, and so forth, thus entailing higher risk for spread of resistant bacteria to other patients.

In other situations, the individual hospital must rely on local surveillance and experience to help set formal or intuitive epidemic thresholds for instituting aggressive containment measures and epidemiologic investigations. The thresholds will probably differ for each hospital and for specific multiply resistant strains. For example, with *Serratia* a low threshold may trigger an investigation because of the "iceberg" effect often seen in patients with urinary catheters or on respirators. In some hospitals, ongoing laboratory studies, such as serotyping or molecular strain typing [145], may be used to help evaluate possible single-strain outbreaks [144] (see Chapter 9). Plasmid outbreaks and multiple-strain outbreaks may be more difficult to identify even with ongoing surveillance, and the mere suspicion of clustering of similarly resistant Enterobacteriaceae may warrant an investigation. Finally, if clusters of resistant organisms occur in the face of barrier precautions, our experience suggests that a chronically colonized patient or an environmental source should be sought vigorously [82].

SPECIFIC ORGANISMS

Enterobacteriaceae

Antibiotic-resistant Enterobacteriaceae are common in hospitals, especially resistant *Klebsiella, Serratia*, and *Enterobacter* [69]. Drug-resistant *Proteus, Providencia*, and *Morganella* are also very common, particularly in geriatric wards and in patients transferred from nursing homes [45,47,82]. The clinical aspects of infections caused by Enterobacteriaceae are described in chapters on urinary tract infection (see Chapter 31), pneumonia (see Chapter 32), wound infection (see Chapter 37), and bacteremia (see Chapter 44). Microbiologic diagnosis of these infections usually poses no problem for the modern laboratory, particularly with the availability of newer diagnostic kits (see Chapter 9).

TABLE 15-8. *Epidemiologic patterns in outbreaks of urinary tract infection by multiply resistant organisms*

	Organism[a]		
Factor	*Klebsiella pneumoniae*	*Serratia marcescens*	*Proteus rettgeri*
Reservoir			
Symptomatic GU infection	++++	±	++
Asymptomatic GU infection	++	++++	+++
Gastrointestinal colonization	++	0	0
Mode of transmission	Hands[b]	Hands	Hands
Spatial clustering of cases prominent	++	++++	++++
Risk factors			
Urinary catheterization	Yes	Yes	Yes
Broad-spectrum antimicrobial exposure	Yes	Yes	Yes
Urinary catheter irrigation	Yes	No	No
GU instrumentation	No	No	Yes

GU, genitourinary.
[a]Scale: 0 (no contribution) to ++++ (maximal contribution).
[b]Contact spread on hands of personnel.
(Adapted from Schaberg DR, Weinstein RA, and Stamm WE. Epidemics of nosocomial urinary tract infection caused by multiply resistant gram-negative bacilli: Epidemiology and control. *J Infect Dis* 176;133:363.)

Predisposing factors for, and the epidemiology of, resistant Enterobacteriaceae have differed somewhat from genus to genus [146] (Table 15-8). Some organisms, such as *Klebsiella*, may be more viable on human skin and thus may have a greater potential for person-to-person spread on the hands of hospital personnel [32,146]. *Serratia* commonly causes asymptomatic colonization of urinary tract and respiratory tract, and chronically colonized patients are often a source for large numbers of cross-infections [82,148]. There have also been several outbreaks described in which environmental contamination with *Serratia*, notably of graduated cylinders and ventilators, led to epidemics of urinary tract infection, peritonitis, or pneumonia [82]. *Enterobacter*, as well as *Serratia, Citrobacter, Pseudomonas*, and some *Proteus* and *Providencia* strains often become resistant to second- and third-generation cephalosporins during therapy [21–23]. This genetic predilection and the ubiquity of *Enterobacter* may explain in part why *Enterobacter* species are a relatively common cause of mediastinitis after open heart surgery despite cephalosporin prophylaxis [22,44,49].

As noted earlier, in some hospitals 15% to 25% or more of all antibiotic-resistant Enterobacteriaceae are cultured from patients at the time of admission. Patients with chronic respiratory or urinary tract infections, those who have frequent admissions, and patients transferred from nursing homes or other hospitals are particularly likely to bring resistant strains into the hospital [47,82]. In several instances, such patients have been the index cases in outbreaks [48,63,149,150].

Since drug-resistant Enterobacteriaceae appear to spread largely from patient to patient on the hands of hospital personnel (Table 15-9), and because colonized or infected patients are usually the major reservoir in the hospital, it has usually been possible in the past to contain resistant Enterobacteriaceae using the precautions described previously [5,82]. However, the more recent problems with emergence of chromosomal mutations that encode resistance to newer cephalosporins and with plasmids that encode novel β-lactamases [151,152] suggest the need to heighten surveillance for such strains, tighten precautions for colonized patients, and possibly consider selective decontamination, as noted previously, in some specially selected outbreak settings [127].

TABLE 15-9. *Epidemiology of endemic antibiotic resistance in nosocomial gram-negative bacilli*

Factor	Relative contribution (%)
Cross-infection	30%–40%
Antibiotic pressures	20%–25%
Community acquisition	20%–25%
Other (environment, food, personnel, air, unknown)	20%

Pseudomonas aeruginosa

Pseudomonas aeruginosa has intrinsic resistance to most available antibiotics, leaving aminoglycosides, antipseudomonal penicillins, newer cephalosporins, imipenem, and fluoroquinolones as treatment options for systemic infection. *Pseudomonas* is ubiquitous in the hospital, frequently colonizing patients before admission and contaminating water and various foods, particularly salads and fresh vegetables [46,66,67,135,153]. Laboratory identification is not difficult, although aminoglycoside susceptibility testing was confounded until the recognition that the divalent cation content of media needs to be carefully controlled.

There has been considerable controversy over whether resistant gram-negative bacilli are less virulent than sensitive strains. In a number of studies using a variety of measures of virulence, such as chills, fever, elevated white cell count, pyuria, and other local findings of infection, there have been no differences detected [85,154]. In a few studies, however, particularly in oncology patients, aminoglycoside-resistant *Pseudomonas* strains have been less prone to cause bacteremia than sensitive strains [31,155].

Several studies have shown that aminoglycoside-resistant *Pseudomonas* may emerge from sensitive populations of the same serotype during treatment [46,47,67,77, 88,135]. In fact, some institutions have found that despite isolating patients with antibiotic-resistant *P. aeruginosa*, the incidence of colonization and infection with these strains has continued to increase [46,47,82,135,154,157], in part paralleling the increasing use of aminoglycoside antibiotics.

In epidemic situations, *P. aeruginosa* has been noted to spread from contaminated common sources to patients as well as from person to person [15,67,68,144]. Such transmission may be more amenable to the control measures outlined previously. However, control of endemic *P. aeruginosa* infections is problematic and may well require more innovative strategies that interfere with the ability of *Pseudomonas* to colonize or invade.

Staphylococcus aureus

Despite aggressive control efforts, resistance of *S. aureus* to methicillin (aminoglycosides, or clindamycin) has been increasing in frequency in the United States since the early 1980s [3,60,100,157,158] (see Table 15-2). Ciprofloxacin resistance has also increased steadily, especially among MRSA (see earlier discussion). In some hospitals, nearly 100% of MRSA isolates are concomitantly resistant to ciprofloxacin [43].

Microbiologic diagnosis of MRSA is facilitated when the potential causes of false-negative tests for methicillin resistance are recognized [3,159]. Methicillin resistance in staphylococci is most commonly due to synthesis of a low-affinity penicillin-binding protein (PBP2a). Expression of resistance by a population of MRSA may not be uniform (heteroresistance), and so specific test conditions are necessary to ensure detection [159]. Conversely, MRSA may be reported erroneously when colonies from mixed cultures of resistant coagulase-negative and sensitive *S. aureus* are not picked carefully. Enterococcal colonies, if picked from blood agar, can give the impression that the enterococci, which can give positive catalase tests, are MRSA.

The epidemiology of drug-resistant isolates of *S. aureus* appears to be similar to that of susceptible strains (see Chapter 41). In addition, particular reservoirs for MRSA include intravenous drug addicts, burn unit patients, nursing home patients, and hospital personnel with dermatitis. In Detroit, MRSA arose as a major community problem in drug addicts who frequently self-prescribed antibiotics to forestall or treat infections related to the illicit use of contaminated needles. When these addicts were admitted to hospitals, waves of nosocomial methicillin-resistant infections followed [100]. In some areas, the growing prevalence of MRSA in hospitals can be traced in part to admission to hospital of colonized patients from nursing homes [160]. Community acquisition of MRSA in patients with no known risk factors for colonization or infection is being recognized more commonly [13].

Once drug-resistant staphylococci have become entrenched in the hospital, eradication is difficult. Control has required accurate laboratory identification, prospective surveillance for colonized and infected patients (including, in some hospitals, periodic culture surveys of high-risk patients), identification of previously colonized patients at readmission, appropriate isolation of all identified patients, search for environmental and personnel sources, and aggressive antibiotic therapy of infected patients (vancomycin with or without rifampin) [3,60,161]. Aggressive attempts to eradicate specific strains from colonized patients or personnel have been variably successful (see Chapter 41). Commonly recommended regimens include combinations of rifampin, TMP–sulfamethoxazole, and ciprofloxacin [162–164], with the caveat that use of a single agent may heighten risk of further resistance; topical mupirocin, vancomycin, or antiseptics have also been used, with mupirocin appearing particularly promising [165–168]. Mupirocin resistance has been reported, however, and may be increasing in institutions where this antibiotic is commonly used [169]. Efforts to eradicate colonization are indicated for personnel who have been epidemiologically linked to spread of resistant strains, for patients whose nursing homes refuse to take them back while positive cultures persist, for patients with recurrent infections, and in some outbreaks. Additional measures to control endemic and epidemic MRSA colonization should be tailored to the individual healthcare setting and guided by surveillance data and available resources. This topic and suggested control measures have been reviewed [170, 171] (see Chapter 41).

Coagulase-Negative Staphylococci

Coagulase-negative staphylococci, formerly believed to be an avirulent part of our normal flora, have become a problem pathogen in patients with implanted prosthetic joints (see Chapter 40), heart valves (see Chapter 39), or neurosurgical shunts (see Chapter 36); in patients with intravascular catheters [36], particularly long-duration central lines [37] such as Hickman catheters (see Chapter 44); and in immunosuppressed patients, particularly those who have received broad-spectrum antibiotics to treat or prevent infection with gram-negative bacilli (see Chapter 45).

Methicillin-resistant coagulase-negative staphylococci may be present in low numbers on the skin of patients and emerge in hospital as predominant flora and potential pathogens, especially after surgical antimicrobial prophylaxis [172], which is very similar to the epidemiology of *Enterobacter* infection [44,49]. Using gentamicin resistance as a marker, we found that resistant coagulase-negative staphylococci are relatively uncommon in healthy nonhospitalized people but are rapidly acquired in the hospital, related to either previous antibiotic exposure or ubiquitous environmental contamination [173]. The resistance was plasmid mediated and could be transferred in vitro or on skin to *S. aureus* [174]. In one study, most nosocomial isolates of gentamicin-resistant *S. aureus* appeared to result from in vivo plasmid spread from resistant coagulase-negative staphylococci [173].

Because drug-resistant coagulase-negative staphylococci often become part of the patient's normal flora and are so ubiquitous [174,175], control is difficult. In patients with indwelling intravascular catheters or patients undergoing implantation of foreign bodies, preventing infections with coagulase-negative staphylococci depends on strict attention to asepsis and, in some situations, antibiotic prophylaxis. More recent observations of wound infection due to dissemination of coagulase-negative strains by colonized surgeons [61] suggest the need to consider this mode of transmission when wound infection rates exceed expected norms.

Finally, the potential impact on hospitals of vancomycin-resistant coagulase-negative staphylococci remains undetermined [176].

Penicillin-Resistant Pneumococci

Although multiply resistant *S. pneumoniae* infections have not been a significant nosocomial problem in the United States, they reached epidemic proportions on crowded pediatric wards in South African hospitals in 1977 to 1978 [134]. During that time, 48 patients, almost all younger than 3 years, had positive blood or cerebrospinal fluid cultures, representing 8.5% of all pneumococcal isolates from these two sites. In addition, > 300 carriers of resistant pneumococci were found. Successful control measures included restriction of unnecessary antibiotic use (because antibiotic exposure increased the risk of colonization), susceptibility testing of all pneumococci, nasopharyngeal culture surveys, respiratory isolation of all infected and colonized patients, and aggressive use of antimicrobials to eradicate carriage.

Corynebacterium jeikeium

The JK strain of *Corynebacterium*, often susceptible only to vancomycin, has been noted to be an increasingly common pathogen in immunocompromised oncology patients, mostly causing bacteremia or wound infections at bone marrow aspiration and intravenous catheter sites [177–179]. JK diphtheroids appear commonly to colonize the skin of hospitalized patients [177,179] but, interestingly, are found more often in men and postmenopausal women, suggesting a possible relation between colonization and sebum content of skin. Because of extensive skin colonization, control of endemic infections with *C. jeikeium*, like control of coagulase-negative staphylococci, may depend in large part on good aseptic technique. In addition, at least one outbreak of JK diphtheroids has been described in which evidence suggested possible person-to-person spread and a role for careful handwashing in preventing infections.

Enterococci

Since the mid-1980s, enterococci have emerged as significant nosocomial pathogens. The most recent NNIS report lists enterococci as the second most common isolate, after *E. coli* [4]. Enterococci are not highly virulent bacteria and tend to cause infections in patients who are elderly, debilitated, or immunocompromised [180]. The increased rate of isolation of enterococci from clinical specimens is probably due partly to increasing numbers of patients with one or more predisposing factors for enterococcal infection.

The widespread use of antibiotics with little or no activity against enterococci may provide selective pressure for enterococcal survival. Enterococci are intrinsically resistant to all cephalosporins, semisynthetic penicillinase-resistant penicillins, erythromycin, and clindamycin. Moreover, since the mid-1970s, enterococci have acquired high-level resistance to penicillin, ampicillin, aminoglycosides, and most recently, vancomycin. For a growing number of strains, no effective antimicrobial regimen is available. The increase in the number of nosocomial enterococcal isolates coupled with increasing enterococcal resistance has led one observer to term multiply-resistant *E. faecium* "the nosocomial pathogen of the 1990s" [181].

Although enterococcal infection has traditionally been considered to originate from a patient's endogenous flora, more recent evidence demonstrates that nosocomial acquisition and spread of enterococci can occur. In one set of studies, the reservoir for gentamicin-resistant enterococci appeared to be the gastrointestinal tract of asymptomatic patients and nursing home transfers, and spread was from person to person on the hands of hospital personnel [182,183]. An outbreak of β-lactamase-producing, gentamicin-resistant *Enterococcus faecalis* in a neonatal ICU was terminated after a persistently colonized nurse was removed from patient care [184]. A contaminated electronic rectal thermometer was implicated as the vehicle of transmission in an outbreak of vancomycin-resistant *E. faecium* [104].

Vancomycin resistance is probably the most worrisome antibiotic resistance to emerge in enterococci [185], for several reasons. First, the incidence of vancomycin resistance in Europe and the United States has increased dramatically since it was first described in France in 1988 [186]. In 1989, 0.3% of enterococcal isolates reported to the NNIS System were resistant to vancomycin [187]. By 1995, >10% of enterococcal strains isolated in both non-ICUs and in ICUs were resistant to vancomycin [188]. A second reason for concern is that most vancomycin-resistant enterococci are concomitantly resistant to moderate or high levels of ampicillin and to high levels of aminoglycosides. Treatment of infections due to these multiply resistant pathogens is often limited to unproven combinations of antibiotics or investigational compounds [104,189]. Third, we and others have found that vancomycin-resistant enterococci can become hospital-acquired skin flora [190,191] as part of the "fecal veneer" that covers ill, hospitalized patients. As skin flora, vancomycin-resistant enterococci may be transmitted more readily between patients and may contaminate blood cultures or cause vascular access site infections. Finally, enterococci may act as a reservoir for vancomycin resistance genes that could then be transferred to other, more virulent bacteria, such as *S. aureus* (see earlier).

In response to these real and theoretic concerns, the Hospital Infection Control Practices Advisory Committee (HICPAC) and the CDC have published detailed recommendations for preventing the spread of vancomycin resistance [192]. These include more prudent use of vancomycin by clinicians, education of hospital staff regarding the problem of vancomycin resistance, surveillance for vancomycin resistance in enterococci and other gram-positive bacteria by the hospital laboratory, and contact isolation of patients identified as colonized or infected with vancomycin-resistant enterococci.

Extensive environmental contamination with vancomycin-resistant enterococci has been reported from several institutions [102,104,184,193]. In one outbreak, patients infected or colonized with an epidemic clone of vancomycin-resistant *E. faecium* were placed in private rooms, and all staff who entered the patient's room were required to wear gloves [193]. However, the outbreak was not controlled until personnel were required to wear gowns in addition to gloves for all patient contact. These data prompted the HICPAC/CDC recommendation that gowns be worn by healthcare workers who have substantial contact with an infected or colonized patient or with environmental surfaces in the patient's room. However, these measures may not be effective in decreasing the incidence of vancomycin-resistant enterococcal colonization or infection among patients in hospitals where this pathogen is well established. In a study we completed in 1996, the use of gloves and gowns was no more effective than the use of gloves alone in controlling the nosocomial spread of vancomycin-resistant enterococci in an ICU where this pathogen was endemic [106]. Moreover, multiple strains types were identified among vancomycin-resistant enterococci that appeared to have been acquired by patients after ICU entry. This suggests a more complex epidemiology than described by analyses of previous single-clone outbreaks—one that may require more elaborate or ingenious strategies to control.

Candidae

The incidence of nosocomial infections due to *Candida* species has risen dramatically in the United States since the late 1970s. Analysis of data collected by the NNIS System from 1980 to 1990 revealed that the rate of nosocomial fungal infections increased from 2.0 to 3.8 infections/1,000 patients discharged [194]; *Candida* species were responsible for 78.3% of reported fungal infections. *Candida* species are the sixth most common nosocomial pathogen isolated at NNIS hospitals that do institution-wide surveillance, and the fourth most commonly reported bloodstream isolate [195]. The increasing incidence of candidal infection is likely related to an increase in the number of immunocompromised patients, more aggressive and invasive therapy of these and other patient populations, and the use of broad-spectrum antibacterial agents.

Although resistance of *Candida* species to amphotericin B, 5-flucytosine, and ketoconazole has been described, the emergence of resistance to fluconazole has attracted the most attention. The high oral bioavailability of this drug combined with its low toxicity make fluconazole an appealing alternative to amphotericin B for selected candidal infections. It is especially used widely for the treatment of patients with acquired immunodeficiency syndrome (AIDS) who have oropharyngeal candidiasis, a disease that is typically relapsing and usually requires chronic suppressive or intermittent antifungal therapy for control [196]. It is not surprising, then, that clinical resistance to fluconazole has been described most frequently among AIDS patients with oropharyngeal candidiasis. Attempts to correlate clinical failure with an elevated fluconazole MIC have been hampered by the absence of a well standardized in vitro susceptibility testing method. However, in AIDS patients with oropharyngeal candidiasis, MICs of fluconazole of approximately 16 μg/ml by the National Committee for Clinical Laboratory Standards method [197] seem to correlate with a poor clinical response to 100 mg of fluconazole per day, and MICs > 64 μg/mL correlate with a poor response to 400 to 800 mg of fluconazole per day [196]. Development of resistance has been related to advanced human immunodeficiency virus infection (CD4 cell count < 50) and to cumulative fluconazole dose [196,198]. Studies in which DNA subtyping of *Candida* has been done have usually reported susceptible and resistant isolates from the same patient to be the same genotype [199–201], although multiple genotypes with different fluconazole MICs in a single patient [202] and acquisition of a new, resistant genotype have been reported [199,201,202]. However, as mentioned earlier, genotyping of fungi and bacteria is not standardized, and variations in the methods used or in the interpretation of results may have led to some of the differences in conclusions in these studies.

Although an elevated fluconazole MIC may be an important predictor of clinical failure in oropharyngeal candidiasis in AIDS patients, it appears to be less predictive of clinical response in other groups of patients and in other candidal infections. A multicenter trial of fluconazole versus amphotericin B for treatment of candidemia in nonneutropenic patients found no correlation between treatment failure and elevated fluconazole MICs, although the number of patients infected with these strains and treated with fluconazole was small [203]. A more accurate predictor of clinical failure with either antifungal agent was incomplete catheter exchange in patients with intravenous catheter-related fungemia [204].

On a broader scale, widespread use of fluconazole may result in a decrease in the prevalence of more susceptible *Candida* species, such as *C. albicans*, and an increase in prevalence of *Candida* species that typically have higher fluconazole MICs, such as *Candida krusei* and *Torulopsis* (*Candida*) *glabrata*. This has been reported in several studies [205–207], and warrants monitoring.

Although common source outbreaks involving candidae have been reported [208,209], most hospitalized patients appear to contract infection with *Candida* strains they already harbor [210–212]. Evidence suggests that in some cases, patients may become colonized with candidal strains that they acquire nosocomially. One series of studies used restriction endonuclease analysis of total genomic DNA to type isolates of *Candida* species found colonizing patients in a bone marrow transplant unit and an ICU of a university hospital [212–215]. Geographic and temporal clustering of patients from whom identical *Candida* strains were isolated suggested that exogenous nosocomial acquisition of *Candida* may have occurred. In one case, *Candida parapsilosis* was cultured from an air-conditioning vent in a room that later housed a patient whose sternal wound was found to be colonized with the same organism [214]. However, more than one molecular typing method may be needed to optimally discriminate among candidal strains. Initial investigation of a cluster of serious *C. albicans* infections used two DNA-based typing methods in conjunction with classic epidemiologic evaluation and identified limited nosocomial spread of a single strain. When the isolates were evaluated by a third molecular typing technique, all strains involved in the cluster appeared unique [216]. Additional studies are needed to identify the most accurate method of typing candidae, and to clarify the epidemiology of these pathogens and the potential for their control in hospitals.

Other Resistant Organisms

A variety of vancomycin-resistant gram-positive bacteria, such as *Leuconostoc, Pediococcus*, and *Lactobacillus* species, have been described [217,218]. Whether the increased use of vancomycin in hospitals will create enough pressure to allow these uncommon, usually avirulent strains to emerge as pathogens, particularly in the highly susceptible, heavily vancomycin-exposed populations such as oncology patients, remains to be seen.

Clindamycin resistance in the *Bacteroides fragilis* group has been a sporadic, relatively unusual problem that is plasmid mediated and has occurred in 0% to 10% of strains in various medical centers [219]. One group described an outbreak of clindamycin-resistant *B. fragilis* on a surgical ward in which 7 (13%) of 52 isolates were affected [220]; 85% of involved patients had received clindamycin or erythromycin before recovery of a resistant strain. The epidemiology of this outbreak is not entirely clear.

Stenotrophomonas (*Xanthomonas*) *maltophilia* is being more commonly recognized as a nosocomial pathogen [221,222]. This bacterium is frequently resistant to extended-spectrum penicillins, cephalosporins, aminoglycosides, fluoroquinolones, and imipenem. Infection and colonization has primarily been reported in ICU and oncology ward patients who have received multiple courses of antibiotics [222–225]. Involvement of the respiratory tract is common, and colonized or infected respiratory secretions or uncontained wound drainage may serve as bacterial reservoirs. One investigation suggested that transient carriage of *S. maltophilia* on the hands of hospital personnel contributed to an ICU outbreak [225]. However, a second, unrelated investigation of hospital-acquired *S. maltophilia* infection and colonization found only limited evidence for horizontal transmission [226]. Further studies to elucidate the epidemiology of this pathogen are needed.

Since the early 1990s, nosocomial transmission of multiply drug-resistant *Mycobacterium tuberculosis* to patients and healthcare workers has been reported from medical facilities in New York City, Miami, and Chicago [228,229] (see Chapter 33). Most outbreaks primarily involved people infected with the human immunodeficiency virus (see Chapter 43). Progression from new infection to active disease was often rapid, and mortality rates were high. Delays in diagnosis, initiation of effective therapy, and isolation of patients, as well as failure to institute recommended engineering controls, all contributed to the spread of infection in many outbreaks. Implementation of 1990 CDC guidelines for the prevention of transmission of tuberculosis in healthcare settings [230] was shown to be effective in terminating several of these outbreaks [229–232]. Newer CDC guidelines [233] are more cumbersome and expensive, and their superiority in preventing nosocomial acquisition of multiply drug-resistant tuberculosis is unproven.

The increasing availability of antiviral agents such as acyclovir presents the problem of acquired drug resistance in herpes virus and other viruses, a problem already arising in AIDS patients. Whether these organisms will become significant nosocomial pathogens remains to be seen.

FUTURE CHALLENGES

The ingenious ways in which microorganisms "learn" to evade our antimicrobial pharmacopeia will no doubt continue to astound, and at times confound, and perplex us. As the pressures on our antimicrobial armamentarium increase, and as our patients are subjected to more invasive procedures and immunosuppressive regimens, we can look forward to greater resistance and more problems with the traditionally avirulent normal flora.

Unfortunately, our control of resistant strains has advanced little since the singular contribution of Semmelweis. Moreover, we still have trouble encouraging and motivating personnel to follow the most basic concepts in asepsis. In fact, our most successful advances are attributable to the development of newer antimicrobials and less infection-prone devices rather than to improvements in application of basic aseptic principles.

At the same time, we need to use advances in microbiologic techniques to obtain a better understanding of the epidemiology of nosocomial resistance, not only in single-strain outbreaks but in the endemic setting and in plasmid and even transposon outbreaks. As we increase our understanding of bacterial [234] and host factors that control colonization with normal flora and lead to overgrowth of resistant bacteria, new approaches may emerge for preventing colonization with nosocomial pathogens, blocking adherence of unwanted resistant strains, or halting progression from colonization to infection.

In the meantime, we believe the key is not to delay in applying the strategies available to us and not to apply measures in too piecemeal a fashion, lest control always lag behind resistance. The growing interchange of resistant bacteria among nursing homes, community hospitals, tertiary care centers, and high-risk outpatient populations emphasizes the need for concerted control efforts.

REFERENCES

1. McGowan JE. Antimicrobial resistance in hospital organisms and its relation to antibiotic use. *Rev Infect Dis* 1983;5:1033.
2. Stamm WE, Weinstein RA, Dixon RE. Comparison of endemic and epidemic nosocomial infections. *Am J Med* 1981;70:393.
3. Haley RW, Hightower AW, Khabbaz RF, et al. The emergence of methicillin-resistant *Staphylococcus aureus* infections in United States hospitals. *Ann Intern Med* 1982;97:297.
4. Schaberg DR, Culver DH, Gaynes RP. Major trends in the microbial etiology of nosocomial infection. *Am J Med* 1991;91(Suppl 3B):72S.
5. Weinstein, RA, Kabins, SA. Strategies for prevention and control of multiple drug-resistant nosocomial infection. *Am J Med* 1981;70:449.
6. Centers for Disease Control and Prevention. Reduced Susceptibility of *Staphylococcus aureus* to vancomycin—Japan, 1996. *MMWR* 1997;46:624.
7. Noble WC, Virani Z, Cree RGA. Co-transfer of vancomycin and other resistance genes from *Enterococcus faecalis* NCTC 12201 to *Staphylococcus aureus*. *FEMS Microbiol Lett* 1992;93:195.
8. Jacoby GA, Archer GL. New mechanisms of bacterial resistance to antimicrobial agents. *N Engl J Med* 1991;324:601.
9. Foster TJ. Plasmid-determined resistance to antimicrobial drugs and toxic metal ions in bacteria. *Microbiol Rev* 1983;47:361.
10. Cairns J, Overbaugh J, Miller S. The origin of mutants. *Nature* 1988; 335:142.
11. Stokes HW, Hall RM. A novel family of potentially mobile DNA elements encoding site-specificic gene-integration functions: integrons. *Mol Microbiol* 1989;3:1669.
12. Embil J, Romotar K, Romance L, et al. Methicillin-resistant *Staphylococcus aureus* in tertiary care institutions on the Canadian prairies 1990–1992. *Infect Control Hosp Epidemiol* 1994;15:646.
13. Layton MC, Hierholzer WJ, Patterson JE. The evolving epidemiology of methicillin-resistant *Staphylococcus aureus* at a university hospital. *Infect Control Hosp Epidemiol* 1995;16:12.
14. Lugeon C, Blanc DS, Wenger A, et al. Molecular epidemiology of methicillin-resistant *Staphylococcus aureus* at a low incidence hospital over a four-year period. *Infect Control Hosp Epidemiol* 1995;16:260.
15. Duncan IBR, Rennie RP, Duncan NH. A long-term study of gentamicin-resistant *Pseudomonas aeruginosa* in a general hospital. *J Antimicrob Chemother* 1981;7:147.
16. Horan TC, White JW, Jarvis WR, et al. Nosocomial infection surveillance, 1984. *MMWR Morb Mortal Wkly Rep* 1986;35:17SS.
17. Jarvis WR, White JW, Munn VP, et al. Nosocomial infection surveillance, 1983. *MMWR Morb Mortal Wkly Rep* 1984;33:9SS. Nosocomial aminoglycoside-resistant gram-negative bacillary infections in the United States, 1975–1982. In: *Programs and abstracts of the twenty-third interscience conference on antimicrobial agents and chemotherapy*. Las Vegas, Nevada, October 24–26, 1983. Washington, DC: American Society for Microbiology, 1983:248.
18. O'Brien TF, Acar JF, Medeiros AA, et al. International comparison of prevalence of resistance to antibiotics. *JAMA* 1978;239:1518.
19. Rennie RP, Duncan IBR. Emergence of gentamicin-resistant *Klebsiella* in a general hospital. *Antimicrob Agents Chemother* 1977;11: 179.
20. Allen JR, Hightower AW, Martin SM, et al. Secular trends in nosocomial infections: 1970–1979. *Am J Med* 1981;70:389.
21. Sanders WE, Sanders CC. Inducible β-lactamases: clinical and epidemiologic implications for use of newer cephalosporins. *Rev Infect Dis* 1988;10:830.
22. Olson B, Weinstein RA, Nathan C, et al. Broad-spectrum beta-lactam resistance in *Enterobacter*: emergence during treatment and mechanisms of resistance. *J Antimicrob Chemother* 1983;11:299.
23. Sanders CC, Moellering RC Jr, Martin RR, et al. Resistance to cefamandole: a collaborative study of emerging clinical problems. *J Infect Dis* 1982;145:118.
24. Chow JW, Fine MJ, Shlaes DM, et al. *Enterobacter* bacteremia: clinical features and emergence of antibiotic resistance during therapy. *Ann Intern Med* 1991;115:585.
25. Burwen DR, Bannerjee SN, Gaynes RP, et al. Ceftazidime resistance among selected nosocomial gram-negative bacilli in the United States. *J Infect Dis* 1994;170:1622.
26. Ballow CH, Schentag JJ. Trends in antibiotic utilization and bacterial resistance: report of the National Nosocomial Resistance Surveillance Group. *Diagn Microbiol Infect Dis* 1991;15:37S.
27. Philippon A, Labia R, Jacoby G. Extended spectrum β-lactamases. *Antimicrob Agents Chemother* 1989;33:1131.
28. Gaynes RP, Culver DH, the National Nosocomial Infection Surveillance (NNIS) System. Resistance to imipenem among selected gram-negative bacilli in the United States. *Infect Control Hosp Epidemiol* 1992;13:10.
29. Ito H, Arakawa Y, Ohsuka S, et al. Plasmid-mediated dissemination of the metallo-β-lactamase gene *blaI* among clinically isolated strains of *Serratia marcescens*. *Antimicrob Agents Chemother* 1995;39:824.
30. Go ES, Urban C, Burns J, et al. Clinical and molecular epidemiology of *Acinetobacter* infections sensitive only to polymyxin B and sulbactam. *Lancet* 1994;344(8933):1329.
31. Greene WH, Moody M, Schimpff S, et al. *Pseudomonas aeruginosa* resistant to carbenicillin and gentamicin. *Ann Intern Med* 1973;79: 684.
32. Hart CA, Gibson MF, Buckles AM. Variation in skin and environmental survival of hospital gentamicin-resistant enterobacteria. *Journal of Hygiene (Cambridge)* 1981;87:277.
33. Huovinen P, Mantyjarvi R, Toivanen P. Trimethoprim resistance in hospitals. *Br Med J* 1982;284:782.
34. Gaynes RP, Culver DH, Horan TC, et al. Trends in methicillin-resistant *Staphylococcus aureus* in United States hospitals. *Infectious Diseases in Clinical Practice* 1993;2:452.
35. Wade JC, Schimpff SC, Newman KA, et al. *Staphylococcus epidermidis*: an increasing cause of infection in patients with granulocytopenia. *Ann Intern Med* 1982;97:503.
36. Baumgart S, Hall SE, Campos JM, et al. Sepsis with coagulase-negative staphylococci in critically ill newborns. *American Journal of Diseases of Children* 1983;137:461.
37. Christensen GD, Bisno AL, Parisi JT, et al. Nosocomial septicemia due to multiply antibiotic-resistant *Staphylococcus epidermidis*. *Ann Intern Med* 1982;96:1.
38. Humphreys H, Mulvill E. Ciprofloxacin-resistant *Staphylococcus aureus*. *Lancet* 1985;2:383.
39. Muder RR, Brennen C, Goetz AM, et al. Association with prior fluoroquinolone therapy of widespread ciprofloxacin resistance among gram-negative isolates in a Veterans Affairs medical center. *Antimicrob Agents Chemother* 1991;35:256.
40. Pascale R, Delangle M, Merrien D, et al. Fluoroquinolone use and fluoroquinolone resistance: is there an association? *Clin Infect Dis* 1994;19:54.
41. Schaeffler S. Methicillin-resistant strains of *Staphylococcus aureus* resistant to quinolones. *J Clin Microbiol* 1989;27:335.
42. Shalit I, Haas H, Berger SA. Susceptibility of *Pseudomonas aeruginosa* to fluoroquinolones following four years of use in a tertiary care hospital. *J Antimicrob Chemother* 1992;30:149.
43. Coronado VG, Edwards JR, Culver DH. Ciprofloxacin resistance among nosocomial *Pseudomonas aeruginosa* and *Staphylococcus aureus* in the United States. *Infect Control Hosp Epidemiol* 1995;16:71.
44. Flynn DM, Weinstein RA, Nathan C, et al. Patients' endogenous flora as the source of "nosocomial" *Enterobacter* in cardiac surgery. *J Infect Dis* 1987;156:363.
45. Gaynes RP, Weinstein RA, Chamberlin W, et al. Antibiotic-resistant flora in nursing home patients admitted to the hospital. *Arch Intern Med* 1985;145:1804.
46. Olson B, Weinstein RA, Nathan C, et al. Occult aminoglycoside resistance in *Pseudomonas aeruginosa*: epidemiology and implications for therapy and control. *J Infect Dis* 1985;152:769.
47. Weinstein RA, Nathan C, Gruensfelder R, Kabins SA. Endemic aminoglycoside resistance in gram-negative bacilli: epidemiology and mechanisms. *J Infect Dis* 1980;141:338.
48. Casewell MW, Dalton MT, Webster M, et al. Gentamicin-resistant *Klebsiella aerogenes* in a urological ward. *Lancet* 1977;2:444.
49. Flynn DM, Weinstein RA, Kabins SA. Infections with gram-negative bacilli in a cardiac surgery intensive care unit: the relative role of *Enterobacter*. *J Hosp Infect* 1988;11:367.

50. Selden R, Lee S, Wang WL, et al. Nosocomial *Klebsiella* infections: intestinal colonization as a reservoir. *Ann Intern Med* 1971;74:657.
51. Jarvis WR. Usefulness of molecular epidemiology for outbreak investigations. *Infect Control Hosp Epidemiol* 1994;15:500.
52. Bingen E. Applications of molecular methods to epidemiologic investigations of nosocomial infections in a pediatric hospital. *Infect Control Hosp Epidemiol* 1994;15:488.
53. Maslow N, Mulligan ME, Arbeit RD. Molecular epidemiology. application of contemporary techniques to the typing of microorganisms. *Clin Infect Dis* 1993;17:153.
54. Tenover FC, Arbeit RD, Goering RV, et al. Interpreting chromosomal DNA restriction patterns produced by pulsed-field gel electrophoresis: criteria for bacterial strain typing. *J Clin Microbiol* 1995;33:2233.
55. Kreiswirth B, Kornblum J, Arbeit RD, et al. Evidence for a clonal origin of methicillin resistance in *Staphylococcus aureus*. *Science* 1993; 259:227.
56. Tenover FC, Arbeit R, Archer G, et al. Comparison of traditional and molecular methods of typing isolates of *Staphylococcus aureus*. *J Clin Microbiol* 1994;32:407.
57. Gilmore DS, Schick DG, Montgomerie JZ. *Pseudomonas aeruginosa* and *Klebsiella pneumoniae* on the perinea of males with spinal cord injuries. *J Clin Microbiol* 1982;16:865.
58. Montgomerie JZ, Morrow JW. *Pseudomonas* colonization in patients with spinal cord injury. *Am J Epidemiol* 1978;108:328.
59. Fainstein V, Rodriguez V, Turck M, et al. Patterns of oropharyngeal and fecal flora in patients with acute leukemia. *J Infect Dis* 1981;144: 10.
60. Craven DE, Reed C, Kollisch N, et al. A large outbreak of infections caused by a strain of *Staphylococcus aureus* resistant to oxacillin and aminoglycosides. *Am J Med* 1981;71:53.
61. Boyce JM, Potter-Bynoe G, Opal SM, et al. A common-source outbreak of *Staphylococcus epidermidis* infections among patients undergoing cardiac surgery. *J Infect Dis* 1990;161:493.
62. Buxton AE, Anderson RL, Werdegar D, et al. Nosocomial respiratory tract infection and colonization with *Acinetobacter calcoaceticus*: epidemiologic characteristics. *Am J Med* 1978;65:507.
63. Graham, DR, Anderson RL, Ariel FE, et al. Epidemic nosocomial meningitis due to *Citrobacter diversus* in neonates. *J Infect Dis* 1981; 144:203.
64. Parry MF, Hutchinson JH, Brown NA, et al. Gram-negative sepsis in neonates: a nursery outbreak due to hand carriage of *Citrobacter diversus*. *Pediatrics* 1980;65:1105.
65. Burke JP, Ingall D, Klein JO, et al. *Proteus mirabilis* infections in a hospital nursery traced to a human carrier. *N Engl J Med* 1971;284:115.
66. Shooter RA. Bowel colonization of hospital patients by *Pseudomonas aeruginosa* and *Escherichia coli*. *Proc R Soc Med* 1971;64:27.
67. Griffith SJ, Nathan C, Selander RK, et al. The epidemiology of *Pseudomonas aeruginosa* in oncology patients in a general hospital. *J Infect Dis* 1989;160:1030.
68. Marrie TJ, Major H, Gurwith M, et al. Prolonged outbreak of nosocomial urinary tract infection with a single strain of *Pseudomonas aeruginosa*. *Can Med Assoc J* 1978;119:593.
69. Wenzel RP, Veazey JM, Townsend TR. Role of the inanimate environment in hospital-acquired infections. In: Cundy KR, Ball W, eds. *Infection control in healthcare facilities: microbiological surveillance*. Baltimore: University Park Press, 1977:71.
70. Feeley TW, DuMoulin GC, Hedley-Whyte J, et al. Aerosol polymyxin and pneumonia in seriously ill patients. *N Engl J Med* 1975;293:471.
71. Levin MH, Olson B, Nathan C, et al. *Pseudomonas* in ICU sinks: relation to patients. *J Clin Pathol* 1984;37:424.
72. Perryman FA, Flournoy DJ. Prevalence of gentamicin-and amikacin-resistant bacteria in sink drains. *J Clin Microbiol* 1980;12:79.
73. Adams BG, Marrie TJ. Hand carriage of aerobic gram-negative rods may not be transient. *Journal of Hygiene (Cambridge)* 1982;89:33.
74. Knittle MA, Eitzman DV, Baer H. Role of hand contamination of personnel in the epidemiology of gram-negative nosocomial infections. *J Pediatr* 1975;86:433.
75. Salzman TC, Clark JJ, Klemm L. Hand contamination of personnel as a mechanism of cross-infection in nosocomial infections with antibiotic-resistant *Escherichia coli* and *Klebsiella aerobacter*. *Antimicrob Agents Chemother* 1968;1967:97.
76. Grieble HG, Bird TJ, Nidea HM, et al. Chute-hydropulping waste disposal system: a reservoir of enteric bacilli and *Pseudomonas* in a modern hospital. *J Infect Dis* 1974;130:602.
77. Gaman W, Cates C, Snelling CF, et al. Emergence of gentamicin- and carbenicillin-resistant *Pseudomonas aeruginosa* in a hospital environment. *Antimicrob Agents Chemother* 1976;9:474.
78. Kauffman CA, Ramundo NC, Williams SG, et al. Surveillance of gentamicin-resistant gram-negative bacilli in a general hospital. *Antimicrob Agents Chemother* 1978;13:918.
79. Chow AW, Taylor PR, Yoshikawa TT, Guze LB. A nosocomial outbreak of infections due to multiply resistant *Proteus mirabilis*: role of intestinal colonization as a major reservoir. *J Infect Dis* 1979;139:621.
80. Graham DR, Correa-Villasenor A, Anderson RL, et al. Epidemic neonatal gentamicin-methicillin-resistant *Staphylococcus aureus* infection associated with nonspecific topical use of gentamicin. *J Pediatr* 1980;97:972.
81. McGowan JE. Do intensive hospital antibiotic control programs prevent the spread of antibiotic resistance? *Infect Control Hosp Epidemiol* 1994;15:478.
82. Gaynes RP, Weinstein RA, Smith J, et al. Control of aminoglycoside resistance by barrier precautions. *Infect Control* 1983;4:221.
83. Meyer RD. Patterns and mechanisms of emergence of resistance to amikacin. *J Infect Dis* 1977;136:449.
84. Noriega ER, Liebowitz RE, Richmond AS, et al. Nosocomial infection caused by gentamicin-resistant, streptomycin-sensitive *Klebsiella*. *J Infect Dis* 1975;131:S45.
85. Roberts NJ, Douglas RG. Gentamicin use and *Pseudomonas* and *Serratia* resistance: effect of a surgical prophylaxis regimen. *Antimicrob Agents Chemother* 1978;13:214.
86. Shulman JA, Terry PM, Hough CE. Colonization with gentamicin-resistant *Pseudomonas aeruginosa*, pyocine type 5, in a burn unit. *J Infect Dis* 1971;124:S18.
87. Mathias RG, Ronald AR, Gurwith MJ, et al. Clinical evaluation of amikacin in treatment of infections due to gram-negative aerobic bacilli. *J Infect Dis* 1976;134:S394.
88. Amirak ID, Williams RJ, Noone P, et al. Amikacin resistance developing in patient with *Pseudomonas aeruginosa* bronchopneumonia. *Lancet* 1977;1:537.
89. Moody MM, deJongh CA, Schimpff SC, et al. Long-term amikacin use: effects on aminoglycoside susceptibility patterns of gram-negative bacilli. *JAMA* 1982;248:1199.
90. Price KE, Kresel PA, Farchione CA, et al. Epidemiological studies of aminoglycoside resistance in the U.S.A. *J Antimicrob Chemother* 1981;8:89.
91. Wormser GP, Tatz J, Donath J. Endemic resistance to amikacin among hospital isolates of gram-negative bacilli: implications for therapy. *Infect Control* 1983;4:93.
92. Houang ET, Greenwood D. Aminoglycoside cross-resistance patterns of gentamicin-resistant bacteria. *J Clin Pathol* 1977;30:738.
93. Mawer SL, Greenwood D. Aminoglycoside resistance emerging during therapy. *Lancet* 1977;1:749.
94. Seal DV, Strangeways JEM. Aminoglycoside resistance due to mutation. *Lancet* 1977;1:856.
95. Meyer KS, Urban C, Eagan JA, et al. Nosocomial outbreak of *Klebsiella* infection resistant to late-generation cephalosporins. *Ann Intern Med* 1993;119:353.
96. Jones RN. The current and future impact of antimicrobial resistance among nosocomial bacterial pathogens. *Diagn Microbiol Infect Dis* 1992;15:3S.
97. Weinstein RA. Endemic emergence of cephalosporin-resistant *Enterobacter*: relation to prior therapy. *Infect Control* 1986;7:120.
98. Murray BE, Rensimer ER, DuPont HL. Emergence of high-level trimethoprim resistance in fecal *Escherichia coli* during oral administration of trimethoprim or trimethoprim–sulfamethoxazole. *N Engl J Med* 1982;306:130.
99. Berntsen CA, McDermott W. Increased transmissibility of staphylococci to patients receiving an antimicrobial drug. *N Engl J Med* 1960; 262:637.
100. Saravolatz LD, Markowitz N, Arking L, et al. Methicillin-resistant *Staphylococcus aureus*: epidemiologic observations during a community-acquired outbreak. *Ann Intern Med* 1982;96:11.
101. Boyle JF, Soumakis SA, Rendo A, et al. Epidemiologic analysis and genotypic characterization of a nosocomial outbreak of vancomycin-resistant enterococci. *J Clin Microbiol* 1993;31:1280.
102. Karanfil LV, Murphy M, Josephson A, et al. A cluster of vancomycin-resistant *Enterococcus faecium* in an intensive care unit. *Infect Control Hosp Epidemiol* 1992;13:195.

103. Rubin LG, Tucci V, Cercenado E, et al. Vancomycin-resistant *Enterococcus faecium* in hospitalized children. *Infect Control Hosp Epidemiol* 1992;13:700.
104. Livornese LL, Dias S, Samel C, et al. Hospital-acquired infection with vancomycin-resistant *Enterococcus faecium* transmitted by electronic thermometers. *Ann Intern Med* 1992;117:112.
105. Edmond MB, Ober JF, Weinbaum DL. Vancomycin-resistant *Enterococcus faecium* bacteremia: risk factors for infection. *Clin Infect Dis* 1995;20:1126.
106. Slaughter S, Hayden MK, Nathan C, et al. A comparison of the effect of universal gown and glove use alone in the acquisition of vancomycin-resistant enterococci in a medical intensive care unit. *Ann Intern Med* 1996;125:448.
107. Elwell LP, Inamine JM, Minshew BH. Common plasmid specifying tobramycin resistance found in two enteric bacteria isolated from burn patients. *Antimicrob Agents Chemother* 1978;13:312.
108. John JF, McKee KT, Twitty JA, et al. Molecular epidemiology of sequential nursery epidemics caused by multiresistant *Klebsiella pneumoniae*. *J Pediatr* 1983;102:825.
109. Markowitz SM, Veazey JM Jr, Macrina FL, et al. Sequential outbreaks of infection due to *Klebsiella pneumoniae* in a neonatal intensive care unit: implication of a conjugative R plasmid. *J Infect Dis* 1980;142:106.
110. Rubens CE, Farrar WE, McGee ZA, et al. Evolution of a plasmid-mediating resistance to multiple antimicrobial agents during a prolonged epidemic of nosocomial infections. *J Infect Dis* 1981;143:170.
111. Rubens CE, McNeill WF, Farrar WE Jr. Evolution of multiple-antibiotic-resistance plasmids mediated by transposable plasmid deoxyribonucleic acid sequences. *J Bacteriol* 1979;140:713.
112. Sadowski PL, Peterson BV, Gerding DN, Cleary PP. Physical characterization of ten R plasmids obtained from an outbreak of nosocomial *Klebsiella pneumoniae* infections. *Antimicrob Agents Chemother* 1979;15:616.
113. Tompkins LS, Plorde JJ, Falkow S. Molecular analysis of R-factors from multiresistant nosocomial isolates. *J Infect Dis* 1980;141:625.
114. Wiener J, Quinn J, Nathan C, et al. Molecular epidemiology of plasmid-mediated ceftazidime resistance (CAZ-R) in *E. coli* and *Klebsiella pneumoniae* in community nursing homes. In: *Abstracts from the thirty-fourth interscience conference on antimicrobial agents and chemotherapy, 1994*. Orlando, October 4–7, 1994. Washington, DC: American Society for Microbiology, 1994:87.
115. Gardner P, Smith DH. Studies on the epidemiology of resistance (R) factors: I. Analysis of *Klebsiella* isolates in a general hospital. II. A prospective study of R-factor transfer in the host. *Ann Intern Med* 1969;71:1.
116. Roe E, Jones RJ, Lowbury EJL. Transfer of antibiotic resistance between *Pseudomonas aeruginosa, Escherichia coli*, and other gram-negative bacilli in burns. *Lancet* 1971;1:149.
117. Kruse H, Sorum H. Transfer of multiple drug resistance plasmids between bacteria of diverse origins in natural microenvironments. *Appl Environ Microbiol* 1994;60:4015.
118. Trieu-Cuot P, Derlot E, Courvalin P. Enhanced conjugative transfer of plasmid DNA from *Escherichia coli* to *Staphylococcus aureus* and *Listeria monocytogenes*. *FEMS Microbiol Lett* 1993;109:19.
119. Bennett SN, McNeil MM, Bland LE, et al. Postoperative infections traced to contamination of an intravenous anesthetic, propofol. *N Engl J Med* 1995;333:147.
120. Maki DG, Hennekens CG, Phillips CW, et al. Nosocomial urinary tract infection with *Serratia marcescens*: an epidemiologic study. *J Infect Dis* 1973;128:579.
121. Haley RW, Cushion NB, Tenover FC, et al. Eradication of endemic methicillin-resistant *Staphylococcus aureus* infections from a neonatal intensive care unit. *J Infect Dis* 1995;171:614.
122. Price DJE, Sleigh JD. Control of infection due to *Klebsiella aerogenes* in a neurosurgical unit by withdrawal of all antibiotics. *Lancet* 1970;2:1213.
123. Gill S, Iyer VN. Nalidixic acid inhibits the conjugal transfer of conjugative N incompatibility group plasmids. *Can J Microbiol* 1982;28:256.
124. Blaser J, Stone BB, Groner MC, et al. Comparative study with enoxacin and netilimicin in a pharmacodynamic model to determine importance of ratio of antibiotic peak concentration to MIC for bacterial activity and emergence of resistance. *Antimicrob Agents Chemother* 1987;31:1054.
125. Nicolau DP, Freeman CD, Belliveau PP, et al. Experience with a once-daily aminoglycoside program administered to 2,184 adult patients. *Antimicrob Agents Chemother* 1995;39:650.
126. Brun-Buisson C, Legrand P, Rauss A, et al. Intestinal decontamination for control of nosocomial multiresistant gram-negative bacilli: study of an outbreak in an intensive care unit. *Ann Intern Med* 1989;110:873.
127. Weinstein RA. Selective intestinal decontamination an infection control measure whose time has come. *Ann Intern Med* 1989;110:853.
128. Sprunt K, Leidy G, Redman W. Abnormal colonization of neonates in an ICU: conversion to normal colonization by pharyngeal implantation of alpha-hemolytic *Streptococcus* strain 215. *Pediatr Res* 1980;14:308.
129. Cook LN, Davis RS, Stover BH. Outbreak of amikacin-resistant Enterobacteriaceae in an intensive care nursery. *Pediatrics* 1980;65:264.
130. Maizels M, Schaeffer AJ. Decreased incidence of bacteriuria associated with periodic instillations of hydrogen peroxide into the urethral catheter drainage bag. *J Urol* 1980;123:841.
131. Thompson RL, Haley CE, Searcy MA, et al. Catheter-associated bacteruria: failure to reduce attack rates using periodic instillation of a disinfectant into urinary drainage systems. *JAMA* 1984;251:747.
132. Makela P, Ojajarvi J, Salminen E. Decontaminating waste-trap. *Lancet* 1972;1:1216.
133. Raz R, Stamm WE. A controlled trial of intravaginal estriol in post-menopausal women with recurrent urinary tract infections. *N Engl J Med* 1993;329:753.
134. Jacobs MR, Koorhof HJ, Robbins-Browne RM, et al. Emergence of multiply resistant pneumococci. *N Engl J Med* 1978;299:735.
135. Olson B, Weinstein RA, Nathan C, et al. Epidemiology of endemic *Pseudomonas aeruginosa*: why infection control efforts have failed. *J Infect Dis* 1984;150:808.
136. Flaherty J, Nathan C, Kabins SA, Weinstein RA. Pilot trial of selective decontamination for prevention of bacterial infection in an intensive care unit. *J Infect Dis* 1990;162:1393.
137. Ledingham IM, Alcock SR, Eastaway AT, et al. Triple regimen of selective decontamination of the digestive tract, systemic cefotaxime, and microbiological surveillance for prevention of acquired infection in intensive care. *Lancet* 1988;1:785.
138. Stoutenbeek CP, vanSaene HK, Miranda DR, et al. Nosocomial gram-negative pneumonia in critically ill patients: a 3-year experience with a novel therapeutic regimen. *Intensive Care Med* 1986;12:419.
139. Stoutenbeek CP, van Saene HK, Zandstra DF. The effect of oral non-absorbable antibiotics on the emergence of resistant bacteria in patients in an intensive care unit. *J Antimicrob Chemother* 1987;19:513.
140. Weiner J, Itokazu G, Nathan C, et al. A randomized, double-blind, placebo-controlled trial of selective digestive decontamination in a medical-surgical intensive care unit. *Clin Infect Dis* 1995;20:861.
141. Bryce EA, Smith JA. Focused microbiological surveillance and gram-negative beta-lactamse-mediated resistance in an intensive care unit. *Infect Control Hosp Epidemiol* 1995;16:331.
142. Gaynes R. Antibiotic resistance in ICUs: a multifaceted problem requiring a multifaceted solution. *Infect Control Hosp Epidemiol* 1995;16:328.
143. Stratton CW, Ratner H, Johnston PE. Focused microbiologic surveillance by specific hospital unit as a sensitive means of defining antimicrobial resistance problems. *Diagn Microbiol Infect Dis* 1992;15:11S.
144. Farmer JJ, Weinstein RA, Zierdt CH, Brokopp CD. Hospital outbreaks caused by *Pseudomonas aeruginosa*: importance of serogroup 011. *J Clin Microbiol* 1982;16:266.
145. Tenover FC, Arbeit RD, Goering RV, et al. How to select and interpret molecular strain typing methods for epidemiological studies of bacterial infections: a review for healthcare epidemiologists. *Infect Control Hosp Epidemiol* 1997;18:426.
146. Schaberg DR, Weinstein RA, Stamm WE. Epidemics of nosocomial urinary tract infection caused by multiply resistant gram-negative bacilli: Epidemiology and control. *J Infect Dis* 1976;133:363.
147. Hart CA, Gibson MF. Comparative epidemiology of gentamicin-resistant enterobacteria: persistence of carriage and infection. *J Clin Pathol* 1982;35:452.
148. Schaberg DR, Alford RH, Anderson R, et al. An outbreak of nosocomial infection due to multiply resistant *Serratia marcescens*: evidence of interhospital spread. *J Infect Dis* 1976;134:181.
149. Edwards LD, Cross A, Levin S, et al. Outbreak of a nosocomial infec-

tion with a strain of *Proteus rettgeri* resistant to many antimicrobials. *Am J Clin Pathol* 1974;61:41.
150. Gerding DN, Buxton AE, Hughes RA, et al. Nosocomial multiply resistant *Klebsiella pneumoniae*: epidemiology of an outbreak of apparent index case origin. *Antimicrob Agents Chemother* 1979;15:608.
151. Jarlier V, Nicolas MH, Fournier G, et al. Extended broad-spectrum betalactamases conferring transferrable resistance to newer beta-lactam agents in Enterobacteriaceae: hospital prevalence and susceptibility patterns. *Rev Infect Dis* 1988;10:867.
152. Labia R, Morand A, Tiwari K, et al. Interactions of new plasmid-mediated β-lactamases with third-generation cephalosporins. *Rev Infect Dis* 1988;10:885.
153. Lowbury EJ, Thom BT, Lilly HA, et al. Sources of infection with *Pseudomonas aeruginosa* in patients with tracheostomy. *J Med Microbiol* 1970;3:39.
154. Meyer RD, Lewis RP, Halter J, et al. Gentamicin-resistant *Pseudomonas aeruginosa* and *Serratia marcescens* in a general hospital. *Lancet* 1976;1:580.
155. Keys TF, Washington JA. Gentamicin-resistant *Pseudomonas aeruginosa*: Mayo Clinic experience, 1970–1976. *Mayo Clin Proc* 1977;52:797.
156. Noone MR, Pitt TL, Bedder M, et al. *Pseudomonas aeruginosa* colonisation in an intensive therapy unit: role of cross-infection and host factors. *Br Med J* 1983;286:341.
157. Panlilio A, Culver DH, Gaynes RP, et al. Prevalence and distribution of methicillin-resistant *Staphylococcus aureus* in the United States. *Infect Control Hosp Epidemiol* 1992;13:582.
158. Semel JD, Trenholme GM, Levin S. Gentamicin- and clindamycin-resistant *Staphylococcus aureus*. *Am J Med Sci* 1980;280:4.
159. Jorgensen JH. Mechanisms of methicillin resistance in *Staphylococcus aureus* and methods for laboratory detection. *Infect Control Hosp Epidemiol* 1991;12:14.
160. Hsu CCS, Macaluso CP, Special L, et al. High rate of methicillin resistance of *Staphylococcus aureus* isolated from hospitalized nursing home patients. *Arch Intern Med* 1988;148:569.
161. Thompson RL, Cabezudo I, Wenzel RP. Epidemiology of nosocomial infections caused by methicillin-resistant *Staphylococcus aureus*. *Ann Intern Med* 1982;97:309.
162. Ellison RT, Judson FN, Peterson LC, et al. Oral rifampin and trimethoprim/sulfamethoxazole therapy in asymptomatic carriers of methicillin-resistant *Staphylococcus aureus* infections. *West J Med* 1984; 140:735.
163. Piercy EZ, Barbaro D, Luby JP, et al. Ciprofloxacin for methicillin-resistant *Staphylococcus aureus* infections. *Antimicrob Agents Chemother* 1989;33:128.
164. Ward T, Winn RE, Hartstein AI, et al. Observations relating to an inter-hospital outbreak of methicillin-resistant *Staphylococcus aureus*: role of antimicrobial therapy in infection control. *Infect Control* 1981; 2:453.
165. Bartzokas CA, Paton JH, Gibson MF, et al. Control and eradication of methicillin-resistant *Staphylococcus aureus* on a surgical unit. *N Engl J Med* 1984;311:1422.
166. Bitar CM, Mayhall CG, Lamb VA, et al. Outbreak due to methicillin- and rifampin-resistant *Staphylococcus aureus*: epidemiology and eradication of the resistant strain from the hospital. *Infect Control* 1987;8:15.
167. Denning DW, Haiduven-Griffiths D. Eradication of low-level methicillin-resistant *Staphylococcus aureus* skin colonization with topical mupirocin. *Infect Control Hosp Epidemiol* 1988;9:261.
168. Hill RLR, Duckworth DJ, Casewell MW. Elimination of nasal carriage of methicillin-resistant *Staphylococcus aureus* with mupirocin during a hospital outbreak. *J Antimicrob Chemother* 1988;22:377.
169. Wise R, Johnson J. Mupirocin resistance. *Lancet* 1991;338:578.
170. Boyce JM, Jackson MM, Pugliese G, et al. Methicillin-resistant *Staphylococcus aureus* (MRSA): a briefing for acute care hospitals and nursing facilities. *Infect Control Hosp Epidemiol* 1994;15:105.
171. Mulligan ME, Murray-Leisure KA, Ribner BS, et al. Methicillin-resistant *Staphylococcus aureus*: a consensus review of the microbiology, pathogenesis, and epidemiology with implications for prevention and management. *Am J Med* 1993;94:313.
172. Kernodle DS, Barg NL, Kaiser AB. Low-level colonization of hospitalized patients with methicillin-resistant coagulase-negative staphylococci and emergence of the organisms during surgical antimicrobial prophylaxis. *Antimicrob Agents Chemother* 1988;32:202.
173. Weinstein RA, Kabins S, Nathan C, et al. Gentamicin-resistant staphylococci as hospital flora: epidemiology and resistance plasmids. *J Infect Dis* 1982;145:374.
174. Jaffe HW, Sweeney HM, Nathan C, et al. Identity and interspecific transfer of gentamicin-resistant plasmids in *Staphylococcus aureus* and *Staphylococcus epidermidis*. *J Infect Dis* 1980;141:738.
175. Bentley DW, Hahn JJ, Lepper MH. Transmission of chloramphenicol-resistant *Staphylococcus epidermidis*: epidemiologic and laboratory studies. *J Infect Dis* 1970;122:365.
176. Schwalbe RS, Stapleton JT, Gilligan PH. Emergence of vancomycin resistance in coagulase-negative staphylococci. *N Engl J Med* 1987; 316:827.
177. Gill VJ, Manning C, Lamson M, et al. Antibiotic-resistant group JK bacteria in hospitals. *J Clin Microbiol* 1981;13:472.
178. Hande KR, Witebsky FG, Brown MS, et al. Sepsis with a new species of *Corynebacterium*. *Ann Intern Med* 1976;85:423.
179. Stamm WE, Tompkins LS, Wagner KF, et al. Infection due to *Corynebacterium* species in marrow transplant patients. *Ann Intern Med* 1979;91:167.
180. Murray BA. The life and times of the enterococcus. *Clin Microbiol Rev* 1990;3:46.
181. Spera RV. Multiply-resistant *Enterococcus faecium*: the nosocomial pathogen of the 1990s. *JAMA* 1992;268:2563.
182. Zervos MJ, Kauffman CA, Therasse PM, et al. Nosocomial infection by gentamicin-resistant *Streptococcus faecalis*. *Ann Intern Med* 1987; 106:687.
183. Zervos MJ, Kauffman CA, Therasse PM, et al. High-level aminoglycoside-resistant enterococci: colonization of nursing home and acute care hospital patients. *Arch Intern Med* 1987;147:1591.
184. Rhinehart E, Smith NE, Wennersten C, et al. Rapid dissemination of β-lactamase-producing, aminoglycoside-resistant *Enterococcus faecalis* among patients and staff on an infant-toddler surgical ward. *N Engl J Med* 1990;323:1814.
185. Murray BE. Editorial response: What can we do about vancomycin-resistant enterococci? *Clin Infect Dis* 1995;20:1134.
186. Leclercq R, Derlot E, Duval J, et al. Plasmid-mediated resistance to vancomycin and teicoplanin in *Enterococcus faecium*. *N Engl J Med* 1988;319:157.
187. Centers for Disease Control and Prevention. Nosocomial enterococci resistant to vancomycin: United States, 1989–1993. *MMWR Morb Mortal Wkly Rep* 1993;42:597.
188. Gaynes R. Nosocomial enterococci resistant to vancomycin: United States, 1989–1994. National Nosocomial Surveillance System, CDC.
189. Lynn W, Wont S, Lacey S, et al. Treatment of peritoneal dialysis-associated peritonitis due to vancomycin-reisistant *Enterococcus faecium* with RP 59500 (quinpristin/dalfopristin). In: *Abstracts from the thirty-fourth interscience conference on antimicrobial agents and chemotherapy, 1994*. Orlando, October 4–7, 1994. Washington, DC: American Society for Microbiology, 1994:145.
190. Beezhold D, Slaughter S, Hayden MK, et al. Prevalence of skin colonization with vancomycin-resistant enterococci (VRE) among hospitalized patients with bacteremia. *Clin Infect Dis* 1997;24:704.
191. Yamaguchi E, Valena F, Smith SM, et al. Colonization pattern of vancomcyin-resistant *Enterococcus faecium*. *Am J Infect Control* 1994; 22:202.
192. Hospital Infection Control Practices Advisory Committee (HICPAC). Recommendations for preventing the spread of vancomycin resistance. *Infect Control Hosp Epidemiol* 1995;16:105.
193. Boyce JM, Opal SM, Chow JW, et al. Outbreak of multidrug-resistant *Enterococcus faecium* with transferable *vanB* class vancomycin resistance. *J Clin Microbiol* 1994;32:1148.
194. Beck-Sagué CM, Jarvis WR, the National Nosocomial Infections Surveillance System. Secular trends in the epidemiology of nosocomial fungal infections in the United States, 1980–1990. *J Infect Dis* 1993; 167:1247.
195. Jarvis WR. Epidemiology of nosocomial fungal infections, with emphasis on *Candida* species. *Clin Infect Dis* 1995;20:1526.
196. Rex JH, Rinaldi MG, Pfaller MA. Resistance of *Candida* species to fluconazole. *Antimicrob Agents Chemother* 1995;39:1.
197. National Committee for Clinical Laboratory Standards. *Reference method for broth dilution antifungal susceptibility testing of yeasts*. Proposed standard M27-P. Villanova, PA: National Committee for Clinical Laboratory Standards, 1992.
198. Troillet N, Durussel C, Billie J, et al. Correlation between in vitro sus-

ceptibility of *Candida albicans* and fluconazole-resistant oropharyngeal candidiasis in HIV-infected patients. *Eur J Clin Microbiol Infect Dis* 1993;12:911.

199. Bart-Delabesse E, Boiron P, Carlotti A, et al. *Candida albicans* genotyping in studies with patients with AIDS developing resistance to fluconazole. *J Clin Microbiol* 1993;31:2933.
200. Millon L, Manteaux A, Reboux G, et al. Fluconazole-resistant recurrent oral candidiasis in human immunodeficiency virus-positive patients: persistence of *Candida albicans* strains with the same genotype. *J Clin Microbiol* 1994;32:1115.
201. Sangeorzan JA, Bradley SF, He S, et al. Epidemiology of oral candidiasis in HIV infected patients: colonization, infection, treatment, and emergence of fluconazole resistance. *Am J Med* 1994;97:339.
202. Pfaller MA, Rhine-Chalberg J, Redding SW, et al. Variations in fluconazole susceptibility and electrophoretic karyotype among oral isolates of *Candida albicans* from patients with AIDS and oral candidiasis. *J Clin Microbiol* 1994;32:59.
203. Rex JH, Bennett JE, Sugar AM, et al. A randomized trial comparing fluconazole with amphotericin B for the treatment of candidemia in patients without neutropenia. *N Engl J Med* 1994;331:1325.
204. Rex JH, Pfaller MA, Barry AL, et al. Antifungal susceptibility testing of isolates from a randomized multicenter trial of fluconazole versus amphotericin B as treatment of nonneutropenic patients with candidemia. *Antimicrob Agents Chemother* 1995;39:40.
205. Price MF, LaRocco MT, Gentry LO. Fluconazole susceptibilities of *Candida* species and distribution of species recovered from blood cultures over a 5-year period. *Antimicrob Agents Chemother* 1994;38:1422.
206. Wingard JR, Merz WG, Rinaldi MG, et al. Association of *Torulopsis glabrata* infections with fluconazole prophylaxis in neutropenic bone marrow transplant patients. *Antimicrob Agents Chemother* 1993;37:1847.
207. Wingard JR, Merz WG, Rinaldi MG, et al. Increase in *Candida krusei* infection among patients with bone marrow transplantation and neutropenia treated prophylactically with fluconazole. *N Engl J Med* 1991;325:1274.
208. Doebbeling BN, Hollis RJ, Isenberg HD, et al. Restriction fragment analysis of a *Candida tropicalis* outbreak of sternal wound infections. *J Clin Microbiol* 1991;29:1268.
209. Weems JJ, Chamberland ME, Ward J, et al. *Candida parapsilosis* fungemia associated with parenteral nutrition and contaminated blood pressure transducers. *J Clin Microbiol* 1987;25:1029.
210. Dembry L, Vazquez JA, Zervos MJ. DNA analysis in the study of the epidemiology of nosocomial candidiasis. *Infect Control Hosp Epidemiol* 1994;15:48.
211. Voss A, Hollis RJ, Pfaller MA, et al. Investigation of the sequence of colonization and candidemia in nonneutropenic patients. *J Clin Microbiol* 1994;32:975.
212. Reagan DR, Pfaller MA, Hollis RJ, et al. Characterization of the sequence of colonization and nosocomial candidemia using DNA fingerprinting and a DNA probe. *J Clin Microbiol* 1990;28:2733.
213. Vazquez JA, Sanchez V, Dmuchowski C, et al. Nosocomial acquisition of *Candida albicans*: an epidemiologic study. *J Infect Dis* 1993;168:195.
212. Sanchez V, Vazquez JA, Barth-Jones D, et al. Nosocomial acquisition of *Candida parapsilosis*: an epidemiologic study. *Am J Med* 1993;94:577.
213. Sanchez V, Vazquez JA, Barth-Jones D, et al. Epidemiology of nosocomial acquisition of *Candida lusitaniae*. *J Clin Microbiol* 1992;30:3005.
216. Voss A, Pfaller MA, Hollis RJ, et al. Investigation of *Candida albicans* transmission in a surgical intensive care unit cluster by using genomic DNA typing methods. *J Clin Microbiol* 1995;33:576.
217. Hoi AB, Branger C, Acar JF. Vancomycin-resistant streptococci or *Leuconostoc* sp. *Antimicrob Agents Chemother* 1985;28:458.
218. Ruoff KL, Kuritzkes DR, Wolfson JS, Ferraro MJ. Vancomycin-resistant gram-positive bacteria isolated from human sources. *J Clin Microbiol* 1988;26:2064.
219. Tally FP, Cuchural GJ, Jacobus NV, et al. Susceptibility of the *Bacteroides fragilis* group in the United States in 1981. *Antimicrob Agents Chemother* 1983;23:536.
220. England AC III, Bond EJ, Livingston H, et al. Epidemiology of clindamycin-resistant *Bacteroides fragilis*. In: *Programs and abstracts of the annual meeting of the American Society for Microbiology*. Atlanta, GA, March 7–12, 1982. Washington, DC: American Society for Microbiology, 1982:87.
221. Sanders CC, Sanders WE Jr. β-Lactam resistance in gram-negative bacteria: global trends and clinical impact. *Clin Infect Dis* 1992;15:824.
222. Marshall WF, Keating MR, Anhalt JP, et al. *Xanthomonas maltophilia*: an emerging nosocomial pathogen. *Mayo Clin Proc* 1989;64:1097.
223. Khadori N, Elting L, Wong E, et al. Nosocomial infections due to *Xanthomonas maltophilia* (*Pseudomonas maltophilia*) in patients with cancer. *Rev Infect Dis* 1990;12:997.
224. Vartivarian SE, Konstantinos PA, Palacios JA, et al. Mucocutaneous and soft tissue infections caused by *Xanthomonas maltophilia*: a new spectrum. *Ann Intern Med* 1994;121:969.
225. Villarino ME, Stevens LE, Schable B, et al. Risk factors for epidemic *Xanthomonas maltophilia* infection/colonization in intensive care unit patients. *Infect Control Hosp Epidemiol* 1992;13:201.
226. Laing FPY, Ramotar K, Read RR, et al. Molecular epidemiology of *Xanthomonas maltophilia* colonization and infection in the hospital environment. *J Clin Microbiol* 1995;33:513.
227. Kenyon TA, Ridzon R, Luskin-Hawk R, et al. Anosocomial outbreak of multidrug-resistant tuberculosis. *Ann Intern Med* 1997;127:32.
228. Edlin BR, Tokars JI, Grieco MH, et al. An outbreak of multidrug-resistant tuberculosis among hospitalized patients with the acquired immunodeficiency syndrome. *N Engl J Med* 1992;326:1514.
229. Beck-Sagué C, Dooley SW, Hutton MD, et al. Hospital outbreak of multidrug-resistant *Mycobacterium tuberculosis* infections. *JAMA* 1992;268:1280.
230. Centers for Disease Control and Prevention. Guidelines for preventing the transmission of tuberculosis in health-care settings, with special focus on HIV-related issues. *MMWR Morb Mortal Wkly Rep* 1990;39(RR-17):1.
231. Maloney S, Pearson M, Gordon M, et al. Efficacy of control measures in preventing nosocomial transmission of multidrug-resistant tuberculosis to patients and healthcare workers. *Ann Intern Med* 1995;122:90.
232. Wenger PN, Otten J, Breeden J, et al. Control of nosocomial transmission of multidrug-resistant Mycobacterium tuberculosis among healthcare workers and HIV-infected patients. *Lancet* 1995;345:235.
233. Centers for Disease Control and Prevention. Guidelines for preventing the transmission of *Mycobacterium tuberculosis* in health-care facilities, 1994. *MMWR Morb Mortal Wkly Rep* 1994;43(RR-13):1.
234. Casewell MS. The different characteristics of antibiotic-resistant and sensitive bacteria. In: Stuart-Harris CH, Harris DM, eds. *The control of antibiotic-resistant bacteria.* London: Academic Press, 1982:77.
235. Yu VL, Oakes CA, Axnick KJ, et al. Patient factors contributing to the emergence of gentamicin-resistant *Serratia marcescens*. *Am J Med* 1979;66:468.

Hospital Infections, Fourth Edition,
edited by John V. Bennett and Philip S. Brachman.
Published by Lippincott–Raven Publishers, Philadelphia, 1998

CHAPTER 16

Molecular Biology of Resistance

Fred C. Tenover and Dennis R. Schaberg

A BRIEF HISTORY OF RESISTANCE MECHANISMS AND THE DISCOVERY OF GENE TRANSFER

The development of antimicrobial agents active against a wide array of microbial pathogens in the 1940s and 1950s enabled physicians to begin to turn the tide against a variety of infectious scourges. However, since the early 1970s, the development and spread of bacterial strains that are resistant to these drugs has emerged as a global problem [1–4]. The development of resistance to antimicrobial agents was not anticipated as a serious problem in the beginning of the antimicrobial era because it was assumed that the only mechanism of resistance was likely to be random mutations leading to altered target sites that would prevent the binding of the drug [5]. However, beginning with the discovery in 1940 of penicillinase (an enzyme that hydrolyzes penicillin, destroying its antibacterial properties), first in *Escherichia coli* [6] then in *Staphylococcus aureus* [7], it became clear that other mechanisms of resistance were likely to be found. Subsequently, active efflux of drugs [8], modification of drug target sites [9], and other mechanisms to inactivate drugs chemically [5] have all been found to mediate resistance to various antibiotics.

In the 1950s, the remarkable finding that multiply antibiotic-resistant strains of *Shigella* were able to transfer the resistance phenotype to other bacterial strains during cell-to-cell mating experiments [10] dramatically changed our understanding of the molecular basis of antimicrobial resistance. Resistance was linked to the presence of extrachromosomal circles of DNA in bacteria called *plasmids*. Subsequently, plasmids have been found in most clinically important bacterial pathogens [11,12].

In the 1960s, bacterial viruses were noted to move antimicrobial resistance genes between strains of staphylococci in a process called *transduction* [13]. In some instances, it appeared that entire plasmids could be moved from one strain of *S. aureus* to another, enhancing the ability of resistance genes to disseminate. In the 1970s, the recognition of transposable elements (i.e., stretches of DNA), often containing antimicrobial resistance genes, that could move from plasmids to bacteriophage [14], or from plasmids to chromosomal locations independent of the usual DNA recombination mechanisms [15], added another dimension to the ability of resistance genes to move among bacteria. This novel mechanism of mobilizing genes among bacterial cells indicated that the likelihood of widespread gene dissemination was high, particularly in environments where antibiotics were present in high concentrations to offer an advantage to those organisms that possessed a resistance mechanism.

The 1980s saw the emergence of another unique genetic element, the integron [16]. *Integrons* are mobile DNA elements that encode enzymes capable of inserting resistance gene cassettes into a stable DNA backbone that can be located either on a plasmid or the chromosome of an organism. The pool of gene cassettes in nature contains a variety of resistance determinants, ranging from aminoglycoside resistance genes to β-lactamase genes [17]. Integrons allow the accumulation and transmission of constellations of resistance determinants within and among diverse species of bacteria. As many as five different resistance genes may be accumulated together in a single integron.

Our understanding of the various mechanisms of antimicrobial resistance has grown tremendously since

F. C. Tenover: Nosocomial Infections Branch, Hospital Infections Program, Centers for Disease Control and Prevention, Atlanta, Georgia 30333.

D. R. Schaberg: Department of Internal Medicine, University of Tennessee at Memphis, Memphis, Tennessee 38163.

the mid-1980s, as has our knowledge of the ways by which genes move among bacteria in the hospital environment. This chapter reviews both the mechanisms of antimicrobial resistance and the modes of resistance gene dissemination in bacteria.

MECHANISMS OF RESISTANCE

Intrinsic Resistance

Some bacteria are intrinsically resistant to antimicrobial agents because they either lack the target site for that drug, or the drug is unable to transit through the organism's cell wall or membrane to reach its site of action [18]. For example, most enterococci are resistant to low levels of aminoglycosides because the drug cannot penetrate the organism's peptidoglycan wall to reach the ribosomes. Only in the presence of cell-wall–active agents, such as penicillin or vancomycin, can aminoglycosides reach their site of action. Intrinsic resistance also includes chromosomally encoded enzymes, such as β-lactamases, that are characteristic of some bacterial species. The AmpC enzyme of *Enterobacter cloacae*, which is inducible and mediates resistance to extended-spectrum cephalosporins and cephamycins (such as cefoxitin and cefotetan), is an example of such an enzyme.

Acquired Resistance

Bacteria that are by nature susceptible to an antimicrobial agent may become resistant by chromosomal mutation, or by the acquisition of new genetic material [18]. For example, point mutations that occur in the chromosomal *rpsL* gene that encodes a ribosomal protein found in *E. coli* [19] and *Mycobacterium tuberculosis* [20] may result in an amino acid change that prevents the binding of streptomycin to the ribosome, resulting in resistance.

The acquisition of new resistance genes carried on plasmids or transposable elements (including integrons) usually results in the synthesis of new proteins in the cell. The known modes of plasmid- and transposon-encoded resistance mechanisms include enzymatically inactivating the antibiotic, altering the target sites for the antibiotic, blocking the transport of the antibiotic into the bacterial cell, enhancing the efflux of the antibiotic out of the cell, and bypassing the metabolic steps inhibited by the antibiotic [21] (Table 16-1). Multiple resistance mechanisms may be present on a single plasmid, transposon, or integron. In addition, organisms may harbor more than one mechanism of resistance for a single class of drugs. Examples of resistance mechanisms for several classes of antimicrobial agents are described in the following sections.

Resistance to β-Lactam Drugs

β-Lactam drugs include penicillins, cephalosporins, monobactams, carbapenems, and a variety of other related compounds. Plasmid-mediated resistance to β-lactam agents most often is a result of β-lactamases, that is, enzymes that hydrolyze the β-lactam ring, detoxifying the drug. The number of different β-lactamases described from gram-negative and gram-positive organisms exceeds 60 [22] and can be divided into several different classes based on chemical structure, substrate profile, isoelectric point, and amino acid sequence. Point mutations in the structural genes of TEM- and SHV-type enzymes may result in amino acid alterations that extend the spectrum of activity of the enzymes that can be inactivated [23,24]. Changes of three, two, or even a single amino acid at specific sites can broaden their spectrum of activity to include hydrolysis of ceftazidime, cefotaxime, ceftriaxone, and aztreonam. In addition, spontaneous mutations that result in changes in the porins of the organism's outer membrane can enhance resistance to ceftazidime [25] and cephamycins, such as cefoxitin [26].

Resistance to β-lactam drugs can also be mediated by changes in the enzymes in the organism's cell wall that are inhibited by penicillin (the penicillin binding proteins) [9]. The changes may be the result of chromosomal mutations or the acquisition of new DNA through transformation, such as is common in *Streptococcus pneumoniae* and *Neisseria meningitidis* [27].

Resistance to Erythromycin and Other Macrolides

Erythromycin resistance in gram-positive bacteria is an example of plasmid-mediated alteration of an antimicrobial-sensitive target. In this instance, the 23S RNA of the 50S ribosome unit is methylated at a specific adenine residue, which prevents binding of macrolides, lincosamides (e.g., clindamycin), and streptogramin-type drugs and leads to high-level resistance [28]. The *erm* genes (for *e*rythromycin *r*RNA *m*ethylase) constitute a family of resistance determinants that have been isolated from many gram-positive species and from *Bacteroides fragilis* [28].

Erythromycin resistance can also be the result of esterification or phosphorylation of the drug [28], and from efflux of the drug out of the cell [29]. The latter mechanism has been reported to occur in both staphylococci and streptococci.

Aminoglycoside Resistance

Aminoglycoside resistance is common in both gram-positive and gram-negative organisms and usually is the result of phosphorylation, acetylation, or adenylylation of

TABLE 16-1. *Examples of bacterial mechanisms of antimicrobial resistance*

Antimicrobial class	Example	Mechanism	Organisms
Aminoglycosides	Gentamicin	Drug modification	Enterobacteriaceae
			Pseudomonas spp.
			Enterococci
			Staphylococci
	Amikacin	Reduced permeability	*Pseudomonas* spp.
β-lactam drugs	Penicillin	β-lactamase	Staphylococci
			Enterococci
			Enterobacteriaceae
			Pseudomonas spp.
			Gonococci
		Altered cell wall	Pneumococci
			Meningococci
Fluoroquinolones	Ciprofloxacin	Altered DNA gyrase	Staphylococci
			Pseudomonas spp.
			Enterobacteriaceae
Glycopeptides	Vancomycin	Altered DNA ligase	Enterococci
Macrolides	Erythromycin	RNA methylase	Staphylococci
			Pneumococci
			Streptococci
Tetracyclines	Doxycycline	Drug efflux	Streptococci
			Enterobacteriaceae
			Staphylococci
			Pseudomonas spp.
Trimethoprim	Trimethoprim	Altered enzymes	Enterobacteriaceae
			Pseudomonas spp.

(Adapted from Neu HC. Overview of mechanisms of bacterial resistance. *Diagn Microbiol Infect Dis* 1989;12: 109S–116S.)

the antimicrobial agent by plasmid- or transposon-encoded enzymes [30]. The nucleotide sequence diversity among the genes that encode the three subclasses of enzymes is higher than would be expected for genes that diverged in recent times, suggesting that although most of the genes share a common ancestral sequence, divergence occurred long ago, making these genes a particularly old group. The enzymes are located at the inner membrane of bacterial cells, and the modified aminoglycoside blocks the transport of the antibiotic into the cell, keeping it from its site of action on the ribosome.

Reduced permeability of the cell envelope, which can occur by spontaneous mutation of the genes that encode the cells' porins, change in the ribosomal target site, and active efflux of drugs out of the cell, also contribute to resistance, particularly in gram-negative organisms [8].

Tetracycline Resistance

Tetracycline resistance is widespread among gram-positive and gram-negative bacterial species and can be the result of drug efflux, target site modification, or permeability [31]. Several tetracycline resistance determinants, such as the *tet(M)* gene, are widely distributed in species as diverse as *Enterococcus faecalis, Neisseria gonorrhoeae, Mycoplasma pneumoniae*, and *B. fragilis* [32]. This resistance gene, and a number of other tetracycline resistance genes, are commonly found on transposable elements, often linked together with chloramphenicol or macrolide resistance determinants.

Glycopeptide Resistance

Vancomycin is the glycopeptide most commonly used to treat gram-positive nosocomial bacterial infections, such as methicillin-resistant *S. aureus* (MRSA), and ampicillin-resistant enterococcal infections. Resistance in enterococci is mediated by a series of plasmid- and transposon-encoded genes that produce altered DNA ligases that result in a cell wall structure that does not bind the drug [33]. Resistance to teicoplanin, another glycopeptide, is also mediated by the *vanA* gene complex. Intrinsic vancomycin resistance is recognized in *Enterococcus gallinarum, Enterococcus flavescens*, and *Enterococcus casseliflavus*, and appears to be a chromosomally mediated trait of these species [34]. Although transfer of the operon containing the *vanA* resistance gene from *E. faecalis* to *S. aureus* has been achieved in vitro [35], high-level vancomycin resistance has yet to be recognized in clinical isolates of staphylococci. Low-level resistance to vancomycin and teicoplanin has been reported in *Staphylococcus haemolyticus* [36].

Trimethoprim and Sulfonamide Resistance

Bypass of inhibited metabolism is exemplified by the resistance to trimethoprim [37] and sulfonamides [38]. This mechanism is based on plasmid- or transposon-encoded enzymes that substitute for the chromosomal enzymes normally inhibited by these drugs. Sulfonamides work through competitive inhibition of the enzyme dihydropteroate synthetase. The plasmid-coded enzyme is smaller and more heat sensitive and requires a thousand times as much sulfonamide to inhibit it as does the chromosomal enzyme [38]. Similarly, some strains resistant to high levels of trimethoprim, an agent that inhibits dihydrofolate reductase, contain a plasmid-mediated gene coding for a new, trimethoprim-resistant dihydrofolate reductase. In each of these instances, the plasmids provide a mechanism whereby products vital to the bacterial cell can be synthesized and the inhibiting effect of the drug bypassed.

Resistance to Multiple Antimicrobial Agents

Resistance to multiple classes of antimicrobial agents, such as chloramphenicol, tetracycline, and fluoroquinolones, in gram-negative and gram-positive organisms is often due to efflux of the drugs out of the bacterial cell [8,39]. There are several genetic determinants that mediate such resistance, including *marA, qacA-qacB*, and *norA* [39]. Many multiresistant organisms that were previously thought to have permeability barriers that limited the access of drugs to their sites of action are now known to contain effective efflux pumps that direct the drug out of the cell before it reaches its internal site of action [8]. Of course, solitary resistance to chloramphenicol, tetracycline, or the fluoroquinolones is also seen, although this is often mediated by mechanisms other than efflux. Quinolone resistance, for example, is frequently mediated by point mutations in the *gyrA* and *gyrB* genes, which decrease binding of the drugs to the target enzyme, DNA gyrase [40].

Antimicrobial Resistance in **M. tuberculosis**

The molecular mechanisms of drug resistance in *M. tuberculosis* are just beginning to be understood. Resistance to rifampin and streptomycin is frequently the result of point mutations in the *rpoB* [41] and *rpsL* [20,42] genes, respectively. However, some resistant strains do not contain these mutations. Isoniazid resistance appears to have multiple causes, including deletions in the *katG* gene [43] and rearrangements in *inhA* gene [44], the latter of which is also linked to ethionamide resistance. Studies of multidrug-resistant strains of *M. tuberculosis* by Morris et al. [45] suggest that although these mutations do occur in clinical isolates, additional mechanisms of isoniazid, rifampin, and streptomycin resistance await discovery.

DISSEMINATION OF RESISTANCE GENES IN NATURE

Bacteria can exchange genetic information by means of transformation, transduction, and conjugation [46]. Resistance determinants can be encoded on an organism's chromosome or on the plasmids, bacteriophages, transposons, or integrons harbored in the cell, all of which may be moved from cell to cell by transformation, transduction, or conjugation. Thus, there is a multitude of pathways by which resistance genes move from one organism to another. Each of the various genetic elements that harbor resistance determinants has unique features.

Plasmids

Plasmids are self-replicating, extrachromosomal segments of DNA that can be found in many species of bacteria and yeast. Plasmids are usually circular and range in size from 2 to 400 kilobases [11,12]. The number of proteins encoded on plasmids can be substantial, with larger plasmids (~300 kilobases) encoding 50 to 75 proteins. The proteins may include enzymes involved in antimicrobial resistance, virulence, or the molecular machinery for plasmid transfer, in addition to those proteins required for plasmid maintenance. Plasmids usually can be acquired or lost by bacteria without affecting basic cellular functions because most of the genetic information necessary for metabolism and growth of the bacterial cell is located on the chromosome. For some plasmids, no phenotypic properties are known, and they are deemed "cryptic."

Plasmids are classified into incompatibility groups based on their ability to coexist with known plasmids in the same bacterial cell [47]. Many of the traditional classification techniques have been replaced with DNA probes and hybridization assays [48]. Plasmids are also categorized on their ability to transfer themselves to other organisms. Those that are self-transmissible from one bacterial cell to another are termed "conjugative" [11]. When a gram-negative bacterial cell contains a conjugative plasmid, a proteinaceous appendage called a "pilus" is synthesized on the outside of the cell; this, together with other plasmid-mediated proteins, enables cell-to-cell transmission of the plasmid DNA [46,49]. Conjugative plasmids of gram-positive bacteria do not use pili for conjugation; rather, direct cell-to-cell contact is required. In some cases, this is facilitated by plasmid-coded proteins (pheromones) that enhance clumping of donor and recipient cells [50]. Both staphylococci and enterococci have been shown to contain conjugal plasmids [50,51].

Nonconjugative plasmids are often smaller in size than conjugative plasmids [12]. Some nonconjugative plasmids can still be transferred to recipient organisms by a process called mobilization, in which a coresident, nonconjugative plasmid takes advantage of the transfer of a conjugative one present in the same cell [49]. In addition, nonconjugative and conjugative plasmids may also be transmitted by bacterial virus vectors through transduction [13,52]. In this process, plasmid DNA instead of phage DNA is packaged in the viral protein coat and, on infection of a suitable recipient cell, the plasmid DNA is released and begins replication in the new host. Because transduction requires that the plasmid DNA be packaged in the protein coat of a bacteriophage, the amount of plasmid DNA that can be transduced is limited to approximately the size of the phage genome [52]. This process operates much more efficiently for the smaller nonconjugative plasmids and appears to be an important mechanism of plasmid exchange in *S. aureus*. In gram-negative bacilli and streptococci, conjugation and mobilization seem to be the most common means of transfer [52,53]. Direct uptake of both conjugative and nonconjugative plasmid DNA by a recipient cell can also occur through transformation. However, even in those naturally transformable species, this mode of plasmid transfer is probably uncommon.

Transposons and Insertion Sequences

A transposon is a segment of DNA that can move as an intact unit from one replicating DNA unit (replicon) to another by mechanisms other than those used in generalized recombination [54]. These sequences can "jump" from plasmid to plasmid, plasmid to bacteriophage, plasmid to chromosome, or the reverse using a "transposase" enzyme that is encoded in the element. Transposons encoding resistance genes to a variety of antimicrobial agents have been described [54]. In theory, any plasmid could gain a transposon if DNA containing the transposon were to coexist in a cell long enough for transposition to occur. Transposons also promote a variety of rearrangements of DNA in adjoining regions, including deletions, inversions, and duplications [55]. Some transposons, particularly those in gram-positive organism, such as enterococci, are conjugative and promote their own transfer from the chromosome of the donor cell to that of the recipient [56]. Such elements have also been recognized in *S. pneumoniae*.

Simpler genetic structures, called insertion sequences, do not contain antimicrobial resistance determinants but promote gene rearrangements and can modify the expression of resistance genes by inserting strong promoter elements upstream of open reading frames [55]. One such element, IS*1*, has been reported to cause increased expression of the bla_{TEM-6} gene, resulting in extended-spectrum β-lactamase activity [57].

Integrons

Integrons are mobile DNA elements that contain "hot spots" of recombination where a variety of antimicrobial resistance gene cassettes can insert mediated by an integrase enzyme [16]. The gene cassettes must contain a key 59-base-pair region at their termini to be recognized by the integrase enzyme (Figure 16-1). The gene cassettes do not contain their own promoters, and thus expression depends on insertion into the integron in the appropriate orientation downstream from a promoter element [58]. The cassettes appear to undergo integration and excision as covalently closed circular molecules [59]. Large, com-

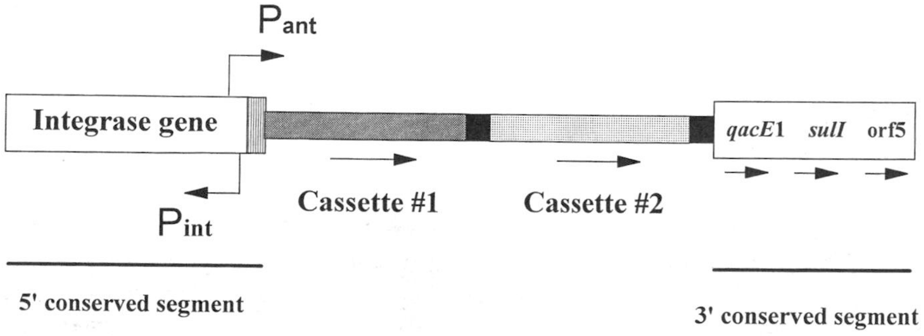

FIGURE 16-1. Schematic representation of an integron showing the 5′ and 3′ conserved regions (open boxes) that encode the integrase gene (5′) and three other genes (3′); two integrated resistance genes labeled cassettes 1 and 2; the 59-base-pair elements that serve as the sites of integration of the cassettes (small black boxes); and the location of the promoters for the integrase gene (P_{int}) and for the integrated cassettes that do not have their own promoters (P_{ant}). The arrows indicate the direction of gene transcription. (Adapted from Collis CM, Hall RM. Expression of antibiotic resistance genes in the integrated cassettes of integrons. *Antimicrob Agents Chemother* 1995;39:155–162; and Lévesque C, Piché L, Larose C, et al. PCR mapping of integrons reveals several novel combinations of resistance genes. *Antimicrob Agents Chemother* 1995;39:185–191.)

plex integrons with as many as five resistance genes have been detected on plasmids in enteric organisms [17]. The proximity of the cassette to the integron's promoter has a major effect on expression, with those genes that are proximal to the promoter showing strong and consistent expression, and those that are distal showing low-level or no expression [60].

Development of Multiresistant Organisms

Multiresistant organism can develop over time by the successive acquisition of resistance genes in a number of different ways (Figure 16-2). These may include spontaneous mutation, acquisition of plasmids and transposons, and insertion of gene cassettes into integrons. Acquisition of plasmids is commonplace and a variety of outbreaks due to dissemination of plasmid-containing isolates are detailed in Chapter 15 of this volume. The secondary spread of plasmids from the epidemic strain to other species was noted by many investigators, including Tompkins et al. [61] in the late 1970s. Dissemination of epidemic plasmids (sometimes referred to as "plasmid outbreaks") continues to plague hospitals as demonstrated by Neuwirth et al., who noted dissemination of an extended-spectrum β-lactamase-producing strain of *Enterobacter aerogenes* in their hospital followed by transfer of the β-lactamase-encoding plasmid to other species of Enterobacteriaceae [62]. Studies by Rubens et al. demonstrate how a gentamicin-resistance determinant originally present on a small nonconjugative plasmid was transposed onto a larger, self-transferable plasmid [15]. Once on the conjugative element, the resistance was efficiently transferred among a variety of genera in the hospital. This process provided a mechanism to assemble new resistance determinants on a preexisting plasmid and appears to be one way that multiresistance plasmids can develop.

ENVIRONMENTAL CONDITIONS THAT FAVOR THE DEVELOPMENT OF RESISTANT ORGANISMS—SELECTIVE PRESSURE

Resistant organisms, particularly those that develop through spontaneous mutation, usually will not survive unless there is an advantage to maintaining the resistance phenotype. The hospital environment, which is rich with antimicrobial agents, can be hostile to antibiotic-susceptible organisms. Thus, resistant organisms have an advantage in this environment. In genetic terms, the presence of antimicrobial agents in the environment is the "selective pressure" that favors the development and spread of resistant strains of bacteria. However, as noted by Murray [2], selective pressures are not unique to hospitals. To control the spread of resistant organisms, the selective pressures provided by both hospital and community must be considered.

The Hospital Environment

The most frequently encountered hospital-acquired pathogens, staphylococci, enterococci, and gram-negative bacilli [63], all have demonstrated the ability to acquire and disseminate resistance genes [5,18]. Intensive use of antimicrobial agents exerts a selective pressure favoring those organisms that have acquired resistance determinants through mutation or genetic exchange [2,18,32]. In addition, antimicrobial therapy alters the normal flora found in many niches of the human body, which may allow colonization with resistant nosocomial

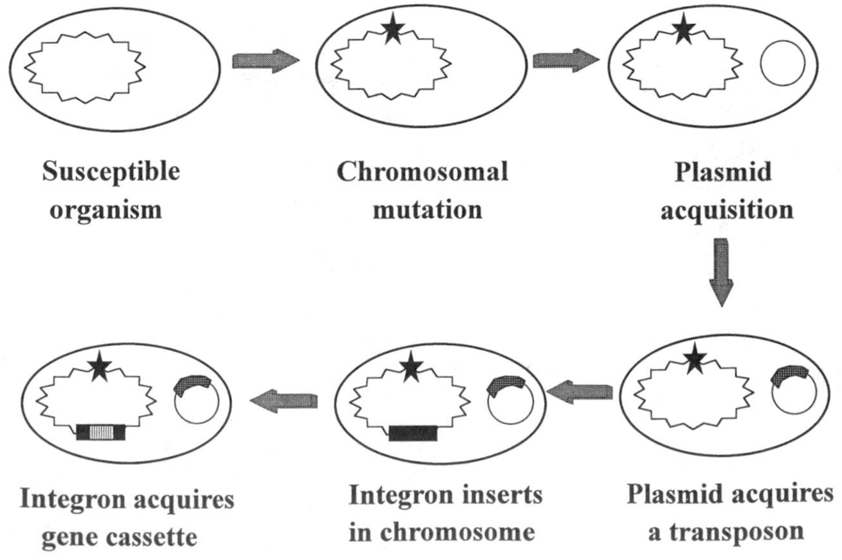

FIGURE 16-2. A schematic diagram showing the stepwise acquisition of antimicrobial resistance genes by a bacterium, beginning with a chromosomal mutation that results in a resistant phenotype (star), followed by acquisition of a plasmid containing a resistance gene, followed by insertion of a transposon containing additional resistance genes into the plasmid, followed by insertion of an integron with resistance genes into the chromosome, and finally insertion of a resistance gene cassette into the integron backbone.

strains. This, in turn, likely contributes to enhanced plasmid transfer among organisms, particularly in the gastrointestinal tract [64]. Plasmid transfer is also readily observed in aqueous reservoirs peculiar to the hospital environment, such as urinary catheter collection bags [65]. Conditions that enhance transfer of plasmids also favor the transmission of transposons, further increasing the dissemination of resistance genes [54]. Immunocompromised patients who are receiving antimicrobial agents and who are hospitalized for prolonged periods provide a reservoir for resistant organisms [66]. In addition, antimicrobial agents find their way into the general inanimate environment, which also contributes to the selective advantage obtained by plasmid-containing organisms. Thus, the hospital environment is conducive to the development and spread of resistant bacteria.

The Community Environment

The use and sometimes misuse [67,68] of antimicrobial agents in the community contributes to the selective pressure that results in resistant nosocomial pathogens, because the gene pools for the organisms are the same [2,5,46]. Selective pressures outside of the hospital, including the use of antibiotics in humans, particularly in children for respiratory infections [69], in animals both therapeutically and as growth promotants, in fish (aquaculture), and on vegetables [3,4], suggests that the development of resistant strains can and does occur almost everywhere. The development and spread of penicillin-resistant strains of *Hemophilus influenzae* [70] and *Neisseria gonorrhoeae* [71] in the 1970s and multiresistant pneumococci in the 1970s and 1980s [72], as well as the descriptions of multiply resistant *Salmonella* and *Shigella* [1,2], should have convinced us that problems with resistant organisms are not confined to the hospital. The two locations often come together, as when patients from nursing homes who harbor MRSA are transferred to acute care community hospitals [73].

EPIDEMIOLOGIC STUDIES OF BACTERIAL RESISTANCE

To study the epidemiology of antimicrobial-resistant bacteria, it is imperative to have strain typing methods that are both discriminatory and reproducible [74]. When an outbreak of a resistant strain is suspected in a hospital, several techniques can be used to confirm that the isolates are clonal (i.e., derived from a common parent). Biochemical patterns and antimicrobial susceptibility test results can provide initial clues to strain identity, but more definitive information, as provided by plasmid fingerprints, pulsed-field gel electrophoresis (PFGE) patterns, or arbitrarily primed polymerase chain reaction (PCR) results, is often necessary.

Plasmid Fingerprinting

Plasmid fingerprinting uses the number and size of extrachromosomal elements within an organism as means of strain identification [75] (Figure 16-3). Most gram-negative nosocomial pathogens contain plasmids [76], as do most staphylococci, making this an effective tool for examination of presumptive outbreaks of bacterial infections. Several techniques, including those described by

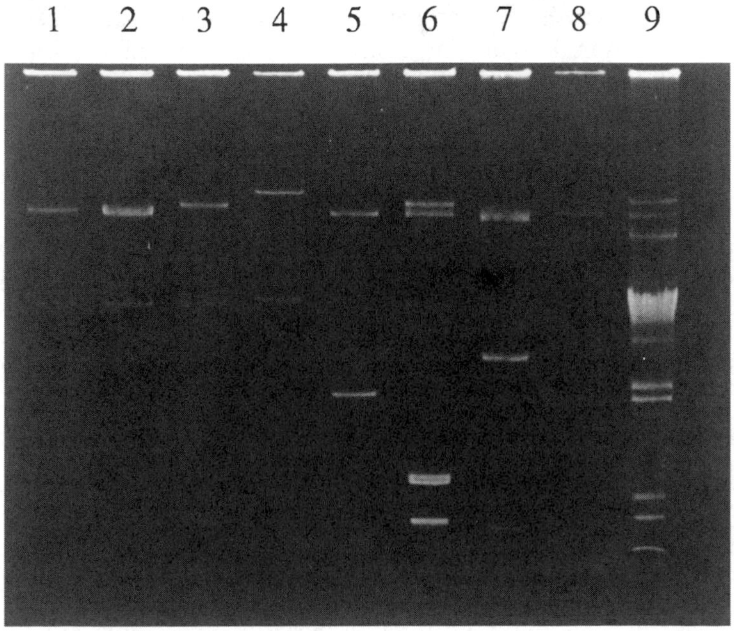

FIGURE 16-3. Example of a plasmid fingerprinting gel showing the various plasmids of *Yersinia enterocolitica*. Isolates in lanes 1 and 2 share the same plasmid. The isolates in lanes 5, 6, and 7 also share a common plasmid, although plasmids of other sizes are also present in these isolates. The latter is an example of spread of an "epidemic" plasmid.

Birnboim and Doly [77], Kado and Liu [78], and Goering and Ruff [79], have proven to be simple and reliable over the years. Even so, some organisms, such as *Serratia* and *Enterobacter* species, are often devoid of plasmids and require further testing.

Pulsed-Field Gel Electrophoresis

Of all of the strain typing methods currently available, PFGE of chromosomal DNA comes the closest to being a universal typing method for bacteria. PFGE uses infrequent cutting restriction endonucleases to cleave the chromosome of an organism into a relatively small number (usually 10 to 25) of fragments (Figure 16-4). The fragments are subjected to electrophoresis through agarose in a special chamber in which the direction of the electrical current is switched frequently according to a preset pattern. This resolves the fragments into discrete patterns that can be easily photographed and analyzed [74,80]. The method of typing has been validated against epidemiologic data collected during outbreak investigations for a large number of bacterial species, and interpretive criteria for analyzing restriction fragment banding patterns have been published [81]. For example, outbreaks of extended-spectrum β-lactamase-producing *Klebsiella pneumoniae* have been successfully typed using PFGE [82].

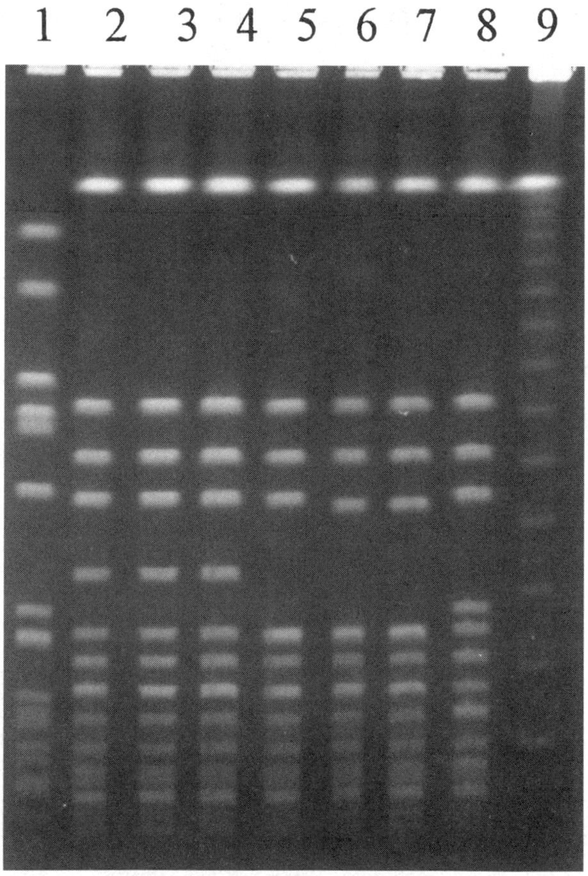

FIGURE 16-4. Example of pulsed-field gel electrophoresis showing eight isolates of *Staphylococcus aureus*. The isolate in lane 1 is epidemiologically unrelated to the remaining seven isolates, which were collected from the same hospital unit. Lanes 2–4 show isolates with indistinguishable patterns, whereas the patterns in lanes 5–8 show minor variations from the outbreak strain but would still be considered "related" to the outbreak strain using published interpretive criteria [81]. This gel demonstrates the variation commonly seen among isolates collected over an extended period of time. Molecular size standards are shown in lane 9.

Arbitrarily Primed Polymerase Chain Reaction

The ability of PCR to amplify large quantities of DNA in short periods of time has been applied to bacterial strain typing in an effort to decease the time necessary to produce epidemiologically useful data regarding outbreaks of resistant organisms [83]. The arbitrarily primed PCR typing procedure can be completed for 40 bacterial isolates in a single day. However, testing is expensive compared with plasmid fingerprinting and PFGE, and the interpretation of the results has yet to be standardized. The reproducibility of the banding patterns for a given strain over time can vary significantly with changes in primer and target DNA concentration, the commercial source of DNA polymerase, and the electrophoretic conditions, all of which must be tightly controlled. Nonetheless, arbitrarily primed PCR has been used successfully to type a variety of bacterial species, including multiresistant isolates of *E. cloacae* from a neonatal intensive care unit [84].

Additional Methods for Laboratory Studies of Resistant Microorganisms

New molecular techniques for characterizing transposons [85] and integrons [86] have enhanced our ability to follow the dissemination of resistant bacteria in hospital settings. The availability of a large battery of DNA hybridization probes and PCR assays [87] has also enhanced our ability to conduct surveys of specific resistance determinants in hospitals [88], which has contributed to our understanding of the evolution of resistance genes over time in the hospital environment [88]. It is now clear that the dissemination of resistance genes occurs on three levels in hospitals. The first level is dissemination of a resistant strain, often on the hands of healthcare workers, or through patient contact with environmental reservoirs of resistant organisms [64,65]. The next level occurs when a resistance plasmid transfers from one organism to another or from one species to another [61,62], which amplifies the extent of the problem and makes epidemiologic studies more complex and the outbreak more difficult to control. The third level involves the acquisition of novel resistance genes by the outbreak strain through generalized recombination, transposition, or insertion of resistance gene cassettes into integrons [32,46]. Examples of this include the acquisition of chloramphenicol resistance by strains of MRSA during an outbreak in a hospital in Seattle [89], or the acquisition of gentamicin-resistance transposons by an epidemic strain of *Pseudomonas aeruginosa* [90]. Furthermore, spontaneous mutation to a resistant phenotype followed by dissemination of the novel strain also occurs, as evidenced by the explosive increase in ciprofloxacin-resistant strains of MRSA reported by Blumberg et al. [91], where the new resistant strains represented > 90% of MRSA isolates over the course of a single year after the introduction of ciprofloxacin in the hospital. The emergence of fluoroquinolone-resistant *E. coli* at a cancer center was also observed after patients started receiving ofloxacin prophylactically to prevent bacterial infection [92]. Thus, spread of a resistant strain, transfer of plasmids, spontaneous mutation, and genetic exchange in the presence of antibiotic selective pressure are the key factors in the development and spread of resistant organisms in the hospital setting.

ORIGIN OF ANTIMICROBIAL RESISTANCE GENES

The exact origin of antimicrobial resistance genes remains a mystery. However, there is evidence that points to two potential origins. First, some resistance genes have probably been acquired by pathogenic species over time from antibiotic-producing bacteria [93]. For example, aminoglycoside-producing streptomycetes contain aminoglycoside-modifying enzymes that protect the host from self-destruction. These genes are similar in sequence to the genes that encode aminoglycoside-modifying enzymes found in resistant clinical isolates of Enterobacteriaceae and *Pseudomonas* species [94], providing a potential link between the two organism groups. The mechanism of exchange is not clear, but may have been transformation.

Other aminoglycoside resistance genes, such as those that encode the 3′-aminoglycoside phosphotransferases (e.g., APH[3′]-VI), encode proteins that resemble a bacterial cell's normal "housekeeping" enzymes, such as the protein kinases that serve as intracellular protein regulators [95]. Some resistance genes may have evolved from genes already present in the cell that served purposes other than protecting the cell from antibiotic exposure.

SUMMARY

Antimicrobial resistance in bacteria comprises a wide variety of biochemical mechanisms and processes that allow microorganisms to grow in the presence of antibiotics. Bacteria are able to transmit this acquired "knowledge" to other species through transformation, transduction, and conjugation. Specialized structures, including transposons and integrons, allow cells to recruit additional genetic information outside of the normal processes of generalized recombination. The web of genetic exchange in bacteria is very broad and even crosses between gram-positive and gram-negative organisms. Finally, there is no barrier between hospital and the community when it comes to resistant organisms. All bacteria can draw on the same gene pool to find ways to cope with the presence of antibiotics in their environment.

REFERENCES

1. Cohen M. Epidemiology of drug resistance: implications for a post-antimicrobial era. *Science* 1992;257:1050–1055.
2. Murray BM. New aspects of antimicrobial resistance and the resulting therapeutic dilemmas. *J Infect Dis* 1991;163:1185–1194.
3. U.S. Congress, Office of Technology Assessment. *Impacts of antibiotic resistant bacteria*. OTA-H-629. Washington, DC: U.S. Government Printing Office; 1995.
4. American Society for Microbiology. *Report of the ASM task force on antibiotic resistance*. Washington, DC: American Society for Microbiology Press; 1995.
5. Davies J. Inactivation of antibiotics and the dissemination of resistance genes. *Science* 1994;264:375–382.
6. Abraham EP, Chain E. An enzyme from bacteria able to destroy penicillin. *Nature* 1940;146:837–839.
7. Kirby WMM. Extraction of a highly potent penicillin inactivator from penicillin resistant staphylococci. *Science* 1944;99:452–455.
8. Nikaido H. Prevention of drug access to bacterial targets: permeability barriers and active efflux. *Science* 1994;264:382–388.
9. Spratt BG. Resistance to antibiotics mediated by target alterations. *Science* 1994;264:388–393.
10. Akiba T, Koyama K, Ishiki Y, et al. On the mechanism of the development of multiple drug resistant clones of *Shigella*. *Japanese Journal of Microbiology* 1960;4:219–222.
11. Falkow S. *Infectious multiple drug resistance*. London: Pion Press; 1975.
12. Bukhari AI, Shapiro JA, Adhya SL, eds. *DNA insertion elements, plasmids, and episomes*. Cold Spring Harbor, NY: Cold Spring Harbor Laboratory; 1977:601–704.
13. Novick RP, Morse SI. In vivo transmission of drug resistance factors between strains of *Staphylococcus aureus*. *J Exp Med* 1967;125:45–59.
14. Berg DE, Davies J, Allet B, et al. Transposition of R factor genes to bacteriophage. *Proc Natl Acad Sci U S A* 1975;72:3628–3632.
15. Rubens CE, McNeil WF, Farrar WE Jr. Transposable plasmid deoxyribonucleic acid sequence in *Pseudomonas aeruginosa* which mediates resistance to gentamicin and four other antimicrobial agents. *J Bacteriol* 1979;139:877–882.
16. Stokes HW, Hall RM. A novel family of potentially mobile DNA elements encoding site-specific gene integration functions: integrons. *Mol Microbiol* 1989;3:1669–1683.
17. Lévesque C, Piché L, Larose C, et al. PCR mapping of integrons reveals several novel combinations of resistance genes. *Antimicrob Agents Chemother* 1995;39:185–191.
18. Neu HC. The crisis in antibiotic resistance. *Science* 1992;257:1064–1073.
19. Funatsu G, Wittmann HG. Location and amino acid replacements in protein S12 isolated from *Escherichia coli* mutants resistant to streptomycin. *J Mol Biol* 1972;68:547–550.
20. Nair J, Rouse DA, Bai G-H, et al. The *rpsL* gene and streptomycin resistance in single and multiple drug-resistant strains of *Mycobacterium tuberculosis*. *Mol Microbiol* 1993;10:521–527.
21. Neu HC. Overview of mechanisms of bacterial resistance. *Diagn Microbiol Infect Dis* 1989;12:109S–116S.
22. Bush K, Jacoby GA, Medeiros AA. A functional classification scheme for β-lactamases and its correlation with molecular structure. *Antimicrob Agents Chemother* 1995;39:1211–1233.

23. Philippon A, Labia R, Jacoby G. Extended-spectrum β-lactamases. *Antimicrob Agents Chemother* 1989;33:1131–1136.
24. Jacoby GA, Medeiros AA. More extended-spectrum betaβ-lactamases. *Antimicrob Agents Chemother* 1991;35:1697–1704.
25. Weber DA, Sanders CC, Bakken JS, Quinn JP. A novel chromosomal TEM derivative and alterations in outer membrane proteins together mediate selective ceftazidime resistance in *Escherichia coli. J Infect Dis* 1990;162:460–465.
26. Pangon B, Bizet C, Buré A, et al. In vivo selection of a cephamycin-resistant, porin-deficient mutant of *Klebsiella pneumoniae* producing a TEM-3 β-lactamase. *J Infect Dis* 1989;159:1005–1006.
27. Spratt BG, Dowson CG, Zhang QY, et al. Campisi J, Cunningham D, Inouye M, Riley M (eds). Mosaic genes, hybrid penicillin-binding proteins, and the origins of penicillin resistance in *Neisseria meningitidis* and *Streptococcus pneumoniae*. In: *Perspectives on cellular regulation: from bacteria to cancer*. New York: Wiley-Liss, Inc. 1991: 73–83.
28. Arthur M, Brisson-Noel A, Courvalin P. Origin and evolution of genes specifying resistance to macrolide, lincosamide, and streptogramin antibiotics: data and hypotheses. *J Antimicrob Chemother* 1987;20: 783–802.
29. Eady EA, Ross JI, Tipper JL, et al. Distribution of genes encoding erythromycin ribosomal methylases and an erythromycin efflux pump in epidemiologically distinct groups of staphylococci. *J Antimicrob Chemother* 1993;31:211–217.
30. Shaw KJ, Rather PN, Hare RS, et al. Molecular genetics of aminoglycoside resistance genes and familial relationships of the aminoglycoside-modifying enzymes. *Microbiol Rev* 1993;57:138–163.
31. Speer BS, Shoemaker NB, Salyers AA. Bacterial resistance to tetracycline: mechanisms, transfer, and clinical significance. *Clin Microbiol Rev* 1992;5:387–399.
32. DeFlaun MF, Levy SB. Genes and their varied hosts. In: Levy SB, Miller RV, eds. *Gene transfer in the environment.* New York: McGraw-Hill; 1991:1–32.
33. Arthur M, Courvalin P. Genetics and mechanisms of glycopeptide resistance in enterococci. *Antimicrob Agents Chemother* 1993;37:1563–1571.
34. Navarro F, Courvalin P. Analysis of genes encoding D-alanine–D-alanine ligase-related enzymes in *Enterococcus casseliflavus* and *Enterococcus flavescens*. *Antimicrob Agents Chemother* 1994;38:1788–1793.
35. Noble WC, Virani Z, Cree RGA. Co-transfer of vancomycin and other resistance genes from *Enterococcus faecalis* NCTC 12201 to *Staphylococcus aureus*. *FEMS Microbiol Lett* 1992;93:195–198.
36. Schwalbe RS, Stapleton JT, Gilligan PH. Emergence of vancomycin resistance in coagulase-negative staphylococci. *N Engl J Med* 1987; 316:927–931.
37. Amyes SGB, Towner KJ. Trimethoprim resistance: epidemiology and molecular aspects. *J Med Microbiol* 1990;31:1–19.
38. Wise EM, Abou-Donia MM. Sulfonamide resistance mechanism in *Escherichia coli*: R plasmids can determine sulfonamide-resistant dihydropteroate synthetases. *Proc Natl Acad Sci U S A* 1975;72:2621.
39. Levy SB. Active efflux mechanisms for antimicrobial resistance. *Antimicrob Agents Chemother* 1992;36:695–703.
40. Nakamura S, Nakamura M, Kojima T, et al. *gyrA* and *gyrB* mutations in quinolone resistant strains of *Escherichia coli*. *Antimicrob Agents Chemother* 1989;33:254–255.
41. Telenti A, Imboden P, Marchesi F, et al. Detection of rifampicin-resistance mutations in *Mycobacterium tuberculosis*. *Lancet* 1993;341: 647–650.
42. Finken M, Kirschner P, Meier A, et al. Molecular basis of streptomycin resistance in *Mycobacterium tuberculosis*: alternations of the ribosomal protein A12 and point mutations within a functional 16S ribosomal RNA pseudoknot. *Mol Microbiol* 1993;9:1239–1246.
43. Zhang Y, Heym B, Allen B, et al. The catalase–peroxidase gene and isoniazid resistance of *Mycobacterium tuberculosis*. *Science* 1992;358: 591–593.
44. Bannerjee A, Dubnau E, Quemard A, et al. inhA, a gene encoding a target for isoniazid and ethionamide in *Mycobacterium tuberculosis*. *Science* 1994;263:227–230.
45. Morris S, Bai GH, Suffys P, et al. Molecular mechanisms of multiple drug resistance in clinical isolates of *Mycobacterium tuberculosis*. *J Infect Dis* 1995;171:954–60.
46. Porter RD. Modes of gene transfer in bacteria. In: Kucherlapi R, Smith GR, eds. *Genetic recombination.* Washington, DC: American Society for Microbiology Press; 1988:1–42.
47. Datta N. Plasmid classification: incompatibility grouping. In: Timmis KN, Pichler A, eds. *Plasmids of medical, environmental, and commercial importance.* Amsterdam: Elsevier/North-Holland Biomedical Press; 1979:47–53.
48. Berquist PL. Incompatibility. In: Hardy KG, ed. *Plasmids: a practical approach*. Oxford: IRL Press; 1987:37–78.
49. Ippen-Ihler K. Bacterial conjugation. In: Levy SB, Miller RV, eds. *Gene transfer in the environment.* New York: McGraw-Hill; 1991:33–72.
50. Dunny G, Brown B, Clewell D. Induced cell aggregation and mating in *Streptococcus faecalis*: evidence for a bacterial sex pheromone. *Proc Natl Acad Sci U S A* 1978;75:3479–3483.
51. Forbes BA, Schaberg DR. Transfer of resistance plasmids from *Staphylococcus epidermidis* to *Staphylococcus aureus*: evidence for conjugative exchange of resistance. *J Bacteriol* 1983;153:627–631.
52. Kokjohn TA. Transduction: mechanism and potential for gene transfer in the environment. In: Levy SB, Miller RV, eds. *Gene transfer in the environment.* New York: McGraw-Hill; 1991:73–98.
53. Mazodier P, Davies J. Gene transfer between distantly related bacteria. *Annu Rev Genet* 1991;25:147–171.
54. Berg DE. Transposable elements in prokaryotes. In: Levy SB, Miller RV, eds. *Gene transfer in the environment.* New York: McGraw-Hill; 1991:99–138.
55. Kleckner N. Translocatable elements in prokaryotes. *Cell* 1977;11: 11–23.
56. Clewell DB, Gawron-Burke C. Conjugative transposons and dissemination of antibiotic resistance in streptococci. *Annu Rev Microbiol* 1986;40:635–659.
57. Goussard S, Sougakoff W, Mabilat C, et al. An IS*1*-like element is responsible for high level synthesis of extended spectrum β-lactamase TEM-6 in Enterobacteriaceae. *Journal of General Microbiology* 1991; 137:2681–2687.
58. Collis CM, Grammaticopoulos G, Briton J, et al. Site specific insertion of gene cassettes into integrons. *Mol Microbiol* 1993;9:41–52.
59. Collis CM, Hall RM. Gene cassettes from the insert region of integrons are excised as covalently close circles. *Mol Microbiol* 1992;6: 2875–2885.
60. Collis CM, Hall RM. Expression of antibiotic resistance genes in the integrated cassettes of integrons. *Antimicrob Agents Chemother* 1995; 39:155–162.
61. Tompkins LS, Plorde JJ, Falkow S. Molecular analysis of R factors from multiresistant nosocomial isolates. *J Infect Dis* 1980;141:625.
62. Neuwirth C, Siebor E, Lopez J, et al. Outbreak of TEM-24-producing *Enterobacter aerogenes* in an intensive care unit and dissemination of the extended-spectrum β-lactamase to other members of the family Enterobacteriaceae. *J Clin Microbiol* 1996;34:76–79.
63. Emori TG, Gaynes RP. An overview of nosocomial infections, including the role of the microbiology laboratory. *Clin Microbiol Rev* 1993; 6:428–42.
64. McGowan JE Jr. Antibiotic resistance in hospital bacteria: current patterns, modes for appearance or spread, and economic impact. *Reviews in Medical Microbiology* 1991;2:161–169.
65. Schaberg DR, Tompkins LS, Rubens CE, et al. R plasmids and nosocomial infection. In: Stuttard C, Royce KR, eds. *Plasmids and transposons: environmental effects and maintenance mechanisms.* New York: Academic Press; 1980:43–55.
66. Kotilainen P, Nikoskelainen J, Huovinen P. Emergence of ciprofloxacin-resistant coagulase-negative staphylococcal skin flora in immunocompromised patients receiving ciprofloxacin. *J Infect Dis* 1990;161: 41–44.
67. Freiden TR, Mangi RJ. Inappropriate use of oral ciprofloxacin. *JAMA* 1990;264:1438–1440.
68. Gonzales R, Sande M. What will it take to stop physicians from prescribing antibiotics in acute bronchitis? *Lancet* 1995;345:665–666.
69. McCaig LF, Hughes JM. Trends in antimicrobial drug prescribing among office-based physicians in the United States. *JAMA* 1995;273: 214–219.
70. Elwell LP, deGraaff J, Seibert D, et al. Plasmid-linked ampicillin resistance in *Haemophilus influenzae* type b. *Infect Immun* 1975;12: 404–410.
71. Phillips I. Beta-lactamase producing penicillin-resistant gonococcus. *Lancet* 1976;2:656–657.
72. Klugman K. Pneumococcal resistance to antibiotics. *Clin Microbiol Rev* 1990;3:171–196.
73. Hsu CCS, Macalusco CP, Special L, et al. High rate of methicillin-

resistance of *Staphylococcus aureus* isolated from hospitalized nursing home patients. *Arch Intern Med* 1988;148:569–570.
74. Arbeit RD. Laboratory procedures for the epidemiologic analysis of microorganisms. In: Murray PR, Baron EJ, Pfaller MA, Tenover FC, Yolken RH, eds. *Manual of clinical microbiology.* 6th ed. Washington, DC: American Society for Microbiology Press; 1995:190–208.
75. Tenover FC. Plasmid fingerprinting: a tool for bacterial strain identification and surveillance of nosocomial and community-acquired infections. *Clin Lab Med* 1985;5:413–436.
76. Schaberg DR, Tompkins LS, Falkow S. Use of agarose gel electrophoresis of plasmid deoxyribonucleic acid to fingerprint gram-negative bacilli. *J Clin Microbiol* 1981;13:1105–1109.
77. Birboim HC, Doly J. A rapid alkaline extraction procedure for screening recombinant plasmid DNA. *Nucleic Acids Res* 1979;7:1513–1523.
78. Kado CI, Liu ST. Rapid procedure for detection and isolation of large and small plasmids. *J Bacteriol* 1981;145:1365–1373.
79. Goering RV, Ruff EA. Comparative analysis of conjugative plasmids mediating gentamicin resistance in *Staphylococcus aureus*. *Antimicrob Agents Chemother* 1983;24:450–452.
80. Swaminathan B, Matar GM. Molecular typing methods: definition, applications, and advantages. In: Persing DH, Smith TF, Tenover FC, White TJ, eds. *Diagnostic molecular microbiology: principles and applications*. Washington, DC: American Society for Microbiology Press; 1993:26–50.
81. Tenover FC, Arbeit RD, Goering RV, et al. Criteria for interpreting pulsed-field gel electrophoresis patterns. *J Clin Microbiol* 1995;33: 2233–2239.
82. Gouby A, Neuwirth C, Bourg G, et al. Epidemiological study by pulsed field gel electrophoresis of an outbreak of extended-spectrum β-lactamase-producing *Klebsiella pneumoniae* in a geriatric hospital. *J Clin Microbiol* 1994;32:301–305.
83. van Belkum A. DNA fingerprinting of medically important microorganisms by use of PCR. *Clin Microbiol Rev* 1994;7:174–184.
84. Grattard F, Pozzetto B, Berthelot P, et al. Arbitrarily primed PCR, ribotyping, and plasmid pattern analysis applied to investigation of a nosocomial outbreak due to *Enterobacter cloacae* in a neonatal intensive care unit. *J Clin Microbiol* 1994;32:596–602.
85. Foster TJ. Analysis of plasmids with transposons. *Methods in Microbiology* 1984;17:197–223.
86. Lévesque C, Roy PH. PCR analysis of integrons. In: Persing DH, Smith TF, Tenover FC, White TJ, eds. *Diagnostic molecular microbiology: principles and applications*. Washington, DC: American Society for Microbiology Press; 1993:590–594.
87. Tenover FC, Popovic T, Olsvik Ø. Genetic methods for detecting antibacterial resistance genes. In: Murray PR, Baron EJ, Pfaller MA, Tenover FC, Yolken RH, eds. *Manual of clinical microbiology.* 6th ed. Washington, DC: American Society for Microbiology Press; 1995: 1368–1378.
88. Flamm RK, Phillips KL, Tenover FC, et al. A survey of clinical isolates of Enterobacteriaceae using a series of DNA probes for aminoglycoside resistance genes. *Mol Cell Probes* 1993;7:139–144.
89. Locksley RM, Cohen ML, Quinn TC, et al. Multiply antibiotic resistant *Staphylococcus aureus*: introduction, transmission, and evolution of nosocomial infection. *Ann Intern Med* 1982;97:317–324.
90. Rubens CE, McNeill WF, Farrar WE. Evolution of multiple antibiotic-resistance plasmids mediated by transposable deoxyribonucleic acid sequences. *J Bacteriol* 1979;140:713–719.
91. Blumberg HM, Rimland D, Carroll DJ, et al. Rapid development of ciprofloxacin resistance in methicillin-susceptible and -resistant *Staphylococcus aureus*. *J Infect Dis* 1991;163:1279–1285.
92. Kern WV, Andriof E, Oethinger M, et al. Emergence of fluoroquinolone-resistant *Escherichia coli* at a cancer center. *Antimicrob Agents Chemother* 1994;38:681–687.
93. Davies J. Another look at antibiotic resistance. *Journal of General Microbiology* 1992;138:1553–1559.
94. Thompson CJ, Gray GS. Nucleotide sequence of a streptomycete aminoglycoside phosphotransferase gene and its relationship to phosphotransferases encoded by resistance plasmids. *Proc Natl Acad Sci USA* 1983;80:5190–5194.
95. Martin P, Jullien E, Courvalin P. Nucleotide sequence of *Acinetobacter baumannii aphA-6* gene: evolutionary and functional implications of sequence homologies with nucleotide-binding proteins, kinases, and other aminoglycoside-modifying enzymes. *Mol Microbiol* 1988;2: 615–625.

Hospital Infections, Fourth Edition,
edited by John V. Bennett and Philip S. Brachman.
Lippincott–Raven Publishers, Philadelphia © 1998

CHAPTER 17

Cost–Benefit Analysis of Infection Control Programs

Robert W. Haley

ECONOMIC ANALYSIS IN INFECTION CONTROL

Economic concerns have taken on increasing importance in infection control since the mid-1970s. The increase in published scientific articles on economic aspects of infection control has followed closely both the proliferation of organized infection control programs and the nationwide expenditures on healthcare in the United States (Figure 17-1). During these years, the growing recognition of the preventive value of organized infection control programs stimulated pressure on hospital administrators to allocate more resources to such programs, while they were simultaneously being pressured to reduce overhead costs to keep their hospitals financially viable. Both their patients and their medical staffs were pressing for more patient care programs, but, although the advocates for prevention were relatively few, their voices were sustained largely by the force of the accreditation process. Faced with having to decide whether to put available financial resources into new patient care programs that generate direct revenue and profit or into infection prevention programs that do not, tough-minded administrators have been understandably reluctant to invest in prevention programs without some reasonable assurance that the programs would be effective in reducing nosocomial infection risks and thereby contribute to the hospital's financial solvency. To compete successfully for resources, the advocates of infection control programs have responded with an increasingly sophisticated array of economic analyses substantiating the economic benefits of their programs. Because the decisions on hospital expenditures are influenced by authorities both in hospitals and in advisory and regulatory agencies outside of hospitals, the economic arguments have been targeted at both the hospital level and at the national or international levels.

Current estimates of the economic impact of nosocomial infections can be found in the concluding section of Chapter 30, under the heading "Adverse Effects of Nosocomial Infections." This chapter focuses on the issues involved in conducting and interpreting studies on the economics of nosocomial infection and infection control.

Types of Economic Analyses

Studies on the economics of nosocomial infections and infection control have been mainly of the following four types: 1) estimates of the costs, and thus the potential benefits through prevention, of nosocomial infections (cost estimates); 2) comparisons of the costs of providing an infection control program and its potential economic benefits (cost–benefit analyses); 3) estimates of the financial savings to be obtained by an infection control program's eliminating unnecessary, often ritualistic, practices in patient care or in their own programs (cost-containment studies); and 4) comparisons of the relative efficiency of alternative strategies for bringing about given improvements in particular patient outcomes (cost-effectiveness analyses). Whereas the distinctions among these different types of analyses have often been blurred, from the frequency with which they have been used and reported, each appears to have been used persuasively in convincing hospital administrators to invest resources in infection control.

This chapter deals primarily with cost estimates and cost–benefit analyses (recognizing, of course, that the first is a necessary component of the second), because they should ultimately prove the most convincing to

R. W. Haley: Department of Internal Medicine, Division of Epidemiology, University of Texas Southwestern Medical Center at Dallas, Dallas, Texas 75235-8874.

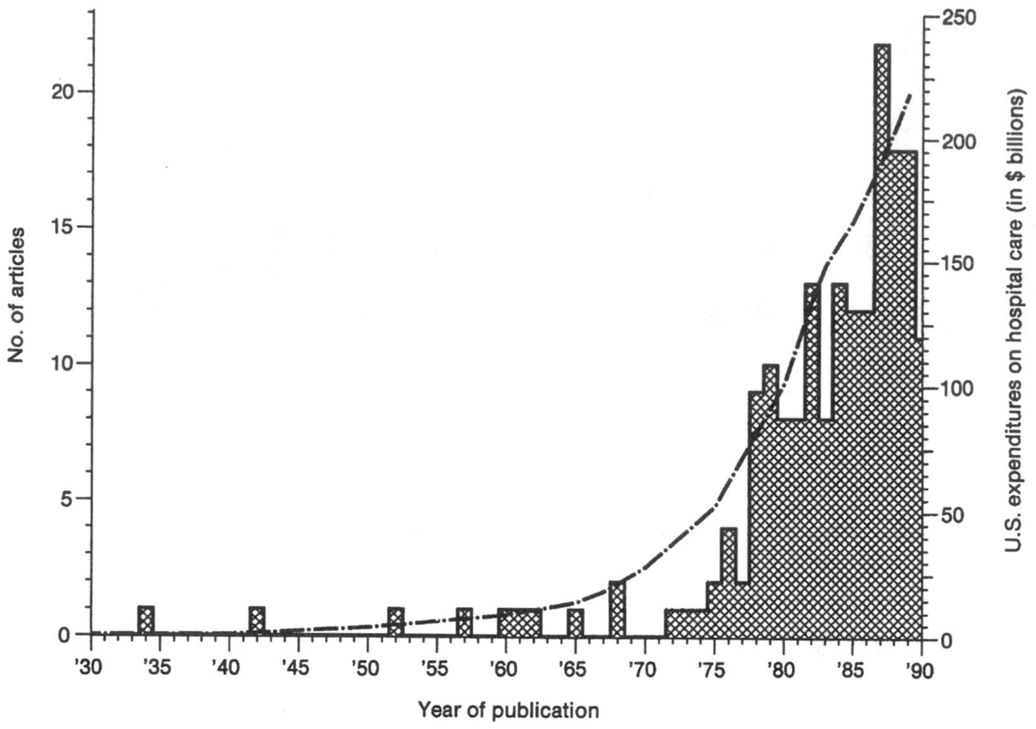

FIGURE 17-1. The increase in the number of articles on the economics of nosocomial infections and infection control in scientific journals (histogram) in relation to the increases in expenditures for hospital care in the United States (broken line). (Hospital care expendItures data from Letsch SW, Levitt KR, Waldo DR. National health expenditures, 1987. *Health Care Finance Review* 1988;10:1019.)

administrators. This is not to discourage cost-containment studies [1–10] and cost-effectiveness studies [11–17] related to infection control, for they also can be useful. Nevertheless, it must be recognized that although the latter two techniques deal with more immediate and tangible financial savings, their ultimate financial impact is substantially less than the potential savings from reductions in nosocomial infections brought about by effective infection surveillance and control programs, which is measured by cost–benefit analysis.

Cost–Benefit Analysis

Cost–benefit analysis is the exercise of estimating, in comparable economic units (usually a particular monetary currency, such as U.S. dollars), all of the costs and benefits of a proposed program regardless of to whom they accrue, over as long a period as is pertinent and practicable [18]. The balance, or ratio, of the costs and benefits provides a measure of the value of the program that can be compared with similar measures for competing programs, even though the programs and health outcomes of the programs are entirely disparate. For example, it would be reasonable to compare the cost–benefit ratio of an infection control program with that of a proposed renal dialysis center or radiologic imaging device. (Note that cost-effectiveness analysis, which compares the costs of alternative strategies for achieving a given outcome, cannot be used to compare programs that affect different outcomes.)

Although the basic concept of cost–benefit analysis seems straightforward, serious methodologic problems surface as soon as one begins to design an analysis of a particular program to influence a specific decision maker. For instance, one must decide whether *all* the costs and benefits are to be included or only those of interest to the particular decision maker to whom the study is directed. A complete cost–benefit analysis would estimate all the costs of nosocomial infections that are to be saved by effective infection control, including the physicians' fees and costs to the patient from time off work, but few published studies have included these because they may be of little strategic interest to hospital administrators. Similarly, one must decide whether to measure hospital charges attributable to nosocomial infection, which are easily obtained from the patient's hospital bill, or actual costs incurred by the hospital as a result of the patient's nosocomial infection, which are far more difficult to obtain, requiring a type of cost-accounting system that exists in few hospitals. Because patient charges are different from hospital costs, can they be compared with the costs incurred by the hospital for supporting its infection control program? These and the other equally troublesome methodologic decisions listed in Tables 17-1 and 17-2 explain the wide variation in the designs and methods used in the published cost–benefit studies of infection control.

It is of interest that cost–benefit analysis is of rather recent origin, its first serious applications appearing in the late 1950s [18]. Consequently, its quantitative methods are still developing. The major advances in its application to infection control have occurred since the early 1980s. It is no wonder, then, that many methodologic questions remain to be answered.

With the financial pressures on hospitals likely to become increasingly intense under managed care, it can be expected that there will be an increasing demand for cost–benefit studies that are more and more convincing to decision makers. It is not unlikely that more sophisticated cost–benefit analyses will compare the cost–benefit ratio of infection control with those of newly proposed patient care services or alternative preventive programs and that the results will be used to direct resources to the programs with the most favorable cost–benefit ratios. This expectation justifies greater attention to the methodologic issues in performing cost–benefit studies of infection control.

METHODOLOGIC ISSUES IN ESTIMATING THE COSTS OF NOSOCOMIAL INFECTIONS

The many methodologic issues that are inherent in the published cost and cost–benefit studies of infection control are listed in Tables 17-1 and 17-2. That there are far more issues in estimating the costs of nosocomial infections than in estimating the costs of the infection control programs may only reflect the fact that the former has been studied more extensively.

The eight main issues in the design of studies to estimate the costs of nosocomial infections are listed in Table 17-1. Within each column of the table, the methodologic choices are not necessarily mutually exclusive and, in many studies, several of them are used simultaneously. The large number of possible combinations of choices across the columns explains the enormous diversity of study designs as well as the considerable difficulty in trying to understand and compare studies. Such a classification of issues is helpful in comparing the results of many studies, because it allows the identification of subtle methodologic differences that can produce large disparities in the final estimates. Besides these eight issues, one must also consider the many methodologic issues common to all epidemiologic studies, including the use of valid definitions for nosocomial infections as well as the complete and accurate ascertainment of infections (see Chapter 5).

Basic Design

The most fundamental issue is whether the study is of cross-sectional or longitudinal design (see Table 17-1). Either can produce valid estimates of the costs of nosocomial infections, but longitudinal studies including an infection control intervention can be more insightful by providing a more convincing estimate of a reduction in the infection rate. Depending on how well the intervention study is designed, an empiric demonstration of a reduction may constitute a more convincing estimate of the economic impact that an infection control program can have than may a hypothetical estimate or one taken

TABLE 17-1. *Methodologic issues in performing cost–benefit studies of infection control: estimating the costs of nosocomial infections*

Basic design	Patient selection	Setting	Scope	Design for attributing extra days and costs	Currency	Summary statistics	Unit of analysis
Cross-sectional	Incidence series	In hospital	Hospital	Crude weighting	Hospital costs	Mean	Patient
Longitudinal	Prevalence series	Postdischarge follow-up	Nation	Direct attribution	Hospital charges	Median	Infection
Demonstration of a change in the infection rate	Epidemics	Readmissions	Developing countries	Comparative attribution	Components of cost or charges	Geometric mean	
	High-cost patients	Outpatient clinics	Site	Randomized trial	Hospital days	Percentage	
			Service		Lost wages	Total	
			Pathogen		Intangibles		
			Surgical procedure		Cost to third parties		
					Adjustments for diagnosis-related group payments		
					Deaths		
					Antimicrobial use		
					Antimicrobial resistance		
					Environmental damage		

TABLE 17-2. *Methodologic issues in performing cost–benefit studies of infection control (IC): estimating the costs of nosocomial infections and IC programs*

Components assessed	Effect on patient care practices	Indirect effects	Revenue from IC services	Issues affecting the estimation of both nosocomial infections and IC programs
IC practitioners Hospital epidemiologist IC Committee Clerical Equipment Maintenance/operations Space Utilities Administrative overhead	Burden on nursing time Expense of supplies used Quantity of supplies used Number of tests (cultures) done Isolation and private rooms	Malpractice losses Hospital marketing	Charging for services	Adjusting for inflation in costs to compare estimates obtained in different years Discounting future costs Providing convenient methods for cost estimates to be used for making economic projections in individual hospitals

from other published studies [19–21]. Most studies on the costs of nosocomial infections, however, are cross-sectional.

Patient Selection

There are four ways in which patients have been selected for estimating the costs of nosocomial infections. These include incidence studies covering either endemic periods or epidemics, prevalence studies, and special cohorts of "high-cost patients."

Incidence Series

In most cost–benefit studies of infection control, the patients constitute an incidence series—that is, all patients admitted or operated on during a defined, usually prolonged, time period. Most of these studies have been based on endemic incidence series, although there is an increasing literature on the costs of epidemics [21–34].

Prevalence Series

At least two studies have used data collected in prevalence studies to estimate the costs of nosocomial infections [35,36]. Although prevalence studies, usually involving surveying every bed in a hospital on a single day, can be done with relatively little effort and expense, the results are difficult to interpret. The difficulty arises from the fact that prevalence is a function of incidence times duration of the illness. Thus, patients found to be in the hospital and to have an active nosocomial infection on the day of a prevalence survey will predictably be the longer-staying patients, those with a higher risk of nosocomial infection, and those with the more long-lasting (more severe) infections. Consequently, in the same patient population the prevalence rate can be expected to be one and a half to two times higher than the incidence rate, and the average prolongation of stay and extra costs attributable to infection will be similarly longer in the prevalence series than in the corresponding incidence series.

In the first economic study from a prevalence study, Freeman et al. [35] estimated that the average length of stay of patients identified as having nosocomial infections identified in a prevalence study was 13.0 days longer than uninfected patients selected from a concurrent incidence series, matched on age, diagnosis, and operative procedure. In a follow-up report, these investigators found that the prolongation of stay due to nosocomial infection, similarly estimated, was 13.3 days for infections identified in the same prevalence series, but only 7.3 days for infections identified in a concurrent incidence series assembled from the same population of patients [37]. They concluded, "Results from prevalence and incidence series must be clearly distinguished because the same events will be perceived differently in the two types of series" [37]. In a later study, Thomann [36], attempting to correct this bias, estimated the incidence rate from his prevalence study by multiplying the prevalence rate by two thirds before projecting the costs. Although this might correct the estimated number and rate of infections, it would not correct for the selection bias in the higher average severity and costliness of the patients selected in the prevalence series.

In general, prevalence studies should not be used for making economic projections because of the uncertainty in trying to correct for the large selection bias inherent in the prevalence survey method. If they are used, conversion models, similar to those for estimating the incidence rate from a prevalence series [38], should be developed.

High-Cost Patients

A particularly enlightening group of patients to study comprises those who suffer the most costly nosocomial infections. Successfully identifying risk factors unique to these more serious infections might lead to the development of intervention strategies that prevent them selectively. Such strategies would be likely to have a particularly high level of cost-effectiveness relative to other infection control measures.

In 1979, Schroeder et al. [39] studied the characteristics of high-cost patients in a general hospital population without regard to nosocomial infection to estimate the implications for a national catastrophic health insurance. The fact that a relatively small percentage of patients with nosocomial infection (25%) account for a disproportionately large share (64% to 86%) of the total extra days and costs of nosocomial infection was demonstrated in three hospitals by Haley et al. [40], and corroborated by Green et al. [41] and Wakefield et al. [42] using different methods. A follow-up analysis of high-cost infections by Pinner et al. [43] found that surgical patients with wound infections after injuries and medical patients with lower respiratory nosocomial infections were likely to have the most costly infections. Numerous studies have shown that multiple nosocomial infections and secondary bacteremia are also associated with more costly infections [37,40,41,44].

Setting

Most of the studies have concentrated on patients whose nosocomial infections were detected while they were in the hospital. Recognizing that many surgical patients are now being discharged from the hospital soon after their operations, some investigators have excluded from surveillance, or from the analysis, all patients who remained in the hospital < 48 hours or, in studies of surgical patients, < 48 hours after the operation [45,46]. As the duration of hospitalization continues to decrease in hospitals in the United States and in some other countries, it will become increasingly important to continue surveillance after discharge to measure some infection rates accurately and without bias, particularly surgical wound infections [47]. For economic studies, however, as long as the objective of the cost–benefit study is to demonstrate the impact of nosocomial infections on the hospital's financial balance, studies can concentrate on detecting patients whose infections begin before discharge, those readmitted to the hospital for treatment of a nosocomial infection, or those seen in an outpatient clinic, if run by the hospital. This would not be adequate, however, for true cost–benefit studies in which *all* the costs are to be enumerated [18].

Scope

The scope of the study—that is, the nature and extent of the target universe to which the investigator wishes to project the cost or cost–benefit projection—varies widely in the published studies. Most commonly, studies have attempted to estimate the costs of nosocomial infections in an individual hospital, but they often make imprecise extrapolations of their findings to nationwide estimates for the United States [20,48–54] and for other countries [2,6,32,44,46,53,55–70].

Some studies have estimated costs for each site of infection [32,40], particularly surgical wound infections [20,34,35,40,44,71–98], nosocomial urinary tract infections [13,20,35,40,89–91,99–104], bacteremia [20,35, 40,90,91,105–108], and pneumonia [11,21,35,40,90,91, 109–111]. Others have reported their estimates stratified by service [40,46,112] or for a particular service, such as the neonatology service [57,113], intensive care units [46,108], orthopedics [77,84], obstetrics [33], or other surgical services [32,34,98]. Estimates for particular pathogens have most commonly focused on infections involving *Staphylococcus aureus* [27,74,114,115].

Design for Attributing Extra Days and Costs

The methodologic issue that has received the most critical attention is the series of design strategies used to estimate how many extra hospital days and how much extra "cost" are *attributable* to nosocomial infections. A classification of these design strategies is shown in Table 17-3. Four basic strategies have been used to estimate attributable days and "costs." The strategies are not mutually exclusive; that is, often investigators have used more than one of them in a particular study, although each usually requires its own separate statistical analysis and possibly even its own separate database [37,42,46,116]. In view of the fact that the imprecise terms used to describe these methods have led to considerable confusion among them, the following discussion explains each method in detail, following the terminology given in Table 17-3.

Crude Weighting

The simplest method is to select some constant that estimates the average extra costs or the average number of extra days to be expected for each nosocomial infection, and use it to weight (multiplying by the constant) the number of nosocomial infections detected in the study to estimate an overall cost of infections in the setting of the

TABLE 17-3. *Classification of types of study designs used to estimate the number of days and costs that are attributable to nosocomial infections*

I. Crude weighting
II. Direct attribution
   A. Clinician's subjective judgment
   B. Variation from a predicted value
   C. Standardized case-review protocol
III. Comparative attribution
   A. Unmatched group comparison
   B. Matching on multiple characteristics
   C. Matching on summary measures of confounding
   D. Stratification with indirect standardization
IV. Randomized trial

study. The constant is usually obtained from a previous study using one of the other attribution methods. A table of constants can be used for more precise weighting of stratified analyses: for example, site-specific cost constants can be used to weight infections stratified by site. Additional constants can be used to project the estimates to wider target universes, such as a nation or the world.

Although this strategy, often referred to as the "back of the envelope" method, is quick, its accuracy is limited by a number of factors, particularly the intrinsic accuracy of the constants and their appropriateness to the set of data being weighted. This method was frequently used in most of the initial cost–benefit studies, particularly those intended to create political urgency for directing resources to preventive services in the United States [48, 50–52,54] and other countries [36,53,59,64–66,117]. It is still used to provide an "economic punch" at the conclusion of epidemiologic descriptions of emerging nosocomial infection problems [33,76,87,99,101,118,119] and in editorials and reviews on the subject [6,12, 120–122]. Perhaps its most important use is in estimating the cost savings to the hospital when infection control measures have brought about a reduction in infection rates [21,33].

Direct Attribution

The second main approach is to attempt to measure directly for each infected patient how many hospital days or costs are attributable to the infection. Three important variations have been used for making attributions by the direct approach.

Clinician's Subjective Judgment

Most often it has been done by having a physician, infection control practitioner, or trained technician visit each infected patient daily to study the medical and nursing record and to speak with the physicians or nurses or examine the patient as needed to decide which days, services, and costs are attributable to the infection [1,29,34, 40,58,79,83,90,91,95–98,116,123]. This method has the advantage of an expert's being at the bedside each day to ferret out whatever evidence is needed to attribute days and costs accurately [116,124]. It has two basic disadvantages. First, it is, to one extent or another, subjective and not amenable to exact replication from study to study [37]. Second, because the physician surveyors have usually been conservative in their judgments, attributing extra days only in the face of definite evidence that the patient would have been discharged absent the infection, they are prone to overlooking attributable services and extra days. Consequently, this method has an inherent tendency to underestimate the attributable days and costs [37,116]

Variation From a Predicted Value

In several studies investigators have obtained an *a priori* estimate of the patient's expected length of stay in the absence of nosocomial infection based on the diagnoses, operations, and other factors, and they have subtracted this reference value from each patient's actual length of stay to estimate the extra hospital days attributable to nosocomial infection [26,40,74,88,90,116,125]. In two studies, the investigators used as the reference durations the average length of stay of all patients, or of all uninfected patients, in the hospital's population at risk [26,74]. In others, the investigators used the published figures for the 50th or 75th percentiles of the distribution of length of stay of all patients in the same region of the country, stratified by age, diagnosis, and operation [126], as the reference value for *otherwise uncomplicated patients* in whom nosocomial infection developed, but they relied on subjective clinical judgments for complicated cases, thus combining design types IIA and IIB [40,90,116]. In a study of surgical wound abscesses, Olson and Allen [88] used the length of postoperative stay up until the onset of the signs and symptoms of the abscess as the expected length of stay in the absence of infection.

The advantages of using predicted values of length of stay is that they can be applied easily, particularly to the large number of otherwise uncomplicated patients in whom nosocomial infections develop, and, as the precision of criteria used widely in routine utilization review increases in the future, the *a priori* estimates may become increasingly precise. There are several disadvantages. First, in many circumstances the *a priori* reference values may not be accurate. Second, the rationale behind choosing the 50th or 75th percentiles is not well established. Choosing the 50th percentile is perhaps too liberal, leading to an overestimate of attributable stay, because it assumes that the distribution of the length of stay of patients who get nosocomial infections is the same as those who do not, whereas the 75th percentile, which may be as much as twice as long as the 50th [37], may be too conservative, leading to an underestimate of the attributable length of stay.

Standardized Case Review Protocol

Clearly, the greatest innovation to the methods of attributing extra days and costs has been the introduction of a standardized case review protocol. Known as the *appropriateness evaluation protocol*, this method was developed as a standardized technique for patient care reviewers to detect unnecessary days of hospitalization [127,128]. In the late 1980s, Wakefield et al. [42,114] adapted the method for use in estimating the number of extra days that are attributable to nosocomial infection. The method involves having trained record reviewers review the medical records of discharged patients who had nosocomial infections and apply standardized criteria for classifying each hospital day into one of three categories: those attributable to the patient's reason for admission (or to noninfectious complications), those attributable to both the reason for admission and nosocomial infection, and those attributable only to nosocomial infection [42]. The days in the last category are the ones that are counted in estimating the costs of nosocomial infection. The method has been subjected to validation and found to produce very high levels of interreviewer agreement [127,128].

The advantages of this method are that it is simple enough to be applied in scientific studies or in routine infection control work; being standardized, it is replicable from setting to setting; it has been validated; and, by incorporating it into routine utilization review screening, it could potentially be applied to large numbers of patients or over long time periods. Its disadvantage is that it relies on the clinical information available in medical records, which are less complete in some hospitals than in others [129,130].

Comparative Attribution

The third main approach is to compare the lengths of stay and costs of patients with nosocomial infection (infected patients) with patients who did not suffer a nosocomial infection (uninfected patients). Investigators who favor this class of methods have referred to it as the *case–control method* or the *epidemiologic approach*. In actuality, the design of these studies is not strictly a case–control design, as the term is currently used in epidemiology [131] (see Chapter 6). In a true case–control study, the subjects are initially selected and classified on the outcome variable and are then studied to determine their exposure to the risk factor. In comparative attribution studies on the costs of nosocomial infections, the patients are selected and classified on the basis of the risk factor (presence or absence of nosocomial infection), and then their lengths of stay or costs (the outcome variable) are compared. This constitutes a cohort, or follow-up, study design rather than a case–control design. Four types of comparative attribution studies have been used to estimate the extra days and costs attributable to nosocomial infections (see Table 17-3).

Unmatched Group Comparison

The earliest, and still the least sophisticated, of the comparative attribution studies involves comparing the lengths of stay or costs of a group of infected patients with those of a group of uninfected patients, the difference between the means or totals of the two groups being accepted as the amount that is attributable to nosocomial infection [37,46,71,73–75,78,81,84,92,94,113,116,132, 133]. From the beginning, most investigators who used this method acknowledged that it overestimates the amount that is actually attributable to infection, because patients in whom nosocomial infections develop are generally more severely ill, and thus are destined for longer hospitalization even if the infection had not occurred [37, 41,46,57,66,80,94,105–107,113,116]. This phenomenon, which pervades all discussion of the comparative attribution methods, will be referred to as the *severity bias*. One indication of its possible presence is the fact that in several studies the preoperative stay of patients who later got wound infections is longer than that of patients who did not get a wound infection [65]. The severity bias causes all unmatched group comparison studies to overestimate substantially the extra days and costs attributable to nosocomial infection. Consequently, this method should never be reported.

Matching on Multiple Characteristics

In an effort to overcome the severity bias, numerous investigators have tried various schemes for matching uninfected patients (controls) to the infected patients (cases) to set up a comparison between groups that have the same predicted length of stay and cost before the infections supervened [32,35,37,41,44,46,57,77,80,82,85,86, 89,90,93,100,105–108,111,112,116,124,134,135]. These studies have been known by the misnomer *matched case–control studies*, when in fact they are *cohort studies with matched exposure groups* (matched infected and uninfected patient groups).

In most of these studies, the investigators have matched the infected and uninfected patients on several parameters. Most commonly, they have chosen one uninfected match for each infected patient, but two or three matched "controls" per "case" have been used to advantage in some studies [37,80]. The number of matching parameters used has varied from one to eight, with four or five being the number most often used. The parameters most commonly used in matching are patients' age (within ±5 years), sex, service, main discharge diagnosis, first listed surgical procedure, and month or year of discharge. Other interesting parameters that have been used uncommonly include the following: the Quetelet index of obesity, smoking, and social class [77]; subjective estimates of the severity of underlying illness from medical record review [45]; the presence or absence of unspecified "major confounding factors" [41]; and the number of valves replaced or the number of coronary vessels bypassed in cardiac surgery [136].

Recognizing that matching on these parameters may not entirely control for the severity bias, some investigators have required the length of stay, or the postoperative stay, of the uninfected patient to be at least as long as that of the infected patient before the onset of the infection

[37,41,105,107,108,111,134], or for all infected and uninfected patients included in the analysis to have stayed ≥ 7 days [89]. Freeman and McGowan [37] demonstrated that, after matching for several of the usual characteristics, this further restriction had a very small, though measurable, impact on the estimated prolongation of stay due to nosocomial infection (only 0.8 days of the average of 13 extra days).

The more matching parameters that are required to accept a match and the more categories contained in each matching variable, the larger the pool of potential uninfected patients that is needed to find matches for all the infected patients. Consequently, in many of these studies a substantial number of the infected patients have had to be excluded from the analysis for lack of a match; in some studies [41,57,91,105,106,111,116], these excluded patients tend to have longer lengths of stay and more severe infections than those who remain in the analysis, but in others this was not so [32,108,135]. This introduces a bias that tends to underestimate the extra days and costs attributable to nosocomial infection. In a carefully matched comparative study of bloodstream infection in a surgical intensive care unit (SICU), Pittet et al. [108] matched on five parameters and still were able to find matched controls for 86 of 97 infected patients. The mortality rates in the included and excluded cases were the same, suggesting the absence of a selection bias. This degree of success was possible because over 3,000 uninfected SICU patients were available for matching with the 97 infected patients.

A related pitfall, referred to previously, is the bias that results from selecting uninfected patients ("controls") from an *incidence* series, matched to infected patients ("cases") who were identified in a *prevalence* study [35]. Because the prevalence study design selectively identifies longer-staying patients with longer-lasting infections, this selection bias causes the comparison of infected patients from a prevalence series with uninfected patients from an incidence series to overestimate the attributable extra stay and costs [37].

In the analysis of matched comparison studies, opinions differ over whether to maintain the matching in the analysis. Examples of statistical techniques used for analyzing matched data include Wilcoxon's signed rank test, McNemar's test, the paired *t* test, and the Mantel-Haenszel technique [137]. Although several studies have used the correct statistical methods for matched data [37,57,85,91,108,116,135], most have analyzed the matched series as if they were unmatched groups of infected and uninfected patients [32,46,57,77,80,82,86,89,93,100,105,106,112]. Failure to maintain the matching may lead to underestimating the true magnitude of the difference and to overestimating its variance, but the errors are usually far less important in matched cohort studies, like matched comparison studies of costs, than for true case–control studies [137].

There are several advantages to the method of matching on multiple characteristics. First, it is relatively easily done on computerized data bases collected by routine surveillance or in outbreak investigations, and the patients' lengths of stay, or postoperative stay, and total hospital bill are easily obtained and merged into the data base. Second, the matching on these convenient parameters clearly does reduce the effects of the severity bias that are more evident in the unmatched comparison studies [116]. Its main disadvantages are the need for rather large pools of uninfected patients from which to select the matches and the selection bias resulting from excluding unmatched infected patients. Another drawback is the difficulty of knowing how much of the severity bias was eliminated by the matching and, conversely, how much overestimation remains uncontrolled in the estimates of the attributable extra stay and costs.

Matching on Summary Measures of Confounding

Despite the widespread use of matching on multiple characteristics, it has been suggested that the usual matching characteristics may not be the ones that best control for the severity bias [124]. It is conceivable that infected and uninfected patients may be perfectly matched on age, sex, diagnosis, operation, and length of stay until onset of infection, and yet the infected patients still have a longer expected stay apart from the additional stay conferred by the infection. This is because, even within the strata defined by the intersection of these usual matching characteristics, it is intuitively apparent that the severity of illness, infection risk, and expected length of stay and cost may differ substantially among patients. If true, these matching parameters will not completely eliminate the effects of the severity bias. In addition, matching on multiple characteristics, with some (such as diagnosis and operation) having thousands of diagnosis or procedure categories, often makes it difficult to obtain enough matches.

These problems have led to a search for summary measures of confounding that control more efficiently for the severity bias. The ideal summary measures should meet the following three conditions: First, they should be truly confounding variables in the analysis of the association of nosocomial infection with length of stay or cost [124]; second, they must have face validity for controlling much of the variance in length of stay due to diagnoses, operations, and severity of illness, but not that attributable to nosocomial infection; and third, they must contain as few categories as possible to maximize the number of infected patients for whom a match can be found. Statistical methods for reducing many confounding variables to a single summary measure have been described [138–140].

The available measure considered the most powerful predictor of length of stay and resource utilization is the system of diagnosis-related groups (DRGs), used in the

United States as the basis for the federal government's paying hospitals to care for its elderly citizens under the Medicare system [141,142]. For the DRG variable to qualify as a useful matching parameter, two conditions would have to be met. First, it would have to be augmented by another simple indicator of patient severity of illness, because DRGs are known to leave some amount of severity uncontrolled [124]. Several measures of severity of illness have been proposed, including complex measures such as the Medical Illness Severity Grouping System (MEDISGRPS) and the Acute Physiology and Chronic Health Evaluation (APACHE) system, and simple ones such as a count of the number of discharge diagnoses (the comorbidity index) [124,143–146]. Second, to qualify as a confounding variable, a parameter must have been shown to be reasonably strongly associated with both the risk factor and the outcome variable in the analysis [147]. Satisfactory resolution of this issue has been frustrated by the lack of large enough data bases containing all of the required variables along with accurately ascertained nosocomial infections.

A reanalysis of the large data base from the Study on the Efficacy of Nosocomial Infection Control (SENIC Project) addressed this problem [124]. The 169,526 patients were divided into two arbitrary groups, and multivariate linear models were fit to each half separately to determine the multivariate association of DRG, number of diagnoses, and their interaction with length of stay and with nosocomial infection. The results, summarized in Table 17-4, support the following conclusions. First, DRG is strongly associated with both length of stay and nosocomial infection, making it a true confounding variable. Second, the number of diagnoses increased the explanatory power of DRGs by ~10% (e.g., an increase in R^2 from 0.31 to 0.34) for both length of stay and nosocomial infection, suggesting that it provides additional control of severity of illness within DRG categories. And third, all these findings were corroborated by the finding of virtually identical results in both halves of the data base and by the additional validation analyses (see Table 17-4). These findings suggest that matching on DRG and the number of diagnoses might be a better way of estimating the extra stay and costs attributable to nosocomial infection in comparative attribution studies using matching or stratification with indirect standardization. Additional studies are needed to compare results obtained by matching on the traditional characteristics with those obtained by matching on DRG and the number of diagnoses.

Boyce et al. [112] reported a study in which they used DRGs along with age (±7 years), sex, urgency of surgery, type of surgery, and number of vessels bypassed or valves replaced as matching parameters in estimating the extra stay and costs attributable to postoperative infections in open-heart surgery. Pittet et al. [108] matched SICU patients with bloodstream infection with uninfected SICU patients on primary diagnosis, age (± 5 years), sex, the control's length of stay at least as long as the infected patients' interval from admission to infection, and number of discharge diagnoses [140]. These appear to be the most thoroughly controlled of the comparative attribution studies using matching on multiple characteristics.

Stratification With Indirect Standardization

In 1982, Fabry et al. [44] reported a study on the costs of nosocomial infections in abdominal surgery in which they used stratification and indirect standardization instead of matching to reduce the severity bias. A similar method was used several years later in a report by Le Coutour et al. [29]. This method attempts to include as many of the uninfected patients as possible in the analysis by stratifying on the confounding parameters instead of matching.

The infected patients and the uninfected patients were separately stratified on the intersection of several confounding variables. Fabry's group [44] used age, surgical procedure, and level of *medical risk*, defined by "infection at entry, heavier surgery and associated chronic condition." Uninfected patients in strata containing no infected patients were excluded from the analysis. Within each of the resulting strata, the mean length of stay (or costs) of the uninfected patients was weighted by the proportional distribution of the infected patients in the strata and summed across strata to derive the *expected* mean length of stay. The difference between this expected mean length of stay and the mean length of stay of the infected patients was considered to be the average extra days attributable to infection.

Le Coutour's group [29] stratified according to whether the patient had an infection on admission, four classes of admitting illness, and a severity of illness measure (described by Le Gall et al. [147]) used for only two classes of admitting illness. Although the stratification table was set up similarly to Fabry and colleagues', Le Coutour et al. calculated the attributable mean length of stay in each stratum by subtracting the means of the infected and uninfected patients, and then calculated a weighted average of the stratum-specific attributable means to obtain an overall estimate of the attributable length of stay per infected patient. This constitutes the calculation of a weighted mean rather than the method of indirect standardization used by Fabry et al.

These two approaches offer the advantage over the matching methods of using all, or almost all, of the information available in the population of uninfected patients for estimating the expected length of stay or "costs," whereas matching uses only one or two uninfected patients per infected patient. The effectiveness of both methods, however, ultimately depends on how well the stratifying parameters, like the matching parameters, control for the severity bias while minimizing the number of strata.

TABLE 17-4. *Values of explained variance from general linear models and contingency tables of the SENIC data base of 169,526 patients from 1975 to 1976 [141],[a] demonstrating that DRGs and the number of diagnoses (coded 1, 2, or 3+) and their interaction constitute true confounding variables in the analysis of nosocomial infection and length of hospital stay*

					Both halves combined[d]	
Dependent variable	Predictors in the models	First half[b]	Second half[b]	Validation analysis[c]	Linear model R^2	Contingency table U
Log(LOS)[e]	DRG only	0.32	0.31	0.30	0.31	
Log(LOS)	Number of diagnoses only	0.07	0.07	0.07	0.07	
Log(LOS)	DRG, number of diagnoses, and their interaction	0.35	0.34	0.32	0.34	
Nosocomial infection[f]	DRG only	0.18	0.16	0.15	0.16	0.27
Nosocomial infection	Number of diagnoses only	0.01	0.01	0.01	0.01	0.02
Nosocomial infection	DRG, number of diagnoses, and their interaction	0.19	0.18	0.16	0.18	0.29

SENIC, Study on the Efficacy of Nosocomial Infection Control; DRGs, diagnosis-related groups.

[a]The 147 DRGs (31%) that contained < 100 patients each were excluded, eliminating 6,979 patients (4%) from the analyses. All linear models were generated with the General Linear Models (GLM) procedure of the Statistical Analysis System (SAS), and were statistically significant at $p < 0.0001$.

[b]The data base was arbitrarily divided into two halves containing 80,805 and 81,742 patients, respectively. The numbers in the table are R^2 values unless otherwise stated.

[c]To validate the models, the coefficients from the first-half model were used to generate predicted values of the dependent variable in the second-half data, and these were regressed on the dependent variable in the second-half data; model R^2 values are reported.

[d]Because the R^2 values obtained in the first and second halves of the data base were similar, final estimates of R^2 from linear models were generated from the complete data base and, for the analyses of nosocomial infection, were compared with the asymmetric uncertainty coefficient (U) from contingency table analyses [174].

[e]Logarithmic transformation of length of stay (LOS).

[f]Coded *1* if the patient had any nosocomial infection and *0* otherwise.

(Reprinted with permission from Haley RW. Measuring the costs of nosocomial infections: methods for estimating economic burden on the hospital. *Am J Med* 1991;91(Suppl 3B):32S–38S.

To clarify the place of this method in the classification of study designs (see Table 17-3), indirect standardization resembles, although it improves on, the comparison of infected patients' length of stay with an *a priori* predicted expected length of stay (design type IIB). The reason it is classified separately is that comparison with a predicted value (design type IIB) is usually applied prospectively in the data collection stage, whereas stratification with indirect standardization (design type IIID) has been applied in the analytic stage.

Randomized Trial

The fourth main approach to estimating the attributable extra stay and costs is to conduct a prospective, randomized clinical trial. How a randomized trial would be designed to address this question most effectively has not to date been addressed in the literature on the economics of nosocomial infection, but a clever clinical trial on prophylactic antibiotic therapy conducted by Stone et al. [95] in the late 1970s deserves serious study. In that trial, the investigators randomized 463 patients undergoing elective stomach, biliary tract, or colon operations into two groups, one receiving cefazolin and the other a placebo intramuscularly 8 to 12 hours and 1 hour preoperatively, in the recovery room after the operation, on the morning after the day of surgery, and on that same afternoon. Infections of the wound or peritoneal cavity developed in 11 (4.7%) of the 232 patients in the cefazolin group and in 36 (15.6%) of the 231 patients in the placebo group. Because the patients were randomly assigned, the lengths of stay and hospital costs of the two groups should have been equal except for those resulting from the difference in the number of infections due to the use of the effective prophylactic antibiotic in the experimental group.

Although the investigators then sacrificed the advantage of the randomized trial methodology by resorting to direct attribution by subjective judgment (design type IIA) to estimate the attributable days and "costs," they supplied the basic data with which the true difference in length of stay between the two groups could be calculated. From the calculations shown in Table 17-5, the patients in the placebo group had 25 more wound and peritoneal infections and spent a total of 428 more postoperative days in the hospital than those in the experimental group, amounting to an average of 17.1 extra postoperative days per infection. Still, however, this figure may be an overestimate because the 11 infections in the experimental group appear to have been less serious on average than the 36 in the placebo group (average excess postoperative days by the clinician's subjective assessment, 13.3 vs. 17.0), possibly due to an ameliorating effect of the prophylactic antibiotic in addition to the demonstrated preventive effect. Against this interpretation, however, is the finding that the average excess postoperative stay estimated by the clinician's subjective judgment was 17.0 days for all 36 infections in the placebo group, agreeing with the figure of 17.1 days for the overall trial, calculated in Table 17-5.

The estimate of 17 extra days per postoperative wound infection is among the highest in the literature. Its derivation from a randomized trial may shed doubt on the much smaller estimates from the many direct and comparative attribution studies, although the higher figure may reflect the mix of more serious surgery studied in this randomized trial. Because of the promise of this method, future designers of randomized antibiotic trials should consider including measurements and analyses to estimate the extra days and costs of wound infections.

Currency

A central concept of cost–benefit analysis is to express both the costs and benefits of a program in a common currency so that they can be meaningfully compared. Although financial currencies are most often used, the costs of nosocomial infections are often expressed in a wide variety of currencies, including true economic costs, hospital charges, components of costs or charges, hospital days, lost wages, intangible costs, costs to third parties, deaths, excessive antimicrobial use and resistance, and, possibly, environmental damage (see Table 17-1). Even though these diverse currencies do not conform to the conventions of cost–benefit analysis, many do seem to have been useful in conveying the seriousness of the problem of nosocomial infections and in focusing attention on the need to reduce infection risks.

Extra Days and Charges

By far the most commonly used currencies in studies estimating the costs of nosocomial infections have been hospital days and hospital charges attributable to nosocomial infections [20,33,35,40,82,98,108,114]. These recur repeatedly in studies because they are the most readily measured variables that get relatively close to what concerns hospital administrators, namely, hospital costs. Patients' length of stay (Julian discharge date minus admission date) can be obtained quickly from diverse sources, such as the hospital's medical records system and patient accounting system, and patients' charges can be obtained from their itemized hospital bills or from the billing system. Extra days has the advantage of appearing to be a "harder" measure that varies less from year to year, whereas extra charges is more inclusive but also more variable because of inflationary pressures. Most often both are reported.

TABLE 17-5. *Estimation of the extra hospital days attributable to postoperative wound and peritoneal infections in a randomized clinical trial of cefazolin in intraabdominal operations*

	Preoperative antibiotics		Preoperative placebo
Total patients[a]	232		231
Average postoperative hospital days[a]	10.9		12.8
Total postoperative hospital days	2,529		2,957
Difference in postoperative hospital days		428	
Postoperative infections[a]	11		36
Difference in post-operative infections		25	
Average extra days per infection		17.1	
Average excess postoperative days per infection[a,b]	13.3		17.0

[a](Data from Stone HH, Haney BB, Kolb LD, et al. Prophylactic and preventive antibiotic therapy: timing, duration and economics. *Ann Surg* 1979;189:691.)

[b]Derived by clinician's subjective judgment (design type IIA).

Components

A number of investigators have attempted to desegregate the total charges due to nosocomial infection [1,29, 32,40,44,46,57,77,92,95,98,107,114,132]. The components of the costs can best be viewed in two major categories: routine and ancillary costs [40]. *Routine costs* are those due to the extra days of hospitalization and are often referred to as the *per diem costs* or *hotel costs*. They include nursing care and other recurring expenses and vary widely among different locations in the hospital (e.g., routine costs are higher in intensive care units than in general ward areas). *Ancillary costs* are those resulting from definable services performed in the treatment of the infection, such as antibiotics, respiratory therapy, microbiologic cultures, other laboratory services, and radiologic examinations. Although the proportional distribution of these components varies among different types of nosocomial infections, overall the routine and ancillary components each account for approximately half of the costs of nosocomial infections [40].

Extra Hospital Costs

An issue of increasing concern to investigators in this area is how to estimate the actual costs to the hospital of nosocomial infection [124]. The review by Finkler [148] pointed out the potential biases inherent in using hospital charges to estimate hospital costs. Briefly, third-party payers tend to underpay, or refuse to pay, for some hospital patients or services and will pay more for others. To maintain financial balance, hospitals tend to shift their charges for underreimbursed costs to those for which they can recover more than their costs. This means that the charges for a given service may be far higher or lower than the hospital's actual cost for delivering it. As a result, depending on the mix of services that are attributable to nosocomial infections, the charges may or may not reflect the hospital's costs accurately.

Realization of this pitfall has led a few investigators to use new methods to generate estimates that are closer to actual hospital costs [32,34,112,114,124,149]. These usually involve itemizing the actual services provided for treatment of the nosocomial infection and weighting each service by a cost weight that reflects the costs to the hospital of the goods and personnel services used to deliver the service. For example, the cost of administering a dose of an antibiotic would include the price paid by the hospital for the dose and the salary and benefits costs of the personnel time required to order, store, dispense, and administer the dose.

Methods for estimating true hospital costs are still crude and the resulting estimates appear little different from those derived from charges, but the advent of more detailed cost-accounting systems in hospitals is likely to provide more accurate estimates of true costs in the future. The alternative approaches have been reviewed in detail [40].

Adjustments for Insurance Reimbursements

In attempting to estimate the impact of nosocomial infections on hospitals' costs, it is potentially important to adjust for reimbursement payments that the hospital might receive specifically for complications such as nosocomial infections. Under fee-for-service reimbursement, hospitals passed their costs for caring for nosocomial infections directly through to the payers who reimbursed them entirely [2,45,91,132]. Under that system, hospitals bore little or none of the costs; instead, they were borne by the third-party payers who passed them on to the public through higher health policy premiums. When the prospective payment system (PPS) using DRGs was introduced into the United States hospital system, several investigators predicted that by reimbursing hospitals a set fee based on the admitting diagnosis, the DRG system would provide little reimbursement for the occurrence of a nosocomial infection [45,48,51,91,121,150, 151]. The added provisions that the costs of complications were built into the *adjusted standard amount* on which DRG payments are based and that patients in some DRGs are moved to higher-paying DRGs when they suffer a complication made it impossible to estimate how much of the costs of nosocomial infections are actually recovered by hospitals through reimbursements. Later studies, however, confirmed empirically that only 5% or so of hospitals' costs for caring for nosocomial infections are returned in added reimbursement under the PPS in all United States hospitals [141], and similar findings were obtained in special settings [27,42,86,112]. These findings indicate that there appears to be a strong financial incentive for hospitals to prevent nosocomial infections under the PPS form of hospital reimbursement.

Indirect Costs

Although almost all of the research has dealt with estimating the direct costs of nosocomial infections, Fabry et al. [44,149] in France and Schäfer [92] in Germany have estimated some of the important indirect costs to patients attributable to nosocomial infections. Among their findings were that, after surgical patients returned home, surgical wound infection prolonged their absence from work an average of 13.8 and 20 days [44,92]. These rather large estimates suggest the need for additional research to document the extent of morbidity and indirect costs due to nosocomial infections.

Deaths

An important cost of nosocomial infection is the occurrence of death. Most of the studies on the mortality related to nosocomial infection have studied matched infected and uninfected patients (design type IIIB), but just as for attributing extra days and economic costs, it is frequently unclear whether the matching has completely controlled for the severity bias in attributing deaths to nosocomial infection [46,105–107,152,153]. In the most thoroughly controlled comparative study, Pittet et al. [108] demonstrated an attributable risk of death from bloodstream infection in a SICU of 35% (mortality rate of 50% in the cases minus 15% in the controls) and a relative risk of 3.3.

An alternative to the comparative design is a longitudinal study observing the reduction in the mortality rate after an infection control intervention. Kelleghan et al. [21] estimated deaths attributable to ventilator-associated pneumonia by demonstrating a reduction in mortality after implementing an effective program to improve the care of ventilated patients. This design can be criticized, however, for the lack of simultaneous controls.

The best estimates of the frequency of deaths due to nosocomial infections came from a combined analysis of data from the National Nosocomial Infections Surveillance (NNIS) System and the SENIC Project [20]. In the NNIS System, the collaborating infection control practitioners followed a protocol to examine every death in a patient with nosocomial infection and make a clinical determination of the extent to which the death was caused by the infection (design type IIA). The findings indicate that 10% of patients with nosocomial infection die in the hospital, which breaks down as follows: In 6%, the death is unrelated to the nosocomial infection; in 3%, the nosocomial infection contributes to, but is not the main cause of, death; and in 1%, nosocomial infection is the main cause of death. By applying these figures to the nationally representative SENIC data, it is estimated that nosocomial infections directly cost more than 20,000 lives per year in United States hospitals and contribute to an additional 60,000 deaths per year [20]. No estimates of the economic costs of premature death from nosocomial infections have been made.

In studies to estimate the economic costs of nosocomial infection, it has been suggested that patients who die in the hospital should be excluded from analysis to avoid underestimating the extra days and costs attributable to the nosocomial infections when length of stay is cut short by death. Whereas some patients' length of stay is clearly shortened by death, other patients linger for long periods with nosocomial infection before dying. In their carefully controlled study, Pittet et al. [108] found that the excess length of hospital stay attributable to bloodstream infection was greater (mean, 26 days) in carefully matched case–control pairs in which the case survived than in all matched pairs (mean, 14 days), thus indicating that it must have been substantially less in pairs with a nonsurviving case. Estimates of the excess hospital costs were also higher in the pairs with a surviving case (mean $40,890) than in all pairs (mean $33,268), again indicating substantially less attributable costs in cases who died. There was no difference in excess SICU stay related to death. These findings indeed indicate that death in the hospital reduces the financial impact of nosocomial infections. Further empiric study of this question in other hospital settings would be useful.

Antimicrobial Use for Treating and Preventing Nosocomial Infection

A substantial body of literature has been generated to analyze the costs of antibiotics used either to prevent or to treat nosocomial infections [1,14,15,81,109,154–161]. Although this might be viewed as only a component of the overall costs of nosocomial infections, this component has arisen as a subject of interest in its own right (see Chapter 14).

Antimicrobial Resistance

Another unique currency in which the costs of nosocomial infections can be expressed is the emergence of antimicrobial resistance [114,162,163]. Under the pressure of broad-spectrum antimicrobial treatment, highly resistant strains of microorganisms emerge in the hospital and become preferentially involved in nosocomial infections (see Chapters 14, 16). As cross-infection spreads these resistant strains among patients, causing more nosocomial infections, resistance becomes increasingly widespread. Through this mechanism, nosocomial infections have greatly increased the costs of hospital care, not only by incurring costs to care for the patients during more prolonged illnesses, but also by requiring the development and increasing use of new, more powerful, and more expensive antimicrobial drugs.

Environmental Damage

A final currency is the impact on the environment of measures taken to prevent nosocomial infections. Daschner [164] has pointed out the enormous amount of waste and environmental pollution that is introduced into the environment as a direct result of efforts to prevent nosocomial infections in hospitals. The major offending elements include disposable equipment and supplies, detergents, washing agents, disinfectants, chlorides, and phosphates. No estimate of the cost to society of environmental damage has been made, but clinical efforts to control infection clearly contribute to this problem. An important role that organized infection control programs can play is in limiting the environmentally damaging products to at least those that actually lead to the reduction in infection risks.

Summary Statistics

In describing the quantitative impact of nosocomial infections, it is necessary to calculate summary statistics that express the central or overall magnitude of the problem. Although the various articles on the subject use standard statistical measures, the choice of summary statistics is controversial and requires careful consideration by future investigators.

The most commonly used summary statistics are the arithmetic mean, the percentage and the total of the estimated attributable extra days or costs. The total extra days (or costs) is used to express the overall impact of the problem in a hospital or country. It is simply the sum of the extra days, or cost, of all of the patients with nosocomial infection in a study or the total from a study projected, or extrapolated, to a larger population.

The percentage is used to indicate the relative magnitude of the extra days and costs to the total hospital days and costs of hospitalization. The most carefully derived percentages were reported by Wakefield et al. [42,114] from their study using direct attribution by standardized case review protocol (design type IIC). As found by other investigators, they reported that fewer than half (38%) of patients with nosocomial infection have their hospital stay prolonged by the infection, but that in those patients whose stay was prolonged, the extra stay constituted half (52%) of their total length of stay, and the magnitude of the prolongation (average of 20 extra days per infection) was more severe than appreciated by calculations of the overall average prolongation of stay.

Whereas the total and percentage are straightforward statistics, the mean has almost always been used incorrectly. The problem arises because the distribution of extra days, or costs, is almost always skewed positively by a relatively few, very high-cost nosocomial infections [40–43]. This skewness causes the arithmetic mean to overestimate the central tendency of the distribution, as discussed thoroughly by Green et al. [41]. For matched comparison studies (design types IIB and IIC), they recommended using either the geometric mean of the *difference* in length of stay (or cost) between the infected and uninfected patients in the matched pairs, or the geometric mean of the *ratio* of the values in the matched pairs. The former retains the advantage that its interpretation is closer to that of the familiar arithmetic mean, whereas the latter conveys the length of stay of the infected patients as a percentage of that of their uninfected matches. The median difference could also be used.

In comparative studies where the matching is preserved in the analysis, the median difference between cases and controls gives a falsely low estimate of the central tendency of the distribution of attributable length of stay or cost (it would be zero), because fewer than half of patients with nosocomial infection have their stay prolonged by nosocomial infection. Therefore, the geometric mean may be preferred if the distribution is found to be skewed. In comparative studies where the matching is not preserved in the analysis, the median length of stay can be used to great advantage [108].

Unit of Analysis

A methodologic issue that has been little noticed is the distinction between analyzing nosocomial infections or patients with nosocomial infection. In the former, the extra days, or costs, attributable to each infection are counted separately, whereas in the latter, the extra days, or costs, of all infections in a given patient are summed for that patient. These will be different to the extent that individual patients have more than one nosocomial infection. On a nationwide basis, 18% of patients with nosocomial infection have more than one episode or site affected [165] and, in another study of three hospitals, 15% had more than one infection [40]. Whereas the average extra days and costs are higher in patients with more than one infection than in those with only one [35,37,40,41,44], the amount that can be separately attributed to a second infection is usually far less than that attributed to the first infection, except when the second infection is nosocomial pneumonia [40]. The importance of knowing the unit of analysis is that estimates of the average extra days and costs are ~15% higher for studies of patients with nosocomial infection than for studies of nosocomial infections [29,40].

ESTIMATING THE COSTS AND THE COST–BENEFIT RATIO OF INFECTION CONTROL PROGRAMS

Despite a great deal of research on measuring the costs of nosocomial infections, less work has been done toward estimating the costs to the hospital for conducting an organized infection control program and the ratio of its costs and benefits. The first study on the costs of infection control was published in 1959 by Gee [166]. Because the study predated recommendations for surveillance and full-time infection control staff, it is no surprise that Gee enumerated the costs of changes in hospital practice that were brought about by starting a new infection control program. These included one-time costs such as construction and physical changes, adding sterilizers and increasing the numbers of thermometers, masks, and gowns and shoe covers, amounting to approximately $43,000 (in 1958 dollars), and recurring costs such as additional personnel in the laboratory, housekeeping, and laundry, and more disposable supplies and equipment and soaps and disinfectants, amounting to approximately $44,000 per year.

Ten years later, using Gee's method, Sperry and Craddock [94] estimated the start-up cost of their program at

$90,000 and annual recurring costs at $60,000, and compared these to the estimated economic benefits of preventing nosocomial infections, under varying assumptions of the percentage (20%, 50%, and 80%) of nosocomial infections prevented by the program. Dividing the costs attributable to their infection control program by the anticipated benefits from preventing infections, they derived the first cost–benefit ratio for an infection control program (incorrectly referred to as a *cost-effectiveness ratio*). They estimated that at 20% preventive efficacy, the costs would outweigh the benefits by 30%, at 50% efficacy, the costs would constitute only 51% of the benefits; and at 80% efficacy, they would constitute only 32% of the benefits. Their estimates of the potential benefits (i.e., the costs of nosocomial infections) were derived by the comparative attribution method (design type IIIA).

As part of the planning of the SENIC Project, Haley [52] derived a cost–benefit analysis that was later used for generating policy support for infection control programs in the United States [54] and internationally [52]. Because that analysis was generated after the beginning of the infection control movement in the 1970s, the cost of the infection control program focused on the salary costs of one infection control nurse, a part-time infection control physician, clerical assistance, and miscellaneous expenses, amounting to $20,000 per 250 hospital beds in 1975 dollars. These infection control program costs were then projected to the universe of United States hospitals, amounting to $71,840,000 nationwide. To estimate the potential benefits from prevention nationwide, the costs of nosocomial infection were estimated with the crude weighting method (design type I), arriving at a nationwide estimate of approximately $1 billion. From these assumptions, the costs of having an infection control program in every United States hospital amounted to ~6% of the costs of all nosocomial infections. Thus, at 6% preventive efficacy, the costs of the program would be exactly balanced by the benefits from infection costs averted; at 20% efficacy, there would be a $155 million nationwide savings; and at 50% efficacy, there would be a half billion dollar savings, all in 1975 dollars.

In 1986, Haley [20] updated the estimates of the costs and benefits of infection control to 1985 dollars and reformatted the analysis to allow infection control staff in individual hospitals to make estimates for their own institutions. On the basis of nationwide figures from the SENIC Project and the NNIS System and infection costs derived by the direct attribution method (design type IIA) updated for inflation, estimates were provided for the ratio of extra days, dollars, and deaths to total hospital beds for use in projecting these numbers to hospitals of varying sizes. Models were given for making cost–benefit calculations for hospitals of any size. Examples were given for assumed levels of preventive efficacy of 6%, 32%, and 50%, and a detailed form was included for estimating a program's level of preventive efficacy from a profile of its surveillance and control program activities and personnel, based on SENIC findings [20].

Subsequently, several investigators have compared the estimated costs and the benefits of their infection control programs with varying degrees of sophistication [6,27, 52,75,87,118,132,149]. The most interesting of these contributions is the analysis by Miller et al. [168]. Using the Haley methods [20] on data from the University of Virginia Hospitals, they estimated the costs of running their infection control program and the actual savings from nosocomial infections prevented, and they used these estimates to derive a fee that should be charged to patients and third-party payers to reimburse hospitals for these preventive services. Although the suggestion does not appear to have been adopted in practice, probably because of the inability to render charges under the United States PPS, the concept is an interesting one that might someday prove useful as hospital reimbursement systems evolve further.

Because relatively little research has been done in the area of estimating the costs and cost–benefit ratios of infection control programs, many methodologic issues remain to be addressed. Some of the more obvious ones are listed in Table 17-2. In estimating the costs of infection control programs, it is important to decide what components of the programs are to be counted. Certainly, all would agree on the salary of the infection control practitioner, the time of the infection control physician and committee, any direct costs for clerical assistance, maintenance and operations costs, and a portion of the hospital's overhead costs (e.g., utilities, space, administrative costs), but there has been little discussion of whether to include the myriad patient care practices that are done wholly or in part to prevent cross-infection (e.g., closed system urinary drainage, isolation and hand-washing costs, prophylactic antibiotic costs, control of outbreaks [117]). The prevailing view appears to be that these costs now constitute a minimal standard of care, regardless of whether there is an organized infection control program, and that the enumeration of the costs of the infection control program should be limited to those costs incurred directly by the infection control practitioners and the infection control committee. Opposing this view, however, is the growing body of articles pointing to the savings produced for the hospital by reductions in wasteful patient care practices initiated to control infection but eliminated at the suggestion of infection control staff [1–10,164]. If savings from phasing out ineffective practices should be credited to infection control, should not the costs of continuing useful practices be counted on the other side?

A potentially useful study would be a complete enumeration of all of the economic costs borne by hospitals to control and prevent nosocomial infections and all of the economic costs to society for nosocomial infections, distinguishing those that are preventable from those that are not. Whereas such a complete cost–benefit study has not been attempted, the progress in the methods for studying the economics of this problem provide a rich base for attempting it [11,13,15,37,42,46,116,117,120, 169]. In view of the rapidly changing economic forces in healthcare, further research of this problem is likely to continue to interest decision makers.

SUMMARY RECOMMENDATIONS FOR HOSPITALS

Infection control personnel wishing to estimate how much nosocomial infections are costing to elevate interest in the problem might consider three alternative study designs. The best crude estimates for the least time expenditure can be obtained by simply multiplying the estimated numbers of nosocomial infections at various sites by the site-specific cost weights (cost per infection) derived from the SENIC study and published by Haley [20] (design type I). Notable examples have been reported by Kelleghan et al. [21]. Probably the most precise measurements within a hospital for the least time commitment involve using the Appropriateness Evaluation Protocol (design type IIC), described for this purpose by Wakefield and colleagues [42,114], perhaps with the hospital's actual cost weights obtained in a detailed cost-accounting system. New approaches for refining the matched comparison method (design type IIIC) [108,112,124] have improved to the point that reasonably unbiased estimates of attributable excess stay, cost, and mortality are now possible, as best illustrated by the studies of Pittet et al. [108] and Boyce et al. [112]; however, completing a valid comparative study remains a laborious task, requiring careful design, a substantial time commitment, and expert statistical analysis.

REFERENCES

1. Beyt BE Jr, Troxler S, Cavaness J. Prospective payment and infection control. *Infect Control* 1985;6:161–164.
2. Daschner F. Economic aspects of hospital infections. *J Hosp Infect* 1982;3:1–4.
3. Daschner FD. Practical aspects for cost reduction in hospital infection control. *Infect Control* 1984;5:32–35.
4. Franck JN. Literature search reveals focus of cost savings. *J Hosp Infect* 1984;5(Suppl A):115–116.
5. Garner JS, Emori TG, Haley RW. Operating room practices for the control of infection in U.S. hospitals, October 1976 to July 1977. *Surg Gynecol Obstet* 1982;155:873–880.
6. Grazebrook J. Hospital-acquired infection: counting the cost of infection. *Nursing Times* 1986;82:24–26.
7. McGowan JE Jr. Cost and benefit: a critical issue for hospital infection control. Fifth Annual National Foundation for Infectious Diseases Lecture. *Am J Infect Control* 1982;10:100–108.
8. Meers PD. Facts and fancies in hospital infection. *Ann Acad Med Singapore* 1966;16:671–675.
9. Pobanz RB. The economic impact of universal precautions on a surgical unit. *Nursing Management* 1942;20:38–40.
10. Valenti WM, Sovie MD, Reifler CB, et al. Cut costs by revising policies and procedures. *Hospitals* 1980;54:84–86.
11. Fedson DS. Prevention and control of influenza in institutional settings. *Hosp Pract* 1989;24:87–91.
12. McGowan JE Jr. Cost and benefit in control of nosocomial infection: methods for analysis. *Rev Infect Dis* 1981;3:790–797.
13. Platt R, Polk BF, Murdock B, et al. Prevention of catheter-associated urinary tract infection: a cost–benefit analysis. *Infect Control Hosp Epidemiol* 1989;10:60–64.
14. Scheife RT, Cox CE, McCabe RE, et al. Norfloxacin vs best parenteral therapy in treatment of moderate to serious, multiply-resistant, nosocomial urinary tract infections: a pharmacoeconomic analysis. *Urology* 1988;32:24–30.
15. Stevenson RC, Blackman SC, Williams CL, et al. Measuring the saving attributable to an antibiotic prescribing policy. *J Hosp Infect* 1988; 11:16–25.
16. Adal KA, Anglim AM, Palumbo CL, et al. The use of high-efficiency particulate air-filter respirators to protect hospital workers from tuberculosis: a cost-effectiveness analysis. *N Engl J Med* 1994;331: 169–173.
17. Croce MA, Fabian TC, Shaw B, et al. Analysis of charges associated with diagnosis of nosocomial pneumonia: can routine bronchoscopy be justified? *J Trauma* 1994;37:721–727.
18. Klarman HE. Application of cost–benefit analysis to the health services and the special case of technologic innovation. *Int J Health Serv* 1974;4:325–352.
19. Haley RW, Culver DH, White JW, et al. The efficacy of infection surveillance and control programs in preventing nosocomial infections in US hospitals. *Am J Epidemiol* 1985;121:182–205.
20. Haley RW. *Managing hospital infection control for cost-effectiveness*. Chicago: American Hospital Association Publishing; 1986.
21. Kelleghan SI, Salemi C, Padilla S, et al. An effective continuous quality improvement approach to the prevention of ventilator-associated pneumonia. *Am J Infect Control* 1993;21:322–330.
22. Van Voris LP, Belshe RB, Shaffer JL. Nosocomial influenza B virus infection in the elderly. *Ann Intern Med* 1982;96:153–158.
23. Hyams PJ, Stuewe MC, Heitzer V. Herpes zoster causing varicella (chickenpox) in hospital employees: cost of a casual attitude. *Am J Infect Control* 1984;12:2–5.
24. Johnston JM, Burke JP. Nosocomial outbreak of hand-foot-and-mouth disease among operating suite personnel. *Infect Control* 1986;7: 172–176.
25. Finn A, Anday E, Talbot GH. An epidemic of adenovirus 7a infection in a neonatal nursery: course, morbidity, and management. *Infect Control Hosp Epidemiol* 1988;9:398–404.
26. Goetz A, Yu VL, O'Donnell WF. Surgical complications related to insertion of penile prostheses with emphasis on infection and cost. *Infect Control Hosp Epidemiol* 1988;9:250–254.
27. Rao N, Jacobs S, Joyce L. Cost-effective eradication of an outbreak of methicillin-resistant *Staphylococcus aureus* in a community teaching hospital. *Infect Control Hosp Epidemiol* 1988;9:255–260.
28. Barnass S, O'Mahony M, Sockett PN, et al. The tangible cost implications of a hospital outbreak of multiply-resistant *Salmonella*. *Epidemiol Infect* 1989;103:227–234.
29. Le Coutour X, Gallet E, Noyer V, et al. The cost of hospital acquired infections. *Agressologie* 1989;30:275–277.
30. Choi M, Yoshikawa TT, Bridge J, et al. Salmonella outbreak in a nursing home. *J Am Geriatr Soc* 1990;38:531–534.
31. Matson DO, Estes MK. Impact of rotavirus infection at a large pediatric hospital. *J Infect Dis* 1990;162:598–604.
32. Coello R, Glenister H, Fereres J, et al. The cost of infection in surgical patients: a case–control study. *J Hosp Infect* 1993;25:239–250.
33. Henderson E, Love EJ. Incidence of hospital-acquired infections associated with caesarean section. *J Hosp Infect* 1995;29:245–255.
34. Kent KC, Bartek S, Kuntz KM, et al. Prospective study of wound complications in continuous infrainguinal incisions after lower limb arterial reconstruction: incidence, risk factors, and cost. *Surgery* 1996;119:378–383.
35. Freeman J, Rosner BA, McGowan JE. Adverse effects of nosocomial infection. *J Infect Dis* 1979;140:732–740.
36. Thomann J. An attempt at evaluating the costs of nosocomial infections. *Agressologie* 1987;28:1221–1225.
37. Freeman J, McGowan JE Jr. Methodologic issues in hospital epidemiology: III. investigating the modifying effects of time and severity of underlying illness on estimates of cost of nosocomial infection. *Rev Infect Dis* 1984;6:285–300.
38. Rhame FS, Sudderth WD. Incidence and prevalence as used in the

analysis of the occurrence of nosocomial infections. *Am J Epidemiol* 1981;113:1.
39. Schroeder SA, Showstack JA, Roberts HE. Frequency and clinical description of high-cost patients in 17 acute-care hospitals. *N Engl J Med* 1979;300:1306–1309.
40. Haley RW, Schaberg DR, Crossley KB, et al. Extra charges and prolongation of stay attributable to nosocomial infections: a prospective interhospital comparison. *Am J Med* 1981;70:51–58.
41. Green MS, Rubinstein E, Amit P. Estimating the effects of nosocomial infections on the length of hospitalization. *J Infect Dis* 1982;145: 667–672.
42. Wakefield DS, Pfaller MA, Hammons GT, et al. Use of the appropriateness evaluation protocol for estimating the incremental costs associated with nosocomial infections. *Med Care* 1987;25:481–488.
43. Pinner RW, Haley RW, Blumenstein BA, et al. High cost nosocomial infections. *Infect Control* 1982;3:143–149.
44. Fabry J, Meynet R, Joron MT, et al. Cost of nosocomial infections: analysis of 512 digestive surgery patients. *World J Surg* 1982;6:362–365.
45. Aber RC. Nosocomial infections—1979. *Del Med J* 1979;51:635–642.
46. de Clercq H, De Decker G, Alexander JP, et al. Cost evaluation of infections in intensive care. *Acta Anaesthesiol Belg* 1983;34:179–189.
47. Weigelt JA, Dryer D, Haley RW. The necessity and efficiency of wound surveillance after discharge. *Arch Surg* 1992;127:77–81.
48. Bennett JV. Human infections: economic implications and prevention. *Ann Intern Med* 89:761–763, 1978;.
49. Brachman PS. Nosocomial infection control: an overview. *Rev Infect Dis* 1981;3:640–648.
50. Brown A, Magnussen MH. Infection control problems: a survey of the Veterans Administration Medical Centers in the northeastern United States. *Mil Med* 1981;146:348–352.
51. Dixon RE. Effect of infections on hospital care. *Ann Intern Med* 1978; 89:749–753.
52. Haley RW. Preliminary cost–benefit analysis of hospital infection control programs (the SENIC Project). In: Daschner F, ed. *Proven and unproven methods in hospital infection control: proceedings of an international workshop at Baiersbronn, September 24–25, 1977.* New York: Gustav Fischer Verlag; 1978:93–95.
53. Kereselidze T, Maglacas AM. Nosocomial infections: what WHO is doing. *J Hosp Infect* 1984;5(Suppl A):7–11.
54. Sencer DJ, Axnick NW. Utilization of cost/benefit analysis in planning prevention programs. *Acta Med Scand* 1975;576(Suppl):123–128.
55. Apostolopoulou E. Nosocomial infections. *Noseleutike* 1990;29:23–29.
56. de Martïn MC, de Cajar S, Abrego G, et al. Economic impact of nosocomial infections on the Metropolitan Hospital Complex of the Social Security Fund (from January through December, 1987). *Rev Med Panama* 1990;15:112–118.
57. Girard R, Fabry J, Meynet R, et al. Costs of nosocomial infection in a neonatal unit. *J Hosp Infect* 1983;4:361–366.
58. Jorup-Rönström C, Britton S. The nosocomial component of medical care: a prospective study on the amount, spectrum and costs of medical disturbances in a department of infectious diseases. *Scand J Infect Dis Suppl* 1982;36:150.
59. Losos J, Trotman M. Estimated economic burden of nosocomial infection. *Can J Public Health* 1984;75:248.
60. Lossa GR, Valzacchi B. Estimation of the cost of hospital infections. *Bol Oficina Sanit Panam* 1986;101:134–140.
61. Martïn DA. Repercussions at the individual and social level of hospital infections. *Rev Enferm* 1985;8:81–85.
62. Norberg B. Hospital infections cost money and suffering. *Vardfacket* 1986;10:24–25.
63. Pastorovä J, Ostrovskä A, Markvart K, et al. Results of a prospective study of the economic importance of nosocomial infections in the surgical department in a type I polyclinic hospital. *Rozhl Chir* 1981;60: 433–438.
64. Piffaut V. Nosocomial infections. Position of the Council of Europe: impact legal, economic and at the social security level. *Agressologie* 1987;28:1133–1135.
65. Prabhakar P, Raje D, Castle D, et al. Nosocomial surgical infections: incidence and cost in a developing country. *Am J Infect Control* 1983; 11:51–56.
66. Suwanakoon P, Silpapojakul K, Watanasri S, et al. Symposium: impact of nosocomial infections on Thailand. *J Med Assoc Thailand* 1988;71(Suppl 3):52–55.
67. Trilla A, Mirö JM. Control of nosocomial infections: who? how? and how much does it cost? *Med Clin (Barc)* 1989;92:217–219.
68. Verbrugh HA, Mintjes-de Groot AJ, Verkooyen RP. Registration and prevention of hospital infections in a general hospital. *Ned Tijdschr Geneeskd* 1990;134:490–495.
69. Williams REO. Infection and the injured patient: lessons and opportunities. *Injury* 1978;9:227–235.
70. Chaudhuri AK. Infection control in hospitals: has its quality-enhancing and cost-effective role been appreciated? *J Hosp Infect* 1993;25:1–6.
71. American College of Surgeons, Committee on Control of Surgical Infections, and Committee on Pre- and Post-operative Care. *Manual on control of infection in surgical patients.* Philadelphia: JB Lippincott; 1976:11–15.
72. Brachman PS, Dan BB, Haley RW, et al. Nosocomial surgical infections: incidence and cost. *Surg Clin North Am* 1980;60:15–25.
73. Brote L, Gillquist J, Tarnvik A. Wound infections in general surgery. *Acta Chir Scand* 1976;142:99–106.
74. Clarke SKR. Sepsis in surgical wounds, with particular reference to *Staphylococcus aureus*. *Br J Surg* 1957;44:592–596.
75. Collier C, Miller DP, Borst M. Community hospital surgeon-specific infection rates. *Infect Control* 1987;8:249–254.
76. Cruse PJE, Foord R. The epidemiology of wound infection: a 10-year prospective study of 62,939 wounds. *Surg Clin North Am* 1980;60: 27–40.
77. Davies TW, Cottingham J. The cost of hospital infection in orthopaedic patients. *J Infect* 1979;1:329–338.
78. Edwards LD. The epidemiology of 2056 remote site infections and 1966 surgical wound infections occurring in 1865 patients: a four year study of 4,923 operations at Rush-Presbyterian-St. Luke's Hospital, Chicago. *Ann Surg* 1976;184:758–766.
79. Eliason EL, McLaughlin C. Post-operative wound complications. *Ann Surg* 1934;100:1159–1176.
80. Fekety FR. The epidemiology of infections in surgical patients. In: Berlin BS, Hilbert M, eds. *Control of infections in hospitals: proceedings of an institute held at the University of Michigan, March 1–3, 1965.* Ann Arbor: University of Michigan School of Public Health; 1965:24–38.
81. Germiniani R. Prevention of infections in surgery: costs and benefits of infections of surgical wounds and of their prevention with antibiotics. *Minerva Chir* 1989;44:789–792.
82. Green JW, Wenzel RP. Postoperative wound infection: a controlled study of the increased duration of hospital stay and direct cost of hospitalization. *Ann Surg* 1977;185:264–268.
83. Kaiser AB, Petracek MR, Lea JW IV, et al. Efficacy of cefazolin, cefamandole, and gentamicin as prophylactic agents in cardiac surgery. *Ann Surg* 1987;206:791–797.
84. Lidgren L, Lindberg L. Duration and costs of hospitalisation because of orthopaedic infections and proposed cooperation between orthopaedic departments and departments of infectious diseases. *Acta Orthop Scand* 1972;43:335–342.
85. Lowenthal J. Sources and sequelae of surgical sepsis. *Br Med J* 1962; 1:1437–1440.
86. Nelson RM, Dries DJ. The economic implications of infection in cardiac surgery. *Ann Thorac Surg* 1987;42:240–246.
87. Olson MM, Lee JT Jr. Continuous, 10-year wound infection surveillance: results, advantages, and unanswered questions. *Arch Surg* 1990; 125:794–803.
88. Olson MM, Allen MO. Nosocomial abscess: results of an eight-year prospective study of 32,284 operations. *Arch Surg* 1989;124:356–361.
89. Rubinstein E, Green M, Modan M, et al. The effects of nosocomial infections on the length and costs of hospital stay. J Antimicrob Chemother 1982;9(Suppl A):93–100.
90. Scheckler WE. Hospital costs of nosocomial infections: a prospective three-month study in a community hospital. *Infect Control* 1980;1: 150–152.
91. Scheckler WE. Septicemia and nosocomial infections in a community hospital. *Ann Intern Med* 1978;89:754–756.
92. Schäfer U. Cost analysis in nosocomial infections: a 1-year study in the surgical department of Riesa District Hospital. *Zentralbl Chir* 1987;112:1552–1560.
93. Simchen E, Sacks T. Infection in war wounds-experience during the 1973 October war in Israel. *Ann Surg* 1975;182:754–761.
94. Sperry HE, Craddock J. It pays to spend money for infection control. *Modern Hospital* 1968;111:124–128.
95. Stone HH, Haney BB, Kolb LD, et al. Prophylactic and preventive antibiotic therapy: timing, duration and economics. *Ann Surg* 1979; 189:691–699.

96. Thoburn R, Fekety FR, Cluff LE, et al. Infections acquired by hospitalized patients. *Arch Intern Med* 1968;121:1–10.
97. Williams REO, McDonald JC, Blowers R. Incidence of surgical wound infection in England and Wales. *Lancet* 1960;2:659–663.
98. Calderone RR, Garland DE, Capen DA, et al. Cost of medical care for postoperative spinal infections. *Orthop Clin North Am* 1996;27:171–182.
99. Cox CE. Nosocomial urinary tract infections. *Urology* 1988;32:210–215.
100. Givens CD, Wenzel RP. Catheter-associated urinary tract infections in surgical patients: a controlled study on the excess morbidity and costs. *J Urol* 1980;124:646–648.
101. Krieger JN, Kaiser DL, Wenzel RP. Nosocomial urinary tract infections: secular trends, treatment and economics in a university hospital. *J Urol* 1983;130:102–106.
102. O'Leary MP. Economic considerations in management of complicated urinary tract infections. *Urology* 1990;35:22–24.
103. Rutledge KA, McDonald HP Jr. Costs and strategies for managing nosocomial urinary tract infections. *Drug Intelligence and Clinical Pharmacology* 1986;20:587–589.
104. Rutledge KA, McDonald HP Jr. Costs of treating simple nosocomial urinary tract infection. *Urology* 1985;26:24–26.
105. Martin MA, Pfaller MA, Wenzel RP. Coagulase-negative staphylococcal bacteremia: mortality and hospital stay. *Ann Intern Med* 1989;110:9–16.
106. Rose R, Hunting KJ, Townsend TR, et al. Morbidity/mortality and economics of hospital-acquired blood stream infections: a controlled study. *South Med J* 1977;70:1267–1269.
107. Spengler RF, Greenough WB. Hospital costs and mortality attributed to nosocomial bacteremias. *JAMA* 1978;240:2455–2458.
108. Pittet D, Tarara D, Wenzel RP. Nosocomial bloodstream infection in critically ill patients: excess length of stay, extra costs, and attributable mortality. *JAMA* 1994;271:1598–1601.
109. Mangi RJ, Ryan J, Berenson C, et al. Cefoperazone versus ceftazidime monotherapy of nosocomial pneumonia. *Am J Med* 1988;85:44–48.
110. Septimus EJ. Nosocomial bacterial pneumonias. *Semin Resp Infect* 1989;4:245–252.
111. Kappstein I, Schulgen G, Beyer U, et al. Prolongation of hospital stay and extra costs due to ventilator-associated pneumonia in an intensive care unit. *Eur J Clin Microbiol Infect Dis* 1992;11:504–508.
112. Boyce JM, Potter-Bynoe G, Dziobek L. Hospital reimbursement patterns among patients with surgical wound infections following open heart surgery. *Infect Control Hosp Epidemiol* 1990;11:89–93.
113. Hemming VG, Overall JC, Britt MR. Nosocomial infections in a newborn intensive-care unit: results of forty-one months of surveillance. *N Engl J Med* 1976;294:1310–1316.
114. Wakefield DS, Helms CM, Massanari RM, et al. Cost of nosocomial infection: relative contributions of laboratory, antibiotic, and per diem costs in serious *Staphylococcus aureus* infections. *Am J Infect Control* 1988;16:185–192.
115. Turnidge J. MRSA: is control worthwhile and feasible? *Med J Aust* 1990;152:225–226.
116. Haley RW, Schaberg DR, Von Allmen SD, et al. Estimating the extra charges and prolongation of hospitalization due to nosocomial infections: a comparison of methods. *J Infect Dis* 1980;141:248–257.
117. Poulsen KB, Bremmelgaard A, Sorensen AI, et al. Estimated costs of postoperative wound infections: a case–control study of marginal hospital and social security costs. *Epidemiol Infect* 1994;113:283–295.
118. Condon RE, Schulte WJ, Malangoni RA, et al. Effectiveness of a surgical wound surveillance program. *Arch Surg* 1983;118:303–307.
119. Mead PB, Pories SE, Hall P, et al. Decreasing the incidence of surgical wound infections: validation of a surveillance-notification program. *Arch Surg* 1986;121:458–461.
120. Fuchs PC. Hospital infection in orthopaedic patients. *J Infect* 1980;2:185–186.
121. Polakavetz SH, Dunne ME, Cook JS. Nosocomial infection: the hidden cost in healthcare. *Hospitals* 1978;52:101–102.
122. Schaffner W. Infection control: time to justify the costs. *Hospitals* 1979;53:125–126.
123. Goodall JWD. Cross-infection in hospital wards: its incidence and prevention. *Lancet* 1952;1:807–812.
124. Haley RW. Measuring the costs of nosocomial infections: methods for estimating economic burden on the hospital. *Am J Med* 1991;91(Suppl 3B):32S–38S.
125. Christakis GT, Fremes SE, Naylor CD, et al. Impact of preoperative risk and perioperative morbidity on ICU stay following coronary bypass surgery. *Cardiovasc Surg* 1996;4:29–35.
126. Commission on Professional and Hospital Activities. *Length of stay in PAS hospitals, United States, regional reports*. Ann Arbor: Commission on Professional and Hospital Activities; 1980.
127. Gertman PM, Restuccia JD. The appropriateness evaluation protocol: a technique for assessing unnecessary days of hospital care. *Med Care* 1981;19:855–871.
128. Rishpon S, Lubacsh S, Epstein LM. Reliability of a method of determining the necessity of hospitalization days in Israel. *Med Care* 1986;24:279–282.
129. Haley RW, Culver DH, Morgan WM, et al. Increased recognition of infectious diseases in U.S. hospitals through increased use of diagnostic tests, 1970–1976. *Am J Epidemiol* 1985;121:168–181.
130. Massanari RM, Wilkerson K, Streed SA, et al. Reliability of reporting nosocomial infections in the discharge abstract and implications for receipt of revenues under prospective reimbursement. *Am J Public Health* 1987;77:561–564.
131. Kleinbaum DG, Kupper LL, Morgenstern H. Typology of observational study designs. In: *Epidemiologic research: principles and quantitative methods*. Belmont, CA: Lifetime Learning Publications; 1982:62–95.
132. Reinarz JA, Megna MJ, Brown GT. Nosocomial infection: time for accountability. In: Gilbert DN, Sanford JP, eds. *Infectious diseases: current topics*. Vol. 1. New York: Grune and Stratton; 1979:219–240.
133. Westwood JCN, Legrace S, Mitchell MA. Hospital-acquired infection: present and future impact and need for positive action. *Can Med Assoc J* 1974;110:769–774.
134. Kappstein I, Schulgen G, Fraedrich G, et al. Added hospital stay due to wound infections following cardiac surgery. *Thorac Cardiovasc Surg* 1992;40:148–151.
135. Vegas AA, Jodra VM, Garcia ML. Nosocomial infection in surgery wards: a controlled study of increased duration of hospital stays and direct cost of hospitalization. *Eur J Epidemiol* 1993;9:504–510.
136. Scheckler WE. Nosocomial infections in a community hospital: 1972 through 1976. *Arch Intern Med* 1978;138:1792–1794.
137. Kleinbaum DG, Kupper LL, Morgenstern H. Matching in epidemiologic studies. In: *Epidemiologic research: principles and quantitative methods*. Belmont, CA: Lifetime Learning Publications; 1982:377–402.
138. Hooton TM, Haley RW, Culver DH, et al. The joint associations of multiple risk factors with the occurrence of nosocomial infection. *Am J Med* 1981;70:960–970.
139. Miettinen OS. Stratification by a multivariate confounder score. *Am J Epidemiol* 1976;104:609–620.
140. Haley RW. Nosocomial infections in surgical patients: developing valid measures of intrinsic patient risk. *Am J Med* 1991;19(Suppl 3B):145S–151S.
141. Haley RW, White JW, Culver DH, et al. The financial incentive for hospitals to prevent nosocomial infections under the prospective payment system: an empirical determination from a nationally representative sample. *JAMA* 1987;257:1611–1614.
142. Wenzel RP. Nosocomial infections, diagnosis-related groups, and study on the efficacy of nosocomial infection control: economic implications for hospitals under the prospective payment system. *Am J Med* 1985;78(Suppl 6B):3–7.
143. Gross PA, Beyt BE Jr, Decker MD, et al. Description of case-mix adjusters by the Severity of Illness Working Group of the Society of Hospital Epidemiologists of America (SHEA). *Infect Control Hosp Epidemiol* 1988;9:309–316.
144. Jencks SF, Dobson A, Willis P, et al. Evaluating and improving the measurement of hospital case mix. *Health Care Finance Review* 1984;Nov/Annual Suppl:1–11.
145. Munoz E, Rosner F, Friedman R, et al. Financial risk, hospital cost, and complications and comorbidities in medical non-complications and comorbidity-stratified diagnosis-related groups. *Am J Med* 1988;84:933–939.
146. Munoz E, Sterman H, Cohen J, et al. Financial risk, hospital cost, complications, and comorbidities in surgical noncomplication- and noncomorbidity-stratified diagnostic related groups. *Ann Surg* 1988;xx:305–309.
147. Le Gall JR, Loirat P, Alperovitch A. Simplified acute physiologic score for intensive care patients. *Lancet* 1983;2:741.
148. Finkler SA. The distinction between cost and charges. *Ann Intern Med* 1982;96:102–109.
149. Lambert DC, Fabry J. Cost–benefit and cost-effectiveness methods

and evaluation of additional costs due to hospital infection. *Agressologie* 1985;26:173–176.

150. Dunk-Richards G. Cost factors associated with hospital acquired infection. *Australian Nursing Journal* 1961;8:36–38.
151. Daschner F. Patient-oriented prevention and control of hospital-acquired infections. *Klin Wochenschr* 1979;57:1203–1208.
152. Gross PA, Van Antwerpen C. Nosocomial infections and hospital deaths: a case–control study. *Am J Med* 1983;75:658–662.
153. Platt R, Polk BF, Murdock B, et al. Mortality associated with nosocomial urinary-tract infection. *N Engl J Med* 1982;307:637–642.
154. Briceland LL, Nightingale CH, Quintiliani R, et al. Antibiotic streamlining from combination therapy to monotherapy utilizing an interdisciplinary approach. *Arch Intern Med* 1988;148:2019–2022.
155. Ehrenkranz NJ. Containing costs of antimicrobials in the hospital: a critical evaluation. *Am J Infect Control* 1989;17:300–310.
156. Guimarães RX, Maluvayshi CH, Hayashi F, et al. Hospital infection: reduction of antibiotics consumption due to the action of the Hospital Infection Control Committee of the Hospital do Servidor Publico Municipal de São Paulo. *Rev Paul Med* 1986;104:274–279.
157. Hemsell DL, Hemsell PG, Heard MC, et al. Piperacillin and a combination of clindamycin and gentamicin for the treatment of hospital and community acquired acute pelvic infections including pelvic abscess. *Surg Gynecol Obstet* 1987;165:223–229.
158. Huckleberry SD. Antibiotic cost-containment. *Drug Intelligence and Clinical Pharmacology* 1986;20:589–591.
159. Neu HC. Antimicrobial activity, bacterial resistance, and antimicrobial pharmacology: is it possible to use new agents cost-effectively? *Am J Med* 1985;78:17–22.
160. Quintiliani R, Cooper BW, Briceland LL, et al. Economic impact of streamlining antibiotic administration. *Am J Med* 1987;82:391–394.
161. Weinstein MC, Read JL, MacKay DN, et al. Cost-effective choice of antimicrobial therapy for serious infections. *J Gen Intern Med* 1986; 1:351–363.
162. Holmberg SD, Solomon SL, Blake PA. Health and economic impacts of antimicrobial resistance. *Rev Infect Dis* 1987;9:1065–1078.
163. Phelps CE. Bug/drug resistance: sometimes less is more. *Med Care* 1989;27:194–203.
164. Daschner F. Cost-effectiveness in hospital infection control: lessons for the 1990s. *J Hosp Infect* 1989;13:325–336.
165. Haley RW, Hooton TM, Culver DH, et al. Nosocomial infections in U.S. hospitals, 1975–1976: estimated frequency by selected characteristics of patients. *Am J Med* 1981;70:947–959.
166. Gee DA. How infection control affects the hospital. *Modern Hospital* 1959;93(9):63–66.
167. Lambert DC. The cost of nosocomial infection and its prevention: projection and limitations of an economic analysis. *Agressologie* 1987; 28:1123–1131.
168. Miller PJ, Farr BM, Gwaltney JM Jr. Economic benefits of an effective infection control program: case study and proposal. *Rev Infect Dis* 1989;11:284–288.
169. Snyder LL, Wiebelhaus P, Boon SE, et al. Methicillin-resistant *Staphylococcus aureus* eradication in a burn center. *J Burn Care Rehabil* 1993;14:164–168.
170. Daschner FD. The cost of hospital-acquired infection. *J Hosp Infect* 1984;5(Suppl A):27–33.
171. Daschner FD, Frank U. Controversies in hospital infection control. *Eur J Clin Microbiol* 1987;6:335–340.
172. Hess D, Burns E, Romagnoli D, et al. Weekly ventilator circuit changes: a strategy to reduce costs without affecting pneumonia rates. *Anesthesiology* 1995;82:903–911.
173. Munoz E, Sterman H, Goldstein J, et al. Financial risk, hospital cost, and complications and comorbidities (CCs) in the non-CC-stratified pulmonary medicine diagnostic-related group Medicare hospital payment system. *Am Rev Respir Dis* 1988;137:998–1001.
174. Agresti A. *Categorical data analysis.* New York: John Wiley & Sons; 1990:24–35.

Hospital Infections, Fourth Edition,
edited by John V. Bennett and Philip S. Brachman.
Lippincott–Raven Publishers, Philadelphia © 1998

CHAPTER 18

Legal Aspects of Hospital Infections

G. Scott Baity, Karen Rose Koppel Kaunitz and Andrew M. Kaunitz

As the sophistication of medical practice along with patient expectations continue to grow, our society's appetite for litigation continues to increase. These synergistic trends have expanded legal liability related to nosocomial infections. Today's human immunodeficiency virus (HIV) epidemic has certainly intensified such liability. By reviewing how liability related to hospital infection may occur, this chapter seeks to help hospitals and clinicians minimize their exposure to legal consequences of these infections.

INTRODUCTION TO LAW AND THE LEGAL SYSTEM

Sources of the law include federal and state constitutions, statutes, administrative law, and judicial decisions (common law). A legal *cause of action* may be created by a constitutional right, a statute, or by common law. A cause of action is composed of several elements, each of which must be proved before the plaintiff (person on whose behalf the suit is filed) can establish legal liability on the part of the defendant (person being sued) [1]. Each cause of action consists of its own distinct elements but, in general, the following must exist before legal liability occurs:

1. The plaintiff must have an interest that is protected by law.
2. There must be a legal duty.
3. A breach of duty by the defendant must be proved.
4. An injury must be shown damage to the protected interest.
5. It must be proved that the breach caused the injury.

G. S. Baity, K. R. K. Kaunitz: Baptist/St. Vincent's Health System, Incorporated, Jacksonville, Florida 32207.

A. M. Kaunitz: Department of Obstetrics and Gynecology, University of Florida Health Science Center, Jacksonville, Florida 32207.

Initially, the burden of proof rests with the plaintiff. The plaintiff must establish each element at least by a preponderance of the evidence. If the plaintiff succeeds in this, the burden shifts to the defendant to offer a legal defense. If liability is established, the plaintiff must then prove damages [1].

In some cases, the court decides that there are no material fact issues and that the required elements of the cause of action do or do not exist (or that a legal defense does exist). In these cases, the court grants summary judgment in favor of the prevailing party, and there is no trial.

Negligence

Malpractice is defined as a tort, or civil wrong, committed by a professional acting in his or her professional capacity. Negligence, the most common allegation (cause of action) in medical malpractice cases, is legally defined as the "omission to do something which a reasonable man, guided by those ordinary considerations which ordinarily regulate human affairs, would do, or the doing of something which a reasonable and prudent man would not do" [2]. Therefore, negligence is a violation of the duty to use care, and it arises where injury results from the failure of the wrongdoer ("tort-feasor") to exercise due care [3]. There are four general elements to establishing a *prima facie* case for negligence: duty, breach, causation, and compensable injury [4]. These elements are met in a negligence action alleging damages due to a hospital infection when the plaintiff (the person bringing the action) establishes that an infection was contracted in the hospital, that the hospital breached its duty to the plaintiff through an act of negligence, and that this negligence caused the infection or the damages sustained [5]. The test for negligence in an infection control case, therefore, might be framed in the following way: "Was the hospital care or lack of care in some way responsible for the infection; and did the hospital act in a reasonable and prudent manner in recognizing, reporting and trying to control the infection?" [6].

Standard of Healthcare and Breach of the Standard

A fundamental component of establishing liability involves delineating which particular duties hospitals and physicians have toward patients. In the healthcare context, these duties translate to the *standard of care*. Once patients have placed themselves under healthcare practitioners' care, those practitioners then have a duty to provide the patients with *reasonable* care. To prevail in negligence actions, plaintiffs must establish that a provider has failed to meet such a standard of care. The standard of care required depends, in turn, on the circumstances of the particular case.

Confusion arises when determining the applicable standard of *reasonable* care in a specific situation, and whether this standard of care has been breached. To make this determination, U.S. negligence law looks to the customs of the medical profession through the use of expert testimony [7–10]. The traditional rule, which was favorable to healthcare providers, held that practices should conform to the standards of other providers in the same locality [11]. Under this *customary practice standard* of the local community, or *locality rule*, a provider's performance was measured against the level of care delivered by reasonably competent persons or institutions of equivalent skill in the same or similar geographic community. The court's sole function, therefore, was to determine whether the providers did something that was not customary or failed to do something that was [12].

The locality rule has been abandoned in most states, in favor of a more national standard of care [12]. This nationwide approach is based on the assumption that there should be one prevailing level of care. Experts frequently disagree, however, as to what constitutes appropriate care in specific situations. Hence, a variety of approaches may be considered to define the standard of care for a given clinical situation.

Standard of Care in Nosocomial Infection Cases

Although hospitals have a duty to protect patients from injury due to infections, courts have never maintained that hospitals guarantee their patients will not acquire nosocomial infections. A hospital, however, may be liable for a patient's infection if it can be shown that the infection was caused by the negligence of the hospital or any of its agents. Hospitals' duties to monitor medical care include conducting infection control reviews. If a plaintiff establishes that an excessive number of infections has occurred at a defendant hospital, the hospital may have to prove that it could not have discovered the pattern any sooner and that, on discovery, measures were immediately undertaken to correct the problem. To minimize the risk of failing to meet the standard of care, hospitals should vigorously educate personnel in aseptic technique and infection control procedures and should institute monitoring mechanisms to establish that proper procedures are indeed being followed.

A spectrum of standards rather than a single standard of infection control applies to hospitals. In determining the standards of care within a hospital, courts have looked to various sources. One source is based on the hospital's own internal rules; these include protocols, procedures manuals, and bylaws. A hospital's failure to follow its own rules and procedures may lead to a liability claim against which it may be particularly difficult to defend:

> . . . [T]he hospital should be very careful to make sure that its own hospital regulations and procedures are followed assiduously. Because these items may be taken as the duties or standards of care incumbent upon a hospital, the failure to perform such duties or to meet such standards of care may allow the plaintiff to show the first two elements of negligence; then he [she] would only have to show that such failure to perform the duty or failure to meet a standard of care was the direct cause of his [her] injury and to show the amount of his [her] damages [13].

In addition to promoting staff compliance with internal regulations, hospitals should establish in their internal manuals procedures that are as practicable as possible.

Accreditation requirements, federal and state laws, and regulations governing hospitals may also establish standards of care. In some instances, they may serve as a substitute for expert testimony. In most states, hospitals are subject to government rules regulating the practice of hospital infection control. These requirements vary considerably from state to state; hence, hospital administrators and counsel should consult their own state's regulations. Some states allow considerable latitude in procedures, providing little guidance. Other states, such as Illinois, set forth explicit requirements for infection control procedures, including requirements for the sterilization of equipment, instruments, utensils, water, and supplies. In some circumstances, regulations even specify the particular methods of sterilization to be used. Courts have sometimes ruled that these regulations establish guidelines for minimum standards of hospital care.

Mere compliance with minimum statutory or regulatory standards and licensure provisions, however, may not preclude liability for negligence. Hospitals may be held to a higher degree of care because of local practices and requirements of good medical practice or because the court rejects an existing standard as inadequate to protect the public.

To summarize, courts look to a variety of sources, including national practices, local or national rules, and guidelines, when determining the standard by which a defendant is judged.

Establishing the Standard of Care

When a plaintiff alleges a defendant has failed to meet a standard of care, the plaintiff must first establish the standard and then prove that it was breached. This proof is normally accomplished by the use of expert testimony. When negligence has been admitted, however, or when the neglect is obvious to a layperson, expert testimony may not be required. Alternatives to expert testimony include the use of medical texts, journals, state and federal laws, regulations, and guidelines (or parameters) to establish the standard. In addition, direct cross-examination of the provider, as well as the doctrine of *res ipsa loquitur* may be used in establishing a standard of care.

Practice Parameters

Practice parameters have arisen on both the state and federal level in response to the clamor for healthcare reform. Although many of these parameters surfaced in the healthcare reform debates of the 1990s, they have been gaining increased recognition since the late 1980s [14].

Practice parameters, or practice protocols, are medical guidelines that "encompass a broad range of strategies designed to assist practitioners in the clinical decision-making process" [15]. More specifically, they are "standardized specifications for care developed by a formal process that incorporates the best scientific evidence of effectiveness with expert opinion" [16]. These guidelines are set by specific areas of the medical profession to advise members of the recommended standard of care to be used in a given situation. For example, the goal of practice parameters established by the Agency for Health Care Policy and Research (AHCPR), a federal agency empowered to establish practice parameters, is "to encourage physicians and other healthcare providers to change their practice behavior by adopting guidelines, thus improving patient care, patient outcomes, and quality of life" [17].

One of the applications of practice guidelines is to help clarify the standard of care in medical malpractice litigation. As alluded to previously, a major difficulty in medical malpractice cases is establishing the appropriate standard of care before "layperson" decision makers. Practice parameters have the potential to reduce such difficulties by establishing a reliable and predictable standard of conduct, relieving the decision maker of the dilemma of balancing the opinions of competing experts. In theory, a physician could rely on the practice parameter as the appropriate standard of care without having to worry whether a judge or jury, in a medical malpractice case, would consider the care administered appropriate. By establishing an unbiased standard of care, the use of practice parameters should "significantly reduce the most vexing problem in malpractice litigation: the battle of the experts" [11]. The only remaining issues to be determined in medical negligence litigation will be whether the practice parameter "is relevant to the case at hand, and whether it is appropriate to use the [parameter] to establish the standard of care" [11].

Practice parameters are not absolute rules of conduct. Therefore, unless the practice parameter was "promulgated by a government body with jurisdiction over medical malpractice and is intended to mandate the standard of care, a deviation from it will not constitute negligence *per se*" [11]. However, because compliance is voluntary, most practice parameter proposals include incentives for physicians', hospitals', and other healthcare workers' participation, such as compliance constituting an absolute or affirmative defense in medical negligence litigation [18,19]. Through this incentive, the conduct of physicians, hospitals, and other healthcare workers can be shaped, thereby improving "patient care, patient outcomes, and quality of life" [17].

The diversity of interests involved in the practice parameters movement "contribute to its momentum" [20]. Active participants include the American Medical Association (AMA), the AHCPR, "state governments, private healthcare researchers, third-party payors, health benefit plan sponsors, medical specialty societies, and voluntary health organizations" [20]. These varied groups consider practice parameters a "means of improving the quality and the affordability of medical care" [20].

The Doctrine of Res Ipsa Loquitur

Res ipsa loquitur, "the thing speaks for itself," is related to strict liability and expert testimony. To use the doctrine of *res ipsa loquitur*, the following three elements must be established:

1. The accident must be of a kind that ordinarily does not occur in the absence of someone's negligence.
2. It must be caused by an agency or instrumentality within the exclusive control of the defendant.
3. It must not have been due to any voluntary action or contribution on the part of the plaintiff [21].

Because infections occur in the absence of negligence, courts have infrequently applied *res ipsa loquitur* when plaintiffs attempt to establish liability for infections [22,23].

Causation, Damages, and Infections Liability

To prevail in a negligence action, a plaintiff must prove that a provider's failure to exercise the required standard of care directly or *proximately* caused the plaintiff's injury [1,24,25]. A defendant's acts are proximate if "in a natural and continuous sequence, unbroken by any efficient intervening cause, [they] produce injury, and without which the result would not have occurred."[1] If a patient can establish that he or she suffered injury due to an infection resulting from hospital or staff negligence, the hospital or its staff may be liable.

Liability is not established on mere proof that a plaintiff contracted an infection. Because nosocomial infections are common, unpredictable, and may be difficult to prevent, courts have recognized that such infections may occur despite reasonable care. For example, in *Simmons v United States* (1983), an abscess developed in a patient because of infection around an intravenous needle site. The court stated that proper prophylactic care (such as using a sterile needle and frequent dressing examination and change) does not eliminate the possibility of an infection developing [26]. Hospital employees, therefore, must be alert to infections and call them to the attention of the attending physician. A provider may not be liable for infection sustained by a patient who is more susceptible to infection than the average patient. For example, in the 1994 case of *Lawlor-Covell v Wack, M.D.*, a leukemia patient with a decreased white blood cell count due to chemotherapy died of an infection. The plaintiffs alleged that the decedent contracted the infection because of the negligence of a hospital worker. The jury found, however, that the defendant did not act negligently, and rendered a defense verdict [27].

Because it is often difficult or impossible to establish that a particular negligent act or omission specifically resulted in infection, patients are rarely awarded damages for hospital-acquired infections. As methods of typing microorganisms improve, however, the ability to trace the specific sources of infections, thereby proving proximate causation, may also improve (see Chapter 9).

Defenses to Negligence

Despite the plaintiff's ability to establish all required elements of a *prima facie* case for medical negligence, the defendant healthcare provider can raise affirmative defenses that, if proven, excuse the defendant from liability.

Examples of affirmative defenses are the statute of limitations, assumption of risk, contributory negligence, release/waiver, and any other matter constituting an avoidance [28]. An affirmative defense is "a response to a plaintiff's claim which attacks the plaintiff's *legal right* to bring an action, as opposed to attacking the truth of the claim" [2]. These legal approaches can avoid or reduce liability even if the plaintiff can establish all the necessary elements of a cause of action. Contributory negligence arises when the plaintiff failed to exercise ordinary care and self-protection, thereby contributing to the injury. The assumption of risk defense prevents a recovery of damages when the plaintiff perceives a risk and still voluntarily exposes himself or herself to it. A release or waiver executed by a patient may relieve the defendant of liability for the results of subsequent treatment. Likewise, the statute of limitations prevents the plaintiff from initiating a lawsuit after a statutorily defined period of time has elapsed. Other defenses that may excuse a defendant from liability include good Samaritan statutes, workers' compensation, and government immunity [1].

Affirmative defenses must be proven at trial, leaving the final verdict to a jury of laypersons. Absolute defenses, in contrast, are statutory-created defenses that take the decision one step further from the jury. Compliance with the requirements of an absolute defense eliminates a defendant's liability. The jury does not have to decide the merits of the absolute defenses requirements, or the comparative fault of the plaintiff and defendant, but merely has to decide the factual issue of whether the defendant *actually* complied with the requirements.

Theories of Liability

Liability for nosocomial infections may be imposed on any healthcare provider, including hospitals, physicians, and nurses [29]. Nosocomial infections occur in an estimated 5% of hospitalized patients in the United States (see Chapters 4, 30). They are believed to add more than $4.5 billion annually in hospital charges [30].

A variety of legal theories may be used to impose liability, including negligence, warranty, and strict tort liability, as well as government statutes and regulations. Hospital liability for negligence arises under two different theories. The first theory is based on the doctrine of *respondeat superior* ("let the master answer"), arising from the negligence of one or more employees or agents. The second theory holds that a hospital corporation itself may be negligent if it fails to perform a legally recognized corporate duty—the corporate negligence theory. If a staff physician, resident, nurse, or other hospital employee is negligent with respect to a patient, negligence may be imputed to the hospital, and the patient may have a cause of action against both the employee and the hospital–employer.

Even if an employer is found to be liable under the principle of agency, the employee who actually committed the tort can also be held personally liable for his or her wrongful act or omission. The plaintiff may sue any such parties separately or all of them together. The plaintiff is not, however, permitted to collect a judgment in full from two or more defendants. If the plaintiff collects the judgment from the employer, the employer may have a right of indemnification from the negligent employee. This right is most likely to be asserted when the employer and employee are insured by different carriers.

[1] *Black's law dictionary*, p. 1225 (quoting *Wisniewski v Great Atlantic & Pac Tea Co.*, 323 A.2d 744, 748 (Pa. Super. Ct. 1974).

Doctrine of Respondeat Superior

Under the theory of *respondeat superior*, a hospital may be liable for the acts or omissions of its employees. In applying this standard on a case-by-case basis, the courts have addressed two concerns regarding the relationship of the parties and the foreseeability of the action.

The first aspect of *respondeat superior* focuses on whether the negligent or tortious act was committed by an employee. Because the theory of *respondeat superior* applies only to the employees, the relationship between the hospital and the person committing the negligent or tortious act determines the liability of the hospital. For example, in the 1968 case of *Lundahl v Rockford Memorial Hospital Assoc.*, a hospital was not held liable for the negligence of a staff physician because "[t]he physician was not employed by the hospital, was not an agent of the hospital, and was not subject to the supervision of the hospital" [31]. Although a hospital is liable, under the theory of *respondeat superior*, for the negligent or tortious actions of its employees and employee–physicians, unlike the broader liability of corporate negligence, *respondeat superior* does not apply to independent physicians: "the mere granting of hospital staff privileges to an independent private physician [does] not establish the degree of authority or control needed to hold the hospital liable for the doctor's actions under the doctrine of *respondeat superior*" [32].

The second aspect of *respondeat superior* relates to whether the negligent or tortious act was committed in the course of the employee's or physician's medical duties. Most courts have held that hospitals are liable only for acts done in the course of the employee's duties. According to *Taylor v Doctor's Hospital (West)*, a 1987 Ohio case, a "hospital is not liable under the doctrine of *respondeat superior* for the intentional, malicious actions of employees performed when the employee acts outside the scope of his or her employment" [33].

Corporate Negligence Theory

The doctrine of corporate negligence extends a hospital's liability to independent contractors (physicians) merely granted staff privileges, a much broader basis of liability than under the theory of *respondeat superior*. Under the doctrine of corporate negligence, a hospital may be liable for negligently hiring or retaining its medical staff and personnel. For example, Florida has codified the doctrine of corporate negligence for hospitals:

> All healthcare facilities, including hospitals and ambulatory surgical centers . . . have a duty to assure . . . the competence of their medical staff and personnel through careful selection and review, and are liable for a failure to exercise due care in fulfilling these duties [34].

The courts' main emphasis in determining if a hospital is liable under the doctrine of corporate negligence is the foreseeability of the result. A court is more likely to find negligence if the hospital knew, or had reason to know, the potential for the offense. Most cases in which a hospital was held liable for the negligence or tortious actions of its employees involved the hospital's failure properly to perform background checks, or act on past allegations.[2]

Apparent (Ostensible) Agency

Apparent agency subjects a hospital to potential liability for the negligence or tortious actions of an independent contractor (physician) because of a perceived agency relationship between them. The following three elements must be proved to establish a *prima facie* case of apparent agency against a hospital:

1. The hospital must have acted or "held out" the physician in a manner that would have led a reasonable person to believe the physician was employed by the hospital;
2. The patient must have actually believed the physician was an employee of the hospital; and
3. The patient must have relied on that belief to his or her detriment (would have acted otherwise without such a belief) [35–37].

To minimize their potential liability related to apparent agency, hospitals should develop ways to advise patients, when appropriate, that their treating physician is not an employee of the hospital.

Corporate Obligations

Hospitals have been found to owe a variety of obligations directly to patients and the public. These obligations include:

1. The duty to furnish and maintain proper equipment, supplies, and services and to exercise reasonable care in the selection and use of such equipment, supplies, and services.
2. The duty to exercise reasonable care in the selection and retention of appropriate personnel.
3. The duty to exercise reasonable care with respect to the maintenance of buildings and grounds, including

[2]See generally *Insinga v LaBella*, 543 So.2d 209 (Fla. 1989) (holding a hospital liable for failing to properly verify the credentials of a person who was granted staff privileges after assuming the identity of a deceased physician); *Copithorne v Framingham Union Hosp.*, 520 N.E.2d 139 (Mass. Sup. Jud. Ct. 1988) (holding a hospital liable for an assault by a staff physician because the physician had been reappointed every year for 17 years in spite of actual notice of at least two previous incidents involving allegations that he head sexually assaulted patients). See also *Scheneck v Gov't of Guam*, 609 F.2d 387 (9th Cir. 1979); *Darling v Charleston Comm. Memorial Hosp.*, 211 N.E.2d 253 (Ill. 1965), *cert. denied*, 383 U.S. 946 (1966); *Elam v College Park Hosp.*, 183 Cal. Rptr. 156 (Cal. Ct. App. 1982).

keeping the environment clean and sanitary with the aim of preventing infection.

4. The duty to comply with policies and procedures that, whether established by the hospital or by outside agencies, have as their objective the safety and well-being of patients and the public [38].

Because such duties include the obligation to promulgate and enforce rules to protect patients from infections, hospitals that fail to establish proper procedures, organizations, and techniques of infection control may be liable. In addition, hospitals may have a duty to monitor infection rates by specific physicians and to intervene if excessively high rates are noted (see Chapter 4).

The Joint Commission on the Accreditation of Healthcare Organizations (JCAHO) mandates the presence of "an effective, hospital wide program for the surveillance, prevention, and control of infection" [29]. A required characteristic is that there are written policies and procedures for infection surveillance, prevention, and control for all patient care department services. Medicare Conditions of Participation for Hospitals constitute federal regulation of hospital infection control programs and state that "the hospital must provide a sanitary environment to avoid sources and transmission of infections and communicable diseases. There must be an active program for the prevention, control, and investigation of infections and communicable diseases" [39].

CLAIMS DATA

According to data published in December, 1994 by the St. Paul's Fire and Marine Insurance Company, improper treatment of infection ranks eighth by frequency in allegations in claims reported by St. Paul's-insured hospitals during 1994, with 168 claims filed at an average cost per claim of $72,958 [40]. Failure to diagnose infection-related illnesses rose from the sixth most costly allegation in 1993 to the fourth most costly allegation in 1994, with the average cost of such claims being $113,120 [41].

MEDICAL STAFF OBLIGATIONS

The medical staff as well as the hospital has an obligation to prevent and control infections. Physician responsibilities include appropriate clinical care; in certain cases, serving as a member of the infection control committee or as a hospital epidemiologist or infection control officer; and, in general, setting a proper example in practicing medical asepsis. Physicians may incur liability for failure to adhere to appropriate standards of care. In addition, as the availability of physicians specializing in infectious disease grows, liability may even be imposed for failure to consult with a specialist.

PATIENT NOTIFICATION OF THE PRESENCE OF INFECTION OR DISEASE

Some lawsuits have involved plaintiffs' allegations that they were not informed of the presence of hospital infections. In *Jones v Sisters of Charity*, a 1915 Texas case, the plaintiff alleged that his wife died from smallpox because the hospital failed to notify her that there was a case of this disease in the hospital. Because strict quarantine was maintained and there was no concealment, the court found for the defendant hospital [42]. In the 1939 case of *Robey v Jewish Hosp. of Brooklyn*, the court took a similar stand when damages for the infection of a newborn infant were alleged. In this case, an expectant mother was not warned of infection currently affecting infants in the hospital; the court ruled, however, that the record failed to show any actionable negligence on the part of the hospital [43]. In *Aetna Casualty and Surety Co. v Pilcher*, a 1968 Arkansas case, the hospital's failure to warn the plaintiff before surgery that pathogens existed in the hospital was not found to be the proximate cause of infection.

Hospitals have an obligation to patients sharing a room with another patient with a contagious disease. It is recommended that physicians treating such patients be informed; the physicians can then determine appropriate care. The patients likewise should be informed of exposure in such situations [44].

NEGLIGENT HANDLING OF PATIENTS

Infections resulting from negligent handling of patients have resulted in liability. For example, in *Larsen v American Medical International*, a nurse who was a hospital patient had an intravenous line inserted in her right arm. Her arm later became infected, leaving her with postphlebitic pain syndrome. Although the patient admitted that she was allergic to many different medications, the jury found that the infection was caused by the hospital negligently placing and maintaining the intravenous line. The jury returned a verdict for the patient in the amount of $135,000 [45].

A patient contracted an infection after a blood sample was taken in the defendant's emergency room in *Jones v Rapides General Hospital*. The patient was diagnosed with fasciitis caused by a gas-producing bacteria of unknown etiology, which required surgery that left disfiguring scars on her forearm. At trial, the plaintiff testified that the emergency room technician who performed the phlebotomy had difficulty locating the vein in the left arm and stuck her twice with the same needle to obtain the sample. The jury returned a verdict in favor of the plaintiff for $35,500, which was later reduced by the appeals court to $2500 because it found no proof of past medical expense [46].

EXPOSURE TO CONTAGIOUS PATIENTS

Hospital licensure regulations in most states require isolation facilities for patients with communicable diseases. Liability may be imposed for failure to isolate patients with communicable diseases or for failure to guard against cross-infection.

Courts have held that defendants are liable should a patient contract an infection after being negligently exposed to a contagious patient. In the case of *Ryan v Frankford Hosp.*, the minor plaintiff, Sean Ryan, was hospitalized and, during his hospitalization, was placed in a room with another minor, Donald Cummings. A sign above the bed of the Cummings child read "Enteric Conditions and/or Precautions." In their complaint, the plaintiffs alleged that at no time throughout Sean Ryan's hospitalization at the defendant hospital were they advised that their child's roommate had a contagious infection, shigellosis. Interaction between the minor plaintiff and infected roommate was encouraged, and meals were served to the two minor patients at the same table. The minor plaintiff was discharged from the hospital on March 29, 1982. On March 22, his pregnant mother, as a result of her contact with Donald Cummings or the minor plaintiff, was admitted to Jeanes Hospital with the diagnosis of shigellosis. Shortly thereafter, she underwent a therapeutic abortion. Court documents show that the case was settled in 1988, but the amount of the settlement was not disclosed [47].

In 1989, five patients in Sequoia Hospital in Redwood City, California, alleged that their infections with hepatitis B virus resulted from an anesthesiologist giving a local anesthetic to patients from a contaminated multidose vial. The anesthesiologist routinely administered lidocaine anesthetic from a 50-ml vial. During this procedure, blood from a hepatitis-infected patient was aspirated into the container. When lidocaine was given to subsequent patients, the hepatitis virus was transmitted. Although many patients were believed to be exposed to the virus, only five agreed to be tested [48].

A hospital may avoid liability when it is not aware of a contagious patient, such as when a physician neglects to notify hospital personnel that a patient was contagious [49,50].

RESTRICTIONS ON INFECTED PATIENTS

The acquired immunodeficiency syndrome (AIDS) epidemic has raised issues regarding the proper scope of infection control measures (see Chapter 43). In *Rhodes v Charter Hospital*, suit was filed against a psychiatric hospital under the Federal Rehabilitation Act alleging a patient was the subject of discrimination because of unnecessarily restrictive infection control procedures by the hospital [51]. The plaintiff alleged he was restricted to his room and not allowed to shower or eat with other patients and that hospital personnel who came in contact with him were fully masked, gowned, and gloved. The case was dismissed on the grounds that damages for mental anguish were unavailable and any action for injunctive relief would be moot [51]. Nonetheless, hospitals should assure that isolation policies have a scientific rationale.

EXPOSURE TO CONTAGIOUS PERSONNEL

Hospitals in most states are required to screen personnel for infectious disease by testing new employees and periodically screening existing personnel (see Chapter 3). Medicare and Medicaid Conditions of Participation require that a continuing process is enforced for inspection and reporting of any hospital employee with an infection who may be in contact with patients, their food, or laundry [52]. The failure to recognize obvious symptoms of an employee's poor health and to remove such an employee from duty may also generate liability. Hospitals must minimize patient contact with staff who are carriers of infection. Detecting, reassigning, and even removing contagious staff from duty, therefore, are all parts of a hospital's duties.

FEAR OF DISEASE CLAIMS

Increasingly, hospitals and physicians are facing claims for "mental distress engendered by the mere *possibility* that [a person] may suffer physical injury in the future" [53]. Examples of such allegations in the healthcare context are "fear of AIDS" claims, which require a particularly close analysis. In most states that allow "fear of AIDS" claims, "[t]he reasonableness of such claims depends not only on the existence of a physical injury, but also on whether the plaintiff was actually exposed to the AIDS virus" [53]. Some states, such as Florida and Tennessee, require the plaintiff to prove "actual exposure to the AIDS virus, not the mere possibility of exposure to HIV, before they will allow recovery for fear of AIDS" [53].[3] Other

[3]See, for example, *Carrol v Sisters of St. Francis Health Services Inc.*, 868 S.W.2d 585 (Tenn. 1983) (holding that a plaintiff may not recover damages for negligent infliction of emotional distress based on the fear of contracting AIDS without presenting evidence of actual exposure to the virus); *Doe v Surgicare of Joilet Inc.*, 643 N.E.2d 1200 (Ill. App. 3rd, Aug. 25, 1994), *reh'g denied* Sept. 21, 1994 (holding that a plaintiff may not recover damages for negligent infliction of emotional distress based on the fear of contracting AIDS without proving actual exposure to the virus); *R.J. v Humana of Florida Inc.*, 625 So.2d 116 (Fla. App. 1993) (dismissing an action for erroneous diagnosis of HIV because the plaintiff failed to show an actual physical impact); *Burke v Sage Products Inc.*, 747 F. Supp. 85 (E.D. Pa. 1990) (holding that a needle prick was not actionable without evidence that the needle was previously used on an AIDS patient); *Hare v State*, 539 N.Y.S.2d 1018 (N.Y. Ct. Cl. 1989), *aff'd* 173 A.D.2d 523 (N.Y. App. 1991) (holding that a plaintiff could not recover for fear of contracting AIDS after being bitten by a patient who was merely rumored to have AIDS); *Barrett v Danbury Hosp.*, 232 Conn. L.J. 242 (Feb. 21, 1995) (holding that a fear of contracting AIDS claim is unreasonable without evidence of actual exposure).

states, such as Maryland and Virginia, do not require actual exposure, but will allow recovery for the "window of anxiety between the time plaintiffs learn of their possible exposure to HIV and the time they receive negative test results" [53].[4] To ensure that such claims are genuine, most jurisdictions still require certain minimum levels of proof, such as:

1. *Exposure*: Was there actual, or only possible, exposure to a hazard?
2. *Injury*: Was there some physical impact, however minimal, that initiated the alleged emotional injury?
3. *Risk:* What is the probability that the claimant will actually contract the feared condition?
4. Fear: Is there a reasonable "window of anxiety" with which to mitigate damages [53]?

CONTAGIOUS PATIENTS SEEKING PREMATURE HOSPITAL DISCHARGE

When a patient who is actively infected with a communicable disease seeks discharge from the hospital against medical advice, the general rule that a patient of sound mind may leave the hospital at any time he or she chooses does not apply. In such cases, hospitals usually have the lawful authority to detain the patient. In fact, many states' public health laws provide the authority to restrain a contagious patient from leaving. Hospital legal counsel and public health authorities should be consulted immediately in such situations.

In addition, hospitals face liability for releasing patients without proper treatment. For example, in *Messot v St. Michael's Medical Center*, a hospital was held negligent for releasing a patient without proper treatment of severe urinary tract infection. The decedent's symptoms were attributed to her HIV status and long-standing diabetes, so she was released rather than treated. The jury returned a verdict of $755,000. Although no charges were filed in this case under the Consolidated Omnibus Budget Reconciliation Act of 1985 (COBRA) or the Emergency Medical Treatment and Active Labor Act of 1985 (EMTALA), hospitals must be especially careful to avoid "dumping" patients (releasing patients before stabilizing them) [54]. Penalties for noncompliance with COBRA/EMTALA by a hospital or physician include being subject to termination of Medicare provider agreements and civil monetary penalties up to $50,000 for each violation [54].

[4]See, for example, *Howard v Alexandria Hosp.*, 429 S.E.2d 22 (Va. 1993) (allowing the plaintiff to seek recovery for fear of contracting AIDS without proof of actual exposure to HIV); *Faya v Almarez*, 620 A.2d 327 (Md. 1993), *digested at*, 26 J. Health & Hosp. L. 246 (1993) (holding that a plaintiff may recover for fear of AIDS during the window of anxiety, even in the absence of actual exposure); *K.A.C. v Benson*, 1995 Minn. App. LEXIS 97 (Feb. 10, 1995) (holding that plaintiffs can recover for fear of AIDS without actual exposure if they are in the zone of danger of contracting HIV, but limiting the recovery to the window of anxiety period).

INFORMED CONSENT

With regard to consent, "every human being of adult years and sound mind has a right to determine what should be done with his own body" [55]. Failure to obtain informed consent may subject the doctor to criminal and civil liability for assault and battery or negligence.

Patients should be fully informed of the risk of medical procedures, including the risk of contracting infection. However, a dissertation on the epidemiology and pathophysiology of nosocomial infections is not required. The doctrine of informed consent requires reasonable disclosure of the available choices with respect to proposed therapy and the dangers inherently and potentially involved in each. In general, this is sufficient compliance with the disclosure rule when the patient has been informed of the possibility of infection and given some idea of the probability of its occurrence under the circumstances. Because in some cases infection is an inevitable risk over which the physician and hospital have no control, some decisions have concluded that there is no legal obligation to warn of its dangers, which are widely known to the public [56–59].

The current trend in decisions, however, indicates that patients are entitled to all relevant information to assess risks associated with their medical care. In *Harwell v Pittman*, the court concluded that the patient was not adequately informed of the material risks of postoperative infection. The plaintiff underwent an elective cholecystectomy without being informed that the risks of infection were greater in his case because of his obesity. The plaintiff alleged that had he been so advised, he would not have consented to the proposed surgery [60].

In general, the responsibility to obtain informed consent rests with the physician. In *Baltzell v Baptist Medical Center*, a woman brought suit against her physician and the hospital, charging that she was subjected to surgical assault when she was not warned of the dangers of infection before undergoing surgery for the removal of a breast lump. The court held that the trial court properly directed a verdict in favor of the hospital in the absence of evidence that the hospital, as opposed to the attending physician, had any duty to inform the patient of risks. The court held that the verdict should not have been directed in favor of the physician, however, because jury issues were raised by the testimony of the plaintiff's expert that the applicable standard of care required that the patient be warned that the surgery in question carried a 5% to 10% risk of staphylococcal infection [61].

To establish patients' awareness of hospital infections, some attorneys have suggested that hospital admission consent forms should state that infections are a risk associated with any hospitalization and that there is no assurance that the patient will not contract an infection. Operative consent forms in many hospitals state that infections are a possible complication of surgical procedures [13].

As discussed in the section on Posttransfusion Infection and Litigation, the patient's risk of contracting from blood products viruses that cause hepatitis or AIDS should be discussed, if appropriate, when obtaining informed consent [62,63].

Human immunodeficiency virus testing has focused attention on informed consent issues. Some argue that hospital general consent forms signed at admission allow physicians to order diagnostic tests necessary to treat the illness. This is based on the argument that specific consent is not customarily obtained before performing blood tests in that consent is implied because of the routine nature of the procedure. Others contend that informed consent before testing is required because a positive test result has significant personal and social consequences and may create psychologic distress, form a basis for discrimination, and affect the availability of health and life insurance. Many states, by law or regulation, require informed consent before testing. A number of states have enacted legislation to allow exceptions to the informed consent requirement in the case of occupational exposures of healthcare workers to individuals who are potentially infected with HIV.

In the absence of law or regulations, common law and ethical principals of informed consent suggest it is prudent to obtain consent before HIV testing. Industry guidelines are uniform in recognizing that consent should be obtained before testing. Hence, liability for failure to obtain consent may be established because a standard of practice has evolved through policy statements of several leading healthcare organizations, including the American Hospital Association (AHA), the United States Centers for Disease Control and Prevention (CDC), and the AMA.

Unless dictated by state law, consent to testing does not need to be in writing. However, it is strongly advisable to document the consent process. Regarding the scope of disclosure for an informed consent, industry guidelines should be consulted. The April, 1987 CDC Guidelines for HIV Antibody Counseling and Testing in *Prevention of HIV Infection and AIDS* (April 30, 1987) states, "Ideally, a person who requests testing or for whom testing is recommended should have a reasonable understanding of the medical and social aspects of HIV infection and the process of post-test counseling before consent." Patients should be told that the test is being done; that it is intended to indicate whether they have been exposed to HIV, the virus that causes AIDS; that the test can give false-negative or false-positive results; and that they have the right to refuse testing. In addition to disclosures regarding the nature, scope, and effects of the testing, some suggest that physicians discuss potential adverse personal social consequences before testing.

After the test, the patient should be counseled by trained personnel regarding interpretation. The American Medical Record Association has issued a pamphlet titled "Guidelines for Handling Health Data on Individuals Tested for HIV Virus," which includes forms for request and consent for testing and a recommended procedure for conducting a confidential screening program (for further information, contact the American Medical Record Association, 875 N. Michigan Avenue, Suite 1850, Chicago, Illinois 60611). Sample forms are also included in a publication prepared in November, 1989 by the AIDS Task Group of the American Academy of Hospital Attorneys of the AHA. They are available from the AHA, 1 North Franklin Street, Chicago, Illinois 60606.

POSTOPERATIVE INFECTIONS

Postoperative wound infections affect at least 920,000 of the 23 million patients who undergo surgery every year in the United States [64]. Not surprisingly, many malpractice claims filed against surgeons involve infections. As in all categories of potential liability, one key element in such suits relates to whether the provider met the standard of care [65,66].

Organisms causing postoperative infection are those frequently present in many healthy individuals. This observation had been used to counter plaintiffs' allegations of negligence in cases involving postoperative infections. For example, in *Roark v St. Paul Fire and Marine Insurance Company*, a staphylococcal infection occurred at the plaintiff's surgical site (see Chapter 41). Evidence established that standard procedures were followed by the hospital to establish the sterility of the supplies and instruments and that the environment met or exceeded national standards. An expert testified that:

> Most individuals who contract a staph infection after surgery had the bacteria on their skin prior to surgery. Since the bacteria is found within the subcutaneous sweat glands and hair follicles of some patients, the organism may survive the cleansing of the skin with antiseptics.

The physician also testified that susceptibility to staphylococcal infection varies from individual to individual. "With the present state of medicine, there is no practical way to determine prior to surgery who may be more susceptible to staph infection or who may be a `carrier' of the staph bacteria." The expert concluded that staphylococcal infections are an unavoidable risk of surgery [67].

OBLIGATION TO INFORM PATIENTS OF NOSOCOMIAL INFECTION

Providers should inform patients when a nosocomial infection has occurred. Courts have become increasingly insistent that physicians have a duty to disclose fully all pertinent facts concerning their patient's condition, even if the physician is convinced that he or she is acting in the patient's best interest by remaining silent [68]. This obligation exists regardless of whether the condition is the result of negligence of the physician, a colleague, or the hospital. Failure to inform patients in such situations may result in liability for fraud (constructive fraud or fraudulent concealment), negligence, or conspiracy. Punitive as well as compensatory damages may be awarded in such situations. In addition, courts have held that allegation of fraud stops the running of the statute of limitations [69].

INFECTIONS DUE TO MEDICAL EQUIPMENT AND DEVICES

Hospitals have an obligation to ensure proper cleaning, handling, storage, and sterilization of equipment and supplies. Hence, infections caused by contaminated instruments, equipment, or appliances may result in liability. Such cases often have involved the use of improperly sterilized needles or unclean catheters.

For example, in *Ernest Chester v Mercy Catholic Medical Center of Southeastern Pennsylvania*, the plaintiff contracted a staphylococcal infection that caused an enlarged heart and mitral valve prolapse. He claimed the infection was caused by improper placement and monitoring of equipment, which allowed the intravenous site to become contaminated. The plaintiff also claimed the infection was not properly diagnosed. An undisclosed settlement was reached in February, 1989 [70].

A physician's assistant, employed by the defendant, used an unsterile needle to administer a tetanus shot to the plaintiff in *Rung v St. Luke's Memorial Hospital Center*. The plaintiff claimed that the physician's assistant's infant son had touched the needle before the injection. She further claimed she had requested a different needle be used, but the defendant's employee assured her there was no need to be concerned. The plaintiff claimed that as a result of this negligent injection, she suffers from chronic infection resulting in permanent loss of the use of her left arm, resulting in permanent pain and suffering. The jury returned a verdict in the plaintiff's favor in the amount of $1,889,700 [71].

In *Brick v Greenbriar Nursing Home*, a Hickman catheter was inserted to administer nutrition to an 82-year-old woman recuperating from colitis. After a nurse was unable to flush the catheter, it broke, and the nurse used adhesive tape to cover the break. The patient contracted a staphylococcal infection of the lungs, and sustained neurologic damage that affected her mobility and ability to care for herself. Although the defendant nursing home claimed that the infection was a known risk of catheter use, and could have occurred without a break, the parties settled before trial for $450,000 [72].

The reuse of disposable, single-use medical devices can be problematic. Some providers have reused devices such as hemodialyzers, transducer domes, balloon-tipped catheters, cardiac catheters, catheter guide wires, biopsy needles, endotracheal tubes, anesthesia face masks, irrigating syringes, and manual resuscitators [73,74]. JCAHO requires that "there are written policies and procedures addressing the reuse of disposable items and these policies and procedures address the reprocessing of disposable items to be reused" [29]. When the devices are explicitly labeled "for single use only," hospitals and physicians bear the burden of proving that reuse poses no threat to the quality of care they provide. Guidelines and protocols regarding reuse procedures should be established, and careful, detailed records should be kept to substantiate that reuse does not jeopardize patient care (see Chapter 24).

ANTIBIOTICS

When antibiotics are used inappropriately, litigation may result. Suits alleging negligence have focused on failure to prescribe indicated antibiotics,[5] failure to screen adequately for sensitivity or properly monitor antibiotics,[6] prescription of antibiotics that are not clinically indicated or are contraindicated [75–77], inappropriate use of antibiotics for surgical prophylaxis,[7] and the subtherapeutic use of antibiotics [78,79] (see Chapter 14). According to data published by St. Paul's Fire and Marine Insurance Company, two of the five most frequent allegations for improper treatment, drug side effects and infection, were related to antibiotic use [80]. It is important to note that the emergence of organisms resistant to multiple antibiotics may increase litigation in this area.

In principle, it may be possible for a patient who contracts a nosocomial infection caused by a resistant organism to recover damages resulting from the organism's resistance, if he or she can prove that the resistance was caused by the physician's or hospital's indiscriminate use of antibiotics. In hospitals where antibiotic usage is not left entirely to the discretion of individual physicians, and the hospital can take affirmative steps to

---

[5]See, for example, *Hellwig v Potluri*, WL 285712 (Ohio 7th Cir. Ct. App. 1991) (holding a defendant emergency-room physician liable for failing to prescribe antibiotics after the plaintiff stepped on a rusty nail); *Griffith v West Suburban Hosp.*, No. 86L-23904 (Cook County Cir.Ct. 1993) *reprinted in* 10 Medical Malpractice Verdicts, Settlements, & Experts 31 (October 1993); *Toler v United States of America* (1993) *reprinted in* 9 Medical Malpractice Verdicts, Settlements, & Experts 32 (September 1993).

[6]See, e.g., *Sims v United States*, 645 F. Supp. 47 (D. Mo. 1986) (holding a physician liable for failing to administer ampicillin which might have prevented a postoperative infection); *Casterline v Streng*, No. EA C 53789 (L.A. County Super. Ct. July 13, 1990) *reprinted in* 10 Medical Malpractice Verdicts, Settlements, & Tactics 261 (August 1990); *Ordonez v Ariz. Board of Regents*, No. 207409 (Pima County Super. Ct. July 1987) *reprinted in* 8 Medical Malpractice Verdicts, Settlements, & Tactics 37 (February 1988).

[7]See *Orbay v Castellanos*, No. 91-36124 (Dade County Super. Ct. May 18, 1993) *reprinted in* 13 Medical Malpractice Verdicts, Settlements, & Experts 373 (October 1993) (holding a dentist liable for failing to prescribe prophylactic antibiotics and failure to obtain a full medical history or medical clearance from a patient at risk of developing bacterial endocarditis).

control the use of antibiotics, legal exposure may extend to the hospital.

Clinical review of hospital antibiotic use may be performed by the medical staff as a whole, by a medical staff committee, or by a hospital clinical department. Such review should assess clinical aspects of infections occurring in hospitalized patients, pharmacy data on antibiotic use, and trends in pathogen resistance reported by the hospital microbiology laboratory. Institutional observations, actions, and recommendations regarding hospital antibiotic use should be documented in writing. Should it be appropriate to restrict the use of a particular antibiotic, this decision should be implemented through the medical staff or departmental chairpersons.

DUTIES TO NONPATIENTS

Providers' obligations extend to persons other than their patients.[8] A duty of reasonable care extends to all employees, volunteers, and visitors on the premises. An individual who visits during regular visiting hours and remains in those parts of the premises open to visitors is an invitee to whom the hospital owes the duty of exercising ordinary care [81]. If a third party contracts an infection from a patient because of the provider's negligence, case law has established that damages may be awarded to the third party [82]. Visitors of isolation patients, for example, should be warned of the risk of contracting the disease, and documentation should be made indicating the visitor was so advised [83].

For example, in *Johnson v West Virginia University Hospitals, Inc.*, a university police officer who was called to help restrain a combative patient was bitten on the forearm [84]. After being bitten, the officer learned that hospital personnel knew the patient had AIDS. The officer sued the hospital for negligence, asserting that the hospital failed to advise him that the patient had AIDS, and that as a result of the exposure to AIDS, he suffered emotional distress [84].[9] The jury returned a verdict in the plaintiff's favor for $1.9 million. The verdict was upheld on appeal because there was an actual exposure (before the patient bit the officer he had bitten himself and there was still blood in his mouth) and the hospital failed to follow its own rules and regulations by posting a warning that the patient had an infectious disease [84].

The duty to protect third parties has been expanded by a Tennessee Supreme Court ruling that imposed liability on a physician for failing to "warn family members who are at risk from a patient's noncontagious disease" [85]. The son of a couple who died of Rocky Mountain spotted fever sued the physician for negligence in not warning his mother that she also was at risk of contracting the disease. The physician argued that because the mother was not his patient and Rocky Mountain spotted fever is not contagious from humans to other humans, there was no duty to warn of the risk of exposure. The Supreme Court found that "those who come in contact with the disease are at risk of infection from ticks carrying the disease," and held that the "existence of the physician–patient relationship is sufficient to impose upon a physician an affirmative duty to warn identifiable third persons in the patient's immediate family against foreseeable risks emanating from a patient's illness" [85].

STRICT LIABILITY OR BREACH OF IMPLIED WARRANTY

Liability is usually based on finding fault, or negligence. Attorneys, however, have sought to assert that providers are liable on a theory of strict liability in tort or breach of implied warranty. Under such theories, a plaintiff need not allege or prove a negligent act or omission to establish liability. These theories originate in the Uniform Commercial Code's section on implied warranty of fitness for a particular purpose. This section provides that when a merchant knows that a product is purchased for a particular use and is relied on to provide the correct product, an implied-in-law warranty arises that the product provided should be suitable for the particular use. Attorneys who wish to apply this theory to healthcare litigation argue that the implied warranty applies to a hospital room and warrants that the room is infection free. This argument, however, has not prevailed to date. Plaintiffs may be more successful by establishing that an implied contract, under which the hospital had infection control obligations, arose between a patient and the hospital at the time of admission.

Although efforts to establish liability without negligence have failed in most cases involving infections, courts have applied strict liability in tort and warranty liability in cases in which a patient contracted viral hepatitis after a blood transfusion.[10]

[8]See *DiMarco v Lynch Holmes-Chester County*, 559 A.2d 530 (Pa. Super. Ct. 1989) (holding that one who renders services to another should recognize, as necessary to protect a third party, he or she may be liable to the third party who is injured in reliance). But see *Kniere v Albany Medical Center Hosp.*, 500 N.Y.S.2d (1986) (declining "to impose a duty upon a hospital to warn the general public that one of its staff members had been exposed to an infectious disease"); *Livingston v Gribetz*, F. Supp. 238 (S.D.N.Y. 1982) (holding that there was no evidence of a duty owed to a nurse who contracted herpetic encephalitis from an infant, despite the pediatrician's failure to institute or monitor proper isolation procedures).

[9]There was testimony that the officer's wife refused to have sex with him, his children and grandchildren did not want to be around him, and his treating psychologist diagnosed him with posttraumatic stress disorder. There was also evidence that he had physical injuries, including sleeplessness, loss of appetite, and other physical manifestations accompanying his emotional distress.

[10]See *Williamson v Memorial Hosp. of Bay County*, 307 So.2d (Fla. 1st Dist. Ct. App. 1975) (stating that hospitals and physicians could only be held liable on the theory of implied warranty for serum hepatitis which the patient contracted, and which was allegedly caused by blood administered to her, only upon showing that the defect in the blood was detectable or removable through the reasonable use of scientific procedures or techniques).

POSTTRANSFUSION INFECTION AND LITIGATION

Liability for negligence may be imposed when a patient contracts an infection from a blood transfusion [86,87]. Infections acquired through blood transfusions include viral hepatitis, syphilis, malaria, toxoplasmosis, brucellosis, cytomegalovirus, and HIV [88]. In general, liability can be established only when a reliable test to detect the particular infection in the donor blood is available. For example, because tests are available to detect the presence of syphilis, failure to identify this infection in donor blood has resulted in liability [89]. Because posttransfusion viral hepatitis is not universally preventable by donor screening, however, contraction of this disease per se does not imply negligence.

Early cases held that a hospital was performing a service rather than a sale in furnishing blood to its patients; therefore, no warranty of fitness was implied [90]. Under this interpretation, hospitals could not incur liability related to administering blood without proof of negligence. As a reaction to difficulty in establishing negligence in posttransfusion cases, some courts have categorized the administration of blood components as the sale of a product, using product liability or implied warranty of fitness theories to impose liability [91,92]. Such decisions prompted virtually every state to enact remedial legislation (blood-shield statutes) that classifies blood transfusion as a service, which precludes strict liability. These statutes limit liability for adverse effects to those unusual cases in which negligence can be demonstrated. In many states, however, these statutes fail to state explicitly that blood banks and hospitals that administer blood components are immune from liability in the absence of negligence [1].

Efforts to apply *res ipsa* usually fail in posttransfusion cases. Because posttransfusion infections ordinarily occur without negligence, the first criterion of the doctrine of *res ipsa loquitur* is not met.[11]

Established blood bank practices, accreditation standards, state and federal statutes, regulations, and guidelines may all play a role in establishing standards of care for transfusion services. Public Health Service (PHS) recommendations for the prevention of HIV infection, for example, might be used by a court seeking to establish the appropriate standard of care.

Hospitals normally are not held responsible for contaminated blood obtained from community blood banks. Nevertheless, hospitals should scrutinize the source from which they obtain blood, ascertaining that the supplier is in fact screening donors in accordance with professional standards.

Considerable posttransfusion infection litigation involves HIV. One survey found that 14 such cases had been settled and 15 were pending [93,94]. Many of these cases concern the failure of blood collection centers to assess HIV risk factors among donors during the early years of the epidemic, before the availability in 1985 of antibody tests for HIV.

Even when a blood supplier has exercised due care, transfusion of HIV-contaminated blood may occur. Because infected patients are unable to recover damages for failure to screen or to defer high-risk donors, in such cases they often turn to other causes of action, such as failure to warn a patient about the risk of transfusion-associated HIV infection before obtaining consent and failure to inform the patient about alternatives to transfusions from the general blood supply, such as directed or autologous donations [95]. Clearly, liability may be imposed on physicians and hospitals for transfusions that result in HIV infections if the transfusions are deemed medically inappropriate or if informed consent is not obtained.[12]

In the spring of 1986, the American Red Cross, the American Association of Blood Banks, and the Council of Community Blood Centers instituted the Look-Back Program to identify and notify all recipients of blood that was known to be or suspected of being HIV positive. Since the implementation of the Look-Back Program, providers may be found liable for the failure to trace recipients. Liability exposure may extend from the patient to any third party, such as the patient's spouse, who might be at risk. Once physicians and hospitals are notified of the potential exposure of one of their former patients, they have a duty to notify the patient and advise further testing. It is prudent to document all efforts to locate the patient, especially if initial tracing efforts are unsuccessful.

Another issue raised by the AIDS epidemic concerns protecting the confidentiality of blood donors' identities. To prove the plaintiff contracted HIV from a blood transfusion, litigants have sought to discover the identity of the donor. Blood banks and hospitals have uniformly opposed the disclosure of the donor's identity, arguing that revealing the identity of donors could undermine the voluntary and confidential nature of the blood supply system. If disclosure were allowed, people might decline to donate blood to avoid being personally involved in subsequent litigation. Theories invoked by hospitals and blood banks to protect blood donors include:

1. The identities of blood donors fall within the scope of the physician–patient privilege and thus are not discoverable.

[11]See *Morse v Riverside Hosp.*, 339 N.E.2d 846, 848 (Ohio 1974) (stating that "no presumption that the hospital is negligent can be drawn solely from the fact that the patient contracted hepatitis following a blood transfusion, and the patient cannot recover damages on the theory of *res ipsa*").

[12]See *Valdiviez v United States*, 884 F.2d 196 (5th Cir. 1989) (holding that a jury could find that a patient could have refused a blood transfusion if informed of the risk). *Accord Doe v Werner*, Milwaukee County Cir. Ct., *reprinted in* AIDS Lit. Rptr., May 27, 1988; *Doe v Johnson, Iowa Methodist*, Polk County Dist. Ct., *reprinted in* AIDS Lit. Rptr., September 9, 1988; *Quintana v United Blood Serv.*, Denver County Dist. Ct., *reprinted in* AIDS Lit. Rptr., June 10, 1988.

2. An order compelling disclosure of donors' names and addresses is an unconstitutional infringement of the donor's fundamental right to privacy.
3. State abuse-of-discovery rules may be applied to protect the identities of blood donors [96].

Courts of Florida, New York, Pennsylvania, Tennessee, Ohio, and Michigan have ruled that privacy and public health interest are more important than the plaintiff's need for the information. In contrast, those who argue on behalf of disclosure have said it is necessary for the administration of justice. The Texas Supreme Court ruled that litigants have the right to confidential donor information because the donor's identity does not fall within the protected physician–patient privilege, the donor's right to privacy is not compelling, and the volunteer blood supply is not unreasonably harmed. The U.S. Supreme Court refused to hear an appeal of this issue. Disclosure of donor information was allowed by courts in Kentucky, Colorado, and Nevada. A Pennsylvania judge ruled that a blood transfusion recipient who acquired AIDS was entitled to learn about, but not to identify, the donor or other recipients.

ROLE OF MEDICAL RECORDS IN HOSPITAL INFECTION LIABILITY

Statutes and regulations concerning medical records vary from state to state. Some states require that the record contain minimum categories of information. Other statutes stipulate that records should be "adequate," "accurate," or "complete." Other jurisdictions set out requirements for medical records in greater detail, addressing such concerns as timeliness, retention procedures, and requirements for maintenance, signature, and filing. In addition to local requirements, Medicare and Medicaid regulations and the standards of the JCAHO should be followed.

Medical records often play a critical role in defending against a charge of negligence [97,98]. Failure to maintain accurate, complete, and current records has frequently enhanced plaintiffs' assertions of negligence. Speculative comments should not be included in the chart, nor should blame be assigned for an outbreak. The notation of "nosocomial infection," for instance, should be written in a chart only after such an infection is confirmed. If a notation in the record is made in error, a line should be drawn through the word or phrase so that it remains legible. The change should then be dated and initialed, and the correction should be noted elsewhere in the record, or in a marginal note explaining the correction. An entry should never be obliterated or removed and replaced with a copy.

Poor medical records often force physicians and hospitals to settle medically defensible malpractice cases [99]. Few things are as damaging as incomplete or inconsistent records, because juries rarely find undocumented recollections credible.

INFECTIONS CONTROL COMMITTEE REPORTS

According to the JCAHO, hospital infection control programs (see Chapter 4) are to include a multidisciplinary committee that "oversees the program for surveillance, prevention, and control of infection" [29]. Plaintiffs' attorneys, not surprisingly, may become interested in the proceedings, records, and reports of these committees. Accordingly, protection of the patient's confidentiality, names of personnel involved in hospital infection surveillance, and the infection control reports themselves have become controversial issues. Whether these records may be disclosed remains unresolved. Courts have sought to balance the desire of infection control personnel to maintain confidentiality with plaintiffs' need for information to support their allegations. In response to court decisions that have found infection control program records discoverable, most states have enacted statutes to protect such records. The protection such statutes offer varies considerably among states, however.

In *In re K.*, the New Hampshire Supreme Court ruled that the defendant hospital's infection control committee minutes and epidemiologist's report were privileged and not subject to disclosure in an action brought by a plaintiff diagnosed with herpes after giving birth at the hospital. The concerns of the plaintiff's husband led the hospital's nurse epidemiologist to conduct an investigation to determine whether the plaintiff could have contracted the infection while in the hospital. The findings were reported to the infection control committee. The state statute provided that records created to evaluate patient care or treatment for quality assurance are privileged. The trial court found that the privilege applied only to committee records related to quality assurance, and because the hospital had separate quality assurance and infection control committees, the records were not privileged. The Supreme Court, however, found the infection control committee was indeed a quality assurance committee and that the reports were privileged, because the infection control committee was serving its quality assurance function when it investigated the source of the plaintiff's infection [100–103].

By avoiding written speculation when recording observations, members of hospital infection control committees can minimize potential medicolegal problems. Members should use equivocal language such as "may have caused" or "may have contributed to," rather than conclusionary language such as "caused" or "contributed to." Such phrases would be more accurate and less damaging to the hospital should litigation occur.

EMPLOYEE HEALTH

Healthcare providers have a duty to protect the health of personnel as well as patients (see Chapter 3). Healthcare workers are exposed to a wide array of health and safety hazards including exposure to biologic agents, physical agents, stress, injury, and chemical agents [104]. Under the common law, employers had a duty to provide reasonably safe working conditions for their employees or to warn of unsafe conditions they might not discover on their own. These requirements have now been codified by administrative agencies such as the Occupational Safety and Health Administration (OSHA).

The OSHA requirements obligate private employers, including healthcare providers, to take all feasible measures necessary to recognize and eliminate significant occupational hazards. In the absence of specific federal and state occupational safety and health laws and regulations, an employer has the "general duty" to provide a safe workplace. The Occupational Safety and Health Act's general duty clause provides that:

> (E)ach employer . . . shall furnish to each of his [her] employees employment and a place of employment which are free of recognized hazards that are causing or are likely to cause death or serious physical harm to his [her] employees [105].

Violations of this provision can result in heavy fines. In addition, under 43 C.F.R. Part 85A, OSHA has broad powers to investigate workplaces and employer records and to conduct medical examinations to ensure that employees have a safe workplace.

In October, 1993, OSHA issued an enforcement policy regarding occupational exposure to *tuberculosis* (TB; see Chapter 33). This enforcement policy emphasized:

1. Control measures, including administrative and engineering controls and personal respiratory protection;
2. Risk assessment and development of a written TB control plan;
3. Early identification and management of persons with TB;
4. Purified protein derivative (PPD) skin testing programs; and
5. Educational programs for healthcare workers [106].

Medical Examination of Prospective Employees

A health inventory on all new employees is critical. It has been recommended that the inventory should include immunization status, past health conditions that might predispose the employee to certain communicable diseases, and any history of certain communicable diseases [107]. The health inventory should be used as a guide to determine on an individual basis whether an examination or laboratory studies are needed.

Surveillance of Personnel and Medical Staff

Hospitals should monitor infectious disease and carrier states in personnel. Special effort should be made to monitor staff in high-risk areas such as nurseries and hemodialysis units [108,109]. As pathogens such as HIV and hepatitis C "continue to invade healthcare settings, a comprehensive surveillance system for healthcare workers is needed now more than ever" (see Chapter 3) [110]. Accordingly, a "consolidated surveillance system to allow hospitals to monitor infectious diseases among healthcare workers is being developed by the Centers for Disease Control and Prevention..." [110].

Regardless of whether a provider knows of any medical staff member infected with HIV, it should take steps to protect its patient population and other healthcare personnel from infection. Providers should rigorously monitor and enforce continued compliance with CDC guidelines to reduce the risk of patients' exposure to HIV and other pathogens from healthcare workers, including physicians. A provider or its medical staff may also choose to adopt a policy under which physicians have responsibility for disclosing to patients any physical impairment that might adversely affect patient care. Such a policy would theoretically compel a physician to disclose to patients that he or she has AIDS or HIV infection. In addition to patient disclosure policy, the hospital or medical staff may consider a policy requiring disclosure of physician HIV or AIDS infection to the hospital itself. For example, some hospitals' medical staff bylaws require that physicians disclose their health status on application for privileges and also require routine disclosure of any changes in their health status while on the medical staff.

Immunization of Personnel

Immunization of personnel is an important component of hospital infection control programs (see Chapter 3). Records of the immunization status of employees should be maintained. The PHS's Immunization Practices Advisory Committee, the AHA's Committee on Infections Within Hospitals, and some medical specialty organizations routinely issue immunization recommendations. A number of states also require specific immunizations.

On December 2, 1991, OSHA announced the issuance of a final standard on bloodborne pathogens to protect healthcare workers against bloodborne diseases (see Chapters 42, 43), including the hepatitis B virus and HIV [111]. The standard, which went into effect March 6, 1992, requires the following:

1. Employers must establish a written exposure control plan that identifies workers with occupational exposure to blood and other potentially infectious mater-

ial and that specifies the means that will be used to protect and train these employees;
2. "Universal Precautions" must be instituted that treat blood and certain body fluids as though they were infectious;
3. Engineering controls, such as puncture-resistant containers for used needles, practices, and personal protective equipment, such as gowns, gloves and masks;
4. Labels and training to alert workers to the risks posed by the bloodborne pathogens;
5. Hepatitis B vaccination must be available at no cost to all employees with potential occupational exposure;
6. Postexposure evaluation and follow-up; and
7. Employers must keep records of exposure incidents, postexposure follow-up, hepatitis B vaccinations, and employee training. Medical records must be kept for the duration of employment plus 30 years [111].

These standards were reviewed in *American Dental Association v Martin*, and were found to be valid when applied to the dental industry and most medical personnel services [112]. Another example of these standards applied to the healthcare industry occurred in 1994, in New York. AmeriCare, a New Hartford, New York healthcare personnel firm, was cited for an alleged violation of OSHA's bloodborne pathogens standard. The reported $44,000 fine was levied because AmeriCare failed to offer hepatitis B vaccinations to employees who had been exposed to blood or other infectious materials. In addition, AmeriCare failed to include all required information in its written exposure control plan [113].

Although OSHA standards require an employer to make the hepatitis B vaccine available to all employees who have occupational exposure, this standard does not require compliance on the part of the employee to any vaccination program [114,115]. It merely requires that the employee has the opportunity to receive the vaccination free of charge. OSHA concluded that mandatory vaccination might present numerous religious and privacy concerns. It specifically stated that "attempting to compel workers to subject themselves to detailed medical examinations, presents the possibility of clashes with legitimate privacy and religious concerns. Health in general is an intensely personal matter" [116].

When Employees Contract Diseases

Diseases acquired on the job by employees are ordinarily covered under state workers' compensation laws. Workers' compensation is normally the claimant's sole remedy, precluding the claimant from filing a negligence action against the employer [117–120]. The employee is entitled to recover without proof of fault or negligence on the part of the employer. The employee usually must establish that his or her illness was contracted on and from the job [121].

In certain circumstances, hospital employees acquiring work-related infections may be eligible for remuneration beyond that provided by the workers' compensation system, if it can be established that an employer was aware of and intentionally disregarded an infection risk in the workplace [120,122,123]. When seeking coverage under workers' compensation laws, a hospital employee alleging he or she contracted an infection on the job must establish that the infection was not acquired outside the working environment. Such an employee may also have to prove that the risk of acquiring the infection as a hospital employee was greater that the general public's risk.

If an employee becomes infected with HIV in the course of employment, workers' compensation benefits are the proper remedy if the worker can demonstrate a "causal connection" between his or her HIV infection and employment. Specifically, the employee would need to establish that an incident occurred on the job involving a documented needle-stick injury, puncture wound, or other exposure to HIV-contaminated blood or body fluids.

Employee Exposure to Blood and Body Fluids

The stigma associated with AIDS has added to the dilemma hospitals face when deciding how to treat workers accidentally exposed to patients' blood and body fluids. Hospitals have faced a similar dilemma for years with workers filing false workers' compensation claims for hepatitis B and back injuries. Workers' compensation laws usually cover infections employees acquire on the job. Employees may try filing claims outside the workers' compensation system for negligent failure to disclose harmful conditions at the workplace, malicious intent to conceal, or failure to use due care in keeping the workplace safe. Should it be determined there is no entitlement to workers' compensation benefits, the provider's hospitalization and medical care benefits program may cover needed care, absent any exclusions from coverage on account of preexisting conditions or on other grounds.

The CDC recommends that after a healthcare worker suffers a parenteral or mucous membrane exposure to blood or other body fluids or has a cutaneous exposure involving large amounts of blood, the source patient should be informed of the incident and should be tested for serologic evidence of HIV infection after informed consent is obtained. If the source patient is positive for HIV or refuses HIV antibody testing, the healthcare worker should be counseled and evaluated clinically and serologically for evidence of HIV infection as soon as possible after the exposure. If the source patient is seronegative, it is advisable that the healthcare worker still be provided a baseline HIV antibody test. The CDC recommends that no further follow-up of the exposed worker is necessary unless the patient is at high risk of HIV infection. Because of heightened employee concern, many hospitals have chosen to make serologic testing available to all workers who are fearful they may have been infected.

If the source patient, after being informed of the incident, refuses HIV testing, the hospital's options depend on state law. In some states, state law forbids testing without written informed consent. In a few states (such as Colorado and Florida), state law expressly allows testing regardless of consent. In at least one state (Maine), one may apply for a court order requiring testing of the source patient.

When an Employer Discovers an Employee Has an Infection

Employers may query how to react when they learn that an employee is infected with HIV. Public relations concerns are often a problem for employers in the health-care field. Employers often face a difficult dilemma and are forced to make a business decision between facing charges of employee discrimination or facing the repercussions stemming from public hysteria.

Once a provider learns an employee is infected with HIV, it should approach the employee and verify this status with sensitivity, in a private and confidential manner. If HIV infection is confirmed, the provider should take appropriate action to protect the employee, other health-care workers, and the patient population, with the assistance of the provider's infection control staff. The provider and employee should attempt to agree on appropriate and reasonable protection measures, following CDC guidelines, which in some circumstances could include limiting tasks to noninvasive procedures, double gloving, and other safety procedures. When an employee does not agree with the procedures that the provider deems necessary, the provider's actions should be fully documented, and disciplinary measures may be considered if the employee will not comply.

WHEN PROVIDERS REFUSE TO CARE FOR CONTAGIOUS PATIENTS

Patients suffering from incurable infections such as Creutzfeld-Jacob disease and HIV have at times encountered difficulty in obtaining care. Historically, private hospitals had no legal obligation to accept nonemergency patients they did not desire. Traditional rules governing a hospital's responsibility in this area, however, have undergone many changes in reaction to legal theories, statutes, and licensing agency regulations. Aside from discrimination, providers must consider other restrictions on their ability to refuse care. As mandated by law in most states and to avoid sanctions and civil liability under the antidumping provisions of the Social Security Act, emergency care must be rendered by hospitals whenever requested.

Denials based on such factors as race or handicap are illegal. Any hospital that receives federal financial assistance bears an obligation under Section 504 of the Federal Rehabilitation Act of 1973 to provide nondiscriminatory treatment. Therefore, discrimination against AIDS patients is currently considered unethical and may be illegal under federal and state laws prohibiting discrimination against handicapped people. These laws provide that hospitalization or treatment cannot be denied to a person merely because that person is handicapped.

Once a hospital admits a patient, it is obligated to provide appropriate care or risk potential liability for abandonment; hence, if the hospital staff refuse to care for a patient with a contagious disease, the hospital has a responsibility to see to it that care is rendered, even if this means a transfer of the patient to another facility where appropriate care will be provided [124].

Although there is generally no duty for a hospital to provide nonemergency services, failure to follow established hospital policy, such as failure to follow hospital admission policies for reasons related to race, sex, age, religion, or national origin, may result in liability under state discrimination statutes. An AIDS patient might allege sexual orientation discrimination if, for example, a hospital treated transfusion-associated AIDS but refused to treat sexually transmitted AIDS.

Discrimination against individuals who are HIV infected because of employee fear of infection may violate federal and state antidiscrimination laws.[13] For example, a hospital was held liable for violating the Americans with Disability Act in *Howe v Hull*, when the hospital's emergency room staff refused to treat a man with AIDS who presented with an allergic reaction to medication. Finding that the patient's HIV status was the motivating factor in the hospital's refusal to admit and treat him, the court held that the refusal to treat him was a discriminatory denial of the opportunity to participate in or benefit from a public accommodation [125]. In *Glanz v Vernick*, an HIV-positive patient was refused elective surgery at a hospital's ear, nose, and throat clinic. The patient sued both the hospital and the physician who refused to operate, alleging that they discriminated against him on the basis of a "handicap," which constituted a violation of the Federal Rehabilitation Act. Holding that the hospital was liable, but the physician was not, the court reasoned that the hospital's receipt of Medicare or Medicaid payments for its services subjected the hospital to the requirements of the Federal Rehabilitation Act. The physician avoided liability in this instance because the hospital billed the patient for Dr. Vernick's services, not the physician himself [126].

---

[13]See, for example, *Trovinger v Mauer*, No. 94C-2239 (N.D. Ill. April 12, 1994) (holding that a physician's refusal to provide appropriate treatment to an HIV-positive patient suffering from "life-threatening hepatitis B" was a violation of Title III of the Americans with Disabilities Act).

Healthcare personnel should not be excused from providing care to patients with infectious diseases. The provider's personnel policies and procedures (or handbook) should specifically address employee insubordination or unreasonable refusals to treat patients.[14] Employee educational programs have been very effective in assuaging the fears of personnel. Employees should be reminded that the hospital provides gowns, gloves, masks, goggles, and the like to protect against transmission of infectious diseases. If an employee, after individual education and counseling, still refuses to perform his or her duties in caring for infected patients, the hospital may either attempt to accommodate the employee by job reassignment or institute disciplinary action for insubordination [127]. In doing this, the hospital will have to act within any relevant limitations imposed by the National Labor Relations Act or collective bargaining agreement.

Medical Staff Issues and AIDS

Physicians' obligation to treat HIV-infected patients should be addressed by hospital and medical staff policies. Some surgeons have publicly announced their refusal to operate on HIV-infected patients. Others argue that patients should be treated based on their clinical condition: If such a patient is judged to be a candidate for cardiac surgery, for example, neither AIDS nor HIV infection should, in and of itself, be considered a contraindication.

Although hospitals cannot require physicians to accept AIDS patients in their private practices, the legal and ethical principles that require employees to provide care to AIDS patients also apply to physicians. In view of hospitals' duty to treat emergency patients and to render appropriate care to admitted patients, they should have policies establishing physicians' obligation to treat. Although such policies should rely on education and counseling, they need to include provisions for withdrawal of staff privileges (after a hearing and appeal) in the case of persistent physician noncompliance. Courts should uphold disciplinary actions based on bylaw provisions where it can be demonstrated that a physician's conduct endangered patient welfare.

The AMA's Council on Ethical and Judicial Affairs, issued in 1987, stated that physicians have an obligation to treat HIV-infected patients. Previous AMA policy held that physicians should have the freedom, except in emergencies, to choose whom to serve. This same earlier policy indicated, however, that during an epidemic, "a physician must continue his [her] labors without regard to the risk of his [her] own health."

Individual state medical organizations have not felt bound by the AMA's recommendations. The Arizona State Board of Medical Examiners, for example, issued a statement that endorses the right of a physician to refuse to treat patients who have AIDS. The Texas Medical Association, in 1987, also determined that physicians could ethically refuse treatment to patients with AIDS.

The Deans of New York medical schools, in December, 1987, announced that refusal of faculty, residents, or medical students to treat AIDS or HIV patients would be grounds for dismissal or other sanctions. The American College of Physicians and the Infectious Disease Society of America, in a March, 1988 statement, indicated that "physicians, other health professionals, and hospitals are obligated to provide competent and humane care to all patients, including patients with AIDS and AIDS-related conditions as well as HIV-infected patients with unrelated medical problems. The denial of appropriate care to patients for any reason is unethical" [128].

Employee Insistence Regarding Precautions

An employee may lawfully refuse to work in proved unsafe conditions and may also insist on wearing safety equipment while working. OSHA does not permit employees to leave the job because of potential unsafe work conditions. Rather, the employees are to inform their employer of the conditions or request an OSHA inspection of the workplace under OSHA guidelines if no action is taken by the employer [129]. If an employee is confronted with a condition presenting a real danger of serious injury or death, he or she may refuse in "good faith" to work [130,131]. For the employee to be protected, the perceived hazard must be such that a reasonable person would believe it to present a real danger of death or serious injury and that the danger was of such an urgent nature that the use of normal channels of solving the problem would be ineffective.

When an employee insists on wearing more protective gear than the employer healthcare provider believes is necessary to prevent disease transmission, the employer is advised to investigate the employee's rationale and then to educate employees regarding appropriate infection control techniques. If, after this process, the employee still insists on following procedures contrary to the recommended approach based on the most recent medical information, legal advice should be sought regarding state law on the subject. Predisciplinary legal consultation is appropriate because some state and federal statutes forbid discrimination against employees for complaining about health hazards, even if there is no actual danger, as long as the employee has a reasonable belief that a danger exists [132].

---

[14] See, for example, *Armstrong v Flowers Hospital, Inc.*, No. 93-6502 (11th Cir. Oct. 3, 1994) (holding that a hospital has the right to discipline or terminate a nurse who refused to treat a patient who was HIV-positive, for fear of contracting the virus); *Doe v Aliquippa Hospital Association*, No. 93-570 (W.D. Pa. Sept. 29, 1994) (holding that a hospital was not required under the Rehabilitation Act of 1973 to take any steps to accommodate an operating room technician who experienced an extreme fear of contracting AIDS).

RESTRICTIONS OF DUTIES OF HEALTH CARE WORKERS

A complaint was filed in 1987 by a nurse at New York Hospital who sought relief from the New York City Commission on Human Rights after a transfer in job assignments. The complaint alleged that the nurse decided she wanted to become pregnant and sought to take advantage of the confidential HIV testing program made available through the hospital's employee health service. After a positive result occurred, the nurse was informed by her employer that she would be transferred out of the surgical intensive care unit to another position in emergency critical care with the same salary and benefits. The nurse declined the transfer and filed the discrimination action. In 1988, an administrative law judge denied prehearing motions challenging the commission's jurisdiction on grounds that the decision to reassign the nurse was made in good faith based on medical judgment [133].

RELEASING INFORMATION REGARDING COMMUNICABLE DISEASE

Ingrained in American society is the deeply held belief that individuals have a right to privacy. This right is tempered, however, by the obligation to disclose information needed by others to protect themselves from injury [134]. In most states, an obligation exists to report communicable diseases to health officials. Individuals or organizations such as hospitals who hold privileged information are expected to protect it from disclosure to those without a legitimate need to know. Statutes mandating the reporting of communicable diseases contain strict confidentiality requirements and are evidence of public policy to protect this information.

According to unpublished data from a national survey of states conducted by the Council of State and Territorial Epidemiologists regarding state and federal laws pertaining to public information including HIV/AIDS surveillance data, and immunization information collected by schools, health departments, or as part of immunization, of 45 responding states, 45 states require mandatory reporting of AIDS, 35 states require mandatory reporting of HIV in adults, and 34 states require mandatory reporting of HIV in infants (Council of State and Territorial Epidemiologists and The National Public Health Surveillance System, unpublished data, 1994). Although mandatory reporting is required by law, most state statutes provide specific safeguards for the confidentiality of all HIV test results. Despite these safeguards, a hot debate continues over mandatory name reporting. According to the *American Medical News*, half of all states currently require physicians to report the name of any individual testing positive for HIV in all circumstances, with a few others requiring name reporting in specific situations [135].

The legal risks associated with divulging a patient's HIV status, whether publicly or to a single person, differ greatly from state to state (see Chapter 43). If a hospital, physician, blood bank, laboratory, school, employer, or insurance company releases information concerning diagnosis of AIDS or a positive HIV test in an individual, it may be subject to liability under various traditional legal theories. A breach of confidentiality can result in civil liabilities for injury under the causes of action of defamation and invasion of privacy. Recognizing the sensitive nature of HIV-related information, many states have enacted statutes establishing the confidentiality of such information as test results, the identity of persons seeking testing, or reports to health departments. These statutes provide for civil or criminal damages for breach of confidentiality. For example, California has a law specifying a $10,000 penalty for divulging a patient's HIV serostatus without his or her permission.

A hospital can be liable for disclosing to a third party that a patient has AIDS or is infected with HIV unless the patient consents to the disclosure or a situation exists that overrides the patient's right of privacy. Healthcare providers have been found liable for posting names of HIV-positive patients on a laboratory bulletin board to allay the fears of technicians, and for disclosing a patient's HIV status to family, friends, or employers [93]. Damages that may be alleged include loss of employment, loss of housing, loss of or inability to obtain insurance, school expulsion, social stigma, harassment, and mental anguish. The disclosure of inaccurate information implying that a person is infected with HIV will be "actionable per se" in most states, implying there is no requirement to prove specific damages.

Unfortunately, healthcare providers can also be sued by an infected third party for failing to disclose an individual's HIV status. In such bedeviling situations, providers may find themselves forced to choose between potential liability for breach of confidentiality and potential liability for wrongful death. Before ordering an HIV test in such a setting, it is advisable to inform the patient that positive results may be reported to third parties [136]. For example, in *Reisner v Regents of the University of California*, a 1995 California case, a 12-year-old patient received a transfusion of HIV-contaminated blood. The physician failed to inform her that she became infected with HIV and failed to warn her of the danger of spreading the disease or how to prevent it. Five years later the doctor informed her, and her sexual partner, that she had AIDS. Shortly thereafter she died of AIDS, and her sexual partner discovered he was HIV positive. The young man sued the doctor and UCLA medical center for negligence for not warning her of her HIV status, which, he argued, resulted in his infection. The court held that the duty to warn a contagious patient to take steps to protect others could be extended to a third party not reasonably ascertainable by the physician, but pointed out that the duty would be discharged by the physician warning the patient of the risk to others and advising him or her how to prevent the spread of the disease [137].

A patient's AIDS diagnosis or HIV infection may be disclosed to hospital personnel who require such information to care for the patient. In addition, the patient's diagnosis may be recorded in the medical record, where only authorized personnel are allowed access to it.

TESTING AND SCREENING ISSUES

Human immunodeficiency virus antibody testing raises a number of legal issues. Healthcare providers have been drawn into the debate about testing all hospitalized patients for HIV. The balancing of the rights of the infected and the rights of the uninfected to exercise self-protection is at the core of this issue. State laws differ on the treatment of this information, and many legislative proposals have been introduced at the state and federal level regarding confidentiality; hence, providers should remain current regarding evolving law in this area. The CDC initially specified that hospitals should not screen patients or healthcare workers. The August 21, 1987, recommendations for prevention of HIV transmission in healthcare settings stated that "decisions regarding the need to establish testing programs for patients should be made by physicians or individual institutions." The following types of abuses in HIV testing were cited by the CDC:

1. Ordering tests for hospitalized patients under false names
2. Failing to inform patients they are being tested or failing to inform patients of the result
3. Failing to report test results to the state health department

Because there are circumstances in which an HIV test may be indicated to care for a patient, a provider may request the test for diagnosis and treatment. If a patient refuses to consent to the test, diagnosis and treatment should continue without the test. The patient's refusal, together with the discussion of risks and consequences of the decision, should be fully documented in the medical record. A national policy of mandatory testing of all hospitalized patients for HIV has been opposed by the AMA, AHA, and public health officials. The fear is that mandatory testing will drive those infected underground, further exacerbating difficulties in controlling the spread of the virus. They point to the observance of universal precautions as a more appropriate course of action. Technical limitations of currently available tests are also relevant here. A negative test does not necessarily prove an absence of HIV infection, and therefore a broad testing program would create a false sense of security in some. In addition, testing is expensive and carries with it obligations for counseling, confidentiality, and reporting that may be challenged as unlawful discrimination. In the absence of state law authorizing testing without a patient's consent, testing is not advisable unless as part of a formal research project or surveillance that provides for the removal of patient-identifying information.

In March, 1989, a nurse was fired for refusing to communicate his HIV test results to his hospital employer. A U.S. District Court ruled that he failed to show he was handicapped or perceived to be handicapped and therefore was not protected under the Vocational Rehabilitation Act of 1973. The plaintiff claimed the hospital requested the test because his roommate of 8 years had recently died of AIDS. He was fired for insubordination after continuing to refuse to be tested. The judge stated the hospital had a "legitimate and nondiscriminatory reason for firing Lockett: the need of a healthcare institution to monitor the health status of employees who have been exposed to infectious diseases, particularly diseases such as AIDS . . . in order to protect patients and co-workers and to accommodate any current or future handicap of the employee" [138].

In 1988, a U.S. District Court ruled that the mandatory employee testing at a Nebraska facility for the mentally retarded violated the Fourth Amendment's ban on unreasonable searches and seizures. The court issued a permanent injunction in the class action filed by some 400 staff members at the Eastern Nebraska Community Office of Retardation. The court stated the medical evidence "is overwhelming that the risk of transmission in the (facility) is trivial to the point of non-existence. Such a theoretical risk does not justify a policy which interferes with the constitutional rights of the staff members." The court went on to suggest that a testing program might be upheld under the Constitution when a risk of transmission "is real and tangible" [139].

RISK MANAGEMENT

Risk management functions encompass activities that are intended to conserve financial resources from loss. The JCAHO mandates that "there is a safety management program that is designed to provide a physical environment free of hazards and to manage staff activities to reduce the risk of human injury" [29]. This program must involve a risk assessment program that evaluates the impact on patient care and safety of the buildings, grounds, equipment, occupants, and internal systems and involves policies and procedures for the timely reporting and resolution of situations that pose an immediate threat to life, health, or property. An effective risk management program consists of risk identification, risk analysis, risk control, and risk financing, including:

1. Reducing financial losses through effective investigation and management of claims

2. A patient representative program
3. Review and coordination of insurance programs
4. Inspection of premises to discover and correct deficiencies in the physical plant
5. Review of policies and procedures to reflect acceptable quality of care
6. Investigation of adverse incidents and reviewing all incident reports
7. Review of patient grievances
8. Educational programs [140]

Risk Management Related to Nosocomial Infections

The risk manager should work closely with the infection control practitioner (ICP) to identify, monitor and control nosocomial infections. A team approach should be used to control the spread of disease and prevent further outbreaks. Such a team approach may benefit from an infection control committee, which fulfills an important link between risk management and infection control. Instances of noncompliance with infection control procedures, such as breaks in sterile technique or equipment contamination, should be reported to the risk manager. The risk manager should be informed of any instances of nosocomial infections that the ICP may be concerned with, such as:

1. Infections that could have been prevented;
2. Infections that were caused by inappropriate care; or
3. Infections that could lead to a malpractice claim.

In addition, high-risk patients (i.e., neonates, elderly, patients in specific units such as the burn or intensive care units, or patients undergoing a specific procedure such as urinary catheterization, mechanical ventilation, or surgical implants) should be identified and a surveillance program should be instituted [106].

Risk Control Related to Nosocomial Infections

The risk manager and ICP should coordinate efforts to ensure that the following types of risk prevention measures are taken:

1. Screening for risk factors, such as nutritional assessments before surgery;
2. Early identification of infected patients to reduce the probability of cross-infection;
3. Establishment of stringent isolation or barrier protection to prevent cross-infections;
4. Availability of adequate infection control devices and supplies in patient care areas;
5. Disposal of filled infectious waste containers in a timely manner in accordance with the hospital's hazardous materials and waste program;
6. Consultation by persons qualified in infection control regarding the purchase of all equipment and supplies used for sterilization, disinfection, and decontamination purposes;
7. Periodic review of cleaning procedures, agents, and schedules used throughout the hospital;
8. Consultation by persons qualified in infection control regarding any major change in cleaning products or techniques;
9. Existence and enforcement of written policies and procedures for the reuses of disposable items and for the shelf life of all stored sterile items;
10. Existence and enforcement of written policies and procedures for the appropriate handling of soiled and clean linen;
11. Existence and enforcement of written guidelines developed specifically for infection control in anesthesia, surgery, and postanesthesia areas throughout the hospital;
12. Orientation for new personnel and continuing education for all personnel regarding infection control; and
13. Close monitoring of personnel for infection and compliance with policies and procedures for removal of infected personnel from direct patient contact [106].

Employee Health and Risk Management

The risk manager should be involved in the process of developing policies and procedures for identifying and limiting the spread of infectious diseases among personnel. Compliance with OSHA regulations on monitoring and investigating bloodborne pathogen exposures and employer follow-up should be reviewed periodically.

Hospital infection control programs take into account problems arising from employee noncompliance and lack of motivation. Other problems resulting from a lack of staff awareness of published recommendations should be identified and solved through education [106].

Ethical Issues and Risk Management

Ethics is defined as the science that deals with moral conduct or human duty, including customs and habits, insofar as these are concerned with good or bad and right or wrong [141]. Ethical issues often compel a choice between competing values. Examples of ethical issues that arise in infection control include:

1. The question of isolating a patient colonized with resistant organisms. This constrains the patient's freedom of movement, but may be necessary to protect the rights of other patients to be treated in an environment without unnecessary risk;

2. Restricting healthcare workers with contagious diseases from patient care; and
3. The ICP may be involved in product evaluation, balancing expensive technologies with cost-containment concerns [142].

Given the complexity of ethical decisions, the following has been offered as an approach to resolve such problems:

1. Collect all relevant background data;
2. Identify the ethical dilemma;
3. Specify alternative courses of action;
4. Choose the alternative that best balances the competing values; and
5. Act on that choice and evaluate the outcome [143].

REFERENCES

1. Southwick A. *The law of hospital and healthcare administration*. Ann Arbor, MI: Health Administration Press, 1988:71–77.
2. *Black's law dictionary*. 6th ed. St. Paul, MN: West Publishing Co., 1990:249.
3. Crook GB. Negligence. 57 Am. Jur.2d *Municipal, school, and state tort liability* § 1 (1988).
4. Restatement (Second) of Torts § 281 (1964).
5. Kraut J. Annotation, *Hospital's liability for exposing patient to extraneous of contagion*, 96 ALR2d 1205 (1964). Rochester, NY: Lawyers Cooperative Publishing Co, 1964 Rochester, NY: Lawyers cooperative Publishing Co.; 1964.
6. Attorneys outline basics of IC malpractice cases. *Hosp Infect Control* 1980;7:32.
7. *Chumbler v McClure*, 505 F.2d 489 (6th Cir. 1974).
8. *MacDonald v United States*, 767 F. Supp. 1295 (M.D. Pa. 1991).
9. *Estate of Smith v Lerner*, 387 N.W.2d 576 (Iowa 1986).
10. *Brannen v Lankenua Hosp.*, 417 A.2d 196 (Pa. 1980).
11. West JC. The legal implications of medical practice guidelines. *Journal of Health and Hospital Law* 1994;27:99.
12. Keaton P. Medical negligence: the standard of care. *Texas Tech Law Review* 1979;10:351.
13. Nottebart HC Jr. Legal aspects of infection control. In: Cundy KR, Ball W, eds. *Infection control in healthcare facilities: microbiological surveillance*. Baltimore, MD: University Park Press, 1977:199.
14. Kaunitz K, Baity GS, Kaunitz A, Congress of the United States, Office of Technology Assessment. *Legal aspects of antibiotic use.* Report to House Committee on Energy and Commerce and Senate Committee on Labor and Human Resources, 1995.
15. Shanz SJ. The emerging status of practice parameters. *Medical Staff Counselor* 1993;7(3):31.
16. Leape LL. Practice guidelines and standards: an overview. *Quality Review Bulletin* 1990;16:42–49.
17. AHCPR outlines clinical guidelines dissemination strategies. *Research Activities* 1993:4.
18. Minn. Stat. § 62J.30(1)(A) (1992).
19. Me. Rev. Stat. Ann. title 24 § 2975(2) (West 1992).
20. Kuc GW. Comment: practice parameters as a shield against physician liability. *Journal of Contemporary Health Law and Policy* 1994;10:439.
21. *Ybarra v Sangard*, 154 P.2d 687 (1944).
22. *Southern Florida Sanitarium and Hosp. v Hodge*, 215 S.2d 753 (Fla. 1986).
23. *Robinson v InterMountain Health Care*, 740 P.2d 262 (Utah Ct. App. 1987).
24. *Kosberg v Washington Hosp. Center, Inc.*, 394 F.2d 947 (D.C. Cir. 1968).
25. Prosser WL. *Handbook of the law of torts*, 3rd ed. St. Paul, MN: West Publishing Co.; 1964:146.
26. *Simmons v United States*, 841 F. Supp. 748 (W. D. La. 1993).
27. *Lawlor-Covell v Wack, M.D.*, No. CV 2890429 (Pima County Super. Ct. 1994).
28. Fed. R. Civ. P. 8(c).
29. Joint Commission on the Accreditation of Healthcare Organizations. *Accreditation manual for hospitals*. Chicago, IL: Joint Commission on the Accreditation of Healthcare Organizations, 1994:121–124.
30. Getting sick in the hospital: drug resistant strep. *Hospital News and Florida Health Care Report* 1995;xx(4):18.
31. *Lundahl v Rockford Memorial Hosp. Ass'n.*, 235 N.E.2d 671 (Ill. Ct. App. 1968).
32. *Albain v Flower Hosp.*, 553 N.E.2d 1038 (Ohio 1990).
33. *Taylor v Doctor's Hosp. (West)*, 486 N.E.2d 1249 (Ohio Ct. App. 1987).
34. Fla. Stat. § 766.110(1) (1992).
35. *Irving v Doctors Hosp. of Lake Worth*, 415 So.2d 55 (Fla. 4th Dist. Ct. App. 1982).
36. *Porter v Sisters of St. Mary*, 756 F.2d 669 (8th Cir. 1985).
37. *Cuker v Hillsborough County Hosp. Auth.*, 605 So.2d 998 (Fla. 2nd Dist. Ct. App.1992).
38. Horty J. Negligence, liability, hospital corporate negligence. In: *Hospital law*. Pittsburgh, PA: Action-Kit for Hospital Law, 1981:2,6.
39. 42 C.F.R. § 482.42 (1986).
40. St. Paul's Fire and Marine Insurance Co. *St. Paul's 1993 annual report to policyholders*. St. Paul, MN: St. Paul's Fire and Marine Insurance Co., 1993:5.
41. St. Paul's Fire and Marine Insurance Co. *St. Paul's 1993 annual report to policyholders: physicians and surgeons update*. St. Paul, MN: St. Paul's Fire and Marine Insurance Co., 1993:3–4.
42. *Jones v Sisters of Charity*, 173 S.W. 639 (Tex. 1915).
43. *Robey v Jewish Hosp. of Brooklyn*, 20 N.E.2d 6 (N.Y. 1939).
44. Practitioner outlines isolation problems. *Hosp Infect Control* 1980;7:70.
45. *Larsen v American Medical Int'l*, No. LC 003 276 (L.A. County Super. Ct. May 1992).
46. *Jones v Rapides Gen. Hosp.*, 598 So.2d 619 (La. 3rd Cir. Ct. App. 1992).
47. *Ryan v Frankford Hosp.*, No. 1754 (Phila. County C.P. Sept. 1983).
48. Hospital Risk Management, Sept. 1989.
49. Attorneys explain liability of hemodialyzer reuse. *Hosp Infect Control* 1982;9:129.
50. Bernstein AH. *A trustee's guide to hospital law*. Chicago, IL: Teach 'Em, Inc., 1981:59.
51. *Rhodes v Charter Hosp.*, CA J89-0062 (S.D. Miss. 1989).
52. 42 C.F.R. § 405.1022(c)(8) (1985).
53. Smith JW. Fear-of-disease claims: are they compensable? *Medical Malpractice: Law and Strategy* 1995;12(4):1–4.
54. 42 U.S.C. § 1395dd (1994); 42 C.F.R. §§ 489.20 & 489.24 (1994).
55. *Schoendorff v Soc y of N.Y. Hosp.*, 105 N.E. 92 (N.Y. 1914).
56. *Butler v Berkeley*, 213 S.E.2d 571 (N.C. Ct. App. 1975).
57. *Tripp v Pate*, 271 S.E.2d 407 (N.C. Ct. App. 1980).
58. *Contreras v St. Luke's Hosp.*, 144 Cal. Rptr. 647 (1st Dist. Ct. App. 1978).
59. *Cobbs v Grant*, 502 P.2d 1 (Cal. 1972).
60. *Harwell v Pittman*, No. 82 CA 0397 (La. 1st Cir. Ct. App. Feb. 22, 1983).
61. *Baltzell v Baptist Medical Ctr.*, 718 S.W.2d 140 (Mo. 1986).
62. *Moore v Underwood Memorial Hosp.*, 371 A.2d 105 (N.J. Super. Ct. 1977).
63. *Sawyer v Methodist Hosp.*, 522 F.2d 1102 (6th Cir. 1975).
64. Wenzel RP. Preoperative antibiotic prophylaxis. *N Engl J Med* 1992; 326:337.
65. *Fluhrer v Ritter*, No. 845-1956 (Nassau County Super. Ct. April 1962).
66. *Barlett v Argonaut Ins. Co.*, 523 S.W.2d 385 (1975).
67. *Roark v St. Paul Fire and Marine Ins. Co.*, 415 So.2d 295 (La. 1982).
68. Chavigny KH, Helm A. Ethical dilemmas and the practice of infection control. *Law, Medicine and Health Care* 1982;10:169.
69. LeBlang TR. Disclosure of injury and illness: responsibilities in the physician–patient relationship. *Law, Medicine and Health Care* 1981; 9:4.
70. *Chester v Mercy Catholic Medical Ctr. of So.E. Pa.*, No. 2555 (Phila. County C.P. May 1984).
71. *Rung v St. Luke's Memorial Hosp. Ctr.*, No. 89-01825 (Oneida County Super. Ct. 1989).
72. *Brick v Greenbriar Nursing Home*, No. 94-00755 (Dade County Cir. Ct. 1994). Reprinted in *Medical Malpractice Verdicts, Settlements, and Experts* 1995;3(3):31–32.

73. Florida Society for Healthcare Risk Management. Reusing disposable devices. ??? *FSHRM Risk Review* 1995;95-1:2.
74. Avitail B, Khan M, Krum D, et al. Repeated use of ablation catheters. a prospective study. *J Am Coll Cardiol* 1993;22:1367.
75. *Haynes v Baton Rouge Gen. Hosp.*, 298 So.2d 149 (1974).
76. *Shirley Burd v Strutin and Urgent Care Medical Ctr., Inc.* (Morris County Super. Ct. November 1992). Reprinted in *Medical Malpractice Verdicts, Settlements, and Experts* 1992;8(11):26.
77. *Lewis v Golden State Memorial Hosp., et al.*, No. NWC 40143 (L.A. County Super. Ct. 1985).
78. *United States v An Article of Drug Consisting of 4,680 Pails...*, 725 F.2d 976 (5th Cir. 1984).
79. *United States v An Article of Drug... Neo-Terramycin*, 540 F. Supp. 363, 367 (N.D. Tex. 1982).
80. St. Paul's Fire and Marine Insurance Co. *St. Paul's 1994 annual report to policyholders*. St. Paul, MN: St. Paul's Fire and Marine Insurance Co., 1994:4–5.
81. Hospitals and Asylums, 40 Am. Jur.2d *Highways, streets and bridges* §§ 14.5, 26, 29, 33, 35 (1968).
82. Annas GJ, et al. Malpractice litigation. In: *The rights of doctors, nurses, and allied health professionals: a health law primer*. New York, NY: Avon, 1981:246.
83. Griffith JL. Advise visitors of risks from isolated patients. *Hosp Infect Control* 1980;7:53.
84. *Johnson v W. Va. Univ. Hosp. Inc.*, No. 19678 (W. Va. Super. Ct. App. Nov. 21, 1991).
85. Doctor must warn family about risk. *American Medical News* 1993; April 26:10.
86. Purver JM. Annotation, *Liability for injury or death from blood transfusion*, 45 A.L.R.3d 1364 (1972).
87. Zitter JM. Annotation, *Liability for hospital, physician, or other individual medical practitioner for injury or death resulting from blood transfusion*, 20 A.L.R.4th 136 (1983).
88. Lasky PC. Principals of liability. In: Lasky PC, ed. *Hospital law manual*. Rockville, MD: Health Law Center, Aspen Systems Corp., 1983: 4, 21 , 37–38, 75.
89. *Giambozi v Peters*, 16 A.2d 833 (Conn. 1940).
90. *Perlmutter v Beth David Hosp.*, 123 N.E.2d 792 (N.Y. 1954), reh'g denied, 125 N.E.2d 869 (N.Y. 1955).
91. *Cunningham v MacNeal Memorial Hosp.*, 266 N.E.2d 897 (Ill. 1970).
92. *Hoffman v Misericordia Hosp. of Phila.*, 267 A.2d 867 (Pa. 1970).
93. Gostin L, et al. The AIDS litigation project. *JAMA* 1980;264:4.
94. Gostin L, et al. *The AIDS litigation project: a national survey of federal, state, and local cases before courts and human rights organizations*. Washington, DC: Department of Health and Human Services, 1990:17–18.
95. *Fridena v Evans*, 622 P.2d 463 (Ariz. 1980).
96. Bollows RC, Capp DJ. Protecting the confidentiality of blood donors identities in AIDS litigation through state abuse of discovery rules. *Journal of Health and Hospital Law* 1989;22(2):37.
97. *Ahrens v Katz*, 595 F. Supp. 1108 (N.D. Ga. 1984).
98. *Pisel v Stamford Hosp.*, 430 A.2d 1 (Conn. 1980).
99. Karp D. How can physicians reduce their malpractice risks? *Hospital Physician* 1984:18.
100. *In re K.*, 561 A.2d 1063 (N.H. 1989).
101. *Accord Smith v Lincoln Gen. Hosp.*, 605 So.2d 1347 (La. 1992).
102. *Sakoski v Memorial Hosp.*, 522 N.E.2d 273 (Ill. 1988).
103. *Cobb County Kennestone Hosp. Auth. v Martin*, 430 S.E.2d 604 (Ga. Ct. App. 1993).
104. Rutala DM, Harmory B. Infection control. *Hospital Epidemiology* 1989;10:261.
105. 29 U.S.C. § 645(a)(1) (1982).
106. Center for Healthcare Environmental Management. *ECRI advisory: final CDC TB guidelines expected by September—OSHA cites hospitals for TB violations*. Plymouth Meeting, PA: ECRI, 1994:1.
107. Centers for Disease Control and Prevention. *Guidelines for the prevention and control of nosocomial infections*. Atlanta, GA: Centers for Disease Control and Prevention, 1981.
108. Centers for Disease Control and Prevention. Guidelines for preventing the transmission of *Mycobacterium tuberculosis* in healthcare facilities—1994. MMWR Morb Mortal Wkly Rep 1994;43(RR-13): 1–6.
109. Williams WW, Centers for Disease Control and Prevention. CDC guidelines for infection control in hospital personnel. In: *Guidelines for prevention and control of nosocomial infections*. Atlanta, GA: Centers for Disease Control and Prevention, 1983.
110. CDC plans to help hospitals track outbreaks of disease among workers. *BNA's Health Law Reporter* 1995;4:59
111. Occupational Safety and Health Administration. *Bloodborne pathogens final standard:* 29 C.F.R. § 1910.1030, Health Care Facility Management 2: ¶ 13,747 (1990).
112. Am. Dental Ass'n v Martin, 984 F.2d 823 (7th Cir. 1993).
113. Bloodborne pathogens. alleged willful bloodborne rule violations draw citation for N.Y. firm. *BNA's Health Law Reporter* 1994;3:1458.
114. *Rules and regulations*, 56 Fed. Reg. 64,153 (1991).
115. Occupational Safety and Health Administration. *Bloodborne pathogens final standard. 29 C.F.R. §§ 1910.1030(f)(2)(iii) and 1910.1030(f)(2)(iv) (1991).*
116. *54 Fed. Reg. 23042, 23045 (1989).*
117. Bd. of Trustees of the Fire and Police Employees Retirement Sys. v Powell, No. 955 (Md. Ct. Spec. App. Mar. 8, 1989).
118. *Sperling v Industrial Comm'n*, No. 67533 (Ill. May 17, 1989).
119. *Gatlin v Truman Medical Ctr.*, 770 S.W.2d 510 (Md. Ct. App. 1989).
120. *Peters v N.Y. City Health and Hosp. Corp.*, No. 22907-89 (Kings City Super. Ct. March 29, 1990).
121. *Chestnut Hill Hosp. v Workmen's Compensation App. Bd.*, 551 A.2d 683 (Pa. Commw. Ct. 1988).
122. *Prego v New York*, 534 N.Y.S.2d 95 (N.Y. Sup. Ct. 1989), *aff'd*, 541 N.Y.S.2d 995 (1990).
123. *Vinokurov v Mt. Sinai Hosp.*, No. 88-31586 (Unemployment Compensation App. Bureau March 29, 1988).
124. *Rhodes v Charter Hosp.*, 730 F. Supp. 1383 (S.D. Miss. 1989).
125. *Howe v Hull*, No. 3:92CV7658 (N.D. Ohio Nov. 21, 1994).
126. *Glanz v Vernick*, 756 F. Supp. 632 (D. Mass. 1991).
127. Stickler BK. Labor law and liability considerations of acquired immune deficiency syndrome. Chicago, IL: Pamphlet; Wood, Lucksinger and Epstein.
128. Health and Public Policy Committee of the American College of Physicians and Infectious Diseases Society of America. *The acquired immunodeficiency syndrome (AIDS) and infection with the human immunodeficiency virus (HIV)*. 1988.
129. 29 C.F.R. § 1977.12(b)(1) (1973).
130. 29 C.F.R. § 1977.12(b)(2) (1973).
131. *Whirlpool Corp. v Marshall*, 445 U.S. 1 (1980).
132. 29 U.S.C.A. § 660(c) (1995).
133. *Doe v New York Hosp.*, No. GA-000350 41487 DN (N.Y. Comm. Human Rights Oct. 3, 1988).
134. *Tarasoff v Regents of the Univ. of Cal.*, 551 P.2d 334 (Cal. 1976).
135. Shelton DL, Cutler D. What's in a name? *American Medical News* 1995;October 16:13.
136. *Burton v Yaeger, Quakertown Community Hosp., et al.*, No. 87-287-03-2 (Bucks County C.P. 1987).
137. *Reisner v Regents of the Univ. of Cal.*, No. B076913 (Cal. Ct. App. Jan. 26, 1995).
138. *Lockett v Hosp. Dist. No. 1*, No. 89-3256 (5th Cir. 1989).
139. *Glover v Encor*, CA 88-1678 (8th Cir. 1989).
140. Rowland HS, Rowland BL. *Hospital risk management: forms, checklists & guidelines* §§ 1.1-1.2 (1989). Rockville, MD: Aspen Publishing, 1989.
141. Herwaldt LA. National issues and future concerns. In: Wenzel RP, ed. *Prevention and control of nosocomial infections*. 2nd ed. Baltimore, MD: Williams and Wilkins, 1993.
142. Perkins HS, Jonson AR. Conflicting duties to patients: the case of a sexually active hepatitis-B carrier. *Ann Intern Med* 1981;94:523–530.
143. Soskolne CL. Ethical decision-making in epidemiology: the case study approach J Clin Epidemiol 1991;44(Suppl):125S–130S.

Hospital Infections, Fourth Edition,
edited by John V. Bennett and Philip S. Brachman.
Lippincott–Raven Publishers, Philadelphia © 1998

CHAPTER 19

Infection Control in Developing Countries

Samuel Ponce-de-León Rosales and M. Sigfrido Rangel-Frausto

The organization of a nosocomial infection control program is never an easy task, and starting it with limited resources, as is the case with most if not all developing countries, requires additional efforts. To achieve the main goal of a program, the interactions of various sorts of persons are necessary, as is a great deal of patience, shrewdness, and hard work. It is also important to be aware that each hospital has its own special culture: every medical center is unique, even though similarities in category, number of beds, or paramedical services might exist. Thus, individual peculiarities must be considered in the effort to adjust the proposals for change to meet the needs of each hospital. Furthermore, one must avoid being in the unfortunate position of trying to change the institution to meet a series of preconceived regulations that may not be appropriate for the hospital. The hospital's infection control program and the hospital epidemiologist must, therefore, be dynamic, yet flexible because a hospital is often very limited in such characteristics. Developing countries have to face two crucial problems: limited resources for healthcare and lack of awareness of the importance of preventing nosocomial infections.

NOSOCOMIAL INFECTIONS IN LATIN AMERICA

Developing countries have to deal with these two cited problems. Thus, it is urgent to improve medical care, which will not happen until money is invested in hospital maintenance and payment of wage increases. National authorities must realize that insufficient resources turn hospitals into high-risk areas that cause complications that would not occur if the patients were cared for properly. This cost is, of course, much higher than the money needed to cover the essential needs of hospitals.

S. Ponce-de-León Rosales, M. S. Rangel-Frausto: Division of Hospital Epidemiology, Instituto Nacional de la Nutricion, Tlalpan, Mexico City 14000, Mexico.

Until recently most developing countries were unaware of the problem of nosocomial infection, and sporadic reports, based almost exclusively on inadequate surveillance, have shown very low incidence rates. This situation is changing rapidly—several countries in Latin America have developed national policies and even national programs on infection control. In Brazil, for example, infection control programs were organized for the first time in 1976, but it was not until 1983 that the Ministry of Health mandated control of nosocomial infections and organized a training program to stimulate the development of Infection Control Committees [1]. In Belo Horizonte, Dr. Starling has started a network of five hospitals where the average rate of nosocomial infections for the past 5 years has been 5.1%, or 9.7/1,000 patient-days. Surgical and severity of illness scores have also been implemented for interhospital comparisons [2,3]. In São Paulo, the effectiveness of infection control has been verified in a 600-hundred-bed federal hospital, through the lowering of infection control rates from 11.8% to 7.4% [4].

Chile has developed a national program, one of the most successful in the region, bringing together a network of hospitals whose infection control practitioners receive training and support from a central office in the Ministry of Health. Infection rates have been lowered to an average of 4.5% [5]. Other countries have begun infection control programs as well [6,7,8,9]. Nosocomial infection rates vary from country to country (Table 19-1). In the case of Mexico, assuming a nosocomial infection average of 10% to 15% [6], ~300,000 to 450,000 episodes of nosocomial infections could occur among the three million patients who have received medical care in hospitals during the past year. Obviously the economic impact of the nosocomial infections in developing countries is proportionately far greater than that in developed countries because budgets are more restricted.

Table 19-2 outlines the main causes of death in Mexico [10] and incorporates a projection of the mortality that could result from the 450,000 episodes of infection just

TABLE 19-1. *Nosocomial infection rates in Latin America*

Country	Type of hospital/unit	Rates (n/100 discharges)	Year	Surveillance	Reference
Brazil	Multicenter	5.1	1994	Incidence	[4]
Chile	Multicenter	4.5	1992	Incidence	[7]
Mexico	Multicenter Study	15	1994	Incidence	[8]
Paraguay	OB/GYN-Pediatrics	12.5	1995	Prevalence	[9]
El Salvador	Neonatology unit	7.8	1994	Incidence	[10]
Panama	Internal Medicine	14	1978–1980	Incidence	[11]
Uruguay	SICU	13.4	1993–1995	Incidence	[12]

SICU, surgical intensive care unit.

mentioned, assuming an associated mortality of 5%. According to our predictions, nosocomial infections could be the fifth most common cause of mortality, a figure that must be similar to those in other developing countries. Thus the incorporation of information about nosocomial infection prevention into routine medical and paramedical personnel training programs and the commitment of major authorities to the resolution of this problem are both essential. Regions with limited resources face another challenge represented by the dispersion of hospitals. According to a survey done by Pan-American Health Organization (PAHO), there are ~20,000 hospitals in Latin America; more than half have < 20 beds and operate without essential services, such as blood banks and intensive care units. It is still possible to organize a control program fitted to such circumstances.

Epidemics of nosocomial infections in Latin America represent another important problem that deserves special mention. There have been reports from some hospitals that the proportion of infections that constitute an epidemic may be as high as 19%, which is more than five times the rates cited by developed countries (which range from 2% to 3.7% [11].

TABLE 19-2. *Mortality rate in Mexico, 1995 (per 100,000 inhabitants)*[a]

Disease	Number	Rate
Cardiovascular diseases	63,609	69.4
Malignant diseases	48,222	52.6
Accidents	35,567	38.0
Diabetes mellitus	33,316	36.4
Nosocomial infections	33,000	35.1
Cerebrovascular disease	23,400	25.5
Liver disease	21,245	23.2
Pneumonia, influenza	19,717	21.5
Homicide, violence	15,615	17.0
Nosocomial bacteremia[b]	13,200	14.1

[a]Nosocomial infections rates are, of course, included in other mortality rates, because nosocomial infections are not routinely reported on death certicates.

[b]Bacteremias are also considered in the total of nosocomial infections.

ORGANIZATION

The organization of a surveillance system is the logical initial step of any infection control program because subsequent changes must be based on the identification of local problems that may be unique and distinctly different from those of other institutions. The selection of a surveillance system among the many existing options should be made after considering the special characteristics of the hospital, the expected goals, and the available resources. In hospitals with limited resources, the program must begin with the surveillance of critical areas, such as emergency room/intensive care units, because these areas are the loci of ≥ 40% of bloodstream and pulmonary infections [12]. Based on the initial results of the surveillance, it is possible to have a realistic idea of the nosocomial infection rate as well as issues of morbidity, mortality, and costs. These data are essential to obtaining adequate financial support for the program from the hospital administration and to deciding which areas within the hospital need more attention.

A CONTROL PROGRAM WITH LIMITED RESOURCES

The regulation of various procedures, as well as the policy of isolation of patients, should be determined according to each hospital's possibilities. Thus, if there are no individual rooms in a given hospital, it is preposterous to rule on the isolation of patients; other possible forms of isolation must be considered. Even in the United States, a situation may not be so simple as to allow choosing between the two isolation systems proposed by the Centers for Disease Control and Prevention (CDC) (category-specific versus disease-specific isolation precautions) [13]. Although, generally speaking, the safer and more practical way to initiate a program is to use category-specific isolation precautions [13,14], hospital limitations might require an intermediate or alternate solution. Furthermore, the possibility of implementing a universal precautions program must be evaluated. Similarly, the acquisition of equipment or material will depend on existing economic resources. New isolation policies have been proposed by the CDC. The new policies, formulated to be simple but more efficient, are based on mechanisms of transmission of infections in the hospital: standard precautions have replaced universal precautions, and three new categories of route of infection, aerial, droplets, and contact, have been substituted for previous categories [15].

All of the recommendations of the program should be based on the actual capabilities of the hospital and its personnel. Even the proposal of a few regulations that cannot be met, for any reason, is risky because the administration of the hospital might consider it unrealistic and therefore impracticable. The hospital's personnel will be willing to collaborate with a specific program only if they are convinced of its feasibility. The problem of tuberculosis deserves particular mention, especially in developing countries, where the high community endemic rates produce a large number of admissions for this disease (see Chapter 33). With hospitals that are lacking the most basic services, adequate isolation is almost impossible, and the risk of transmission to healthcare workers is very high. At the National Institute of Nutrition in Mexico City, the purified protein derivative skin test conversion rate is ~17% year, almost twice as high as the rate reported for endemic areas in the United States [16].

The continuing education program directed at controlling and preventing hospital-acquired infections must first be addressed to nurses. This approach has several advantages because nurses are the medical care workers with the greatest contact with patients as well as those with the greatest risk of transmission of organisms. They are, therefore a very important link in the pathway for interrupting infection transmission.

It is commonly recognized that nurses are one of the most receptive and enthusiastic groups of professionals within the hospital and are willing to follow control practices. This fact can be inferred from data obtained from hand-washing studies [17]. Moreover, nurses are present everywhere in the hospital and participate in practically every procedure within the institution. Wherever a patient is exposed to a high-risk procedure, it is of utmost importance that nurses be trained in its adequate execution. If they are aware of the importance of their participation, the recommended procedures will be followed correctly, thus guaranteeing the success of the program.

IMPLEMENTING THE PROGRAM

There are several measures that may be considered as specific recommendations for an infection control program. One of the most important measures addresses the relationship of the hospital epidemiologist with other hospital personnel. The hospital epidemiologist or the infection control team is frequently involved in situations in which the clinical staff might feel threatened. For example, the investigation of an epidemic in a specific department will obviously affect physicians and nurses who might be fearful of being blamed for the problem. The epidemiologist must convince everybody that his or her goal is not to focus on guilt or innocence, but instead to solve a problem in the best possible way and, with their collaboration, to prevent its recurrence. On the contrary, if the epidemiologist has an aggressive attitude toward the personnel, not only will he or she not receive their support, but there is also the enhanced likelihood of their concealing future problems. The epidemiologist's specific goal at the beginning of a control program must be to gain confidence, not to give orders.

Several countries are aware of the relationship of antibiotic use and the emergence of antibiotic-resistant nosocomial infections [18–20]. One strategy to improve awareness concerning optimal antibiotic use is to incorporate into the monthly report of the Infection Control Committee information about the susceptibility of the microorganisms isolated from nosocomial infections. Along with this information one could also suggest policies on the proper use of antibiotics. Another approach is to restrict information about the susceptibility pattern of the isolates obtained in the hospital, so that clinicians can prescribe only those antibiotics that are authorized by the infectious diseases department or the nosocomial infection committee.

ECONOMICS

In developing countries starting up infection control programs must be a priority; to wait for better economic times that may never come is preposterous. But the organization of an infection control program does need economic support, which ideally should come from the hospital administration itself. The hospital itself has to be responsible for most of the expenses of the infection control department as well as for the preventable infections contracted during hospitalization. The best way to convince the hospital administration of the advantages of supporting the program is to disseminate information about morbidity and mortality rates related to nosocomial infection and to illustrate their economic impact. This information can be obtained from the experience of other hospitals or from CDC studies [21–23].

It is, however, much more compelling to submit information about the incidence and magnitude of the problem in the hospital itself, which can be produced from general data. The purpose is to show the importance of nosocomial infections in terms of human suffering as well as economic impact. One should emphasize the fact that the situation can be modified favorably with the proposed program [24], which will be comparatively less expensive. It is very important not to promise a dramatic change in a short time but to consider a reasonable length of time in which to see favorable changes [25]. Other sources of economic support are industry-supported studies on the usefulness of specific products for the control of nosocomial infections, such as soaps, disinfectants, or disposable devices. In developing countries, lack of money is sometimes used as an excuse not to begin an infection control program, so it is very important to understand that beginning by focusing on the essential is an activity that will bring about worthwhile results.

An important aspect of the proper functioning and development of such a program is the support of people who are politically prominent in the hospital. The best way to obtain their support is to encourage their participation in the program as advisers or members of the Infection Control Committee; once they are involved, they will become natural allies and will see that their collaboration is needed to ensure the success of the program.

THE TEAM IN INFECTION CONTROL

The nurse-epidemiologist model, which has been successfully used in the United States, may not be the most effective approach in countries with different healthcare systems. The professional relationships and physician, nurse, laboratory, and auxiliary health personnel ratios must be considered in selecting the healthcare professional who will be responsible for epidemiological activities and the administration of the program [26]. As previously mentioned, however, nurses offer important advantages over other healthcare workers.

The best nurses to retain for an infection control program are those who have expressed their interest in it. Personnel who have been selected arbitrarily, without evidence of a real interest in the area, might abandon the program after receiving special training, a situation that consumes a great deal of time and money. There is always a risk of abandonment, but it is lower among those people who have an interest in the program. Ideally, selected nurses should be sensitive and courteous with a level of training above the average, because they will need to establish a special nurse-physician relationship, different from the usual clinical role, and will frequently be required to discuss or propose changes in the attitudes of hospital personnel. Simultaneously, the training of infection control practitioners can be augmented by ensuring their attendance at regional and national meetings or at local continuing education courses.

Because the Infection Control Committee has to provide basic support for the hospital epidemiologist, its members must have a genuine interest in the activity (see Chapter 4). Even though it is useful for the Infection Control Committee members to have relevant academic and political positions, it is more important that they be able to devote enough time to the program. It is better to invite very busy persons to be part-time advisers than to select them as permanent members of the committee because their frequent absences would obstruct the progress of the program.

INTERNAL AFFAIRS

The activities of the infection control program need to be disseminated throughout the hospital in a comprehensible language, emphasizing aspects that are relevant to particular departments in the hospital. For example, the results of the surveillance system may be summarized for every service, with an effort to individualize as much as possible (see Chapter 5). The policies and regulations, as well as results of achievements and difficulties, may be communicated extensively in hospital sessions and summarized in a written document.

Communication with the head of a department in which an epidemic has occurred or a special problem has been detected is important. Once the problem is confirmed, the best approach is to speak directly with the head of the affected service, before discussing the problem widely with hospital authorities or taking any action to resolve it. The personal approach is more effective than an impersonal written communication. Generally speaking, personal intervention is the best approach to any problem; however, there are situations that may be solved with a simple telephone call and many others that are routine and may be communicated by memo. Obviously, the method used to communicate a problem will depend on its seriousness and the people it affects. If in doubt, however, make an appointment to meet directly with the person involved.

COMMITTEE MEETINGS

Most committees meet once a month. It is most practical to have a well-thought-out agenda for each meeting, and it is a good idea to begin by discussing the continuing problems not resolved in previous meetings. Then the results of surveillance over the course of the month could be presented, comparing the data with information garnered from previous months. Last, the committee should address new problems and suggest solutions.

ORGANIZING THE INFECTION CONTROL PROGRAM

The greatest problem in the organization of an infection control program is integration of its components to establish supervision and feedback among participants, with the purpose of achieving steady progress. In the past, programs have been centralized, with the hospital epidemiologist, infection control practitioner, and hospital Infection Control Committee responsible directly or indirectly for the maintenance of the system. Because most programs have only one part-time epidemiologist and one infection control nurse, it could be very useful to stimulate the formation of "satellite infection control programs" under the supervision of the hospital committee. This is especially important in critical areas where the head nurse and head physician have their own meetings and could report directly to the hospital infection control staff. This approach could help make surveillance easier and engage the personnel of such areas more deeply in the program [27]—an economical solution for infectious control programs with limited resources.

Figure 19-1 is a schematic view of an infection control program in which each participant is at the same time supervised and supervisor of the other participants. Even though the responsibility for the maintenance of the system belongs to the hospital epidemiologist, all of its members should be considered fundamental to the organization and responsible for its accomplishments. This attitude favors efficiency but is not spontaneous; rather, it will be necessary to create a favorable atmosphere in establishing this supervision system, which will allow for the evaluation of everyone's work.

The supervision system gives specific tasks to several members. The hospital epidemiologist is directly responsible for the organization and development of surveillance activities, which are routinely carried out by infection control practitioners. He or she also revises and analyzes the results of surveillance along with other members of the program and writes a report for the Infection Control Committee, from which to develop guidelines, regulations, or policies. These proposals will have to be followed and observed not only by hospital personnel but also by patients and visitors to the hospital. Obviously, such guidelines are designed to modify habits and attitudes and ultimately to produce changes in nosocomial infection rates. The resulting modifications in infection rates are evaluated by the epidemiologist and practitioners, who in turn study the feasibility of the committee's proposals. They will also monitor the way in which guidelines are followed by personnel, patients, and visitors, thus closing the circle. This sequence must exist in every infection program; it emphasizes the interdependence and evaluation of each member's performance.

Within this general scheme, it is important to point out that the routine work may become uninteresting for the people who do it. To avoid loss of interest in weekly surveillance activities, certain measures need to be implemented. The routine, of course, is broken when epidemic outbreaks are detected, since they imply a special and intense activity for the epidemiologist and infection control practitioners, who will find renewed interest in their work. However, epidemics are intermittent and should not be necessary to maintain interest in everyday work. Instead, it is much better to be continually stimulated, and one of the best ways to achieve this is through educational activities. The involvement of practitioners in an education program provides training of newcomers and continually motivates all program members to reach a better performance level.

Figure 19-1 shows the levels where education programs should be brought in. Infection control practitioners may be responsible for continuing education programs for nurses and physicians interested in this work as well as for hospital personnel; they also are responsible for training new hospital personnel or even outsiders. Ideally, the hospital epidemiologist supervises the courses and oversees the training of medical residents in this area. Medical residents may participate in the infection control program, as may those students in fellowship training in infectious diseases or those in a Master of Science degree course in epidemiology. Any participation by local residents will surely enhance the value of the program.

Another vital aspect of hospital epidemiology is the development of a quality control program that will allow for the objective evaluation of every member of the infection control program. There are few reports on the sensitivity and comparative effectiveness of the various surveillance systems that do not contemplate the evaluation of the program itself [28,29]. Once the sensitivity of a specific surveillance system is known, the program can be properly evaluated in terms of fulfillment of its goals, such as the number of problems solved, the degree of reduction of infection rates, and the ability to detect epidemics.

The lack of validation of infection control systems is a generalized problem not exclusive to developing countries. To address this issue, surveillance over a few months conducted in conjunction with a team of experts

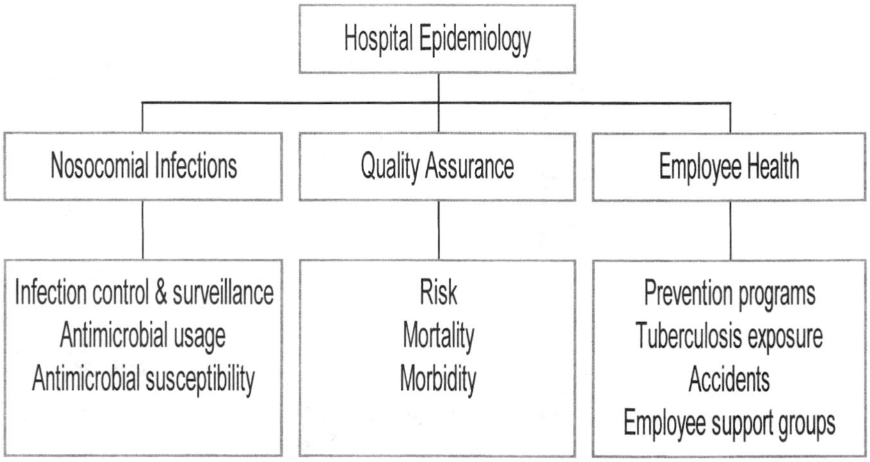

FIGURE 19-1. Components of an infection control program. Each of the members of each program should be supervised and act as supervisor.

will produce reliable results of high quality. It is also necessary to check the surveillance system's accuracy at least once a year, through short prevalence studies to detect false-positive or false-negative cases reported, and to improve the reliability of program evaluation. These periodic short studies should be very easy to execute. For instance, the selection of a sample of patients hospitalized during a 1-week period would be sufficient. The infections detected with the kardex system could be compared with the retrospective review [28]. The sample should be designed on sound statistical bases.

Research projects that are directly related to the surveillance system are a tool for evaluating the control program, including proposed regulations. An example would be the design of a research protocol to analyze the results of a specialized nursing team's handling of parenteral feeding catheters in view of the high incidence of bacteremia among patients with these catheters. Research protocols could also be designed to evaluate the risks, costs, and benefits of new proposals compared against existing ones.

Overall infection rates can be reduced in most hospitals. Even if infection control programs become more efficient, however, nosocomial infection rates cannot be lowered to < 5% without incurring excessive costs. This is what is called the irreducible minimum [30]. In recent times, developing countries have begun to recognize the significance of nosocomial infections. However, because of economic limitations, health is not a priority in most of these countries. Thus, we have to work with limited resources, often providing inferior services, which, in the long run, are more expensive than paying close attention to avoiding the problems in the first place. This situation will become critical in the short term as a consequence of continuing economic problems. As a result of the globalization of the economy, the government and local hospital services could be left far behind, especially if large private hospital corporations extend to developing countries, underscoring the inequities of medical care in these impoverished places in the developing world.

REFERENCES

1. Pannuti C, Grinbaum R. An overview of nosocomial infection in Brazil. *Infect Control Hosp Epidemiol* 1995;16:170–174.
2. Starling CEF, Pinheiro SMC, Almeida FF, Couto BRGM. *NNISS methodology in Brazilian hospitals: five years of experience.* (Report of the infection control team, Belo Horizonte, Minais Gerais). Brazil: Assoc Brasileira do Infectologia, 1995.
3. Starling CEF, Pinheiro SMC, Couto BRGM. Assessment of severity of illness in intensive care units: a new ASIS average severity index score [Abstract M75]. Proceedings of the fifth annual SHEA meeting, San Diego, April 2–4, 1995. *Infect Control Hosp Epidemiol* 1995;16 (part 2):45.
4. Wey S. Infection control in a country with annual inflation of 3,600%. *Infect Control Hosp Epidemiol* 1995;16:175–178.
5. Otaiza F. Programs of prevention and control for nosocomial infections in Chile [in Spanish]. In: *Development and fortification of local health systems* [in Spanish]. Washington D.C.: Pan American Health Organization, 1991:141–162.
6. Ponce de León S. Nosocomial infections: characteristics of the problem, as reported by the National Institute of Nutrition in Mexico [in Spanish]. *Salud Pública Méx* 1986;28:29–36.
7. Montiel T, Recalde S, Arrechea A, Vega M. Intrahospital infections and the use of antibiotics. In: *Programa y resúmenes del 1er Congreso Panamericano de Control de Infecciones y Epidemiología Hospitalaria y IV Congreso Chileno de Control de Infecciones,* [in Spanish], Viña del Mar, Chile, December 4–7, 1995.
8. Herig E, Juliet C, Lohse MT. Impact of intrahospital infection surveillance on a neonatal unit [in Spanish]. In: *Programa y resúmenes del 1er Congreso Panamericano de Control de Infecciones y Epidemiología hospitalaria y IV Congreso Chileno de Control de Infecciones,* [in Spanish]. Viña del Mar, Chile, December 4–7, 1995.
9. González MC, Binagui V, Wider I, Pedreira W, Bagnulo H. Surveillance of interhospital infection in a surgical intensive care unit. In: *Programa y resúmenes del 1er Congreso Panamericano de Control de Infecciones y Epidemiología Hospitalaria y IV Congreso Chileno de Control de Infecciones,* Viña del Mar, Chile, December 4–7, 1995.
10. Ponce de León S. The needs of developing countries and the resources required. *J Hosp Infect* 1991;18(A):376–381.
11. Zaidi M, Sifuentes J, Bobadilla M, et al. Epidemic of *Serratia marcescens* bacteremia and meningitis in a neonatal unit in Mexico City. *Infect Control Hosp Epidemiol* 1989;10:14–20.
12. Wenzel RP, Osterman CA, Donowitz LG, et al. Identification of procedure-related nosocomial infections in high-risk patients. *Rev Infect Dis* 1981;3:701–707.
13. Garner JS, Simmons BP. CDC guidelines for isolation precautions in hospitals. *Infect Control Hosp Epidemiol* 1983;4(suppl):245–325.
14. Saravolatz LD, Arking L. Isolation guidelines—A or B? [Editorial]. *Infect Control Hosp Epidemiol* 1984;5:269–270.
15. Centers for Disease Control and Prevention. *Guideline for isolation precautions in hospitals.* Federal Register 1994;55552–55570.
16. Vázquez de la Serena A, Romero-Oliveros C, Báez-Martínez RM, et al. High frequency of PPD transmission among healthcare workers [in Spanish]. *Enferm Infecc Microbiol Clin* 1995;15:313.
17. Albert RK, Condie F. Handwashing patterns in medical intensive care units. *N Engl J Med* 1981;304:1465–1460.
18. Marinero JA, Sotello Y. Infection control in El Salvador: the Hospital Rosales experience. *Infect Control Hosp Epidemiol* 1987;8:495–500.
19. Goldmann DA, Otaiza F, Ponce de León S, Faingezicht G. Infection Control in Latin America. *Infect Control Hosp Epidemiol* 1988;9:291.
20. Rangel Frausto S, Sifuentes J, González R, Ponce de León S, Ruíz-Palacios G. Multiresistant gram-negative nosocomial infections associated to a common plasmid: a case control study [Abstract 1005]. *Abstracts of the 1991 ICAAC.* Chicago: *Am Soc Microbiol* 1991:266.
21. Wenzel RP, Osterman CA, Hunting KJ. Hospital-acquired infections. II. Infection rates by service and common procedures in a university hospital. *Am J Epidemiol* 1976;4:645–650.
22. Rose R, Hunting KJ, Towsend TR, Wenzel RP. Morbidity/mortality and economics of hospital acquired bloodstream infections: a controlled study. *South Med J* 1977;70:267–269.
23. Eickhoff TC. Hospital epidemiology: an emerging discipline, In: Remington JS, Swartz MN, eds. *Current clinical topics in infectious diseases.* New York: McGraw-Hill 1984:24.
24. Haley RW, Culver DH, White JW, Morgan WM, Emory TG. The nationwide nosocomial infection rate. *Am J Epidemiol* 1985;2:59–67.
25. Wenzel RP, Schaffner W. Infection control: a progress report [Editorial]. *Infect Control* 1985;6:9–10.
26. Western KA, St. John RK, Shearer LA. Hospital infection control: an international perspective. *Infect Control Hosp Epidemiol* 1982;3: 453–454.
27. Ford-Jones EL, Mindorff CM, Gold R. Satellite Infection Control Committees within the hospital: decentralizing for action. *Infect Control Hosp Epidemiol* 1989;10:368–370.
28. Wenzel RP, Osterman CA, Hunting KJ. Hospital acquired infections. I. Surveillance in a university hospital. *Am J Epidemiol* 1976;3:25–60.
29. Tager IB, Gingsberg MB, Simchen E, Miao L, Holbrook K, Faich GA. Rationale and methods for a state-wide prospective surveillance system for the identification and prevention of nosocomial infections. *Rev Infect Dis* 1980;3:683–693.
30. Ayliffe GAJ, Path FRC. Nosocomial infection: the irreducible minimum. *Infect Control Hosp Epidemiol* 1986;7:92–95.

Part II

Functional Areas of Concern

Hospital Infections, Fourth Edition,
edited by John V. Bennett and Philip S. Brachman.
Lippincott–Raven Publishers, Philadelphia © 1998

CHAPTER 20

The Inanimate Environment

Frank S. Rhame

Concern about the infection hazard of environmental microorganisms arises because of our close interaction with the environment and its high content of microorganisms, including important human pathogens. Microbes are remarkably efficient at becoming dispersed to virtually all unprotected sites. Where there is moisture and organic material, proliferation to large numbers occurs. Even on dry, infertile surfaces, microbes survive in various relatively inactive states. Unfortunately, though it is easy to establish the presence of microorganisms in the environment, it is difficult to assess their role in causing human disease. Evaluating the evidence in this matter is the fundamental subject of this chapter.

The scope of this chapter is determined partly by logic and partly by tradition. The title itself is a misnomer: if the environment were inanimate, it would not require discussion. The major focus is on those normally nonsterile items that may serve as *fomites,* or vectors of infectious agents [1].[1] Consideration is extended to items that are often sterilized, even though the need to do so is arguable (e.g., the internal surfaces of respirator and anesthesia breathing circuits, water in humidifier reservoirs [2], endoscopes that are to be passed through nonsterile cavities, and reusable pressure transducer heads) [3]. Items that clearly must be sterile are not discussed. Some inclusion distinctions are quite arbitrary. Pus, while it is in a patient's wound or on the unwashed hands of a hospital worker, would not be considered part of the inanimate environment, but as soon as it is deposited on a surface, it would. Skin is not considered in this chapter, but airborne squamae are. Finally, elements traditionally considered environmental are also included, such as potted plants, cut flowers, insects, and problems associated with animal visitation in the hospital. In this chapter there will also be discussion of the ultimate concern about the inanimate environment, ultraclean protective environments for immunosuppressed patients; sections on disinfection and sterilization; and a discussion of routine microbiologic monitoring of inanimate objects in the hospital.

The simplistic dichotomous view that we can apply to sterilization (i.e., an item is sterile or it is not) is not applicable to the factors under discussion. Instead, we must contend with the difficulty of determining the appropriate degree of contamination. In some cases standards exist (e.g., dialysis water) but for the most part no standards have been set, and there is little rational basis for setting them. Setting such standards is made more difficult because microbiologic classification of environmental organisms is not as well developed as for organisms from clinical specimens.

There are paradoxes associated with microbiologic content of the environment. Some objects may be sterile as a by-product of manufacture. For instance, the protected outside surfaces of intravenous bottle stoppers are usually sterile, although manufacturers do not make the claim of sterility because it is burdensome to prove it to regulatory agencies. There are items that are not marketed as sterile but that usually are sterile (and arguably should be). When contaminated, these items have been responsible for outbreaks: elastic bandages have caused *Rhizopus* [4] and *Clostridium perfringens* [5] skin infections; wooden tongue depressors have led to *Rhizopus* skin infections in preterm babies [6]; contaminated blood collection tubes have caused pseudobacteremias [7,8] and true bacteremias; and contaminated hand-care products have been implicated as a cause of infection [9,10]. Clinicians often perceive products that come in closed containers as sterile and use them as such even when they are not so marketed.

F. S. Rhame: Division of Epidemiology, University of Minnesota School of Public Health, Abbott Northwestern Hospital, Minneapolis, Minnesota 55407-3799.

[1] The word *fomite,* although it is in disfavor among some researchers, remains quite useful. A fomite is an inanimate object that may be contaminated with microorganisms and serve in their transmission. The origin of the term fomites is the Latin plural of *Fomes*, the genus of fungus that was used as tinder. The dried fungus is porous and thus was considered "capable of absorbing and retaining contagious effluvia."

Most would find surprising the frequency of contamination of oral medications (especially those of animal origin), ointments, nasal sprays, and lotions [11].

The fomites discussed in this chapter include many entities for which no infection-causing potential has been established. Questions concerning the proper management of these items frequently confront infection control personnel. Even those skeptical of the infection-causing potential of environmental surfaces and ordinary objects used in the care of patients advocate processing and cleaning methods that may have a considerable financial impact. At times, procedures rest on aesthetic considerations. Carpets may not usually constitute an infection hazard, but fecal stains are unacceptable. Health care professionals may be convinced that microorganisms on the walls and floors play no role in causing human disease, but the lay public's perception is exactly the contrary. In an era of increasing attention to marketing, visible dirt is undesirable. When standards have been set, formally or informally, they are often based on the recognition of what reductions in microbial content can be consistently achieved with moderate resource use, rather than on what levels prevent infection.

The fact that there are outbreaks of nosocomial infection stemming from contaminated inanimate objects is often invoked as a basis for concern about endemic nosocomial infection attributable to the inanimate environment. But publication bias brings forth the atypical. A single outbreak does not provide a basis for concern about environmental contamination.

ENVIRONMENTALLY ALTERED MICROORGANISMS

It seems paradoxical that environmental objects can frequently be contaminated by human pathogens while only rarely contributing to human infection. A potential explanation lies in the concept of environmentally damaged organisms. This concept has been rigorously demonstrated for *Streptococcus pyogenes* by Perry et al. and Rammelkamp and colleagues [12–14]. In a classic series of experiments, they studied streptococcal transmission in army barracks. Air, dust, and personal effects such as blankets were more often contaminated by streptococci when recruits had streptococcal illness or pharyngeal colonization. However, recruits who had been issued freshly laundered, *Streptococcus*-free blankets acquired streptococcal infection or pharyngeal colonization just as often as barracks mates issued highly contaminated blankets [12]. The authors then directly assessed the infectious potential of naturally contaminated barracks dust. Dust samples, dispersed in small enclosures, produced between 3,500 and 56,600 streptococci/m^3 air but did not result in pharyngeal colonization or infection in volunteers within the enclosures. Six volunteers had 17 direct inoculations of dust containing 1,800 to 42,000 streptococci onto the posterior pharynx. There resulted only transient colonization lasting ≤ 30 minutes [12].

In contrast, fresh oropharyngeal secretions mixed with sterile dust and dried 4 to 8 hours produced streptococcal pharyngitis in two of eight volunteers after inoculation. Two of the remaining six volunteers developed pharyngitis on subsequent inoculation of smaller numbers of streptococci directly transferred on swabs of nasopharyngeal sections [14]. The designation of this phenomenon as *environmental damage* reflects a rather anthropocentric perspective. Streptococci presumably shift their metabolism to meet their needs. The physiologic basis of bacterial adaptation to desiccation has been explored [15] and involves substantial changes in internal constituents.

The loss of human pathogenicity associated with adaptation to the environment has been established for desiccated *S. pyogenes.* It seems plausible that other species have different adaptations to various environmental situations that would also reduce their pathogenicity for humans. For some organisms, however, it is reasonable to speculate that the required adaptations are less debilitating. "Water bacteria" in moist environments might be in metabolic states less different from their most pathogenic state. In contrast, *Legionella* spp in their inanimate reservoir are hazardous, but person-to-person transmission does not take place. Viruses are either viable or not. *Clostridium difficile* as an environmental spore is more durable; if the spore is an infectious form for humans, environmental damage would not be relevant. These matters are, at present, largely unexplored.

EPISTEMOLOGY

With the foregoing generalities in mind, we confront the methodologic inadequacies that characterize most published studies asserting a causative role of inanimate objects in human disease. Evidence suggesting that a fomite has a role in causing disease due to a particular pathogen can be divided into seven categories. They are ordered here by the rigor with which they establish the point.

1. *The organism can survive after inoculation onto the fomite.* This is the weakest form of evidence, yet good journals allocate space to these studies, which sometimes gain widespread attention from the press. A case in point is the demonstration that herpes simplex virus can survive when inoculated on hot-tub seats [16]. The finding was published despite the cogent words of the accompanying editorial [17], which pointed out the inconclusiveness of the observation.
2. *The pathogen can be cultured from in-use fomites.* A vast set of publications report the recovery of human pathogens from healthcare items. These demonstrations are a necessary but insufficient element in the assertion that a fomite causes infection. When the

pathogen is present more frequently or in higher concentration in association with infected humans, this element is only marginally strengthened because the association is as likely to be due to the patient's infecting the environment as vice versa [18]. When the pathogen cannot be cultured, other markers may be used (e.g., hepatitis B surface antigen in the case of hepatitis B [19]). When it is suspected that environmental adaptation may lessen pathogenicity, it is desirable that the detection method simulate the natural infection (e.g., animal inoculation).

3. *The pathogen can proliferate in the fomite.* Whether proliferation must be confirmed is largely a function of the size of the inoculum required to cause infection. For instance, this element is important in the case of contaminated intravenous solutions: most intravenous fluid contamination is at low concentrations, and humans ordinarily tolerate a few organisms given intravenously. For intravenous fluid contamination to be a hazard, the organisms must have the ability and time to proliferate. In general, contaminated objects do not cause infection in immunocompetent persons unless the contaminating organism can proliferate in the contaminated environment or the contamination is heavy and occurs shortly before exposure. However, immunocompromised persons may be more susceptible to becoming infected from such contaminated objects.
4. *Some fraction of acquisition cannot be accounted for by other recognized methods of transmission.* An example of this type of evidence is found in the last of a series of studies that began with the classic demonstration of the importance of hands and contact in nursery acquisition by newborns of *Staphylococcus aureus.* In the final study of the series, Mortimer and colleagues [20] went to great lengths to eliminate contact transmission in a nursery in which index babies were colonized by *S. aureus.* At least nine of 158 contact-protected babies became colonized. This finding, and the recovery of *S. aureus* on settle plates, was taken as evidence that air was the vector of transmission. A more recent example was seen during a nursing-home outbreak of Norwalk agent diarrhea. Thirteen ill employees were very unlikely to have had stool contact. The authors suggested that airborne spread had occurred [21].
   This element may appear to be present simply because of the vicissitudes of biologic systems. It is inevitable that it will be difficult to account for all transmissions by any given mechanism. Implication of a fomite by exclusion of alternatives should be considered weak evidence unless a large fraction of transmissions cannot otherwise be explained.
5. *Retrospective case-control studies show an association between exposure to the fomite and infection.* The association must be verified by less frequent exposure in a comparison unaffected population. Such findings are strengthened when contamination can be confirmed microbiologically. The most common type of study reliably implicating a fomite in endemic or epidemic nosocomial infection is a case-control study of this type. Case-control methodology is discussed in Chapters 1 and 6.
6. Prospective observational studies may be possible when more than one similar type of "fomite" is in use. Such observations can be made without the need to randomize exposures.
7. *Prospective studies allocating exposure to the fomite to a subset of patients show an association between the exposure and infection.* Microbiological confirmation of contamination assists in establishing a causal relationship. Ideally, the exposed group is selected randomly. There are two scenarios to consider: fomite A versus nothing when it is not important in patient care (e.g., potted plants), and fomite A versus fomite B when it is necessary in patient care (e.g., two or more different types of thermometers, endoscopes, etc.). Only evidence from categories 5, 6, and 7 should be considered strong enough to securely implicate a fomite.

Strain analysis and molecular markers of clonality, so helpful in many areas of epidemiology [22], are less useful in this epistemology (see Chapter 9). Strain differences can negate evidence in category 2. However, strain analysis usually doesn't substitute for evidence in categories 5, 6, or 7. For instance, most hospital outbreaks of vancomycin-resistant *Enterococcus* or *C. difficile* have been due to a particular strain. Strain homogeneity, compared with extra-hospital isolates, can establish that the cases among patients are nosocomial in origin. But finding the outbreak strain in the environment doesn't establish its causal role. The transmissions could result from hand carriage or some other person-to-person contact and the infected patients could be contaminating the environment. Only when the direction is clear (there is no likely way for patients to contaminate a hot water tank with *Legionella*, for instance) can establishing strain identity between patient's and fomite isolates establish environmental causality. There is one last distinctive aspect of the application of strain identification techniques to environmentally caused outbreaks. A bona fide outbreak may arise from heterogeneous strains, since environmental isolates are generally heterogeneous. For instance, nosocomial *Aspergillus* isolates in an outbreak due to a defect in air filtration will reflect the heterogeneity of environmental isolates [23].

AIR

There has probably been concern about air as a vehicle for transmission of infection for as long as there has been recognition of the transmissibility of disease. Surely more data have been generated for this mode of transmission than for any other. Entire books have been devoted to the subject [24,25], suggesting that concise summarization is difficult. For much of human history, air was considered the primary carrier of contagion. The word "malaria" reflects the recognition that proximity to swamps increased the risk of illness (the ancients were correct, in a sense, since mosquitoes fly). However, the advent of scientific medicine caused the pendulum to swing too far in the opposite direction. By 1910, no illness was any longer thought to be airborne. Large droplets travel up to 1 to 2 m through the air but are not borne on it.[2] Large-droplet transmission is instead considered a type of contact spread [26] (see Chapter 1). Only at the time of World War II did a more balanced view become established. Much of the subsequent work on air as a vector was done in the context of studies of biological warfare.

Although there are many concerns about air as a means of nosocomial transmission [27], the trend has been away from concern. There were six articles dealing with airborne spread of infection presented at the initial International Conference on Nosocomial Infections in 1970, and an estimate was made in 1970 by Brachman [28] that between 10% and 20% of endemic nosocomial infections resulted from the airborne route. At the second International Conference on Nosocomial Infections in 1982, however, there was only one presentation about airborne organisms [29], and it dealt with the operating room. At the third International Conference in 1990, except for measles virus transmission, the topic was not discussed.

Air may be sampled volumetrically or on settling plates (see Chapter 9). Volumetric sampling produces quantitative data that are more readily conceptualized and seems more relevant to situations in which a pathogen is inhaled. It is the standard for rigorous studies. However, settling plates may be more appropriate to infections that result from settling organisms (e.g., wound infections), and such sampling can be performed without special equipment or expertise [30]. Unfortunately, there are few side-by-side surveys of air using volumetric and settling methods. In one study of air fungal content, 15-minute pairs compared volumetric sampling of 0.42 m^3 air with settling on a 100-mm plate (79 cm^2) [31]. A total of 127 sample pairs yielded total recoveries of 12,900 cfu and 1,031 cfu, respectively, establishing one advantage for volumetric sampling. Furthermore, of the organisms captured by volumetric sampling, 9.2% were *Aspergillus* spp, while only 5.5% of the settling organisms were in that relatively buoyant genus, pointing out one of the complexities of interpreting settle plate results.

Assessment of the organism content of air is difficult because the concentration of certain organisms in the air is small compared with the volumes that can be conveniently assessed, producing considerable sampling error. Furthermore, there is tremendous variation in the microbial content of air, depending on location in the hospital, ventilation systems, concurrent human activity, and proximity to sources of organisms. For a review of available air sampling methods, see Chapter 9 and Burge [32].

There are few broad surveys of hospital air with complete microbial identification. In one set of studies, Greene and colleagues [33,34] found a mean organism count of 350 to 700 organisms/m^3. The highest counts were in laundry-handling areas, followed closely by other storage and disposal areas. The lowest counts were in operating and delivery rooms. Approximately one third of the organisms recovered were gram-positive cocci, another one third were gram-positive bacilli, and the remainder were gram-negative bacilli or fungi. Gram-positive cocci constituted a higher proportion of the organisms in operating rooms, gram-positive bacilli (presumably mostly *Bacillus* species) made up a higher proportion of the organisms in the laundry and waste storage areas, and gram-negative bacilli were found in relatively high numbers in corridors.

More detailed consideration of air as a means of transmission is best made by considering the specific organism. There is convincing evidence for airborne transmission of varicella-zoster virus, smallpox, influenza, measles, *Mycobacterium tuberculosis*, *Brucella* spp, *Pseudomonas pseudomallei*, *Coxiella burnetii*, *Chlamydia psittaci*, *Francisella tularensis*, *Bacillus anthracis*, *Legionella* spp, *Yersinia pestis*, *Pneumocystis carinii*, *Aspergillus* spp, and other filamentous fungi. Additional organisms probably achieve airborne transmission, for example, mumps, rubella, *Mycobacterium avium* complex, *S. aureus*. And still other organisms possibly do so [27]. For most pathogens, humans (not the environment) are the source of contagion. Control of airborne transmission in hospitals consists mainly of promptly identifying infectious patients and placing them in isolation rooms. Influenza control during community outbreaks is a bit more complicated because of the high prevalence of infectious patients and personnel and because infectious persons may have subtle or no respiratory symptoms [35]. Preventing nosocomial influenza during community influenza outbreaks is one of the few solid rationales for human traffic control within hospitals.

Staphylococcus Aureus

There is a solid theoretic basis for concern about the importance of airborne transmission of *S. aureus* (see Chapter 41). Noble [36], probably the most avid student of this matter, summarizes information bearing on the origin of airborne *S. aureus* as follows. Humans liberate ~ 3×10^8 squamae per day. Because the size distribution

[2] In the context of infection transmission, airborne means "borne on the air" rather than "transported through the air."

of airborne particles containing *S. aureus* (~ 4 to 25 μm in diameter] is nearly that of squamae and well above the diameter of naked, single *S. aureus* cells (~ 1 μm in diameter), it is presumed that most or all airborne *S. aureus* organisms are carried on these skin flakes. Since particles of this size become impacted on the nasal turbinates, a closed loop may exist: proliferation of *S. aureus* on the nasal mucosa, hand transfer of *S. aureus* to the skin, liberation on squamae, airborne transport of squamae, and impaction on the nasal mucosa. Hospital air contains ~ 0.7 *S. aureus* particles/m^3 [37].

Outbreaks of *S. aureus* (and *S. pyogenes*) surgical wound infection have been solidly linked to airborne spread from dispersers in the operating room (see Chapter 37). In this context, surgical gowns make direct contact improbable and masks make droplet spread improbable. However, the importance of air as a medium for endemic *S. aureus* transmission in other settings is less clear. The strongest positive evidence is that of Mortimer and co-workers [20], who studied acquisition of staphylococcal colonization in newborn infants housed in a special nursery that was also used for the care of known colonized infants. Extraordinary measures were undertaken to eliminate contact transfer of *S. aureus* from the index babies to the study babies. Nevertheless, at least nine of 158 newborns became colonized. The authors offered as evidence that these acquisitions were airborne the following points. Contact transmission did not occur; index strains of *S. aureus* were recovered on settling plates throughout the nursery; the infants were ≥ 2 m apart, making large-droplet transmission unlikely; and the study infants tended to be colonized in the nose first, whereas in previous studies infants acquiring *S. aureus* by physical transfer tended to be colonized at the umbilicus first.

Wenzel and colleagues [38] have critically analyzed nine additional articles published between 1966 and 1976 that purport to establish airborne transmission of *S. aureus*. None of these additional studies provides even strongly suggestive evidence of airborne spread. A bit of negative evidence with respect to endemic operating room acquisition of *S. aureus* came from the National Academy of Sciences–National Research Council study [39] of the influence of ultraviolet radiation on postoperative wound infection (see Chapter 27). In the study, high-intensity ultraviolet light in the operating room reduced airborne bacterial counts, as measured on settling plates, by 52% or 63%, depending on the ultraviolet intensity used. At neither intensity was there a similar reduction in postoperative wound infection rates.

Gram-negative Bacilli

Volumetric sampling of ordinary hospital air with recovery of pathogenic *Enterobacteriaceae* and nonfermenters has been rare. Available studies tend to focus on specialized areas of the hospital (especially operating rooms), use settling-plate methods, assess outbreak situations, or provide incomplete microbiologic identification. *Klebsiella* [40], *Pseudomonas* [41], and other gram-negative organisms can be recovered from hospital air, but the best correlation with acquisition by patients is via handborne rather than airborne organisms [42].

Clinicians have been particularly concerned about the spread of *Pseudomonas aeruginosa* and *Burkholderia cepacia* from or to hospitalized patients with cystic fibrosis. Molecular strain identification techniques establish that institutional person-to-person transmission occurs [43,44], but they do not identify the mechanism. *P. aeruginosa* has been recovered on settling plates near patients with cystic fibrosis [45]. Institution of isolation protocols has been associated with reduced transmission rates. However, the potential interactions between patients with cystic fibrosis are many, and air is not established as a path of transmission.

Two studies have described an association between airborne gram-negative bacilli and endemic nosocomial infection. The first and more convincing situation resulted from a very unusual circumstance. The newly constructed Hines Veterans Administration Hospital had a novel chute hydropulping waste disposal system that introduced malodorous bacteria-laden air throughout the hospital. Air sampling near the system demonstrated > 5,600 cfu of *Pseudomonas* organisms and *Enterobacteriaceae* (unfortunately, the relative amounts were unspecified) per cubic meter [46]. Concurrent continuous infection surveillance indicated that the nosocomial bacteremia rate approximately doubled coincident with moving to the new hospital and fell to the baseline level after the chute hydropulping system was closed.

In a second study, carried out over a 5-year interval by Kelsen and McGuckin [47], there was a significant positive correlation between the monthly rate of nosocomial respiratory tract infection in patients hospitalized in an intensive care unit and the average bacterial content of the air. During periods of heavy air contamination, the authors found an unusually high concentration of airborne gram-negative bacilli, ranging up to a *P. aeruginosa* content of 1,050 cfu per cubic meter and a *Klebsiella* content of 315 cfu per cubic meter. As the authors point out, the association may not imply that airborne gram-negative rods directly cause nosocomial respiratory tract disease; it is possible that airborne bacteria seeded nebulizers [48] or another intermediate reservoir. The association may have resulted from a third factor affecting both bacterial content of the air and the nosocomial infection rate. Finally, it is possible that the air may reflect patients' illnesses rather than the reverse.

Ultimately, the best evidence that endemic nosocomial infection does not often result from airborne gram-negative bacilli probably arises from the repeated failure to recover such organisms in air cultures obtained during epidemic investigations. Although these situations may be atypical, as negative evidence they are convincing, since this may be expected to be the situation most likely to produce positive air cultures. The widespread belief that gram-negative bacilli do not survive for prolonged periods when airborne, if true, may provide additional evidence. Here the experimental support is more tenuous than one might wish. Under certain conditions of humidity, temperature, and physiologic state, *Escherichia coli* can sustain up to 100% survival for $^1/_2$ hour in microaerosols [49,50]. In general, *E. coli* survives better when aerosols are generated using broth cultures of organisms in relatively inactive states.

In summary, although there is insufficient evidence that airborne gram-negative bacilli constitute a source of endemic nosocomial infection to warrant changes in our current practices, situations that lead to high airborne concentrations of gram-negative bacilli should be avoided. Such situations include the use of aerosol-generating room humidifiers, which have been shown to cause considerable dissemination of *Pseudomonas* [51] and *Acinetobacter* [52].

Legionella

The original legionnaires' outbreak included cases of "Broad Street pneumonia," found among persons who remained outside the implicated hotel. These cases are presumed to establish airborne *Legionella pneumophilia* transmission, but they were not definitely proved to be due to *L. pneumophilia*. Subsequent outbreak cases have been attributed to cooling tower contamination. Few of these studies have included long-term follow-up after cooling tower decontamination nor have they demonstrated an association through strain identification. Although airborne transmission may take place, for nosocomial legionellosis, the emphasis should be on control of contamination in the potable water supply, as discussed in the section on water transmission.

Aspergillus

Several lines of evidence strongly suggest that airborne *Aspergillus fumigatus* spores cause aspergillosis in immunosuppressed patients [53].

1. *Aspergillus* spores are always present in unfiltered air, and the organism is highly adapted to airborne spread.
2. Most nosocomial aspergillosis appears first as pneumonia or nasopharyngeal infection. Even if there is an intermediate step of nasopharyngeal colonization, airborne spores would be the ultimate source.
3. Two hospitals have reported a decline in endemic nosocomial aspergillosis coincident with moving to new facilities with improved air filtration systems.
4. In all reported outbreaks of nosocomial aspergillosis, there has been an implicated airborne source of transmission stemming from a breakdown in the heating, ventilation, and air conditioning system; a breech of the building shell; or an in-hospital source of fungal spores.
5. Nosocomial aspergillosis arising in a patient cared for in a high-efficiency particulate air (HEPA) filtered room has not been described in print [54].
6. In one hospital, reductions in airborne *Aspergillus* spores coincided with a lowered rate of nosocomial aspergillosis in bone marrow transplant recipients.

It is likely that many other fungal organisms, such as *Mucor, Fusarium,* and *Pseudoallescheria,* also are transmitted to patients through the air.

Occasionally water reaches organic material within the hospital by penetration of the building shell, plumbing leakage, or condensation on chilled water lines or the inner surfaces of cold outside walls. Fungal growth may result within several days. Hospitals must act vigorously to stop the water leakage and promptly achieve drying. If growth of hazardous fungi has occurred, careful remediation is required.

Notwithstanding the occasional episode of in-hospital fungal growth, the majority of spores in hospital air derive from outdoor air. Spores gain entrance into the hospital because of incomplete filtration—infiltrating around improperly seated filters, around window casings (especially when there is perpendicular wind), through entrances or via loading docks, and on the clothes of personnel and visitors. The better the filtration (i.e., the lower the spore counts), the more important the other sources of spores become. Spores may settle over time and be re-aerosolized during manipulations of the heating, ventilation, and air conditioning systems; while cleaning, or during renovation that produces "minibursts" of spores. Explosive demolition produces very high *Aspergillus* counts. Excavation can do so as well, and renovation may [55] or may not [56].

Special efforts are required to protect bone marrow transplant (BMT) recipients (discussed later herein). Other patients are also highly susceptible to aspergillosis, including lymphoma and leukemia patients, solid organ transplant recipients, solid tumor chemotherapy patients, other recipients of cytotoxic therapy, patients with the acquired immunodeficiency syndrome, and steroid-treated patients. While special units for BMT patients are warranted, the potential for competition in room assignment and issues concerning where one draws the line for the remaining groups of patients make it desirable to achieve low spore counts throughout the hospital. In BMT units counts of < 0.02 pathogenic *Aspergillus* spp organisms/m^3 and, in the remainder of the hospital, counts of $< 0.05/m^3$ can be achieved without undue burden.

Human Immunodeficiency Virus

There has been anxiety about airborne human immunodeficiency virus (HIV) transmission, especially in the operating room and the autopsy department (see Chapter 43). This anxiety persists partly because of the potential for aerosol generation by mechanical saws [57] or other activities. Clearly, splatter of blood and tissue happens in these locations, and scrupulous attention should be paid to barriers for the surgeon or prosector. The available studies do not, unfortunately, adequately distinguish between those droplets and tissue fragments that travel < 2 m in smooth arcs to the ground and aerosols (droplet nuclei) that remain airborne and threaten persons at a greater distance from the aerosol generation point. The hepatitis B precedent would suggest that only operating room or autopsy personnel in direct contact with blood are at risk. Special devices to protect against airborne HIV transmission are not warranted.

Laser Plumes

Surgical lasers generate visible smoke that could, in theory, contain viable airborne organisms [58]. Although infection transmission has not been verified, safety guidelines have been published [59].

WATER

Potable Water

Achievement of potability of water is a major public health activity, the discussion of which is beyond the scope of this book. Standard works may be consulted for details of water treatment and examination [60]. Verification of ordinary potability is of importance to infection control personnel only in hospitals with private water supplies, where verification of water quality is a hospital's responsibility. It should be noted that federal drinking water regulations call for only one microbiologic assessment [61]: a coliform count (acceptable levels depend on sampling frequency but must average < 1 per 100 ml). Even for community water, this sole criterion is probably inadequate, considering the variety of water sources, potential contaminants, and uses of water [62]. The European Community standards also include a limit on the total viable count [63]. Except for legionellosis (discussed later), there is only one report of nosocomial infection arising from drinking water [64]; thus further consideration of water in this chapter focuses on specialized uses in the hospital.

Potable water supply systems must be protected by vacuum breakers or other devices to keep water from being sucked back into the system during unusual events. To save expense, some building designers plan separate potable and nonpotable water systems. These systems must never be interconnected. Common sense requires that the potable water system be used for all hand washing, bathing of patients, cooking, washing of foods and utensils for cooking and eating, food preparation or processing, and laundry. Given the few valid uses for nonpotable water in the hospital and the difficulty in forever preventing cross-connection, the value of designing hospitals with separate nonpotable water systems is questionable.

Dialysis Water

Detailed standards for hemodialysis water have been prepared by the Association for the Advancement of Medical Instrumentation (AAMI) and accepted by the American National Standards Institution [65]. The standard specifies that water used to prepare dialysate shall have a total microbial count of < 200 per ml and the dialysate itself shall have < 2,000 microbes per ml (see Chapter 24). The rationale for the standard lies in studies carried out in the 1970s that indicated that pyrogenic reactions did not occur when dialysate had < 2,000 organisms per milliliter [66,67]. Bacteria do not cross an intact dialysis membrane, but endotoxin may. The viable bacterial concentration is a rough measure of the endotoxin concentration. The rationale for the stricter (< 200 organisms per ml) standard for water used to prepare dialysate is that organism multiplication may take place within the dialyzer. This is a more important problem for recirculating systems than for single-pass systems [68], a distinction not recognized in the AAMI standard. In recirculating systems, dialyzed materials can provide nutrition to contaminating bacteria. There are many types of water treatment devices for use in preparing dialysate. A brief discussion is available in Appendix B to the AAMI standard [69]. A more detailed discussion is available in a Food and Drug Administration (FDA) technical report [70].

Hydrotherapy Pools and Tanks

A number of features of hydrotherapy tanks have generated concern that they may transmit infection. Patients using them may have active infection, which may introduce hazardous bacteria and organic debris; patients may be incontinent of feces; warm temperature, water agitation, and a high number of successive patients per unit volume of water reduce available chlorine; the internal channels of agitators are difficult to disinfect; and highly contaminated water may be brought into close contact with potential portals of entry, such as pressure sores, Foley catheters, or percutaneous devices (see Chapter

44). One outbreak of *P. aeruginosa* wound infections has been reliably linked to these tanks [71]. Since a wide variety of other human pathogens, such as coliforms, staphylococci, and fungi, have been isolated from immersion tanks [72], there is a broader potential of transmission.

Indeed, in a burn center, where the infection potential of hydrotherapy tanks may be most severe, Mayhall and colleagues [73] have reported a bacteremia outbreak due to *Enterobacter cloacae,* which may have been associated with hydrotherapy transmission. To the extent that hydrotherapy tanks are similar to hot tubs and whirlpool spas, there is a more ominous possibility. Contamination of these water sources has resulted in *P. aeruginosa* folliculitis [74], urinary tract infections [75], and even pneumonia [76]. The danger from in-hospital hydrotherapy tanks is probably mitigated by higher standards of disinfection. In the outbreaks of community-acquired *P. aeruginosa* skin infections, even rudimentary standards of water maintenance were not in effect [74].

The Centers for Disease Control and Prevention (CDC) published recommendations for disinfection of hydrotherapy pools and tanks in 1974 [77]. For immersion tanks, the CDC recommended maintaining a free chlorine residual of 15 mg/L with a pH of 7.2 to 7.6, draining tanks between each patient's use, scrubbing out the tank with a germicidal detergent, and circulating chlorine solution through the agitator of the tank for ≥ 15 minutes at the end of each treatment day. For hydrotherapy pools, the CDC favored continuous filtration and the maintenance of free chlorine residuals of 0.4 to 0.6 mg/L. In the absence of continuous filtration, the CDC recommended potassium iodide and chloramine.

High-Purity Water

Distillation apparatus, reverse osmosis devices, and ion-exchange resin beds are all subject to contamination. Some hospital personnel erroneously assume this type of water is sterile. Distilled water, even if subsequently sterilized, may contain endotoxin. Febrile reactions caused by exposure to items rinsed in endotoxin-containing distilled water have occurred [78].

Water Bacteria

So-called water bacteria are organisms that proliferate in relatively pure water. The most adept species is *B. cepacia.* Carson and colleagues [79] found *B. cepacia* strains that could multiply to the levels of 10^7/ml and remain at these high levels for weeks in distilled water of very high resistivity. *P. aeruginosa* follows closely behind in this ability [80]. Furthermore, *P. aeruginosa* strains adapted to distilled water are relatively resistant to disinfectants [81]. *Acinetobacter calcoaceticus* seems particularly well adapted to highly aerated water sources. An enrichment technique for isolation of *Acinetobacter* from environmental samples using vigorous aeration has been described [82]. This feature of *Acinetobacter* presumably accounts for its increased relative frequency of citation as a cause of humidifier or other respiratory device contamination [83,84]. Other water bacteria include *Flavobacterium meningosepticum* [85], other *Pseudomonas* species, *Acromobacter* species, *Aeromonas hydrophila*, *Flavimonas* [86], and certain nontuberculous mycobacteria [87]. These last-named organisms are also relatively resistant to various disinfectants [88], including formaldehyde [89]. Among the water bacteria, *P. aeruginosa* and *Acinetobacter* [90] are unusual in that they also are common colonizers of healthy humans. Unprotected wet areas in a hospital should be considered contaminated with one or more water bacteria. These sources include tap water, drains and sinks, water baths, shower heads, flower water, ice machines, and water carafes.

Legionella

Among the important nosocomial pathogens, *Legionellaceae* are the agents for which environmental sources are the most securely established. Person-to-person transmission of *L. pneumophila* is either very rare or nonexistent [91]. Nosocomial *L. pneumophila* pneumonia has been strongly associated with hot-water distribution systems and, perhaps, cooling towers (see Chapter 32). *Legionella micdadei* appears to have a similar epidemiology [92]. Outbreaks of *Legionella dumoffii* surgical wound infections due to tap water contamination of fresh wounds appear to be a more atypical problem [93].

Muder and co-workers [94] have critically reviewed the mechanisms of transmission of *L. pneumophila.* Most of the initial outbreak reports, particularly those outbreaks occurring in nonhospital settings, were associated with adjacent excavation or contaminated air-handling-system cooling towers. However, more recent hospital outbreaks have been securely linked to contamination of hot water systems. At the Wadsworth Veterans Administration Hospital in Los Angeles, where a large outbreak of nosocomial legionellosis took place over a period of several years, improvements in the air-handling system preceded efforts to eliminate *Legionella* from the water system. Only the latter endeavor was followed by a reduction in the number of cases of infection [95]. Many additional reports have attributed cessation of nosocomial cases of infection to reductions in the presence in hot-water systems of *L. pneumophila.* Unfortunately, with few exceptions [96], follow-up has been of more than one year's duration, and case ascertainment is unsure.

The way in which *L. pneumophila* contamination of hot water systems produces nosocomial pneumonia is not established. Presumably, inhalation of freshly aerosolized droplets predominates, although inhalation of particles (droplet nuclei) airborne from distant sources, aspiration of colonizing pharyngeal organisms, ingestion of drinking water, or contaminated respiratory therapy devices all remain possibilities [97]. An association of cases with the use of contaminated shower heads has been found in some [98,99], but not the majority, of investigations.

L. pneumophila contamination of hot water distribution systems is variably present in hospitals; Vickers et al. [100] found it in 9 of 15 Pennsylvania hospitals. Systems more likely to be contaminated were older and tended to be in a vertical configuration, perhaps because of a greater tendency to have accumulated scale. Systems set at > 60°C were less likely to be contaminated. Given the exacting nutritional requirements of the *Legionellaceae*, it is not usual for this contamination to be widespread. A potential explanation is the promotion of *Legionella* growth by other bacteria [101] or their ability to survive within amoebas [102]. In one investigation, shower heads contaminated with *L. pneumophila* were more likely to harbor amoebas [99]. These associations may ultimately permit indirect *Legionella* decontamination.

The need to keep hospital hot water systems free of *Legionellaceae* and the role of routine culture confirmation of the presence of organisms are unresolved. Until recently, CDC personnel opposed culturing hospital water not associated with cases of infection [103]. In 1995 an ambivalent stance was adopted [104]. Nosocomial *Legionella* pneumonia often goes unrecognized unless the possibility is avidly investigated [97], making it difficult for any hospital to be complacent about its *Legionella* situation. There is at least one cited case of a hospital with a contaminated potable water system and fairly secure evidence of the absence of nosocomial legionellosis [105], but such reports are rare. Yu [106] has advocated a 1-year quarterly cycle of hospital water cultures in hospitals where identification of nosocomial *Legionella* pneumonia cases is uncertain. The availability of commercial media for *Legionella* cultivation makes such surveillance relatively simple, although some expertise is required for confirmation of recovered isolates. Vigorously swabbing scale from shower heads is more sensitive than culture of flushed water, but detailed protocols for routine culture programs are lacking. Shower head scale and water from the base of hot water storage tanks should be included in surveillance. Hospitals recovering *L. pneumophila* and, perhaps, *L. micdadei* should strengthen clinical case ascertainment methods.

Hospitals with nosocomial *Legionella* pneumonia cases and contaminated hot water systems must strive to eliminate the latter. Superheating the water (to as high as 77°C [170°F]) provides an immediate solution but may cause scalding of patients or personnel. Instituting long-term solutions is more difficult. Persistent colonization of hospital potable water systems by *L. pneumophila* arises, at least in part, because the organism can tolerate low levels of chlorine for relatively long periods of time [107]. Hyperchlorination damages some plumbing system components, and raising the pH aggravates scale formation [108]. Other possible ways to eliminate colonization include use of instantaneous steam water heaters, ultraviolet light, and ozonation [101].

Eyewash Stations

Clinical laboratories have eyewash stations for emergency eye flushing. These often go unused for months. There have been recent reports that water in these stations becomes contaminated with *Acanthamoeba* and other amoebas [109] capable of causing chronic destructive keratitis. Although no such infections have been reported, a weekly flush reduces the contamination.

Walls, Floors, and Other Smooth Surfaces

Maki and his infection control group [18] performed a landmark study assessing the relationship between organisms on environmental surfaces and nosocomial infection. During 1979, the University of Wisconsin Hospital moved to a new facility. There was no change in the rate of nosocomial infection at any patient care site or due to any pathogen associated with this change. Cultures of floors, walls, and other surfaces (as well as air, water, faucets, and sink drains) showed very similar organism profiles in the old facility and, after 6 to 12 months of occupancy, in the new facility. In contrast, corresponding cultures taken in the new facility before occupancy were relatively devoid of common nosocomial pathogens. The constancy of infection rates provides strong evidence that the association between hospital environmental organism content and nosocomial infection arises because patients infect the environment, not vice versa. It is important to realize some limitations of the Maki study. The two pathogens for which environmental content is of primary importance (*Aspergillus* and *Legionella*) were not assessed, and the environmental cultures were not processed for anaerobes (e.g., *C. difficile*) or viruses.

This study virtually rules out the environment as a significant vector for the assessed organism-object combinations and severely undercuts the rationale for concern about other combinations in the absence of specific data to the contrary. In fact, one is forced to question seriously even such relatively modest recommendations as the use of antimicrobial detergents in hospital cleaning, terminal disinfection of isolation rooms, special cleaning of objects removed from isolation rooms, and the wearing of gowns and gloves when entering the room of patients in isolation when no contact with patients is anticipated.

Respiratory Syncytial Virus

One pathogen clearly transmissible in the hospital by fomites is respiratory syncytial virus (RSV) (see Chapter

32). Indirect evidence suggests that RSV transmission happens through contact; inoculation of RSV onto nasal or eye membranes causes infection quite efficiently [110]. Moreover, this virus survives for several hours on smooth surfaces [111]. Direct evidence of fomite transmission is now available [112]. Volunteers entering a hospital room that had just been vacated by an RSV-infected patient, after handling objects in the room and touching their eyes and nose, became infected with RSV more than half as often as volunteers who cuddled RSV-infected babies. Volunteers sitting in the same room with an RSV-infected baby did not contract the illness. The relative importance of hand and fomite transmission is unknown, but it is of interest that RSV survives approximately ten times better on smooth surfaces than on skin [111].

Clostridium Difficile

Strain analysis techniques have unequivocally established that in-hospital transmission of *C. difficile* can take place (see Chapter 34) [113]. Variation in hospital *C. difficile* transmission would provide a satisfactory explanation for the apparently wide variation in rates of *C. difficile* colitis in different hospitals. As is the case for many nosocomial pathogens, increased environmental presence of *C. difficile* is associated with infected patients. In their excellent review, McFarland and Stamm [114] found five supportive studies. With regard to environmental concerns, what distinguishes *C. difficile* is its ability to form spores, with the consequent prolonged survival of the organism in the environment and the plausibility that the spores retain full infectiousness. However, a controlled study of glove use suggested that most *C. difficile* transmissions arise from carriage by hand [115]. The same group has used restriction endonuclease strain analysis to establish that *C. difficile* acquisition does not geographically cluster within wards and is not more likely to be transmitted to a subsequent bed occupant [116]. No special environmental cleaning techniques for *C. difficile* contamination have been formally advocated.

Hepatitis B Virus

Concern about environmental hepatitis B virus (HBV) transmission arises from several lines of evidence. Clinical laboratories and hemodialysis units, areas frequently contaminated by blood, were foci of HBV transmission throughout the 1970s (see Chapters 23 and 24). Many of the ward-acquired, and an even larger fraction of the laboratory-acquired, HBV cases occurred without recognized percutaneous inoculation of blood. A decline in the incidence of hepatitis among healthcare workers began in the mid-1970s (before the introduction of HBV vaccine), when concern about blood contact became widespread [117]. Approximately 30% to 40% of community-acquired cases of HBV cannot be ascribed to sexual contact, needle sharing, or therapeutic blood component exposure [118]. Hepatitis B surface antigen (HBsAg) may be antigenically detected on surfaces in hospital areas likely to have been blood-contaminated [19]. Surfaces not visibly contaminated with blood may also yield HBsAg. Even today, blood contamination can frequently be found on items related to the care of patients [119]. In blood, HBV remains viable for ≤ 1 week after desiccation at room temperature [120], although it is not difficult to inactivate with disinfectant [121]. Very high dilutions of HBV-containing blood can transmit hepatitis B.

These lines of evidence do not establish a role of the environment in HBV transmission. Coincident with efforts to eliminate or decontaminate environmental blood was the adoption of segregation of HBsAg-positive patients in dialysis and more widespread recognition of the hazard of needle sticks. Nevertheless, when contaminated objects have been in close proximity to a portal of entry, such as the finger platform of an automatic finger stick device, HBV transmission by inanimate objects has been verified [122].

To clean blood spills, the CDC most recently recommended the use of any chemical germicide that is approved by the U.S. Environmental Protection Agency (EPA) as a "hospital disinfectant" and is tuberculocidal [123]. Since no contact time was specified, the recommendation is not that a tuberculocidal standard be met. Nevertheless, OHSA may arbitrarily enforce the germicide choice strictly. In areas where large blood spills are commonplace, such as around operating room tables, even this recommendation seems excessive. As long as such units have specialized cleaning protocols and good protective equipment, any hospital disinfectant should suffice. With large spills of cultured or concentrated agents in the laboratory, the contaminated area should be flooded with germicide before cleaning. Otherwise, the area should be cleaned and then decontaminated.

Viral Hemorrhagic Fever

The CDC regards environmental surfaces to be a potential vector of viral hemorrhagic fever transmission. The 1980 recommendations [124] for the treatment of patients with Lassa fever and other acute viral hemorrhagic fevers included special isolation units with exhaust air filtration, use of a chemical toilet, disinfection of all items taken from the patient's room, and disinfection of the vacated room with gaseous formalin or paraldehyde. The CDC 1988 revision [125] restricted concern to patients with confirmed or suspected hemorrhagic fever due to the agents of Lassa, Marburg, or Ebola or Crimean-Congo hemorrhagic fever. A 1995 CDC statement [126] recommends the use of a negative pressure room with an anteroom and HEPA respirators for entering the room of patients with prominent cough, vomiting, diarrhea, or hemorrhage; minimizing laboratory testing; autoclaving, incinerating, or using bleach in washing linen; use of a chemical toilet or bleach disinfection of excretions and fluids before discarding them in the sewer; incineration or decontamination of solid medical waste; and special handling of laboratory specimens.

OTHER ENVIRONMENTAL FACTORS

Carpets

Carpeting a floor increases the microbiologic content per unit of floor surface by approximately four orders of magnitude [127]. Contaminating organisms include *S. aureus, E. coli* and, more rarely, *Pseudomonas.* After removal of carpeting from hospital environments, the carpet content of *S. aureus* remains stable for more than a month and of other organisms for ≤ 6 months. In the best-controlled study, however, the total bacterial content of air was apparently unaffected by the presence or absence of carpet in the sampled area [128]. For areas with carpets, the air content was also not significantly influenced by vacuuming frequency (daily, every other day, or every third day) [128]. Unfortunately, these studies were carried out before the widespread adoption of large, self-propelled, high-pressure cleaner-extractors, which do create transient increases in air fungal content.

The infection hazard of carpets may be more important when patients have direct contact with carpeting (e.g., in pediatric areas) or when patients use wheelchairs. Wet machine cleaning has been associated with *Aspergillus flavus* proliferation. However, it has yet to be demonstrated that any nosocomial infection has arisen from a carpet. In recent years, manufacturers have marketed carpets with antimicrobial substances. As yet, these have not been rigorously assessed in independent studies.

Air-Fluidized Beds

Designed to prevent pressure sores by "flotation," air-fluidized beds have features posing a potential for infection transmission. Flotation is accomplished by driving air up through a 25-cm-deep layer of silicon-coated, soda lime glass microspheres 50 to 150 μm in diameter. The microspheres are held in the bed by a monofilament polyester filter sheet with openings of ~37 μm, through which the microspheres cannot pass. Disinfection of the beds is accomplished by sieving out clumps of beads and organic debris, then operating the bed at high temperature and air flow to inactivate organisms by heat, abrasion [129], and desiccation.

Initial anxieties about the infection hazard from air-fluidized beds have largely dissipated. Beds spiked with *Staphylococcus epidermidis, P. aeruginosa,* and *Bacillus subtilis* did not cause airborne dissemination of these organisms, even shortly after inoculation [130]. The air over beds contaminated by use did not contain more organisms than control air over ordinary beds [131]. A single report of infection transmission, due to *Enterococci*, has appeared [132], suggesting that attention to proper decontamination of these beds is important. There remains the theoretic possibility that the air fluidization process renders airborne those organisms that usually remain harmlessly attached to surfaces (e.g., *M. tuberculosis*), and a study of the beds in the most heavily contaminated contexts has not been undertaken.

Soap

Given the emphasis on hand washing, it is surprising that the problem of soap contamination is not better studied. That the problem is largely theoretic is suggested by the paucity of reported outbreaks attributed to contaminated soap. The outbreak most often cited [133] is relatively unconvincing. Recently, however, clinical illness has been securely attributed to an antiseptic soap [10]. It is reasonable to postulate that it is advantageous to wash the hands with sterile soap (liquid or leaf) dispensed from forearm or leg-operated dispensers that are resistant to contamination. The use of contaminated hand lotion has been implicated in a *P. aeruginosa* outbreak [9].

Data confirming the expected contamination of in-use bar soap have been widely disseminated in the promotion of dispensed liquid soap [134]. However, data comparing the microbial burden on hands washed using a contaminated soap bar with that using uncontaminated nonmedicated soap are unavailable. At the least, it seems prudent to reduce the microbial content of soaps by using disposable liquid soap containers, thoroughly cleaning reusable liquid soap containers or, if bar soap is used, purchasing small bars and providing soap racks that permit water drainage. The relative merits of these alternatives await additional study.

Flowers

Flowers pose two theoretic infection hazards. Vase water inevitably contains large concentrations of potential nosocomial pathogens [135], and decaying organic matter in the dirt of potted plants provides a substrate for fungal growth. Although there are no convincing data establishing vase water as a seat of nosocomial infections, many hospitals bar flowers in water and potted plants from the rooms of immunosuppressed patients and from intensive care units. If vase water were to be disposed of gently and patients, personnel, and visitors washed their hands after touching the water, little danger should arise. Unfortunately, achieving uniform compliance with these precautions is improbable.

Animals

Sanctioned animal contact with hospital patients is of several types: blind or disabled patients or personnel may be accompanied by Seeing Eye or other service animals, pets may be brought to patients, animals may be used to entertain patients or provide pet therapy, and research animals may be housed in areas near patient care units. Although Q fever is the only zoonosis shown to have been associated with epidemics in healthcare facilities, more than 100 organisms infect both humans and other animals [136]. Knowledge of transmission mechanisms of these organisms suggests several prudent measures.

Persons handling Seeing Eye or other dogs should be sure that the dogs are vaccinated against rabies, appear to be free of ectoparasites, and are healthy (in particular, ringworm should not be present). Arrangements should be made for walking the dogs and assuming responsibility for disposal of animal excreta. Pregnant ewes used in research centers have been the source of outbreaks of Q fever [137]. Hospitalized patients have not been affected in these outbreaks; however, airborne transmission to personnel having no direct contact with pregnant ewes has occurred. Although the hazard appears to be most severe at or near parturition [138], it seems prudent to bar all contact between patients and pregnant ewes and to ensure that pregnant ewes used for research are never, even during transportation, in areas from which airborne spread to patients can take place. More stringent recommendations for protection of personnel working with pregnant ewes have been published [139].

Certain animal contacts with children seem inadvisable in any circumstance. Reptiles cannot be reliably certified to be free of salmonellosis, wild carnivores (e.g., skunks, ferrets, raccoons) and bats pose an unacceptably high risk of rabies, and birds of virtually any species may transmit *C. psittaci.* Any contact with animal urine should be followed by hand washing and, if appropriate, more extensive disinfection procedures because of the possibility of leptospirosis. Contact with mouse or hamster urine is also hazardous to the immunocompromised patient because of the possibility of transmission of lymphocytic choriomeningitis virus.

Linen

Laundry processing and the protection of laundry workers is discussed in Chapter 21. This section highlights the hazards to patients. Considering how heavily contaminated soiled linen is [140], it is remarkable how rarely it causes infection. Laundry workers, who have prolonged close contact with soiled linen, seem to be at risk only as a result of exposure to blood-contaminated sharp implements, hepatitis A [141] and other enteric pathogens [142], or unusually infectious organisms, such as *C. burnetii.* None of these dangers represents a meaningful hazard to patients. It seems prudent to handle soiled linen gently to reduce the dispersal of microorganisms in areas dedicated to the care of patients. Beyond that, there is little basis for employing special procedures. Given the improbability that soiled laundry reposing in a partially filled hamper adds organisms to the environment (much less causes infection), it is difficult to understand the emphasis that hospital inspection agencies have previously placed on closing soiled-linen hampers.

Clean laundry, even after cold water processing, contains few pathogenic organisms. Sheets have a total aerobic colony-forming unit count of ~ 0.2 cfu per cubic centimeter, and terry cloth items have ~ 2 cfu per cubic centimeter. The profile of contaminating organisms (*Bacillus* spp, 58%; coagulase-negative staphylococci, 25%; *Corynebacterium* spp, 18%] after cleaning is markedly different from the prewash profile. Pathogenic species are rarely found in washed linen. The proper handling of clean linen during transportation and storage is probably the most important determinant of the microbial content at the time of use. Meyer and colleagues [143] studied newborn intensive care unit laundry that had been washed at 75°C (167°F), dried at 96°C (205°F), and carefully handled. Rodac contact plates showed no organisms one third of the time and >10 colonies per contact plate only 9% of the time. Linen near the top of the stack had a higher incidence of positivity and a greater number of colonies per plate than linen in the middle of the stack, suggesting that handling was the source of transfer of organisms.

Nosocomial *Bacillus cereus* infection has been attributed to clean linen [144,145]. The reported outbreak consisted of *B. cereus* umbilical colonization without clinical signs of infection in normal neonates and neonates in a special baby care unit. The source was considered to be contaminated clean diapers because the implicated *B. cereus* type was found in washed diapers and in the laundry machine. Since the implicated *B. cereus* type was also recovered from the hands of nursing staff, this attribution is unconvincing. Other reports of nosocomial infection due to clean linen—tinea pedis in a nursing home [146], staphylococcal disease in newborns [147], and urinary tract infection [148]—are likewise not persuasive.

The final revision of the American Hospital Association's *Infection Control in the Hospital* [149] recommended autoclaving linen for patients "particularly susceptible to infections," such as burned patients, and for the nursery. The American Academy of Pediatrics [150] supported this recommendation until they softened their stance in 1983 [151]. No consensus body has such a recommendation at present. One line of argument against autoclaving linen arises after consideration of the panoply of techniques required to maintain sterility until the linen reaches the point of use. Applying these procedures to autoclaved linen would be burdensome and costly. Only one rationale for autoclaving laundry seems plausible. Laundry dried in unfiltered air becomes contaminated by *A. fumigatus,* and in specialized patient care units with a very low fungal spore content and low air change rates, a few introduced spores can contribute a substantial portion of the ambient spores [152].

ULTRACLEAN PROTECTIVE ENVIRONMENTS

The ultimate expression of concern that environmental organisms pose an infection hazard is the ultraclean protective environment. When fully developed, these environments have HEPA air filtration with horizontal or vertical laminar airflow; sterile food or food with a low organism content; frequent disinfection of walls, floors, and other environmental surfaces; sterile linen and drinking water; toilet water disinfection; sterile booties, gowns, caps, and gloves for personnel and visitors entering the room; and elaborate protective garb for patients leaving the room. Patients placed in such an environment are generally given oral nonabsorbable, topical, or systemic antimicrobials. This package of protective measures has been termed a *total protective environment*, *life island*, *protected environment*, or *barrier isolation.*

It has long been recognized that these special efforts can produce environmental surfaces and ambient air with markedly diminished organism content [153]. More important, a meta-analysis [154] of random allocation trials of various forms of ultraclean protective environments suggested that this package of techniques produces a statistically significant reduction in the incidence of infection. Of 10 trials [155–164], five showed a statistically significant reduction in overall, severe, or fatal infections. Of the remaining studies, three showed a trend to fewer infections in the protected patients, and one did not report infection rates. This infection prevention effect was generally noted after the second week, a finding in agreement with the view that there is a lag between becoming colonized with a nosocomial pathogen and subsequent infection.

However, the use of ultraprotective environments remains controversial for a number of reasons.

1. *Expense.* In new hospital construction, the capital cost of laminar airflow rooms is not great, especially when amortized over the life of a building. Modular units are commercially available. However, depending on what additional features are incorporated into the protective package, substantial ongoing expenses may be incurred.
2. *Deleterious effects.* During periods of severe illness, seeing only masked and gowned people, being served relatively unpalatable food, remaining confined to a small room, and consuming foul-tasting, diarrheagenic antibiotics aggravates the psychologic stress of having a potentially fatal condition. Premature withdrawal from protected environments, however, may predispose to gut colonization and subsequent disease caused by environmental pathogens.
3. *Difficulty in apportioning benefit among the various features of protected environments.* With few exceptions [162], the available studies deal with the impact of the total package versus conventional treatment of patients. If infections are prevented, it is difficult to factor out which component is responsible. It is even possible that the beneficial effect results from enhanced adherence to standard infection control procedures (e.g., vascular access cannula or Foley catheter management) rather than the protected environment per se.
4. *Doubts about study design.* Diagnosis of infection in very immunosuppressed patients with highly complicated profiles leads to problems. The physicians providing direct care of the patients, who are in the best position to make an assessment, are also the least blinded with respect to the study group. All of these studies are described as using random allocation. However, the vicissitudes of room availability at the time of admission and the many factors involved in assignment of patients to rooms make true randomization awkward. Only six of the studies provide detailed information about comparability of the groups of patients. And the studies conducted by the M. D. Anderson Hospital [155,160] have a troublesome design feature: the protected patients received more intensive chemotherapy. The investigators proceeded on the unproved but logical assumption that subsequent courses of induction could be more intensive in patients with no history of infection. The improved survival may have resulted from the more intensive therapy, which may not have been possible to administer to the control patients, who had been infected more often.
5. *Doubts about the larger significance of a real difference in infection rates.* In many of the studies, the lower infection rate provided only a brief postponement of death; longevity was most strongly influenced by the severity of the underlying illness. The reduction in infection, if real, may be most meaningful for patients treated with potentially curative therapies, such as children with acute lymphocytic leukemia or patients undergoing bone marrow transplantation.

Clearly, special efforts are warranted to lower the airborne fungal spore concentration in the rooms of highly immunosuppressed patients [165]. It is important to consider separately several features of air purification systems. Top-of-the-line bag filters probably remove nearly all fungal spores, but many hospitals prefer HEPA filters because they add relatively little capital expense and meet standards more directly related to microbial filtration. The

CDC has recommended HEPA filtration [104]. It may be desirable to place duct insulation outside the ducts [166]. Placing filters at the point of entrance of air into a patient's room permits safe local maintenance while the room is otherwise unoccupied and accommodates malfunction or maintenance of the central system. Sealing the room and placing it at positive pressure reduces infiltration of spores from the outside or adjacent hospital areas. Increasing the air change rate minimizes the potential exposure of a patient to infiltrating or introduced spores [152].

Air change rates of ≥ 10 per hour are desirable for BMT patients. Rates above 15 to 25 per hour are best accommodated by placing fans and filters next to the rooms, since the caliber of ducts conveying air to and from central systems would have to be too large. Laminar airflow (a misnomer, since objects in a room cause considerable turbulence) units are best thought of as ultrahigh air change rates. Air change rates of 100 to 400 changes per hour can be achieved. Attention to in-room air flow patterns [167] may lead to improvements in the safety of patients without requiring extra resources.

There are concerns associated with other efforts to eliminate a patient's exposure to environmental organisms. Food with low organism content is unpalatable. Organisms on surfaces that do not come in contact with the patient probably are harmless. Elimination of environmental organisms can be very difficult. In one ultraprotective unit, there was a prolonged struggle to eliminate an unusual *Pseudomonas* species from toilet bowl water. Notably, although the organism was present for 20 months, no instance of infection or colonization due to the organism was identified [168].

Except for fungal spore control, ultraprotective environments are not yet an established infection control measure. Even their advocates do not believe they are truly indicated except for patients undergoing bone marrow transplantation or intensive chemotherapy likely to produce > 25 days of granulocytopenia [169]. What is critically needed is analysis of the relative benefit of the components of the protective package.

DISINFECTION AND STERILIZATION

Definitions

Sterilization means the complete elimination or rendering nonviable of all microorganisms, including all spores. Nonviable is best taken to mean the irreversible loss of the ability to propagate indefinitely [170]. Ultraviolet light, although lethal, does not interrupt germination and temporary growth. Conversely, organisms seemingly killed by mercury can be resurrected by compounds that displace mercury from sulfhydryl groups. Disinfection is divided into three levels [171]. *High-level disinfection* means the elimination of all viruses and vegetative microorganisms and most, but not necessarily all, bacterial or fungal spores. *Intermediate disinfection* means the elimination of all vegetative pathogenic bacteria, including *M. tuberculosis,* but not necessarily all viruses (nonenveloped and smaller viruses are more resistant to disinfection) or spores. Inactivation of *M. tuberculosis* is used in this definition not primarily because of concern about *M. tuberculosis* contamination. Mycobactericidal capacity is used because the organism is relatively resistant to disinfection compared with other vegetative bacteria, and a procedure to assess mycobactericidal activity has been established by the Association of Official Analytical Chemists (AOAC) [172]. But even the AOAC procedure has been challenged [173]. Whether the AOAC procedure should be made more stringent or whether the original procedure suffices (since it was used as a surrogate indication of increased disinfectant capacity) is unresolved. *Low-level disinfection,* roughly equivalent to *sanitization,* means the elimination of most pathogenic bacteria. *Cleaning* means the removal of all visible debris. All items should be scrupulously cleaned before disinfection, since disinfecting methods may not penetrate debris. *Antisepsis* is the application of compounds to skins or mucous membranes to reduce microorganism content substantially.

Although the foregoing definitions correspond best to practical use requirements, the EPA, the main regulatory agency for disinfectants and sterilants until 1993, used a noncongruent classification of chemical germicides. *Sporicides* meet an AOAC standard for spore destruction [172]. They achieve sterilization or high-level disinfection depending on contact time. *Hospital disinfectants* inactivate *Salmonella choleraesuis*, *S. aureus*, and *P. aeruginosa* in highly specified AOAC tests [172]. *Disinfectants* and *sanitizers* meet other tests. The EPA registration categories made no reference to effectiveness against *M. tuberculosis*, the critical distinction between intermediate- and low-level disinfectants, or to effectiveness in inactivating all viruses, the critical distinction between high- and intermediate-level disinfection. The FDA is now the regulatory agency for germicides that are sterilants or used for high-level disinfection. Its criteria for labeling are sufficiently stringent that few germicides have achieved sanction.

Kinetics of Microbial Killing

It is generally assumed, although not always supported by experimental evidence, that most microbial inactivation processes follow a "one hit" killing curve. This presumption is equivalent to asserting that all the organisms in the population are equally susceptible to the process. These presumptions can be restated mathematically as follows. The number of microorganisms killed is proportional to the number present, and the proportion does not change as the population of remaining organisms decreases. When the logarithm of the concentration of organisms is displayed on the vertical scale and time on the horizontal scale, this relationship results in the familiar straight-line killing curve. The slope of the killing curve is the measure of the rapidity of organism destruction. It is often expressed as the *decimal reduction time,* the time interval required to bring the concentration of organisms to one tenth its previous concentration (i.e., 90% destruction). The difficulty in validating one-hit kinetics arises because of technical obstacles to experimentally ruling out the possibility that a very small fraction of the starting population of organisms is more resistant to killing. The potential difficulty in killing the last few (possibly more resistant) contaminating organisms is one basis for the overkill present in most sterility standards.

The preceding kinetics analysis establishes the importance of exposure time in accomplishing microbial destruction. A perfectly acceptable disinfection process will fail if not applied for sufficient time. If extremely high numbers of organisms must be inactivated with a very high probability that no survivors remain (e.g., manufacture of some vaccine), prolonged exposure times may be required. Furthermore, a given process may be sanitizing, disinfecting, or sterilizing, depending on the length of time it is applied.

Microbial Safety Index

The kinetics analysis also establishes that the operational assessment of sterility is a probabilistic assertion, not an all-or-nothing phenomenon [174]. This fact has led to the recommendation that the label *sterile* be supplemented by a microbial safety index (MSI) [175], defined as the absolute value of the logarithm of the probability that the item is contaminated.

For example, an item with an MSI of 3 would have a probability of 1 in 1,000 of containing a viable microorganism. As a practical matter, establishing that an item in a lot has an MSI in excess of 3 is extremely difficult by direct microbiologic assessment. With even the most rigorous culture technique, it is difficult to avoid introducing contamination at a level much less than 1 per 1,000 cultured items. Furthermore, the mathematics of sterility testing is unfavorable. For instance, to establish with 95% confidence that a lot containing 10,000 items is contaminated at a rate of less than 1 per 1,000, almost 3,000 of the items must be cultured and found sterile.

Administrative Issues

The Food and Drug Administration requires that reusable medical devices be sold with specific instructions regarding reprocessing methods [171]. The use of alternate methods may invalidate a warranty or create a medicolegal dilemma. The latter problem arises if a product failure damages a patient. The manufacturer may try to shift liability to the hospital because the product was not used according to instructions. Manufacturers may thus escape the stringency of strict liability for product failure.

These same considerations apply to reprocessing disposable items. Through the early 1980s, relevant standard-setting organizations lined up fairly solidly against reprocessing disposable items. The CDC recommended in 1982 that "no disposable object designed for sterile, single use should be resterilized" [176]. This restriction was rescinded in 1985 [177]. Through 1984, the Joint Commission on Accreditation of Healthcare Organizations (JCAHO) flatly opposed any reprocessing. However, the current JCAHO standards are less restrictive, merely requiring hospitals to have written policies that address reprocessing methods [178].

A 1977 FDA policy guide assigned full responsibility to the hospital when disposable medical devices are reused [179]. However, the FDA guide explicitly sanctioned the reuse of disposable items when the facility can establish that the item can be cleaned and sterilized adequately, that its "physical characteristics or quality are not adversely affected by their reprocessing" and, somewhat redundantly, that the product remains safe and effective for its intended use. None of these statements addresses the resterilization of an unused item. Occasionally, an item is removed from its package or else the package is damaged, but the item has not been used. Consistency requires that these items also be resterilized.

A key question, begged by all the aforementioned bodies, is "How does one determine whether an item is disposable?" At present, the manufacturer makes the determination. An item is disposable if it comes in a package labeled with the words *disposable*, *single use only*, or the like. Some manufacturers have added such language to packages of products previously marketed with resterilization instructions. Indeed, manufacturers have little incentive, at least in the short term, to do otherwise. Labeling an item as disposable minimizes liability and maximizes sales volume.

The most compelling case for reuse of disposable items has been made for dialyzers [180–182] (see Chapter 24). First use of hollow-fiber dialyzers may be more often associated with mechanical failure and systemic reactions (fever, chest pain, transient fall in white blood cell count) due to chemicals leaching out of the membrane or increased complement activation by new dialysis membranes. Some first-use-type reactions continue to occur, however, with reused dialyzers [183]. Other items may be very expensive and capable of withstanding reprocessing methods. Since resterilization of an item costs a hospital between $10 and $20, depending on the time required to clean and package it and the sterilization method used, the impetus to reuse exists only for expensive items. A detailed protocol for reuse of specific items has been successfully employed [184].

The JCAHO requires written hospital policies regarding decontamination and sterilization activities, the performance of sterilizing equipment, and the shelf life of all stored sterile items [178]. The CDC guidelines recommend weekly biologic monitoring of all sterilizers [177]. When an implantable device is sterilized, a biologic indicator should be used and found sterile before the device is implanted. A chemical indicator should be visible on the outside of all sterilized packages. Careful follow-up of unconverted indicators should be undertaken, since investigation often turns up significant problems [185].

Choice of Sterilization or Disinfection Level

Support continues for Spaulding's classification scheme indicating the level of sterilization or disinfection required for various items [171,177,186]. *Critical* items enter tissue or the vascular space. *Semicritical* items come into contact with mucous membranes or nonintact skin. *Noncritical* items touch intact skin. Critical items are generally held to require sterilization, semicritical items to require high-level disinfection, and noncritical items to require intermediate- or low-level disinfection [171,176,187]. Virtually all germicides are effective against HIV [188].

High-level disinfection is, in fact, rather difficult to achieve. Most germicides require 20 to 45 minutes to attain tuberculobactericidal activity, exposure times well in excess of common usage [189]. Furthermore, if a device really has to be at a state of high-level disinfection at the time of subsequent use on another patient, it would have to be subject to sterile water rinsing, manipulation using sterile technique, air drying with filtered air, and protective wrapping. Such precautions are rarely part of hospital practice [189]. Nor are they called for in many specialty societies' published guidelines for the reprocessing of semicritical items [190]. This amounts to an acknowledgment that organisms carried over from the previous patient are the primary target of reprocessing techniques. This is a rational emphasis provided that the disinfected device is protected from "water bacteria" by complete drying and from gross recontamination or hand contact before subsequent usage.

The assertion that all semicritical items must be processed by high-level disinfection is difficult to justify. To make this claim is to suggest that items coming into contact with mucous membranes can be contaminated with no more than a few bacterial or fungal spores. High-level disinfection seems unwarranted for items that will touch normally contaminated mucous membranes, such as the mouth or the colon. The distinction made between mouthpieces, for which some authorities have recommended high-level disinfection [189], and silverware is difficult to understand. For items in contact with the gut, elimination of carryover enteric pathogens is the goal. Unfortunately, assessment of the ability to inactivate small nonenveloped viruses, which are the most resistant enteric pathogens, is not routinely available.

The evolution of the category of intermediate-level disinfection is intriguing. It was not included in the CDC guidelines published through 1983 [191]. The category was defined in the 1985 CDC revision [177], although there were no specific recommendations for how to achieve it nor distinctions made between items requiring low- versus intermediate-level disinfection. In 1987, Rutala and Weber's table combined low- and intermediate-level disinfection [192]. In the 1990 Association for Practitioners in Infection Control (APIC) [193] guideline, the categories were separated and specific indications given for each. Both were described with *maximum* exposure times, suggesting that the briefest contact with the disinfectant suffices. Unfortunately, although the difficulty in achieving and maintaining high-level disinfection establishes the usefulness of a less-intensive disinfection level, there remains practically no rigorous study or body of evidence providing a foundation for the category of intermediate-level disinfection.

Special issues regarding certain devices should be recognized. Nebulizers produce, by design, particles that become deposited in the alveoli. Accordingly, nebulizer cups and solutions intended for nebulization must be sterile. Endoscopic retrograde cholangiopancreatography is potentially much more hazardous than all other forms of endoscopy as a result of the vulnerability of partially obstructed biliary tracts to infection and the severe nature of acute cholangitis. Contamination of the biliary tract can arise if the water channel in an endoscope used for the procedure holds contaminated water. When water is expelled from the catheter, then drawn back into the suction channel, organisms introduced into the suction channel can be picked up by the cannula before introduction above the ampulla of Vater.

Tonometers pose special difficulties. Numerous adenovirus outbreaks have resulted from inadequate disinfection procedures [194,195]. Adenoviruses, which are small and lipid free, are relatively difficult to disinfect. Furthermore, tonometer tips are expensive, harmed by many disinfectants, and used frequently. In addition, pneumotonometer tips have a cavity that can retain germicides with the potential for subsequent damage of a patient's cornea. The American Academy of Ophthalmology's recommendations for simple alcohol wiping do not achieve even intermediate-level disinfection [196]. The CDC, in turn, has recommended disinfection procedures in excess of those ordinarily associated with intermediate-level disinfection [194]. Automated reprocessing machines have also produced disinfection failures [197]. Standards for evaluating these machines have been published [198].

Table 20-1 presents the sterilization and disinfection levels used at the University of Minnesota Hospital and Clinic. In general, *sterilization* is required for items that enter tissue, the vascular system, or the biliary tract; items that penetrate the vagina of a woman in labor or after rupture of membranes; objects that can be kept sterile to the point of contact with normally sterile mucous membranes (e.g., the bladder); and the blood-contacting surfaces of blood recirculating machines. *High-level disinfection* is essential for items that come into contact with normally sterile mucous membranes but cannot be kept sterile to the point of membrane contact (e.g., the bronchi); instruments that come into contact with mucous membranes with minimal flora (e.g., conjunctiva); dialysis machine surfaces in contact with dialysate; and channels through which biopsy forceps or other instruments requiring sterilization must pass. *Intermediate-level disinfection* is required for items that touch normally nonsterile mucous membranes (except the vagina after rupture of membranes) and those that come into contact with nonintact skin. *Low-level disinfection* is necessary for articles that normally need only cleaning but because of special circumstances require disinfection, items that may be mouthed by infants, objects that are used repeatedly in the mouth of a single patient, hydrotherapy tanks and infant bathtubs, and items that ordinarily need only cleaning if they have become contaminated by blood or other infectious material.

The requirements outlined in the table are less stringent than many have advocated but are probably more rigorous than those actually put into practice in many institutions. The major variation from standard practice is the use of intermediate-level disinfection for many devices that contact normally nonsterile membranes. Intermediate-level disinfection (discussed later) is also defined more rigorously. Many of the distinctions in the table are arbitrary and reflect what can be practically accomplished. Rigid endoscopes can be steam-auto-

TABLE 20-1. *Minimum sterilization/disinfection level requirements for various items*

Sterilization	Arthroscope
	Cardiac catheter
	Culdoscope
	Cystoscope
	Dental: forceps, scalpels, bone chisels, scalers, and other instruments; burrs, hand pieces, antiretraction valves, other intraoral devices attached to air or water lines, prophylaxis angles, ultrasonic scaler tips, air/water syringe tips, saliva ejectors, air evacuator tips, prophylaxis cups and brushes
	Dermabrasion wheel
	Endoscopic biopsy forceps, cannulas, papillotomes, guide wires
	Endoscope, rigid
	Implantable device
	Intravascular device
	Needle
	Peritoneoscope
	Surgical instrument
	Transducer head
	Ureteroscope
	Urinary catheter
	Urological laser
	Vaginal speculum (for use after rupture of membranes)
High-level disinfection	Bronchoscope
	Cryoprobe
	Dental: mirrors, amalgam condensers
	Dialysis machine surfaces in contact with dialysate
	Endoscope, flexible fiberoptic or video
	Endotracheal tube
	Laryngeal blades
	Maschiadscope
	Prostate ultrasound probe
	Sinuscope
	Tonometer tip
Intermediate-level disinfection	Anoscope
	Bite blocks (between patients)
	Breast pump surfaces in contact with milk
	Breathing circuit
	Dental: items to be handled in the laboratory, such as impressions, bite registrations, fixed and removable prosthesis, orthodontic appliances
	Ear speculum and ear-examining instruments
	EEG/EKG electrode
	Electric razor head
	Laryngeal mirror
	Mouthpiece, anesthesia or pulmonary function testing
	Nasal speculum
	Thermometer (between patients)
	Transesophageal electrode
	Vaginal speculum (except during labor or after rupture of membranes)
	Vaginal ultrasound probe
	Ventilation bag connector
Low-level disinfection	Bathtub, infant
	Bite blocks, radiation therapy (between uses by a single patient)
	Hydrotherapy tanks
	Infant furniture
	Thermometers (between uses by a single patient)
	Toy, infant
Cleaning—between all patients	Bathtubs, ceramic
	Bedpans
	Bed rails
	Earphones
	Food utensil
	Nasal gas administration hood, dental
Cleaning—when visibly soiled	Blood pressure cuff
	Electric razor body
	Examination table
	Shampoo tray

claved so they are sterilized. A laryngeal blade passes the epiglottis to a sterile mucous membrane (and may penetrate or lacerate tissue) and is subjected to high-level disinfection, while a laryngeal mirror is subjected to only intermediate-level disinfection. Dental items are upgraded beyond the general scheme because of a consensus set of recommendations [199].

Many endoscopy systems, ultrasound probes, and other semicritical items are now marketed with disposable sheaths. In theory, the underlying item should need no reprocessing whatsoever after the sheath is discarded. Unfortunately, there is relatively little independent assessment of the integrity and durability of these sheaths. Clearly, if a defect in the sheath is detected after use or if the underlying item is visibly contaminated with a patient's secretions, the item should be reprocessed as if it had been used without a sheath. Otherwise it is probably sufficient to reprocess the item using low-level disinfection.

Steam Sterilization

Steam sterilization is highly reliable and is the method of choice when the device can tolerate the procedure. Nevertheless, there are subtleties to its use that sometimes go unrecognized. Steam is more than an efficient conveyor of heat. The water molecules participate in the denaturation of proteins and the disruption of other complex molecules. Accordingly, it is essential that steam reach all the surfaces to be sterilized. In gravity displacement autoclaves, the introduced steam, which is less dense than air, forces air down and out through the autoclave drain. Devices with depressions that are not placed on their side or that have curved lumens will not be completely exposed to steam. The AAMI standard for 132°C (270°F) sterilization assumes that this problem can be overcome by extending the cycle to 10 minutes [69]. Unfortunately, if steam does not reach the surface, this is equivalent to dry heat, a process that is generally held to require 2 hours of exposure. The penetration of steam into wrapped packages, porous materials, or in overpacked chambers is also not secure in gravity displacement autoclaves. These problems are mitigated in vacuum displacement autoclaves, which are evacuated before the introduction of steam. Pulsed vacuum autoclaves are even more efficient, since they go through several cycles of vacuum and steam replacement, thus more reliably eliminating air.

Flash autoclaving also has attendant problems. The term itself is used variably to refer to short-duration, high-temperature steam autoclaving; the autoclaving of devices without wrapping; gravity displacement autoclaving; or some combination of the foregoing procedures. There is doubtlessly a need for rapid sterilization of low-inventory instruments that inadvertently become contaminated during surgery or highly tailored implantable items for which it is difficult to maintain a complete sterile inventory. Recent evidence suggests that the widely accepted 3-minute standard for 132°C (270°F) autoclaving should be extended to 4 minutes [200]. Anxieties about the low margin of safety from the 3-minute autoclaving underlie the CDC's recommendation [177] that the 3-minute cycle is not sufficient for implantable objects. The CDC did not specify any minimum duration for implantable objects, although the AAMI suggests that 10 minutes will suffice [69].

The duration of sterilization cycles at standard sterilization temperatures (121°C [250°F]) for liquids is also somewhat arbitrary. In this situation, steam is conveying only heat; thus, by extension from the standard 30-minute cycle for solid objects, longer times should be required for large volumes of liquids. The fact that most standards recommend < 30 minutes or, for volumes in excess of 1 L, only 45 minutes, probably reflects the low organism burden of most such materials before sterilization.

Selection and Use of Germicides

There are many physical techniques and chemical agents that are useful in various contexts for disinfection or sterilization [201]. A summary of methods appropriate for various uses has been updated periodically and was last published by the CDC in 1983 [176,191]. Unfortunately, the CDC was forced to refrain from tying recommendations closely to particular products. The substituted CDC environmental guideline published in 1985 [177] discussed disinfectants and sterilants in a more general way. Revisions of the initial CDC summary have appeared [193,202]; they are presented in the APIC's "Guideline for Selection and Use of Disinfectants," written by Rutala [186]. Given the increase in type and composition of medical devices and the great variety of disinfection methods, this tabular approach is an oversimplification. The object categories overlap and are not comprehensive. And the descriptions of methods are largely references to manufacturers' recommendations for germicide concentrations, temperatures, and exposure times.

The APIC guideline [186] contains a superb discussion of the mechanisms of action, advantages and disadvantages, and tips on use of various disinfection methods. Besides the level of sterilization or disinfection, selection of a method necessitates considering its impact on the integrity of the device to be reprocessed, the possible affects on the warranty of the product and liability exposure, and occupational safety. Ethylene oxide, formaldehyde, and glutaraldehyde all pose potential risks to personnel. A proposed federal glutaraldehyde exposure standard, 0.2 parts per million (ppm) ceiling, will preclude glutaraldehyde use without evacuation hoods, personnel protection devices, or special enclosed reprocessors [203]. Whatever technique is selected, the manufacturer's instructions should be used to determine contact times and other use parameters. The disinfectant must be in contact with all relevant surfaces for the entire specified contact time.

It is commonly recommended that a particular product be purchased based on reference to standard guidelines, scientific literature, and manufacturers' recommendations. At a practical level, however, it is very difficult to use the first two. There is such a profusion of products that the standard recommendations [177,186] do not have enough specificity. Furthermore, manufacturers regularly modify their formulations and freely assert that flaws described in scientific publications [173,204] have been corrected. Thus, users are forced to rely on manufacturers' information. The only effectively regulated statement from manufacturers is that found on the label applied to the actual product.

The EPA has required that companies generate data underlying a claim that a product is a sporicide, hospital disinfectant (i.e., meets AOAC standards for disinfection of *S. aureus*, *P. aeruginosa*, and *S. choleraesuis*), or tuberculocide. The label has to specify the dilution, exposure time, and any other conditions required to achieve these disinfection. Reliance on the label is tricky for several reasons: the EPA or FDA can only irregularly independently verify manufacturers' claims [177,205,206], independent testing has revealed failures to meet standards [207], some disinfectant types may be inherently deficient [193], translating the EPA/FDA categories into the high-, intermediate-, and low-level disinfection system is somewhat arbitrary, and manufacturers do not always put all relevant information on the label. A manufacturer's written statement that a given product passes certain AOAC tests is important even if it is not independently verified.

Notwithstanding all the difficulties attending reliance on the EPA-registered product label and other written statements by manufacturers, most users must depend on them in product selection. At the University of Minnesota Hospital and Clinic, sterilization is considered achievable by any germicide that passes the AOAC test as a sporicide when it is used at the dilution, temperature, and exposure time required for sporicidal activity. In addition, steam, ethylene oxide, and dry heat are believed to produce sterilization. When a liquid germicide is used for sterilization, the item to be sterilized must be rinsed in sterile water, thoroughly dried, and enclosed in a sterile package.

High-level disinfection is considered possible using any germicide that passes AOAC tests as a sporicide and a tuberculocide when used at a dilution, temperature, and time required to produce tuberculocidal activity. After high-level disinfection, rinsing in tap water followed by thorough drying and low touch handling is permitted. In addition, high-level disinfection is considered feasible with use of sodium hypochlorite at 10,000 ppm for 5 minutes and 1,000 ppm for 20 minutes and pasteurization at 75°C (170°F) for 30 minutes or at 90°C (195°F) for 10 minutes [208]. Intermediate-level disinfection is believed to be effected by any germicide that passes AOAC tests as a hospital disinfectant and a tuberculocide when used at the concentration and temperature required to produce tuberculocidal activity with an exposure time of ≥ 10 minutes. Also accepted are sodium hypochlorite at 1,000 ppm and ethanol or isopropyl alcohol at 70% to 90% at an exposure time of 10 minutes. There is no actual evidence of effectiveness for the 10-minute exposure time. Finally, low-level disinfection is considered achievable through the use of any germicide that passes AOAC tests as a hospital disinfectant when used at the label concentration and temperature required to produce hospital disinfection—sodium hypochlorite at 100 ppm and ethanol or isopropyl alcohol at 70% to 90%. There is no specified minimum exposure time for low-level disinfection; merely wiping with the disinfectant is thought to be sufficient.

Creutzfeldt-Jakob Agent

The Creutzfeldt-Jakob agent and other prions are transmissible proteins in conformations that irreversibly autocatalize conversion of the native proteins to the nonfunctional conformation. They are unusually resistant to inactivation. Transmission to humans has happened from stereotactic instruments, pituitary-derived growth hormone, corneal transplants, and dura mater grafts. Sporadic cases in histopathology technicians has provoked anxiety about transmission to healthcare workers [209, 210]. Critical and semicritical items previously in contact with brain tissue from Creutzfeldt-Jakob patients should be autoclaved for 1 hour at 132°C (270°F), immersed for 1 hour in 1 N sodium hydroxide, or both [211]. Although blood and spinal fluid have been found to transmit prions experimentally, there is no practical way to apply disinfecting methods to all the surfaces these body substances can come into contact with. Given the frequency with which Creutzfeldt-Jakob disease remains undiagnosed, the potential for transmission by tissues other than brain, and the paucity of adequate disinfection methods, there is currently no practical way to accommodate fully the potential for transmission of this agent.

ENVIRONMENTAL SAMPLING

Routine Microbiologic Surveillance of Inanimate Objects

Environmental sampling accounted for a large fraction of nosocomial infection control efforts in the United States through 1970. As late as 1976, 74% of hospitals with 50 beds or more conducted routine environmental culturing [212]. This activity was conducted despite explicit statements by the CDC in 1970 [213] and the American Hospital Association in 1973 [214] recommending sharp circumscription of such routine culturing. These statements advocated abandonment of the practice of routinely culturing floors, walls, linens, and air but left open the possibility of conducting epidemiologically indicated cultures, spot-checking critical hospital equipment items (e.g., respiratory care equipment), undertaking routine microbial evaluation of hospital-prepared infant formula, and verifying sterilization procedures. Only the last procedure, however, was deemed necessary (see Chapter 9).

Possible grounds for routine culturing of inanimate objects include prevention of infection, education of personnel, and responding to the guidelines put forth by a number of organizations and government agencies. To contribute to the prevention of infection, the culture must at least have an interpretable result. When sterility is the goal, interpretation is possible. Culturing may also be of value, however, when the need for sterility is not established (e.g., infant formula, dialysis water). Perhaps the best operational definition of interpretability is that certain results lead to specific actions. An additional, less commonly articulated criterion is that the cultured object have a high enough probability of contamination, with a severe enough consequence if contaminated, to justify the culture. Routine culturing of purchased sterile supplies is not justified because of the very low chance of a positive culture.

The educational value of culturing inanimate objects is limited but may be a valid adjunct to other teaching efforts. Care must be taken to prevent such efforts from growing beyond the bounds of a specific educational objective. Responding to the guidelines of various organizations quickly becomes an arcane and ineffectual exercise. First, these organizations have considerably varied standings. One *must* comply with the rules of regulatory agencies such as the FDA, the federal and state Occupational Health and Safety Administration, or the Federal End Stage Renal Dialysis (ESRD) program. Any hospital with a training program must meet the standards of the JCAHO. However, compliance is less essential in terms of the recommendations of the many respected government (e.g., the CDC) and nongovernment (e.g., the AAMI) agencies.

A second problem in formulating a hospital's response to these various guidelines is that the statements themselves are sometimes frankly inconsistent. For instance, the CDC's "Draft Guideline for Prevention of Intravascular Device–Related Infections" [215] made no mention of culturing hospital-compounded infusion solutions at a time when the JCAHO seemed to require such culturing. A third problem, ambiguity, is illustrated by the JCAHO statement on monitoring parenteral medication. Through 1991 (but not thereafter), solutions "manufactured" in the hospital were supposed to "be examined on a sampling basis." We can only asssume that the intent was to subject solutions to microbiologic examination.

A fourth problem is the lack of regular updating. Although some agencies, such as the JCAHO and AAMI, have instituted formal updating that includes specific rescission of previous statements, others have actually disbanded (e.g., the National Coordinating Committee on Large-Volume Parenterals (NCCLVP) sponsored by the USP and FDA [216]). A fifth complexity involves interlocking use of these dicta. The AAMI dialysis water–culturing protocol is explicitly intended to be flexible. However, the federal ESRD program requires exact compliance [217]. The American Society of Hospital Pharmacists has formally accepted the NCCLVP recommendations, giving them a longevity beyond that of their creator [216]. Despite these complexities, infection control personnel must consider the statements of these bodies in making decisions about culturing inanimate objects. If nothing else, these statements can assume substantial medicolegal importance.

A general problem that arises in considering culturing protocols for any product is determining when in the preparation-use sequence to perform the culture. It is logistically simpler to obtain the culture at the point of preparation, and the impetus to culture implements and objects used in the care of patients often comes from the quality control effort of the department preparing them. However, more relevant to patients' care is the status of the item at the time of its actual use. If cultures are positive at the end of the preparation-use sequence, efforts may be undertaken to determine the sources of contamination.

Some unusual biologic items probably should be routinely cultured. Organs, including corneas, bone, kidneys, livers, hearts, pancreases, and bone marrow for transplantation (especially if highly processed), may become contaminated in procurement, transportation, or storage. Positive cultures can have therapeutic implications in addition to suggesting the need for improvements in sterilization techniques. A biologic product that probably does not need routine culture is banked, expressed human milk intended for prompt ingestion by the donor's offspring. It is administered orally and inevitably is frequently contaminated [218]. However, standards for donor selection, milk pasteurization, and microbiologic screening in other contexts have been published [219]. Consensus on two possible recommendations—routine culturing of hospital water for *Legionella* and of air for fungi—may yet emerge. Routine culturing of air should be relevant only in hospitals with highly immunosuppressed patients.

Dialysis Water

The AAMI standard for culturing dialysis water (presented earlier) has been endorsed by the CDC [177]. Sampling should be conducted at least monthly. It is preferable to sample system water just before a disinfection cycle. Machine water should be taken from different machines to ensure that all defects are identified.

Hospital-Compounded Pharmacy Products

At present there is confusion regarding whether the production, mixing, or aliquoting of sterile materials by hospital pharmacies should be considered compounding or manufacturing. Preparations for individual patients clearly fall into the former category. Batches made in advance for many patients may be interpreted as being of the latter type. The implications are considerable. Compounding is governed by state boards of pharmacy and is subject to less stringent requirements. Manufacturing is regulated by the FDA and, thus, must comply with Good Manufacturing Practice [220]. These standards, like JCAHO standards, are broadly phrased but are taken to require detailed compliance. With respect to sterility, these requirements call for culturing two items from batches of < 20 items, 10% of lots of 20 to 200 items, and 20 units of larger lots [220]; detailed culturing procedures that include 14 days of observation for most items [220]; and quarantine of an entire batch until the sterility testing is completed [220]. These stipulations would be burdensome for hospital pharmacies.

Additional considerations apply to infusion solutions. A 1980 NCCLVP statement "endorses the concept of hospital pharmacies using sterility testing of IV admixtures as a method for monitoring the performances of pharmacy equipment and personnel" [216]. The rationale is worded to avoid the demand that sterility testing be completed before administering the solutions. The JCAHO eliminated an apparent requirement for culturing of parenteral medications and solutions in 1992.

These recommendations may be challenged on several grounds. The bulk of infusion-caused infection arises from organisms ascending along the tissue-cannula interface rather than by fluid contamination (see Chapter 44). Much of the contamination of in-use infusion fluid probably arises during administration rather than compounding. Even the need for sterility of infusion fluid is arguable. Most in-use fluid contamination is present at very low concentrations, is due to relatively nonpathogenic strains, and has not been proved to be associated with illness. The least irrational program of infusion fluid culturing would focus on the in-use product, would use culture methods that do not yield positive cultures with very low levels of contamination, and would involve organism speciation to identify properly the few hazardous species capable of proliferating in the product.

Respiratory Therapy and Anesthesia Equipment

The current CDC "Guideline for the Prevention of Nosocomial Pneumonia" [104] does not contain a recommendation for or against culturing respiratory therapy equipment. No recent organizational statement favors it. Advocates of routine culturing of breathing circuits must surmount two counter arguments: first, that there is no secure demonstration that small numbers of organisms on internal surfaces of breathing circuits cause disease and, second, that in-use breathing circuits frequently become contaminated with the patient's organisms even if the circuits start out sterile [221]. Most reports of infection caused by contamination of breathing circuits are not convincing. In others, it is not possible to be sure the contamination was of tubing rather than of a nebulizer or that the tubing was thoroughly dried after reprocessing [222]. Any program of routine culturing of these items should cope with the logistic problem of examining the most relevant specimens–those actually in use.

Laminar Airflow Hoods

Since HEPA filters do develop leaks, routine periodic evaluation is indicated. However, dioctyl phthalate testing is more reliable than using settling plates or other microbiologic assessments [223]. Through 1991 the JCAHO required microbiologic monitoring, but in 1992 the requirement was abridged to call for "a suitable area for manipulation of parenteral medications."

Formula

Through 1977, successive editions of *Standards and Recommendations for Hospital Care of Newborn Infants,* published by the American Academy of Pediatrics [150], recommended routine culturing of hospital-manufactured formula obtained from nursing units. Plate counts exceeding 25 organisms per milliliter were deemed to indicate that technique was faulty and immediate corrective action required. The CDC supported this measure in 1982 [176]. A 1983 American Academy of Pediatrics and American College of Obstetricians and Gynecologists publication, *Guidelines for Perinatal Care* [151], has superseded the former series, and it is silent with respect to culturing hospital-manufactured formula. Similarly, subsequent statements by the American Hospital Association [149] and the JCAHO contain no reference to this issue. Abandonment of this widely accepted practice—even by those skeptical of environmental culturing [224]—probably reflects a perception that most hospitals have switched to commercially prepared formulas. Although this is true of routine infant care, there is an increase in the development of hospital-prepared specialized enteral feedings, for which specific guidelines may need to be developed.

Clearly, it is necessary for infant formula and adult enteral supplements to be free of enteric pathogens and organisms capable of generating enterotoxins (e.g., *S. aureus*). It seems desirable that formula also be free of high concentrations of potent nosocomial pathogens. Neonatal *Klebsiella* bacteremia has followed oral ingestion of *Klebsiella*-contaminated breast milk [225]. *Enterobacter sakazakii* diarrhea with bacteremia in neonates has resulted from imbibing contaminated powdered milk [226]. Freedom from *Aspergillus flavus* is probably desirable for all foodstuffs because of the potential of aflatoxin production. Nonetheless, previous recommendations do not call for organism identification, and it is unclear that even large numbers of organisms, excluding those mentioned previously, constitute any hazard.

Establishing protocols for culturing formula leads to many questions:

1. *Which of the many formulas hospitals now make must meet the standard?* The usual age cutoff for infants is 1 year, but it is likely that a contaminated enteral formula poses a greater hazard to an immunocompromised adult than to a relatively healthy 11-month-old baby.
2. *What culture methods should be used?* Since dry formula powder may contain high concentrations of spores, culture techniques that promote thermophilic organism growth frequently produce excessive counts from nonhazardous formulas.
3. *If counts exceed 25 cfu per milliliter, what actions should be taken?* Hospitals producing many small batches of highly individualized enteral formulas find it very burdensome to use sterile blenders and, when possible, sterile formula components. Blenders are often difficult to sanitize because of the crevices in the blade housing. Many specialized supplements rapidly lose nutritional value at 100°C (212°F), precluding postpreparation treatment.

The least arbitrary routine culturing program would focus on formula to be given to the most debilitated neonates or other patients, would use culturing methods yielding only human pathogens—perhaps only enteric pathogens—and would be considered only a marginal supplement to general sanitary measures.

REFERENCES

1. Anonymous. *Oxford English dictionary*. Glasgow: Oxford University Press, 1971.
2. Cahill CK, Heath J. Sterile water used for humidification in low-flow oxygen therapy: Is it necessary? *Am J Infect Control* 1990;18:13.
3. Beck-Sague CM, Jarvis WR. Epidemic bloodstream infections associated with pressure transducers: a persistent problem. *Infect Control Hosp Epidemiol* 1989;10:54.
4. Mead JH, Lupton GP, Dillavon CL, Odom RB. Cutaneous *Rhizopus* infection: occurrence as a postoperative complication associated with an elasticized adhesive dressing. *JAMA* 1979;242:272.
5. Pearson RD, Valenti WM, Steigbigel RT. *Clostridium perfringens* wound infection associated with elastic bandages. *JAMA* 1980;244:1128.
6. Mitchell SJ, Gray J, Morgan MEI, Hocking MD, Durbin GM. Nosocomial infection with *Rhizopus microsporus* in preterm infants: association with wooden tongue depressors. *Lancet* 1996;348:441.
7. Hoffman PC, et al. False-positive blood cultures: association with non-sterile blood collection tubes. *JAMA* 1976;236:2073.
8. Semel JD, et al. *Pseudomonas maltophilia* pseudosepticemia. *Am J Med* 1978;64:403.
9. Becks VE, Lorenzoni NM. *Pseudomonas aeruginosa* outbreak in a neonatal intensive care unit: a possible link to contaminated hand lotion. *Am J Infect Control* 1995;23:396.
10. Parrott PL, et al. *Pseudomonas aeruginosa* peritonitis associated with contaminated poloxamer-iodine solution. *Lancet* 1982;2:683.
11. Kallings LO. Contamination of therapeutic agents. In: *Proceedings of the International Conference on Nosocomial Infections*. Chicago: American Hospital Association, 1970:241–245.
12. Perry WD, et al. Transmission of group-A streptococci. I. The role of contaminated bedding. *Am J Hyg* 1957;66:85.
13. Perry WD, Siegel AC, Rammelkamp CH Jr. Transmission of group-A streptococci. II. The role of contaminated dust. *Am J Hyg* 1957;66:96.
14. Rammelkamp CH Jr, et al. Transmission of group-A streptococci. III. The effect of drying on the infectivity of the organism for man. *J Hyg (London)* 1958;56:280.
15. LeRudulier D, et al. Molecular biology of osmoregulation. *Science* 1984;224:1064.
16. Nerurkar LS, West F, Madden DL, Sever JL. Survival of herpes simplex virus in water specimens collected from hot tubs in spa facilities and on plastic surfaces. *JAMA* 1983;250:3081.
17. Douglas JM, Corey L. Fomites and herpes simplex viruses: a case for nonvenereal transmission? *JAMA* 1983;250:3093.
18. Maki DG, Alvarado CJ, Hassemer CA, Zilz MA. Relation of the inanimate hospital environment to endemic nosocomial infections. *N Engl J Med* 1982;307:1562.
19. Lauer JL, Van Drunen NA, Washburn JW, Balfour HH Jr. Transmission of hepatitis B virus in clinical laboratory areas. *J Infect Dis* 1979;140:512.
20. Mortimer EA Jr, Wolinsky E, Gonzaga AJ, Rammelkamp CH Jr. Role of airborne transmission in staphylococcal infections. *Br Med J* 1966;1:319.
21. Gellert GA, et al. An outbreak of acute gastroenteritis caused by a small round structured virus in a geriatric convalescent facility. *Infect Control Hosp Epidemiol* 1990;11:459.
22. Maslow J, Mulligan ME. Epidemiologic typing systems. *Infect Control Hosp Epidemiol* 1996;17:595.
23. Rodriguez E, De Meeus T, Mallie M, et al. Multicentric epidemiological study of *Aspergillus fumigatus* isolates by multilocus enzyme electrophoresis. *J Clin Microbiol* 1996;34:2559.
24. Kundsin RB, ed. Airborne contagion. *Ann N Y Acad Sci* 1980;353:1.
25. Muilenberg ML, Burge HA. *Aerobiology*. Boca Raton: Lewis Publishers, 1996.
26. Eickhoff TC. Airborne disease: including chemical and biological warfare. *Am J Epidemiol* 1996;144:S39.
27. Eickhoff TC. Airborne nosocomial infection: a contemporary perspective. *Infect Control Hosp Epidemiol* 1994;15:663.
28. Brachman PS. Nosocomial infection: airborne or not? In: *Proceedings of the International Conference on Nosocomial Infections*. Chicago: American Hospital Association, 1970:189–192.
29. Lidwell OM. Airborne bacteria and surgical infection. *Am J Med* 1981;70:693.
30. Iwen PC, Davis JC, Reed EC, Winfield BA, Hinrichs SH. Airborne fungal spore monitoring in a protective environment during hospital construction and correlation with an outbreak of invasive aspergillosis. *Infect Control Hosp Epidemiol* 1994;15:303.
31. Sayer WJ, Shean DB, Ghosseiri J. Estimation of airborne fungal flora by the Andersen sampler versus the gravity settling culture plate. I. Isolation frequency and number of colonies. *J Allergy* 1969;48:214.
32. Burge HA. *Bioaerosols*. Boca Raton: Lewis Publishers, 1995.
33. Greene VW, Vesley D, Bond RG, Michaelsen GS. Microbiological contamination of hospital air. I. Quantitative studies. *Appl Microbiol* 1962;10:561.
34. Greene VW, Vesley D, Bond RG, Michaelsen GS. Microbiological studies of hospital air. II. Qualitative studies. *Appl Microbiol* 1962;10:567.
35. Bean B, et al. Influenza B: hospital activity during a community epidemic. *Diagn Microbiol Infect Dis* 1983;1:177.
36. Noble WC. Dispersal of microorganisms from skin. In: *Microbiology of human skin*, 2nd ed. London: Lloyd-Luke Ltd., 1981:79–85.
37. Shaffer JG, Key ID. A three-year study of carpeting in a general hospital. *Health Lab Sci* 1969;6:215.
38. Wenzel RP, Veazey JM Jr, Townsend TR. Role of the inanimate environment in hospital-acquired infections. In: Cundy KR, Ball W, eds. *Infection control in healthcare facilities: microbiological surveillance*. Baltimore: University Park Press, 1977:71–98.
39. Committee on Trauma, Division of Medical Sciences, National Academy of Sciences–National Research Council. Postoperative wound infections: the influence of ultraviolet irradiation of the operating room and of various other factors. *Ann Surg* 1964;160 (suppl):1.
40. Turner AG, Craddock JG. *Klebsiella* in a thoracic ICU. *Hospitals* 1973;47:79.
41. Dexter F. *Pseudomonas aeruginosa* in a regional burn center. *J Hyg* 1971;69:179.

42. Bauer TM, et al. An epidemiological study assessing the relative importance of airborne and direct contact transmission of microorganisms in a medical intensive care unit. *J Hosp Infect* 1990;15:301.
43. Cheng K, Smyth RL, Govan JRW, et al. Spread of β-lactam-resistant *Pseudomonas aeruginosa* in a cystic fibrosis clinic. *Lancet* 1996;348: 639.
44. LiPuma JJ,et al. Person-to-person transmission of *Pseudomonas cepacia* between patients with cystic fibrosis. *Lancet* 1990;336:1094.
45. Blessing-Moore J, Maybury B, Lewiston N, Yeager A. Mucosal droplet spread of *Pseudomonas aeruginosa* from cough of patients with cystic fibrosis. *Thorax* 1979;34:429.
46. Grieble HG, Bird TJ, Nidea HM, Miller CA. Chute-hydropulping waste disposal system: a reservoir of enteric bacilli and *Pseudomonas* in a modern hospital. *J Infect Dis* 1974;130:602.
47. Kelsen SG, McGuckin M. The role of airborne bacteria in the contamination of fine-particle nebulizers and the development of nosocomial pneumonia. *Ann N Y Acad Sci* 1980;353:218.
48. Kelsen SG, McGuckin M, Kelsen DP, Cherniak NS. Airborne contamination of fine-particle nebulizers. *JAMA* 1977;237:2311.
49. Dark FA, Callow DS. The effect of growth conditions on the survival of airborne *E. coli*. In: Hers JF, Winkler KC, eds. *Airborne transmission and airborne infection*. New York: Wiley, 1973:97–99.
50. Marthi B, Fieland VP, Walter M, Seidler RJ. Survival of bacteria during aerosolization. *Appl Environ Microbiol* 1990;56:3463.
51. Grieble HG, et al. Fine-particle humidifiers: source of *Pseudomonas aeruginosa* infections in a respiratory-disease unit. *N Engl J Med* 1970;282:531.
52. Smith PW, Massanari RM. Room humidifiers as the source of *Acinetobacter* infections. *JAMA* 1977;237:795.
53. Rhame FS, Streifel AJ, Kersey JH Jr, McGlave PB. Extrinsic risk factors for pneumonia in the patient at risk. *Am J Med* 1984;76(5A):42.
54. Barnes RA, Rogers TR. Control of an outbreak of nosocomial aspergillosis by laminar air-flow isolation. *J Hosp Infect* 1989;14:89.
55. Kennedy HF, Michie JR, Richardson MD. Air sampling for *Aspergillus* spp. during building activity in a paediatric hospital ward. *J Hosp Infect* 1995;31:322.
56. Goodley JM, Clayton YM, Hay RJ. Environmental sampling for aspergilli during building construction on a hospital site. *J Hosp Infect* 1994;26:27.
57. Green FHY, Yoshida K. Characteristics of aerosols generated during autopsy procedures and their potential role as carriers of infectious agents. *Appl Occup Environ Hyg* 1990;5:853.
58. McKinley IB Jr, Ludlow MO. Hazards of laser smoke during endodontic therapy. *J Endodont* 1994;20:558.
59. Association of Operating Room Nurses. Proposed recommended practices: laser safety in the practice setting. *AORN J* 1993;57:720.
60. American Public Health Association. *Standard methods for the examination of water and wastewater*, 17th ed. Washington, D.C.: American Public Health Association, 1989.
61. U.S. Environmental Protection Agency. National interim primary drinking water regulations. *Federal Register,* 1975;40:59566.
62. Geldreich EE. Current status of microbiological water quality criteria. *ASM News* 1981;47:23.
63. European Community Council directive no. 80/778/EEC of 15 July 1980 relating to the quality of water intended for human consumption. *Off J Eur Commun* 1980;L229:11.
64. Picard B, Goullet P. Seasonal prevalence of nosocomial *Aeromonas hydrophila* infection related to aeromonas in hospital water. *J Hosp Infect* 1987;10:152.
65. Association for the Advancement of Medical Instrumentation. *American national standard for hemodialysis systems*. Arlington: Association for the Advancement of Medical Instrumentation, 1981.
66. Dawids SG, Vejlsgaard R. Bacteriological and clinical evaluation of different dialysate delivery systems. *Acta Med Scand* 1976;199:151.
67. Favero MS, et al. Gram-negative bacteria in hemodialysis systems. *Health Lab Sci* 1975;12:321.
68. Lauer JL, et al. The bacteriological quality of hemodialysis solution as related to several environmental factors. *Nephron* 1975;15:87.
69. Association for the Advancement of Medical Instrumentation. *Sterilization*. Arlington: Association for the Advancement of Medical Instrumentation, 1990. (*Standards and recommended practices*, vol. 2).
70. Kesmaviam P, Luehmann D, Shapiro F, Comty C. Investigation of the risks and hazards associated with hemodialysis systems. Washington, D.C.: FDA Bureau of Medical Devices, 1980. (Technical report, contract no. 223–78–5046).
71. McGuckin MB, Thorpe RJ, Abrutyn E. An outbreak of *Pseudomonas aeruginosa* wound infections related to Hubbard tank treatments. *Arch Phys Med Rehabil* 1981;62:283.
72. Turner AG, Higgins MM, Craddock JG. Disinfection of immersion tanks (Hubbard) in a hospital burn unit. *Arch Environ Health* 1974;28: 101.
73. Mayhall CG, Lamb VA, Gayle WE Jr, Haynes BW Jr. *Enterobacter cloacae* septicemia in a burn center: epidemiology and control of an outbreak. *J Infect Dis* 1979;139:166.
74. Gustafson TL, Bank JD, Hutcheson RH Jr., Schaffner W. *Pseudomonas* folliculitis: an outbreak and review. *Rev Infect Dis* 1983;5:1.
75. Salmen P, Dwyer DM, Vorse H, Kruse W. Whirlpool-associated *Pseudomonas aeruginosa* urinary tract infections. *JAMA* 1983;260: 2025.
76. Rose HD, et al. *Pseudomonas* pneumonia associated with use of a home whirlpool spa. *JAMA* 1983;250:2027.
77. Centers for Disease Control and Prevention. *Disinfection of hydrotherapy pools and tanks*. Atlanta: Hospital Infections Program, Center for Infectious Diseases, Centers for Disease Control and Prevention, 1974;reprinted 1982.
78. Centers for Disease Control and Prevention. Endotoxic reactions associated with the reuse of cardiac catheters—Massachusetts. *MMWR* 1979;28:25.
79. Carson LA, Favero MS, Bond WW, Petersen NJ. Morphological, biochemical, and growth characteristics of *Pseudomonas cepacia* from distilled water. *Appl Microbiol* 1973;25:476.
80. Favero MS, Carson LA, Bond WW, Petersen NJ. *Pseudomonas aeroginosa*: growth in distilled water from hospitals. *Science* 1971; 173:836.
81. Carson LA, Favero MS, Bond WW, Petersen NJ. Factors affecting comparative resistance of naturally occurring and subcultured *Pseudomonas aeruginosa* to disinfectants. *Appl Microbiol* 1972;23:863.
82. Baumann P. Isolation of *Acinetobacter* from soil and water. *J Bacteriol* 1968;96:39.
83. Contant J, et al. Investigation of an outbreak of *Acinetobacter calcoaceticus* var. *anitratus* infections in an adult intensive care unit. *Am J Infect Control* 1990;18:288.
84. Gervich DH, Grout CS. An outbreak of nosocomial *Acinetobacter* infections from humidifiers. *Am J Infect Control* 1985;13:210.
85. Ratner H. *Flavobacterium meningosepticum*. *Infect Control Hosp Epidemiol* 1984;5:237.
86. Decker CF, Simon GL, Keiser JF. *Flavimonas oryzihabitans* (*Pseudomonas oryzihabitans*; CDC Group Ve-2) bacteremia in the immunocompromised host. *Arch Intern Med* 1991;151:603.
87. DuMoulin GC, Stottmeier KD. Waterborne mycobacteria: an increasing threat to health. *ASM News* 1986;52:525.
88. Carson LA, Petersen NJ, Favero MS, Aguero SM. Growth characteristics of atypical mycobacteria in water and their comparative resistance to disinfectants. *Appl Environ Microbiol* 1978;36:839.
89. Hays PS, McGiboney DL, Band JD, Feeley JC. Resistance of *Mycobacterium chelonei*–like organisms to formaldehyde. *Appl Environ Microbiol* 1982;43:722.
90. Bergogne-Baérézin E, Joly-Guillou ML, Vieu JF. Epidemiology of nosocomial infections due to *Acinetobacter calcoaceticus*. *J Hosp Infect* 1987;10:105.
91. Yu VL, Zuravleff JJ, Gavlik L, Magnussen MH. Lack of evidence for person-to-person transmission of Legionnaires' disease. *J Infect Dis* 1983;147:362.
92. Doebbeling BN, et al. Nosocomial *Legionella micdadei* pneumonia: 10 years experience and a case-control study. *J Hosp Infect* 1989;13:289.
93. Lowry PW, et al. A cluster of *Legionella* sternal-wound infections due to postoperative topical exposure to contaminated tap water. *N Engl J Med* 1991;324:109.
94. Muder RR, Yu VL, Woo AH. Mode of transmission of *Legionella pneumophila*: a critical review. *Arch Intern Med* 1986;146:1607.
95. Shands KN, et al. Potable water as a source of Legionnaires' disease. *JAMA* 1985;253:1412.
96. Helms CM, et al. Legionnaires' disease associated with a hospital water system: a five-year progress report on continuous hyperchlorination. *JAMA* 1988;259:2423.
97. Muder RR, et al. Nosocomial Legionnaire's disease uncovered in a prospective study: implications for underdiagnosis. *JAMA* 1983;249: 3184.
98. Brady MT. Nosocomial Legionnaires' disease in a children's hospital. *J Pediatr* 1989;115:46.

99. Breiman RF, et al. Association of shower use with Legionnaires' disease. *JAMA* 1990;263:2924.
100. Vickers RM, et al. Determinants of *Legionella pneumophila* contamination of water distribution systems: 15-hospital prospective study. *Infect Control Hosp Epidemiol* 1987;8:357.
101. Muraca PW, Yu VL, Stout JE. Environmental aspects of Legionnaires' disease. *J Am Water Works Assoc* 1988;80:78.
102. Barbaree JM, et al. Isolation of protozoa from water associated with a legionellosis outbreak and demonstration of intracellular multiplication of *Legionella pneumophila*. *Appl Environ Microbiol* 1986;51:422.
103. Centers for Disease Control and Prevention. Should hospital water be checked for *Legionella*? *Hosp Infect Control* 1983;10:125.
104. Tablan OC, Anderson LJ, Arden NH, et al. Guideline for prevention of nosocomial pneumonia. *Am J Infect Control* 1994;22:247.
105. Plouffe JF, et al. Subtypes of *Legionella pneumophila* serogroup 1 associated with different attack rates. *Lancet* 1983;2:649.
106. Yu VL. Nosocomial legionellosis: current epidemiological issues In: Remington JS, Swartz MN, eds. *Current clinical topics in infectious disease*, 7th ed. New York: McGraw-Hill, 1986:239–253.
107. Kuchta JM, et al. Susceptibility of *Legionella pneumophila* to chlorine in tap water. *Appl Environ Microbiol* 1983;46:1134.
108. States SJ, et al. Chlorine, pH, and control of *Legionella* in hospital plumbing systems. *JAMA* 1989;261:1882.
109. Bier JW, Sawyer TK. Amoebae isolated from laboratory eyewash stations. *Curr Microbiol* 1990;20:349.
110. Hall CB, Douglas RG Jr, Schnabel KC, Geiman JM. Infectivity of respiratory syncytial virus by various routes of inoculation. *Infect Immun* 1981;33:779.
111. Hall CB, Douglas RG Jr, Geiman JM. Possible transmission by fomites of respiratory syncytial virus. *J Infect Dis* 1980;141:98.
112. Hall CB, Douglas RG Jr. Modes of transmission of respiratory syncytial virus. *J Pediatr* 1981;99:100.
113. Wust J, Sullivan NM, Hardegger U, Wilkins TD. Investigation of an outbreak of antibiotic-associated colitis by various typing methods. *J Clin Microbiol* 1982;16:1096.
114. McFarland LV, Stamm WE. Review of *Clostridium difficile*–associated diseases. *Am J Infect Control* 1986;14:99.
115. Johnson S, et al. Prospective, controlled study of vinyl glove use to interrupt *Clostridium difficile* nosocomial transmission. *Am J Med* 1990;88:137.
116. Johnson S, et al. Nosocomial *Clostridium difficile* colonisation and disease. *Lancet* 1990;336:97.
117. Osterholm MT, Garayalde SM. Clinical viral hepatitis B among Minnesota hospital personnel. *JAMA* 1985;254:3207.
118. Alter MJ, et al. The changing epidemiology of hepatitis B in the United States: need for alternative vaccination strategies. *JAMA* 1990;263:9.
119. Forester G, Joline C, Wormser GP. Blood contamination of tourniquets used in routine phlebotomy. *Am J Infect Control* 1990;18:386.
120. Bond WW, et al. Survival of hepatitis B virus after drying and storage for one week. *Lancet* 1981;1:550.
121. Bond WW, Favero MS, Petersen NJ, Ebert JW. Inactivation of hepatitis B virus by intermediate-to-high-level disinfectant chemicals. *J Clin Microbiol* 1983;18:535.
122. Douvin C, et al. An outbreak of hepatitis B in an endocrinology unit traced to a capillary-blood-sampling device. *N Engl J Med* 1990;322:57.
123. Centers for Disease Control and Prevention. Recommendations for prevention of HIV transmission in health-care settings. *MMWR* 1987;36(no. 2S):1S.
124. Centers for Disease Control and Prevention. Recommendations for initial management of suspected or confirmed cases of Lassa fever. *MMWR* 1980;28(suppl):52.
125. Centers for Disease Control and Prevention. Management of patients with suspected viral hemorrhagic fever. *MMWR* 1988;37(no. S-3):1.
126. Centers for Disease Control and Prevention. Update: management of patients with suspected viral hemorrhagic fever—United States. *MMWR* 1995;44:475.
127. Anderson RL. Biological evaluation of carpeting. *Appl Microbiol* 1969;18:180.
128. Shaffer JG. Microbiology of hospital carpeting. *Health Lab Sci* 1966;3:73.
129. Winters WD. A new perspective of microbial survival and dissemination in a prospectively contaminated air-fluidized bed model. *Am J Infect Control* 1990;18:307.
130. Vesley D, Hankinson SE, Lauer JL. Microbial survival and dissemination associated with an air-fluidized therapy unit. *Am J Infect Control* 1986;14:35.
131. Bolyard EA, Townsend TR, Horan T. Airborne contamination associated with in-use air-fluidized beds: a descriptive study. *Am J Infect Control* 1987;15:75.
132. Freeman R, Gould FK, Ryan DW, Chamberlain J, Sisson PR. Nosocomial infection due to *Enterococci* attributed to a fluidized microsphere bed: the value of pyrolysis mass spectrometry. *J Hosp Infect* 1994;27:187.
133. Morse LJ, et al. Septicemia due to *Klebsiella pneumoniae* originating from a hand-cream dispenser. *N Engl J Med* 1967;277:472.
134. Heinze JE. Bar soap and liquid soap [Letter]. *JAMA* 1984;251:3222.
135. Kates SG, McGinley KJ, Larson EL, Leyden JJ. Indigenous multiresistant bacteria from flowers in hospital and nonhospital environments. *Am J Infect Control* 1991;19:156.
136. Acha PN, Szyfres B. *Zoonoses and communicable diseases common to man and animals*. Washington, D.C.: Pan American Health Organization, 1980. (Scientific Publication No. 354.)
137. Hall CJ, et al. Laboratory outbreak of Q fever acquired from sheep. *Lancet* 1982;1:1004.
138. Abinanit FR, Welsh HH, Lennette EH, Brunetti O. Q fever studies. XVI. Some aspects of the experimental infection induced in sheep by the intratracheal route of inoculation. *Am J Hyg* 1953;57:170.
139. Bernard KW, Parham GL, Winkler WG, Melmick CG. Q fever control measures: recommendations for research facilities using sheep. *Infect Control Hosp Epidemiol* 1982;3:461.
140. Blaser MJ, et al. Killing of fabric-associated bacteria in hospital laundry by low-temperature washing. *J Infect Dis* 1984;149:48.
141. Centers for Disease Control and Prevention. Outbreak of viral hepatitis in the staff of a pediatric ward—California. *MMWR* 1977;26:77.
142. Standaert SM, Hutcheson RH, Schaffner W. Nosocomial transmission of *Salmonella* gastroenteritis to laundry workers in a nursing home. *Infect Control Hosp Epidemiol* 1994;15:22.
143. Meyer CL, et al. Should linen in newborn intensive care units be autoclaved? *Pediatrics* 1981;67:362.
144. Birch BR, et al. *Bacillus cereus* cross-infection in a maternity unit. *J Hosp Infect* 1981;2:349.
145. Public Health Laboratory Service. *Bacillus cereus* infections in hospitals. *Communicable Dis Rep* 1990;44:3.
146. English MP, Wethered RR, Duncan EHL. Studies in the epidemiology of tinea pedis. VIII. Fungal infection in a long-stay hospital. *Br Med J* 1967;3:136.
147. Gonzaga AJ, Mortimer EA Jr., Wolinsky E, Rammelkamp CH Jr. Transmission of staphylococci by fomites. *JAMA* 1964;189:711.
148. Kirby WMM, Corpron DO, Tanner DC. Urinary tract infections caused by antibiotic-resistant coliform bacilli. *JAMA* 1956;162:1.
149. American Hospital Association. Infection control in the hospital, 4th ed. Chicago: American Hospital Association, 1979.
150. American Academy of Pediatrics. *Standards and recommendations for hospital care of newborn infants*, 6th ed. Evanston, Ill.: American Academy of Pediatrics, 1977.
151. American Academy of Pediatrics and American College of Obstetricians and Gynecologists. *Guidelines for perinatal care*. Evanston, Ill.: American Academy of Pediatrics, 1983.
152. Rhame FS. Endemic nosocomial filamentous fungal disease: a proposed structure for conceptualizing and studying the environmental hazard. *Infect Control Hosp Epidemiol* 1986;7(suppl):124.
153. Solberg CO, et al. Laminar airflow protection in bone marrow transplantation. *Appl Microbiol* 1971;21:209.
154. Rhame FS. The inanimate environment. In: Bennett JV, Brachman PS, Eds. *Hospital infections*, 2nd ed. Boston: Little, Brown, 1986:223–249.
155. Bodey GP, Rodriguez V, Cabanillas F, Freireich EJ. Protected environment–prophylactic antibiotic program for malignant lymphoma: randomized trial during chemotherapy to induce remission. *Am J Med* 1979;66:74.
156. Buckner CD, et al. Protective environment for marrow transplant recipients: a prospective study. *Ann Intern Med* 1978;89:893.
157. Dietrich M, et al. Protective isolation and antimicrobial decontamination in patients with high susceptibility to infection: a prospective cooperative study of gnotobiotic care in acute leukemia patients. I. Clinical results. *Infection* 1977;5:107.
158. Klastersky J, Debusscher L, Weerts D, Daneau D. Use of oral antibi-

otics in protected environment units: clinical effectiveness and role in the emergence of antibiotic-resistant strains. *Pathol Biol [Paris]* 1974; 22:5.

159. Levine AS, et al. Protected environments and prophylactic antibiotics: a prospective controlled study of their utility in the therapy of acute leukemia. *N Engl J Med* 1973;288:477.
160. Rodriguez V, et al. Randomized trial of protected environment–prophylactic antibiotics in 145 adults with acute leukemia. *Medicine* 1978;57:253.
161. Schimpff SC, et al. Infection prevention in nonlymphocytic leukemia: laminar air flow room reverse isolation with oral, nonabsorbable antibiotic prophylaxis. *Ann Intern Med* 1975;82:351.
162. Schimpff SC, et al. Comparison of basic infection prevention techniques with standard room reverse isolation or with reverse isolation plus added air filtration. *Leuk Res* 1978;2:231.
163. Storb R, et al. Graft-versus-host disease and survival in patients with aplastic anemia treated by marrow grafts from HLA-identical siblings: beneficial effect of a protective environment. *N Engl J Med* 1983;308: 302.
164. Yates JW, Holland JF. A controlled study of isolation and endogenous microbial suppression in acute myelocytic leukemia patients. *Cancer* 1973;32:1490.
165. Rhame FS. Nosocomial aspergillosis: how much protection for which patients? *Infect Control Hosp Epidemiol* 1989;10:296.
166. Fox BC, et al. Heavy contamination of operating room air by *Penicillium* species: identification of the source and attempts at decontamination. *Am J Infect Control* 1990;18:300.
167. Marshall JW, Vincent JH, Kuehn TH, Brosseau LM. Studies of ventilation efficiency in a protective isolation room by the use of a scale model. *Infect Control Hosp Epidemiol* 1996;17:5.
168. Newman KA, et al. Persistent isolation of an unusual *Pseudomonas* species from a phenolic disinfectant system. *Infect Control Hosp Epidemiol* 1984;5:219.
169. Pizzo PA. The value of protective isolation in preventing nosocomial infections in high risk patients. *Am J Med* 1981;70:631.
170. Davis BD. Growth and death of bacteria. In: Davis BD, Dulbecco R, Eisen HN, and Ginsberg HS, eds. *Microbiology*, 4th ed. Philadelphia: Lippincott, 1990:57–63.
171. Favero MS, Bond WW. Chemical disinfection of medical and surgical materials. In: Block SS, ed. *Sterilization and preservation*, 4th ed. Philadelphia: Lea & Febiger, 1991:617–641.
172. Helrich K, ed. *Official methods of analysis of the Association of Official Analytical Chemists*, 15th ed. Arlington: Association of Official Analytical Chemists, 1990.
173. Cole EC, et al. Effect of methodology, dilution, and exposure time on the tuberculocidal activity of glutaraldehyde-based disinfectants. *Appl Environ Microbiol* 1990;56:1813.
174. Kelsen JC. The myth of surgical sterility. *Lancet* 1972;2:1301.
175. Campbell RW. Sterile is a sterile word. *Radiat Phys Chem* 1980;15:121.
176. Simmons BP. Guideline for hospital environmental control. *Infect Control Hosp Epidemiol* 1981;2:131. (Revision of July 1982 available from CDC, Atlanta, Ga., 30333.)
177. Garner JS, Favero MS. CDC guidelines for the prevention and control of nosocomial infections: guideline for handwashing and hospital environmental control, 1985. *Am J Infect Control* 1986;14:110. (Also available as HHS Publication No. 99–1117.)
178. Joint Commission on Accreditation of Healthcare Organizations. *Accreditation manual for hospitals, 1996*. Oakbrook Terrace, Ill.: Joint Commission on Accreditation of Healthcare Organizations, 1996.
179. Food and Drug Administration. Devices: reuse of medical disposal devices. In: *Food and Drug Administration Compliance Policy Guide No. 7124.23*. Washington, D.C.: Executive Director of Field Operations, Division of Field Operations, 1977.
180. Alter MJ, et al. Reuse of hemodialyzers: results of nationwide surveillance for adverse effects. *JAMA* 1988;260:2073.
181. Gordon SM, Tipple M, Bland LA, Jarvis WR. Pyrogenic reactions associated with the reuse of disposable hollow-fiber hemodialyzers. *JAMA* 1988;260:2077.
182. Pollak VE. Adverse effects and pyrogenic reactions during hemodialysis. *JAMA* 1988;260:2106.
183. Centers for Disease Control and Prevention. Update: acute allergic reactions associated with reprocessed hemodialyzers—United States, 1989–1990. *MMWR* 1991;40:147.
184. Dunnigan A, et al. Success of re-use of cardiac electrode catheters. *Am J Cardiol* 1987;60:807.
185. Alvarado CJ, Stolz SM, Maki DG. Nosocomial *P. aeruginosa* infections from contaminated endoscopes. In: *ASM International Symposium on Chemical Germicides* [Abstract 39]. Madison: University of Wisconsin, 1990.
186. Rutala WA and the 1994, 1995, and 1996 APIC Guidelines Committee. APIC guideline for selection and use of disinfectants. *Am J Infect Control* 1996;24:313.
187. Rutala DR, Rutala WA, Weber DJ, Thomman CA. Infection risks associated with spirometry. *Infect Control Hosp Epidemiol* 1991;12:89.
188. Sattar SA, Springthorpe VS. Survival and disinfectant inactivation of the human immunodeficiency virus: a critical review. *Rev Infect Dis* 1991;13:430.
189. Rutala WA, Clontz EP, Weber DJ, Hoffmann KK. Disinfection practices for endoscopes and other semicritical items. *Infect Control Hosp Epidemiol* 1991;12:282.
190. Society of Gastroenterology Nurses and Associates. *Recommended guidelines for infection control in gastrointestinal endoscopy settings*. Rochester, NY: Society of Gastroenterology Nurses and Associates, 1990.
191. Simmons BP. CDC guidelines for the prevention and control of nosocomial infections. *Am J Infect Control* 1983;11:97.
192. Rutala WA, Weber DJ. Environmental issues and nosocomial infections. In: Farber BF, ed. *Infection control in intensive care*. New York: Churchill Livingstone, 1987:131–171.
193. Rutala WA. APIC guideline for selection and use of disinfectants. *Am J Infect Control* 1990;18:99.
194. Centers for Disease Control and Prevention. Epidemic keratoconjunctivitis in an ophthalmology clinic—California. *MMWR* 1990;39:598.
195. Koo D, et al. Epidemic keratoconjunctivitis in a university medical center ophthalmology clinic; need for re-evaluation of the design and disinfection of instruments. *Infect Control Hosp Epidemiol* 1989;10: 547.
196. American Academy of Ophthalmology. *Updated recommendations for ophthalmic practice in relation to the human immunodeficiency virus*. San Francisco: American Academy of Ophthalmology, 1988.
197. Centers for Disease Control and Prevention. Nosocomial infection and pseudoinfection from contaminated endoscopes and bronchoscopes—Wisconsin and Missouri. *MMWR* 1991;40:675.201. Also in Block SS, ed. *Disinfection, sterilization and preservation*, 3rd ed. Philadelphia: Lea & Febiger, 1983.
198. Reichert M. Automatic washers/disinfectors for flexible endoscopes. *Infect Control Hosp Epidemiol* 1991;12:497.
199. Centers for Disease Control and Prevention. Recommended infection-control practices for dentistry, 1993. *MMWR* 1993;42(no.RR-8):1.
200. Vesley D, Langholz AC, Rohlfing SR, Foltz WE. Fluorimetric detection of a *Bacillus stearothermophilus* spore-bound enzyme, alpha-D-glucosidase, for rapid indication of flash sterilization failure. *J Environ Microbiol* (in press).
202. Rutala WA. Disinfection, sterilization, and waste disposal. In: Wenzel RP, ed. *Prevention and control of nosocomial infections*. Baltimore: Williams & Wilkins, 1987:257–282.
203. Occupational Health and Safety Agency. Glutaraldehyde. *Federal Register*, 1989;54:2464.
204. Rutala WA, Cole EC. Ineffectiveness of hospital disinfectants against bacteria: a collaborative study. *Infect Control Hosp Epidemiol* 1987;8:501.
205. Groschell DHM. Caveat emptor: Do your disinfectants work? *Infect Control Hosp Epidemiol* 1983;4:144.
206. United States General Accounting Office. *Disinfectants: EPA lacks assurance they work*. Gaithersburg, Md.: GAO, 1990:64.
207. Rutala WA, Cole EC, Wannamaker NS, Weber DJ. Inactivation of *Mycobacterium tuberculosis* and *Mycobacterium bovis* by 14 hospital disinfectants. *Am J Med* 1991;91(suppl 3B):3B–267S.
208. Best M, Sattar SA, Springthorpe VS, Kennedy ME. Efficacies of selected disinfectant against *Mycobacterium tuberculosis*. *J Clin Microbiol* 1990;28:2234.
209. Miller DC. Creutzfeldt-Jakob disease in histopathology technicians. *N Engl J Med* 1988;318:853.
210. Sitwell L, et al. Creutzfeldt-Jakob disease in histopathology technicians. *N Engl J Med* 1988;318:854.
211. Steelman VM. Creutzfeld-Jakob disease: recommendations for infection control. *Am J Infect Control* 1994;22:312.
212. Mallison GF, Haley RW. Microbiological sampling of the inanimate environment in U.S. hospitals, 1976–1977. *Am J Med* 1980;70:941.
213. Centers for Disease Control and Prevention. *Microbial environmen-*

tal surveillance in the hospital. (National Nosocomial Infections Study report). Atlanta: Centers for Disease Control and Prevention, 1970.
214. American Hospital Association. Statement on microbiological sampling in the hospital. *Hospitals* 1974;48:125.
215. United States. Department of Health and Human Services. Draft guideline for prevention of intravascular device–related infections. *Federal Register* September 27, 1995;60:49978–50006.
216. National Coordinating Committee on Large-Volume Parenterals. Recommended guidelines for quality assurance in hospital centralized intravenous admixture services. *Am J Hosp Pharm* 1980;37:645.
217. Department of Health and Human Services. Standards for the reuse of hemodialysis filters and other dialysis supplies. *Federal Register* 1987;52:36926.
218. Pejaver KR, Toonisi MA, Carg AK, Al-Hifzi I. Is expressed breast milk from home safe? A survey from a neonatal intensive-care unit. *Infect Control Hosp Epidemiol* 1996;17:356.
219. Arnold LDW, Tully MR, eds. Human Milk Banking Association of North America: guidelines for the establishment and operation of donor human milk bank. 1993.
220. United States Pharmacopeial Convention, Inc. *The United States Pharmacopeia XXII, The National Formulary XVII.* Rockville, Md.: USP, 1989.
221. Craven DE, Goularte TA, Make BJ. Contaminated condensate in mechanical ventilation circuits: a risk factor for nosocomial pneumonia? *Am Rev Respir Dis* 1984;129:625.
222. Cefai C, Richards J, Gould FK, McPeake P. An outbreak of *Acinetobacter* respiratory tract infection from incomplete disinfection of ventilatory equipment. *J Hosp Infect* 1990;15:177.
223. National Sanitation Foundation. *Standard No. 49 for class II (laminar flow) biohazard cabinetry.* Ann Arbor: National Sanitation Foundation, 1976:B4.
224. McGowan JE Jr. Environmental factors in nosocomial infection: a selective focus. *Rev Infect Dis* 1981;3:760.
225. Donowitz LG, Marsik FJ, Fisher KA, Wenzel RP. Contaminated breast milk: a source of *Klebsiella* bacteremia in a newborn intensive care unit. *Rev Infect Dis* 1981;3:716.
226. Simmons BP, et al. *Enterobacter sakazakii* infections in neonates associated with intrinsic contamination of a powdered infant formula. *Infect Control Hosp Epidemiol* 1989;10:398.

Hospital Infections, Fourth Edition,
edited by John V. Bennett and Philip S. Brachman.
Lippincott–Raven Publishers, Philadelphia © 1998

CHAPTER 21

Central Services, Linens, and Laundry

Gina Pugliese and Cynthia A. Hubbard

The central service department (CSD), also referred to as the processing or central supply department, is responsible for cleaning, preparing, processing, storing, and distributing medical and surgical supplies and equipment, both sterile and nonsterile, required for diagnosis of disease and treatment and care of patients. In carrying out these functions, the CSD staff is responsible for removing or destroying potentially infectious contamination on reusable devices and distributing both reusable and single-use items to various sites within the hospital.

The importance of this role in the prevention of nosocomial infections is clear: reusable medical devices improperly handled, disinfected, or sterilized provide a source of contamination and increase the risk of transmission of infection to both patients and the staff involved in reprocessing procedures [1]. As such, all reusable equipment and devices that have come in contact with a patient's blood or body fluids should be considered potentially infectious and must be decontaminated and reprocessed before being used again [2,3].

Hospitals have found it preferable to handle the cleaning, disinfection, and sterilization procedures for all reusable supplies and equipment in a central, specially designed and equipped location for efficiency of operations and economic reasons and to maintain high quality control standards [4]. There must be specific written policies and procedures for all aspects of reprocessing, storage, and distribution, and they must be followed consistently throughout the facility [5,6]. These policies and procedures should also specify methods for monitoring disinfection and sterilization, assuring continued sterility of both hospital-sterilized and commercially prepared sterile items, recalling items that are potentially contaminated and for which removal from use is indicated, and reprocessing when clinically necessary disposable items that are reused [5,6].

G. Pugliese: Associate Faculty, Rush University College of Nursing, Chicago, Illinois 60657.

C. A. Hubbard: Lerch Bates Hospital Group, Incorporated, Littleton, Colorado 80122.

WORKERS' SAFETY

Workers in the CSD are at risk of injury and infection from exposure to contaminated supplies that are returned to the CSD for reprocessing. The Occupational Safety and Health Administration's bloodborne pathogen standard applies to workers in the CSD who are exposed to contaminated equipment [7]. To comply with this standard, written policies and procedures should specify the steps that are to be taken to reduce the risk of injury and infection to workers exposed to potentially contaminated equipment. These policies will include providing appropriate personal protective clothing and equipment and designing work practices to reduce the risk of injury during handling of contaminated sharp instruments which pose the greatest risk of transmission of bloodborne pathogens. In addition, the employer must provide hepatitis B vaccination, postexposure medical evaluation and follow-up, and specific education and training.

COLLECTION AND TRANSPORT OF CONTAMINATED DEVICES

Precleaning reusable supplies and equipment in areas dedicated to the care of patients, other than for removal of gross soil, is difficult to accomplish in a safe manner with personnel not attired or equipped for this procedure. It is often more efficient and cost-effective to use the facilities of the CSD when available. Therefore, items for reprocessing should be removed from the area of use and placed in a designated holding area (i.e., soiled utility room) for pickup and timely return to the CSD. Soiled instruments and devices from the operating room may be precleaned and decontaminated in designated and specially equipped areas by trained and experienced personnel, to remove gross soil and to render them safe for handling before transport to a central processing area, where they will be prepared and packaged before sterilization [8,9].

All soiled reusable supplies and equipment should be collected, contained, and transported to the CSD in a manner that reduces risk of contamination of personnel and the environment. Containers or bags used for holding and transporting soiled items should be clearly marked to indicate that the items are contaminated. Sharp items should be handled with caution and collected and transported in specially labeled, puncture-resistant containers. Transport of bulk soiled supplies should be made on carts or mechanical conveyors used only for that purpose. A dedicated soiled cart lift from the operating room to the CSD is recommended when architecturally feasible [4].

DESIGN OF THE CSD

The CSD should have adequate space to carry out its responsibilities and process the needed inventories. Soiled and contaminated supplies and procedures must be physically separated from those that are clean or sterile. This separation is accomplished by a facility design (walls or partitions) that segregates the functional work areas and management of work flow and controls traffic [5,6,8]. The ideal design provides four separate functional areas: soiled receiving and decontamination, sterile assembly and processing, clean or sterile supply and equipment storage, and distribution [10]. Additional functional areas may be required for surgical linen pack preparation and staging of surgical case carts or supply exchange carts. Administrative areas, janitors' closets, conveniently located hand-washing facilities, and appropriate staff space (lockers, changing areas) are also necessary [4].

Proper ventilation, humidity, and temperature control is necessary to hold in check the bioburden and environmental contamination, to provide appropriate hydration for packaging materials, and to ensure comfortable working conditions. The ventilation system should be designed so that air flows into relatively soiled areas from clean adjoining spaces, with the appropriate number of air exchanges per hour [8,10]. Air movement in the soiled areas should be under negative pressure in relation to adjacent areas [10]. Air movement in the sterile processing areas and the clean and/or sterile supply storage areas should be under positive pressure in relation to adjacent areas [8,10]. All air from soiled processing areas should be vented to the outside or to a partial recirculating system [8,10].

New hospital and facility renovation designs should provide efficient transport between the CSD and the receiving dock, general stores, laundry, operating rooms, emergency rooms, and major areas of patient care. The location, type, and number of elevators and other materials-handling conveyances, as well as traffic patterns, should be planned to maintain separation of supply transport from patients, staff, and visitors [10]. Manual transport of supplies by hospital personnel is the most frequently used method of transferring supplies to and from the CSD. Depending on the type, size, and design of the healthcare facility, automated materials-handling systems (pneumatic tubes, automated box conveyors, or automated guided vehicle systems) may be indicated for efficient materials handling. However, automated or semi-automated systems must be properly sized, designed, and managed to be effective.

DECONTAMINATION

The decontamination process should take place in an environment designed, maintained, and controlled to ensure the safety and efficacy of the process and to protect staff from exposure to infectious materials or toxic and hazardous substances. All CSD personnel assigned to the decontaminated area must be properly trained to carry out carefully the decontamination procedures designed to render items safe for subsequent handling and further processing. To reduce the risk of exposure to potentially infectious blood and body fluids during decontamination procedures, personnel should wear protective apparel, such as gowns, gloves, masks, eyewear, or face shields. The criteria for selection of the appropriate type of protective apparel should address the probability of splashing, splattering, and soiling of clothing and exposed skin or mucous membranes [7].

Reprocessing procedures for reusable items include cleaning; decontamination; low-level, intermediate, or high-level disinfection; and sterilization. The specific processes indicated for an item will depend on its intended use. The process begins with removal of items from their protective packaging or containers and sorting as to the type of reprocessing procedures required. The cleaning recommendations, selection and use of cleaning equipment, chemicals, and exposure times suggested by the device manufacturers should be followed, to prevent damage to the items or risk to the staff during the process [1,2].

Reusable items must first be thoroughly cleaned. Organic materials, such as blood, may contain high concentrations of microorganisms, may inactivate some chemical germicides, and may protect microorganisms from the disinfection or sterilization process [1,11]. For most noncritical items that either do not ordinarily touch patients or touch only intact skin, such as blood pressure cuffs, careful washing with a detergent or disinfectant-detergent, rinsing, and thorough drying is all that is necessary [1,4].

In the circumstance where contaminated reusable equipment is sent from the healthcare facility to another organization (for example, a special treatment bed leased from a vendor or equipment sent for repair), it should be decontaminated before removal from the healthcare facility. If it is not possible to decontaminate equipment before sending it for repair, it should be labeled appropriately (with a biohazard designation), identifying the portions that remain contaminated [7,12].

The cleaning process may be accomplished manually or mechanically and depends on the characteristics of the device being cleaned. Presoaking or prerinsing of items requiring further reprocessing may be indicated if protein residues have been allowed to dry on the items. All jointed instruments should be opened and equipment that is easily disassembled should be taken apart to facilitate the cleaning and decontamination process. Presoaking is accomplished in cool water or through exposure to a protein and blood-dissolving enzyme solution. Care must be taken to avoid splashing or aerosolization of solutions, and personnel should be properly attired [4,11].

Manual cleaning is indicated for many noncritical reusable items, such as bulky or electric equipment and some delicate or complex devices or instruments. Manual cleaning requires multiple sinks and adequate counter space. Care should be taken during handling and manual cleaning of all sharp items to avoid injury.

Mechanical cleaning is an efficient and effective process and should be used for all items that will not be damaged by this process and, whenever possible, for cleaning of sharp objects. Equipment used for mechanical cleaning, decontamination, disinfection, or sterilization includes ultrasonic cleaners, washer disinfectors, washer sterilizers, pasteurizers, cart washers, and scope disinfectors. The specific equipment used will depend on the type, volume, and material specifications of the devices and the processing outcomes desired [4,11].

Following the cleaning and decontamination procedures, semicritical and critical items require further disinfection or sterilization processing. Semicritical items, such as endoscopes or endotracheal tubes, that touch mucous membranes and do not penetrate body surfaces should receive high-level disinfection. Critical items, such as surgical instruments, that enter normally sterile tissue or the vascular system or through which blood flows should be subjected to a sterilization procedure before each use [1,4,11].

The chemicals for high-level disinfection or sterilization in the decontamination area must be used in the concentrations and manner suggested by the manufacturer. It is also recommended that the hospital's infection control program review all products used, to ensure that they are appropriate for the intended outcome [13]. Specific guidelines for disinfection and sterilization are described in Chapter 20 and by Garner and Favero [1]. Waste generated during the decontamination process will normally be considered part of the regulated medical waste stream. As such, it must be placed into appropriately marked waste containers to differentiate it from non-biohazardous waste [7,14].

ASSEMBLY AND STERILE PROCESSING

The work area in the CSD should be designed to allow for separation of procedures in the decontamination area from those in the clean area. Devices that have been cleaned in the decontamination area are inspected and tested before packaging or sterilization to ensure their cleanliness and proper functioning. The CSD should be equipped to routinely test before reuse the function of clean equipment used in the care of patients, such as suction machines. Routine preventive maintenance and equipment repair should be designated to the appropriate department [4,12].

The packaging of items requiring sterilization should be selected according to the size, shape, and weight of the device and should be appropriate for the sterilization process used [15–17]. Only materials that provide penetration and removal of the sterilant, maintain a barrier to microorganisms, and allow sterile presentation of package contents should be used. Appropriate materials include 180- to 240-thread-count woven textiles, sterilization containers, and nonwoven, disposable materials [4].

Reliable sterilization depends on the contact of the sterilant with all surfaces of the device. Therefore, disassembly and arrangement of instruments in a tray, packaging, sterilizer loading, and air evacuation are important considerations in the sterilization process and should be monitored [8,9,15,16]. Sterilization methods used in hospitals at present include thermal (steam) and chemical (ethylene oxide, hydrogen peroxide vapor with a plasma phase [gas plasma], vapor phase hydrogen peroxide, formaldehyde, glutaraldehyde, peracetic acid) processes. Environmental monitoring to detect levels of personnel exposure to chemicals such as ethylene oxide is recommended to ensure a safe working environment [17]. Guidelines for selection and use of specific sterilizing processes are described in Chapter 20.

Sterilizers should be validated on installation and their performance reassessed by engineering studies on a yearly basis. All sterilizers should be tested with live bacterial spores at least weekly or with each load [5,6]. Sterilizers should be monitored with commercial preparations of live bacterial spore monitors specifically intended for each type of sterilizer (i.e., *Bacillus stearothermophilus* for steam sterilizers and *Bacillus subtilis* for ethylene oxide and dry-heat sterilizers) [1]. Chemical indicators should be used with each package sterilized. When implantable or intravascular materials undergo sterilization, live spore controls should be used with each load, and the results of the spore tests should be obtained before the items are used [9,17]. The use of flash sterilizers should be limited to those urgent situations in which the requirements of patient care preclude the use of other sterilization methods [9,16].

Records must be kept of all sterilizer preventive maintenance and performance verification procedures. If bacterial spores are not killed during routine spore testing, the sterilizer should be checked for proper use and function and the spore test repeated. Items other than implantable objects do not need to be recalled because of a single positive spore test unless the sterilizer or sterilization procedure is defective, as indicated by the other mechanical or chemical sterilization monitors [1]. If the spore test remains positive, use of the sterilizer should be discontinued until it is serviced, and all items from the load should be recalled and reprocessed. Recall is expedited when each package is labeled with a control number that indicates the sterilizer used, the cycle, the date of sterilization, and expiration information [4,9,16].

SURGICAL TEXTILE PACKS

Textile packs used as gowning and draping material during sterile procedures should be prepared under controlled conditions to minimize the lint in the environment and within the pack [4,16]. Many hospitals transport clean textiles to the CSD, where they are inspected, packaged, and then sterilized. Pack construction must not inhibit steam penetration, and it is recommended that the size and weight of packs should be no larger than 30×30×50 cm (12×12×20 inches) and 12 pounds, respectively. The maximum density must not exceed 7.2 pounds per cubic foot [8].

STORAGE OF STERILE SUPPLIES

All sterile packs should be handled as little as possible to minimize the opportunity for microbial contamination of the contents. Storage areas for clean and sterile items should be designed and maintained to limit traffic, encourage easy identification of items, facilitate stock rotation, promote cleanliness, and protect the packages. Three conditions can directly compromise the sterile integrity of a package: moisture, soil, and physical damage by penetration. Proper humidity and temperature control are thus essential to maintaining package integrity [4,9,17,19].

Clean and sterile supplies are generally stored on carts or fixed wall shelving. Both open and closed shelving systems are used. The system design should facilitate routine cleaning of the storage units and the environment without compromising the sterile integrity of the packages. Sterile supplies should not be stored in outside shipping cartons; rather, they should be removed from these cartons and stored in washable storage containers. Shelving systems should be designed so that packages are placed at least 8 inches from the floor, 2 inches from outside walls, and 18 inches from ceiling fixtures, such as sprinklers. Sterile items should always be stored away from sources of water, windows, doors, exposed pipes, and vents. Items on the top shelf should also be protected from contaminants that may fall from the ceiling, ceiling fixtures, or ventilation system [4,7].

SAFE STORAGE TIMES FOR STERILE ITEMS

Shelf-life policies for CSD-sterilized items and other devices commercially sterilized should be determined by the healthcare facility's infection control program. Consideration must be given to the type of packaging materials used, storage conditions, and handling practices of the staff. Storage of hospital-sterilized packages without contamination (under open and closed clean-storage conditions) has been documented for periods of ≤ 50 weeks [20]. The packaging materials in this study included nonbarrier woven textiles, barrier nonwoven materials, and polypropylene peel pouches. Dust covers provided no advantage in extending the shelf life of sterile packs. Thus, shelf life may be considered to depend on events rather than on time.

Some hospitals still prefer to designate specific times when sterile packs are outdated. Policies and procedures should indicate the method to be used for designation of shelf life and the system for stock rotation. Inventory levels should be kept low so that packages are not damaged by overcrowding and do not become obsolete. If an event-related designation is used, procedures should specify those circumstances that would indicate an item should not be used, for example, package wrappings that are torn, punctured, or wet [1,4,8,15].

REUSE OF SINGLE-USE ITEMS

The reuse of devices intended by the manufacturer to be for a single patient's use only (disposable) is a controversial topic. Each facility must address this issue in view of the needs of its population, information about risks associated with reprocessing of specific devices, manufacturers' warnings, and liability from equipment malfunction from the reprocessing procedure. Policies and procedures should address the facility's position on reprocessing of disposable items and should detail protocols for reprocessing of such items [4,8,17]. Additional information on the reuse of single-use items is described in Chapters 20 and 24.

QUALITY CONTROL

Infection prevention and control education must be provided for all CSD staff. Compliance with the policies and procedures should be verified by ongoing quality audits. Appropriate follow-up and corrective action should be taken when monitoring reveals a failure to follow recommended practices. All quality control and monitoring activities should be documented.

LINENS AND LAUNDRY

Soiled healthcare linens, like other used patient care items, can be a potential source of human pathogens and require appropriate handling and processing to lessen the risk of cross-transmission of potentially infectious organisms. Appropriate procedures are also necessary to minimize the risk of dermal irritation or related illness from exposure to residual chemicals used in the laundering process [21,22].

Although soiled linen has been found to contain large numbers of pathogenic microorganisms, reports of transmission of infections to patients are rare. Reports suggesting linen as a source of infections among patients have been limited to staphylococcal, streptococcal, and *Bacillus cereus* colonization and infections of newborns [23–25] and antibiotic-resistant organisms causing urinary tract infections in catheterized patients [26]. It is unlikely that the linen was the actual source of the infection in these cases because the organisms causing infections were also found on other patient care items and on the hands of healthcare personnel. Instead, the linen may have become contaminated from contact with an infected patient or healthcare worker or with the contaminated hands of a worker. This finding of the lack of risk from contaminated inanimate items, such as linen, is in agreement with the results of numerous epidemiologic studies that have shown that the source of organisms causing nosocomial infections is most frequently animate (human). Additional information on the inanimate environment as a source of nosocomial pathogens is described in Chapter 20.

One other report in the literature, of an outbreak of tinea pedis (ringworm of the feet) in a residential care hospital, suggests that the source of infection was linen. However, improperly washed linens belonging to patients, including socks, and the communal ownership of socks and towels were more likely to have contributed to this outbreak [27]. Infections in workers handling soiled linen are also rarely reported and are frequently the result of improper handling. Reports among workers of infections related handling soiled linen over the past 30 years have included Q fever [28], salmonellosis [29–31], fungal infections [32], scabies [33], hepatitis A [34], and smallpox [35].

Although there may have been other episodes of infections related to linens not recognized or reported in the scientific literature, the paucity of such reports suggests that the risk of actual disease transmission is rare, even among workers who have direct and frequent contact with soiled linens as part of their daily routine. The low risk of infection may be related to adherence to appropriate handling and processing procedures designed to reduce the risk of transmission of infectious agents to patients and workers who come in contact with soiled linen [7,36].

The Centers for Disease Control and Prevention (CDC) has recognized that the risk of disease transmission associated with soiled linen is negligible and has published guidelines recommending hygienic and common-sense handling, storage, and processing rather than rigid rules and regulations [1,2]. These guidelines were reemphasized in the CDC's universal precautions guidelines for prevention of transmission of bloodborne pathogens [2,3]. The most practical application of universal precautions is to handle and process any patient's linen soiled with blood, body fluids, secretions, or excretions in the same manner, regardless of the source. The bloodborne pathogen standard put out by OSHA also applies to workers handling soiled laundry and contains specific requirements for identifying, bagging, and handling all contaminated laundry and protective clothing that must be worn to prevent occupational exposure [7].

Collection

Soiled linen used for patients should be collected and handled with minimum agitation, to prevent contamination of the air and persons handling the linen. Special care should be taken with those items visibly soiled with blood or body fluids to prevent contamination of workers. If the linen is heavily soiled, protective barriers (such as gloves) may be necessary. However, in some situations, a relatively clean or lightly soiled item can serve as a barrier by using it to collect a heavily soiled item or portion of an item in such a way (either by folding or rolling) as to keep the visibly or heavily soiled areas contained in the center of the bundle. This technique can also serve to prevent contamination of the worker and soaking through of the laundry bag. All soiled linen should be bagged at the location where it was used. The collection bag should be of sufficient quality to contain the wet or soiled linen and prevent leakage during transport. Both cloth and plastic laundry bags are available. However, the type of bag used should depend on the amount and type of soil present. Cloth laundry bags are adequate for the majority of linens. For linen soaked with blood or body fluids, such as that from some surgical or trauma patients, some facilities prefer the use of plastic bags. However, cloth bags, which can be washed and reused, are cheaper than the cost associated with single-use plastic bags and cut down the unnecessary generation of disposable waste. To meet the intent of the OSHA standard, the hospital may select any type of bag or container for contaminated laundry that will prevent soak-through or leakage of fluids to the exterior of the bag [7].

In the past, linen from isolation patients was handled differently from other patients' linen [37]. Isolation linen was double-bagged, with the inner bag made of a water-soluble material that could be placed directly into the washer, eliminating presorting of the contents and minimizing handling by laundry workers. This practice was based on the belief that all isolation linen posed a greater risk of disease transmission than linen coming from other areas. Two recent studies comparing double-bagged isolation linen with single-bagged linen from nonisolation patients found no significant difference in the level of bacterial contamination of either the outside of the bags or the linen inside the bag [38,39].

In fact, it was noted in one of these studies that nonisolation linen was more often grossly soiled with feces, urine, and blood, and that the degree of soiling was more closely related to whether the patient was incontinent or to the type of procedures being performed than to the patient's isolation status [39]. There is thus no infection control advantage to double-bagging linen unless the primary bag leaks. In addition, the use of water-soluble bags is generally not necessary for a number of reasons [40]. First, it adds to the cost of bagging and processing. Second, water-soluble bags dissolve only in hot water, which cannot be used in the initial flush of the laundry cycle if one is to achieve effective stain removal. Third, if the stains are not properly removed, they can render the item unsuitable for further use. Finally, because laundry in water-soluble bags is not sorted before washing, instruments and other items inadvertently left in the laundry can cause damage to the laundry equipment, the linen itself, and also the laundry workers sorting the linen after washing.

Care should be taken during collection and bagging to ensure that all nonlinen items, such as instruments, needles, or plastic underpads, are removed. The greatest risk to healthcare workers of acquiring bloodborne infections, such as hepatitis B virus and human immunodeficiency virus infections, is from accidental punctures or injuries from sharp items that are contaminated with the blood of infected patients [2,3]. All personnel should be trained in the proper procedures for handling and disposing of needles and other sharp objects.

The Occupational Safety and Health Administration does not require special "biohazard" labeling of laundry if universal precautions are used for handling all soiled laundry. In this case, the healthcare facility may choose any type of labeling or color-coding of laundry bags if all employees recognize the labeling as requiring compliance with universal precautions [7]. If a hospital sends its laundry to an off-site facility (e.g., a commercial laundry), alternative labeling may also be used if the off-site laundry facility uses universal precautions for all laundry. In situations where off-site laundry facilities do not follow universal precautions for all laundry, specific labeling with the biohazard symbol is required by OSHA.

Transportation and Storage

Clean and soiled linen should be separated during storage and transport. Separation may be maintained if the container used to transport soiled linen is properly cleaned before its use to transport clean linen, the clean linen is wrapped properly, or transportation of clean and soiled linen is done in separate containers [36]. The precise length of time that soiled linen can remain bagged and stored before washing is not based on a risk of disease transmission but rather on concerns for stain removal and aesthetics. After the soiled linen is properly collected, reasonable schedules should be developed for transport and processing.

The linings of hard-surfaced carts should be cleaned frequently. If soiled linen is transported in carts with cloth liners or in cloth bags on rolling hampers, the cloth liners and bags should be washed daily. The individual cloth bags used to bag soiled linen require the same processing as their contents each time the bags are used. If laundry chutes are used, all soiled linen should be bagged and the laundry chute should discharge into the soiled linen collection area [1,10,41]. Clean linen should be properly protected during storage and transport to prevent contamination. Although protection is recommended during transport and storage of bulk supplies on clean linen carts, once clean linen is distributed for individual use, additional protection is not necessary.

Sorting and Handling

All workers who sort and handle soiled linen should wear protective apparel to lower the risk of contamination of exposed areas of the skin and soiling of clothing [7]. Appropriate protective apparel may include gloves and gowns or aprons. Protective eyewear is generally not necessary because splashing of blood or body fluids is unlikely in the laundry setting. Hands should be washed after gloves are removed, and reusable protective apparel, such as gowns, should be washed after use. Personnel should also be instructed in the principles of personal hygiene, including frequent hand washing; for this reason hand-washing facilities must be conveniently located. Because all linen is handled and sorted in a similar manner with appropriate protective apparel, prewashing of linen to reduce microbial contamination before handling is unnecessary for prevention of infections.

Plant Facilities

A separate room should be provided for receiving and holding soiled linen until it is ready for pickup. Processing of linen may be done within the facility, in a separate building on or off site, or in a commercial or shared laundry. The soiled linen-processing facility, when it is located in the hospital, should be separated from the clean linen storage and processing areas, from patients' rooms, from food preparation and storage areas, and from areas where clean supplies or equipment is stored [10]. The laundry facility should also be designed, equipped, and ventilated to minimize mixing of air from clean and soiled operations. Functional separation of clean and soiled areas may be achieved by a physical barrier, negative pressure system in the soiled area, or positive airflow from the clean to the soiled area [36]. Hand-washing facilities should be available in each area where clean or soiled linen is handled or processed [10].

Processing and Laundering

There are no standards on acceptable levels of microbial contamination of clean linen. This is in part due to the variability of microbial survival depending on the degree of soiling, laundering techniques, and the ability of the microbes to adhere to various fabrics [42]. There is a significant reduction in microbial counts during the laundering process, as part of the mechanical action and dilution of washing and rinsing [43,44]. Detergents, which act as surfactants, loosen and lift the soil from the laundry and enhance the penetration of the textile fiber by water, which assists with the removal of foreign substances, including microbes [22]. Hot water also destroys microorganisms, and a temperature of ≥ 71°C (160°F) for a minimum of 25 minutes is recommended for hot-water washing [1,2]. The addition of other chemicals, such as chlorine bleach, reduces bacterial counts further [43].

One of the last steps in the washing process is the addition of a mild acidic agent, referred to as a sour, to neutralize the alkalinity from the fabrics, water, and detergent. This shift in pH from ~ 12 to 5 inactivates some microorganisms and lessens the risk of skin irritation [43]. Moreover, the addition of fabric softeners or bacteriostats in the final rinse leaves a residue on the fabric that inhibits bacterial growth.

Recent studies have shown that a satisfactory reduction of microbial contamination can be achieved at lower water temperatures (< 70°C) when washing formulations, wash cycles, and, in particular, the use of bleach is carefully controlled [42,43,45,46]. Although some recontamination of washed linens may occur during removal from the washing machine, the high temperatures achieved during drying and ironing are also effective in minimizing any microbial contamination.

Both the CDC guidelines and OSHA's standard recommend that soiled linen not be sorted or rinsed in areas dedicated to the care of patients [1,2,7]. These recommendations were intended for processing of linens that are routinely soiled with blood, body fluids, and other substances. In some healthcare settings, patients' linens and clothing are not routinely soiled with blood or body fluids. For example, in ambulatory care settings, such as psychiatric units, patients' clothing is often washed in designated locations near patient care areas by the staff or even by the patients themselves as part of their activities of daily living. In these situations, guidelines should be developed to ensure that staff and patients are instructed on appropriate processing procedures.

Sterilization of Linens

It is recommended that surgical gowns and drapes that come in contact with the operating field be rendered sterile [18]. Reusable gowns and linens are sterilized by steam autoclaving after laundering. The need for sterile nursery linens to prevent infections has never been established and is no longer recommended [47]. However, thorough rinsing after washing nursery linens is essential to reduce the risk of skin irritation from residual chemicals.

Disposable Linens

Both disposable and reusable patients' linens are available in the healthcare setting. Certain disposable items are considered more cost-effective by some hospitals, including small articles that carry a proportionately higher handling charge when recycled, such as caps, masks, shoe covers, washcloths, diapers, underpads, and some wrappers. In choosing between disposable and reusable patient care items, necessary considerations include not only cost but also accessibility, life expectancy of a reusable article, availability of laundering facilities, storage space for disposable items, delivery capabilities, size and type of hospital, and the cost of disposal.

REFERENCES

1. Garner JS, Favero MS. *Guideline for handwashing and hospital environmental control.* Washington, D.C.: U.S. Government Printing Office 1985;544–436;24441.
2. Centers for Disease Control and Prevention. Recommendations for prevention of HIV transmission in healthcare settings. *MMWR* 1987; 36(suppl 2S):3S.
3. Centers for Disease Control and Prevention. Update: universal precautions for prevention of transmission of HIV, HBV, and other bloodborne pathogens in the health setting. *MMWR* 1988;37:377.
4. American Society for Healthcare Central Services. *Training manual for central service technicians.* Chicago: American Hospital Association, 1993.
5. Joint Commission on Accreditation of Healthcare Organizations. *Stan-*

dards. Oak Brook Terrace, Ill.: Joint Commission of Accreditation of Healthcare Organizations, 1995. (*Accreditation manual for hospitals*, vol. 1.)
6. Joint Commission on Accreditation of Healthcare Organizations. *Scoring guidelines*. Oak Brook Terrace, Ill.: Joint Commission on Accreditation of Healthcare Organizations, 1995. (*Accreditation manual for hospitals*, vol. 2.)
7. Department of Labor, Occupational Safety and Health Association. Occupational exposure to bloodborne pathogens: final rule. *Federal Register* December 6, 1991:56(235):64004–64182.
8. Association for the Advancement of Medical Instrumentation. *Sterilization. I. Good hospital practices*. Arlington: Association for the Advancement of Medical Instrumentation, 1995. (*AAMI standards and recommended practices*, vol 1.)
9. *AORN standards and recommended practices (1995): sterilization and disinfection*. Denver: Association of Operating Room Nurses, 1995.
10. American Institute of Architects and U.S. Department of Health and Human Services. *Guidelines for construction and equipment of hospital and medical facilities*. Washington, D.C.: American Institute of Architects Press, 1993.
11. American Society for Healthcare Central Services. *Recommended practices for central service. Decontamination*. Chicago: American Hospital Association, 1991.
12. American Society for Healthcare Central Services. *Recommended practices for central service. Patient care equipment*. Chicago: American Hospital Association, 1993.
13. Rutala WA, Gergen MF, Weber DJ. Sporicidal activity of chemical sterilants used in hospitals. *Infect Control Hosp Epidemiol* 1993;14:713–718.
14. Sierocinski DM, Gore RJ. OSHA and the decontamination area. *J Healthcare Materials Manage* 1993;11:5.
15. *AORN standards and recommended practices (1995): selection and use of packaging material*. Denver: Association of Operating Room Nurses, 1995.
16. American Society for Healthcare Central Services. *Recommended practices for central service. Sterilization*. Chicago: American Hospital Association, 1989.
17. Association for the Advancement of Medical Instrumentation. *American national standard good hospital practice: ethylene oxide sterilization and sterility assurance*. Arlington: Association for the Advancement of Medical Instrumentation, 1992.
18. *AORN standards and recommended practices (1995):* aseptic barrier materials for surgical gowns and drapes. Denver: Association of Operating Room Nurses, 1995.
19. American Society for Healthcare Central Services. *Recommended practices for central service*. VII. *Sterile storage, inventory control and distribution*. Chicago: American Hospital Association, 1989.
20. Klapes NA, Greene VW, Langholz AC, et al. Effect of long-term storage on sterile status of devices in surgical packs. *Infect Control Hosp Epidemiol* 1987;8:7.
21. Armstrong RW. Pentachlorophenol poisoning in a nursery for newborn infants. II. Epidemiologic and toxicologic studies. *J Pediatr* 1969;75:317.
22. Riggs CL, Sherrill JC. *Textile laundering technology*. Hallandale, Fla.: Textile Rental Services Association of America, 1979.
23. Birch BR. *Bacillus cereus* cross infection in a maternity unit. *J Hosp Infect* 1981;2:349.
24. Gonzaga AJ, Mortimer EA, Wolinski E Jr., Rammelkamp CH. Transmission of staphlococci by fomites. *JAMA* 1964;189:711.
25. Brunton WAT. Infection and hospital laundry. *Lancet* 1995;345:1574–1575.
26. Kirby WMM, Corpron DO, Tanner DC. Urinary tract infections caused by antibiotic-resistant coliform bacilli. *JAMA* 1956;162:1.
27. English MP, Wethered RR, Duncan EHL. Studies of the epidemiology of tinea pedis. VII. Fungal infection in a long-stay hospital. *Br Med J* 1967;3:136.
28. Oliphant JW, Gordon DA, Meis A, Parker RR. Q fever in laundry workers, presumably transmitted from contaminated clothing. *Am J Hyg* 1949;49:76.
29. Standaert SM, Hutcheson RH, Schaffner WA. Nosocomial transmission of salmonella gastroenteritis to laundry workers in a nursing home. *Infect Control Hosp Epidemiol* 1994;15:22–26.
30. *Salmonella typhi. Can Epidemiol Bull* 1972;16:128.
31. Steere AC, Hall WJ, Wells JG, et al. Person-to-person spread of *Salmonella typhimurium* after a hospital common source outbreak. *Lancet* 1975;1:319.
32. Shah PC, Krajden S, Kane J, Summerbell RC. Tinea corporis caused by *Microsporum canis*: report of a nosocomial outbreak. *Eur J Epidemiol* 1988;4:33.
33. Thomas MD, Giedinghagen DH, Hoff GL. Brief report: an outbreak of scabies among employees in a hospital-associated commercial laundry. *Infect Control Hosp Epidemiol* 1987;8:427.
34. Centers for Disease Control and Prevention. Outbreak of viral hepatitis in the staff of a pediatric ward—California. *MMWR* 1977;28:77.
35. Anonymous. Smallpox [Editorial]. *Br Med J* 1951;1:288.
36. Joint Committee on Healthcare Laundry Guidelines. *1993 Guidelines for healthcare linen service*. Hallandale, Fla.: Textile Rental Service Association of America, 1988.
37. Garner JS, Simmons BP. CDC guideline for isolation precautions in hospitals. *Infect Control Hosp Epidemiol* 1983;4(suppl):245.
38. Maki DG, Alvarado C, Hassemen BS. Double-bagging of items from isolation rooms is unnecessary as infection control measure: a comparative study of surface contamination with single- and double-bagging. *Infect Control Hosp Epidemiol* 1986;7:535.
39. Weinstein SA, Gantz NM, Pelletier C, Hilbert D. Bacterial surface contamination of patients' linen: isolation precautions versus standard care. *Am J Infect Control* 1989;17:264.
40. Pugliese G. Isolating and double-bagging laundry: Is it really necessary? *Health Facilities Manage* 1989;2:16.
41. Hughes HG. Chutes in hospitals. *J Can Hosp Assoc* 1964;41:56.
42. Smith JA, Neil KR, Davidson CG, Davidson RW. Effect of water temperature on bacterial killing in laundry. *Infect Control Hosp Epidemiol* 1987;8:204.
43. Blaser MJ. Killing of fabric-associated bacteria in hospital laundry by low temperature washing. *J Infect Dis* 1984;149:48.
44. Walter WG, Schillinger JE. Bacterial survival in laundered fabrics. *Appl Microbiol* 1975;29:368.
45. Battles DR, Vesley D. Wash water temperature and sanitation in the hospital laundry. *J Environ Health* 1981;43:244.
46. Christian RR, Manchester JT, Mellor MT. Bacteriologic quality of fabrics washed at lower-than-standard temperatures in a hospital laundry facility. *Appl Environ Microbiol* 1983;45:591.
47. American Academy of Pediatrics, American College of Obstetricians and Gynecologists. *Guidelines for perinatal care*, 3rd ed. Elk Grove Village, Ill.: American Academy of Pediatrics, 1992.

Hospital Infections, Fourth Edition,
edited by John V. Bennett and Philip S. Brachman.
Published by Lippincott–Raven Publishers, Philadelphia, 1998

CHAPTER 22

Foodborne Disease Prevention in Healthcare Facilities

Laurence Slutsker, Margarita E. Villarino, William R. Jarvis, and Joy Goulding

Foodborne disease outbreaks may occur when food becomes contaminated with pathogenic organisms or toxins. When these contaminants are bacterial pathogens, mishandling of food may permit proliferation of these organisms and subsequently cause illness when ingested by susceptible persons. Food service departments at hospitals and other healthcare facilities, such as nursing homes, must cope with problems associated with handling large amounts of raw food, serving many meals throughout the day, preparing and handling food for a variety of diets, and delays in serving. These challenges in food preparation and delivery in healthcare facilities are compounded by the necessity of serving many patients who are at high risk of contracting foodborne disease. Because of these problems, prevention of foodborne disease should be a high priority in healthcare facilities.

Foodborne disease outbreaks related to food service in healthcare facilities may affect patients [1–9], personnel [10,11], and visitors [12,13] and may involve food prepared in the facility itself [1,2,4], or food prepared elsewhere but served in the healthcare facility [14,15]. Generally, hospitalized persons are more likely than nonhospitalized persons to acquire disease when exposed to foodborne agents and to develop serious side effects associated with such diseases. This is most likely due to host factors (e.g., malignancy, achlorhydria, advanced age, diabetes mellitus, and acquired immunodeficiency syndrome [AIDS]) or iatrogenic factors (e.g., use of antibiotics, immunosuppressive agents, or antacids and gastric surgery). Small inocula of enteric pathogens that might be innocuous to most healthy people can cause disease and even death in highly susceptible patients.

Secondary transmission of foodborne pathogens may also come about when patients or healthcare facility personnel become infected and, in turn, expose other patients or personnel as a consequence of poor personal hygiene or improper patient care techniques. Epidemics resulting from person-to-person transmission occur most often in nurseries, pediatric wards, and nursing homes, where fecal-oral spread may be facilitated by difficulties in maintaining good hygiene [16]. Secondary transmission may involve persons within the healthcare facility (patients, personnel, and visitors), and others (such as family members) outside the hospital setting. Foodborne disease outbreaks affecting large numbers of hospital personnel have led to staffing problems and may hinder delivery of optimal care [11,12]. With assumptions made about the values of indirect costs, the cost of a hospital-based outbreak has been estimated to be as high as $400,000 [17].

The problems of food or dietetic services in healthcare facilities generally parallel those of large restaurants and catering firms but may be even more complex [18]. Healthcare facilities' food services typically operate 12 to 18 hours daily, 7 days per week. Similar to large restaurants, such institutions purchase and rapidly process quantities of food that require large working surfaces, numerous utensils, and many working hands. They also must adhere to tight schedules, rapidly preparing and storing a large variety of foods. In addition, food services in such facilities have unique problems created by the need for a wide assortment of special diets, including enteral feedings. Meals and supplemental feedings must be provided from a central kitchen and sometimes from

L. Slutsker: Foodborne and Diarrheal Diseases Branch
M. E. Villarino: National Center for Infectious Diseases, Hospital Infections Program
W. R. Jarvis: Hospital Infections Program
J. Goulding: Division of Bacterial and Mycotic Diseases, National Center for Infectious Diseases, Centers for Disease Control and Prevention, Atlanta, Georgia 30333

decentralized kitchens on wards. Finally, food must often be transported from a central preparation area throughout the institution. If food is not held at appropriate temperatures, delays between preparation and service present opportunities for proliferation of foodborne pathogens.

EPIDEMIOLOGIC ASPECTS OF FOODBORNE DISEASES

The epidemiology of foodborne disease outbreaks in the United Kingdom and the United States has been reviewed extensively elsewhere [19–22]. In Scotland, during the 9-year period from 1978 to 1987, some 48 foodborne outbreaks were reported from hospitals, compared with 50 outbreaks during the previous 4 years (1973 to 1977) [19]. The decline in the overall incidence of food poisoning outbreaks was attributed to an increased recognition by dietary departments of the principles of food temperature control. Reductions were seen in the number of outbreaks caused by *Clostridium perfringens* and *Staphylococcus* species, while the number of outbreaks of salmonellosis rose. The average number of persons affected per outbreak of salmonellosis increased from 36 in 1973 to 81 in 1987. In contrast, in England and Wales during 1978 to 1987, a total of 248 outbreaks of salmonellosis were reported in hospitals, compared with 522 outbreaks reported during 1968 to 1977 [20]. This decline might have been a result of improved food-handling practices; environmental health officers in the United Kingdom have expanded the monitoring of hospital food service departments since 1977.

In the United States, from all foodborne outbreaks reported to the Centers for Disease Control and Prevention (CDC) during 1975 to 1992, the bacterial agents most frequently identified were *Salmonella*, *Staphylococcus aureus*, *C. botulinum*, and *C. perfringens* (Table 22-1). In healthcare facilities, *Salmonella* and *C. perfringens* are more significant than *C. botulinum* and *S. aureus*. Transmission of all four of these common foodborne bacterial pathogens was typically associated with certain food vehicles; likely sources of contamination varied for the different pathogens (Table 22-1). The number of reported foodborne outbreaks in known locations during 1975 to 1992, and the associated cases and deaths in hospitals, nursing homes, and other known locations, are shown in Table 22-2. Of these, hospitals and nursing homes accounted for 3.3% of the outbreaks, 4.8% of the cases, and 28.9% of the deaths.

Only 123 foodborne disease outbreaks in hospitals were reported during this 17-year period. However, because foodborne disease outbreaks must be recognized, investigated, and reported to state health departments before being reported to the CDC, it is highly likely that foodborne outbreaks are underreported nationally. During 1975 to 1992, reported outbreaks in hospitals and nursing homes were significantly more likely to be caused by bacterial agents (n=143) than by viruses, parasites, or chemicals (n=16) (Table 22-3). Nonetheless, viral [13,23] and parasitic [24] foodborne outbreaks have been reported from healthcare facilities.

It is important to investigate foodborne disease outbreaks in hospitals, to define sources, modes of spread, and methods for prevention and control of nosocomial foodborne disease. Of 233 hospital-based outbreaks of infection investigated by the CDC from 1956 to 1979, gastroenteritis was the most common cause; typical organisms were *Salmonella* and enteropathogenic *Escherichia coli* [25]. In adult patients, contaminated food vehicles were frequently implicated in salmonellosis outbreaks. Outbreaks attributed to cross-infection, such as gastroenteritis in nurseries due to *E. coli* or *Salmonella*, were more difficult to recognize and control than were foodborne outbreaks. Most cross-infection outbreaks were recognized because the infecting pathogen was unusual or distinguished by a unique antimicrobial resis-

TABLE 22-1. *Foods commonly involved and reported cause of contamination in foodborne outbreaks of bacterial etiology, United States, 1975–1992*

			Usual reported cause of contamination			
Cause	Numbers of outbreaks	Typical foods	Improper holding	Inadequate cooling	Poor hygiene	Contaminated equipment
Salmonella	1,270	Poultry, eggs, beef, pork, ice cream	+	++	+	+
Staphylococcus aureus	355	Ham, poultry, pastries, beef	++	–	+	–
Clostridium botulinum	260	Vegetables, fish	+	++	–	–
Clostridium perfringens	206	Beef, poultry, Mexican food	++	+	–	–
Shigella	118	Salads	+	–	++	–
Bacillus cereus	77	Fried rice, Chinese food	++	+	–	–
Campylobacter jejuni	80	Milk	+	+	–	+
Vibrio parahaemolyticus	26	Shellfish	+	++	–	–

–, less frequent cause; +, frequent cause; ++, most frequent cause.
(From Centers for Disease Control and Prevention, Foodborne Disease Surveillance.)

TABLE 22-2. *Reported foodborne outbreaks, cases, and deaths in hospitals, nursing homes, and other known locations, 1975–1992*

	Hospitals		Nursing homes		Other known locations	
	Total	Confirmed cause	Total	Confirmed cause	Total	Confirmed cause
No. of outbreaks	123	67	168	92	8,631	3,225
No.of cases	6,638	3,941	6,783	3,665	268,009	135,035
No.of deaths	11	7	86	82	235	215
Deaths/1,000 cases	1.7	1.8	12.7	22.4	0.9	1.6

(From Centers for Disease Control and Prevention, Foodborne Disease Surveillance.)

tance pattern. In England and Wales from 1978 to 1987, 71 (30%) of 235 reported outbreaks of salmonellosis in hospitals were attributed to cross-infection, compared with 57 (24%) outbreaks attributed to foodborne transmission [20]. However, foodborne outbreaks affected more persons (n=1,862) than did those due to cross-infection (n=558). Since 1979, CDC investigation of such outbreaks has been uncommon.

In the United States during 1975 to 1992, there were 336 reported deaths associated with foodborne disease outbreaks with known place of preparation (Table 22-4). Eighty-six (26%) took place in nursing homes and 11 (3%) in hospitals. Of the 97 deaths in hospitals and nursing homes, 72 (74%) were due to *Salmonella*. In the United States, isolation rates of *Salmonella* serotype Enteritidis have been increasing since 1976 [26]. From 1985 to 1991, some 380 S. Enteritidis outbreaks were reported to the CDC, involving 13,056 ill persons, 1,512 hospitalizations, and 50 deaths [27]. Of these outbreaks, 59 (16%) were in nursing homes or hospitals, accounting for 1,512 illnesses (12%) and 45 (90%) of deaths. Of 167 outbreaks in which a food vehicle was identified, 137 (82%) implicated fresh eggs in the shell. During this same period, nine (60%) of 15 reported nursing home outbreaks with a known vehicle implicated dishes containing shell eggs. Four (8%) of the 49 *S. enteritidis* outbreaks reported from January to October 31, 1990, occurred in hospitals or nursing homes, compared with 20 (26%) of 77 such outbreaks in 1989 [28]. This decline in hospital- and nursing home-associated *S. enteritidis* outbreaks may reflect efforts to improve food safety in these settings (e.g., by using pasteurized eggs).

Surveillance data can help elucidate the relative importance of various factors that contribute to the occurrence of foodborne disease outbreaks. During 1975–1992, food-handling errors were noted in 212 reported foodborne outbreaks in hospitals or nursing homes. Holding food at improper temperatures was the most common such error. Other important errors included inadequate cooking, poor personal hygiene of

TABLE 22-3. *Confirmed causes of reported foodborne outbreaks related to hospitals, nursing homes, and other known locations, United States, 1975–1992*

	Hospitals		Nursing homes		Other known locations	
	Number of outbreaks	% of total[a]	Number of outbreaks	% of total[a]	Number of outbreaks	% of total[a]
Bacterial						
Salmonella	35	52	61	66	1,157	36
Staphylococcus aureus	5	8	14	15	332	10
Clostridium perfringens	7	11	8	9	202	6
Shigella	3	5	1	1	112	4
Bacillus cereus	1	2	2	2	74	2
Campylobacter jejuni	1	2	3	3	74	2
Other bacteria	1	2	1	1	304	9
Subtotal	53	79	90	98	2,255	70
Viral	1	2	0	0	166	5
Parasitic	1	2	1	1	116	4
Chemical						
Scombroid	8	12	0	0	244	8
Ciguatera	0	0	0	0	211	7
Other	4	6	1	1	233	7
Subtotal	12	18	1	1	688	21
Total	67	100	92	100	3,225	100

[a]Percentages may sum to >100% because of rounding.
(From Centers for Disease Control and Prevention, Foodborne Disease Surveillance.)

TABLE 22-4. *Causes of deaths associated with foodborne diseases outbreaks in hospitals, nursing homes, and other known locations, United States, 1975–1992*

Cause	Total deaths	Deaths in hospital outbreaks		Deaths in nursing home outbreaks		Deaths in other known locations	
		No.	% of total	No.	% of total	No.	% of total
Salmonella	121	2	2	70	58	49	41
Clostridium perfringens	11	5	45	3	27	3	27
Staphylococcus aureus	4	0	0	2	50	2	50
Escherichia coli	4	0	0	4	100	0	0
Other known cause	168	0	0	3	2	165	98
Unknown cause	28	4	14	4	14	20	71
Total	336	11	3	86	24	239	71

(From Centers for Disease Control and Prevention, Foodborne Disease Surveillance.)

food-handlers, use of food from unsafe sources, and use of contaminated equipment. Training personnel in proper food-handling practices can eliminate these errors and prevent outbreaks.

Food served from a health-care facility kitchen can be contaminated before, during, or after preparation. When purchased, raw poultry and red meat might already be contaminated with organisms (e.g., *Salmonella*, *C. perfringens*, *Campylobacter jejuni* or, more rarely, *E. coli* 0157:H7). In a 1988 survey of broiler chicken specimens from 195 poultry-processing plants, the prevalence of *Salmonella* contamination was 21% of 15,391 specimens [29]. *Campylobacter jejuni* typically is present in >50% of poultry carcasses at the point of sale [30]. Raw fish and shellfish can be contaminated with such pathogens as *Vibrio parahaemolyticus*, *C. perfringens*, and *V. vulnificus*. Shell eggs may be contaminated with *S. enteritidis*, either externally through fecal contamination or internally through transovarian transmission [31,32]. During processing, food also may become contaminated with organisms through contact with dirty hands, infected aerosols spread through coughing or sneezing, and contaminated equipment, such as meat slicers or working surfaces [33]. Finally, bacteria may grow while food is stored (e.g., when cooked foods are stored in direct contact with raw foods or when foods are held at inadequate temperatures). *Listeria monocytogenes* can survive and grow in food even with adequate refrigeration [34].

FOODS AND THE IMMUNOCOMPROMISED HOST

Patients in healthcare facilities are more susceptible to certain foodborne infections than the general population. The elderly, the immunosuppressed, and persons with chronic underlying diseases are generally at higher risk of infection and associated morbidity and mortality. In particular, outbreaks of foodborne disease in nursing homes can be associated with serious morbidity and mortality; therefore, efforts to provide the safest possible food to the elderly in nursing homes should be maximized.

Among persons in hospitals and nursing homes, increased susceptibility to foodborne infections may be caused by associated physiologic changes or therapy of underlying disease. Although the gastrointestinal tract is normally resistant to colonization, this resistance can be substantially diminished by antimicrobial therapy, mucositis from cancer treatments, decreased stomach acidity, impaired intestinal motility, and diminished mucosal, humoral, and cellular immunity. Even in numbers smaller than the usual infective dose, ingested microorganisms may cause systemic infection in these patients.

Because *E. coli*, *Klebsiella* spp, and *Pseudomonas aeruginosa* can contaminate fresh fruits, salads, and vegetables [35], these foods should not be served to neutropenic patients [36]. Another potential contaminant of fresh vegetables is *L. monocytogenes*, a gram-positive bacterium that particularly affects the elderly, pregnant women, and the severely immunosuppressed [34]. In one *L. monocytogenes* outbreak involving 20 patients from eight hospitals, raw vegetables served in hospital meals may have been contaminated; 10 (50%) of these patients were immunosuppressed [37]. Dairy products and any raw food of animal origin also may be contaminated with *Listeria*, *Salmonella*, or *E. coli* 0157:H7. Outbreaks of *E. coli* O157:H7 and *Salmonella* in nursing homes have been particularly devastating. In two such *E. coli* O157:H7 outbreaks, 15 deaths occurred [1,38]. In an outbreak of *S. enteritidis* in a nursing home, 25 of 104 affected patients died [39].

Human immunodeficiency virus (HIV)-infected persons are at increased risk of infection with bacterial foodborne pathogens (see Chapter 43). Among persons with AIDS, the reported incidence of laboratory-confirmed salmonellosis was 20 times that reported for persons without AIDS [40]. Compared with immunocompetent persons, those with AIDS and salmonellosis are more likely to have initial and recurrent bloodstream infections [41,42]. The reported incidence of campylobacteriosis among persons with AIDS in Los Angeles County between 1983 and 1987 was 39 times higher than the rate in the general population [43]. Similarly, the incidence of listeriosis among persons with HIV infection is estimated to be 60 times that of the general population; among persons with AIDS, the relative risk is more than 140 times greater [44]. Ingestion of contaminated foods is likely to be an important source of enteric infections in persons with AIDS. All immunocompetent persons should cook raw foods of animal origin thoroughly and avoid eating raw shellfish, raw milk, raw meat, and raw eggs [45–47]. Dietary departments in health facilities should follow these recommendations for all hospitalized patients, particularly those who are immunocompromised.

Enteral feeding solutions are used frequently to provide nutritional support to seriously ill patients with a functional digestive tract. These solutions are often prepared in food service departments. Enteral feedings contaminated by bacteria can cause severe nosocomial infections [48–50]; therefore, infection control practices for their preparation and administration should be reviewed and implemented [51]. A high incidence of microbial contamination of enteral nutrition, including powdered feeds requiring reconstitution, has been described [47,48, 50,52–56]. Contamination also can occur during assembly of a delivery system on the ward [57] or by bacteria colonizing the nasogastric tube or ascending from the patient's gut [58].

Factors contributing to the microbial contamination of enteral feeding solutions include the composition of the feeding solution, the lack of preservatives, the number of manipulations involved in the feeding process, the mode and duration of administration, and the timing of sampling [50]. *Enterobacter sakazakii* outbreaks in neonates have been traced to both extrinsically and intrinsically contaminated powdered infant formula [49,54]. Although contamination is most frequently the result of manipulation during preparation, adherence to appropriate food-handling practices is essential to minimize bacterial contamination during preparation and administration and bacterial growth during storage. Monitoring by public health authorities of recommended manufacturing procedures and of the regulations governing the bacterial content of powdered feeds has been suggested [50].

TABLE 22-5. *Summary of requirements and recommendations of the Joint Commission on Accreditation of Healthcare Organizations (JCAHO) and the Association for Professionals in Infection Control, Inc. (APIC) for food (dietetic) services*

JCAHO	APIC
Dietetic services shall meet the nutritional needs of patients through the following standards:	Infection control activities of the food service department should include:
1. Organization to provide optimal nutritional care and quality of service	1. Development of purchasing specifications that meet standards of safety and sanitation for food, equipment, and cleaning supplies
2. Appropriate training of personnel	2. Maintenance and cleaning of work areas, storage areas, and equipment in accordance with state and local health department standards
3. Written policies and procedures	3. Development of written standards for safe food-handling; cleaning and sanitizing of trays, utensils, and tableware; and disposing of dietary waste
4. Safe, sanitary, and timely provision of food to meet nutritional requirements	4. Compliance with local health department regulations for storage, handling, and disposal of garbage
5. Diet in accord with care provider's order and appropriate recording of dietetic information in patient's chart	5. Educational programs for personnel in food preparation and personal hygiene
6. Appropriate quality control mechanisms	
7. Regular evaluation of quality and appropriateness in accordance with JCAHO quality assurance characteristics	

(Data adapted from Joint Commission on Accreditation of Healthcare Organizations. *Accreditation manual for hospitals.* 1991. Chicago: Joint Commission on Accreditation of Healthcare Organizations, 1990; and Association for Practitioners in Infection Control. *APIC infection control and applied epidemiology: principles and practice.* St. Louis: Mosby–Year Book, Inc., 1996.)

PREVENTION OF FOODBORNE TRANSMISSION IN HEALTH CARE FACILITIES

Requirements and recommendations concerning food services are provided to hospitals and other healthcare facilities from the Joint Commission on Accreditation of Healthcare Organizations (JCAHO) and the Association for Professionals in Infection Control and Epidemiology, Inc. (APIC) (Table 22-5). Responsibilities for the inspection and certification of food service facilities in health-care organizations vary by state. Accreditation by JCAHO does not assure regular food service inspection or food-handler training. The infection control committee of each health-care facility has an important responsibility in the prevention of foodborne disease. This committee is responsible for cooperating with the food services department in developing written policies and procedures and for reviewing these policies at least annually [59].

To prevent foodborne disease, both the JCAHO requirements and the APIC recommendations focus prevention efforts by hospitals and other health-care institutions in two areas: food hygiene (i.e., food preparation, storage, and distribution) and health and hygiene of food service personnel. Both of these areas need to be reinforced by specific training of food service workers in the basic principles of food safety. New personnel should receive prompt training in good food-handling practices. Food service personnel from all work shifts should receive regular in-service training stressing the prevention of foodborne diseases and appropriate food-handling practices.

General approaches to limiting contamination and destroying or inhibiting the growth of potential foodborne pathogens have been reviewed elsewhere [60,61]. Healthcare facilities should consult a dietitian with special training in food service sanitation, a sanitarian, or both about formulating and monitoring food-handling operations and procedures. In addition, local or state health departments should be consulted about regulations and standards concerning food service personnel, food sanitation, and waste disposal.

Food Hygiene

Two factors are critical in preventing bacterial foodborne disease: holding food at appropriate temperatures (that is, either above 60°C (140°F) or below 5°C (41°F)) and avoiding cross-contamination of cooked food by raw food or by infected food-handling personnel [62]. In addition, pasteurized milk and pasteurized egg products should be used in place of raw milk and shell eggs. Food must be purchased from reliable sources; commercially filled unopened packages should be used when possible. Microbial contaminants on some raw foods may be kept from multiplying during processing by proper storage, thawing of meat products in refrigerators (under 5°C [41°F]), or adequate heat treatment. Because work surfaces, knives, slicers, pots, pans, and other kitchen equipment can convey bacteria from contaminated food to other foods, food contact surfaces of equipment and utensils must be cleaned and decontaminated between preparation of food items. Items such as slicers must be easy to disassemble to ensure proper cleaning.

Workers should be trained to operate and maintain equipment properly. Hand washing by food service personnel is an essential component of food hygiene. All workers must thoroughly wash their hands after handling raw poultry, meat, fish, fruits, and vegetables; after contact with unclean equipment and work surfaces, soiled clothing, washrags, and other items; and, most important, after using the bathroom. Spilled food should be cleaned up immediately. Equipment and the kitchen layout should be designed to promote rapid processing to minimize chances for cross-contamination; to avoid producing aerosols, sprays, or splashing during processing; and to facilitate cleaning and sanitizing operations [61]. Contamination by insects, rodents, sewage backflow, or drips must be prevented by screening, proper storage (including separating raw meat from processed foods), and adequate plumbing. Garbage from hospital kitchens and wards should be enclosed, protected from insects and rodents, and transported or disposed of in a sanitary manner, according to state and local regulations.

Cross-contamination can be minimized by adopting standard techniques for cleaning work surfaces and kitchen utensils and by ensuring that raw foods are processed in areas of the kitchen and on work surfaces that are not subsequently used for cooked foods. Separate cutting boards may not be required when the boards in use are nonabsorbent and can be cleaned and sanitized adequately between usage for different food categories. Dishwashing and utensil-washing equipment and techniques that sanitize service ware and prevent recontamination should be used to ensure sanitary provision of food. Disposable containers and utensils should be properly discarded after one use. Food hygiene procedures should be reviewed periodically and whenever physical changes are made in the kitchen or new equipment is put into use.

Foodborne disease outbreaks have resulted from poor planning and a lack of understanding of appropriate food-handling practices (e.g., not allowing enough time before cooking for poultry to thaw or assuming that thawing is complete). This problem can result in undercooking and can be compounded by keeping undercooked food in the oven after the heat has been shut off, providing ideal incubation conditions for bacteria that survived the initial cooking. Potentially harmful bacteria in foods must be destroyed by thorough cooking or reheating to the proper internal temperatures for the appropriate length of time. For example, meat and poultry should generally be cooked to heat all parts of the food to ≥ 68°C (155°F) for 15 seconds [62]. Internal meat temperatures should be measured by bayonet-type thermometers. Periodically, the internal temperature of foods in serving lines should be checked.

A common error resulting in foodborne disease outbreaks is storage of food at inappropriate temperatures; this error is most often identified in staphylococcal food poisoning outbreaks and in short- and long-incubation *Bacillus cereus*, *C. perfringens*, and *Salmonella* outbreaks. In some outbreaks, even when refrigerator temperatures have been adequate, the center temperature of perishable foods was warm enough to permit bacteria to grow or toxin to be produced because the foods were in inadequate holding containers. When cooked foods are kept at room temperature (or are refrigerated in large quantities) for a period of ≥ 4 hours, certain pathogens remaining in the food may be able to multiply to sufficient levels or produce enough toxin to cause disease. Cooked foods have been kept too long at room temperature because of inadequate refrigerator space and failure to perceive the importance of refrigeration. In general, cooked food that requires refrigeration should be cooled from 60°C (140°F) to 21°C (70°F) within 2 hours and from 21°C (70°F) to ≤ 5°C (41°F) within 4 hours; storage temperature should not exceed 5°C (41°F). Food should be placed in shallow containers such that the food is no more than 4 inches deep.

Storage is a particular problem when food must be delivered from a central kitchen to peripheral areas of the health-care facility or other buildings either by truck or on food carts. Procedures for transporting food must include a means of keeping hot foods hot and cold foods cold. Thermometers used to measure holding temperatures should be standard equipment in such conveyances. Standby equipment should be on hand or alternative plans formulated to handle emergency conditions arising from equipment failure. Food delivered to a kitchen or ward should be properly stored to prevent growth of bacteria, and it should be distributed with minimum handling by ward personnel. In the event that ward personnel must handle food, they should be carefully supervised to ensure that the same high standards required of kitchen personnel are maintained.

In the past, problems have arisen because of preferences for raw or undercooked foods. Substitution of pasteurized egg products for fresh eggs in nursing homes and hospitals is strongly recommended. Several outbreaks have been traced to blenders used for both raw eggs and pureed foods. Requiring the use of separate blenders to scramble eggs and to puree cooked foods would reduce the risk of cross-contamination. Routine disassembly and sanitation of blenders after blending raw eggs also is important. Avoiding consumption of raw milk is important in preventing outbreaks caused by *Salmonella* and *C. jejuni*.

Health and Hygiene of Food Service Personnel

Supervision of food service personnel requires attention to work habits, personal hygiene, and health. The hands of food service personnel may be colonized or infected with microorganisms, such as *S. aureus*, or may become contaminated by organisms from raw foods (*Salmonella*, *C. jejuni*, or *C. perfringens*) or human excreta (*Salmonella*, *Shigella* spp, Norwalk and Norwalk-like agents, or hepatitis A virus). These organisms may then contaminate food. Although thorough cooking of food just before consumption will eradicate the risk of many illnesses, staphylococcal food poisoning will not be eliminated because staphylococcal enterotoxins are heat-stable.

Hand-washing facilities should be conveniently located to permit use by employees in food preparation and utensil-washing areas and in or immediately adjacent to toilet facilities. Each hand-washing facility should be provided with a continuous supply of clean water; a supply of hand-cleaning liquid, powder, or bar soap; and individual sanitary towels, a continuous towel system supplied with a clean towel, or a heated-air hand-drying device. Common hand-drying towels are prohibited. If disposable towels are used, a waste receptacle should be located next to the hand-washing facility.

Various strategies have been used to monitor the health of food service personnel, including periodic stool examinations for certain pathogens. However, such measures may not be effective. One stool culture is not sufficient to detect the small number of organisms in the stool of an infected person who does not have diarrhea. For example, one rectal swab detected only 47% of chronic *Salmonella* serotype Derby carriers, and seven consecutive daily swabs were needed to detect 95% of known carriers [63]. Such extensive culturing is impractical and costly. Periodic stool cultures of food-handlers may miss persons who excrete organisms intermittently or who become infected during the interval between cultures. In Jordan, a large outbreak of nosocomial salmonellosis caused by an asymptomatic infected food-handler occurred despite the institution of routine quarterly stool cultures for kitchen employees [64].

In addition, cultures of nose and throat secretions and feces may reveal potential foodborne pathogens, such as *S. aureus*, but this carriage may be of no danger to others: *S. aureus* carriers do not usually disseminate the organisms. Laboratory monitoring of food-handlers could actually be counterproductive by instilling a false sense of security. Negative culture reports could be interpreted by the employee to indicate that he or she is not capable of contaminating food. From the management standpoint, laboratory monitoring of food-handlers may convey the false impression that food safety is being enhanced. Thus, routine laboratory testing of food service personnel should not be performed [65].

The proper approach to managing the personal aspects of hygiene is to establish and pursue a policy of training food service managers and workers. The health-care facility infection control committee should ensure a program comprising a comprehensive training course in the appropriate languages for all new employees at the onset of employment and in-service training at regular intervals for all food service personnel (see Chapter 3). As appropriate to the workers' level of responsibility, such courses should cover the basic principles of personal hygiene, emphasizing the need for good hand-washing practices; the importance of informing supervisors of acute intestinal diseases, boils, and any skin infection, particularly on the fingers and hands; the proper inspection, handling, preparation, serving, and storing of food; the proper cleaning and safe operation of equipment; general food service sanitation safety; the proper method of waste disposal; portion control; the writing of modified diets using the diet manual or handbook; diet instruction; and the recording of pertinent dietetic information in each patient's medical record [66]. In addition to training, a liberal medical leave policy will ensure that employees are not penalized financially when they report that they are ill.

SURVEILLANCE AND CONTROL

The responsibility for preventing, detecting, and investigating foodborne disease outbreaks rests with the healthcare facility infection control committee and the infection control practitioner (see Chapter 2). They can begin by carefully reviewing the results of recent hospital kitchen inspections by the local health department and the food safety training program currently in place for kitchen staff. In addition, they can ensure that, whenever possible, pasteurized eggs are used instead of shell eggs and verify that the risks of using a common blender to mix raw eggs and other foods are well understood by all employees. It is important that the infection control committee meet with the kitchen staff and communicate to them that food safety is of the highest priority.

Surveillance for illness among the kitchen staff may prevent some foodborne outbreaks and also may provide an early warning when such an outbreak occurs, because they, too, eat the food. A monitoring procedure should be established to ensure that food service personnel are free from open skin lesions. Designated infection control staff should be informed of acute illnesses among food service workers that could potentially be transmitted by food. It is important that an atmosphere be created that does not penalize food-handlers for reporting illness. Any work restriction policy should encourage personnel to report their illnesses or exposures and not penalize them with loss of wages, benefits, or job status [67].

Appropriate culture specimens should be obtained and processed during such illnesses. In cases of acute diarrhea, rectal swab or fecal specimens promptly inoculated onto appropriate laboratory media are recommended. Workers should not be permitted to return to their assigned jobs until their diarrhea has resolved and two stool cultures obtained ≥ 24 hours apart show negative results (see Chapter 34). If antimicrobial agents are used, follow-up cultures should be obtained after treatment has been completed. Personnel with boils, open sores, or cellulitis of the fingers, hands, and face should be excluded until they are adequately treated. The infection control practitioner's judgment should prevail in deciding when the worker can return to work.

Routine surveillance of patients and employees should detect any episodes of gastrointestinal disease related to the health-care institution's food service. Temporal clustering of such episodes should alert the infection control personnel to the possibility of an outbreak. Prompt investigation and reporting of outbreaks to the appropriate health authorities are essential to identifying and correcting food-handling error(s), preventing additional primary and secondary transmission of disease, and limiting outbreaks caused by commercially distributed foods.

REFERENCES

1. Carter AO, Borczyk AA, Carlson JAK, et al. A severe outbreak of *Escherichia coli* O157:H7-associated hemorrhagic colitis in a nursing home. *N Engl J Med* 1987;317:1496–1500.
2. Centers for Disease Control and Prevention. Foodborne nosocomial outbreak of *Salmonella reading*—Connecticut. *MMWR* 1990;40:804–806.
3. Giannella RA, Brasile L. A hospital foodborne outbreak of diarrhea caused by *Bacillus cereus*: clinical, epidemiologic, and microbiologic studies. *J Infect Dis* 1979;139:366–370.
4. Telzak EE, Budnick LD, Greenberg MSZ, et al. A nosocomial outbreak of *Salmonella enteritidis* infection due to the consumption of raw eggs. *N Engl J Med* 1990;323:394–397.
5. Thomas M, Noah ND. Hospital outbreak of *Clostridium perfringens* food poisoning. *Lancet* 1977;1:1046–1048.
6. Yamagishi T, Sakamoto K, Sakurai S, et al. A nosocomial outbreak of food poisoning caused by enterotoxigenic *Clostridium perfringens*. *Microbiol Immunol* 1983;27:291–296.
7. Pavia AT, Nichols CR, Green DP, et al. Hemolytic-uremic syndrome during an outbreak of *Escherichia coli* O157:H7 infections in institutions for the mentally retarded: clinical and epidemiologic observations. *J Pediatr* 1990;116:544–551.
8. Standaert SM, Hutcheson RH, Schaffner W. Nosocomial transmission of *Salmonella* gastroenteritis to laundry workers in a nursing home. *Infect Control Hosp Epidemiol* 1994;15:22–26.
9. Holtby I, Stendon P. Food poisoning in two homes for the elderly. *Communicable Dis Rep* 1992;2:R125–126.
10. Khatib R, Naber M, Shellum N, et al. A common source outbreak of gastroenteritis in a teaching hospital. *Infect Control Hosp Epidemiol* 1994;15:534–535.
11. Centers for Disease Control and Prevention. Shigellosis in children's hospital—Pennsylvania. *MMWR* 1979;28:498–499.
12. Centers for Disease Control and Prevention. Hospital-associated outbreak of *Shigella dysenteriae* type 2—Maryland. *MMWR* 1983;32: 250–252.
13. Meyers JD, Frederic JR, Tithen WS, Bryan JA. Foodborne hepatitis A in a general hospital: epidemiologic study of an outbreak attributed to sandwiches. *JAMA* 1975;231:1049–1053.
14. Centers for Disease Control and Prevention. Multistate outbreak of salmonellosis caused by precooked roast beef. *MMWR* 1981;30:391–392.
15. Spitalny KC, Okowitz EN, Vogt RL. Salmonellosis outbreaks at a Vermont hospital. *South Med J* 1984;77:168–172.
16. Linnemann CC Jr., Cannon CG, Stancek JL, et al. Prolonged hospital epidemic of salmonellosis: use of trimethoprim-sulfamethoxazole for control. *Infect Control Hosp Epidemiol* 1985;6:221–225.
17. Yule BF, MacLeod AF, Sharp JCM, Forbes GI. Costing of a hospital-based outbreak of poultry-borne salmonellosis. *Epidemiol Infect* 1988; 100:35-42
18. Anonymous. Food poisoning in hospitals [Editorial]. *Lancet* 1980;1: 576.
19. Collier PW, Sharp JC, MacLeod AF, et al. Food poisoning in hospitals in Scotland, 1978–1987. *Epidemiol Infect* 1988;101:661–667.
20. Joseph CA, Palmer SR. Outbreaks of *Salmonella* infection in hospitals in England and Wales, 1978–1987. *Br Med J* 1989;298:1161–1164.
21. Archer DL, Young FK. Contemporary issues: diseases with a food vector. *Clin Microbiol Rev* 1988;1:377–398.
22. Bean NH, Griffin PM, Goulding JS, Ivey CB. Foodborne disease outbreaks in the United States, 1973–1987. *J Food Protect* 1990;53: 711–730.
23. Stevenson P, McCann R, Duthie R, Glenn E, Ganguli L. A hospital outbreak due to Norwalk virus. *J Hosp Infect* 1994;26:261–272.
24. Levine WC, Smart JF, Archer DL, et al. Foodborne disease outbreaks in nursing homes, 1975 to 1987. *JAMA* 1991;266:2105–2109.
25. Stamm WE, Weinstein RA, Dixon RE. Comparison of endemic and epidemic nosocomial infections. *Am J Med* 1981;70:393–397.
26. Tauxe RV. *Salmonella*: a postmodern pathogen. *J Food Protect* 1991; 54:563–568.
27. Mishu B, Koehler J, Lee LA, et al. Outbreaks of *Salmonella enteritidis* infections in the United States, 1985–1991. *J Infect Dis* 1994;169: 547–552.
28. CDC. Update: *Salmonella enteritidis* infections and shell eggs—United States, 1990. *MMWR* 1990;39:909–912.
29. Lee L, Threatt VL, Puhr ND, et al. Antimicrobial-resistant *Salmonella* spp. isolated from healthy broiler chickens after slaughter. *J Am Vet Med Assoc* 1993;202:752–755.
30. Tauxe RV. Epidemiology of *Campylobacter jejuni* infections in the United States and other industrialized nations. In: Nachamkin T, Blaser MJ, Tompkins LS, eds. Campylobacter jejuni: *current status and future trends*. Washington, DC: American Society for Microbiology, 1992: 9–19.
31. St. Louis ME, Morse DL, Potter ME, et al. The emergence of grade A eggs as a major source of *Salmonella enteritidis* infection. *JAMA* 1988; 259:2103–2107.

32. Gast RK, Beard CW. Production of *Salmonella enteritidis* contaminated eggs by experimentally infected hens. *Avian Dis* 1990;34:438–446.
33. Jordan MC, Powell KE, Corothers TE, Murray RJ. Salmonellosis among restaurant patrons: the incisive role of a meat slicer. *Am J Public Health* 1973;63:982–985.
34. Schucat A, Swaminathan B, Broome C. Epidemiology of human listeriosis. *Clin Microbiol Rev* 1991;4:169–183.
35. Shooter RA, Cooke EM, Faiers MC, et al. Isolation of *Escherichia coli, Pseudomonas aeruginosa*, and *Klebsiella* from food in hospitals, canteens, and schools. *Lancet* 1971;2:390–392.
36. Remington JS, Schimpff SC. Please don't eat the salads. *N Engl J Med* 1981;304:433–435.
37. Ho JL, Shands KN, Fredland G, et al. An outbreak of type 4b *Listeria monocytogenes* infection involving patients from eight Boston hospitals. *Arch Intern Med* 1986;146:520–524.
38. Ryan CA, Tauxe RV, Hosek GW, et al. *Escherichia coli* O157:H7 diarrhea in a nursing home: clinical, epidemiological, and pathological findings. *J Infect Dis* 1986;154:631–638.
39. Centers for Disease Control and Prevention. Salmonellosis—Baltimore, Maryland. *MMWR* 1970;19:340.
40. Celum CL, Chaisson RE, Rutherford GW, Bernhart JL, Echenberg DF. Incidence of salmonellosis in patients with AIDS. *J Infect Dis* 1987;156:998–1002.
41. Gruenewald R, Blum S, Chan J. Relationship between human immunodeficiency virus infection and salmonellosis in 20- to 59-year-old residents of New York City. *Clin Infect Dis* 1994;18:358–363.
42. Sperber SJ, Schleupner CJ. Salmonellosis during infections with human immunodeficiency virus. *Rev Infect Dis* 1987;9:925–934.
43. Sorvillo FJ, Lieb LE, Waterman SH. Incidence of campylobacteriosis among patients with AIDS in Los Angeles County. *J Acquir Immune Defic Syndr* 1991;4:598–602.
44. Jurado RL, Farley MM, Pereira E, et al. Increased risk of meningitis and bacteremia due to *Listeria monocytogenes* in patients with human immunodeficiency virus infection. *Clin Infect Dis* 1993;17:224–227.
45. Archer DL. Food counseling for persons infected with HIV: strategy for defensive living. *Public Health Rep* 1989;104:196–198.
46. Griffin PM, Tauxe RV. Food counseling for patients with AIDS [Letter]. *J Infect Dis* 1988;158:668.
47. Angulo FK, Swerdlow DL. Bacterial enteric infections in persons infected with human immunodeficiency virus. *Clin Infect Dis* 1995;21 (suppl 1):S84–93.
48. Thurn J, Crossley K, Gerdts A, Maki M, Johnson J. Enteral hyperalimentation as a source of nosocomial infection. *J Hosp Infect* 1990;15:203–217.
49. Caswell MW, Cooper JE, Webster M. Enteral feeds contaminated with *Enterobacter cloacae* as a cause of septicemia. *Br Med J* 1981;282:973.
50. Noriega FR, Kotloff KL, Martin MA, Schwalber RS. Nosocomial bacteremia caused by *Enterobacter sakazakii* and *Leuconostoc mesenteroides* resulting from extrinsic contamination of infant formula. *Pediatr Infect Dis* 1990;9:447–449.
51. Levy J. Enteral nutrition: an increasingly recognized cause of nosocomial bloodstream infection. *Infect Control Hosp Epidemiol* 1989;10:395–397.
52. Anderson KR, Norris DJ, Godfrey LB, et al. Bacterial contamination of tube feeding formula. *J Parenter Enter Nutr* 1984;8:673–678.
53. Patchell CJ, Anderton A, MacDonald A, et al. Bacterial contamination of enteral feeds. *Arch Dis Child* 1994;70:327–330.
54. Moe G. Enteral feeding and infection in the immunocompromised patient. *Nutr Clin Pract* 1991;6:55–64.
55. Simmons BP, Gelfand MS, Haas M, et al. *Enterobacter sakazakii* infections in neonates associated with intrinsic contamination of a powdered infant formula. *Infect Control Hosp Epidemiol* 1989;10:398.
56. U.S. Food and Drug Administration. *Bacterial contamination of enteral formula products*. Washington, D.C.: Public Health Service, Food and Drug Administration Bulletin, 1988.
57. Anderton A, Aidov KE. The effect of handling procedures on microbial contamination of enteral feeds. *J Hosp Infect* 1988;11:364—372.
58. de Leeuw I, Van Alsenoy L. Bacterial contamination of the feeding bag during catheter jejunostomy: exogenous or endogenous origin? *J Parenter Enter Nutr* 1984;9:591–592.
59. Joint Commission on Accreditation of Healthcare Organizations. *Accreditation manual for hospitals, 1991*. Chicago: Joint Commission on Accreditation of Healthcare Organizations, 1990.
60. Bryan FL. Prevention of foodborne diseases in food-service establishments. *J Environ Health* 1979;41:198–206.
61. Bryan FL. Factors that contribute to outbreaks of foodborne disease. *J Food Protect* 1978;41:816–827.
62. U.S. Department of Health and Human Services. *Food code, 1993*. Washington, D.C.: Public Health Service, Food and Drug Administration, 1993.
63. McCall CE, Martin WT, Boring JR. Efficiency of cultures of rectal swabs and faecal specimens in detecting *Salmonella* carriers: correlation with number of salmonellas excreted. *J Hyg (London)* 1966;64:261–269.
64. Khuri-Bulos NA, Khalaf MA, Shehabi A, Shami K. Foodhandler-associated *Salmonella* outbreak in a university hospital despite routine surveillance cultures of kitchen employees. *Infect Control Hosp Epidemiol* 1994;15:311–314.
65. World Health Organization. *Health surveillance and management procedures for foodhandling personnel*. Geneva, Switzerland: World Health Organization, 1989. (WHO Technical Report Series, no. 785.)
66. Association for Practitioners in Infection Control. *APIC infection control and applied epidemiology: principles and practice*. St. Louis: Mosby-Year Book, Inc., 1996.
67. Williams WW. Guideline for infection control in hospital personnel. *Infect Control Hosp Epidemiol* 1983;4(suppl 4):326–349.

Hospital Infections, Fourth Edition,
edited by John V. Bennett and Philip S. Brachman.
Lippincott–Raven Publishers, Philadelphia © 1998

CHAPTER 23

Clinical Laboratory–Acquired Infections

Michael L. Wilson and L. Barth Reller

Clinical laboratories are an area of special concern in hospital infection control. Laboratory workers may be exposed to infectious agents during all steps of collection, transport, processing, and analysis of patients' specimens. The clinical microbiology staff, in particular, are at risk of occupational infection, since the clinical specimens submitted for culture are likely to contain infectious agents and the process of isolation and culture generates large numbers of pathogenic microorganisms.

The goals of this chapter are to provide an overview of the epidemiology of laboratory-acquired infections, to highlight those infections of special concern to clinical laboratories, and to make specific recommendations for the prevention and control of laboratory-acquired infections. Not discussed in this chapter are the individual problems of clinical virology, research, anatomic pathology, commercial reference laboratories, and laboratories involved in the production or processing of large volumes of pathogenic microorganisms. The reader is referred to Collins' monograph for an extensive review of the subject of laboratory-acquired infections [1]. The role of the clinical microbiology laboratory in infection surveillance, investigation of endemic and epidemic hospital infections, and the control of nosocomial infections is discussed in Chapters 5, 6, and 9, respectively.

INCIDENCE, CAUSATIVE AGENTS, AND COST

The true incidence of laboratory-acquired infections is unknown. Early data were derived from surveys, personal communications, and literature reports, and thus incidence rates cannot be calculated using those data [2–6]. The only available modern data are derived from surveys, which also cannot be used to calculate true incidence rates. One of these surveys [7] reported an annual incidence of three laboratory-acquired infections per 1,000 employees, and another [8] cited annual incidences of 1.4 and 3.5 per 1,000 employees among workers in hospital-based and public health laboratories, respectively. Despite the limitations of the published data, it seems reasonable that the annual incidence of laboratory-acquired infections is between one and 5 per 1,000 employees. There is some evidence that the annual incidence is declining [2], particularly for hepatitis B virus (HBV) infections [9], owing to hepatitis B immunization and adoption of universal precautions [10].

In years past, the most common laboratory-acquired infections were brucellosis, Q fever, typhoid fever, hepatitis B, tularemia, and tuberculosis [3,4]. More recent data show that the infections now most commonly acquired in clinical laboratories are hepatitis B, shigellosis, and tuberculosis [7,11–14]. Other agents continue to pose a hazard to laboratory workers, however, as demonstrated by continuing reports of laboratory-acquired brucellosis [12,14,15], salmonellosis [13,16–19], and meningococcemia [20,21].

The cost to healthcare systems for these infections is unknown. In one report [8], each laboratory-acquired infection resulted in an average of 1.2 lost work days for hospital-based laboratories and 1.3 lost work days for public health laboratories. The latter figure, however, does not include the 48 work days lost when one employee was hospitalized for a laboratory-acquired infection.

An accurate estimate of the cost to healthcare systems may not be possible without additional data or further studies, but it is clear that the cost to an infected individual can be high. It is estimated that 200 to 300 healthcare workers die each year as a consequence of chronic HBV infection [22]. Since the risk to laboratorians of acquiring HBV equals or exceeds that of other healthcare workers [23,24], it seems reasonable that a substantial proportion of these deaths occur among laboratorians. There are also fatal laboratory-acquired infections caused by other path-

M. L. Wilson: University of Colorado School of Medicine, Denver, Colorado 80204-4507.

L. B. Reller: Departments of Pathology and Medicine, Duke University School of Medicine and Medical Center, Durham, North Carolina 27710.

ogens [17,21]. Laboratory-acquired infection with human immunodeficiency virus (HIV), resulting in acquired immunodeficiency syndrome, has been reported in laboratory workers [25–27], who account for ~25% of reported occupational transmissions.

SOURCES OF INFECTION

Pike [2,3] and others [7,8,28,29] have attempted to determine which laboratory procedures, accidents, or other exposures to infectious agents are the source of laboratory-acquired infections (Table 23-1). These data indicate that the source of infection is unknown in ≤ 20% of cases and that the infected individual is known only to have worked with the agent in the past in another 21% of cases [3]. Thus, the exact source, procedure, or breach in technique can be identified in just over half of cases. Among the recognized sources are accidents, which account for 18% of cases. The kinds of accidents that lead to laboratory-acquired infections are listed in Table 23-2.

Laboratory accidents associated with exposure to infectious materials include creation of aerosols from spatters or spills; exposure of skin defects (cuts, abrasions, ulcers, dermatitis, etc.), conjunctivas, or mucosal surfaces; accidental aspiration or ingestion; and traumatic implantation [3]. Needle-stick injuries and cuts with broken glass and other sharp objects account for up to half of accidents associated with laboratory-acquired infections [2,3,30,31]. The microbiological hazards associated with injuries from needle sticks and sharp objects have recently been reviewed [30,31]. Surprisingly, accidental ingestion or aspiration of infectious materials via mouth pipetting continues to be a source of laboratory-acquired infections [30,31], despite the fact that such behavior is proscribed in all laboratories [32–34].

Aerosol droplets vary in size, with larger droplets rapidly settling onto exposed surfaces. These droplets may carry infectious agents and can thus contaminate environmental surfaces. Smaller droplets remain suspended in the air for a longer period of time and, under the appropriate environmental conditions, can remain suspended indefinitely. Aerosols with droplets measuring < 5 mm in diameter can be inhaled directly into alveoli; those measuring ~ 1 mm are the most likely to be retained within alveoli [35]. Many common laboratory procedures have been shown to produce aerosols in this size range [36–39]. Both *Mycobacterium tuberculosis* and atypical mycobacteria may be transmitted by the aerosol route [40].

Laboratory personnel have among the highest rates of needle-stick injuries [31,41]. In general, most needle-stick injuries occur during disposal of used needles, assembly or disassembly of intravenous infusion sets, administration of parenteral injections or infusion therapy, drawing of blood, recapping of needles, or handling of waste that contains needles [31,41–43]. Recapping needles is particularly hazardous, causing 12% to 30% of needle-stick injuries [31,41]. It should be noted, however, that not recapping needles may also be hazardous [44]. The epidemiology of needle-stick injuries among laboratory personnel has not been studied, but since activities such as intravenous infusion and handling infusion sets are not carried out in laboratories, recapping needles and handling waste are likely to be the most common causes of needle-stick injuries among laboratory personnel.

TABLE 23-1. *Sources of laboratory-acquired infections in the United States and abroad*

Proved or probable source	Number of infections	Percentage of total
Working with agent	827	21.1
Unknown and other	783	20.0
Known accident	703	17.9
Animal or arthropod	659	16.8
Aerosol	522	13.3
Patient's specimen	287	7.3
Human autopsy	75	1.9
Discarded glassware	46	1.2
Intentional infection	19	0.5
Total	3,921	100.0

(Adapted from Pike RM. Laboratory-associated infections: summary and analysis of 3,921 cases. *Health Lab Sci* 1976; 13:105–114.)

TABLE 23-2. *Kinds of laboratory accident resulting in infection*

Known accident	Number of infections	Percentage of total
Spill or spatter	188	26.7
Needle stick	177	25.2
Broken glass injury	112	15.9
Bite or scratch	95	13.5
Mouth pipetting	92	13.1
Other	39	5.5
Total	703	99.9

(Adapted from Pike RM. Laboratory-associated infections: summary and analysis of 3,921 cases. *Health Lab Sci* 1976; 13:105–114.)

INFECTIOUS AGENTS OF SPECIAL CONCERN IN CLINICAL LABORATORIES

The risk of acquiring infections in a clinical laboratory is dependent upon several factors, the most important of which is the likelihood of exposure to an infectious agent [45]. The probability that such an exposure will result in infection is dependent upon inoculum size, viability of the infectious agent, the immune status of the exposed individual, and the availability of effective postexposure prophylactic therapy.

Human Immunodeficiency Virus

At least one million Americans are infected with HIV (see Chapter 43). More than 50% of infected persons have developed the acquired immunodeficiency syndrome; of this group, 62% have now died [46,47]. The prevalence of HIV-infected patients varies between regions, cities, and even hospitals within a given city. Seropositivity rates also vary by age, gender, race, and socioeconomic group; these rates range from 0.9% to 22% in different populations [48–52]. A survey from Seattle showed that the HIV antibody was present in 3% of all serum or plasma specimens submitted to the clinical chemistry laboratory at an urban teaching hospital [53]. Thus, a significant proportion of clinical specimens may be infected with HIV, and all clinical laboratory personnel can expect to eventually work with HIV-infected clinical specimens.

Transmission of HIV during an occupational exposure occurs as a result of contact of infected material with nonintact skin or mucosal surfaces or as a result of traumatic implantation of infectious material [25,26]. It is estimated that the risk of acquiring HIV infection after a single cutaneous exposure to infected blood is low, < 1% [54], and that the risk of infection from a needle-stick injury is ~ 0.3% to 0.5% [27,55–57]. Although both types of exposure are common among some healthcare workers [58], the frequency of such exposures among laboratory personnel has not been reported. Based on the epidemiology of HBV infection among laboratory personnel [24,30], however, it is likely that these personnel are among those healthcare workers most commonly exposed to HIV-infected specimens. The prevalence of HBV serological markers among clinical laboratory workers that handle blood or serum matches or exceeds that of other healthcare workers, including nurses and surgeons [59].

Although an effective postexposure treatment protocol exists [54,60], prevention of HIV infection among healthcare workers depends mainly upon prevention of exposure to the virus. Guidelines for preventing HIV exposure in the workplace have been published; they are based on the principle of universal (sometimes now referred to as "standard" precautions) [25,61,62] (see Chapter 13). These guidelines are also useful in preventing occupational exposure to other bloodborne pathogens, particularly HBV. The guidelines are based on a common-sense approach to infection control. Although direct evidence that use of universal precautions has prevented cases of HIV or HBV infection is not available, there is evidence that occupational exposures to HIV in patients' specimens has been reduced when universal precautions are used [10,45,63]. Even though the cost of implementing universal precautions is substantial (and may have been significantly underestimated heretofore [64,65]), universal precautions provide the most rational approach to minimizing the risk of acquiring bloodborne pathogens [45,53,63].

Hepatitis B Virus

Despite the availability of safe and effective vaccines and of effective postexposure treatment regimens, HBV infection (see Chapter 42) remains one of the most common hospital-acquired infections [7,14,28]. Surveys have repeatedly shown that laboratorians are among the most frequently infected healthcare workers [7,13, 23,66], with seropositivity rates between two and twenty-seven times that of the general population [59,66–70]. It is estimated that of the 300,000 new cases of HBV infection in the United States each year, 1% to 6% (6,000 to 18,000) occur in healthcare workers [9,71]. One report estimates that 12% of HBV-infected patients require hospitalization, indicating that each year 720 to 2,160 healthcare workers may require hospitalization for HBV infections [9].

Since the incidence of HBV infection in a given population of patients may be high, and is often underestimated, and since compliance with barrier precautions is often inconsistent, the easiest way to prevent occupational HBV infection is by vaccination (see Chapter 3). Although it is reported that the incidence of laboratory-acquired HBV infection has decreased since the vaccine was introduced in 1982 [9,13,72], ≤ 50% of healthcare workers have not received complete vaccinations [71,73]. Since 1992, the Occupational Safety and Health Administration has required that all employers have an exposure plan [74]. As part of this plan, employees are categorized as to the likelihood of occupational exposure to blood; those with such exposure are to be provided with HBV vaccination at no cost to the employee [74].

Employers should focus vaccination strategies on those employees most likely to be exposed, since vaccinating employees with little or no risk of occupational exposure diverts resources from those employees who are at the highest risk [73]. Similarly, there is no compelling evidence to routinely perform postvaccination testing or provide booster doses; employers should not divert resources for either purpose [73]. Until all healthcare workers are willing to complete HBV vaccination, HBV is likely to remain a serious infection control issue in healthcare settings. Requiring HBV vaccination as a condition of employment may be the simplest way to ensure compliance.

Most laboratory-acquired HBV infections probably are not acquired via needle-stick injuries or cuts with infected instruments, but rather by clinically inapparent cutaneous or mucosal exposure to blood or blood products [23,68,70,75]. Therefore, rigid adherence to published guidelines for prevention of HIV and HBV infection via universal precautions should be followed by all laboratory personnel. Percutaneous exposure is not limited to those employees working directly with body fluids. One outbreak of laboratory-acquired HBV infection occurred among clerical employees whose only risk factor was exposure to HBV-contaminated computer requisitions [76]; in another study, the highest prevalence of seropositivity in a laboratory was among persons employed as glassware washers [77].

Hepatitis C Virus

Hepatitis C virus (HCV) (see Chapter 42) is transmitted via the same routes as HBV. Unlike HBV, HCV is not as readily transmitted via needle-stick injury; estimates of the risk of transmission following needle-stick injury are in the range of 0% to 10% [60,78–80]. Nonetheless, exposure is to be avoided, since ≥ 50% of HCV-infected persons progress to chronic liver disease, and cirrhosis or hepatocellular carcinoma or both will develop in many of them. As with HBV and HIV, HCV infection is highly prevalent in some populations of patients, such as injection drug-users. [81].

Mycobacterium Tuberculosis

Employees involved in the processing of clinical specimens or cultures from patients with tuberculosis (see Chapter 33) are at a much greater risk of acquiring tuberculosis than is the general population [11,13,14,82]. Once thought to be controlled in the United States, tuberculosis has reemerged as an important public health problem. Two issues are of particular importance to laboratory employees: the increasing incidence of tuberculosis and the development of strains that are resistant to several or all first-line chemotherapeutic agents. All healthcare facilities should have a comprehensive plan for the prevention, control, and treatment of tuberculosis [83,84].

Bacteria and Fungi

Bacterial infections of special concern to laboratory personnel are primarily those caused by highly virulent pathogens, such as *Brucella* and *Francisella tularensis* [3,15] and the enteric pathogens *Shigella* and *Salmonella* [16–19]. Infections caused by *Shigella* (see Chapter 34) now are the most common laboratory-acquired bacterial infections in both the United States and Great Britain [7,14]. Fungal pathogens of significance to laboratory employees include *Coccidioides immitis*, *Blastomyces dermatitidis*, and *Histoplasma capsulatum* [85]. Recommendations for the safe processing of clinical specimens and cultures suspected of containing any of these agents are given later herein.

PREVENTION OF LABORATORY-ACQUIRED INFECTIONS

Each clinical laboratory must develop policies and procedures to prevent, document, and treat laboratory-acquired infections. The laboratory director, in conjunction with a designated laboratory safety officer, should take the lead role in developing and implementing these policies and should integrate them into the laboratory procedure manual [1,32–34,86,87]. All employees should receive the appropriate education and training necessary to perform their job safely. They should be aware of hazards associated with various infectious agents, how to prevent the risk of exposure to each agent, and exactly what should be done should an exposure take place. Immunization against HBV should be required for laboratory workers [9,22,59,88,89]. Initial and follow-up tuberculin skin tests should be given according to current guidelines [84,87,90]. Finally, a method for maintaining compliance with these policies and procedures must be implemented, along with the appropriate documentation, counseling, and, if necessary, disciplinary action to ensure that employees work safely.

Biosafety Levels

The Centers for Disease Control and Prevention (CDC) and National Institutes of Health have published a document defining four biosafety levels based on "the potential hazard of the agent and the laboratory function or activity" [32]. Laboratory design, equipment, and procedures necessary to achieve each biosafety level are detailed in that document. Most common pathogens may be handled under biosafety level 2 conditions. Cultures suspected of containing *Brucella*, *F. tularensis*, *M. tuberculosis*, *C. immitis*, *B. dermatitidis*, or *H. capsulatum* should be processed only under biosafety level 3 conditions. Biosafety level 4 conditions are not needed in general clinical microbiology laboratories.

Universal Precautions

Special policies and procedures are necessary for the safe handling and disposal of certain highly virulent pathogens. Rigorous adherence to universal precautions is sufficient to lessen or eliminate the risk of acquiring an

TABLE 23-3. *Universal precautions for prevention of transmission of HIV, HBV, and other bloodborne pathogens in healthcare settings*

1. All healthcare workers should routinely use appropriate barrier precautions to prevent skin and mucous membrane exposure when contact with blood or other body fluids of any patient is anticipated. Gloves should be worn for touching blood and body fluids, mucous membranes, or nonintact skin of all patients; for handling items or surfaces soiled with blood or body fluids; and for performing venipuncture and other vascular access procedures. Gloves should be changed after contact with each patient. Masks and protective eyewear or face shields should be worn during procedures that are likely to generate droplets of blood or other body fluids to prevent exposure of mucous membranes of the mouth, nose, and eyes. Gowns or aprons should be worn during procedures that are likely to generate splashes of blood or other body fluids.
2. Hands and other skin surfaces should be washed immediately and thoroughly if contaminated with blood or other body fluids. Hands should be washed immediately after gloves are removed.
3. All healthcare workers should take precautions to prevent injuries caused by needles, scalpels, and other sharp instruments or devices during procedures; when cleaning used instruments; during disposal of used needles; and when handling sharp instruments after procedures. To prevent needle-stick injuries, needles should not be recapped, purposely bent or broken by hand, removed from disposable syringes, or otherwise manipulated by hand. After they are used, disposable syringes and needles, scalpel blades, and other sharp items should be placed in puncture-resistant containers for disposal; the puncture-resistant containers should be located as close as practical to the use area. Large-bore reusable needles should be placed in a puncture-resistant container for transport to the reprocessing area.
4. Although saliva has not been implicated in HIV transmission, to minimize the need for emergency mouth-to-mouth resuscitation, mouthpieces, resuscitation bags, or other ventilation devices should be available for use in areas in which the need for resuscitation is predictable.
5. Healthcare workers who have exudative lesions or weeping dermatitis should refrain from all direct care of patients and from handling equipment used in the care of patients until the condition resolves.
6. Pregnant healthcare workers are not known to be at greater risk of contracting HIV infection than healthcare workers who are not pregnant; however, if a healthcare worker develops HIV infection during pregnancy, the infant is at risk of infection resulting from perinatal transmission. Because of this risk, pregnant healthcare workers should be especially familiar with and strictly adhere to precautions to minimize the risk of HIV transmission.

TABLE 23-4. *Universal precautions for workers in diagnostic pathology laboratories*

1. All specimens of blood and body fluids should be put in a well-constructed container with a secure lid to prevent leaking during transport. Care should be taken when collecting each specimen to avoid contaminating the outside of the container and of the laboratory form accompanying the specimen.
2. All persons processing blood and body-fluid specimens (e.g., removing tops from vacuum tubes) should wear gloves. Masks and protective eyewear should be worn if mucous membrane contact with blood or body fluids is anticipated. Gloves should be changed and hands washed after completion of specimen processing.
3. For routine procedures, such as histologic and pathologic studies or microbiologic culturing, a biological safety cabinet is not necessary. However, biological safety cabinets (class I or II) should be used whenever procedures are conducted that have a high potential for generating droplets, including activities such as blending, sonicating, and vigorous mixing.
4. Mechanical pipetting devices should be used for manipulating all liquids in the laboratory. Mouth pipetting must not be done.
5. Use of needles and syringes should be limited to situations in which there is no alternative, and the recommendations for preventing injuries with needles outlined under universal precautions in healthcare settings (Table 23-3) should be followed.
6. Laboratory work surfaces should be decontaminated with an appropriate chemical germicide after a spill of blood or other body fluids and when work activities are completed.
7. Contaminated materials used in laboratory tests should be decontaminated before reprocessing or be placed in bags and disposed of in accordance with institutional policies for disposal of infective waste.
8. Scientific equipment that has been contaminated with blood or other body fluids should be decontaminated and cleaned before being repaired in the laboratory or transported to the manufacturer.
9. All persons should wash their hands after completing laboratory activities and should remove protective clothing before leaving the laboratory.

infection from most patients' specimens processed in clinical laboratories. Implementation of universal precautions will be successful only if laboratory administrators and workers integrate CDC recommendations into routine laboratory operations and make every reasonable attempt to maintain and enforce such policies. Universal precautions have been shown to decrease the number of occupational exposures to blood and other body fluids among one group of healthcare workers [10,63]. The CDC recommendations for universal precautions for all healthcare workers and clinical laboratories are given in Tables 23-3 and 23-4, respectively.

Standard Microbiological Practices

When used in conjunction with universal precautions, the following practices should be effective in preventing most laboratory-acquired infections. These or equivalent procedures should be routine practice in all clinical laboratories [33,34,45,61–63,91–97].

TABLE 23-5. *A 10-step program for training laboratory workers in biohazard safety*

1.	Universal precautions for handling blood and body fluids
2.	Aseptic technique and procedures
3.	Personal hygiene and protective equipment
4.	Criteria for biosafety levels 1–4
5.	Effective use of biological safety cabinets classes I–III
6.	Safe use of centrifuges and autoclaves
7.	Decontamination, disinfection, and sterilization
8.	Handling, packaging, and disposal of biohazardous waste
9.	Packaging, transporting, and shipping biohazardous waste
10.	Reporting incidents and accidents

(Modified from U.S. National Research Council, Committee on Hazardous Biological Substances in the Laboratory. *Biosafety in the laboratory: prudent practices for the handling and disposal of infectious materials.* Washington, D.C.: National Academy of Sciences, 1989.)

Laboratory Access

Only trained personnel should be allowed in a laboratory under ordinary circumstances. Maintenance personnel, delivery persons, and other visitors with a legitimate reason for being in the laboratory should either be escorted or be closely supervised to prevent unnecessary exposure to infectious agents. Laboratory trainees, house staff, and other students should also be supervised closely. Children should not be allowed in laboratories.

Personnel Policies

All personnel should have training commensurate with the level of expertise needed to safely perform all necessary procedures. Suggested topics for such training are given in Table 23-5 [34]. All personnel should receive the necessary continuing education and training to ensure job safety. Employee job appraisals should document lapses in safety, techniques, or other behaviors that could result in occupational exposure to infectious agents. Persons exhibiting such behavior should be counseled and/or retrained.

Laboratory Facility

Laboratories should be designed to minimize traffic and unnecessary access to work areas. Laboratory furniture should be sturdy and easy to clean, and the laboratories themselves should be uncluttered and easy to clean. Foot-, knee-, or elbow-operated hand-washing sinks should be available and located near laboratory exits. The laboratory facility should be designed and constructed to meet criteria recommended for the appropriate biosafety level [32].

Hygiene for Workers

Eating, drinking, smoking, and applying cosmetics should be strictly prohibited within the laboratory [32]. All personnel should wear and button full-length white laboratory coats while in the laboratory. Laboratory coats should not be worn outside the laboratory. Personnel and visitors should wash their hands before leaving the laboratory. Food and other personal items should not be stored in refrigerators or freezers used to store clinical specimens or cultures. Refrigerators, freezers, and microwave ovens used to store or prepare food must be located outside the laboratory.

Clinical Specimens

Specimens must be labeled with the patient's full name, hospital identification number and the date drawn. Specimens received in damaged, leaking or contaminated containers should not be processed; the person who collected the specimen should be notified and the specimen recollected.

Microbiological Techniques

Mouth pipetting should be **strictly** prohibited, and mechanical pipetting devices should be immediately available within the laboratory. All procedures should be carefully performed to prevent the formation of aerosols; procedures that generate aerosols should be performed in a biological safety cabinet. Cylindrical electric burners are preferable to flame burners for sterilizing inoculating loops or needles and the tips of other small instruments. If flame burners are used, care should be taken to avoid spattering. This can be achieved by slowly drawing loops or needles through the flame with the loop entering the flame last. Cool inoculating loops and needles should be used when touching plates, colonies, or broth cultures. Work surfaces should be decontaminated at least once a day with an acceptable germicide. Work surfaces should also be decontaminated after spills (discussed later). Infectious wastes and patients' specimens should be disinfected before disposal (see later herein). Needles, blades, and other sharp items should be disposed of in rigid, tamper-resistant, puncture-proof, marked containers. Materials removed from the laboratory should be free of infectious hazard. Clinical specimens, cultures, or other potentially infectious materials should be packaged, labeled, and shipped according to federal regulations [34,98].

Safety Procedure Manual

Every laboratory should have an up-to-date safety manual as an integral part of the laboratory procedure manual. The following information should be included.

1. A designated laboratory safety officer and explicit instructions as to how to get in contact with that individual in the event of an accident or exposure. This officer should lead the educational program for biohazard safety (Table 23-5).
2. Synopsis of safety components of good laboratory practice and hospital policies for infection control, including universal precautions.
3. A program for the prevention of transmission of *M. tuberculosis* to laboratory workers, developed in accordance with current recommendations [99].
4. Location of necessary emergency equipment and spill cleanup kits.
5. Detailed procedures for cleanup of spills.
6. Instructions for the effective use of biological safety cabinets.
7. Procedures for safe use of centrifuges and autoclaves.
8. Vaccination policies.
9. Procedures for postexposure treatment, prophylaxis, and counseling.

SAFETY IN HANDLING ACCIDENTS, USING EQUIPMENT, AND DISPOSING OF WASTES

Procedures for Spills and Accidents

Because of the high concentration of microorganisms in patients' specimens and cultures in clinical laboratories, special procedures must be used to disinfect spills and other laboratory accidents [34,87,97,100]. The current CDC recommendation is to use "chemical germicides that are approved for use as 'hospital germicides' and are tuberculocidal when used at recommended dilutions" [55,73]. This recommendation applies to all types of spills or other laboratory accidents.

Written procedures should be in the laboratory safety manual. Employees should be trained to safely decontaminate and clean up spills involving those microorganisms cultured or studied in their laboratory. All necessary disinfectants and cleaning supplies must be readily available in the laboratory. Because spills may occur at any stage of the transport, plating, processing, or storage of microbiological cultures, specific protocols should be available for spills occurring at each stage and for spills involving common-place moderate-risk microorganisms and those of higher risk, such as *M. tuberculosis*.

The hazard associated with a spill is dependent upon the nature of the spilled agent, the volume of material spilled, the concentration of the agent within the material, and where the spill takes place. Spills involving microorganisms such as *M. tuberculosis*, *F. tularensis*, *Brucella* spp, *C. immitis*, or *H. capsulatum* may pose a major hazard to laboratory workers. Spills of large volumes of moderate-risk microorganisms or those occurring in such a manner that aerosols might be generated should also be treated as a major hazard to laboratory workers.

Procedures Used for Routine Spills of Small Volumes of Moderate-risk Microorganisms

1. The affected area should immediately be flooded with a suitable disinfectant and covered with paper towels.
2. Other workers should be warned to avoid the contaminated area.
3. Personnel should wear gloves and use an autoclavable dustpan and squeegee or forceps to pick up solid materials.
4. Any remaining fluids or other materials should be wiped up with paper towels.
5. Contaminated materials should be disposed of as infectious waste.
6. Unless the laboratory worker is injured or otherwise exposed during the spill or cleanup, no other specific action need be taken.

Procedures for Spills of Large Volumes of Moderate-risk Agents or Highly Pathogenic Agents Outside a Biological Safety Cabinet

1. Employees should hold their breath, immediately evacuate the room, and close the door.
2. Employees should assist others as needed to protect them from potential exposure.
3. Other personnel should be warned to avoid the contaminated area. Personnel in adjacent areas should be warned of any potential hazard to their safety.
4. Contaminated clothing and protective equipment should be removed and discarded as biohazardous waste.
5. Employees should thoroughly wash exposed skin surfaces.
6. The laboratory safety officer and director should be immediately notified.
7. Biological safety cabinets should be left running to help decrease the concentration of aerosols in the contaminated room.
8. If the spill occurs in a room under negative pressure, ≥30 minutes should pass before personnel reenter the affected room.
9. If the spill occurs in a room not under negative pressure, the cleanup should begin immediately.

10. Protective clothing, including a cap, mask, long-sleeved gown, shoe covers, and gloves, should be worn.
11. An appropriate disinfectant should be allowed to run into the spill from the sides. Disinfectant poured directly on the spills may generate aerosols.
12. The area should be covered with paper towels and allowed to stand for 20 minutes.
13. An autoclavable dustpan and squeegee or forceps should be used to clean up pieces of broken glass and other sharp objects.
14. Remaining liquids should be wiped up with paper towels.
15. All materials, including protective clothing, should be discarded as biohazardous waste.

Procedures for Spills in Biological Safety Cabinets

1. Biological safety cabinets (BSCs) should be allowed to operate to minimize further risk to laboratory workers.
2. Cleanup should begin immediately.
3. Gloves, mask, and a gown should be worn during the cleanup.
4. Work surfaces and any catch pans or basins should be flooded with an adequate volume of disinfectant.
5. The flooded area should be allowed to stand for 20 minutes.
6. During this time, the BSC walls, work surfaces, and any equipment within the BSC should be cleaned with a germicidal disinfectant (phenolic or iodophor compounds). Flammable organic solvents, such as alcohols, should not be used, as these compounds may reach dangerous concentrations within certain BSCs.
7. All contaminated materials and fluids should be disposed of as biohazardous waste.
8. Catch pans and basins should be cleaned per the manufacturer's recommendations.
9. High-efficiency particulate air (HEPA) filters and other components of the BSC should not be cleaned or disinfected by laboratory personnel. This is not necessary with most spills and should be done only by factory-trained and certified personnel. Major spills or those involving high-risk agents may necessitate formaldehyde decontamination of the BSC. Such decontamination should be performed only by qualified personnel.

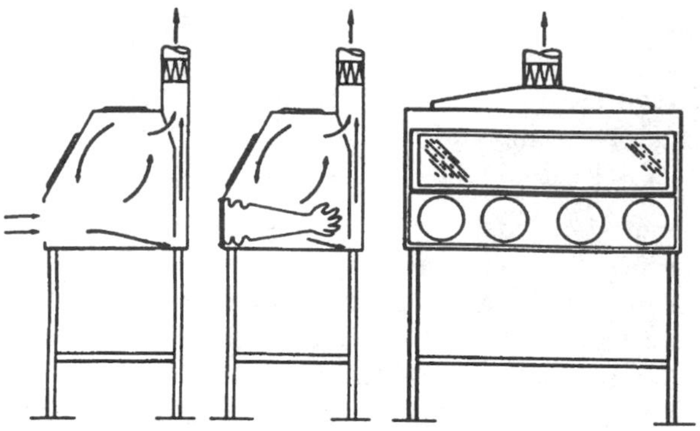

FIGURE 23-1. Design of class I biological safety cabinet.

Laboratory Equipment

Laboratory safety and diagnostic equipment must be of the proper type and should be tested and maintained according to the manufacturer's recommendations. Equally important is its proper use by laboratory personnel. All personnel should be instructed as to the proper use, care, and maintenance of laboratory equipment.

Biological Safety Cabinets

Biological safety cabinets are essential for the safe handling of infectious agents. Different BSCs are available; which one to use depends primarily upon the infectious agents to be handled [100]. Class I BSCs (Figure 23-1) have an open front into which room air flows. All of the exhaust air is discharged through HEPA filters to the outside environment. Although Class I BSCs protect the user from exposure to agents within the cabinet, they do not protect materials within the cabinet against conta-

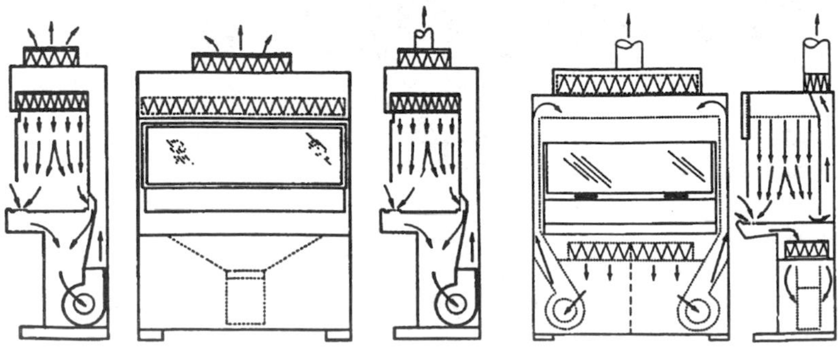

FIGURE 23-2. Design of class II biological safety cabinets types A and B.

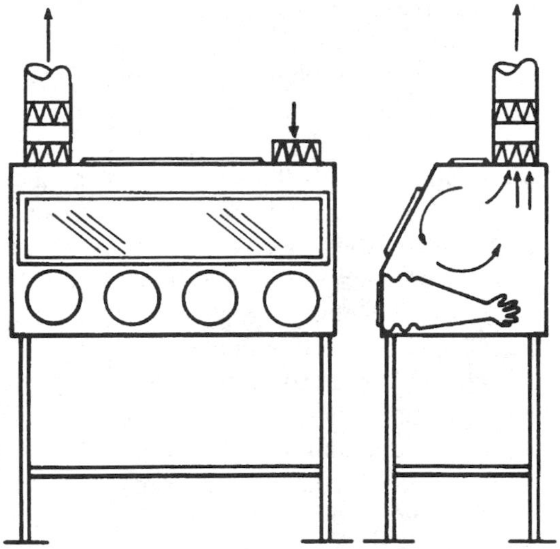

FIGURE 23-3. Design of class III biological safety cabinet.

mination; Class I BSCs are unsuitable for use in clinical microbiology laboratories [34].

Class II BSCs (Figure 23-2) also have an open front into which room air flows. These BSCs differ from Class I BSCs in that a portion of the exhausted air passing through HEPA filters is recirculated into the cabinet. The filtered air is then used to protect clinical specimens or cultures from contamination. Two basic types of Class II BSCs are available. Class II type A BSCs are the most commonly used in clinical laboratories and are sufficient for meeting biosafety level 2 or 3 criteria. Class II type B BSCs may also be used for this purpose but usually are more expensive to purchase and to operate [34,100]. Class III (Figure 23-3) BSCs provide the greatest protection to laboratory personnel, but their use is usually restricted to working with highly virulent pathogens in biosafety level 4 laboratories.

Laboratory workers must remember that BSCs are not chemical fume hoods. Toxic, noxious, or flammable chemicals must not be used in these hoods, since the recirculation of exhaust air may allow these chemicals to reach dangerously high levels in the cabinet. Biological safety cabinets should be installed, tested, and maintained only by qualified personnel. Regular testing and certification of BSCs is essential to assure the safety of users. Laboratory personnel should be instructed in the proper use of BSCs and should be aware of their limitations in controlling aerosols. Personnel working in BSCs can adversely affect the ability of cabinets to contain infectious aerosols [95]. Users should consult with the manufacturer as to the potential effect of this and other factors (such as use of equipment within BSCs) before using a BSC. Finally, personnel should be aware that cabinet function depends upon proper airflow patterns and that changes in airflow patterns because of alterations in building air supplies, temporary shutdowns for repairs, and so forth may adversely affect the function of BSCs.

Centrifuges

Centrifuges used to process clinical specimens or cultures should be equipped with sealable, autoclavable, breakage-resistant cups to prevent contamination of the centrifuge and the release of aerosols should centrifuge tubes break during processing. These cups must be removable from the centrifuge rotor so that they can be cleaned and autoclaved.

Autoclaves

An autoclave should be readily accessible to clinical laboratories. Routine maintenance, testing, and cleaning is essential. Autoclaves should be tested for their ability to kill standard bacterial spores [34]. It should be emphasized that autoclave tape indicates that an object has been autoclaved, but not necessarily sterilized [96,97].

Laboratory and Protective Equipment

Other laboratory equipment should be of a type and design that allows for easy cleaning and disinfection. Safety equipment for the cleanup and disinfection of laboratory spills should be readily available. Proper gloves, gowns, masks, and shoe covers should be handy.

Both latex and vinyl disposable gloves have been shown to vary widely in their permeability [91,93]. It has been found that washing and reusing gloves is inadvisable and that the proportion of hands contaminated with test microorganisms after gloves are removed varies from 5% to 50% [92]. Therefore, healthcare workers should wash their hands after removing gloves. The issue of wearing two pairs of gloves ("double-gloving") is more contentious. Although it is logical to assume that two barriers offer more protection than one, concerns about loss of tactile sensation and dexterity have led to recommendations against double-gloving during routine laboratory procedures [93]. Wearing two pairs of gloves for autopsies and in other situations where large amounts of blood are present has been recommended [33].

Disposal of Infectious Materials

Materials contaminated with infectious agents must be disposed of properly to protect healthcare personnel as well as the general public [34,96]. Safe disposal of infectious materials begins at the source where these materials are generated. The following procedures are recommended for the safe disposal of infectious materials and waste [34,96].

1. Adequate waste bins and containers for disposal of sharp objects must be readily available.
2. Waste bins should be lined with two autoclavable bags.
3. All containers should be clearly marked.
4. Laboratory and maintenance personnel should avoid physical contact with these materials; leaking containers should be treated as spills.
5. Infectious materials should be transported in or on carts that can be easily cleaned and disinfected.
6. Infectious materials should be autoclaved before disposal; double-bagging and overfilling should be avoided, since these practices limit the effectiveness of autoclaving as a means of sterilization.
7. Regular monitoring of the adequacy of autoclave sterilization should be part of routine laboratory quality control procedures.

PREVENTION, POSTEXPOSURE TREATMENT, AND FOLLOW-UP

Vaccination

Recommendations for vaccinations for healthcare workers have recently been reviewed [22] and specific recommendations have been made by the CDC [88,89]. Laboratory workers may or may not have contact with patients, but they should still follow the suggestions for all healthcare workers. It should be strongly emphasized that all healthcare workers should be vaccinated against hepatitis B [88]. Such vaccination should probably be given during the training years, since the risk of occupational exposure to HBV appears to be greatest during that period [89]. Since the licensure of a hepatitis B vaccine in 1982, ~80% of the 2.5 million persons vaccinated for HBV have been healthcare workers [9]. Moreover, the recent 75% decline in hepatitis B associated with healthcare employment is thought to be a direct result of immunization with hepatitis B vaccine and wider use of universal precautions [9].

Before employment, all hospital workers should provide evidence of immunity to rubella. Persons lacking protective antibody to rubella virus should be vaccinated. Influenza, measles, mumps, and polio vaccines and tetanus-diphtheria toxoid immunization should comply with current guidelines from the Immunization Practices Advisory Committee of the U.S. Public Health Service and should be coordinated with personnel health services (see Chapter 3) in the hospital [22, 88,89].

Postexposure Treatment and Prophylaxis

Specific treatment, prophylaxis, and counseling should be available for all healthcare workers after exposure to an infectious agent. Such policies and procedures should be made in consultation with the hospital infection control committee. Clinical laboratories should include such policies as part of their laboratory safety and procedure manuals. Specific recommendations have been formulated for exposure to many infectious agents [60,88]; the reader is referred to Chapter 3 for additional information.

Of special importance to clinical laboratory workers are the recommendations for hepatitis B prophylaxis after percutaneous (needle-stick or injury from sharp object) exposure to blood (see Chapter 42). Hepatitis B immune globulin should be given immediately, followed by HBV vaccine for individuals who have not been vaccinated or who lack adequate anti-HB surface antigen or anti-HB core antigen. Guidelines for the prevention of laboratory-acquired HCV infection are the same as for HBV infection. It is not known whether postexposure prophylaxis with immune globulin is beneficial [60]. Exposed employees should be tested for HCV at the time of exposure and again 4 months later; exposed employees should be followed closely for clinical signs and symptoms of acute hepatitis [60]. An HCV vaccine does not yet exist.

Laboratory workers with percutaneous exposure to blood or body fluid samples from patients are also at risk of infection with HIV. Persons with such exposures in the work place should be informed that post-exposure prophylaxis is associated with a decreased risk for HIV seroconversion [101–102]. Although post-exposure prophylaxis with zidovudine alone has been reported to fail [103], use of the drug in this setting has also been associated with a significant decrease in the risk for HIV seroconversion [101–103]. The efficacy of combining other antiretroviral drugs with zidovudine for post-exposure prophylaxis has yet to be studied in a prospective clinical trial. Nonetheless, the U.S. Public Health Service recommends post-exposure prophylaxis with a regimen including zidovudine [102] (see Chapter 43).

Personnel working in mycobacteriology laboratories, and those involved in the processing or disposal of materials likely to be contaminated with mycobacteria, should receive a pre-employment Mantoux tuberculin skin test with purified protein derivative [90,99]. Persons without signs and symptoms of pulmonary tuberculosis and who have had a previously positive reaction or who have completed either adequate preventive therapy or therapy for active disease that can be documented should not receive skin tests [84]. Subsequent skin testing of purified protein derivative–negative laboratory workers should be done annually and also immediately and again 3 months later after an exposure [84,87]. Exposed persons with skin-test reactions ≥ 5 mm or with symptoms suggestive of tuberculosis should be evaluated for active pulmonary tuberculosis (see Chapter 33). Those with skin-test conversions but without active disease should be considered for preventive therapy; persons with active disease should receive antituberculous chemotherapy in accordance with current recommendations [84,99].

Postexposure Investigation

Laboratory exposure of an employee to a pathogen should prompt an immediate investigation into the reason(s) for the exposure. The investigation should include a review of relevant microbiological practices, laboratory policies and procedures, and equipment and facilities. For example, when an employee who works in a mycobacterial laboratory converts a skin test or develops active pulmonary tuberculosis, BSC and air handling systems should be checked, serviced, and balanced by qualified personnel. If the investigation does not provide a satisfactory explanation for the source of the exposure, then it may be necessary to broaden the investigation. Using the same example, an employee who works in a mycobacteriology laboratory but has other responsibilities outside the laboratory (e.g., phlebotomy) could conceivably have been exposed to a patient with active tuberculosis. If no source of exposure is found, the investigation should be expanded, as appropriate, to include potential sources of exposure outside the healthcare facility (e.g., family members).

CONCLUSIONS

Although the incidence of laboratory-acquired infections appears to be declining, infections still occur at a low rate and are associated with significant morbidity and mortality. Infections caused by hepatitis B and HIV are of particular concern. Laboratory personnel should make every attempt to follow recommended guidelines, policies, and procedures designed to minimize the risk of working with infectious materials. Each laboratory must be designed and constructed in such a way as to minimize accidents and facilitate cleanups. It must contain proper and well-maintained safety and diagnostic equipment. Most important, however, is the proper training and supervision of laboratory personnel and adherence to policies and procedures designed to provide a safe working environment. It is the obligation of laboratory directors and administrators to provide such an environment.

REFERENCES

1. Collins CH. *Laboratory-acquired infections*, 3rd ed. London: Butterworth Heinemann, 1993.
2. Pike RM. Laboratory-associated infections: incidence, fatalities, causes, and prevention. *Annu Rev Microbiol* 1979;33:41–66.
3. Pike RM. Laboratory-associated infections: summary and analysis of 3,921 cases. *Health Lab Sci* 1976;13:105–114.
4. Pike RM. Past and present hazards of working with infectious agents. *Arch Pathol Lab Med* 1978;102:333–336.
5. Harrington JM. Health and safety in medical laboratories. *Bull WHO* 1982;60:9–16.
6. Sewell DL. Laboratory-associated infections and biosafety. *Clin Microbiol Rev* 1995;8:389–405.
7. Jacobson JT, Orlob RB, Clayton JL. Infections acquired in clinical laboratories in Utah. *J Clin Microbiol* 1985;21:486–489.
8. Vesley D, Hartmann HM. Laboratory-acquired infections and injuries in clinical laboratories: a 1986 survey. *Am J Public Health* 1988;78: 1213–1215.
9. Alter MJ, Hadler SC, Margolis HS, et al. The changing epidemiology of hepatitis B in the United States: need for alternative vaccination strategies. *JAMA* 1990;263:1218–1222.
10. Fahey BJ, Koziol DE, Banks SM, et al. Frequency of nonparenteral occupational exposures to blood and body fluids before and after universal precautions training. *Am J Med* 1991;90:145–153.
11. Grist NR. Infections in British clinical laboratories 1980–1. *J Clin Pathol* 1983;36:121–126.
12. Grist NR, Emslie JAN. Infections in British clinical laboratories, 1984–5. *J Clin Pathol* 1987;40:826–829.
13. Grist NR, Emslie JAN. Association of Clinical Pathologists surveys of infections in British clinical laboratories, 1970–1989. *J Clin Pathol* 1994;47:391–394.
14. Harrington JM, Shannon HS. Incidence of tuberculosis, hepatitis, brucellosis, and shigellosis in British medical workers. *Br Med J* 1976;1: 759–762.
15. Staszkiewicz J, Lewis CM, Colville J, et al. Outbreak of *Brucella melitensis* among microbiology laboratory workers in a community hospital. *J Clin Microbiol* 1991;29:287–290.
16. Blaser MJ, Hickman FW, Farmer JJ III, et al. *Salmonella typhi*: the laboratory as a reservoir of infection. *J Infect Dis* 1980;142:934–938.
17. Blaser MJ, Lofgren JP. Fatal salmonellosis originating in a clinical microbiology laboratory. *J Clin Microbiol* 1981;13:855–858.
18. Holmes MB, Johnson DL, Fiumara NJ, et al. Acquisition of typhoid fever from proficiency-testing specimens. *N Engl J Med* 1980;303: 519–521.
19. Steckelberg JM, Terrell CL, Edson RS. Laboratory-acquired *Salmonella typhimurium* enteritis: association with erythema nodosum and reactive arthritis. *Am J Med* 1988;85:705–707.
20. Bhatti AR, DiNinno VL, Ashton FE, et al. A laboratory-acquired infection with *Neisseria meningitidis*. *J Infect* 1982;4:247–252.
21. Centers for Disease Control and Prevention. Laboratory-acquired meningococcemia—California and Massachusetts. *MMWR* 1991;40: 46–47,55.
22. Williams WW, Preblud SR, Reichelderfer PS, et al. Vaccines of importance in the hospital setting: problems and development. *Infect Dis Clin North Am* 1989;3:701–722.
23. Leers W-D, Kouroupis GM. Prevalence of hepatitis B antibodies in hospital personnel. *Can Med Assoc J* 1975;113:844–847.
24. Pattison CP, Maynard JE, Berquist KR, et al. Epidemiology of hepatitis B in hospital personnel. *Am J Epidemiol* 1975;101:59–64.
25. Centers for Disease Control and Prevention. Guidelines for prevention of transmission of human immunodeficiency virus and hepatitis B virus to health-care and public-safety workers. *MMWR* 1989;38(no. S-6):1–37.
26. Centers for Disease Control and Prevention. Surveillance for occupationally acquired HIV—United States, 1981–1992. *MMWR* 1992;41: 823–825.
27. Marcus R, Centers for Disease Control Cooperative Needlestick Surveillance Group. Surveillance of healthcare workers exposed to blood from patients infected with the human immunodeficiency virus. *N Engl J Med* 1988;319:1118–1122.
28. Evans MR, Henderson DK, Bennett JE. Potential for laboratory exposures to biohazardous agents found in blood. *Am J Public Health* 1990;80:423–427.
29. Miller CD, Songer JR, Sullivan JF. A twenty-five-year review of laboratory-acquired human infections at the National Animal Disease Center. *Am Ind Hyg Assoc J* 1987;48:271–275.
30. Collins CH, Kennedy DA. Microbiological hazards of occupational needlestick and "sharps" injuries. *J Appl Bacteriol* 1987;62:385–402.

31. McCormick RD, Maki DG. Epidemiology of needle-stick injuries in hospital personnel. *Am J Med* 1981;70:928–932.
32. Centers for Disease Control and Prevention, National Institutes of Health. *Biosafety in microbiological and biomedical laboratories*, 3rd ed. Atlanta: U.S. Department of Health and Human Services, Public Health Service, Centers for Disease Control, and Bethesda: National Institutes of Health, 1993.
33. National Committee for Clinical Laboratory Standards. *Protection of laboratory workers from infectious disease transmitted by blood, body fluids and tissue*, 2nd ed. Villanova, Penn.: NCCLS, 1991. (Tentative Guideline. NCCLS Document M29-T2.)
34. U.S. National Research Council, Committee on Hazardous Biological Substances in the Laboratory. *Biosafety in the laboratory: prudent practices for the handling and disposal of infectious materials*. Washington, D.C.: National Academy of Sciences, 1989.
35. Brown JH, Cook KM, Ney FG, et al. Influence of particle size upon the retention of particulate matter in the human lung. *Am J Public Health* 1950;40:450–458.
36. Kenny MT, Sabel FL. Particle size distribution of *Serratia marcescens* aerosols created during common laboratory procedures and simulated laboratory accidents. *Appl Microbiol* 1968;16:1146–1155.
37. Stern EL, Johnson JW, Vesley D, et al. Aerosol production associated with clinical laboratory procedures. *Am J Clin Pathol* 1974;62: 591–600.
38. Tomlinson AJH. Infected air-borne particles liberated on opening screwcapped bottles. *Br Med J* 1957;1:15–17.
39. Wedum AG. Laboratory safety in research with infectious aerosols. *Public Health Rep* 1964;79:619–633.
40. Loudon RG, Bumgarner LR, Lacy J, et al. Aerial transmission of mycobacteria. *Am Rev Respir Dis* 1969;100:165–171.
41. Jagger J, Hunt EH, Brand-Elnaggar J, et al. Rates of needle-stick injury caused by various devices in a university hospital. *N Engl J Med* 1988;319:284–288.
42. Weltman AC, Short LJ, Mendelson MH, et al. Disposal-related sharps injuries at a New York City teaching hospital. *Infect Control Hosp Epidemiol* 1995;16:268–274.
43. Anglim AM, Collmer JE, Loving TJ, et al. An outbreak of needlestick injuries in hospital employees due to needles piercing infectious waste containers. *Infect Control Hosp Epidemiol* 1995;16:570–576.
44. Jagger J, Hunt EH, Pearson RD. Recapping used needles: Is it worse than the alternative? *J Infect Dis* 1990;162:784–785.
45. Klein RS. Universal precautions for preventing occupational exposures to human immunodeficiency virus type 1. *Am J Med* 1991;90:141–144.
46. Centers for Disease Control and Prevention. HIV prevalence estimates and AIDS case projections for the United States: report based upon a workshop. *MMWR* 1990;39(no. RR-16):1–18.
47. Division of HIV/AIDS Prevention, National Center for Prevention Services, Centers for Disease Control. First 500,000 AIDS cases—United States, 1995. *MMWR* 1995;44:849–853.
48. Hoff R, Berardi VP, Weiblen BJ, et al. Seroprevalence of human immunodeficiency virus among childbearing women: estimation by testing samples of blood from newborns. *N Engl J Med* 1988;318:525–530.
49. Kelen GD, DiGiovanna T, Bisson L, et al. Human immunodeficiency virus infection in emergency department patients: epidemiology, clinical presentations, and risk to healthcare workers. The Johns Hopkins experience. *JAMA* 1989;262:516–522.
50. Kelen GD, Fritz S, Qaqish B, et al. Unrecognized human immunodeficiency virus infection in emergency department patients. *N Engl J Med* 1988;318:1645–1650.
51. St. Louis ME, Rauch KJ, Petersen LR, et al. Seroprevalence rates of human immunodeficiency virus infection at sentinel hospitals in the United States. *N Engl J Med* 1990;323:213–218.
52. Kelen GD, Hexter DA, Hansen KN, et al. Trends in human immunodeficiency virus (HIV) infection among a patient population of an inner-city emergency department: implications for emergency department–based screening programs for HIV infection. *Clin Infect Dis* 1995;21:867–875.
53. Handsfield HH, Cummings J, Swenson PD. Prevalence of antibody to human immunodeficiency virus and hepatitis B surface antigen in blood samples submitted to a hospital laboratory: implications for handling specimens. *JAMA* 1987;258:3395–3397.
54. Centers for Disease Control and Prevention. Public health service statement on management of occupational exposure to human immunodeficiency virus, including considerations regarding zidovudine postexposure use. *MMWR* 1990;39(no. RR-1):1–14.
55. Henderson DK, Fahey BJ, Willy M, et al. Risk for occupational transmission of human immunodeficiency virus type 1 (HIV-1) associated with clinical exposures: a prospective evaluation. *Ann Intern Med* 1990;113:740–746.
56. Wormser GP, Rabkin CS, Joline C. Frequency of nosocomial transmission of HIV infection among healthcare workers [Letter]. *N Engl J Med* 1988;319:307–308.
57. Gerberding JL. Incidence and prevalence of human immunodeficiency virus, hepatitis B virus, hepatitis C virus, and cytomegalovirus among healthcare personnel at risk for blood exposure: final report from a longitudinal study. *J Infect Dis* 1994;170:1410–1417.
58. Mangione CM, Gerberding JL, Cummings SR. Occupational exposure to HIV: frequency and rates of under reporting of percutaneous and mucocutaneous exposures by medical housestaff. *Am J Med* 1991; 90:85–90.
59. West DJ. The risk of hepatitis B infection among health professionals in the United States: a review. *Am J Med Sci* 1984;287:26–33.
60. Diekema DJ, Doebbeling BN. Employee health and infection control. *Infect Control Hosp Epidemiol* 1995;16:292–301.
61. Centers for Disease Control and Prevention. Recommendations for prevention of HIV transmission in health-care settings. *MMWR* 1987; 36(suppl 2S):3S–18S.
62. Centers for Disease Control and Prevention. Update: universal precautions for prevention of transmission of human immunodeficiency virus, hepatitis B virus, and other bloodborne pathogens in health-care settings. *MMWR* 1988;37:377–382,387–388.
63. Wong ES, Stotka JL, Chinchilli VM, et al. Are universal precautions effective in reducing the number of occupational exposures among healthcare workers? A prospective study of physicians on a medical service. *JAMA* 1991;265:1123–1128.
64. Bachner P. The epidemiology of fear: scientific, social, and political responses to the occupational risk of blood-borne infection. *Arch Pathol Lab Med* 1990;114:319–323.
65. Doebbeling BN, Wenzel RP. The direct costs of universal precautions in a teaching hospital. *JAMA* 1990;264:2083–2087.
66. Skinhøj P, Søeby M. Viral hepatitis in Danish healthcare personnel, 1974–8. *J Clin Pathol* 1981;34:408–411.
67. Hirschowitz BI, Dasher CA, Whitt FJ, et al. Hepatitis B antigen and antibody and tests of liver function: a prospective study of 310 laboratory workers. *Am J Clin Pathol* 1980;73:63–68.
68. Levy BS, Harris JC, Smith JL, et al. Hepatitis B in ward and clinical laboratory employees of a general hospital. *Am J Epidemiol* 1977;106: 330–335.
69. Osterholm M, Andrews JS. Viral hepatitis in hospital personnel in Minnesota: report of a statewide survey. *Minn Med* 1979;62:683–689.
70. Pantelick EL, Steere AC, Lewis HD, et al. Hepatitis B infection in hospital personnel during an eight-year period: policies for screening and pregnancy in high risk areas. *Am J Med* 1981;70:924–7.
71. Kane MA, Alter MJ, Hadler SC, et al. Hepatitis B infection in the United States: recent trends and future strategies for control. *Am J Med* 1989;87(suppl 3A):11S–13S.
72. Lanphear BP, Linnemann CC, Cannon CG, et al. Decline of clinical hepatitis B in workers at a general hospital: relation to increasing vaccine-induced immunity. *Clin Infect Dis* 1993;16:10–14.
73. Agerton TB, Mahoney FJ, Polish LB, et al. Impact of the bloodborne pathogens standard on vaccination of healthcare workers with hepatitis B vaccine. *Infect Control Hosp Epidemiol* 1995;16:287–291.
74. U.S. Department of Labor, Occupational Safety and Health Administration. Occupational exposure to bloodborne pathogens: final rule. *Federal Register*, 1991;56:64175–64182.
75. Lauer JL, VanDrunen NA, Washburn, JW, et al. Transmission of hepatitis B virus in clinical laboratory areas. *J Infect Dis* 1979;140:513–516.
76. Pattison CP, Boyer KM, Maynard JE, et al. Epidemic hepatitis in a clinical laboratory: possible association with computer card handling. *JAMA* 1974;230:854–857.
77. Anderson RA, Woodfield DG. Hepatitis B virus infections in laboratory staff. *N Z Med J* 1982;95:69–71.
78. Kiyosawa K, Sodeyama T, Tanaka E, et al. Hepatitis C in hospital employees with needlestick injuries. *Ann Intern Med* 1991;115: 367–369.
79. Puro V, Petrosillo N, Ippolito G, et al. Occupational hepatitis C virus

infection in Italian healthcare workers. *Am J Public Health* 1995;85: 1272–1275.
80. Suzuki K, Mizokami M, Lau JYN, et al. Confirmation of hepatitis C virus transmission through needlestick accidents by molecular evolutionary analysis. *J Infect Dis* 1994;170:1575–1578.
81. Kelen GD, Green GB, Purcell RH, et al. Hepatitis B and hepatitis C in emergency department patients. *N Engl J Med* 1992;326:1399–1404.
82. Reid DD. Incidence of tuberculosis among workers in medical laboratories. *Br Med J* 1957;2:10–14.
83. Centers for Disease Control and Prevention. Essential components of a tuberculosis prevention and control program: screening for tuberculosis and tuberculosis infection in high-risk populations. Recommendations of the Advisory Council for the Elimination of Tuberculosis. *MMWR* 1995;44(no. RR-11):1–34.
84. Centers for Disease Control and Prevention. Guidelines for preventing the transmission of tuberculosis in health-care settings with special focus on HIV-related issues. *MMWR* 1990;39(no. RR-17):1–29.
85. Standard PG, Kaufman L. Safety considerations in handling exoantigen extracts from pathogenic fungi. *J Clin Microbiol* 1982;15:663–667.
86. Harrington JM, Shannon HS. Survey of safety and healthcare in British medical laboratories. *Br Med J* 1977;1:626–628.
87. Kent PT, Kubica GP. *Public health mycobacteriology: a guide for the level III laboratory*. Atlanta: U.S. Department of Health and Human Services, Public Health Service, Centers for Disease Control, 1985
88. Centers for Disease Control and Prevention. Protection against viral hepatitis: recommendations of the immunization practices advisory committee (ACIP). *MMWR* 1990;39(no. RR-2):1–26.
89. Centers for Disease Control and Prevention. Public health burden of vaccine-preventable diseases among adults: standards for adult immunization practice. *MMWR* 1990;39:725–729.
90. Klein JO. Management of infections in hospital employees. *Am J Med* 1981;70:919–923.
91. DeGroot-Kosolcharoen J, Jones JM. Permeability of latex and vinyl gloves to water and blood. *Am J Infect Control* 1989;17:196–201.
92. Doebbeling BN, Pfaller MA, Houston AK, et al. Removal of nosocomial pathogens from the contaminated glove: implications for glove reuse and handwashing. *Ann Intern Med* 1988;109:394–398.
93. Kotilainen HR, Brinker JP, Avato JL, et al. Latex and vinyl examination gloves: quality control procedures and implications for healthcare workers. *Arch Intern Med* 1989;149:2749–2753.
94. Kubica GP: Your tuberculosis laboratory: Are you really safe from infection? *Clin Microbiol Newslett* 1990;12:85–87.
95. Macher JM, First MW. Effects of airflow rates and operator activity on containment of bacterial aerosols in a class II safety cabinet. *Appl Environ Microbiol* 1984;48:481–485.
96. Reinhardt PA, Gordon JG. *Infectious and medical waste management*. Chelsea, Mich.: Lewis Publishers, 1991.
97. Vesley D, Lauer JL. Decontamination, sterilization, disinfection, and antisepsis. In: Fleming DO, Richardson JH, Tulis JJ, Vesley D, eds. *Laboratory safety: principles and practices*, 2nd. ed. Washington, D.C.: American Society for Microbiology, 1995:219–237.
98. McVicar JW, Suen J. Packaging and shipping biological materials. In: Fleming DO, Richardson JH, Tulis JJ, Vesley D, eds. *Laboratory safety: principles and practices*, 2nd. ed. Washington, American Society for Microbiology, 1995:239–246.
99. Centers for Disease Control and Prevention. Guidelines for preventing the transmission of *Mycobacterium tuberculosis* in health-care facilities, 1994. *MMWR* 1994;43(no. RR-13):1–132.
100. Kruse RH, Puckett WH, Richardson JH. Biological safety cabinetry. *Clin Microbiol Rev* 1991;4:207–241.
101. Centers for Disease Control and Prevention. Case-control study of HIV serpcpnversion in health-care workers after percutaneous exposure to HIV-infected blood—France, United Kingdom, and United States, January 1988–August 1994. *MMWR* 1995;44:929–933.
102. Centers for Disease Control and Prevention. Update: provisional Public Health Service recommendations for chemoprophylaxis after occupational exposure to HIV. *MMWR* 1996;45:468–472.
103. Tokars JI, Marcus R, Culver DH, et al. Surveillance of HIV infection and zidovudine use among healthcare workers after occupational exposure to HIV-infected blood. *Ann Intern Med* 1993;118:913–919.

Hospital Infections, Fourth Edition,
edited by John V. Bennett and Philip S. Brachman.
Published by Lippincott–Raven Publishers, Philadelphia, 1998

CHAPTER 24

Dialysis-Associated Infections and Their Control

Martin S. Favero, Miriam J. Alter, Jerome I. Tokars, and Matthew J. Arduino

The number of patients who have end-stage renal disease and are treated by maintenance dialysis has increased dramatically in the past 30 years. In 1967, ~ 1,000 patients were undergoing maintenance or long-term hemodialysis. In 1973, when full Medicare coverage was extended to persons with end-stage renal diseases, ~ 11,000 patients were undergoing dialysis in independent or hospital-based centers and in homes in the United States. At the end of 1995, there were ~ 235,000 patients undergoing maintenance dialysis and 56,400 staff members in 2,672 dialysis centers throughout the United States. The end-stage renal disease program is administered by the Healthcare Financing Administration (HCFA) of the Department of Health and Human Services. It is the only Medicare entitlement that is based on the diagnosis of a medical condition.

The technology for performing dialysis, and the potential for complications, has changed significantly over the years. In the early 1960s, hemodialysis was used almost exclusively for the treatment of acute renal failure. Subsequently, the development of the arteriovenous shunt and certain other ancillary technologic advances in dialysis equipment expanded the use of hemodialysis to maintenance therapy for end-stage renal disease. In the 1970s, the primary mode for dialysis treatment was hemodialysis performed with various types of artificial kidney machines. Subsequently, the use of peritoneal dialysis, accomplished by automated machines or by intermittent cycling, developed. In the past 15 years, continuous ambulatory peritoneal dialysis (CAPD) and variations of this technique have become popular because patients can perform this procedure at home or while working and do not require lengthy dialysis treatments at a center. At the end of 1995, 17% of all dialysis patients were treated with some form of peritoneal dialysis.

Dialysis patients have a compromised immune system and other disorders that place them at higher than normal risk of infectious diseases. This chapter describes the major infectious diseases and several toxic complications due to chemical contamination that can be acquired in the dialysis center setting, the important epidemiologic and environmental microbiologic considerations, and infection control strategies. We rely in part on two sources of data compiled by the Centers for Disease Control and Prevention (CDC). The first includes outbreak investigations in dialysis centers conducted by the CDC. In this chapter we list 36 outbreak investigations: 17 involved bacterial infections or pyrogenic reactions, 10 were viral infections, eight were toxic chemical complications, and one was an allergic complication of dialysis. National surveillance studies are a second source of data. The CDC conducted national surveys of the incidence and prevalence of hepatitis B virus in the early 1970s. Subsequently, the National Surveillance of Dialysis-Associated Diseases in the United States was undertaken by the CDC in collaboration with the HCFA in the years 1976, 1980, and 1982 to 1995. Data were collected on hemodialysis practices, infection control precautions, and on the occurrence of certain hemodialysis-associated diseases.

BACTERIAL AND CHEMICAL CONTAMINANTS IN HEMODIALYSIS SYSTEMS

A typical hemodialysis system consists of a water supply, a system for mixing water and concentrated dialysis

M. S. Favero: Advanced Sterilization Products, Johnson & Johnson Medical Incorporated, Irvine, California 92618.
M. J. Alter: Hepatitis Branch
J. I. Tokars: Hospital Infections Program, National Center for Infectious Diseases
M. J. Arduino: Hospital Infections Program, Centers for Disease Control and Prevention, Atlanta, Georgia 30333.

fluid, and a machine to pump the dialysis fluid through the artificial kidney (commonly referred to as the hemodialyzer or dialyzer). The dialyzer is connected to the patient's circulatory system and blood is pumped through it to accomplish dialysis through a membrane to remove waste products from the patient's blood.

Bacterial Contamination of Water

Technical development and clinical use of hemodialysis delivery systems improved dramatically in the late 1960s and early 1970s. However, a number of microbiologic parameters were not accounted for in the design of many hemodialysis machines and their respective water supply systems. There are many situations where certain types of gram-negative water bacteria can persist and actively multiply in the aqueous environments associated with hemodialysis equipment. This can result in the production of massive levels of gram-negative bacteria, which can directly or indirectly affect patients through septicemia or endotoxemia [1,2].

A number of factors can influence microbial contamination of fluids associated with hemodialysis systems (Table 24-1). The gram-negative water bacteria can be significant contaminants in hemodialysis systems (Table 24-2), and virtually all disinfection strategies for fluid water distribution lines and dialysis machines are targeted to this group of bacteria.

Gram-negative water bacteria are capable of multiplying rapidly in all types of waters, even those containing relatively small amounts of organic matter, such as water treated by distillation, softening, deionization, or reverse osmosis. These organisms can attain levels ranging from 10^5 to 10^7 per milliliter of water and, under certain circumstances, can be a health hazard for patients undergoing dialysis; they constitute a direct threat of bacteremia, and they contain bacterial endotoxin (lipopolysaccharide) that can cause pyrogenic reactions [3–6]. It should be emphasized that virtually any gram-negative water bac-

TABLE 24-1. *Factors influencing microbial contamination in hemodialysis systems*

Factors	Comments
Water supply	
Source of community water	
Groundwater	Contains endotoxin and bacteria
Surface water	Contains high levels of endotoxin and bacteria
Water treatment at dialysis center	
None	Not recommended
Filtration	
Prefilter	Particulate filter to protect equipment; does not remove microorganisms
Absolute filter (depth or membrane)	Removes bacteria, but unless changed frequently or disinfected, bacteria will accumulate and grow through filter; acts as significant reservoir of bacteria and endotoxin
Activated carbon filter	Removes organics and available chlorine or chloramine; significant reservoir of water bacteria and endotoxin
Water treatment devices	
Ion-exchange softener	Both softeners and deionizers are significant reservoirs of bacteria and do not remove endotoxin
Deionization	
Reverse osmosis	Removes bacteria and endotoxin, but must be disinfected; operates at high water pressure
Ultraviolet light	Kills some bacteria, but there is no residual, and ultraviolet-resistant bacteria can develop
Ultrafilter	Removes bacteria and endotoxin; operates on normal line pressure; can be positioned distal to deionizer; must be disinfected
Water and dialysate distribution system	
Distribution pipes	
Size	Oversized diameter and length decrease fluid flow and increase bacteria reservoir for both treated water and centrally prepared dialysate
Construction	Rough joints, dead ends, and unused branches can act as bacterial reservoirs
Elevation	Outlet taps should be located at highest elevation to prevent loss of disinfectant
Storage tanks	Undesirable because they act as reservoir of water bacteria; if present, they must be routinely scrubbed and disinfected
Dialysis machines	
Single-pass	Disinfectant should have contact with all parts of machine that are exposed to water or dialysis fluid
Recirculating single-pass or recirculating (batch)	Recirculating pumps and machine design allow for massive contamination levels if not properly disinfected; overnight chemical germicide treatment recommended

TABLE 24-2. *Types of water microorganisms that have been found in dialysis systems*

Gram-negative water bacteria
Pseudomonas
Flavobacterium
Acinetobacter
Alcaligenes
Achromobacter
Aeromonas
Serratia
Xanthomonas
Nontuberculous mycobacteria
Mycobacterium chelonei
M. fortuitum
M. gordonae
M. scrofulaceum
M. kansaii
M. avium
M. intracellularis

terium that can grow in water systems represents a potential problem in a hemodialysis unit. These bacteria adhere to surfaces, form biofilms (glycocalyxes), and are virtually impossible to eradicate [7,8]. In fact, control strategies are designed to reduce levels of microbial contamination in water and dialysis fluid to relatively low levels but not to completely eradicate them.

Gram-negative water bacteria can grow even more rapidly in treated water mixed with dialysis concentrate. This mixture results in dialysis fluid that is a balanced salt solution and growth medium almost as rich in nutrients as conventional nutrient broth [2,4]. Gram-negative water bacteria growing in distilled, deionized, or reverse-osmosis-treated water can reach levels of 10^5 to 10^7 organisms per milliliter, but these cell populations are not visibly turbid. On the other hand, these same bacteria growing in dialysis fluids can achieve levels of 10^8 to 10^9 organisms per milliliter and are often associated with noticeable turbidity.

Nontuberculous mycobacteria also can multiply in water (Table 24-2). Although they do not contain bacterial endotoxin, they are comparatively resistant to chemical germicides and, as will be discussed later, have been responsible for infections due to inadequately disinfected dialyzers that are reprocessed and inadequately disinfected peritoneal dialysis machines [1].

The strategy for controlling massive accumulations of gram-negative water bacteria and nontuberculous mycobacteria in dialysis systems primarily involves preventing their growth. This can be accomplished by proper disinfection of water treatment systems and hemodialysis machines. Gram-negative water bacteria and their associated lipopolysaccharides (bacterial endotoxins) and nontuberculous mycobacteria ultimately come from the community water supply, and levels of these bacteria can be amplified, depending on the water treatment systems, dialysate distribution systems, type of dialysis machine, and method of disinfection [9–11] (Table 24-1). Each of these components is discussed separately in some detail.

Water Supply

Dialysis centers use water from a public supply, which may be derived from either surface or groundwaters. The source of the water may be important in terms of bacterial endotoxin content, because surface waters frequently contain endotoxin from gram-negative water bacteria as well as from certain types of blue-green algae. Endotoxin levels are not substantially reduced by conventional municipal water treatment processes and can be high enough to cause pyrogenic reactions in patients undergoing dialysis [12].

Essentially all public water supplies are contaminated with water bacteria; consequently, a dialysis center's water treatment and distribution systems and dialysis machines are challenged repeatedly with continuous inoculation of these ubiquitous bacteria. Even adequately chlorinated water supplies commonly contain low levels of these microorganisms. Whereas chlorine and other disinfectants added to the city water may prevent high levels of contamination, the presence of these chemicals in dialysis fluids is undesirable because of adverse effects on patients undergoing dialysis [13]. Furthermore, the dialysis water treatment systems described here effectively remove chlorine, allowing for the unrestricted growth of water microorganisms.

Water Treatment Systems

Water used for the production of dialysis fluid must be treated to remove chemical contaminants. The Association for the Advancement of Medical Instrumentation (AAMI) has published guidelines for the chemical and bacteriologic quality of water used to prepare dialysis fluid [14]. Depending on the area of the United States, a variety of different water treatment systems are used, but most of them are associated with amplification of water bacteria (Table 24-1). The most common type of treatment is ion exchange using water softeners and deionizers. However, neither of these components removes endotoxins or bacteria, and both provide sites for significant bacterial multiplication [15]. An effective means of treating water for dialysis is reverse osmosis. Water treatment systems relying on reverse osmosis or deionization are used in 99% of U.S. dialysis centers [16–18]. Reverse osmosis possesses the singular advantage of being able to remove both bacterial endotoxins and bacteria from supply water. However, low numbers of gram-negative and nontuberculous mycobacteria water bacteria can either penetrate this barrier or, by other means, colonize the downstream portion of the reverse-osmosis unit. Consequently, reverse-osmosis systems must be disinfected routinely.

There are a variety of filters that are marketed to control bacterial contamination in water and dialysis fluids. Most of these are inadequate, especially if they are not routinely disinfected or changed frequently. Particulate filters, commonly called prefilters, operate by depth filtration and do not remove bacteria or bacterial endotoxins. These filters can become colonized with gram-negative water bacteria, resulting in amplification of the levels of both bacteria and endotoxin in the filter effluent. Absolute filters, including the membrane types, temporarily remove bacteria from passing water. However, some of these filters tend to clog, and gram-negative water bacteria can "grow through" the filter matrix and colonize the downstream surface of the filters within a couple of days. Moreover, absolute filters do not reduce levels of endotoxin in the effluent water. These types of filters should be changed regularly in accordance with the manufacturer's directions and disinfected in the same manner and at the same time as the dialysis system.

Activated carbon filters are used to remove certain organic chemicals and available chlorine from water, but they also significantly raise the level of water bacteria and do not remove bacterial endotoxins. Ultraviolet (UV) irradiation is sometimes used to reduce bacterial contamination in water. However, this approach is not recommended [1,4], because certain populations of gram-negative water bacteria appear to be far more resistant to UV radiation than others, resulting in instances in which significant numbers of bacteria survive theoretically adequate treatment. This problem is accentuated in recirculating dialysis systems, where repeated exposures to UV radiation are used to ensure adequate disinfection. Resistance to UV radiation is enhanced because of the multiplication of those microorganisms surviving initial exposure. In addition, bacterial endotoxins are not affected.

As mentioned previously, an effective means of treating water for dialysis is the correct use of a reverse-osmosis unit. We recommend using a water treatment system that produces chemically adequate water without massive levels of microbial contamination. Such a system is well suited for hard water and follows a specific procedure [19]. Community-supplied water is passed through a set of prefilters, a softener, carbon filters, and a particulate filter and then through a reverse-osmosis unit and a deionization unit. Through these phases, the water becomes progressively more pure chemically, but the level of bacterial contamination increases. To compensate, an ultrafilter is included in the final step of the process to remove bacteria and bacterial endotoxins.

The ultrafilter consists of membranes similar to those of a reverse-osmosis unit, or it may have a polysulfone membrane. It can be operated at ordinary waterline pressure. This entire system can be augmented with other source water treatment devices, depending on the chemical quality of the water in question. If this system is adequately disinfected, the microbial content of water should be well within the recommended guidelines discussed under Monitoring of Water and Dialysis Fluid.

Distribution Systems

Dialysis centers use one of two general systems for delivering dialysis fluids to individual dialysis machines. In the first type, incoming supply water is treated and distributed to individual free-standing dialysis stations. At each station, the water is mixed with a dialysate concentrate by automatic proportioning. A second type of system, usually found in large dialysis centers, involves the automatic mixing of treated water and dialysate concentrate at a central location, followed by distribution of the warmed dialysis fluid through pipes to individual dialysis stations. In both designs, the distribution system consists of plastic pipes (usually polyvinyl chloride) and appurtenances.

These distribution systems can contribute to microbial contamination in two ways. First, they frequently use larger-diameter and longer pipes than are necessary to handle the required fluid flow. This slows the fluid velocity and amplifies both the total fluid volume and the wetted surface area of the system. Gram-negative bacteria in fluids remaining in pipes overnight multiply rapidly and colonize the wetted surfaces of the pipes, producing bacterial populations and endotoxin quantities in proportion to the volume and surface area. Such colonization results in formation of protective biofilm by the bacteria, which is difficult to remove and protects the bacteria from disinfection [20].

Because pipes can constitute a source of water bacteria in a distribution system, routine disinfection should be performed at least weekly. To ensure that the disinfectant cannot drain from pipes by gravity before sufficient contact time has passed, distribution systems should be designed with all outlet taps at equal elevation and at the highest point of the system. Furthermore, the system should be free of rough joints, dead-end pipes, and unused branches and taps. Fluid trapped in such stagnant areas can serve as reservoirs of bacteria capable of continuously inoculating the entire volume of the system [6].

Incorporation of a storage tank in a distribution system greatly increases the volume of fluid and surface area available to act as reservoirs for the multiplication of water bacteria. Storage tanks should not be used in dialysis systems unless they are frequently drained and adequately disinfected, including scrubbing of the sides of the tank to remove bacterial biofilm. It is also recommended that an ultrafilter be used distal to the storage tank.

Hemodialysis Machines

In the United States at present, virtually all centers use single-pass hemodialysis machines. In the 1970s, most machines were of the recirculating or recirculating single-pass type. The nature of their design contributed to a relatively high level of gram-negative bacterial contamination in dialysis fluid. Single-pass dialysis machines tend to respond to adequate cleaning and disinfection procedures and, in general, have lower levels of bacterial contamination in their dialysis fluid than do recirculating machines. Levels of contamination in single-pass machines depend primarily on the bacteriologic quality of the incoming water and on the method of machine disinfection [1,3,4].

A common error in disinfecting single-pass systems is introducing the disinfectant in the same manner and through the same port as the dialysate concentrate. By so doing, the pipes and tubing of the incoming water are not exposed to a disinfectant; thus, the environment is such that bacteria can readily colonize and proliferate, acting as a constant reservoir of contamination. For adequate disinfection of a single-pass system, the disinfectant must reach all parts of the system's fluid pathways.

Dialyzers

The dialyzer (artificial kidney) usually does not contribute significantly to bacterial contamination of the dialysate. Most dialysis centers use hollow-fiber dialyzers rather than plate (parallel flow) dialyzers or coil dialyzers [16–18]; hollow-fiber dialyzers do not amplify bacterial contamination in the dialysis systems. Most centers (73% in 1993) also reprocess dialyzers for reuse on the same patient [21]. Improper reprocessing techniques have been associated with outbreaks of bacteremia and pyrogenic reactions in dialysis patients (Table 24-1). This subject will be discussed further in the section Hemodialyzer Reuse.

Disinfection of Hemodialysis Systems

The objective of a disinfection procedure for a dialysis system is to inactivate bacteria in the fluid pathways associated with the dialysis system and to prevent these organisms from growing to significant levels once the system is in operation. Routine disinfection of isolated components of a dialysis system frequently produces inadequate results, and the hazard to the patient persists. Consequently, the total dialysis system (water treatment system, distribution system, and dialysis machine) needs to be considered when selecting and applying disinfection procedures.

Chlorine-based disinfectants, such as sodium hypochlorite solutions, are convenient and effective in most parts of the dialysis system when used at the manufacturer's recommended concentration. Also, the test for residual available chlorine to confirm adequate rinsing is simple and sensitive. However, because of the corrosive nature of chlorine, the disinfectant is normally rinsed from the system after a short exposure time (20 to 30 minutes). This practice commonly negates the disinfection procedure because the rinse water invariably contains gram-negative water bacteria that immediately resume multiplication. If permitted to stand overnight, the water will contain significant microbial contamination levels.

Therefore, chlorine disinfectants are most effective when applied just before the startup of the dialysis system rather than at the end of daily operation. In some large centers, where there are many shifts, it may be reasonable to use sodium hypochlorite disinfection between shifts (this may not be necessary with some single-pass machines if the levels of bacterial contamination are within AAMI limits) and formaldehyde, peroxyacetic acid, or glutaraldehyde disinfection at the end of the day. The latter formulations are commercially available and are designed for use with dialysis machines.

Aqueous formaldehyde, peroxyacetic acid, or glutaraldehyde solutions can produce good disinfection results. They are not as corrosive as hypochlorite solutions and can be allowed to remain in the dialysis system for long periods when the system is not operational, thereby preventing the growth of bacteria in the system. Formaldehyde has good penetrating characteristics but is considered an environmental hazard and potential carcinogen and is associated with irritating qualities that are objectionable to staff members. There are commercial tests available (e.g., Formalert, Organon Teknika, Durham, NC) that are sensitive for testing for formaldehyde in water at concentrations as low as 1 part per million.[1]

Commercially available glutaraldehyde-based disinfectants and a peroxyacetic acid disinfectant for dialysis systems, when used according to the manufacturer's recommendations, are not corrosive to machines and are good germicides [22,23]. Some dialysis systems use hot-water disinfection for the control of microbial contamination. In this type of system, water heated to > 800°C (176°F) is passed through all proportioning, distribution, and patient-monitoring devices before use. This system is excellent for controlling bacterial contamination [1].

Monitoring of Water and Dialysis Fluid

Bacteriologic assays of water and dialysis fluids should be performed at least once a month. It has been recommended that the levels of microbial contamination in

[1]Trade names are used for identification only and do not imply endorsement by the Public Health Service or by the U.S. Department of Health and Human Services.

water used to prepare dialysis fluid not exceed 200 cfu/ml and that contamination levels not exceed 2,000 cfu/ml in dialysis fluids [14,24] (Table 24-3). These particular numbers are based on bacteriologic assays conducted in the course of epidemiologic investigations; they are not considered absolute and should be used as broad guidelines.

The bacteriologic assay is quantitative rather than qualitative, and a standard technique for enumeration should be used. Water samples should be collected at a point as close as possible to where water enters the dialysate concentrate–proportioning unit. Samples should be collected at least monthly. More samples should be collected when bacteriologic counts exceed 200 cfu/ml and after disinfection changes have been instituted. Dialysis fluid samples should be collected during or at the termination of dialysis, close to where the dialysis fluid either enters or leaves the dialyzer. These types of samples should also be taken at least once monthly and after suspected pyrogenic reactions or changes in the water treatment system or disinfection protocols.

Samples should be assayed within 30 minutes or refrigerated at (4°C) and assayed within 24 hours of collection. Total viable counts (standard plate counts) are the objective of the assays, and conventional laboratory procedures, such as the pour plate, spread plate, or membrane filter technique, can be used; calibrated loops should not be used because they sample a small volume and are inaccurate. Although standard methods—agar, blood agar, and trypticase soy agar—were considered equivalent in the earlier recommendations of the AAMI, it has since been shown that a good portion of the gram-negative bacterial flora of bicarbonate dialysis fluid requires a small amount of sodium chloride for optimal growth. Consequently, trypticase soy agar is now considered the culture medium of choice. Colonies should be counted after 48 hours of incubation at 35° to 37°C (95° to 98.6°F) [8,14,24,25].

In the event of an outbreak investigation, the assay may need to be qualitative as well as quantitative, and sometimes there is concern about nontuberculous mycobacteria in water (Table 24-2). In such cases, plates should be incubated for 5 to 14 days. If centers reprocess dialyzers for reuse on the same patient, water used to rinse dialyzers and prepare dialyzer disinfectants also should be assayed at least monthly in the manner described previously. It is recommended that microbial or endotoxin contamination not exceed 200 cfu/ml or 1 ng (5 endotoxin units)/ml, respectively [8,26] (Table 24-3).

TABLE 24-3. *Microbiologic and endotoxin standards for dialysis fluids*

Type of fluid	Bacteria	Endotoxin
Water used to prepare dialysate	< 200 cfu/ml	No standard
Dialysate	< 2,000 cfu/ml	No standard
Water used to rinse and reprocess dialyzers	< 200 cfu/ml or	< 1 ng/ml
Water used to prepare dialyzer disinfectant	< 200 cfu/ml or	< 1 ng/ml

PYROGENIC REACTIONS AND SEPTICEMIA

Pyrogenic reactions and gram-negative sepsis are the most common complications associated with high levels of gram-negative bacterial contamination of dialysis fluid. Pyrogenic reactions can result from either the passage of bacterial endotoxin (lipopolysaccharide) in the dialysis fluid across the dialyzer membrane [27–29] or the transmembrane stimulation of cytokine production in the patient's blood by endotoxins in the dialysis fluid [30,31]. In other instances, endotoxins can enter the bloodstream directly with fluids that are contaminated with gram-negative bacteria [32,33]. Studies indicate that patients on long-term hemodialysis have an enhanced cytokine response compared with nonhemodialysis patients, and this may account for the high rate of fatal sepsis among uremic patients [34].

The higher the level of bacteria and endotoxin in dialysis fluid, the higher the probability that bacteria or endotoxin will pass through the dialysis membrane or stimulate cytokine production. In one outbreak of febrile reactions among patients undergoing dialysis, the attack rates were directly proportional to the level of bacterial contamination in the dialysis fluid [4]. Prospective studies also have confirmed a lower pyrogenic reaction rate among patients when they underwent dialysis with dialysis fluid that had been filtered and from which most bacteria had been removed compared with patients who underwent dialysis with dialysis fluid that was highly contaminated (mean 19,000 cfu/ml) [35–37].

In 1993, 21% of the hemodialysis centers in the United States reported at least one pyrogenic reaction in the absence of septicemia in patients undergoing dialysis [21]. An active surveillance system is essential for early detection and control of these complications. Clinical reactions should be defined as they occur, since this may be the first clue that a problem exists. In addition, the dialysis system should be bacteriologically monitored periodically by the methods already described. A list of outbreaks of bacteremia and pyrogenic reactions investigated by the CDC are presented in Table 24-4.

Surveillance of Pyrogenic Reactions and Infections

Pyrogenic reactions in patients undergoing dialysis are associated with shaking chills, fever, and hypotension. Depending on the type of dialysis system and the level of initial contamination, the onset of an elevated temperature and chills can occur 1 to 5 hours after the initiation

TABLE 24-4. *Outbreaks of dialysis-associated illnesses investigated by the Centers for Disease Control and Prevention*

Description [reference]	Cause(s) of outbreak	Corrective measure(s) recommended
Chemical contamination of dialysate		
Hemolytic anemia in 41 patients [13]	Chloramines in city water not removed completely by carbon filter	Larger carbon filters connected in series; monitoring of chloramines after filter for each patient shift
Decreased hemoglobin in three pediatric patients [133]	Disinfectant not adequately rinsed from fluid distribution system	Thoroughly rinse germicide from system; use appropriate residual test kit
Severe hypotension in nine patients [134]	Dialysate contaminated with sodium azide from new ultrafilters	Rinse system after modification or installation of new components
Aluminum intoxication in 27 patients [135]	Exhausted deionization tanks unable to remove aluminum from city water	Monitor deionization tanks daily; install reverse-osmosis system
Formaldehyde intoxication in five patients; one death [136]	Disinfectant not properly rinsed from fluid distribution system	Eliminate stagnant flow areas; test for residual germicide
Aluminum intoxication in 27 patients; three deaths [74]	Aluminum pump was used to transfer acid concentrate to treatment area	Use components that do not leach harmful substances into dialysis fluids
Fluoride intoxication in eight patients; one death [75]	Excess fluoride in city water; no water treatment by center	Install reverse-osmosis system
Fluoride intoxication in nine patients; three deaths [137]	Exhausted deionization tanks discharged a bolus of fluoride	Deionization tanks should be monitored by resistivity meters with audible and visual alarms
Bacteremia/pyrogenic reaction not related to hemodialyzer reuse		
Pyrogenic reactions in 49 patients [12]	Untreated city water contained high levels of endotoxin	Install reverse-osmosis system
Pyrogenic reactions in 45 patients [6]	Inadequate disinfection of fluid distribution system	Increase disinfection frequency and germicide contact time
Pyrogenic reactions in 14 patients; two bacteremias; one death [7]	Reverse-osmosis water storage tank contaminated with bacteria	Remove or properly disinfect and maintain storage tank
Pyrogenic reactions in six patients; seven bacteremia [138]	Inadequate disinfection of water distribution system and dialysis machines; improper microbial assay procedure	Use correct microbial assay procedure; disinfect water distribution system and dialysis machines according to manufacturer's recommendations
Bacteremia in 35 patients with central vein catheters [139]	Central vein catheters used as primary access; median duration of infected catheters was 311 days; improper aseptic techniques	Use central vein catheters only when necessary; use appropriate aseptic techniques when inserting catheters and for catheter care
Bacteremia/pyrogenic reaction related to hemodialyzer reuse		
Mycobacterial infections in 27 patients [9]	Inadequate concentration of dialyzer disinfectant	Increase formaldehyde dialyzer disinfectant concentration to 4%
Mycobacterial infection in five high-flux dialysis patients; two deaths [45]	Inadequate concentration of dialyzer disinfectant treatment system	Use higher disinfectant concentration and more frequent disinfection of water
Bacteremia and pyrogenic reactions six patients [140]	Dialyzer disinfectant diluted to improper concentration	Use disinfectant at recommended dilution and verify concentration
Bacteremia in six patients [CDC unpublished data]	Inadequate concentration of dialyzer disinfectant; water used for reuse did not meet AAMI standards	Use AAMI quality of water; ensure proper germicide concentration in dialyzer
Bacteremia and pyrogenic reactions in six patients [141]	Inadequate mixing of dialyzer disinfectant	Thoroughly mix disinfectant and verify proper concentration
Bacteremia in 33 patients at two dialysis centers [33]	Dialyzer disinfectant created holes in dialyzer membrane	Change disinfectant (removed from marketplace by manufacturer)
Bacteremia in six patients; all blood isolates had similar plasmid profiles [142]	Dialyzers contaminated during removal and cleaning of headers with gauze; staff not routinely changing gloves; dialyzers not processed for several hours after disassembly and cleaning	Do not use gauze or similar material to remove clots from header; change gloves frequently; process dialyzers immediately after rinsing and cleaning
Pyrogenic reactions in three high-flux dialysis patients [143]	Dialyzer reprocessed with two disinfectants; water reused	Do not disinfect dialyzers with multiple germicides
Pyrogenic reactions during high-flux dialysis [CDC unpublished data]	Dialyzers rinsed with city water; water for reuse did not meet AAMI standards	Do not rinse or clean dialyzers with city water; disinfect water treatment system more frequently
Pyrogenic reactions in 18 patients [40]	Dialyzers rinsed with city water containing high levels of endotoxin; water for reuse did not meet AAMI standards	Do not rinse or clean dialyzers with city water; disinfect water treatment system more frequently

TABLE 24-4. *Continued.*

Description [reference]	Cause(s) of outbreak	Corrective measure(s) recommended
Pyrogenic reactions in 22 patients [144]	Water for reuse did not meet AAMI standards; improper microbial assay technique	Use correct microbial assay procedure; disinfect water distribution system
Acute allergic-type reactions		
Acute allergic reactions in hundreds of patients using reprocessed dialyzers in ≥ 31 centers [66]	Related to use of angiotensin-converting enzyme inhibitors and possibly to chemicals used in cleaning dialyzer or inadequate germicide rinsing out of dialyzer	No specific recommendation
Transmission of viral agents		
26 patients seroconverted to HBsAg positive during a 10-mo period [85]	Leakage of coil dialyzer membranes and use of recirculating bath dialysis machines	Separation of HBsAg-positive patients and equipment from other patients
19 patients and one staff member seroconverted to HBsAg positive during a 14-mo period [145]	No specific cause determined; false-positive HBsAg results caused some susceptible patients to be dialyzed with infected patients	Laboratory confirmation of HBsAg-positive results; strict adherence to glove use and use of separate equipment
24 patients and six staff members seroconverted to HBsAg positive during a 10-mo period [86]	Staff not wearing gloves; surfaces not properly disinfected; improper handling of needles/sharp items, resulting in many staff needle sticks	Separation of HBsAg-positive patients and equipment from other patients; proper precautions by staff (e.g. gloves; handling of needles/sharp objects)
13 patients and one staff member seroconverted to HBsAg positive during a 1-mo period [146]	Extrinsic contamination of intravenous medication being prepared adjacent to area where blood work handled	Separate medication preparation area and blood processing for diagnostic tests
10 patients seroconverted to HBsAg positive in 1-mo period [81]	Extrinsic contamination of multidose medication vial shared by HBsAg-positive and susceptible patients	No sharing of supplies, equipment, and medications between patients
Eight patients seroconverted to HBsAg positive during a 5-mo period [CDC, unpublished data]	Sporadic screening for HBsAg; HBsAg carriers not separated; major bleeding incident with environmental contamination	Monthly screening of patients for HBsAg; separation of positive patients with dedicated equipment and staff; vaccination of all those susceptible
Seven patients seroconverted to HBsAg positive during a 3-mo period [147]	Same staff were caring for both HBsAg-positive and -negative patients	Separation of HBsAg-positive patients from other patients; same staff should not care for both HBsAg-positive and -negative patients on same shift
Eight patients seroconverted to HBsAg positive during 1-mo period [148]	Not consistently using pressure transducer filters; same staff cared for HBsAg-positive and -negative patients	Use pressure transducer filters and replace after each use; same staff should not care for HBsAg-positive and -negative patients on same shift
36 patients with liver enzyme elevations indicative of NANB hepatitis; other causes excluded [149]	Environmental contamination with blood	Monthly liver enzyme screening; proper precautions (i.e., wearing gloves) by staff
35 patients with liver enzyme elevations indicative of NANB hepatitis during a 22-mo period; 82% of probable cases anti-HCV positive [122]	Inconsistent use of universal precautions, especially hand washing and glove use	Strict compliance with aseptic technique and universal precautions

of dialysis, and these symptoms are usually associated with a decrease in systolic blood pressure of ≥ 30 mm Hg. Other less frequently noted but characteristic symptoms include headache, myalgia, nausea, and vomiting. We define a case of pyrogenic reaction as the onset of objective chills (visible rigors) or fever (oral temperature ≥ 37.8°C (100°F)) or both in a patient who was afebrile (oral temperature ≤ 37.0°C (98.6°F)) and who had no signs or symptoms of infection before the dialysis treatment [1].

Differentiating gram-negative bacterial sepsis from a pyrogenic reaction can be difficult, since the initial signs and symptoms of the two conditions are identical. The most reliable means of detecting sepsis is by culturing blood samples taken at the time of the reaction. However, since the results of these cultures take ≥ 18 to 24 hours to obtain, and since therapy for sepsis should not be withheld for this length of time, other less reliable criteria must be used.

Many pyrogenic reactions are not associated with bacteremia, and the preceding signs and symptoms generally abate within a few hours after dialysis has been stopped. With gram-negative bacterial sepsis, fever and chills may persist, and hypotension is more refractory to therapy [12,32]. The early detection of pyrogenic reactions or gram-negative sepsis depends on a thorough understanding of the signs and symptoms of these entities by the dialysis staff and on the careful charting of the patient's symptoms as well as changes in blood pressure and temperature. The following diagnostic procedures are recommended for patients who meet the criteria of a pyrogenic reaction.

1. A thorough physical examination to rule out other causes of chills and fever (e.g., pneumonia, shunt or fistula infection, urinary tract infection).
2. Cultures of blood samples taken at the time of reactions and cultures of any additional body fluids or secretions indicated by the physical examination as likely sources of infection.
3. Collection of dialysis fluid from the dialyzer (downstream side) for quantitative and qualitative bacteriologic assays.

Hemodialyzer Reuse

In the early 1960s, the most common dialyzer used in dialysis centers was the Kiil plate dialyzer, which was cleaned and disinfected after each use and supplied with a new set of cuprophan membranes. The dialyzer housing, however, was reused each time. With the development of disposable coil and hollow-fiber dialyzers, use of the Kiil dialyzer was discontinued. Disposable dialyzers are medical devices that are supplied in a sterile state and are intended by the manufacturer for one-time use. In recent years, as a cost-saving effort, more centers are reusing dialyzers on the same patient after employing an appropriate disinfection procedure. Although it has been the subject of controversy, this is now standard practice in the dialysis community. From 1976 to 1983, the percentage of dialysis centers in the United States that reported reuse of disposable dialyzers increased from 18% to 52%. This percentage has continued to rise: in 1993, 73% of centers reported that they reused disposable dialyzers on one or more patients, and 73% of all hemodialysis patients were reportedly in dialyzer reuse programs [21]. In 1993 the average number of times a dialysis center reused dialyzers was 15 (range, 2 to 60). The mean number of times a disposable dialyzer was reused was 33 (range, five to 149).

Dialysis centers most likely to report reuse of dialyzers were those with larger populations of patients (> 40), those located in free-standing facilities, and those operated for profit compared with centers with smaller populations, those located in hospitals, and those not operated for profit [16,18,21]. The CDC's surveillance project has not shown a correlation between hepatitis B virus incidence or the prevalence of anti-hepatitis C virus and dialyzer reuse. However, a study has shown a statistically significant association between reuse of dialyzers disinfected with glutaraldehyde or peracetic acid/hydrogen peroxide and higher death rates at dialysis centers [38]. It is uncertain whether this association indicates a causal relationship between reuse and a higher death rate or whether the association was due to unmeasured confounding factors.

In 1986, the U.S. Public Health Service (PHS) subsumed the AAMI's guidelines for reusing hemodialyzers [39] and recommended them as PHS guidance to the HCFA, which, in turn, made them conditions for participation in Medicare/Medicaid. In effect, the AAMI guidelines, which became PHS guidance, resulted in HCFA regulations. In general, if the procedures involved in reprocessing hemodialyzers are performed according to established and strict protocols, there do not appear to be harmful effects on patients. However, the practice of reusing disposable hemodialyzers should not be considered risk-free.

Outbreaks of infections and pyrogenic reactions associated with user error have occurred. Many of these episodes were the result of inadequate reprocessing procedures, such as the use of incorrect concentrations of chemical germicides and failure to maintain standards for water quality [40]. In addition, in 1986, 6 dialysis centers reported outbreaks of pyrogenic reactions and septicemia that were associated with the use of a new germicide, the active ingredient of which was chlorine dioxide. That germicide, although efficacious for disinfecting dialyzers, appeared to degrade the integrity of cellulosic dialyzer membranes to such an extent that leaks in the membranes developed [33,41]. Centers that reported using this germicide employed manual reprocessing systems, and most of these centers reused their dialyzers more than 20 times.

In each of 3 successive years (1985 to 1988), reprocessing dialyzers in a manual reprocessing system was shown consistently to be significantly associated with a higher reported frequency of pyrogenic reactions, even with the use of other germicides, and was not necessarily related to the absolute number of reuses [16,42]. We believe that dialyzer membrane defects may go undetected when manual reprocessing systems are used, because testing for dialyzer membrane integrity, such as by an air-pressure leak test, is generally not performed with this type of system [43]. It is worth emphasizing that adverse reactions associated with reuse of dialyzers are accentuated in dialysis centers that are having problems and that, for the most part, only a small number of centers are experiencing an increased risk with dialyzers that are reused more than 20 times or that include a manual reprocessing system. In 1993, there was only a modest and nonsignificant association between dialyzer reuse and reporting of pyrogenic reactions at U.S. hemodialysis centers [21].

The procedures used in dialysis centers for reprocessing hemodialyzers usually cannot be classified as sterilization procedures (see Chapter 20) but rather constitute high-level disinfection [8,44]. In 1983, most centers in the United States used 2% aqueous formaldehyde with a contact time of ~ 36 hours for high-level disinfection of disposable dialyzers [16]. Although this procedure may be satisfactory against the presumed microbiologic challenge of gram-negative water bacteria, it is inadequate for the highly germicide-resistant nontuberculous mycobacteria (Table 24-2).

The CDC investigated an outbreak of infections caused by nontuberculous mycobacteria during which 27 cases of infection were documented among 140 patients [9]. The source of the nontuberculous mycobacteria appeared to be the water used in processing the dialyzers. It was evident that 2% formaldehyde did not effectively inactivate populations of these mycobacteria within 36 hours. It was subsequently shown that 4% formaldehyde with a minimum contact time of 24 hours can inactivate high numbers of nontuberculous mycobacteria; as a consequence, 4% formaldehyde is recommended as a minimum solution for disinfection of dialyzers [8,43,44]. We would point out, however, that the use of formaldehyde for reprocessing dialyzers is considered environmentally hazardous to patients and staff members, and that this disinfectant is a chemical solution obtained from chemical supply houses rather than a formulation specifically designed for dialyzer disinfection. A number of chemical germicides specifically formulated for this purpose have been shown to be effective and are approved by the Food and Drug Administration for reprocessing hemodialyzers.

A similar outbreak of systemic mycobacterial infections in five dialysis patients, resulting in two deaths, occurred when high-flux dialyzers were contaminated with mycobacteria during manual reprocessing and were then disinfected with a commercial dialyzer disinfectant prepared at a concentration that did not ensure complete inactivation of mycobacteria [45]. These two outbreaks of infection in dialysis patients emphasize the need to use dialyzer disinfectants at concentrations that are effective against the more chemically resistant microorganisms, such as mycobacteria.

Pyrogenic reactions in dialysis patients caused by reprocessing dialyzers with water that does not meet AAMI standards (Table 24-4) have been frequently associated with epidemics investigated by the CDC. In most cases, the water used to rinse dialyzers or to prepare dialyzer disinfectants exceeded allowable AAMI microbial or endotoxin standards, because the water distribution system was not disinfected frequently, the disinfectant was improperly prepared, or routine microbiologic assays were improperly performed.

High-flux Dialysis

High-flux dialysis is a very efficient hemodialysis treatment that uses dialyzer membranes with hydraulic permeabilities five to 10 times greater than those of conventional dialyzer membranes. By using highly permeable membranes in dialyzers that have larger membrane surface areas than conventional dialyzers, dialysis treatment times can be reduced from 4 to 5 hours to 2 to 3 hours. In 1988, 23% of the hemodialysis centers in the United States reported using high-flux dialyzer membranes on at least some patients [21]. Because high-flux membranes are so permeable, there is concern that bacteria or endotoxin in the dialysate may penetrate these membranes, causing infections or pyrogenic reactions in the patient.

Another concern is that high-flux dialysis requires the use of bicarbonate dialysate, which, unlike the acetate-based dialysate used almost exclusively since the 1970s, is prepared from a concentrate that can support rapid bacterial growth. Acetate dialysate is prepared from a single concentrate with such a high salt molarity (4.8 mol/L) that most bacteria cannot grow in it. Bicarbonate dialysate, however, must be prepared from two concentrates, an acid concentrate with a pH of 2.8 that is not conducive to bacterial growth and a bicarbonate concentrate with a relatively neutral pH and a salt molarity of 1.2 mol/L. Because the bicarbonate concentration will support rapid bacterial growth [46], its use can increase bacterial and endotoxin concentrations in the dialysate and, in theory, may contribute to an increase in pyrogenic reactions, especially when it is used during high-flux dialysis.

Some of this concern may be justified. In recent years, surveillance data have shown a significant association between use of high-flux dialysis and reporting of pyrogenic reactions during dialysis [16–18,21]. However, a prospective study of pyrogenic reactions in patients receiving more than 27,000 conventional, high-efficiency, or high-flux dialysis treatments with a bicarbonate dialysate containing high concentrations of bacteria and endotoxin found no association between pyrogenic reactions and the type of dialysis treatment [36]. Although there seem to be conflicting data on the relationship between high-flux dialysis and pyrogenic reactions, centers providing high-flux dialysis should be especially mindful of ensuring that dialysate meets AAMI microbial standards (Table 24-3).

OTHER BACTERIAL INFECTIONS

Vascular Access Site Infections

Hemodialysis procedures depend on direct and repeated access to large blood vessels that can provide rapid extracorporeal blood flow. Hemodialysis vascular access methods are divided into those that provide for acute access, which would include external plastic arteriovenous shunts or fistulas and hemodialysis catheters, and those that provide for permanent vascular access, such as native arteriovenous fistulas or synthetic arteriovenous grafts [47] (see Chapters 44 and 46). Although the external arteriovenous shunts were the foundation on which modern dialysis grew, in recent years their use has been limited to patients who require temporary access.

The material used for these shunts can be biologic or synthetic. The arteriovenous fistula is believed to provide the best long-term access to circulation with the least number of complications. Vascular access site infections may account for 15% to 20% of all access complications. In general, the length of time that a catheter is left in place and the duration of cannulation can be important predisposing factors to infection. In addition, the type of fistula, nature of the access site dressing, number of needle access episodes, movement of the site, and personal hygiene of the patient may play a role in the acquisition of infection. Bacteremia can occur either by migration of bacteria down the outer surface of the catheter or by contamination of the lumen of the catheter during attachment or detachment during dialysis.

Infections of the vascular access site can lead to sepsis, septic pulmonary emboli, endocarditis, and meningitis. No controlled prospective studies have been performed; thus, reported rates of access site infections among hemodialysis patients vary. Although the most common pathogens are *Staphylococcus aureus* and *S. epidermidis*, gram-negative bacteria can also be responsible for access site infections, especially if the site is in the lower extremities of the patient. Transmission of these types of bacterial infections among patients or from staff members to patients in the hemodialysis center is primarily due to cross-contamination, which results in colonization and subsequent infection in a subset of these patients. Transmission can be controlled by appropriate handwashing and gloving techniques and good puncture procedures [48–53].

For many years, central (subclavian or jugular) catheters have been used for temporary venous access for hemodialysis. Recent technical improvements have made it feasible to use these catheters for permanent access, usually in patients for whom other access is unavailable [53]. However, central catheters have high rates of failure due to thrombosis and infection. In 1991, the CDC investigated 35 bloodstream infections among 68 patients receiving hemodialysis through central catheters; one patient died, and one developed endocarditis and required aortic valve replacement [54]. In 1993, 73% of U.S. hemodialysis centers used permanent central catheters on at least one patient [21].

Infections Associated with Peritoneal Dialysis

As mentioned earlier, 17% of patients with end-stage renal disease in the United States were treated by peritoneal dialysis at the end of 1994. In peritoneal dialysis, the patient's peritoneal membrane is used to dialyze waste products from the patient's blood. In the mid-1970s, the development of automated peritoneal dialysis systems made intermittent peritoneal dialysis a viable alternative to hemodialysis for long-term treatment of patients with end-stage renal disease. This approach has been replaced by CAPD, continuous-cycling peritoneal dialysis (CCPD), or chronic intermittent peritoneal dialysis (CIPD), in which presterilized dialysis fluid either is introduced by gravity or is cycled into a patient's peritoneal cavity. In CAPD, a plastic bag is filled with sterile dialysis fluid, which is administered by the patient, who has a surgically implanted catheter. The exchanges are done every 4 hours, and the patient can be mobile between exchanges [55]. The most persistent problem for patients treated by peritoneal dialysis is peritonitis [56,57].

To prevent the growth of pathogenic microorganisms that cause this infection, automated peritoneal dialysis machines must be cleaned and maintained properly. The machines are designed to sterilize and desalinize large quantities of tap water for subsequent mixture with a dialysate concentrate. In theory, the incidence of peritonitis should be low, because the machine functions as a closed system. However, the machines may themselves provide a reservoir for pathogens that cause peritonitis. Several outbreaks of bacterial peritonitis among patients receiving intermittent peritoneal dialysis have been reported, and the etiologic agents have included *Mycobacterium chelonei*–like organisms and *Pseudomonas cepacia* [58,59]. Both organisms can grow in water; investigation of these outbreaks revealed that machines were inadequately cleaned and disinfected, and the product water and dialysis fluid contained the microorganisms responsible for peritonitis [60].

In addition, one group of organisms, the nontuberculous mycobacteria (such as *M. chelonei*), are significantly and extraordinarily resistant to commonly used disinfectants [61]. Berkelman and colleagues [62] have recommended a set of guidelines that can ensure the production of sterile dialysis fluid and reduce the likelihood of outbreaks of peritonitis for dialysis centers using automated peritoneal dialysis machines. The precise details and protocols differ with each machine type, and the reader is referred to the guidelines for a more complete discussion [62]. It should be noted that the use of these automated machines, for all practical purposes, has been discontinued in the United States, and this information is cited for completeness as well as for historical considerations.

With CAPD, CCPD, and CIPD, catheter-related infections and peritonitis remain the most common cause of morbidity among peritoneal dialysis patients, contribute significantly to the cost of this treatment, and are the primary reason for the abandonment of peritoneal dialysis. Incidence rates for peritonitis vary widely among centers and with different techniques. Rates of peritonitis in patients using CAPD declined from 4.6 episodes per treatment year in 1978 to 1.7 in 1982 and appears to have leveled off to ~1.9. The use of CCPD and CIPD in centers with experienced staff has resulted in substantially reduced infection rates compared with CAPD. The weak link with peritoneal dialysis and the present catheter technology is the associated risk of tunnel or exit site infections. These infections occur at a rate of 0.7 episodes per patient per year [57,63].

Clinical symptoms of peritoneal infection usually appear 12 to 36 hours after bacterial contamination of the peritoneal cavity. These symptoms include nausea, vomiting, and abdominal pain. Later, vague abdominal tenderness may progress to severe, diffuse, or localized pain associated with fever, abdominal distention, and gastrointestinal dysfunction. The clinical diagnosis should be confirmed by bacteriologic analysis of the peritoneal fluid. Cloudy peritoneal fluid is often the first sign of infection.

The etiologic agents of peritonitis associated with conventional peritoneal dialysis are usually *S. epidermidis*, *S. aureus*, and other gram-positive bacteria, which collectively account for 55% to 80% of cases; 17% to 30% of cases are caused by gram-negative organisms such as *Enterobacteriaceae*, *P. aeruginosa*, *P. cepacia*, and *Acinetobacter* species; in a few cases (10%), peritonitis is caused by fungi, yeast, mycobacteria, and anaerobic bacteria. Approximately 10% of cases will show culture-negative results [57,64].

The primary strategy for control of peritonitis is to prevent contamination of the dialysis fluid that enters the peritoneal cavity and to prevent tunnel and exit site infections. The prevention method involves (a) aseptic manipulation of the sterile disposable plastic lines leading into the abdominal catheter that deliver the dialysis fluid into the peritoneal cavity and (b) a system for aseptic connection of the tubing containing the sterile dialysis fluid and the patient's catheter [1].

NONINFECTIOUS COMPLICATIONS

First-Use and Allergic Reactions

A variety of symptoms attributed to hypersensitivity reactions may arise during dialysis. Symptoms variously reported include increased or decreased blood pressure, dyspnea, cough, conjunctival injection, flushing, urticaria, headache, and pains in the chest, back, and limbs [65]. Such symptoms are more common during the first use of a dialyzer and have been termed the "first-use syndrome." These reactions are seen more frequently with cuprophan dialyzers; some may be attributable to residual ethylene oxide in dialyzers. During 1992 to 1993, such reactions were reported by 24% to 27% of dialysis centers and were most strongly associated with use of cuprophan and regenerated cellulose membranes [21].

In 1990 several outbreaks of anaphylactoid reactions associated with angiotensin-converting enzyme inhibitors were reported (Table 24-4). Reactions occurred within 10 minutes of initiating dialysis and included nausea, abdominal cramps, burning, flushing, swelling of the face or tongue, angioedema, shortness of breath, and hypotension. One outbreak was linked to reuse of dialyzers [66], but other reports implicated polyacrylonitrile dialyzers in the reactions [67–70]. In 1992 the Food and Drug Administration issued a safety alert regarding anaphylactoid reactions in patients on angiotensin-converting enzyme inhibitors, especially those patients using polyacrylonitrile dialyzers [71].

Dialysis Dementia

Dialysis encephalopathy, or dialysis dementia, is a disorder that affects dialysis patients who, for a variety of reasons, are subjected to water that has a relatively high content of aluminum, such as community water supplies treated with alum. This complication was first described in 1972 by Alfrey and co-workers [72], and the role of aluminum as a significant contributing factor in this disorder was established by Schreeder and associates [73] in an epidemiologic study. In this study they showed that patients were at increased risk of dialysis dementia when the aluminum content of water used to prepare dialysate was high (>100 ng/L). Case definitions of dialysis encephalopathy include three different groups of objective findings: speech impairment (stuttering, stammering, dysnomia, hypofluency, mutism), seizure disorder (generalized tonic-clonic, focal, or multifocal seizures), motor disturbance (myoclonic jerks, motor apraxia, immobility).

The incidence of dialysis dementia reported by hemodialysis centers to the CDC declined from 0.4% in the years 1980 and 1983 to 1985 to 0.1% (129 cases) in 1990, with a case-fatality rate of 21% [17]. Although it is not clear what was responsible for this decrease, we believe it may be related to heightened awareness in the dialysis community of the requirement for good water treatment systems. In 1980, only 26% of hemodialysis centers in the United States reported that they employed a reverse-osmosis system, either alone or with deionization in their water treatment systems. By 1988, 91% of the centers were using reverse osmosis alone or in combination with deionization as an integral part of their water treatment system [16]. Control of dialysis dementia revolves around adequate water treatment systems and invariably requires the use of reverse osmosis, either alone or with deionization.

It is also important to ensure that all components of the water treatment and dialysis fluid preparation and delivery systems be compatible with all fluid with which they are in contact in order to eliminate the possibility of leaching of harmful substances. In one outbreak, 58 of 85 (68%) dialysis patients at a dialysis center were found to have acute or chronic aluminum intoxication that resulted in three deaths. Investigation revealed that the acidified portion (pH=2.7) of the bicarbonate-based dialysate solution was passed through a pump with an aluminum housing and that aluminum was leached out of the pump and into the dialysate solution in concentrations exceeding 200 parts per million and was present in the dialysis fluid [74].

Toxic Reactions

Chemicals in water or as residuals in dialysis fluid can affect dialysis patients. Certain chemicals in water may not be toxic when ingested by humans, but the hemodialysis patient may be exposed directly to 150 L of water per treatment. Two examples will illustrate this problem. Occasionally, suppliers of community water change their water disinfection patterns by increasing chlorine dosages or using chloramines. These changes usually take place without the knowledge of the dialysis staff. Chloramines in water used to prepare dialysis fluid must be removed or the patient will experience acute hemolysis. If the correct water treatment system (activated carbon) is not present or operating in the dialysis center, patients will be exposed to this chemical. In one instance, a dialysis center changed from acetate to bicarbonate dialysate, adding an additional reverse-osmosis unit and tanks for preparation and dilution of the dialysate. No changes were made to increase the capacity of the carbon filter, and within a few weeks, ~ 100 of the center's dialysis patients were exposed to chloramine-contaminated dialysate when the undersized carbon filters failed. A total of 41 patients required transfusion to treat hemolytic anemia caused by the chloramine exposure [13].

Another example of chemical intoxication occurred when a city water treatment plant accidentally fed excessive levels of fluoride into the community water supply, resulting in the death of one dialysis patient and acute illness in several other patients in a hemodialysis center receiving this community water supply. The center's water treatment system was not adequate to remove excessive amounts of fluoride from water [75]. In both of the preceding examples, a properly designed water treatment system—consisting of adequate carbon filtration for the fluid flow and volume plus the use of reverse osmosis, deionization, and ultrafiltration—would have prevented toxic reactions. There have also been instances in which a disinfectant, such as formaldehyde, was not sufficiently removed from dialysis systems, and patients were exposed to the chemical. This exposure can be prevented by monitoring the system for complete rinsing using a chemical assay sensitive to the chemical.

Recently there was a most unusual outbreak of toxic reactions. In February and March of 1996, 100 of 131 patients at a dialysis center in Brazil showed signs of liver disease, visual disturbances, and nausea and vomiting. By January 1997, 48 had died from hepatic failure. It was discovered that the water used to prepare dialysis fluid came from a water reservoir that had had a recent algae/or cyanobacteria (blue-green algae) bloom. The water received inadequate treatment by the municipal water supplier as well as the dialysis center. Cyanobacteria are present in bodies of water worldwide. Some species can produce neurotoxins or hepatotoxins that can be fatal to animals who drink water with a heavy growth or bloom of cyanobacteria. In the investigation of this outbreak undertaken by the CDC, a cyanobacterial toxin, Microcystin-LR, was detected in water from the reservoir, treated water at the dialysis center, and case patients' serum and liver tissue. This is the first report of parenteral exposure to cyanobacterial toxins among humans. The outbreak would have been prevented by proper water treatment at the municipal and dialysis center level. (CDC, unpublished data; E. Jochimsen, personal communication). A summary of toxic reactions in hemodialysis patients that have been investigated by the CDC is given in Table 24-4.

BLOODBORNE VIRUSES: VIRAL HEPATITIS AND ACQUIRED IMMUNODEFICIENCY SYNDROME

Shortly after the art and science of hemodialysis was institutionalized, it was recognized that both patients and staff members were at risk of acquiring viral hepatitis. The development and use of specific serologic testing identified hepatitis B virus (HBV), and later hepatitis C virus (HCV) as those forms most likely to be transmitted within the hemodialysis environment. Other bloodborne pathogens that should be considered potentially transmissible in hemodialysis centers include hepatitis delta virus (HDV) and human immunodeficiency virus (HIV). Hepatitis A virus, which is spread by the fecal-oral route and rarely by blood, has not been associated with hemodialysis (Table 24-4).

Since HBV is the bloodborne virus most efficiently transmitted via dialysis, long-standing precautions developed for and shown to be effective in its control are used, in part, as a model for the prevention of transmission of other bloodborne infections. The primary rationale is that infection control practices that effectively curb the transmission of HBV would also be effective against other bloodborne viruses, such as HCV and HIV, because their efficiency of transmission is much less than that of HBV (see Chapters 42, 43).

Viral Hepatitis

Modes of Transmission

Hepatitis B

Hepatitis B virus is transmitted by percutaneous or mucosal exposure to infectious blood or body fluids that contain blood. Hepatitis B surface antigen (HBsAg)–positive persons who are also positive for hepatitis B e antigen have an extraordinary level of HBV circulating in their blood, $\sim 10^8$ virions per milliliter. With virus titers this high, body fluids containing serum or blood may also contain appreciable levels of HBV; HBV can be present on environmental surfaces in the absence of any visible blood and still contain 10^2 to 10^3 infectious virions per milliliter [76]. Furthermore, HBV is relatively stable in the environment and has been shown to remain viable for ≥7 days on environmental surfaces at room temperature [77]. Thus, wherever there is a good deal of blood exposure, the risk of HBV transmission can be high if proper control measures are not practiced. This is especially true in a hemodialysis center.

In the past, HBV infection could be acquired by patients in a dialysis unit by transfusion of infectious blood or blood products. This is very unlikely now, since all blood is screened for HBsAg and antibody to hepatitis B core antigen (anti-HBc). Dialysis patients, once infected, frequently become chronically infected but asymptomatic and are sources of HBV contamination for many environmental surfaces. Given the extraordinarily high level of HBV in blood, the various modes of HBV transmission can be categorized, based on efficiency, as follows.

1. Direct percutaneous inoculation of HBV by needle from contaminated blood, serum, or plasma.
2. Percutaneous transfer of blood, serum, or plasma, such as may occur through cuts, scratches, abrasions, or other breaks in the skin.
3. Transfer of infected blood, serum, or plasma onto mucosal surfaces such as may occur through inadvertent introduction of these materials into the mouth or eyes.
4. Introduction of other known infectious secretions, such as saliva and peritoneal fluid, onto mucosal surfaces.
5. Indirect transfer of HBV from blood, serum, or plasma by means of environmental surfaces.

TABLE 24-5. *Routes of HBV transmission in hemodialysis centers*

Route	Comment
Transfused blood and blood	Uncommon for HBV owing to HBsAg and anti-HBc screening of donors
Patient to staff member	Transmitted by needle stick/sharp item injuries and inapparent percutaneous exposures
Patient to dialysis system to staff member	Transmitted by HBV-contaminated blood on devices, tubes, and environmental surfaces
Patient to dialysis system external surfaces to staff member's hands to another patient	Frequently touched dialysis machines or associated environmental surfaces may be reservoirs of HBV; transmitted by staff with contaminated gloves or hands
Staff member to patient	Has never been reported in a dialysis center

There is no epidemiologic or laboratory evidence of airborne transmission of HBV [78,79], and no disease is transmitted by the intestinal route. Splashes of infectious blood that enter the oral cavity may result in HBV infection, because the virus enters the vascular system through the buccal cavity but not the intestinal tract. Hepatitis B virus can be transmitted by a number of routes in a hemodialysis center; these routes are listed in Table 24-5. Staff members may become infected with HBV through accidental needle punctures or breaks in their skin or mucous membranes. These staff members have frequent and continuous contact with blood and blood-contaminated surfaces. Dialysis patients may acquire HBV infection in several ways, including (a) internally contaminated dialysis equipment, such as venous pressure gauges or venous pressure isolators or filters (used to prevent reflux of blood into gauges) that are not routinely changed after each use; (b) injections (by contamination of the site of injection or the material being injected); and (c) breaks in the skin or mucous membranes that have contact with blood-contaminated objects. Patients who are dialyzed in centers that routinely reuse dialyzers are not at increased risk of HBV infection [80].

There is no documentation that HBV has been transmitted from infected hemodialysis staff members to dialysis patients. Hypothetically, such transmission is possible but not likely, because infectious blood and body fluids of dialysis personnel are not readily accessible to patients. However, dialysis staff members may physically carry HBV from infected patients to susceptible patients by means of contaminated hands, gloves, and other objects. Environmental surfaces in the hemodialysis center can also play a role in HBV transmission. It has been shown that HBsAg, which is considered a "footprint" of HBV, can be detected on environmental surfaces (especially those often touched) in dialysis centers [76]. For example, HBsAg has been detected on clamps, scissors, dialysis machine control knobs, doorknobs, and other surfaces. If these surfaces or objects are not cleaned or disinfected frequently and are shared among patients using the same or neighboring machines, an almost unnoticeable infection transmission route is created. Although dialysis staff members may routinely change gloves after caring for each patient, a new pair of gloves can become contaminated when the staff member touches surfaces previously contaminated with blood from an HBsAg-positive patient. HBV can be transmitted from patient to patient when a staff member, wearing the contaminated gloves, searches for the patient's best site of injection by applying finger pressure or by otherwise contaminating that site before injection. Staff members, when donning a pair of new gloves, should refrain from touching any environmental surfaces before performing the injection on the patient.

Other environmental sources of contamination include shared items, such as multiple dose medication vials, which can become contaminated with blood and serve as sources of patient-to-patient transmission [81]. It is this potential for the environmentally mediated mode of virus transmission, rather than any phenomenon dealing with internal contamination of dialysis machines, that is the basis for the infection control strategies recommended for preventing HBV transmission in dialysis centers.

Surveillance data from the CDC showed that between 1972 and 1974 the incidence of HBsAg positivity among patients and staff increased by >100%, to 6.2% and 5.2%, respectively [82,83]. In a separate survey of 15 hemodialysis centers during the same 2-year period, Szmuness and colleagues [84] showed that the point prevalence of a positive test for HBsAg was 16.8% among patients and 2.4% among staff. During this time, HBV infection in dialysis units had become highly endemic, and outbreaks were common because of the presence of chronically infected patients who were asymptomatic, the absence of sufficient disease and serologic surveillance systems to detect these chronic infections, and the lack of infection control measures to prevent transmission [85–88].

Subsequently, infection control strategies were developed that incorporated precautions for preventing exposures to blood and body fluids among both patients and staff with several extra precautions (89). As will be discussed later, these extra precautions included routinely testing all dialysis patients and staff members for HBsAg, dialyzing HBsAg-positive patients in separate areas or rooms in the dialysis center using dedicated dialysis machines and staff, and not including HBsAg-positive patients in dialyzer reuse programs.

Continued nationwide surveillance by the CDC found that by 1983 the incidence of HBV infection had declined to 0.5% among both patients and staff members [90]. Over the same period, the proportion of centers using separation practices increased significantly from 75% to 86%, and the proportion of centers that screened patients monthly for HBsAg increased from 57% to 84%. In addition, the risk of acquiring HBV infection for patients was shown to be highest in those centers that provided dialysis to HBsAg-positive patients but did not separate such patients by room and machine. Other investigators also have shown that segregation of HBsAg-positive patients and their equipment reduces the incidence of HBV infection in hemodialysis units [91,92]. The success of separation practices in preventing the transmission of HBV can be linked to other control recommendations, including routine serologic surveillance.

Routine serologic surveillance facilitates the rapid identification of patients who become HBsAg-positive, which allows for immediate implementation of isolation procedures before cross-infection can occur. Although the nationwide incidence of HBV infection among hemodialysis patients for the years 1988 to 1993 was extremely low (0.1% to 0.2%) [21], an increasing number of centers have reported to the CDC episodes of HBV transmission among their patients. During a 5-month period in 1994 alone, five hepatitis B outbreaks in centers offering long-term hemodialysis were investigated by the CDC and/or state and local health authorities [93]. All were the result of failure to follow one or more recommended infection control practices for the prevention of HBV transmission in these settings, including failure to routinely screen patients for HBsAg or review results of testing to detect infected patients; assignment of staff to the simultaneous care of infected and susceptible patients; and sharing of supplies, particularly multidose medication vials, among patients.

These same factors have typically been responsible for most other hemodialysis-associated outbreaks of hepatitis B reported in the past [81,94]. In addition, few patients in these centers have received hepatitis B vaccine. Although hepatitis B vaccine has been recommended for all hemodialysis patients since it became available in 1982 and has been shown to reduce the costs of serologic screening [95], only 29% of patients had received the vaccine by 1993 [21]. As the outbreaks discussed here demonstrate, the generally low incidence of HBV infection among hemodialysis patients does not preclude the need to maintain infection control measures that were specifically formulated to prevent the transmission of bloodborne pathogens in these settings.

Hepatitis C

Hepatitis C virus is the etiologic agent of most cases of parenterally transmitted non-A, non-B (NANB) hepatitis worldwide [96,97]. Commercially available enzyme immunoassays detect antibody to HCV (anti-HCV) in an average 70% to 90% of patients with parenterally transmitted NANB hepatitis [98,99]. However, interpretation of the results of these assays that screen for anti-HCV is limited by several factors: (a) they will not detect anti-HCV in ~10% of persons infected with HCV; (b) they do not distinguish between acute and chronic or past infection; (c) in the acute phase of hepatitis C, there may be a prolonged interval between onset of illness and seroconversion; and (d) in populations with a low prevalence of infection, the rate of false positivity for anti-HCV is high. As with any screening test, the proportion of repeatedly reactive enzyme immunoassay results that are falsely positive varies with the prevalence of infection in the population screened. Although no true confirmatory test has been developed, supplemental tests for specificity are available.

The recombinant immunoblot assay (RIBA, Ortho Diagnostic Systems, Raritan, NJ, U.S.A.) and the MATRIX HCV assay (Abbott Laboratories, North Chicago, IL, U.S.A.) use different formats and expression systems to evaluate repeatedly reactive results obtained from the screening assays [100,101]. The diagnosis of HCV infection also is possible by detecting HCV RNA using polymerase chain reaction techniques to amplify reverse-transcribed cDNA [102]. Hepatitis C virus RNA can be detected many weeks before the appearance of viral antibodies, and in some persons it may be the only evidence of HCV infection. However, improper manipulation and storage of samples may affect the detectability of HCV RNA, and the extraction and handling of the viral RNA is easily subject to contamination, resulting in false-positive results. Currently, the polymerase chain reaction is available only as a research-based technique and is not suitable as a routine diagnostic test.

The transmission of HCV by direct percutaneous exposure to blood has been well documented, and persons traditionally considered at increased risk of acquiring HCV infection have included blood and blood product recipients, injection drug users, persons with occupational exposure to blood, and hemodialysis patients. These groups, however, have accounted for only half of the hepatitis C cases reported in the United States [103]. Exposure to a sexual partner or household contact who has had hepatitis and heterosexual activity with multiple partners also have been associated with acquiring hepatitis C [104, 105]. Although such exposures account for 10% to 15% of cases, the magnitude of risk and the circumstances under which these exposures result in transmission are not well defined.

Worldwide, the average reported prevalence of anti-HCV among hemodialysis patients is 20%, with a range of 1% to 47% [106,107]. In the United States, anti-HCV prevalence rates among hemodialysis patients have been reported to range from 10% to 36% [108,109]. The staff members of hemodialysis centers have rates of anti-HCV comparable to those (1% to 2%) reported among other healthcare workers [106]. The incidence of HCV infection in hemodialysis patients has been evaluated in two studies. Using first-generation anti-HCV testing, Niu and colleagues observed an incidence of 4.6% during one 18-month period, for an annual incidence of ~3% [108]; none of the patients who seroconverted had received transfusions in the interim or were injection drug users. An incidence of 4.9% per patient-year was found by Chan and colleagues using both second-generation anti-HCV testing and the polymerase chain reaction for the detection of HCV RNA [110]. This study was conducted before the introduction of anti-HCV screening of blood donors, and all of the patients who seroconverted had received transfusions.

Several studies have examined risk factors associated with anti-HCV positivity among hemodialysis patients, including history of blood transfusion, volume of blood transfused, number of years on dialysis, and history of injection drug use [108,110–117]. Although a history of ever having received a blood transfusion was found to be significantly associated with anti-HCV positivity in only two studies [111,112], these and others [110,115] found that anti-HCV-positive patients had received more units than had anti-HCV-negative patients. In addition, as the number of units transfused increased, the prevalence of anti-HCV positivity also increased, from an average of 14% to an average of 32% [111,114,115]. Other studies, however, found no association between anti-HCV positivity and a history of ever having received a blood transfusion or volume of blood received [108,115,116,117]. Furthermore, the rate of anti-HCV positivity among hemodialysis patients with no history of blood transfusion ranged from 9% to 22%, substantially higher than the rates observed in blood donor or general population controls [111,113,115,116].

Increasing years on dialysis was the risk factor most consistently reported as being independently associated with higher rates of anti-HCV positivity [108,115, 117,118]. As the number of years patients had been on dialysis increased, their prevalence of anti-HCV positivity also increased, from an average of 12% to an average of 37%. This relationship was found even for patients with no history of blood transfusion, and in three studies it was shown to be independent of injection drug use as well [108,114,117].

Most persons who become infected with HCV remain persistently infected; no effective neutralizing immune response or protective antibody has been identified [99, 118]. Comparative nucleotide sequence analysis of different HCV isolates indicates the existence of multiple HCV genotypes [119]. Animal transmission experiments suggest that antibody elicited by infection with one genotype fails to cross-neutralize heterologous virus genotypes. In addition, within an infected person, HCV consists of a population of closely related yet heterogeneous sequences, called quasi-species, and antibodies elicited by one sequence are not recognized by other sequences.

Thus, a large reservoir of potentially infectious patients exists in the hemodialysis environment. However, HCV circulates at low titers in infected serum, and its ability to survive in the environment is questionable. Although studies that address survival and transmission of HCV in the environment have not been done, rapid degradation of the virus seems to occur when serum samples containing virus are left at room temperature [120].

In spite of this finding, the studies just described, as well as investigations of dialysis-associated outbreaks of NANB hepatitis and hepatitis C [121,122], suggest that HCV can be transmitted between patients in the dialysis center, possibly because of lapses in infection control practices, including sharing of instruments and supplies and improper cleaning practices. NANB hepatitis was added to the CDC's nationwide surveillance of dialysis-associated diseases in 1982. Until 1990, a test for anti-HCV was not available, and surveillance depended on the clinical diagnosis of NANB hepatitis. Patients and staff members were considered to have NANB hepatitis if they had clinical signs or symptoms and/or two test results of elevated liver enzymes ≥ 1 week apart and if other causes of hepatitis had been excluded. From 1982 through 1993, the reported incidence of NANB hepatitis declined among hemodialysis patients from 1.7% to 0.6% and among staff members from 0.5% to 0.1% [21]. Whether these rates accurately reflect the true frequency with which patients and staff acquired NANB hepatitis is unknown, because the criteria applied to distinguish this type of hepatitis from other causes of liver disease varied considerably from center to center.

The downward trend in the rates of NANB hepatitis, particularly among patients, may be explained in part by a decline in the rate of transfusion-associated disease. Transfusion-associated NANB hepatitis declined substantially after 1985 [103]. Most of this decline occurred before surrogate testing of blood donors began and was temporally associated with changes in the donor population resulting from self-exclusion of persons at high-risk of HIV infection and exclusion of HIV-antibody-positive donors, as well as with changes in transfusion practices. The reemphasis on universal precautions also may have contributed to the decline in rates among both patients and staff.

Beginning in 1992, the prevalence of anti-HCV among patients and staff members was ascertained in the CDC annual surveys, although complete information on patients and staff has been available from only a small sample of the centers participating. The reported prevalence of anti-HCV has been 8% to 10% among patients and 1.6% among staff. Centers with the highest incidence of NANB hepatitis among their patients during the previous three years reported the highest prevalence among patients of anti-HCV [21]. Because of the limitations of the anti-HCV test, new disease acquisition will continue to be monitored using a diagnosis of NANB hepatitis that does not depend on anti-HCV testing.

Delta Hepatitis

Delta hepatitis is caused by the HDV, a relatively small virus with defective RNA that causes infection only in persons with active HBV infection [123]. Delta hepatitis is a severe disease with a relatively high mortality rate as a result of acute infection and a high likelihood of the development of chronic disease. Delta hepatitis is endemic in certain areas of the Middle East and the Amazon Basin, but worldwide it is associated with certain high-risk groups, including injection drug users and recipients of multiple blood transfusions or plasma products.

Hepatitis D virus infection may occur as either co-infection with HBV or superinfection of an HBV carrier. Since HDV depends on an HBV-infected host for replication, prevention of HBV infection by either pre-exposure or postexposure prophylaxis will prevent HDV infection for a person susceptible to HBV. The prevalence of HDV infection in the United States is relatively low, but transmission of HDV between hemodialysis patients has been reported [124]. In addition, HDV exists in extraordinarily high concentrations in the circulating blood of infected persons. It has been reported that the concentration exceeds that of HBV by one to three orders of magnitude. Consequently, efficient transmission from patient to patient in a dialysis center is possible.

Infection Control Strategies

The recommendations for preventing the transmission of all bloodborne pathogens in the hemodialysis setting are summarized in Table 24-6 and are a combination of universal or barrier precautions to prevent transmission from patients to staff and precautions unique to the dialysis environment to prevent transmission from patient to patient (see Chapter 13). In this context they go beyond the concept of controlling only bloodborne pathogens and are also effective in preventing the transmission of bacte-

TABLE 24-6. *Recommendations for preventing the transmission of bloodborne pathogens in hemodialysis centers*

1. Standard precautions (formally referred to as universal precautions), including appropriate use of gloves, gowns, other barriers and hand washing.
2. No sharing of instruments, medications, or supplies between any patients regardless of serologic status.
3. Centralized area for medication preparation and distribution.
4. Clear separation of areas established to handle clean and contaminated items.
5. Routine cleaning and disinfection of equipment and reusable devices.
6. Routine cleaning using standard housekeeping protocols for floors and other environmental surfaces.

rial pathogens such as *S. aureus*, enterococci, and antibiotic-resistant gram-negative bacteria.

Patients should have specific dialysis stations assigned to them, and chairs and beds should be cleaned after each use. Sharing of ancillary supply equipment, such as trays, blood pressure cuffs, clamps, scissors, and other nondisposable items should be avoided. Nondisposable items should be cleaned or appropriately disinfected between uses. Medications should be prepared and distributed from a centralized area. Medication carts should not be used. Clean and contaminated areas should be separated; for example, handling and storage of medications and hand washing should not be done in the same area or an area adjacent to that where blood samples or used equipment are handled.

Disposable gloves should be worn by staff members for their own protection when handling patients or dialysis equipment and accessories. Gloves should be worn when taking blood pressure, injecting saline or heparin, or touching dialysis machine knobs to adjust flow rates. For the patient's protection, the staff member should use a fresh pair of gloves and wash their hands between treating each patient, to prevent cross-contamination. Gloves also should be used when handling blood specimens. Staff members should not smoke, eat, or drink in the dialysis treatment area or in the laboratory. There should be a separate lounge for this purpose. However, all patients may be served meals. The glasses, dishes, and other utensils may be cleaned in the usual manner by the hospital staff. No special care of these items is needed.

Staff members may wish to wear protective eyeglasses and masks for procedures in which spurting or spattering of blood may occur, such as cleaning of dialyzers and centrifugation of blood. Staff members should wear gowns, scrub suits, or the equivalent while working in the unit and should change out of this clothing at the end of each day. At the end of each dialysis treatment or dialysis shift, nondisposable equipment should be cleaned and disinfected or sterilized. Special attention should be given to cleaning control knobs on the dialysis machines and other surfaces that are frequently touched and potentially contaminated with patients' blood.

Crowding of patients and overtaxing of staff members may increase the likelihood of virus transmission in dialysis units. To minimize such transmission, each patient's station, with its attendant equipment, should occupy sufficient space to permit easy movement of a staff member completely around the patient without interfering with the neighboring station. This will allow for adequate cleaning and proper care of patients.

The patient's dialysis records should incorporate the lot number of all blood and blood products used; all mishaps, such as needle sticks, blood leaks, and blood spills; and dialysis machine malfunctions; the location name or number of the dialysis machine used for each dialysis session; and the names of staff members who connect and disconnect the patient to and from a machine. In addition, logs should be maintained to record all hepatitis serologic results; records of all accidental needle punctures and similar accidents sustained by staff members and patients, including time, place, names of patients and staff members involved; and prophylactic measures, if any, that were taken.

For the prevention of HBV infection, extra precautions center around hepatitis B vaccination, serologic and disease surveillance of the patients and staff members, and separation of HBsAg-positive patients from susceptible patients. Routine testing for HBsAg and antibody to HBsAg (anti-HBs) should be performed to identify patients and staff members as potential sources of infection (i.e., HBsAg-positive), as immune (anti-HBs positive at a level of 10 milli-international units per milliliter [mIU/ml]), or as susceptible (negative for HBsAg and anti-HBs). Patients and staff members should be screened for HBsAg and anti-HBs when they enter the unit to determine their serologic status. HBsAg positivity in staff members does not preclude employment in a dialysis center, and these individuals may be assigned to care for any patient. After baseline testing, the type and frequency of screening depends on the serologic and vaccination status of the

TABLE 24-7. *Recommendations for serologic surveillance for HBV among patients and staff of hemodialysis centers*

	Vaccination/serologic status		
Screening test	Vaccine nonresponder or susceptible[a]	Vaccine responder or natural immunity[b]	Chronic HBV infection[c]
Patients			
HBsAg	Every mo	None	Every yr
Anti-HBs	Every 6 mo	Every yr	If HBsAg status becomes negative
Staff			
HBsAg	Every 6 mo	None	Every yr
Anti-HBs	Every 6 mo	None	If HBsAg status becomes negative

[a]Anti-HBs <10 mIU/ml.
[b]Anti-HBs ≥ 10 mIU/ml.
[c]HBsAg positive for ≥ 6 mo.

patient or staff member [125] (Table 24-7). The frequency of testing patients and staff members who become infected with HBV (positive for HBsAg and immunoglobulin M anti-HBc) should be based on clinical indications. Only when these persons become HBsAg-negative should they be tested for anti-HBs. Patients and staff members who remain HBsAg-positive for ≥ 6 months should continue to be tested annually for HBsAg, since a small percentage of HBsAg carriers may become HBsAg-negative.

Hepatitis B vaccination is an essential component of prevention in hemodialysis centers. All susceptible patients and staff should receive hepatitis B vaccine (Table 24-8). Susceptible patients and staff who have not yet received hepatitis B vaccine, are in the process of being vaccinated, or have not adequately responded to vaccination should continue to be tested regularly for HBsAg and anti-HBs (Table 24-7). Unvaccinated patients who have anti-HBs on two consecutive tests at a level of ≥ 10 mIU/ml need be tested only annually to verify their immune status. If anti-HBs levels decrease to < 10 mIU/ml, such persons should be considered susceptible and should be vaccinated. Unvaccinated staff members who have anti-HBs on two consecutive tests at a level of ≥ 10 mIU/ml are considered immune and do not need any further routine testing for anti-HBs.

Patients who are initially positive for anti-HBs as a result of vaccination but in whom the level of anti-HBs becomes undetectable should receive a booster dose of the hepatitis B vaccine; staff members who have an adequate response to the vaccine, however, need no further routine testing or booster doses, even if anti-HBs subsequently declines below detectable levels. HBsAg-positive patients should undergo dialysis in a separate room designated only for HBsAg-positive patients. They should use separate machines, equipment, and supplies, and, most important, staff members should not care for both HBsAg-positive and susceptible patients on the same shift or at the same time.

If a separate room is not available, these HBsAg-positive patients should be separated from HBV-seronegative patients in an area removed from the mainstream of activity and should undergo dialysis on dedicated machines. Anti-HBs-positive patients may undergo dialysis in the same area as HBsAg-positive patients, or they may serve as a geographic buffer between HBsAg-positive and seronegative patients; in either instance they may be cared for by the same staff member. If use of separate machines is not possible, the machines can be disinfected using conventional protocols, and the external surfaces can be cleaned or disinfected using soap and water or a detergent germicide.

TABLE 24-8. *Recommended doses and schedules of currently licensed hepatitis B vaccines for adults*

Group	Vaccine	
	Recombivax HB[a]	Engerix-B[ab]
Dialysis patients	40 μg (1 ml)[c]	40 μg (2 ml)[d]
Healthy adults older than 19 yr	10 μg (1 ml)	20 μg (1 ml)

[a]Usual schedule: three doses at 0, 1, and 6 mo.
[b]Alternative schedule: four doses at 0, 1, 2, and 12 mo.
[c]Special formulation for dialysis patients.
[d]Two 1.0-ml doses given at one site in a four-dose schedule at 0, 1, 2, and 6 mo.

Although there is no evidence that patients or staff members in centers that reuse hemodialyzers are at greater risk of acquiring HBV infection [21,42,80], it might be prudent not to allow HBsAg-positive patients to participate in dialyzer reuse programs. Hepatitis B virus can be present at a high concentration in blood, and handling dialyzers used on HBsAg-positive patients during the reprocessing procedures might place staff members at risk of HBV infection.

Some investigators have proposed that recommendations to prevent HCV transmission similar to those for the prevention of HBV infection be implemented in hemodialysis centers. However, the contrasts between HCV and HBV make it difficult to support a proposal that would implement a patient isolation and separation protocol for hepatitis C similar to that devised for hepatitis B. Because HCV circulates in low titers, it is transmitted much less efficiently than is HBV. There are no tests for HCV that can distinguish infectious from noninfectious patients in the clinical setting, as there are for HBV, and placing all anti-HCV positive patients together might enhance their chance of becoming reinfected with the same strain or with another strain. Although the specific factors responsible for transmission of HCV within the dialysis environment have not been identified, available data suggest that such transmission can be prevented by strict adherence to those precautions outlined in Table 24-6. Hemodialysis patients with hepatitis C do not have to be dialyzed in a separate room or on dedicated machines, and they may participate in reuse programs [107]. All patients should be monitored monthly for alanine aminotransferase and aspartate aminotransferase to detect any type of NANB hepatitis, including hepatitis C; clustering of new cases may indicate a problem with infection control practices, and elevations in liver enzymes are more sensitive indicators of acute HCV infection than is detection of anti-HCV. Routine screening of patients or staff members for anti-HCV is not necessary for infection control.

Hemodialysis centers may wish to conduct serologic surveys of their patient and staff populations to determine the prevalence of the virus in their center and, in the case of patients or staff members diagnosed with hepatitis C, to determine medical treatment. In addition, if liver enzyme screening indicates the occurrence of an epidemic of NANB hepatitis in the hemodialysis center, anti-HCV screening of serum samples collected both during and subsequent to the outbreak may be of value. However, since the anti-HCV test cannot distinguish between infectious and noninfectious persons, its usefulness for infection control in hemodialysis centers is limited.

For delta hepatitis, serologic tests to measure HDV and its antibody are commercially available, but because of the low prevalence of this infection in the United States, routine screening of dialysis patients or staff members for HDV infection is not warranted. However, if a patient is known to be infected with HDV or there appears to be evidence of transmission of HDV in a dialysis center, screening for delta antigen and its antibody would be warranted. Patients who are infected with HDV should be separated from all other dialysis patients, especially those who are HBsAg-positive. Patients infected with HDV should undergo dialysis in separate areas and on dedicated machines. Since the transmission of this virus is very similar to that of HBV, the precautions described earlier should be practiced.

Cleaning, Disinfection, and Sterilization

In single-pass artificial kidney machines, the internal fluid pathways that supply dialysis fluid to the dialyzer are not subject to contamination with blood. Although the fluid pathways that exhaust dialysis fluid from the dialyzer may become contaminated with blood in the event of a dialyzer leak, it is unlikely that this blood contamination will reach a subsequent patient. In the absence of microbiologic or epidemiologic evidence incriminating these fluid pathways, disinfection and rinsing procedures should be designed to control microbial contamination problems other than those associated with hepatitis.

For dialysis machines that use a dialysate recirculating system (such as some ultrafiltration control machines), a blood leak in a dialyzer, especially a massive leak, can result in contamination of a number of surfaces that will contact the dialysis fluid of subsequent patients. However, the procedures involved in draining the dialysis fluid, subsequent rinsing, and disinfection that are normally practiced after each use will lower the level of contamination to below infectious levels. In addition, an intact dialyzer membrane will not allow passage of bacteria or viruses. Consequently, if a blood leak does occur with either type of dialysis machine, the standard disinfection procedure used for machines in the dialysis center to control bacterial contamination is appropriate.

External surfaces of the dialysis machine should be cleaned or disinfected after each treatment of a patient. Venous pressure isolators or transducer filters should be used to prevent blood contamination of venous pressure monitors. These isolators or filters should not be reused. Blood and other specimens, such as peritoneal fluid, from all patients should be handled with care. Peritoneal fluid can contain high levels of HBV and should be handled in the same manner as the patient's blood. Consequently, if the center performs peritoneal dialysis, the same criteria for separating HBsAg-positive patients who are undergoing hemodialysis apply to those undergoing peritoneal dialysis.

In general, housekeeping in the dialysis center has two tasks: (a) to remove soil and waste on a regular basis, thereby preventing the accumulation and concentration of potentially infectious material in the patient/staff environment, and (b) to maintain an environment that is conducive to better care of patients. These two purposes are of particular importance in a hemodialysis center because of the critical nature of the procedures performed. The requirement for aseptic access to a patient's blood supply at least twice in each dialysis procedure makes the hemodialysis unit more similar to a surgical suite than to a conventional hospital room. Yet, because of crowding and the presence of complex hemodialysis machines with multiple wires, tubes, and hoses, the dialysis unit frequently receives inferior cleaning. If good housekeeping is to be achieved, work space must be adequate, and the staff should be given special instructions and training regarding the cleaning of hemodialysis equipment and stations. Although allotted space is often limited and cannot be changed, much can be done to use it more efficiently. Elimination of unneeded items, orderly arrangement of required items, and removal of excess lengths of tubes, hoses, and wires from the floor are steps that can provide more accessibility for cleaning.

Disposable materials should be placed in bags thick enough that they do not leak or else be double-bagged. Bags should not be overfilled, requiring the staff to compact the contents by hand to make room for additional waste. Since bags may become contaminated on the outside before they leave the unit, they should be placed in another bag in a "clean" area in the unit before they are picked up. All used needles and syringes should be discarded in puncture-proof containers without being separated. Wastes from a hemodialysis center that are actually or potentially contaminated with blood should be considered infectious and handled accordingly. Eventually, these items of solid waste should be disposed of properly in an incinerator or sanitary landfill, depending on local ordinances.

Good cleaning and adequate disinfection procedures are an important part of a hemodialysis center's efforts to control and prevent cross-contamination (see Chapter 20). Although many of the procedures do not differ from those recommended for medical devices in hospitals and for inanimate surfaces [126], the hemodialysis environment is unique, because there is an extraordinary amount of blood contamination. There should be a thorough mechanical cleaning step before any sterilization or disinfection process and, depending on the compatibility of materials (especially medical devices), sterilization should be chosen over disinfection.

Hepatitis B virus has not been grown on tissue cultures, and, without a viral assay system, studies on the precise resistance of this virus to various chemical germicides and heat have not been performed. In the absence of firm data, some investigators have considered HBV to be extremely resistant and have recommended unreasonably long decontamination and sterilization protocols and use of corrosive chemicals. These recommendations are counterproductive because they are not needed and health professionals do not use them. It should be kept in mind that the HBV is a virus, and its resistance to heat and chemical germicides, at best, may reach the resistance of some other viruses and bacteria but certainly not that of the bacterial endospore. Furthermore, studies have shown that HBV is not resistant to commonly used high-level and intermediate-level disinfectants [128].

Standard protocols for sterilization, disinfection, and decontamination are adequate processing for any items or devices contaminated with blood containing bloodborne viruses, including HBV. For example, any of the standard sterilization systems can be used to inactivate HBV, including standard steam autoclave cycles of 121°C (249.8°F) for 15 minutes, ethylene oxide gas, and low-temperature hydrogen peroxide plasma. Any of these sterilization systems represent a significant overkill. In most instances, decontamination, not sterilization, is needed. For example, in the hemodialysis unit, blood spills can be adequately decontaminated without using special procedures and corrosive chemical germicides. Immediately after a blood spill, the area should be thoroughly cleaned with a cloth soaked in an appropriate hospital disinfectant. The staff member doing the cleaning should wear gloves, and the cloth should be placed in a bucket. After all visible blood is cleaned, a new cloth or towel should be used for a second application of disinfectant. When cleaning frequently touched environmental surfaces in a dialysis unit to prevent cross-contamination, staff members should use a good detergent or detergent germicide. Antiseptics, such as formulations with povidone-iodine, hexachlorophene, or chlorhexidine, should not be used, because they are formulated for use on skin and are not designed for use on hard surfaces.

Acquired Immunodeficiency Syndrome

When acquired immunodeficiency syndrome (AIDS) was described in 1981 and it was subsequently determined that its epidemiology was similar to that of HBV infection, concern increased for dialysis patients who were infected with HIV. However, as the national HIV/AIDS epidemic progressed and it became evident that HIV was significantly less efficiently transmitted than HBV, presumably because of the substantial difference in the amount of infectious virus circulating in the blood of infected individuals, it became clear that standard infection control strategies using basic barrier precautions (universal precautions) could prevent transmission of HIV from patients to staff members as well as from patient to patient (see Chapter 13). Routine testing of dialysis patients or staff members for anti-HIV is not necessary for infection control.

Anti-HIV testing for treatment of patients, antimicrobial prophylaxis, and other reasons, however, may be desirable. Testing for anti-HIV among patients who may be considered at risk because of a long history of blood transfusions, especially in the years before donor blood was screened in the United States, is encouraged. The purpose of these tests is not for infection control within the dialysis center but to prevent HIV transmission between HIV-infected patients and their sexual or needle-sharing partners.

Patients with HIV infection can be treated with either hemodialysis or peritoneal dialysis, and they need not be isolated from other patients, either in separate rooms or by using dedicated machines. The type of dialysis treatment should be based on the needs of the patient. The basic barrier precautions described earlier (universal precautions) are sufficient to prevent HIV transmission in this setting (see Chapter 13). Disinfection and sterilization strategies routinely practiced in dialysis centers are adequate to prevent the risk of HIV transmission [1].

From 1985 to 1993, the percentage of centers that reported providing dialysis for patients with HIV infection increased from 11% to 34%. The number of patients receiving dialysis who were known to be infected with HIV increased from 0.3% in 1985 to 1.5% in 1992 and 1993 [21]. An HIV serosurvey among hemodialysis patients at 28 dialysis centers found that none of 254 seronegative patients became HIV positive during a 1-year follow-up period [130]. There have been reports of transmission of HIV from patient to patient in developing countries [130,131]. Breaks in infection control measures, especially sharing of syringes or needles, appear to be the most likely modes of transmission in these outbreaks. Other than the needle-stick incident described in the next paragraph, transmission of HIV has not been reported from a U.S. hemodialysis center.

To date, there has been one report of HIV transmission from an infected dialysis patient to a dialysis staff member. The worker sustained a needle stick while performing dialysis on a patient who was known to be HIV-positive and was undergoing dialysis in a private room. The dialysis worker had no known HIV risk factors, was negative for anti-HIV at time of the exposure, and subsequently seroconverted to anti-HIV positive [CDC, unpublished data].

In summary, based on current information, HIV-infected patients can undergo dialysis in centers without being isolated or separated from other patients and can take part in dialyzer reuse programs. Standard barrier precautions (universal precautions) are sufficient to prevent HIV transmission from patient to patient or from patient to staff member.

REFERENCES

1. Favero MS, Alter MJ, Bland LA. Nosocomial infections associated with hemodialysis. In: Mayhall CG, ed. *Hospital epidemiology and infection control*. Baltimore: Williams and Wilkins, 1995:693–714.
2. Bland LA, Favero MS. *Microbial contamination control strategies for hemodialysis systems, Oakbrook Terrace, IL*. Oakbrook Terrace, Ill.: Joint Commission on Accreditation of Healthcare Organizations, 1989;3:30–36. (Plant, Technology and Safety Management Series.)
3. Favero MS, Carson LA, Bond WW, Petersen NJ. Factors that influence microbial contamination of fluids associated with hemodialysis machines. *Appl Microbiol* 1974;28:822–830.
4. Favero MS, Petersen NJ, Carson LA, Bond WW, Hindman SH. Gram-negative water bacteria in hemodialysis systems. *Health Lab Sci* 1975; 12:321–334.
5. Carson LA, Petersen NJ, Favero MS. Use of the limulus amoebocyte lysate assay system for detection of bacterial endotoxin in fluids associated with hemodialysis procedures. In: Cohen E, ed. *Biomedical applications of the horseshoe crab* (limulidae). New York: Alan R. Liss, 1979:453–464.
6. Petersen NJ, Boyer KM, Carson LA, Favero MS. Pyrogenic reactions from inadequate disinfection of a dialysis fluid distribution system. *Dial Transpl* 1978;7:52–57.
7. Favero MS, Petersen NJ, Boyer KM, Carson LA, Bond WW. Microbial contamination of renal dialysis systems and associated health risks. *Trans Am Soc Artif Intern Organs* 1974;20:175–183.
8. Favero MS, Bland LA. Microbiologic principles applied to reprocessing hemodialyzers. In: Deane N, Wineman RJ, Bemis JA, eds. *Guide to reprocessing of hemodialyzers*. Boston: Martinus Nijhoff, 1986:63–73.
9. Bolan C, Reingold AL, Carson LA, et al. Infections with *Mycobacterium chelonei* in patients receiving dialysis and using processed hemodialyzers. *J Infect Dis* 1985;152:1013–1019.
10. Carson LA, Bland LA, Cusick LB, et al. Prevalence of nontuberculous mycobacteria in water supplies of hemodialysis centers. *Appl Environ Microbiol* 1988;54:3122–3125.
11. Carson LA, Bland LA, Cusick LB, Collin S, Favero MS, Bolan G. Factors affecting endotoxin levels in fluids associated with hemodialysis procedures. In: Novitsky TJ, Watson SW, eds. *Detection of bacterial endotoxins with the limulus amebocyte lysate test*. New York: Alan R. Liss, 1987:223–234.
12. Hindman SH, Favero MS, Carson LA, Petersen NJ, Schonberger LB, Solano JT. Pyrogenic reactions during hemodialysis caused by extramural endotoxin. *Lancet* 1975;2:732–734.
13. Tipple MA, Shusterman N, Bland LA, et al. Illness in hemodialysis patients after exposure to chloramine contaminated dialysate. *ASAIO Trans* 1991;37:588–591.
14. Association for the Advancement of Medical Instrumentation. *American national standard for hemodialysis systems: ANSI/AAMI RD5-1992*. Arlington: Association for the Advancement of Medical Instrumentation, 1992.
15. Stamm JM, Engelhard WE, Parsons JE. Microbiological study of water softener resins. *Appl Microbiol* 1969;18:376–386.
16. Alter MJ, Favero MS, Miller JK, Coleman PJ, Bland LA. National surveillance of dialysis-associated diseases in the United States, 1988. *ASAIO Trans* 1990;36:107–118.
17. Tokars JI, Alter MJ, Favero MS, Moyer LA, Bland LA. National surveillance of hemodialysis associated diseases in the United States, 1990. *ASAIO J* 1993;39:71–80.
18. Tokars JI, Alter MJ, Favero MS, Moyer LA, Bland LA. National surveillance of hemodialysis associated diseases in the United States, 1991. *ASAIO J* 1993;39:966–975.
19. Favero MS. Microbiological contaminants. In: *Proceedings of the Association for the Advancement of Medical Instrumentation Technology Assessment Conference: issues in hemodialysis*, Arlington: AAMI, 1981:30–33.
20. Anderson RL, Holland BW, Carr JK, Bond WW, Favero MS. Effect of disinfectants on pseudomonads colonized on the interior surface of PVC pipes. *Am J Public Health* 1990;80:17–21.
21. Tokars JI, Alter MJ, Favero MS, Moyer LA, Miller E, Bland LA. National surveillance of dialysis-associated diseases in the United States, 1993. *ASAIO J* 1996;42:219–229.
22. Petersen NJ, Carson LA, Doto IL, Aguero SM, Favero MS. Microbiologic evaluation of a new glutaraldehyde-based disinfectant for hemodialysis systems. *Trans Am Soc Artif Intern Organs* 1982;28:287–290.
23. Townsend TR, Siok-Bi W, Bartlett J. Disinfection of hemodialysis machines. *Dial Transpl* 1985;14:274–287.
24. Favero MS, Petersen NJ. Microbiologic guidelines for hemodialysis systems. *Dial Transpl* 1977;6:34–36.
25. Arduino MJ, Bland LA, Aguero SM, Carson L, Ridgeway M, Favero MS. Comparison of microbiologic assay methods for hemodialysis fluids. *J Clin Microbiol* 1991;29:592–594.
26. Bland LA, Favero MS. Microbiologic and endotoxin considerations in hemodialyzer reprocessing. In: *Dialysis*. Arlington: 1993:293–300. (*AAMI standards and recommended practices*, vol 3.)
27. Gazenfeldt-Gazit E, Elaihou HE. Endotoxin antibodies in patients on maintenance hemodialysis. *Isr J Med Sci* 1969;5:1032–1036.
28. Lonnemann G, Behme TC, Lenzner B, et al. Permeability of dialyzer membranes to TNF-α inducing substances derived from water bacteria. *Kidney Int* 1992;42:61–68.
29. Laude-Sharpe M, Canoff M, Simard L, Pusineri C, Kazatchkine M, Haeffner-Cavaillon N. Induction of IL-1 during hemodialysis: transmembrane passage of intact endotoxin (LPS). *Kidney Int* 1990;38: 1089–1094.
30. Henderson LW, Koch KM, Dinarello CA, Shaldon S. Hemodialysis hypotension: the interleukin hypothesis. *Blood Purif* 1983;1:3–8.
31. Port FK, VanDerKerkhove KM, Kunkel SL, Kluger MJ. The role of dialysate in the stimulation of interleukin-1 production during clinical hemodialysis. *Am J Kidney Dis* 1987;10:118–122.
32. Kantor RJ, Carson LA, Graham DR, Petersen NJ, Favero MS. Outbreak of pyrogenic reactions at a dialysis center: association with infusion of heparinized saline solution. *Am J Med* 1983;74:449–456.
33. Murphy J, Parker T, Carson L, Bland L, Solomon S. Outbreaks of bacteremia in hemodialysis patients associated with alteration of dialyzer membranes following chemical disinfection [Abstract]. *ASAIO Trans* 1987;16:51.
34. Powell AC, Bland LA, Oettinger CW, et al. Enhanced release of TNF-α, but not IL-1β, from uremic blood after endotoxin stimulation. *Lymphokine Cytokine Res* 1991;10:343–346.
35. Pegues DA, Oettinger CU, Bland LA, et al. A prospective study of pyrogenic reactions in hemodialysis patients using bicarbonate dialysis fluids filtered to remove bacteria and endotoxin. *J Am Soc Nephrol* 1992;3:1002–1007.
36. Gordon SM, Oettinger CW, Bland LA, et al. Pyrogenic reactions in patients receiving conventional, high-efficiency or high-flux hemodialysis with bicarbonate dialysate containing high concentrations of bacteria and endotoxin. *J Am Soc Nephrol* 1992;2:1436–1444.
37. Oliver JC, Bland LA, Oettinger CW, et al. Bacteria and endotoxin removal from bicarbonate dialysis fluids for use in conventional, high efficiency and high flux hemodialysis. *Artif Organs* 1992;16:141–145.
38. Held PJ, Wolfe RA, Gaylin DS, et al. Analysis of the association of dialyzer reuse practices and patient outcomes. *Am J Kidney Dis* 1994; 23:692–708.
39. Association for the Advancement of Medical Instrumentation. *American national standard for reuse of hemodialyzers: ANSI/AAMI RD47-1993*. Arlington: Association for the Advancement of Medical Instrumentation, 1993.
40. Gordon S, Tipple M, Bland L, Jarvis W. Pyrogenic reactions associated with the reuse of disposable hollow fiber hemodialyzers. *JAMA* 1988;260:2077–2081.
41. Centers for Disease Control. Bacteremia associated with reuse of disposable hollow-fiber hemodialyzers. *MMWR* 1986;35:417–418.
42. Alter MJ, Favero MS, Miller JK, Coleman PJ, Bland LA. Reuse of hemodialyzers: results of nationwide surveillance for adverse effects. *JAMA* 1988;260:2073–2076.
43. Bland L, Alter M, Favero M, Carson L, Cusick L. Hemodialyzer reuse: practices in the United States and implications for infection control. *ASAIO Trans* 1985;31:556–559.
44. Favero MS. Distinguishing between high level disinfection, reprocessing, and sterilization. In: Association for the Advancement of Medical Instrumentation. *Reuse of disposables: implications for qual-*

ity healthcare and cost containment. Arlington: Association for the Advancement of Medical Instrumentation, 1983:19–20. (Technical assessment report no. 6.)
45. Lowry P, Beck-Sague CM, Bland LA, et al. *Mycobacterium chelonei* infections among patients receiving high-flux dialysis in a hemodialysis clinic in California. *J Infect Dis* 1990;161:85–90.
46. Bland LA, Ridgeway MR, Aguero SM, Carson LA, Favero MS. Potential bacteriologic and endotoxin hazards associated with liquid bicarbonate concentration. *ASAIO Trans* 1987;33:542–545.
47. Bell PRF, Veitch PS. Vascular access for hemodialysis. In: Jacobson HR, Striker GE, Klahr S, eds. *The principles and practice of nephrology*. Philadelphia: BC Decker, 1991:26–44.
48. Mehta S. Statistical summary of clinical results of vascular access procedures for hemodialysis. In: Jacobson HR, Striker GE, Klahr S, eds. *The principles and practice of nephrology*. Philadelphia: BC Decker, 1991:145–157.
49. Whelchel JD. Central venous hemodialysis access catheters: a review of technical considerations and complications. In: Sommer BG, Henry ML, eds. *Vascular access for hemodialysis*, vol. 2. WL Gore and Associates and Precept Press, 1991:123–138.
50. Goldstein MB. Prevention of sepsis from central vein dialysis catheters. *Semin Dial* 1992;5:106–108.
51. Counts CS. Potential complications of the internal vascular access: implications for nursing care. *Dial Transpl* 1993;22:75–79.
52. Dryden MS, Samson A, Ludlam HA, Wing AJ. Infective complications associated with the use of the Quinton Permacath for long-term central vascular access in hemodialysis. *J Hosp Infect* 1991;19(4):257–262.
53. Carlisle EJF, Blake P, McCarthy F, Vas S, Uldall R. Septicemia in long-term jugular hemodialysis catheters: eradicating infection by changing the catheter over a guidewire. *Int J Artif Organs* 1991;14:150–153.
54. Welbel SF, Williams D, Ray B, et al. Central venous catheter–associated bloodstream infections in a dialysis unit, Texas. In: *Abstracts of the 1993 Epidemic Intelligence Service Conference*. Washington, D.C.: Department of Health and Human Services, 1993:59.
55. Nolph KD, ed. *Peritoneal dialysis*, 2nd ed. Boston: Marinus Nijhoff, 1985.
56. Peterson P, Matzke G, Keane WF. Current concepts in the management of peritonitis in patients undergoing continuous ambulatory peritoneal dialysis. *Rev Infect Dis* 1987;9:604–612.
57. Walshe JJ, Morse GD. Infectious complications of peritoneal dialysis. In: Nissenson AR, Fine RN, Gentile DE, eds. *Clinical dialysis*. Norwalk, Conn.: Appleton, 1990:301–318.
58. Band JD, Ward JI, Fraser DW, et al. Peritonitis due to a *Mycobacterium chelonei*–like organism associated with intermittent chronic peritoneal dialysis. *J Infect Dis* 1982;145:9–17.
59. Berkelman RL, Godley J, Weber JA, et al. *Pseudomonas cepacia* peritonitis associated with contamination of automatic peritoneal dialysis machines. *Ann Intern Med* 1982;96:456–458.
60. Petersen NJ, Carson LA, Favero MS. Microbiological quality of water in an automatic peritoneal dialysis system. *Dial Transpl* 1977;6:38–40,86.
61. Carson LA, Petersen NJ, Favero MS, Aguero SM. Growth characteristics of atypical mycobacteria in water and their comparative resistance to disinfection. *Appl Environ Microbiol* 1978;36:839–846.
62. Berkelman RL, Band JD, Petersen NJ. Recommendations for the care of automated peritoneal dialysis machines: Can the risk of peritonitis be reduced? *Infect Control Hosp Epidemiol* 1984;5:85–87.
63. Copley JB. Prevention of peritoneal dialysis catheter-related infections. *Am J Kidney Dis* 1987;10:401–407.
64. Vas S. Microbiologic aspects of chronic ambulatory peritoneal dialysis. *Kidney Int* 1983;23:83–92.
65. Cheung AK. Membrane biocompatibility. In: Nissenson AR, Fine RN, Gentile DE, eds. *Clinical dialysis*, 2nd ed. University of California, Los Angeles: Appleton & Lange, 1990:69–96.
66. Pegues DA, Beck-Sague CM, Woollen SW, et al. Anaphylactoid reactions associated with reuse of hollow-fiber hemodialyzers and ACE inhibitors. *Kidney Int* 1992;42:1232–1237.
67. Teileans C, Madhoun P, Lenaers M, Schandene L. Anaphylactic reactions during hemodialysis on AN69 membranes in patients receiving ACE inhibitors. *Kidney Int* 1990;38:982–984.
68. Verresen L, Waer M, Vanrenterghem Y, Michielsen P. Angiotensin converting enzyme inhibitors and anaphylactoid reactions to high-flux membrane dialysis. *Lancet* 1990;336:1360–1362.
69. van Es A, Henny FC, Lobatto S. Angiotensin-converting enzyme inhibitors and anaphylactic reactions to high-flux membrane dialysis [Letter]. *Lancet* 1991;337(8733):112–113.
70. Jadoul M, Struyven J, Stragier A, Van Ypersele De Strihou C. Angiotensin-converting enzyme inhibitors and anaphylactic reactions to high-flux membrane dialysis [Letter]. *Lancet* 1991;337:112.
71. FDA. Anaphylactoid reactions associated with ACE inhibitors and dialyzer membranes. *FDA Safety Alert*, March 6, 1992.
72. Alfrey AC, Mishell JM, Burks J, et al. Syndrome of dyspraxia and multifocal seizures associated with chronic hemodialysis. *Trans Am Soc Artif Intern Organs* 1972;18:257–267.
73. Schreeder MT, Favero MS, Hughes JR, Petersen NJ, Bennett PH, Maynard JE. Dialysis encephalopathy and aluminum exposure: an epidemiologic analysis. *J Chronic Dis* 1983;36:581–593.
74. Burwen DR, Olsen SM, Bland LA, Arduino MJ, Reid MH, Jarvis WR. Epidemic aluminum intoxication in hemodialysis patients traced to use of an aluminum pump. *Kidney Int* 1995;48:469–474.
75. Centers for Disease Control and Prevention. Fluoride intoxication in a dialysis unit–Maryland. *MMWR* 1980;29:134–136.
76. Favero MS, Maynard JE, Petersen NJ, et al. Hepatitis B antigen on environmental surfaces [Letter]. *Lancet* 1973;2:1455.
77. Bond WW, Favero MS, Petersen NJ, Gravelle CRR, Ebert JW, Maynard JE. Survival of hepatitis B virus after drying and storage for one week. *Lancet* 1981;1:550–551.
78. Petersen NJ. An assessment of the airborne route in hepatitis B transmission. *Ann N Y Acad Sci* 1980;353:157–166.
79. Favero MS, Bolyard EA. Microbiologic considerations, disinfection and sterilization strategies and the potential for airborne transmission of bloodborne pathogens. *Surg Clin North Am* 1995;75(6):1071–1089.
80. Favero MS, Deane N, Leger RT, Sosin AE. Effect of multiple use of dialyzers on hepatitis B incidence in patients and staff. *JAMA* 1981; 245:166–167.
81. Alter MJ, Ahtone J, Maynard JE. Hepatitis B virus transmission associated with a multiple-dose vial in a hemodialysis unit. *Ann Intern Med* 1983;99:330–333.
82. Snydman DR, Bryan JA, Hanson B, et al. Hemodialysis-associated hepatitis in the United States—1972. *J Infect Dis* 1975;132:109–113.
83. Snydman DR, Bregman D, Bryan JA. Hemodialysis-associated hepatitis in the United States, 1974. *J Infect Dis* 1977;135:687–691.
84. Szmuness W, Prince AM, Grady GF, et al. Hepatitis B infection: a point prevalence study in 15 U.S. dialysis centers. *JAMA* 1974;227: 901–906.
85. Snydman DR, Bryan JA, London WT, et al. Transmission of hepatitis B associated with hemodialysis: role of malfunction (blood leaks) in dialysis machines. *J Infect Dis* 1976;134:562–570.
86. Snydman DR, Bryan JA, Macon EJ, Gregg MB. Hemodialysis-associated hepatitis: report of an epidemic with further evidence on mechanisms of transmission. *Am J Epidemiol* 1976;104:563–570.
87. Kantor RJ, Hadler SC, Schreeder MT, Berquist KR, Favero MS. Outbreak of hepatitis B in a dialysis unit, complicated by false positive HBsAg test results. *Dial Transpl* 1979;8:232–235.
88. Carl M, Francis DP, Maynard JE. A common-source outbreak of hepatitis B in a hemodialysis unit. *Dial Transpl* 1983;12:222–229.
89. Centers for Disease Control and Prevention. *Control measures for hepatitis B in dialysis centers*. Atlanta: Centers for Disease Control, 1977. (Viral Hepatitis Investigation and Control Series).
90. Alter MJ, Favero MS, Maynard JE. Impact of infection control strategies on the incidence of dialysis-associated hepatitis in the United States. *J Infect Dis* 1986;153:1149–1151.
91. Marmion BP, Burrell CJ, Tonkin RW, Dickson J. Dialysis-associated hepatitis in Edinburgh: 1969–1978. *Rev Infect Dis* 1982;4:619–637.
92. Najem GR, Louria DB, Thind IS, et al. Control of hepatitis B infection: the role of surveillance and an isolation hemodialysis center. *JAMA* 1981;245:153–157.
93. Centers for Disease Control and Prevention. Outbreaks of hepatitis B virus infection among hemodialysis patients—California, Nebraska, and Texas, 1994. *MMWR* 1996;45:285–289.
94. Niu MT, Penberthy LT, Alter MJ, Armstrong CW, Miller GB, Hadler SC. Hemodialysis-associated hepatitis B: report of an outbreak. *Dial Transpl* 1989;18:542–555.
95. Alter MJ, Favero MS, Francis DP. Cost benefit of vaccination for hepatitis B in hemodialysis centers. *J Infect Dis* 1983;148:770–771.
96. Choo QL, Kuo G, Weiner AJ, Overby LR, Bradley DW, Houghton M. Isolation of a cDNA clone derived from a bloodborne non-A, non-B viral hepatitis genome. *Science* 1989;244:359–362.
97. Kuo G, Choo QL, Alter HJ, et al. An assay for circulating antibodies to a major etiologic virus of human non-A, non-B hepatitis. *Science* 1989;244:362–364.

98. Esteban JI, Gonzalez A, Hernandez JM, et al. Evaluation of antibodies to hepatitis C virus in a study of transfusion-associated hepatitis. *N Engl J Med* 1990;323:1107–1112.
99. Alter MJ, Margolis HS, Krawczynski K, et al. The natural history of community-acquired hepatitis C in the United States. *N Engl J Med* 1992;327:1899–1905.
100. Kleinman S, Alter H, Busch M, et al. Increased detection of hepatitis C virus (HCV)–infected blood donors by a multiple-antigen HCV enzyme immunoassay. *Transfusion* 1992;32:805–813.
101. Mimms L, Vallari D, Ducharme L, Holland P, Kuramoto IK, Zeldis J. Specificity of anti-HCV ELISA assessed by reactivity to three immunodominant HCV regions. *Lancet* 1990;336:1590–1591.
102. Houghton M, Weiner A, Han J, Kuo G, Choo QL. Molecular biology of the hepatitis C viruses: implications for diagnosis, development and control of viral disease. *Hepatology* 1991;14:381–388.
103. Alter MJ, Hadler SC, Judson FN, et al. Risk factors for acute non-A, non-B hepatitis in the United States and association with hepatitis C virus infection. *JAMA* 1990;264:2231–2235.
104. Alter MJ, Gerety RJ, Smallwood L, et al. Sporadic non-A, non-B hepatitis: frequency and epidemiology in an urban United States population. *J Infect Dis* 1982;145:886–893.
105. Alter MJ, Coleman PJ, Alexander WJ, et al. Importance of heterosexual activity in the transmission of hepatitis B and non-A, non-B hepatitis. *JAMA* 1989;262:1201–1205.
106. Alter MJ. Epidemiology of hepatitis C in the west. *Semin Liver Dis* 1995;15:5–14.
107. Moyer LA, Alter MJ. Hepatitis C virus in the hemodialysis setting: a review with recommendations for control. *Semin Dial* 1994;7:124–127.
108. Niu MT, Coleman PJ, Alter MJ. Multicenter study of hepatitis C virus infection in chronic hemodialysis patients and hemodialysis center staff members. *Am J Kidney Dis* 1993;22:568–573.
109. Zeldis JB, Depner TA, Kuramoto, et al. The prevalence of hepatitis C virus antibodies among hemodialysis patients. *Ann Intern Med* 1990; 112:958–960.
110. Chan TM, Lok AS, Cheng IK, et al. Prevalence of hepatitis C virus infection in hemodialysis patients: a longitudinal study comparing the results of RNA and antibody assays. *Hepatology* 1993;17:5–8.
111. Oguchi H, Miyasaka M, Tokunaga S, et al. Hepatitis virus infection (HBV and HCV) in eleven Japanese hemodialysis units. *Clin Nephrol* 1992;38:36–43.
112. Fujiyama S, Kawano S, Sato S, et al. Prevalence of hepatitis C virus antibodies in hemodialysis patients and dialysis staff. *Hepatogastroenterology* 1992;39:161–165.
113. Hayashi J, Nakashima K, Kajiyama W, et al. Prevalence of antibody to hepatitis C virus in hemodialysis patients. *Am J Epidemiol* 1991;134: 651–657.
114. Selgas R, Martinez-Zapico R, Bajo MA, et al. Prevalence of hepatitis C antibodies (HCV) in a dialysis population at one center. *Perit Dial Int* 1992;12:28–30.
115. Hepatitis C virus antibodies in haemodialysis patients [Letter]. *Lancet* 1990;335:1409.
116. Yamaguchi K, Nishimura Y, Fukuoka N, et al. Hepatitis C virus antibodies in haemodialysis patients [Letter]. *Lancet* 1990;335:1409–1410.
117. Hardy NM, Sandroni S, Danielson S, Wilson WJ. Antibody to hepatitis C virus increases with time on hemodialysis. *Clin Nephrol* 1992; 38:44–48.
118. Farci P, Alter HJ, Govindarajan S, et al. Lack of protective immunity against reinfection with hepatitis C virus. *Science* 1992;258:135–140.
119. Bukh J, Miller RH, Purcell RH. Genetic heterogeneity of hepatitis C virus: quasispecies and genotypes. *Semin Liver Dis* 1995;15:41–63.
120. Cuypers HTM, Bresters D, Winkel IN, et al. Storage conditions of blood samples and primer selection affect the yield of cDNA polymerase chain reaction products of hepatitis C virus. *J Clin Microbiol* 1992;30:3220–3224.
121. Niu MT, Alter MJ, Kristensen C, Margolis HS. Outbreak of hemodialysis-associated non-A, non-B hepatitis and correlation with antibody to hepatitis C virus. *Am J Kidney Dis* 1992;19:345–352.
122. Marchesi D, Arici C, Poletti E, et al. Outbreak of non-A, non-B hepatitis in center haemodialysis patients: a retrospective analysis. *Nephrol Dial Transpl* 1988;3:795–799.
123. Polish LB, Gallagher M, Fields HA, Hadler SC. Delta hepatitis: molecular biology and clinical and epidemiological features. *Clin Microbiol Rev* 1993;6:211–229.
124. Lettau LA, Alfred HJ, Glew RH, et al. Nosocomial transmission of delta hepatitis. *Ann Intern Med* 1986;104:631–635.
125. Moyer LA, Alter MJ, Favero MS. Hemodialysis-associated hepatitis B: revised recommendations for serologic screening. *Semin Dial* 1990;3:201–204.
126. Favero MS, Bond WW. Chemical disinfection of medical and surgical materials. In: Block SS, ed. *Disinfection, sterilization, and preservation*, 4th ed. Philadelphia: Lea & Febiger, 1991:617–641.
127. Bond WW, Favero MS, Petersen NJ, Ebert JW. Inactivation of hepatitis B virus by intermediate- to high-level disinfection chemicals. *J Clin Microbiol* 1983;18:535–538.
128. Tokars JI, Alter MJ, Miller E, Moyer LA, Favero MS. National surveillance of dialysis-associated diseases in the United States, 1994. *ASAIO J* 1997;43:108–119.
129. Marcus R, Favero MS, Banerjee S, et al. HIV prevalence and incidence among patients undergoing chronic hemodialysis. *Am J Med* 1991;90:614–619.
130. Velandia M, Fridkin S, Cardena V, et al. Transmission of HIV in dialysis centre. *Lancet* 1995;345:1417–1422.
131. Anonymous. Argentinian doctors accused of spreading AIDS. *Br Med J* 1993;307(6904):584.
132. Gordon SM, Bland LA, Alexander SR, Newman HF, Arduino MJ, Jarvis WR. Hemolysis associated with hydrogen peroxide at a pediatric facility. *Am J Nephrol* 1990;10:123–127.
133. Gordon SM, Drachman J, Bland LA, Reid MH, Favero MS, Jarvis WR. Epidemic hypotension in a dialysis center caused by sodium azide. *Kidney Int* 1990;37:110–115.
134. Centers for Disease Control. *Dialysis dementia from aluminum*. Atlanta: Centers for Disease Control and Prevention, 1982. (Epidemic investigation report EPI 81-39, June 10, 1982.)
135. Centers for Disease Control and Prevention. *Formaldehyde intoxication associated with hemodialysis, California*. Atlanta: Centers for Disease Control and Prevention, 1984. (Epidemic investigation report EPI 81-73, May 7, 1984.)
136. Arnow PM, Bland LA, Garcia-Houchins S, Fridkin S, Fellner SK. An outbreak of fatal fluoride intoxication in a longterm hemodialysis unit. *Ann Intern Med* 1994;121:339–344.
137. Centers for Disease Control and Prevention. *Pyrogenic reactions and gram-negative bacteremia in patients in a hemodialysis center*. Atlanta: Centers for Disease Control and Prevention, 1991. (Epidemic investigation report EPI 91-37, October 17, 1991.)
138. Centers for Disease Control and Prevention. *Bacteremia in hemodialysis patients*. Atlanta: Centers for Disease Control and Prevention, 1992. (Epidemic investigation report EPI 92-10, March 26, 1992.)
139. Centers for Disease Control and Prevention. *Clusters of bacteremia and pyrogenic reactions in hemodialysis patients*. Atlanta: Centers for Disease Control and Prevention, 1987. (Epidemic investigation report EPI 86-65, April 22, 1987.)
140. Beck-Sague CM, Jarvis WR, Bland LA, Arduino MJ, Aguero SM, Verosic G. Outbreak of gram-negative bacteremia and pyrogenic reactions in a hemodialysis center. *Am J Nephrol* 1990;10:397–403.
141. Welbel SF, Schoendorf K, Bland LA, et al. An outbreak of gram-negative bloodstream infections in chronic hemodialysis patients. *Am J Nephrol* 1995;15:1–4.
142. Centers for Disease Control and Prevention. *Pyrogenic reactions in patients undergoing high-flux hemodialysis, California*. Atlanta: Centers for Disease Control and Prevention, 1987. (Epidemic investigation report EPI 86-80, June 1, 1987.)
143. Rudnick JR, Arduino MJ, Bland LA, et al. Pyrogenic reactions associated with hemodialysis reuse. *Artif Organs* 1995;19:289–294.
144. Kantor RJ, Hadler SC, Schreeder MT, Berquist KR, Favero MS. Outbreak of hepatitis B in a dialysis unit, complicated by false positive HBsAg test results. *Dial Transpl* 1979;8:232–235.
145. Carl M, Francis DP, Maynard JE. A common source outbreak of hepatitis B in a hemodialysis unit. *Dial Transpl* 1983;12:222–229.
146. Niu MT, Penberthy LT, Alter MJ, Armstrong CW, Miller GB, Hadler SC. Hemodialysis-associated hepatitis B: report of an outbreak. *Dial Transpl* 1989;18:542–555.
147. Centers for Disease Control and Prevention. *Outbreak of hepatitis B in a dialysis center*. Atlanta: Centers for Disease Control and Prevention, 1993 (Epidemic investigation report EPI 91-17, January 22, 1993.)
148. Centers for Disease Control and Prevention. *Non-A, non-B hepatitis in a dialysis center, Nashville, Tennessee*. Phoenix: Centers for Disease Control and Prevention, 1979. (Epidemic investigation report EPI-78-96-2, April 16, 1979.)

Hospital Infections, Fourth Edition,
edited by John V. Bennett and Philip S. Brachman.
Lippincott–Raven Publishers, Philadelphia © 1998

CHAPTER 25

The Intensive Care Unit

Didier Pittet and Stephan J. Harbarth

The care of critically ill patients in special high-technology units is a primary component of modern medicine. Although the efficacy of critical care has been established for only a few conditions, intensive care units (ICUs) are found in 95% of acute-care hospitals in the United States. Invasive diagnostic and therapeutic procedures are essential for the diagnosis and treatment of critically ill patients. However, life support systems disrupt normal host defense mechanisms. Given the severity of the illnesses affecting patients in ICUs, it is not surprising that mortality rates can exceed 25%. In addition, more than one third of the patients admitted to ICUs experience unexpected complications of medical care. The mortality rate in the group of patients with complications exceeds 40% [1]. Nosocomial infection is one of the most common medical complications affecting patients in ICUs. Although ICUs make up only 5% of hospital beds and care for < 10% of hospitalized patients, infections acquired in these units account for > 20% of nosocomial infections [2–5]. Fortunately, systematic studies of the determinants of nosocomial infections, surveillance for infections, and adherence to protocols for preventing infections have been effective in reducing the risk for patients admitted to ICUs.

ICU-ACQUIRED INFECTIONS

Pathogenesis

The dynamics of ICU-acquired infections are complex and depend on the contribution of the host's underlying conditions, the infectious agents, and the unique environment of the ICU. The following discussion will consider the role of each component in the development of infection.

D. Pittet: Division of Infectious Diseases
S. J. Harbarth: Infection Control Program, Division of Infectious Diseases, Geneva University Hospital, CH-1211 Geneva 14, Switzerland.

Host Defenses

The ability of patients in ICUs to ward off infections is seriously compromised. Natural host defense mechanisms might be impaired by underlying diseases or as a result of medical and surgical interventions. All patients admitted to an ICU will have at least one, and often several, vascular cannulas that break the normal skin barriers and establish direct access between the external environment and the bloodstream. Natural chemical barriers in the stomach are neutralized by administering H2 blockers or antacids that reduce acidity and allow growth of enteric flora. Physiologic mechanisms for evacuating and cleansing hollow organs are disrupted and circumvented by insertion of endotracheal tubes, nasogastric tubes, and urinary catheters.

Specific host defense mechanisms also might be impaired by the underlying diseases. Patients with malignant disorders might have abnormal immune responses as a result of their disease or stemming from therapies that diminish the number of effective phagocyte cells and blunt the normal immune response. Patients admitted to ICUs who are at the extremes of age exhibit selected impairments in natural and specific defense mechanisms that increase the risk of nosocomial infection.

Because of the precarious condition of patients in the ICU, normal food intake is often suspended. The prevalence of malnutrition has been estimated to be as high as 10% to 50% in some U.S. hospitals [6–8], and undernutrition in ICUs is almost universal. Moreover, conditions present in ICU patients might increase the level of malnutrition by increasing metabolic demands. Injured tissue, perfusion deficits, and infection cause fever and tachycardia through mechanisms mediated by hormones, cytokines, and bacterial products, such as endotoxin. The physiologic response to these mediators is an increase in oxygen consumption stemming from an increase in metabolic demand. This response results in breakdown of muscle to meet the body's demand for energy. The lean body mass declines, resulting in deficits in substrates necessary for recovery.

Although its clinical significance in hospitals is not well established, undernutrition has been associated with increased length of stay [9,10], surgical complications [9–11], and delayed wound healing [12]. Several studies suggest that poor nutritional status is a predisposing factor for nosocomial infections such as pneumonia, urinary tract infection, postoperative wound infections, and bacteremia [13–16]. Supplemental nutritional support, on the other hand, has been reported to facilitate weaning from mechanical ventilation and to improve prognoses [15].

Host resistance might be impaired in patients who experience major trauma. In a study by Schimpff and colleagues [17], nosocomial infection developed in 48% of patients with severe trauma, in contrast to only 3% of those with minor injuries whose length of stay in the ICU was equal to that of the patients with major injuries.

Important alterations in T- and B-cell function affecting host defense and resistance to infection are found in critically ill and traumatized patients. Alterations in T-cell activation and cytokine production are frequently associated with trauma and hemorrhage [18]. Injury and blood loss result in activation of CD8 T-cell populations capable of altering bacterial antigen-specific B-cell repertoires and suppressing the function of other T cells. The production of antibodies directed to bacterial antigens, and required for protection against extracellular bacterial infection, is diminished in models of critical illness, primarily because of the disappearance of bacterial antigen-specific B-cell clone precursors at systemic, pulmonary, and intestinal sites [19].

Medical Devices

The results of the European Prevalence of Infection in Intensive Care (EPIC) study [20] highlighted the relative importance of medical devices as risk factors for infections compared with other factors. Factors were collected from >10,000 ICU patients, of whom 2,064 had ICU-acquired infections. Among the seven independent risk factors identified, four were associated with medical devices commonly used in intensive care: central venous catheter (odds ratio [OR]=1.35, 95% confidence interval [95% CI]=1.6 to 1.57), pulmonary artery catheter (OR =1.20, 95% CI=1.01 to 1.43), urinary catheter (OR =1.41, 95% CI=1.19 to 1.69), and mechanical ventilation (OR=1.75, 95% CI=1.51 to 2.03). Other independent risk factors for ICU-acquired infections were stress ulcer prophylaxis (OR=1.38, 95% CI=1.2 to 1.6), the presence of trauma on admission (OR=2.07, 95% CI =1.75 to 2.44), and the length of ICU stay. The latter constituted the strongest predictor of infection and showed a linear increase in the odds for infection with time spent in the ICU [20].

In a recently published study [21], Mermel and colleagues analyzed intravenous catheter use by calculating device-days by the total number of patient-days for each ICU in their institution. They found significant differences in the use of intravascular catheters among different ICUs and among different catheter types. Arterial catheters, central lines, and Swan-Ganz catheters were most often used in surgical intensive car units (SICUs) and least often used in pediatric intensive care units (PICUs). This finding may reflect more prudent and judicious use of these catheter types in the PICU or merely the fact that the majority of surgery patients have their devices put in for hemodynamic monitoring shortly after major surgery rather than for medication administration per se. The authors ask for further studies to correlate catheter use with ventilator use, severity of illness, and risk of infection and ultimately to determine the relationship between catheter use and the patient's outcome [21].

Underlying Diseases

ICUs, by design, serve patients with severe illnesses that compromise host defense. Each patient must be assessed individually to determine how the underlying illness might interfere with host defense mechanisms. A simple assessment of the severity of underlying illness was developed by McCabe and Jackson [22], who stratified patients according to whether the underlying disease was fatal, ultimately fatal, or nonfatal. Subsequent studies by Britt and colleagues [23] have demonstrated the utility of this simple assessment for estimating the risk of nosocomial bacteremias. Numerous studies have found increasing rates of infections among patients with more severe illnesses. These observations were confirmed in the Study on the Efficacy of Nosocomial Infection Control Project [24].

Although McCabe's classification has been useful, it was not designed to assess patients admitted to ICUs. Several severity-of-illness scoring systems have been proposed to estimate a patient's risk of death in ICUs objectively. Models to assess critically ill patients have been revised to improve accuracy in predicting survival [25–28]; some include methods for updating mortality predictions over time [29,30]. Customized [31] or modified [32] versions of the three most frequently used scoring systems have been recently proposed to obtain satisfactory estimates of the probability of death in ICU patients with sepsis.

Knaus and colleagues [32] have proposed a sepsis severity scoring system that modifies the Acute Physiology and Chronic Health Evaluation (APACHE) III score to estimate the 28-day mortality risk for patients with sepsis syndrome—which has been renamed severe sepsis [33]. The model was derived using retrospective analysis of data collection from several large databases. The results of their investigation indicated that acute physiologic abnormalities are the most important prognostic factors influencing outcome. Additional weight assigned to some physiologic variables beyond the weights accorded in the APACHE III scoring system increased the explanatory power of 28-day mortality risk. These findings have been confirmed in a cohort of 1,052 critically ill patients with clinically suspected or microbiologically documented severe sepsis [34]. Severity of illness (assessed using the Simplified Acute Physiology Score II score), the number of acute organ failures, and the characteristics of underlying disease predicted a patient's survival.

To identify ICU patients who are at particularly high risk of nosocomial infection, Gross and colleagues [35] evaluated 148 patients who were admitted to a combined medical ICU/coronary care unit and who stayed in the unit for ≥ 3 days. They found that 75 patients (51%) had three or more active co-morbidities at the time of admission. Furthermore, the length of stay, noninfectious complications, and nosocomial infections were all significantly correlated with the number of preexisting co-morbidities. Their results highlight the fact that preexisting host conditions are important in the development of nosocomial infections. In addition, they suggest that in clinical trials or for comparisons of infection rates between units or hospitals, patients must be stratified according to co-morbidities because many of the outcome indicators are significantly affected by the number of preexisting conditions. If these results are confirmed, patients at high risk of infection could be identified prospectively based on the number of active co-morbidities present on admission. More intensive surveillance and prevention strategies could be targeted at the patients at highest risk of nosocomial infections.

Infectious Agents and Antimicrobial Resistance

In ICUs, where antibiotics are used more frequently and in larger amounts than in almost any other unit in the hospital, antimicrobial resistance ensures the survival of some nosocomial pathogens. Moreover, the close proximity of patients facilitates transfer of resistant organisms from patient to patient. The predominant pathogens found in the ICUs participating in the National Nosocomial Infection Surveillance (NNIS) program are *Pseudomonas aeruginosa* (accounting for 13% of all isolates), *Staphyloccocus aureus* (12%), coagulase-negative staphylococci (10%), *Enterococcus* spp (9%), *Enterobacter* spp (8%), and *Candida* spp (10%) [36]. It is noteworthy that trends in the pathogens responsible for nosocomial infections in the ICU have shown an increase in infections due to coagulase-negative staphylococci, *S. aureus*, *Candida* spp, *E. faecalis*, *E. faecium*, and *E. cloacae* [37]. The emergence of these pathogens is due, at least in part, to patterns of antibiotic use and selection pressure throughout the 1980s and to the development of antibiotic resistance among these isolates. At present, > 60% of nosocomial isolates of coagulase-negative staphylococci and > 20% of *S. aureus* isolates from ICUs are resistant to methicillin [37,38]. Methicillin-resistant *S. aureus* (MRSA) strains are already accounting for ≥ 30% of *S. aureus* isolates in European ICUs [20] and are a growing problem, especially in southern Europe, where the incidence and rates of antibiotic resistance are alarmingly high with a prevalence of methicillin resistance among *S. aureus* isolates of ≤ 50% [20,39] (see Chapter 41).

Organisms such as *Klebsiella* spp are an important source of transferable antibiotic resistance [40], and outbreaks of nosocomial infections caused by multiresistant *Enterobacteriaceae* have been reported [5,41,42]. Brun-Buisson and colleagues described an outbreak of infections caused by *Klebsiella pneumoniae* that successively involved three ICUs within the same hospital [5]. The resistance was plasmid-mediated and emerged in association with an increase in the use of cephalosporins and amikacin (see Chapter 15). The identical pattern of antimicrobial susceptibility was observed in *Escherichia coli* and *Citrobacter freundii* isolates collected from surrounding symptom-free patients. Numerous other reports have demonstrated spread of antibiotic resistance from ICUs to other hospital units [43–45]. Another nosocomial pathogen that is increasingly colonizing and infecting patients in the hospital environment is *Stenotrophomonas maltophilia* (formerly *Xanthomonas maltophilia*). Patients with debilitating conditions are at especially high risk of acquiring pneumonia or bacteremia with this pathogen [46,47]. The wide use of broad-spectrum antibiotics may be one of the promoting factors of colonization and infection with *Stenotrophomonas maltophilia* [46].

Axelrod and Talbot [48] studied risk factors associated with the acquisition of gentamicin resistance by enterococci in a general hospital. The most significant factors were length of hospitalization, number and duration of antibiotics received, and admission to ICUs. Edmond and colleagues described an outbreak of vancomycin-resistant *Enterococcus faecium* bacteremia in an oncology ward [49]. Gastrointestinal colonization with vancomycin-resistant *E. faecium* and the use of antimicrobial agents with significant activity against anaerobes were found to be risk factors for the development of vancomycin-resistant *E. faecium* bacteremia. De Champs and colleagues [50] prospectively studied colonization of ICU patients with *Enterobacteriaceae* that produced expanded-spectrum β-lactamases. Ten of the 56 patients admitted during the 6-month study period became colonized or infected. Colonization was associated with longer stays in the ICU. The number of colonized patients decreased after the antibiotic policy was changed.

The relationship between antibiotic resistance and antibiotic use in ICUs has been studied in a large, multicenter study (Intensive Care Antimicrobial Resistance

Epidemiology Project) conducted in 1994 by the Hospital Infection Program of the Centers for Disease Control and Prevention (CDC) and the Rollins School of Public Health, Emory University [51]. Preliminary results confirm that dramatic differences exist in the pattern of antimicrobial usage and antimicrobial resistance between different hospitals. However, the usage of antimicrobials showed important variations between institutions facing similar prevalences of highly resistant organisms, confirming that efforts to control resistance should focus on both antimicrobial use and infection control practices. Studies of the epidemiology of extended spectrum β-lactamase-resistant nosocomial *K. pneumoniae* highlighted the importance of interhospital spread, stressing the interrelationship of hospitals when attempting to control antimicrobial resistance [52].

The value of the use of combination therapy and cycling of antimicrobial therapy in delaying the emergence of resistance needs to be systematically studied in controlled trials (see Chapter 15). Guidelines for the duration of antibiotic prophylaxis and therapy must be implemented in critical care settings, where measures to optimize use of antimicrobials have special importance.

Sources of Colonization

Host colonization is a prerequisite for the development of infection. This process involves adherence of organisms to epithelial or mucosal cells, proliferation, and persistence at the site of attachment. Although the factors promoting the progression from colonization to infection are not well understood, almost 50% of the ICU-acquired infections are preceded by host colonization with the same microorganism. Factors associated with microbial colonization are similar to those associated with development of infection. These risk factors include the duration of hospitalization and length of stay in the ICU, invasive devices, prolonged antibiotic therapy, and elimination of normal pharyngeal or bowel flora through the use of broad-spectrum antimicrobial agents. Other factors promoting colonization of patients in ICUs include disruption of normal mechanical defense mechanisms (i.e., the bronchial mucociliary "escalator") by drugs and tracheal intubation, changes in protective antibacterial secretions (i.e., lysozyme, lactoferrin, saliva, and gastric acid) in response to stress and therapeutic agents, and disruption of "colonization resistance."

A vast literature exists regarding the development of colonization and subsequent infection (see Chapter 1). A few important studies are summarized. The classic article [53] of Johanson and associates, written in 1969, showed that severe illness predisposes to oropharyngeal colonization with gram-negative bacilli. In 1974, Schimpff and colleagues [17] suggested that in critically ill patients, the origin of infection is usually the endogenous flora. Several studies have subsequently confirmed that patients are rapidly colonized by gram-negative bacteria after admission to ICUs [54–56] and later develop infection with the same organisms [57–60]. Kerver and colleagues [61] showed that the oropharyngeal cavity and lower respiratory tract of 60% of patients on mechanical ventilation were colonized by ICU-acquired organisms after 5 days in the ICU. After 10 days, 100% of the patients were colonized. In 66% of the respiratory tract infections, colonization with the pathogen preceded infection.

Flynn and co-workers [62] prospectively studied colonization in patients undergoing cardiac surgery compared with those who underwent coronary angioplasty. Whereas none of the latter became colonized with gram-negative organisms, the majority of surgical patients were colonized with *Enterobacter* spp. Colonization with *Enterobacter* spp was correlated with antibiotic prophylaxis, and *Enterobacter* spp infection developed in 14% of the colonized patients. Moreover, phage typing methods confirmed that the patients' newly acquired endogenous flora was the most important source of infection. In a related study, the same authors found that in almost 25% of patients colonized with *Enterobacter*, *Pseudomonas*, and *Serratia* species clinical infection [63] developed.

Candida infections in ICU patients have become increasingly important; infections mainly evolve from endogenous colonization facilitated by the use of broad-spectrum antibiotics [64–66]. It has been confirmed that sequential spread of candidal colonization from the abdominal cavity to other body sites takes place before candidemia occurs [64]. In heavily colonized surgical ICU patients, *Candida* spp colonization was patient-specific and always preceded infection with a genotypically identical strain [67]. The degree of *Candida* spp colonization constituted the strongest independent risk factor for infection [68].

The central role of gastric colonization in the pathogenesis of nosocomial infection and pneumonia has been called into question. Based on studying sequences of colonization in ICU patients, Bonten et al. [69] concluded that the stomach is unlikely to be an important source of pathogens leading to nosocomial pneumonia, as diagnosed by bronchoalveolar lavage (BAL) or protected specimen brush (PSB). Furthermore, the initial site and route of colonization might not be the same for all microorganisms [69]. These results were confirmed in a large, adequately designed, prospective observational cohort study conducted in two medical intensive care units (MICU), where specimens for culture were taken daily from nares, oropharynx, trachea, and stomach from the time of admission to the first signs of nosocomial pneumonia [70]. The stomach was an uncommon source of microorganisms that cause pneumonia in ventilated patients. Preventive regimens should thus be mainly directed against colonization of the oropharynx and trachea.

Epidemiology

Infection Sites and Types of ICU

The frequency with which infections occur at different sites in the ICU and hospital-wide is illustrated in Figure 25-1. Urinary tract infections predominate in general wards, whereas the most common nosocomial infections in ICUs are lower respiratory tract infections [71]. We previously reported differences in the incidence of nosocomial infections in different types of ICUs [72]. Overall rates of nosocomial infections, identified through concurrent surveillance by trained epidemiology technicians at the University of Iowa Hospitals and Clinics (UIHC) during the years 1983 to 1989, ranged between 11 and 16 infections per 1,000 patient-days, compared with 36 to 54 per 1,000 patient-days in the SICU, 23 to 47 per 1,000 patient-days in the MICU, and 14 to 32 per 1,000 patient-days in the PICU. These data illustrate several important points.

First, rates of infection tended to be higher in the SICU than in the MICU, confirming the findings of Craven and colleagues [73], and rates in the adult ICUs were higher than in the PICU over the study period. Second, in all three units, the lower respiratory tract was the most common site of infection. Lower respiratory tract infections accounted for ~ 40% of infections in the SICU, 37% to 54% of those in the MICU, and 20% to 50% of those in the PICU throughout the period of the study. High rates of pulmonary infections relative to other infection sites are unique to critical care units, where patients are frequently admitted because of respiratory distress and require endotracheal intubation. When rates of lower respiratory tract infections have been compared over shorter increments of time (i.e., by month) wide variations have been noted. Observations in these units suggested that the level of skilled nursing care relative to patient census may be an important determinant of this variation.

Although primary bacteremia and infections stemming from the presence of vascular cannulas were less common than lower respiratory tract infections, the morbidity and mortality rates associated with these infections are high. The rates of bloodstream infections have increased in all three types of ICUs over the 7 years reported (1982 to 1989) at UIHC [72]; this trend was in accordance with that observed hospital-wide [74]. Although the PICU has had lower overall rates of infection than the MICU and the SICU, the rates of primary bacteremia and vascular cannula–associated infections have been comparable. Consequently, these infections made up a higher percentage of infections in the PICU than in the MICU and SICU. In fact, from 1988 to 1989 primary bacteremias and cannula-associated infections accounted for 12.3% and 14.3% of nosocomial infections, respectively, in the PICU, compared with 5.7% and 6.0%, respectively, in the SICU and 4.8% and 4.3%, respectively, in the MICU [72].

In summary, rates of nosocomial infections vary considerably within hospitals by type of ICU. Rates are generally lower in cardiac care units [3] and higher in neonatal, surgical, trauma, and burn units, reflecting the greater risk of infection of patients admitted to these latter types of units [38]. In 1992, a total of 1,417 ICUs in 17 countries in Western Europe participated in a 1-day point prevalence EPIC study [20]. The overall rate of ICU-acquired nosocomial infection was 20.6% (2,064/10,038). Rates of ICU-acquired infection markedly varied from country to country, ranging from 9.7% to 31.6%. Trends toward higher ICU-acquired infection rates paralleled trends toward higher mortality rates in this large study. These differences are more likely to reflect differences in critical care practice and selection of patients rather than real differences in quality of care. These results certainly reflect the importance for controlling for case mix when interpreting and comparing rates of nosocomial infections, in particular, when comparisons between units or countries have to be made.

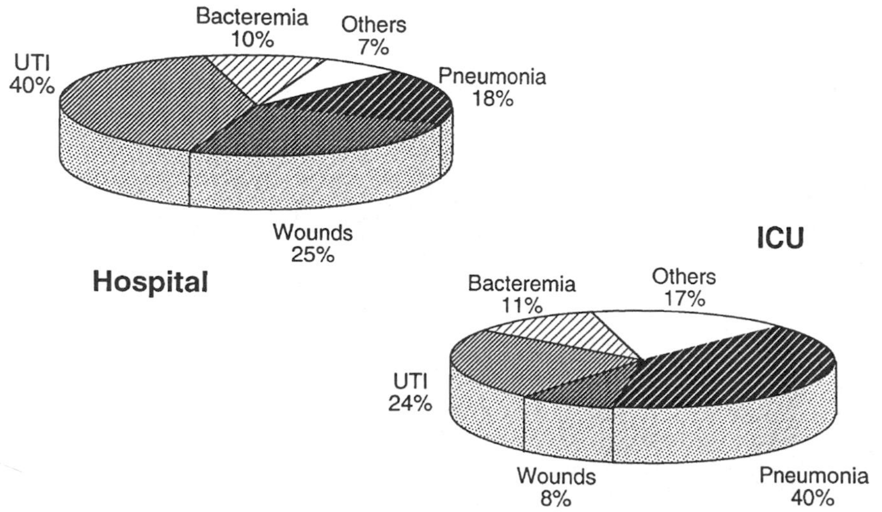

FIGURE 25-1. Relative proportions of nosocomial infections at different sites in the ICU and hospital wide.

The Agent

Bacteria, fungi, and viruses have been reported as causative agents in nosocomial infections. To illustrate the major trends in the microbial etiology of nosocomial infections responsible for disease in ICUs and in other hospital wards, we report data from the NNIS System from 1986 to 1992. These data reflect a large geographic sample of the United States and are representative of ICUs in all types of hospitals around the country and the industrialized world [75,76]. Data are also compared with those abtained in the EPIC study [20].

Table 25-1 lists the most common nosocomial pathogens by site from U.S. ICUs and hospital-wide data and from Western European ICUs. The leading pathogens causing nosocomial bacteremia and surgical wound infections were staphylococci and enterococci. *Pseudomonas aeruginosa* was the most commonly listed pathogen causing respiratory tract infection. *Candida* spp and *E. coli* were the most prevalent isolates of urinary tract infections in the ICU setting. Overall, in contrast to the 1970s, major shifts in the etiology of nosocomial infections have occurred in the decade of the 1980s and early 1990s. Gram-positive infections and fungal infections are becoming more common, and gram-negative organisms are becoming increasingly resistant to available antibiotics. Taken as a whole, the shifts are away from more easily treated pathogens toward more resistant pathogens with fewer options for therapy [37].

TABLE 25-1. *Leading nosocomial pathogens by site and frequency*

Sites	Pathogens	NNIS, hospital wide[a] (%)	NNIS, ICU[a] (%)	EPIC, ICU[b] (%)
Blood	CNS	28	28	34
	S. aureus	16	16	22
	Enterococci	8	12	11
	Candida spp	8	10	9
	E. coli	6	—	7
	Enterobacter spp	—	5	—
Surgical wound	*S. aureus*	17	12	27
	Enterococci	13	16	18
	CNS	13	14	14
	E. coli	9	—	13
	P. aeruginosa	8	9	22
	Enterobacter spp	—	10	8
Respiratory tract	*P. aeruginosa*	17	21	30
	S. aureus	16	17	32
	Enterobacter spp	10	11	7
	S. pneumoniae	6	—	—
	H. influenzae	6	—	—
	Acinetobacter spp	—	6	10
	K. pneumoniae	—	6	8
Urinary tract	*E. coli*	26	17	22
	Enterococci	16	13	15
	P. aeruginosa	12	11	19
	Candida spp	9	25	21
	K. pneumoniae	6	—	—
	Enterobacter spp	—	6	—

CNS, coagulase-negative staphylococci.

[a](Adapted with permission from Jarvis WR, Martone W. Predominant pathogens in hospital infections. *J Antimicro Chemother* 1992;29(suppl A):19–24.)

[b](Adapted from Vincent JL, Bihari DJ, Suter PM. The prevalence of nosocomial infection in intensive care units in Europe: results of the European Prevalence of Infection in Intensive Care (EPIC) Study. *JAMA* 1995;274:639–644, and from Suter PM, personal communication.)

Clusters of Infections in the ICU

Although < 10% of hospitalized patients are treated in ICUs, many outbreaks of nosocomial infections occur in these units [3]. At the University of Virginia Hospital, 10 of 11 outbreaks identified from 1978 to 1982 took place in ICUs, and eight of the outbreaks involved bloodstream infections. Similarly to the outbreak of polymicrobial bloodstream infections described by Ponce de Leon and colleagues [77], these outbreaks were frequently related to breaks in technique or disregard for infection control guidelines. Other epidemics were associated with specific strains of bacteria and may or may not have been confined to a specific anatomic site [42,78]. These outbreaks were usually related to a contaminated inanimate or animate reservoir from which the organism was transmitted to the patients.

A literature search for outbreaks occurring in ICUs from 1983 to 1995 identified more than 50 clusters of infections. Extensive reviews have been published already [72,79]. Overall, ~ 40% of the outbreaks were caused by gram-negative bacilli and nearly another third by gram-positive bacteria. Table 25-2 summarizes important features of selected outbreaks [42,78,80–104]. Leading pathogens of outbreaks in the ICU setting were MRSA, *Acinetobacter* spp, *Enterobacter* spp, and *Pseudomonas* spp.

Although there were unique factors in each epidemic, several generalizations can be made. Epidemics associated with specific pathogens were often associated with bacteria that were relatively resistant to antibiotics, relatively virulent when compared with normal endogenous and environmental flora [82], capable of withstanding variations in environmental conditions [83], and transmitted by hand from patient to patient. Pathogens that exemplify these characteristics include *S. aureus* and *Serratia*, *Klebsiella*, and *Enterobacter* species. Epidemics caused by unusual organisms, such as *Acinetobacter* spp, were often associated with contaminated equipment or with changes in the environment [99]. Outbreaks of infection were more frequently reported from neonatal intensive care units (NICUs) than from other types of ICUs [79]. It is important to remember that new equipment or a new procedure may introduce a new reservoir or mode of transmission into the ICU [100].

TABLE 25-2. *Selected outbreaks in different ICUs*

Unit	Organism	Sites of infection or colonization	Transmission	No. of patients	Duration	Reference
General ICU	*Acinetobacter baumannii*	Multiple sites	Environmental contamination	31	13 mo	[104]
General ICU	*Acinetobacter baumannii*	Multiple sites	Respirator tubes, hand contact	4	3 wk	[78]
SICU	*Acinetobacter baumannii*	Multiple sites	Environmental contamination	59	12 mo	[235]
Burn unit	*Acinetobacter calcoaceticus*	Burn wounds, pneumonia	Patients' mattresses	43	21 mo	[91]
SICU and MICU	*Acinetobacter calcoaceticus*	Pneumonia	Gloves, nebulizer	19	2 mo	[99]
NICU	Adenovirus	Pulmonary infection	ND	11	ND	[236]
General ICU	*Bacillus cereus*	Respiratory tract	Ventilatory equipment	62	7 mo	[101]
MICU	*Candida parapsilosis*	Multiple sites	Hospital environment	5	ND	[237]
NICU	*Candida tropicalis*	Fungemia	Cross-infection	6	5 mo	[98]
NICU	*Enterobacter cloacae*	Multiple sites	Cross-contamination	14	9 mo	[42]
NICU	*Enterobacter cloacae*	Respiratory tract	Cross-contamination	22	ND	[95]
General ICU	*Enterococcus faecium*	Multiple sites	ND	6	6 mo	[238]
General ICU	*Enterococcus faecium*	Bacteremia	Electronic thermometer	9	3 mo	[239]
NICU	Hepatitis A	Viraemia, hepatitis	Vertical transmission	10	1 mo	[240]
General ICU	*Klebsiella pneumoniae*	Multiple sites	ND	74	3 mo	[241]
SICU/MICU	*Klebsiella pneumoniae*	Multiple sites	Hospital environment	52	19 mo	[82]
General ICU	MRSA	Pneumonia	ND	ND	1 yr	[94]
General ICU	MRSA	Multiple sites	Cross-contamination	117	6 mo	[242]
MICU	MRSA	Bacteremia	Cross-contamination	14	9 mo	[243]
General ICU	*Pseudomonas cepacia*	Respiratory tract	Electronic ventilator probes	117	18 mo	[83]
General ICU	*Pseudomonas cepacia*	Pneumonia	Nebulized albuterol therapy	42	ND	[100]
General ICU	*Salmonella wien*	Bacteremia, diarrhea	Cross-infection	27	5 mo	[244]
General ICU	*Serratia marcescens*	Bacteremia	ND	ND	1 mo	[97]
General ICU	*S. pyogenes*	Bacteremia	Cross-infection	3	ND	[87]
NICU	*Trichosporon beigelii*	Multiple sites	ND	3	3 mo	[245]

ND, not documented.

Clinical Aspects of Infections in the ICU

Critically ill patients are highly susceptible to nosocomial infections. The importance of medical devices in catheter-associated urinary tract infections (see Chapter 31), intravascular device–associated infections (see Chapter 44), and ventilator-associated pneumonia (see Chapter 32) is discussed elsewhere. Only selected aspects of infections seen in patients admitted to an ICU will be discussed in this section.

Pneumonia

Pneumonia is the second most common nosocomial infection overall and the most common nosocomial infection in ICUs, accounting for 15% to 20% of all nosocomial infections and 25% to 45% of those in intensive care units, respectively (Figure 25-1; see Chapter 30). Additionally, pneumonia is associated with a high crude mortality rate and an attributable mortality rate ≤ 27% in mechanically ventilated patients [105]. These patients, including those who have suffered severe trauma and those who have had major surgery, are at increased risk of subsequent lower respiratory tract infections [106–109]. Exogenous infection is rare, but, on occasion, medication nebulizers, the endotracheal tube lumen and other respiratory therapy equipment, and contaminated hospital water can serve as sources for the inoculation of microorganisms into the lung [110,111].

Although mechanical ventilation is not a necessary prerequisite for the development of ICU-acquired pneumonia, it substantially increases the risk of lower respiratory tract infection [107,112]. Indeed, Langer and colleagues found that the incidence of pneumonia is directly related to the duration of respiratory support, and the daily rate of acquisition is constant during the first 8 to 10 days of mechanical ventilation [113]. Pneumonia developed in ~ 5% of patients with each additional day of mechanical ventilation.

Cultures of the lower respiratory tract are important in the diagnosis of ICU-acquired pneumonia. Because the oropharynx of critically ill patients is frequently colonized with potentially pathogenic bacteria, care must be taken to avoid contaminating cultures of the lower airways. Retrieval of culture specimens by bronchoscope using either a PSB or BAL has been helpful for this purpose [114–116] (see Chapter 32).

Other techniques that have been studied include protected BAL [116], nonbronchoscopic ("blind") BAL, and blind PSB [117–119]. Middleton et al. [120] compared four of the different methods for diagnosing nosocomial pneumonia in ventilated patients and established that the semiquantitative cultures of blind endotracheal aspirates provided information similar to that derived by PSB or BAL [120]. This remarkable disclosure needs to be validated in further studies of larger populations. In any case, the use of either PSB or BAL should be strongly encouraged to increase the accuracy of the difficult diagnosis of ventilator-associated pneumonia [116,121].

Early-Onset Pneumonia

In a prospective survey of 1,107 patients, Mandelli and colleagues [122] reported that > 50% of ICU-acquired pneumonias appeared within the first 4 days after admission to the unit. In a later prospective multicenter study, these investigators found that 441 of 1,304 admissions were complicated by pneumonia and that 54% of the infections were diagnosed within 4 days of admission [123]. Impairment of reflexes that protect the airways was the most important risk factor for early-onset pneumonia. Aspiration of oropharyngeal flora was the presumed mode of inoculation. Mandelli and colleagues [122] suggested that this entity be called early-onset pneumonia because the pathogenesis and primary causative agents differed from pneumonias arising later in the ICU stay. Because the pathogens causing aspiration pneumonia reflect the oropharyngeal microbial flora at the time of aspiration, the pathogens that bring about early-onset pneumonia are more likely to reflect normal oral flora or pathogens responsible for community-acquired pneumonia (*S. aureus*, *Streptococcus pneumoniae*, and *Hemophilus influenzae*). In patients with multiple traumatic injuries, severe abdominal and thoracic trauma was identified as the strongest independent risk factor for early-onset pneumonia. Age of > 40 and duration of mechanical ventilation of < 24 hours during the first 4 days of hospitalization were additional independent risk factors for infection [124].

Nosocomial Tracheobronchitis

Nosocomial tracheobronchitis, a recently recognized clinical entity, is defined by the presence of fever, purulent sputum, a significant number of polymorphonuclear leukocytes on the gram-stain smear, and positive sputum culture in patients who have no radiographic evidence of pneumonia [41,59]. Although there is no consensus in the literature regarding the need for treatment, most physicians treat tracheobronchitis to prevent subsequent pneumonia. Further studies are under way to define whether tracheobronchitis actually plays a role in the pathogenesis of nosocomial pneumonia.

Sinusitis

Sinusitis frequently complicates nasotracheal or nasogastric intubation (2% to 25%) [125–129]. Mechanical obstruction of the maxillary sinuses usually initiates the process [125], with subsequent spread to the ethmoid and sphenoid sinuses. Fever, leukocytosis, and purulent nasal discharge suggest the diagnosis, but their absence does not exclude it [128,130]. Conventional sinus radiographs and computed tomography scans are useful, but sinus aspirate allows confirmation of the diagnosis and identification of the causative agents. In contrast to community-acquired sinusitis, gram-negative organisms have predominated in this context. *Pseudomonas* and *Klebsiella* species and *Enterobacteriaceae* have been the pathogens most commonly recovered [125,126,131,132]. In addition, *S. aureus* and *Candida* spp have also been frequently encountered, and polymicrobial infection has been documented in 40% to 100% of cases [126,127, 129]. Nasotracheal intubation is associated with a significantly higher risk of infection than orotracheal intubation [125,132] (see Chapter 46). Complications include pansinusitis [125,128], orbital cellulitis, brain abscess, osteomyelitis [127], secondary bloodstream infection [126], and nosocomial pneumonia. Treatment requires removal of the device and intravenous antibiotic therapy, including coverage for *Pseudomonas* spp.

In summary, the existing studies establish that sinusitis joins pneumonia, catheter sepsis, and urinary tract infections as one of the "four horsemen" of clinically important nosocomial infections in critically ill patients. Therefore, a sinus computed tomography scan is a necessary component of the evaluation of intubated patients with fever or signs of sepsis from unknown origin [129,133]. Sinus aspiration is essential to confirm the diagnosis, direct antimicrobial therapy, and help drainage.

Systemic Inflammatory Response Syndrome, Sepsis, and Severe Sepsis

Sepsis and septic shock are commonly used terms. The current theory is that they represent increasingly severe stages of the same disorder. These stages do not necessarily imply increasing severity of infection, rather an increasing severity of the systemic response to infection [134]. Although the term sepsis syndrome, as originally described by Bone and colleagues, identified a population of patients at risk of acute respiratory distress syndrome (ARDS) and death [135], in common usage it now appears both confusing and ambiguous. Newer categories and more precise definitions have evolved from discussions at one American College of Chest Physicians/Society of Critical Care Medicine Consensus Conference [33]. Specifically, the term systemic inflammatory response syndrome (SIRS) was chosen to imply a clinical response arising from a nonspecific insult. It includes four criteria: hypothermia or hyperthermia, tachycardia, tachypnea, and leukocytosis or leukopenia. Sepsis is now defined as the presence of SIRS associated with a confirmed infectious process [33]. Discarding the term sepsis syndrome, members of the consensus conference defined severe sepsis as the presence of sepsis with either hypotension or systemic manifestations of end-organ hypoperfusion, including but not restricted to lactic acidosis, oliguria, or altered mental status. Septic shock was defined as sepsis with hypotension despite adequate fluid resuscitation.

The first studies reporting the incidence and epidemiology of SIRS, sepsis, and septic shock have been published [136,137]. The incidence of SIRS was very high in critically ill surgical patients [137] and was not associated with either significantly higher mortality rates or longer length of ICU or hospital stay, in contrast to sepsis or severe sepsis. The large prospective study by Rangel-Frausto et al. [136] provided strong epidemiologic evidence for the theory that patients with SIRS and three or four positive inclusion criteria (SIRS III or IV) are likely to show signs of sepsis and have higher rates of organ dysfunction and mortality. In any category, 44% to 71% of patients had progressed from a low stage of biologic response syndrome to the higher stage. Other patients progressed through more than two stages within a 24-hour window. Positive blood culture rates, end-organ failure rates, and mortality rates rose with each subsequent stage of systemic inflammatory response. In summary, this study supports the presumption of a clinical progression from SIRS III or IV to sepsis, severe sepsis, and septic shock. Identification of patients at earlier stages of the process of infection based on easily available parameters may help prevent further complications in this critically ill population. Further studies need to be conducted before recommendations for systematic recording of advanced SIRS can be made.

Multiple Organ Dysfunction Syndrome

With better methods for hemodynamic monitoring and support, the primary cause of death in critically ill patients with infection has shifted from shock to multiple organ failure or dysfunction syndrome (MODS). This new terminology has been considered adequate by the previously mentioned consensus conference to describe the dynamic process of organ dysfunction, which presents a continuum of physiologic derangement and not a steady state described by the concept of organ failure [138]. The mortality rate associated with MODS is very high (60% to 80%), even with aggressive treatment, and correlates with the number of organs involved [139].

The association of organ failure with infection has been noted since the earliest descriptions of the syndrome. This relationship between infection and MODS was clearly established by Fry and colleagues [140] in a study of 553 consecutive patients who underwent major operative procedures or who sustained severe trauma. Thirty-eight patients developed MODS, 24 (63%) of whom had uncontrolled infections. The most common primary sites of infection were pleuropulmonary and intraabdominal.

But infection is not a necessary prerequisite for the development of MODS. Some conditions, such as pancreatitis, ARDS, or multiple trauma, in which MODS can evolve are not necessarily associated with an untreated focus of infection [141,142]. Furthermore, recent investigations have shown that MODS can be reproduced experimentally by the infusion of a spectrum of endogenously derived mediators of inflammation [143]. Therefore, some authorities restate the problem of MODS as a primarily uncontrolled inflammatory response or the result of uncontrolled inflammation [143,144].

Different mechanisms of action have been proposed to explain the pathogenesis of MODS. Some authors have suggested that organ failure is a sign of occult, usually intraabdominal infection [145,146]. Marshall and colleagues [60] confirmed the importance of the gastrointestinal tract as a reservoir of pathogens. In 33 of 41 surgical patients in whom MODS developed, pathologic gastrointestinal tract colonization preceded MODS in critically ill surgical patients. *Escherichia coli*, *Bacteroides fragilis*, and enterococci were the predominant pathogens isolated. Whereas the intestinal flora was responsible for most of the initial infections, *Candida* species, coagulase-negative staphylococci, and *P. aeruginosa* were the most common ICU-acquired organisms. Moreover, death among patients with MODS was more strongly correlated with infections caused by *Candida* species and coagulase-negative staphylococci than with infections caused by other organisms. Finally, some investigators have suggested that exploratory laparotomy or laparoscopy is helpful for both disease diagnosis and treatment of patients with MODS who have no recognized site of infection [145,147].

As more patients with MODS without clinical or radiographic evidence of intraabdominal sepsis were studied, however, it became obvious that a large number of them did not have intraabdominal infections. Thus, with the development of more sophisticated and reliable noninvasive imaging techniques, the presence of MODS does not mandate laparotomy when there is no clinical or radiographic evidence suggesting intraabdominal disease [143,144].

Bacterial translocation and endotoxin release have been proposed as pathogenetic mechanisms of MODS of gastrointestinal origin. Bacterial translocation across the gastrointestinal mucosa has been confirmed in animals and humans with shock [148,149]. Positive blood cultures were obtained from patients in shock before the restitution of blood pressure, thereby excluding reperfusion injury as the cause. Rush and colleagues [149] found a relationship between the rates of positive blood cultures and the severity of hypotension in 50 severely injured patients. In another study, 13 (39%) of 33 consecutive patients with cardiac arrest and cardiopulmonary complications had positive blood cultures within 12 hours of the arrest [148]. In 12 of the 13 patients, the same organisms were recovered from blood and feces, suggesting that mesenteric ischemia may predispose patients to bloodstream infection of gastrointestinal origin. Another recently published study showed that among 96 patients surviving cardiac arrest for >24 hours, 23 (24%) showed signs of pneumonia [150]. Gram-positive cocci represented 57% of the isolates. Nine of the 23 patients in the group with pneumonia died.

Another interesting approach to explaining MODS is the so-called macrophage hypothesis. According to this theory, excessive or prolonged activation of macrophages ultimately results in excessive production, surface expression, and liberation of cytokines, which exert deleterious local and systemic effects [143]. The clinical correlate of this hypothesis is the uncontrolled inflammatory response. and it does not necessarily require the presence of infection.

One explanation that overlaps and interacts with the macrophage hypothesis of MODS, is the "microcirculating hypothesis." This theory proposes that organ injury is related to ischemia or vascular endothelial injury. The potential mechanisms of injury are inadequate tissue and cellular oxygen delivery [151], the ischemia-reperfusion phenomenon [152], and tissue injury due to endothelial leukocyte interactions [153]. In this scheme, neutrophil adherence to endothelial cells is a prerequisite for endothelial and subsequent tissue injury [143]. Experimental studies document that shock or ischemia-reperfusion-mediated endothelial cell and organ injury can be corrected by preventing neutrophil adhesion to endothelial cells [154,155].

In summary, there has been an enormous amount of clinical and experimental information generated during the past decade on the pathophysiology and potential therapy of MODS. The major breakthrough has been the idea that MODS can occur without concomitant infection. Thus, there is an urgent demand to restrict the use of multiple broad-spectrum antibiotics in patients with MODS and to use narrow-spectrum antibiotics for documented infection only. Extensive workup is, however, frequently necessary to disprove the role of infection in MODS.

Other ICU-Specific Infectious Problems

Acalculous cholecystitis, also called postoperative cholecystitis, commonly complicates both abdominal and nonabdominal surgery in critically ill patients [156,157]. *Pseudomonas aeruginosa*, *E. coli*, and *Enterobacter* spp are the most commonly isolated pathogens. Severe complications can occur, including gangrene of the gallbladder, perforation, secondary peritonitis, intrahepatic abscesses, and ipsilateral empyema [158]. Abdominal ultrasound has been found to be a reliable method of early detection of acalculous cholecystitis and for follow-up of possible complications [159]. Diagnostic laparoscopy might be another accurate method to establish the early diagnosis [160]. Treatment of acalculous cholecystitis requires surgery and appropriate antimicrobial therapy. Other important ICU-specific problems include *Pneumocystis carinii* pneumonia in patients with the acquired immunodeficiency syndrome, toxic shock syndrome, meningitis, and antibiotic-associated colitis, which are discussed in Chapters 34, 36, 37, 41, and 43, respectively.

The differentiation of the causes of fever in ICU patients is a daily challenge for physicians. Not all fevers are the result of infections; nosocomial fever often does not signal nosocomial infection and may augur a wide variety of other conditions [161]. The most common causes of noninfectious fever are listed in Table 25-3.

Control and Prevention of Nosocomial Infections

Surveillance

Two types of measures are needed to control nosocomial infections. Engineering controls are those controls that are incorporated into the structural design of the unit or equipment and over which there is limited human control (see Chapter 20). Administrative controls are guidelines that must be learned and executed by healthcare workers (see Chapter 3). The latter are effective only if appropriate changes in behavior are incorporated into the routine activities of healthcare workers. We recently experienced a cluster of cases of invasive pulmonary aspergillosis in nonimmunocompromised patients associated with room air filter replacement [162]. Such fatal infection could have been prevented by the establishment and application of guidelines for this procedure.

Engineering Controls

The contribution of the design of critical care units to the control of nosocomial infection is difficult to evalu-

TABLE 25-3. *Noninfectious fever in ICU patients*

Atelectasis
ARDS
Central fever in head trauma patients
Chemical aspiration
Congestive heart failure
Deep venous thrombosis
Drug fever
Pancreatitis
Postoperative fever (during the first 72 hr after surgery)
Pulmonary fibroproliferation or embolism
Resorption of hematomas

ate. However, it seems prudent to consider several issues when remodeling or designing new units.

1. Adequate space around beds is important for placement of support and monitoring equipment, allowing staff access to both the patient and the equipment.
2. Individualized cubicles for each patient may also be important in reducing transmission of pathogens in the unit; the nurse-to-patient ratio should, however, not be affected by geographical distribution.
3. Sinks should be located in convenient places to facilitate hand washing by healthcare workers and to interrupt the most important mode of microbial transmission in the ICU. Separate, designated sinks should be provided for cleaning equipment.
4. All ICUs should be equipped with one or more class A isolation rooms [163]. Class A isolation rooms include an anteroom for gowning and hand washing (see Chapter 13). Additional rooms for isolation precautions are necessary in units where patients are located in large open rooms.
5. Consideration should also be given to functional activities in the unit. Attention to traffic patterns and the location of clean and dirty utilities and janitors' closets may reduce opportunities for cross-contamination. Clean function and storage should be physically separate from dirty function and waste disposal (see Chapter 21). Housekeeping facilities and equipment should be designated for the specific unit and stored separately from clean and dirty utilities.

Although guidelines for constructing and equipping ICUs seem prudent and might be helpful in controlling infections [164], several well-designed studies failed to find improvement in the rates of nosocomial infections after the units were moved into new structures [165]. Studies of postoperative wound infection rates after improvements in the structural design of ICUs have yielded conflicting results. Some investigators have reported lower infection rates, whereas others did not find a significant improvement. Huebner and colleagues [166] conducted a 2-year prospective study after transferring an ICU into a new structure that provided more space and more isolation rooms for infected or colonized patients. They reported that the overall rate of nosocomial infections did not change appreciably after the move.

Administrative Controls for Medical Equipment

Medical technology is changing rapidly, and new diagnostic and therapeutic devices are constantly being introduced into ICUs. In many instances, the efficacy of the devices has not been adequately evaluated, and the effect of the devices on the incidence of nosocomial infections is unknown. For example, vendors seeking to introduce new catheters alleged to have antimicrobial activity should be challenged to provide data on the efficacy of their product. Cleaning protocols for invasive devices should be provided by the industry and be reviewed by infection control practitioners or hospital epidemiologists to ensure the adequacy of the recommendations. Sufficient numbers of frequently used instruments should be available to allow time for cleaning, disinfection, or sterilization. An increase in the initial outlay for equipment may reduce costs and morbidity in the long term. The routine application of guidelines for the appropriate use of medical devices contributes significantly to the control of nosocomial infections. Guidelines for the use and control of urinary tract catheters (see Chapter 31), intravascular devices (see Chapter 44), respiratory devices (see Chapter 32), and other products have been published by the CDC.

Administrative Controls for healthcare Personnel

Staffing and Training

For the patient to benefit from technologic advances in medical care, healthcare workers must be well trained in state-of-the-art intensive care. Studies have documented that cooperation among critical care personnel can directly influence outcomes from intensive care, suggesting that the use of invasive technologies is important but not sufficient for good care of patients. Therefore, healthcare workers in ICUs should be involved in continuous postgraduate medical education to learn new technologies and the proper use of new medical devices and procedures. They also need periodic updates on new disease entities peculiar to patients in ICUs, including the psychologic problems associated with hospitalization in an ICU. Finally, the level of stress in ICUs exceeds that of most other areas of the hospital. As a result, rates of employee turnover are high in special care units. Loss of highly skilled medical care workers requires extensive training of replacement workers, including in-depth training on infection control procedures. Changes in staff and unrecognized modifications in infection control procedures might contribute to epidemics of nosocomial infections.

The extent and severity of illnesses afflicting patients in ICUs demand a high level of nursing care, and the high rate of nosocomial infections mandates strict application of rigid barrier nursing techniques to control transmission (see Chapter 13). Breakdown in these techniques during periods of understaffing or overcrowding has been associated with outbreaks of nosocomial infection [167]. A nurse-to-patient staffing ratio of 1:1 has been recommended to reduce lapses in techniques that lead to person-to-person transmission of pathogens within ICUs [168]. A study by Fridkin and colleagues underlines the importance of an adequate nurse-to-patient ratio [169]. In this study, a low nurse-to-patient ratio was found to be an independent risk factor for bloodstream infections in SICU patients associated with the use of central venous catheters. The authors conclude that reductions in nursing staff below a critical level may cause an increase in such bloodstream infections in ICUs by making adequate catheter care difficult [169].

It is important that workers in ICUs understand their responsibility in preventing transmission of infectious diseases. This responsibility includes prevention of spread of pathogens from patient to patient and from the healthcare worker to the patient. Therefore, it is important that the hospital provide adequate staffing to cover medical absences and personal benefits that will not punish employees who are responsible enough to avoid working when ill (see Chapter 3).

Monitoring Quality of Care

The effectiveness of administrative controls will depend on compliance with established guidelines. Therefore, the performance and behavior of healthcare providers should be monitored. Failure to comply with guidelines, whether on the part of physicians, nurses, or other support personnel, should be addressed promptly to prevent the establishment of bad habits that impose unnecessary risks on patients (see Chapter 2). Monitoring the quality of medical care in ICUs is important, albeit controversial, given the complexity of the conditions of the patients and the procedures performed in these units [170,171]. Few studies have been published regarding the assessment of the quality of care in ICUs. In a study conducted by Fernandez-Segoviano et al. [172], the clinical and pathologic diagnoses from 100 patients who came to autopsy were compared as measures of quality of care. In 77% of the patients, the major clinical diagnoses were confirmed by autopsy. But it is worth noting that myocardial infarction and peritonitis were the most commonly missed diagnoses.

Administrative Controls for Patients

Because of the risk of infection and other complications in ICUs, only patients who will benefit from high-intensity, high-risk care should be admitted to ICUs, and patients should be discharged from the ICU as soon as possible to lower the risk of nosocomial infection. Unfortunately, there is little published information to assist the physician in those important decisions. Surveillance for nosocomial infections, monitoring rates of infection, and reporting results to personnel are important to ensure the quality of medical care in ICUs (see Chapter 5). Properly conducted surveillance can identify behavioral, environmental, or treatment factors that, when corrected, will diminish endemic rates of infection in the unit. Additional benefits of concurrent surveillance include early identification and intervention in epidemics.

Practical Aspects of Infection Control in the ICU

Methods for preventing nosocomial infections are numerous. The principles are the same throughout the hospital, and many are discussed elsewhere in the text. Only selected measures of prime importance in the ICU will be discussed in this section.

Patient Isolation

More than 50% of patients admitted to ICUs are colonized at the time of admission with the organism responsible for subsequent infections. Patients who are readmitted to the hospital may carry and transmit resistant organisms acquired during previous hospitalizations. Not infrequently, unrecognized infection contributes to the decision for entry into the unit. The early diagnosis of potentially transmissible disease requires vigilance on the part of ICU physicians. Patients with suspected infections should be appropriately segregated at the time of admission. The level of isolation should account for each of the following factors: the site of infection, the mode of transmission, the amount of secretions or excretions, and the virulence and antimicrobial susceptibilities of the causative agent. The isolation guidelines published by the CDC are useful in this respect (see Chapter 13).

Discussion of specific isolation techniques are beyond the scope of this chapter. It should be recognized that as the duration of stay increases, the frequency of colonization with resistant microflora also grows. Patients become animate reservoirs that facilitate transmission to susceptible incoming patients (see Chapter 1). It may be wise, therefore, to separate long-stay patients from the short-stay patients who make up the major portion of the population in the unit. This segregation may be accomplished by moving chronically ill patients to single rooms or relocating groups of patients to a physically separate part of the unit. A dedicated nursing staff for the long-term patients would provide an added barrier to transmission, but this is frequently impossible to implement. Adequate hand washing or hand antisepsis certainly constitutes the most appropriate, least expensive, and highly effective measure, but lack of compliance is an issue.

Frequent transfers of patients through various units and levels of care increase the risk of transmission of resistant organisms throughout the hospital. Moreover, colonized patients are important animate reservoirs of resistant microorganisms during interinstitutional transfers and probably account for the spread of MRSA [89,94] (see Chapter 41). To control the spread of resistant organisms, it is extremely important to document information regarding carriage of antibiotic-resistant microflora in the patient's medical record and to report it to receiving units and facilities.

Hand Washing

Routine hand washing before and between contact with patients is the most important feature of infection control. Virtually all medical care workers are aware of and agree with this concept [173,174]. It is dismaying, therefore, to see repeated reports of low levels of compliance with this simple and inexpensive technique. In ICUs, compliance usually does not exceed 40%. Several reasons have been suggested to account for this low level of compliance, including lack of priority over other required procedures, insufficient time to accomplish hand washing, inconvenient placement of hand-washing sinks or other hand-washing tools, allergy or intolerance to the hand-washing solutions, lack of leadership on the part of the senior medical staff, and lack of personal commitment to the routine of hand washing (see Chapters 13, 20).

In a study published by Doebbeling and co-workers [173], a hand-disinfection system using an antimicrobial agent (chlorhexidine) reduced the rate of nosocomial infections more effectively than one using alcohol and soap. The improvement may be explained at least in part by better compliance with hand-washing instructions when chlorhexidine was used [173]. Better compliance was associated with a significant decrease in the incidence of ICU-acquired infections in this study (adjusted incidence density ratio of 0.73, 95% CI=0.59 to 0.9).

Barrier Precautions

There is currently little evidence that the addition of gloves in the routine intensive care setting has any benefit over regular hand washing in controlling infections. However, well-designed studies are extremely difficult to conduct. Major arguments against the routine use of gloves in ICUs rely on the fact that healthcare workers frequently do not remove gloves when moving from patient to patient and forget to wash their hands after glove removal.

Whereas a number of studies investigated the role of very sophisticated forms of protective isolation in reducing high rates of nosocomial infections in patients with profound granulocytopenia or full-thickness burns, only a few have evaluated whether simple protective isolation would be beneficial for ICU patients. Klein and co-workers [175] conducted a prospective, randomized trial in a pediatric ICU. In this well-designed study, the authors tested the benefit of simple barrier precautions (disposable gown and gloves) on both colonization and subsequent infection. Colonization with ICU bacterial strains occurred an average of 5 days later in isolated patients (simple barrier precautions, n=32). The daily rate of infection for isolated patients was 2.2 times lower than among patients provided standard care (n=38, p=0.007).

Although previous studies have reported conflicting results concerning the value of protective isolation in ICU patients, gowns and gloves may be effective in dealing with selected high-risk patients. Further studies are necessary to determine the cost-effectiveness of this approach in the general ICU population. To draw definitive conclusions regarding the effectiveness of this approach, compliance with isolation precautions should also be evaluated. Only a few studies have analyzed compliance with isolation precautions [175–177], and most reported < 50% compliance, despite the fact that healthcare workers were aware that they were under observation [176].

The use of special clothing in ICUs is frequently discussed but has little documentation or support. Carriage of potential pathogens on the gowns and uniforms of healthcare workers in special care units has been repeatedly studied. Isolation of microorganisms from clothing has been confirmed, and carriage increases with time. However, evidence that clothing is important in the transmission of nosocomial pathogens has been convincingly documented in only a few instances. It appears prudent to avoid contamination of uniforms with organisms, but there is no evidence that the addition of special surgical scrubs or caps lowers the rates of nosocomial infections.

Special Units, Special Problems

Each subspecialty unit uses unique medical and administrative methods in the care of patients that are, in turn, associated with special risks. Consequently, each unit develops unique endemic and epidemic nosocomial infection problems. The variation in risk of nosocomial infection will be recognized only with active surveillance systems in each unit. In a study evaluating infection reports from 66 hospitals between 1986 and 1990, the rate and distribution of infections by site and pathogen were shown to vary considerably by ICU type [36]. Effective surveillance allows for early interception of problems and the development of efficacious, focused interventions.

New Therapeutic Approaches

Selective Digestive Decontamination

Since many nosocomial infections are believed to arise from endogenous flora in the oropharyngeal and gastrointestinal tract, innovations in prevention have focused on the control (decontamination) of potential pathogens with oral antimicrobial therapy (see Chapter 15). The aim of selective digestive decontamination (SDD) is to prevent overgrowth of pathogenic gram-negative aerobic bacilli and yeasts by using oral nonabsorbable antibiotics that preserve the endogenous anaerobic flora [178].

In addition to its potential, but very controversial role in preventing ICU-acquired infections, SDD was thought to be of benefit in controlling endotoxemia arising from bowel flora and phenomena associated with endotoxin release, such as MODS, ARDS, and renal failure [179]. However, controversy still exists concerning the use of this therapy because the antibiotics may enhance the release of endotoxins by killing bacteria in the bowel. In a study published by Bion et al. [180], SDD reduced gram-negative pulmonary colonization but failed to clear endotoxemia in patients undergoing elective liver transplantation. The authors conclude that this inability of SDD to affect endotoxemia may be one possible explanation for the failure of SDD to enhance survival rates in many studies.

Another role for SDD may be in the control of nosocomial outbreaks. Brun-Buisson and colleagues [41] reported that intestinal decontamination by oral nonabsorbable antibiotics was important in resolving an outbreak of infection with multiresistant *Enterobacteriaceae* in an MICU. In units where routine infection control measures fail to control outbreaks [62], careful application of SDD, including the selection of appropriate oral antimicrobial agents and diligent monitoring for the emergence of new resistant strains, might be an important adjunct to conventional infection control procedures.

In summary, the use of SDD remains one of the most controversial issues in critical care medicine. Thus, in spite of the data from many clinical trials, it seems difficult to recommend confidently that SDD be either abandoned or used routinely in the ICU setting. It may be premature to ignore the potential benefits of SDD, because the results of most clinical trials have been encouraging in terms of reducing infection rates. Although additional studies are clearly needed, it may not be practical to design and execute a multicenter clinical trial that is properly controlled and large enough to solve this dilemma. For the present, use of SDD is more a question of philosophy and art rather than an exact science [181]. We believe that SDD should be restricted to well-controlled clinical studies among homogeneous subgroups of patients at high risk of nosocomial pneumonia or to situations in which efficacy and cost-effectiveness have been established. In any of these cases, surveillance for antimicrobial resistance must be done. Table 25-4 summarizes situations in which SDD may be beneficial.

TABLE 25-4. *Possible indications for selective decontamination in patients admitted to ICUs*

- Neutropenia
- Multiple trauma
- Outbreak of multiresistant gram-negative bacilli
- Esophageal resection
- Hepatic, renal, and pancreatic transplantation
- Prolonged ICU stay

New Therapy for Sepsis

Endotoxin release by gram-negative bacteria contributes to the clinical manifestations of sepsis in febrile patients. Consequently, a number of clinical trials have been conducted using either hyperimmune serum or anti-endotoxin antibodies for the treatment of gram-negative bacteremia. The initial study by Ziegler and associates [182] was a multicenter, double-blind trial of antiserum prepared by immunizing donors with a "J5" mutant of E. coli 0111. Although treatment with the antiserum was associated with reversal of profound shock, little effect on mortality was reported, and no protective antibody titer could be detected. Following this first report, efforts have been made to produce human antiserum by active immunization with other core endotoxin antigens and to produce monoclonal antibodies of murine or human origin.

Two controlled trials investigated the value of E5, a monoclonal antibody of murine origin [183,184]. The more recently published, second large controlled clinical study of E5 yielded negative results [184]. Among the primary group of patients with clinical symptoms of sepsis and documented gram-negative infection, treatment with E5 had no effect on the mortality rate over a 30-day period of observation. The 30-day mortality rate was slightly higher in the E5 group than in the placebo group. When some secondary outcome parameters, such as resolution of major organ failures, were analyzed, treatment with E5 showed evidence of being beneficial. In addition, E5 resulted in the prevention of adult respiratory distress syndrome and central nervous system organ failure. Nevertheless, it is not clear if further clinical studies of this particular immunotherapeutic agent are warranted, since a number of compounds are now under investigation that appear to be much more effective as endotoxin-neutralizing agents. These compounds include bactericidal permeability–increasing protein [185], cationic antimicrobial protein [186], limulus anti-lipopolysaccharide factor [187], and other novel agents [188].

In addition, a number of large multicenter trials designed to assess the value of HA-1A, a monoclonal antibody directed against the lipid A portion of endotoxins, have been published during the past half decade [189–192]. Taken together, the results of these clinical studies have not been encouraging, producing equivocal results at best. After a first promising publication [189], which was the subject of great controversy, a second multicenter Centroxin-HA-IA Efficacy in Septic Shock (CHESS) trial was terminated after an interim analysis of 1,500 patients found high mortality rates in patients without gram-negative bacteremia who received HA-1A. A French cohort study confirmed the suspicion that HA-1A was developed without reproducible and independently confirmed preclinical results and that rigorous standards were not maintained in evaluating the trial data of the first HA-1A trial [191–193].

Interleukin-1 receptor antagonist (IL-1ra) is a naturally occurring human protein produced by macrophages and other cells in response to IL-1, endotoxin, and other microbial products. Recombinant human IL-1ra prevented death in animal models of endotoxemia and *E. coli* bacteremia [194,195]. Results from two clinical trials have been encouraging and indicate that the outcome of patients with bacterial sepsis might be affected favorably [196,197].

Tumor necrosis factor (TNF), a cytokine produced by activated macrophage, is a primary mediator of the deleterious effects of endotoxin in animals and humans. It plays a major role in the pathogenesis of the septic shock syndrome [198–202]. Plasma TNF levels also rise in the context of a large variety of severe infections [203–205]. Anti-TNF therapies appear to attenuate the injurious effects of TNF. Anti-TNF antibodies protect animals from death caused by endotoxin and gram-negative and gram-positive bacteria and might provide a more general therapy for sepsis than anti-endotoxin antibodies [206–212]. Two phase III studies have already evaluated a murine monoclonal antibody against TNF. The study performed by the North American TNF Sepsis study group revealed a trend toward reduction in mortality rates associated with TNF-antibody therapy [213,214]. Further clinical trials are under way to investigate the efficacy and safety of human TNF receptor antagonists. Preliminary results seem promising.

The value of corticosteroids in the treatment of gram-negative septicemia has been the subject of controversy. In view of the results of a recently published meta-analysis [215] that failed to find a beneficial effect of corticosteroids in the treatment of septic shock and ARDS, this approach cannot be recommended. The authors of this meta-analysis conclude that current evidence provides no support for the use of corticosteroids in patients with sepsis or septic shock and suggests that their use may even be harmful [215]. In these studies, however, large doses of steroids were given at the time of study entry. In patients with septic shock and laboratory test evidence of adrenal insufficiency, repeated doses of corticosteroids might be beneficial; appropriately designed clinical trials should, however, be conducted to test this hypothesis.

Nitric oxide synthase inhibitors have been shown to reverse hypovolemic shock in some experimental studies [216]; in other studies such inhibition had detrimental hemodynamic effects [217,218]. Taking into account these controversial data, nitric oxide synthase inhibitors should be tested only very carefully in well-controlled clinical trials to determine whether they are of benefit for hemodynamic support [219].

Preemptive Therapy

Continued progress in supportive care will be associated with new infections and disease processes. *Candida* infections have become increasingly important, in particular, among critically ill surgical patients [66,220]. Infections mainly evolve from endogenous colonization facilitated by the use of broad-spectrum antibiotics [65,68, 221]. The intensity of *Candida* spp colonization constitutes a strong predictor of subsequent severe infection [64,68,221]. Recognizing the high morbidity and mortality rates associated with those infections [64,65,68,222], an aggressive approach to suspected *Candida* infections seems justified. Preemptive therapy in patients at high risk of infection would need to be tested in prospective, controlled, randomized clinical trials [66,223–225]. These infections constitute an example of what could be the future for other conditions that compromise the benefit of intensive care in critically ill patients.

High Mortality Rates and Impact of Infections

Nosocomial infections in the ICU are harmful for the patients and expensive for society. Recently published data indicate that nosocomial pneumonia and bacteremia are associated with a two- to threefold increased risk of death in critically ill patients [105,107,226–231]. Clinical signs of sepsis—in the absence of positive blood cultures—were associated with an increased risk of death (OR=3.50, 95% CI=1.71 to 7.18) after adjustment for other confounding factors (age, severity of illness, presence of organ failure) in the recently published EPIC study [20]. Thus, in contrast to a widespread theory, a significant proportion of patients in the ICU more die due to nosocomial infection than the infection that brought them into the hospital.

Crude mortality rates in patients who acquire nosocomial infections in the ICU are estimated to vary between 10% and 80%. The term attributable mortality defines the mortality directly associated with the infection, apart from the mortality attributable to underlying conditions. In ICU patients, underlying conditions apart from nosocomial infection that may affect the outcome mainly include preexisting co-morbidities, severity of acute physiologic disturbance, and complications arising from these conditions [232]. Assessing preexisting co-morbidities at the time of admission to the ICU significantly improved the prediction of mortality from bacteremic sepsis compared with using the APACHE II score alone [233].

Assessment of mortality attributable to nosocomial infections in the ICU setting is difficult and not straightforward because nosocomial infections and mortality attributable to other causes share common risk factors that may confound the cause-and-effect relationship. Thus, it is sometimes difficult to estimate whether the critically ill patient would have survived in the absence of a nosocomial infection [231]. The most reliable and often used approach to estimate the attributable mortality of nosocomial infections in ICU patients is to conduct a matched case-control study. In this type of study design, cases are defined as patients in whom nosocomial infections develop during their ICU stay. These case patients are subsequently compared with noninfected controls. Case and control patients are usually matched for age, the time of the year, the underlying diseases, and additional variables that may contribute to excessive mortality rates or extra lengths of ICU stay independent of the infection itself. Control patients are selected among the ICU population according to matching variables, if possible in a stepwise fashion [222,230].

In brief, the attributable morbidity or mortality due to nosocomial infection defines excess rates of morbidity or mortality due to the infection. The attributable mortality is determined by subtracting the crude mortality rate of the cases from the crude mortality rate of the closely matched controls. Similarly, the excess length of ICU or hospital stay defines differences in the length of ICU and hospital stay after the infection. Table 25-5 summarizes estimates of high mortality rates, extra lengths of stay, and associated additional costs attributable to nosocomial bloodstream infection and pneumonia in ICU populations.

The economic burden associated with nosocomial infection varies from institution to institution and from country to country; for example, the extra costs associated with nosocomial bloodstream infection acquired in a surgical ICU in the United States averaged $40,000 per survivor [230]. In addition, attributable mortality can be higher for infections caused by multiply resistant microorganisms [105]. The relative risk of death following nosocomial infection is even higher in patients with less severe underlying disease, probably because patients with very severe underlying conditions are already carrying a higher mortality risk [229,231].

In a large cohort of critically ill patients with sepsis confirmed by positive blood cultures—bacteremic sepsis—with a precise follow-up to hospital discharge, we identified easily obtained clinical and biochemical variables that independently predict mortality at pivotal times [234]. Of the 5,457 patients admitted to the ICU, sepsis developed in 176, with confirmed positive blood cultures (3.2 per 100 admissions). The fatality rate was 35% at 28 days after the onset of sepsis; in-hospital mortality was 43%. Independent predictors of mortality at onset of sepsis were previous antibiotic therapy, hypothermia, requirement for mechanical ventilation, and onset-of-sepsis APACHE II score. Vital organ dysfunction developing after the onset of sepsis influenced the outcome markedly.

The best two independent prognostic factors were the APACHE II score at the onset of sepsis (OR=1.13 per unit, 95% CI 1.08 to 1.17) and the number of organ dysfunctions developing thereafter (OR=2.39, 95% CI 2.02 to 2.82). Thus, in ICU patients with sepsis and positive blood cultures, outcome can be predicted by the severity of illness at onset of sepsis and the number of vital organ dysfunctions developing subsequently. In critically ill patients with bloodstream infection, those factors had a more significant impact on the prognosis than microbiologic characteristics [234]. These findings have been confirmed in patients with severe sepsis, whether or not the infection was microbiologically documented, both in a large prospective study at a single institution [136] and in a cohort of 11,828 patients admitted to 170 adult ICUs in France [34].

Effective infection control measures may substantially decrease the cost of hospitalization by reducing the direct

TABLE 25-5. *Excess mortality rates and costs of nosocomial infections in ICUs*

References	Clinical diagnosis	Setting	Crude mortality	Attributable mortality	Risk ratio (95% CI)	Impact (extra days/$)
Fagon et al. [105]	Pneumonia	ICU	26/48 (54%)	27%	2.5 (1.31—4.61)	13 days
Craig and Connelly [226]	Pneumonia	ICU/hospital	11/54 (20%)	15%	NR	11 days
Leu et al. [107]	Pneumonia	ICU/hospital	15/74 (20%)	7%	NR	9 days
Kappstein et al. [246]	Pneumonia	ICU	NR	NR	NR	10/8,800
Pittet et al. [230]	Bacteremia	ICU	43/86 (50%)	35%	3.31 (1.78—6.15)	14/40,000
Smith et al. [227]	Bacteremia	ICU	28/34 (82%)	28%	NR	NR
Garo and Boles [247]	Pneumonia/ bacteremia	ICU	10/31 (32%)	22%	NR	21/3,441
Bueno Cavanillas et al. [229]	Pneumonia/ bacteremia	ICU	43/279 (16%)	NR	2.5 (1.47—4.16)	NR

NR, not reported.

costs of diagnosing and treating nosocomial infection and associated complications, by shortening the time in the ICU and the overall hospital stay, and by improving patients' survival (see Chapter 17).

Comments

Considerable progress has been made in providing intensive care and life support to patients who are acutely ill. Unfortunately, each new technologic advance is accompanied by potential risks for the patient, including that of nosocomial infections. Clinical research is needed to address the benefits and risks associated with these new interventions. To achieve these objectives, collaboration is needed among critical care physicians, epidemiologists, and infection control practitioners to design appropriate studies, interventions, and policies. Because of problems associated with small sample size and individual institutions, the generation of useful information will be expedited by the development of multicenter studies evaluating benefits and risks. The challenge is to avoid undoing the benefits of intensive care by minimizing risk of complications.

REFERENCES

1. Abramson NS, Wald KS, Grenvik AN, Robinson D, Snyder J. Adverse occurrences in intensive care units. *JAMA* 1980;244:1582–1584.
2. Donowitz LG, Wenzel RP, Hoyt JW. High risk of hospital-acquired infection in the ICU patient. *Crit Care Med* 1982;10:355–357.
3. Wenzel RP, Thompson RL, Landry SM, et al. Hospital-acquired infections in intensive care unit patients: an overview with emphasis on epidemics. *Infect Control Hosp Epidemiol* 1983;4:371–375.
4. Donowitz LG. High risk of nosocomial infection in the pediatric critical care patient. *Crit Care Med* 1986;14:26–28.
5. Brun-Buisson C, Legrand P, Philippon A, Montravers F, Ansquer M, Duval J. Transferable enzymatic resistance to third-generation cephalosporins during nosocomial outbreak of multiresistant *Klebsiella pneumoniae*. *Lancet* 1987;2:302–306.
6. Bistrian BR, Blackburn GL, Vitale J, Cochran D, Naylor J. Prevalence of malnutrition in general medicine patients. *JAMA* 1976;235:1567–1570.
7. Apelgren KN, Rombeau JL, Miller RA, Waters LN, Carson SN, Twomey P. Malnutrition in Veterans Administration surgical patients. *Arch Surg* 1981;116:1059–1061.
8. O'Leary JP, Dunn GD, Basil S. Incidence of malnutrition among patients admitted to a VA hospital. *South Med J* 1982;75:1095–1098.
9. Askanazi J, Hensle TW, Starker PM. Effect of immediate postoperative nutritional support on length of hospitalization. *Ann Surg* 1986; 203:236–239.
10. Rich MW, Keller AJ, Schechtman KB, Marshall WG Jr., Kouchoukos NT. Increased complications and prolonged hospital stay in elderly cardiac surgical patients with low serum albumin. *Am J Cardiol* 1989; 63:714–718.
11. Buzby GP, Mullen JL, Matthews DC, Hobbs CL, Rosato EF. Prognostic nutritional index in gastrointestinal surgery. *Am J Surg* 1980;139: 160–167.
12. Temple WJ, Voitk AJ, Snelling CFT, Crispin JS. Effect of nutrition, diet and suture material on long term wound healing. *Ann Surg* 1975; 182:93–97.
13. Pingleton SK. Enteral nutrition and infection in the intensive care unit. *Semin Respir Infect* 1990;5:185–190.
14. Isaack H, Mbise RL, Hirji KF. Nosocomial bacterial infections among children with severe protein energy malnutrition. *East Afr Med J* 1992;69:433–436.
15. Christman JW, McCain RW. A sensible approach to the nutritional support of mechanically ventilated critically ill patients. *Intensive Care Med* 1993;19:129–136.
16. Minard G, Kudsk KA. Effect of route of feeding on the incidence of septic complications in critically ill patients. *Semin Respir Infect* 1994;9:228–231.
17. Schimpff SC, Miller RM, Polkavetz S, Hornick R. Infection in the severely traumatized patient. *Ann Surg* 1974;179:352–357.
18. Hoch RC, Rodriguez R, Manning T, et al. Effects of accidental trauma on cytokine and endotoxin production. *Crit Care Med* 1993;21: 839–845.
19. Abraham E. T- and B-cell function and their roles in resistance to infection. *New Horiz* 1993;1:28–36.
20. Vincent JL, Bihari DJ, Suter PM. The prevalence of nosocomial infection in intensive care units in Europe: results of the European Prevalence of Infection in Intensive Care (EPIC) Study. *JAMA* 1995;274: 639–644.
21. Mermel L, Pearson K, Parenteau S. Intravenous catheter use in intensive care units [Abstract]. Presented at the Society of Healthcare Epidemiology of America Meeting, March 20–22, 1994, New Orleans, Louisiana.
22. McCabe WR, Jackson GG. Gram-negative bacteremia I. Etiology and ecology. *Arch Intern Med* 1962;110:847–855.
23. Britt MR, Schleupner CJ, Matsumiya S. Severity of underlying disease as a predictor of nosocomial infection. *JAMA* 1978;239:1047–1051.
24. Haley RW, Hooton TM, Culver DH, et al. Nosocomial infections in U.S. hospitals, 1975–1976: estimated frequency by selected characteristics of patients. *Am J Med* 1981;70:947–959.
25. Knaus WA, Draper EA, Wagner DP, Zimmerman JE. APACHE II: a severity of disease classification system. *Crit Care Med* 1985;13: 818–829.
26. Le Gall JR, Lemeshow S, Saulnier F. A new Simplified Acute Physiology Score (SAPS II) based on a European/North American multicenter study. *JAMA* 1993;270:2957–2963.
27. Lemeshow S, Teres D, Klar J, Avrunin JS, Gehlbach SH, Rapoport J. Mortality Probability Models (MPM II) based on an international cohort of intensive care unit patients. *JAMA* 1993;270:2478–2486.
28. Knaus WA, Wagner DP, Draper EA, et al. The APACHE III prognostic system: risk prediction of hospital mortality for critically ill hospitalized adults. *Chest* 1991;100:1619–1636.
29. Wagner DP, Knaus WA, Harrell FE, Zimmerman JE, Watts C. Daily prognostic estimates for critically ill adults in intensive care units: results from a prospective, multicenter, inception cohort analysis. *Crit Care Med* 1994;22:1359–1372.
30. Lemeshow S, Klar J, Teres D, et al. Mortality probability models for patients in the intensive care unit for 48 or 72 hours: a prospective, multicenter study. *Crit Care Med* 1994;22:1351–1358.
31. Le Gall JR, Lemeshow S, Leleu G, et al. Customized probability models for early severe sepsis in adult intensive care patients. *JAMA* 1995; 273:644–650.
32. Knaus WA, Harrell FE, Fisher CJ, et al. The clinical evaluation of new drugs for sepsis: a prospective study design based on survival analysis. *JAMA* 1993;270:1233–1241.
33. American College of Chest Physicians/Society of Critical Care Medicine Consensus Conference. Definitions for sepsis and organ failure and guidelines for the use of innovative therapies in sepsis. *Crit Care Med* 1992;20:864–874.
34. Brun-Buisson C, Doyon F, Carlet J, et al. Incidence, risk factors, and outcome of severe sepsis and septic shock in adults: a multicenter prospective study in intensive care units. *JAMA* 1995;274:968–974.
35. Gross PA, DeMauro PJ, Van Antwerpen C, Wallenstein S, Chiang S. Number of comorbidities as a predictor of nosocomial infection acquisition. *Infect Control Hosp Epidemiol* 1988;9:497–500.
36. Jarvis WR, Edwards JR, Culver DH, et al. Nosocomial infection rates in adult and pediatric intensive care units in the United States: National Nosocomial Infections Surveillance System. *Am J Med* 1991;91:185S–191S.
37. Schaberg DR, Culver DH, Gaynes RP. Major trends in the microbial etiology of nosocomial infection. *Am J Med* 1991;91:72S–75S.
38. Martin MA. Nosocomial infections in intensive care units: an overview of their epidemiology, outcome, and prevention. *New Horiz* 1993;1:162–171.

39. Voss A, Milatovic D, Wallrauch-Schwarz C, Rosdahl VT, Braveny I. Methicillin-resistant *Staphylococcus aureus* in Europe. *Eur J Clin Microbiol Infect Dis* 1994;13:50–55.
40. Casewell MW, Phillips I. Aspects of the plasmid-mediated antibiotic resistance and epidemiology of *Klebsiella* species. *Am J Med* 1981; 70:459–462.
41. Brun-Buisson C, Legrand P, Rauss A. Intestinal decontamination for control of nosocomial multiresistant gram-negative bacilli: study of an outbreak in an intensive care unit. *Ann Intern Med* 1989;110:873–881.
42. Verweij PE, van Belkum A, Melchers WJ, Voss A, Hoogkamp Korstanje JA, Meis JF. Interrepeat fingerprinting of third-generation cephalosporin-resistant *Enterobacter cloacae* isolated during an outbreak in a neonatal intensive care unit. *Infect Control Hosp Epidemiol* 1995;16:25–29.
43. Price DJ, Sleigh J. Control of infection due to *Klebsiella aerogenes* in a neurosurgical unit by withdrawal of all antibiotics. *Lancet* 1970;2: 1213–1215.
44. Jarlier V, Nicolas MH, Fournier G, Philippon A. Extended broad-spectrum beta-lactamases conferring transferable resistance to newer beta-lactam agents in *Enterobacteriaceae*: hospital prevalence and susceptibility patterns. *Rev Infect Dis* 1988;10:867–878.
45. Sirot J, Chanal C, Petit A, Sirot D, Labia R, Gerbaud G. *Klebsiella pneumoniae* and other *Enterobacteriaceae* producing novel plasmid-mediated beta-lactamases markedly active against third- generation cephalosporins: epidemiologic studies. *Rev Infect Dis* 1988;10:850–859.
46. Laing FP, Ramotar K, Read RR, et al. Molecular epidemiology of *Xanthomonas maltophilia* colonization and infection in the hospital environment. *J Clin Microbiol* 1995;33:513–518.
47. VanCouwenberghe C, Cohen S. Analysis of epidemic and endemic isolates of *Xanthomonas maltophilia* by contour-clamped homogeneous electric field gel electrophoresis. *Infect Control Hosp Epidemiol* 1994;15:691–696.
48. Axelrod P, Talbot GH. Risk factors for acquisition of gentamicin-resistant enterococci: a multivariate analysis. *Arch Intern Med* 1989;149: 1397–1401.
49. Edmond MB, Ober JF, Weinbaum DL, Wenzel RP, Pfaller MA. Vancomycin-resistant *Enterococcus faecium* bacteremia: risk factors for infection. *Clin Infect Dis* 1995;20:1126–1133.
50. De Champs C, Sauvant MP, Chanal C, et al. Prospective survey of colonization and infection caused by expanded-spectrum-beta-lactamase-producing members of the family *Enterobacteriaceae* in an intensive care unit. *J Clin Microbiol* 1989;27:2887–2890.
51. Monnet D. Relationship between antibiotic resistance and antibiotic use. Presented at the 35th Interscience Conference on Antimicrobial Agents and Chemotherapy, San Francisco, September 17–20, 1995.
52. Monnet D, Edwards J, Gaynes R. Extended spectrum beta-lactam-resistant nosocomial *Klebsiella pneumoniae* (ESB-KP): epidemiologic evidence of interhospital transmission [Abstract]. *Infect Control Hosp Epidemiol* 1994;15:P23.
53. Johanson WG, Pierce AK, Sanford J. Changing pharyngeal bacterial flora of hospitalized patients: emergence of gram-negative bacilli. *N Engl J Med* 1969;281:1137–1140.
54. Atherton ST, White D. Stomach as source of bacteria colonising respiratory tract during artificial ventilation. *Lancet* 1978;2:968–969.
55. Hartenauer U, Weilemann LS, Bodmann KF, Ritzerfeld WW, Asmus S, Koch EM. Comparative clinical trial of ceftazidime and imipenem/cilastatin in patients with severe nosocomial pneumonias and septicaemias. *J Hosp Infect* 1990;15(suppl A):61–64.
56. Donaldson SG, Azizi SQ, Dal Nogare AR. Characteristics of aerobic gram negative bacteria colonizing critically ill patients. *Am Rev Respir Dis* 1995;144:202–207.
57. Kerver AJ, Rommes JH, Mevissen Verhage EA, et al. Prevention of colonization and infection in critically ill patients: a prospective randomized study. *Crit Care Med* 1988;16:1087–1093.
58. LaForce F. Hospital-acquired gram-negative rod pneumonias: an overview. *Am J Med* 1981;70:664–669.
59. Heyland DK, Cook DJ, Jaeschke R, Griffith L, Lee HN, Guyatt GH. Selective decontamination of the digestive tract: an overview. *Chest* 1994;105:1221–1229.
60. Marshall JC, Christou NV, Meakins JL. The gastrointestinal tract: the "undrained abscess" of multiple organ failure. *Ann Surg* 1993;218: 111–119.
61. Kerver AJ, Rommes JH, Mevissen Verhage EA, et al. Colonization and infection in surgical intensive care patients: a prospective study. *Intensive Care Med* 1987;13:347–351.
62. Flynn DM, Weinstein RA, Nathan C, Gaston MA, Kabins S. Patients' endogenous flora as the source of "nosocomial" *Enterobacter* in cardiac surgery. *J Infect Dis* 1987;156:363–368.
63. Flynn DM, Weinstein RA, Kabins S. Infections with gram-negative bacilli in a cardiac surgery intensive care unit: the relative role of enterobacter. *J Hosp Infect* 1988;11(suppl A):367–373.
64. Solomkin JS, Flohr AB, Quie PG, Simmons RL. The role of *Candida* in intraperitoneal infections. *Surgery* 1980;88:524–530.
65. Wey SB, Mori M, Pfaller MA, Woolson RF, Wenzel RP. Risk factors for hospital-acquired candidemia: a matched case-control study. *Arch Intern Med* 1989;149:2349–2353.
66. Pittet D, Garbino J. Fungal infections in the critically ill. *Curr Opin Crit Care* 1995;1:369–380.
67. Pittet D, Monod M, Filthuth I, Frenk E, Suter PM, Auckenthaler R. Contour-clamped homogeneous electric field gel electrophoresis as a powerful epidemiologic tool in yeast infections. *Am J Med* 1991;91: 256S–263S.
68. Pittet D, Monod M, Suter PM, Frenk E, Auckenthaler R. *Candida* colonization and subsequent infections in critically ill surgical patients. *Ann Surg* 1994;220:751–758.
69. Bonten MJ, Gaillard CA, van Tiel FH, Smeets HG, van der Geest S, Stobberingh EE. The stomach is not a source for colonization of the upper respiratory tract and pneumonia in ICU patients. *Chest* 1994; 105:878–884.
70. George DL, Falk PS, Meduri GU, et al. The epidemiology of nosocomial pneumonia in medical intensive care unit patients: a prospective study based on protected bronchoscopic sampling. *Amer J Resp Crit Care Med* (in press).
71. Widmer AF. Infection control and prevention strategies in the ICU. *Intensive Care Med* 1994;20(suppl 4):S7–11.
72. Pittet D, Herwaldt LA, Massanari RM. The intensive care unit. In: Brachman PS, Bennett JV, eds. *Hospital infections*. Boston: Little, Brown and Company, 1992:405–439.
73. Craven DE, Kunches LM, Lichtenberg DA. Nosocomial infection and fatality in medical surgical intensive care unit patients. *Arch Intern Med* 1988;148:1161–1168.
74. Pittet D, Wenzel RP. Nosocomial bloodstream infections: secular trends in rates, mortality, and contribution to total hospital deaths. *Arch Intern Med* 1995;155:1177–1184.
75. Emori TG, Gaynes RP. An overview of nosocomial infections, including the role of the microbiology laboratory. *Clin Microbiol Rev* 1993; 6:428–442.
76. Weinstein RA. Epidemiology and control of nosocomial infections in adult intensive care units. *Am J Med* 1991;91:179S–184S.
77. Ponce de Leon S, Critchley S, Wenzel RP. Polymicrobial bloodstream infections related to prolonged vascular catheterization. *Crit Care Med* 1984;12:856–859.
78. Struelens MJ, Carlier E, Maes N, Serruys E, Quint WG, van Belkum A. Nosocomial colonization and infection with multiresistant *Acinetobacter baumannii*: outbreak delineation using DNA macrorestriction analysis and PCR-fingerprinting. *J Hosp Infect* 1993;25:15–32.
79. Pittet D. Epidémies en réanimation: réservoirs et modes de transmission. *Réan Urg* 1994;31:91–119.
80. Burnie JP, Odds FC, Lee W, Webster C, Williams JD. Outbreak of systemic *Candida albicans* in intensive care unit caused by cross infection. *Br Med J* 1985;290:746–748.
81. Gordts B. Epidemic of multiresistant *Staphylococcus aureus* in an intensive care unit. *Acta Anaesthesiol Belg* 1983;34:175–178.
82. Meyer KS, Urban C, Eagan JA, Berger BJ, Rahal JJ. Nosocomial outbreak of *Klebsiella* infection resistant to late-generation cephalosporins. *Ann Intern Med* 1993;119:353–358.
83. Weems JJ. Nosocomial outbreak of *Pseudomonas cepacia* associated with contamination of reusable electronic ventilator temperature probes. *Infect Control Hosp Epidemiol* 1993;14:583–586.
84. Hartstein AI, Rashad AL, Liebler JM, et al. Multiple intensive care unit outbreak of *Acinetobacter calcoaceticus* subspecies *anitratus respirato*. *Am J Med* 1988;85:624–631.
85. Henderson DK, Baptiste R, Parrillo J, Gill VJ. Indolent epidemic of *Pseudomonas cepacia* bacteremia and pseudobacteremia in an intensive care unit traced to a contaminated blood gas analyzer. *Am J Med* 1988;84:75–81.

86. Hussain Z, Kuhn M, Lannigan R, Austin TW. Microbiological investigation of an outbreak of bacteraemia due to *Streptococcus faecalis* in an intensive care unit. *J Hosp Infect* 1988;12:263–271.
87. Nicolle LE, Hume K, Sims H, Rosenal T, Sandham D. An outbreak of group A streptococcal bacteremia in an intensive care unit. *Infect Control* 1986;7:177–180.
88. Pien FD, Bruce AE. Nosocomial *Ewingella americana* bacteremia in an intensive care unit. *Arch Intern Med* 1986;146:111–112.
89. Ransjo U, Malm M, Hambraeus A, Artursson G, Hedlund A. Methicillin-resistant *Staphylococcus aureus* in two burn units: clinical significance and epidemiological control. *J Hosp Infect* 1989;13: 355–365.
90. Ribner BS, Landry MN, Kidd K, Peninger M, Riddick J. Outbreak of multiply resistant *Staphylococcus aureus* in a pediatric intensive care unit after consolidation with a surgical intensive care unit. *Am J Infect Control* 1989;17:244–249.
91. Sherertz RJ, Sullivan ML. An outbreak of infections with *Acinetobacter calcoaceticus* in burn patients: contamination of patients' mattresses. *J Infect Dis* 1985;151:252–258.
92. Vandenbroucke-Grauls CM, Kerver AJ, Rommes JH, Jansen R, den DC, Verhoef J. Endemic *Acinetobacter anitratus* in a surgical intensive care unit: mechanical ventilators as reservoir. *Eur J Clin Microbiol Infect Dis* 1988;7:485–489.
93. Villarino ME, Jarvis WR, O'Hara C, Bresnahan J, Clark N. Epidemic of *Serratia marcescens* bacteremia in a cardiac intensive care unit. *J Clin Microbiol* 1989;27:2433–2436.
94. Lingnau W, Allerberger F. Control of an outbreak of methicillin-resistant *Staphylococcus aureus* (MRSA) by hygienic measures in a general intensive care unit. *Infection* 1994;22(suppl 2):S135–S139.
95. Grattard F, Pozzetto B, Berthelot P, et al. Arbitrarily primed PCR, ribotyping, and plasmid pattern analysis applied to investigation of a nosocomial outbreak due to *Enterobacter cloacae* in a neonatal intensive care unit. *J Clin Microbiol* 1994;32:596–602.
96. Siegman Igra Y, Bar Yosef S, Gorea A, Avram J. Nosocomial *acinetobacter* meningitis secondary to invasive procedures: report of 25 cases and review. *Clin Infect Dis* 1993;17:843–849.
97. Volkow Fernandez P, Ponce de Leon Rosales S, Sifuentes Osornio J, Calva Mercado JJ, Ruiz Palacios GM, Cerbon MA. An epidemic of primary bacteremia due to an endemic strain of *Serratia marcescens* in an intensive care unit. *Salud Publica Mex* 1993;35:440–447.
98. Finkelstein R, Reinhertz G, Hashman N, Merzbach D. Outbreak of *Candida tropicalis* fungemia in a neonatal intensive care unit. *Infect Control Hosp Epidemiol* 1993;14:587–590.
99. Patterson JE, Vecchio J, Pantelick EL, et al. Association of contaminated gloves with transmission of *Acinetobacter calcoaceticus* var. *anitratus* in an intensive care unit. *Am J Med* 1991;91:479–483.
100. Hamill RJ, Houston ED, Georghiou PR, et al. An outbreak of *Burkholderia* (formerly *Pseudomonas*) *cepacia* respiratory tract colonization and infection associated with nebulized albuterol therapy. *Ann Intern Med* 1995;122:762–766.
101. Bryce EA, Smith JA, Tweeddale M, Andruschak BJ, Maxwell MR. Dissemination of *Bacillus cereus* in an intensive care unit. *Infect Control Hosp Epidemiol* 1993;14:459–462.
102. Pagani L, Luzzaro F, Ronza P, et al. Outbreak of extended-spectrum beta-lactamase producing *Serratia marcescens* in an intensive care unit. *FEMS Immunol Med Microbiol* 1994;10:39–46.
103. Jumaa P, Chattopadhyay B. Outbreak of gentamicin, ciprofloxacin-resistant *Pseudomonas aeruginosa* in an intensive care unit, traced to contaminated quivers. *J Hosp Infect* 1994;28:209–218.
104. Tankovic J, Legrand P, De Gatines G, Chemineau V, Brun Buisson C, Duval J. Characterization of a hospital outbreak of imipenem-resistant *Acinetobacter baumannii* by phenotypic and genotypic typing methods. *J Clin Microbiol* 1994;32:2677–2681.
105. Fagon JY, Chastre J, Hance AJ, Montravers P, Novara A, Gibert C. Nosocomial pneumonia in ventilated patients: a cohort study evaluating attributable mortality and hospital stay. *Am J Med* 1993;94: 281–288.
106. Garibaldi RA, Britt MR, Coleman ML, Reading JC, Pace NL. Risk factors for postoperative pneumonia. *JAMA* 1981;70:677–680.
107. Leu HS, Kaiser DL, Mori M, Woolson RF, Wenzel RP. Hospital-acquired pneumonia: attributable mortality and morbidity. *Am J Epidemiol* 1989;129:1258–1267.
108. Rello J, Quintana E, Ausina V, et al. Incidence, etiology, and outcome of nosocomial pneumonia in mechanically ventilated patients. *Chest* 1991;100:439–444.
109. Rello J, Ausina V, Castella J, Net A, Prats G. Nosocomial respiratory tract infections in multiple trauma patients: influence of level of consciousness with implications for therapy. *Chest* 1992;102:525–529.
110. Weber DJ, Wilson MB, Rutala WA, Thomann CA. Manual ventilation bags as a source for bacterial colonization of intubated patients. *Am Rev Respir Dis* 1990;142:892–894.
111. Carratala J, Gudiol F, Pallares R, et al. Risk factors for nosocomial *Legionella pneumophila* pneumonia. *Am J Respir Crit Care Med* 1994;149:625–629.
112. Craven DE, Kunches LM, Kilinsky V, Lichtenberg DA, Make BJ, McCabe W. Risk factors for pneumonia and fatality in patients receiving continuous mechanical ventilation. *Am Rev Respir Dis* 1986;133: 792–796.
113. Langer M, Mosconi P, Cigada M, Mandelli M, et al. Long-term respiratory support and risk of pneumonia in critically ill patients. *Am Rev Respir Dis* 1989;140:302–305.
114. Jimenez P, Torres A, Rodriguez-Roisin R, et al. Incidence and etiology of pneumonia acquired during mechanical ventilation. *Crit Care Med* 1989;17:882–885.
115. Chastre J, Fagon JY, Soler P, Bornet M, et al. Diagnosis of nosocomial bacterial pneumonia in intubated patients undergoing ventilation: comparison of the usefulness of bronchoalveolar lavage and the protected specimen brush. *Am J Med* 1988;85:499–506.
116. Meduri GU, Wunderink RG, Leeper KV, Beals DH. Management of bacterial pneumonia in ventilated patients: protected bronchoalveolar lavage as a diagnostic tool. *Chest* 1992;101:500–508.
117. Pugin J, Auckenthaler R, Mili N, Janssens JP, Lew PD, Suter PM. Diagnosis of ventilator-associated pneumonia by bacteriologic analysis of bronchoscopic and nonbronchoscopic "blind" bronchoalveolar lavage fluid. *Am Rev Respir Dis* 1991;143:1121–1129.
118. Rouby JJ, Martin De Lassale E, Poete P, et al. Nosocomial bronchopneumonia in the critically ill: histologic and bacteriologic aspects. *Am Rev Respir Dis* 1992;146:1059–1066.
119. Jorda R, Parras F, Ibanez J, Reina J, Bergada J, Raurich JM. Diagnosis of nosocomial pneumonia in mechanically ventilated patients by the blind protected telescoping catheter. *Intensive Care Med* 1993;19: 377–382.
120. Middleton R, Broughton WA, Kirkpatrick MB. Comparison of four methods for assessing airway bacteriology in intubated, mechanically ventilated patients. *Am J Med Sci* 1992;304:239–245.
121. Chastre J, Fagon JY. Invasive diagnostic testing should be routinely used to manage ventilated patients with suspected pneumonia. *Am J Respir Crit Care Med* 1994;150:570–574.
122. Mandelli M, Mosconi P, Langer M, Cigada M. Is pneumonia developing in patients in intensive care always a typical "nosocomial" infection? *Lancet* 1986;2:1094.
123. Langer M, Cigada M, Mandelli M, Mosconi P, Tognoni G, et al. Early onset pneumonia: a multicenter study in intensive care units. *Intensive Care Med* 1987;13:342.
124. Antonelli M, Moro ML, Capelli O, et al. Risk factors for early onset pneumonia in trauma patients. *Chest* 1994;105:224–228.
125. Caplan ES, Hoyt NJ. Nosocomial sinusitis. *JAMA* 1982;247:639–641.
126. Deutschman CS, Wilton P, Sinow J, Dibbell D Jr., Konstantinides FN, Cerra FB. Paranasal sinusitis associated with nasotracheal intubation: a frequently unrecognized and treatable source of sepsis. *Crit Care Med* 1986;14:111–114.
127. Seiden AM. Sinusitis in the critical care patient. *New Horiz* 1993;1: 261–270.
128. Rouby JJ, Laurent P, Gosnach M, et al. Risk factors and clinical relevance of nosocomial maxillary sinusitis in the critically ill. *Am J Respir Crit Care Med* 1994;150:776–783.
129. Mayhall CG. Nosocomial sinusitis in the intensive care unit. *Curr Opin Crit Care* 1996;2:366–370.
130. Lum Cheong RS, Cornwell EE. Suppurative sinusitis in critically ill patients: a case report and review of the literature. *J Natl Med Assoc* 1992;84:1057–1059.
131. Holzapfel L, Chevret S, Madinier G, et al. Influence of long-term oro- or nasotracheal intubation on nosocomial maxillary sinusitis and pneumonia: results of a prospective, randomized, clinical trial. *Crit Care Med* 1993;21:1132–1138.
132. Bach A, Boehrer H, Schmidt H, Geiss HK. Nosocomial sinusitis in

ventilated patients: nasotracheal versus orotracheal intubation. *Anaesthesia* 1992;47:335–339.
133. Heffner JE. Nosocomial sinusitis: den of multiresistant thieves? *Am J Respir Crit Care Med* 1994;150:608–609.
134. Bone RC. Toward an epidemiology and natural history of SIRS (systemic inflammatory response syndrome). *JAMA* 1992;268:3452–3455.
135. Bone RC, Fisher CJ Jr., Clemmer TP, Slotman GJ, Metz CA, Balk R. Sepsis syndrome: a valid clinical entity. Methylprednisolone Severe Sepsis Study Group. *Crit Care Med* 1989;17:389–393.
136. Rangel-Frausto SM, Pittet D, Costigan M, Hwang TS, Davis CS, Wenzel RP. The natural history of the systemic inflammatory response syndrome (SIRS): a prospective study. *JAMA* 1995;273:117–123.
137. Pittet D, Rangel-Frausto SM, Li N, et al. Systemic inflammatory response syndrome, sepsis, severe sepsis, and septic shock: incidence, morbidities and outcome in surgical ICU patients. *Intensive Care Med* 1995;21:302–309.
138. Marshall JC, Christou NV, Horn R. The multiple organ dysfunction (MOD) score: a reliable descriptor of a complex clinical outcome. *Crit Care Med* 1992;20:S80.
139. Knaus WA, Draper EA, Wagner DP, Zimmerman JE. Prognosis in acute organ-system failure. *Ann Surg* 1985;202:685–693.
140. Fry DE, Pearlstein L, Fulton RL, Polk HC. Multiple system organ failure: the role of uncontrolled infection. *Arch Surg* 1980;115: 136–142.
141. Bell RC, Coalson JJ, Smith JD, Johanson WG Jr. Multiple organ system failure and infection in adult respiratory distress syndrome. *Ann Intern Med* 1983;99:293–298.
142. Faist E, Bave AE, Dittmer H, Heberer G. Multiple organ failure in polytrauma patients. *J Trauma* 1983;23:775–787.
143. Deitch EA. Multiple organ failure: pathophysiology and potential future therapy. *Ann Surg* 1992;216:117–134.
144. Livingston DH, Mosenthal AC, Deitch EA. Sepsis and multiple organ dysfunction syndrome: a clinical-mechanistic overview. *New Horiz* 1995;3:257–266.
145. Polk HCJ, Shields CL. Remote organ failure: a valid sign of occult intra-abdominal infection. *Surgery* 1977;81:310–313.
146. Marshall JC, Christou NV, Horn R, Meakins JL. The microbiology of multiple organ failure: the proximal gastrointestinal tract as an occult reservoir of pathogens. *Arch Surg* 1995;123:309–315.
147. Carrico CJ, Meakins JL, Marshall JC. Multiple-organ-failure syndrome. The gastrointestinal tract: the "motor" of MOF? *Arch Surg* 1986;121:197–208.
148. Gaussorgues P, Gueugniaud PY, Vedrinne JM, Salord F, Mercatello A, Robert D. Bacteremia following cardiac arrest and cardiopulmonary resuscitation. *Intensive Care Med* 1988;14:575–577.
149. Rush BF Jr., Sori AJ, Murphy TF, Smith S, Flanagan JJ Jr., Machiedo GW. Endotoxemia and bacteremia during hemorrhagic shock: the link between trauma and sepsis? *Ann Surg* 1988;207:549–554.
150. Rello J, Vallés J, Jubert A, Ferrer A, Domingo C, Artigas A. Lower respiratory tract infections following cardiac arrest and cardiopulmonary resuscitation. *Clin Infect Dis* 1995;21:310–314.
151. Cain SM, Curtis SE. Experimental models of pathologic oxygen supply dependency. *Crit Care Med* 1991;19:603–612.
152. Reilly PM, Schiller HJ, Bulkley GB. Pharmacologic approach to tissue injury mediated by free radicals and other reactive oxygen metabolites. *Am J Surg* 1991;161:488–503.
153. Law MM, Cryer HG, Abraham E. Elevated levels of soluble ICAM-1 correlate with the development of multiple organ failure in severely injured trauma patients. *J Trauma* 1994;37:100–109.
154. Carlos TM, Harlan JM. Leukocyte-endothelial adhesion molecules. *Blood* 1994;84:2068–2101.
155. Mulligan MS, Jones ML, Vaporciyan AA, Howard MC, Ward PA. Protective effects of IL-4 and IL-10 against immune complex-induced lung injury. *J Immunol* 1993;151:5666–5674.
156. Boland G, Lee MJ, Mueller PR. Acute cholecystitis in the intensive care unit. *New Horiz* 1993;1:246–260.
157. Shapiro MJ, Luchtefeld WB, Kurzweil S, Kaminski DL, Durham RM, Mazuski JE. Acute acalculous cholecystitis in the critically ill. *Am Surg* 1994;60:335–339.
158. Raunest J, Imhof M, Rauen U, Ohmann C, Thon KP, Burrig KF. Acute cholecystitis: a complication in severely injured intensive care patients. *J Trauma* 1992;32:433–440.
159. Imhof M, Raunest J, Ohmann C, Roher HD. Acute acalculous cholecystitis complicating trauma: a prospective sonographic study. *World J Surg* 1992;16:1160–1165.
160. Brandt CP, Priebe PP, Jacobs DG. Value of laparoscopy in trauma ICU patients with suspected acute acalculous cholecystitis. *Surg Endosc* 1994;8:361–364.
161. Arbo MJ, Fine MJ, Hanusa BH, Sefcik T, Kapoor WN. Fever of nosocomial origin: etiology, risk factors, and outcomes. *Am J Med* 1993; 95:505–512.
162. Pittet D, Huguenin T, Dharan S, et al. Unusual cause of lethal pulmonary aspergillosis in patients with chronic obstructive pulmonary disease. *Am J Respir Crit Care Med* 1996;154:541–544.
163. Preston GA, Larson EL, Stamm W. The effect of private isolation rooms on patient care practices, colonization and infection in an intensive care unit. *Am J Med* 1981;70:641–645.
164. Society of Critical Care Medicine. Guidelines for intensive care unit design. Guidelines/Practice Parameters Committee of the American College of Critical Care Medicine, Society of Critical Care Medicine. *Crit Care Med* 1995;23:582–588.
165. Maki DG, Alvarado CJ, Hassemer CA, Zilz MA. Relation of the inanimate hospital environment to endemic nosocomial infection. *N Engl J Med* 1982;307:1562–1566.
166. Huebner J, Frank U, Kappstein I, et al. Influence of architectural design on nosocomial infections in intensive care units: a prospective 2-year analysis. *Intensive Care Med* 1989;15:179–183.
167. Haley RW, Bregman D. The role of understaffing and overcrowding in recurrent outbreaks of staphylococcal infection in a neonatal special-care unit. *J Infect Dis* 1982;145:875–885.
168. Wenzel RP, Osterman CA, Donowitz LG, et al. Identification of procedure-related nosocomial infections in high-risk patients. *Rev Infect Dis* 1981;3:701–707.
169. Fridkin SK, Pear SM, Williamson T, Galgiani JN, Jarvis WR. The role of understaffing in central venous catheter–associated bloodstream infections. *Infect Control Hosp Epidemiol* 1996;17:150–158.
170. Boyd O, Grounds M. Can standardized mortality ratio be used to compare quality of intensive care unit performance? [Letter]. *Crit Care Med* 1994;22:1706–1709.
171. Pollack MM, Cuerdon TT, Patel KM, Ruttimann UE, Getson PR, Levetown M. Impact of quality-of-care factors on pediatric intensive care unit mortality. *JAMA* 1994;272:941–946.
172. Fernandez-Segoviano P, Lazaro A, Esteban A, Rubio JM, Iruretagoyena JR. Autopsy as quality assurance in the intensive care unit. *Crit Care Med* 1988;16:683–685.
173. Doebbeling BN, Stanley GL, Sheetz CT, et al. Comparative efficacy of alternative hand-washing agents in reducing nosocomial infections in intensive care units. *N Engl J Med* 1992;327:88–93.
174. Jarvis WR. Handwashing: the Semmelweis lesson forgotten? *Lancet* 1994;344:1311–1312.
175. Klein BS, Perloff WH, Maki D. Reduction of nosocomial infection during pediatric intensive care by protective isolation. *N Engl J Med* 1989;320:1714–1721.
176. Graham M. Frequency and duration of handwashing in an intensive care unit. *Am J Infect Control* 1990;18:77–81.
177. Leclair JM, Freeman J, Sullivan BF, Crowley CM, Goldmann D. Prevention of nosocomial respiratory syncytial virus infections through compliance with glove and gown isolation precautions. *N Engl J Med* 1987;317:329–334.
178. Tetteroo GW, Wagenvoort JH, Castelein A, Tilanus HW, Ince C, Bruining HA. Selective decontamination to reduce gram-negative colonisation and infections after oesophageal resection. *Lancet* 1990;335: 704–707.
179. Ramsey G. Endotoxaemia in multiple organ failure: a secondary role for SDD? In: van Saene HFK, ed. *Update in intensive care and emergency medicine*, vol 7. Berlin: Springer-Verlag. 1989:135–142.
180. Bion JF, Badger I, Crosby HA, et al. Selective decontamination of the digestive tract reduces gram-negative pulmonary colonization but not systemic endotoxemia in patients undergoing elective liver transplantation. *Crit Care Med* 1994;22:40–49.
181. Wells CL. Editorial response to a decade of experience with selective decontamination of the digestive tract as prophylaxis for infections in patients in the intensive care unit: What have we learned? *Clin Infect Dis* 1993;17:1055–1057.
182. Ziegler EJ, McCutchan JA, Fierer J, et al. Treatment of gram-negative bacteremia and shock with human antiserum to a mutant *Escherichia coli*. *N Engl J Med* 1982;307:1225–1230.
183. Greenman RL, Schein RMH, Martin MA, et al. A controlled clinical trial of E5 murine monoclonal IgM antibody to endotoxin in the treatment of gram-negative sepsis. *JAMA* 1991;266:1097–1102.

184. Bone RC, Balk RA, Fein AM, et al. A second large controlled clinical study of E5, a monoclonal antibody to endotoxin: results of a prospective, multicenter, randomized, controlled trial. *Crit Care Med* 1995; 23:994–1006.
185. Kohn FR, Kung AH. Role of endotoxin in acute inflammation induced by gram-negative bacteria: specific inhibition of lipopolysaccharide-mediated responses with an amino-terminal fragment of bactericidal/permeability-increasing protein. *Infect Immun* 1995;63:333–339.
186. Larrick JW, Hirata M, Zheng H, et al. A novel granulocyte-derived peptide with lipopolysaccharide-neutralizing activity. *J Immunol* 1994; 152:231–240.
187. Nelson D, Kuppermann N, Fleisher GR, et al. Recombinant endotoxin neutralizing protein improves survival from *Escherichia coli* sepsis in rats. *Crit Care Med* 1995;23:92–98.
188. Wang SC, Rossignol DP, Christ WJ, et al. Suppression of lipopolysaccharide-induced macrophage nitric oxide and cytokine production in vitro by a novel lipopolysaccharide antagonist. *Surgery* 1994;116: 339–346.
189. Ziegler EJ, Fisher CJ Jr., Sprung CL, et al. Treatment of gram-negative bacteremia and septic shock with HA-1A human monoclonal antibody against endotoxin: a randomized, double-blind, placebo-controlled trial. The HA-1A sepsis study group. *N Engl J Med* 1991;324:429–436.
190. Quezado ZM, Natanson C, Alling DW, et al. A controlled trial of HA-1A in a canine model of gram-negative septic shock. *JAMA* 1993;269: 2221–2227.
191. National Committee for the Evaluation of Centoxin. The French national registry of HA-1A (centoxin) in septic shock: a cohort study of 600 patients. The National Committee for the Evaluation of Centoxin. *Arch Intern Med* 1994;154:2484–2491.
192. McCloskey RV, Straube RC, Sanders C, Smith SM, Smith CR. Treatment of septic shock with human monoclonal antibody HA-1A: a randomized, double-blind, placebo-controlled trial. CHESS Trial Study Group. *Ann Intern Med* 1994;121:1–5.
193. Quezado ZM, Natanson C, Hoffman WD. Looking back on HA-1A. *Arch Intern Med* 1994;154:2393.
194. Carter DB, Deibel MR Jr., Dunn CJ, et al. Purification, cloning, expression and biological characterization of an interleukin-1 receptor antagonist protein. *Nature* 1990;344:633–638.
195. Fischer E, Marano MA, Van Zee KJ, et al. Interleukin-1 receptor blockade improves survival and hemodynamic performance in *Escherichia coli* septic shock, but fails to alter host responses to sublethal endotoxemia. *J Clin Invest* 1992;89:1551–1557.
196. Fisher CJ Jr., Slotman GJ, Opal SM, et al. Initial evaluation of human recombinant interleukin-1 receptor antagonist in the treatment of sepsis syndrome: a randomized, open-label, placebo-controlled multicenter trial. The IL-1ra Sepsis Syndrome Study Group. *Crit Care Med* 1994;22:12–21.
197. Fisher CJ Jr., Dhainaut JF, Opal SM, et al. Recombinant human interleukin 1 receptor antagonist in the treatment of patients with sepsis syndrome: results from a randomized, double-blind, placebo-controlled trial. Phase III RHIL-1ra Sepsis Syndrome Study Group. *JAMA* 1994;271:1836–1843.
198. Tracey KJ, Vlassara H, Cerami A. Cachectin/tumour necrosis factor. *Lancet* 1989;1:1122–1126.
199. Suffredini AF, Fromm RE, Parker MM, et al. The cardiovascular response of normal humans to the administration of endotoxin. *N Engl J Med* 1989;321:280–287.
200. van der Poll T, Buller HR, ten Cate H, et al. Activation of coagulation after administration of tumor necrosis factor to normal subjects. *N Engl J Med* 1990;322:1622–1627.
201. Doherty GM, Lange JR, Langstein HN, Alexander HR, Buresh CM, Norton JA. Evidence for IFN-gamma as a mediator of the lethality of endotoxin and tumor necrosis factor-alpha. *J Immunol* 1992;149: 1666–1670.
202. Zivot JB, Hoffman WD. Pathogenic effects of endotoxin. *New Horiz* 1995;3:267–275.
203. Girardin E, Grau GE, Dayer JM, Roux-Lombard P, Lambert PH. Tumor necrosis factor and interleukin-1 in the serum of children with severe infectious purpura. *N Engl J Med* 1988;319:397–400.
204. Grau GE, Taylor TE, Molyneux ME, et al. Tumor necrosis factor and disease severity in children with falciparum malaria. *N Engl J Med* 1989;320:1586–1591.
205. Kwiatkowski D, Hill AV, Sambou I, et al. TNF concentration in fatal cerebral, non-fatal cerebral, and uncomplicated plasmodium falciparum malaria. *Lancet* 1990;336:1201–1204.
206. Tracey KJ, Fong Y, Hesse DG. Anti-cachectin/TNF monoclonal antibodies prevent septic shock during lethal bacteremia. *Nature* 1987; 330:662–664.
207. Opal SM, Cross AS, Kelly NM, et al. Efficacy of a monoclonal antibody directed against tumor necrosis factor in protecting neutropenic rats from lethal infection with *Pseudomonas aeruginosa*. *J Infect Dis* 1990;161:1148–1152.
208. Jesmok G, Lindsey C, Duerr M, Fournel M, Emerson T Jr. Efficacy of monoclonal antibody against human recombinant tumor necrosis factor in *E. coli*–challenged swine. *Am J Pathol* 1992;141:1197–1207.
209. Walsh CJ, Sugerman HJ, Mullen PG, et al. Monoclonal antibody to tumor necrosis factor alpha attenuates cardiopulmonary dysfunction in porcine gram-negative sepsis. *Arch Surg* 1992;127:138–144;discussion 144–145.
210. Hinshaw LB, Emerson TE Jr., Taylor FB Jr., et al. Lethal *Staphylococcus aureus*–induced shock in primates: prevention of death with anti-TNF antibody. *J Trauma* 1992;33:568–573.
211. Emerson TE Jr., Lindsey DC, Jesmok GJ, Duerr ML, Fournel MA. Efficacy of monoclonal antibody against tumor necrosis factor alpha in an endotoxemic baboon model. *Circ Shock* 1992;38:75–84.
212. Cornelissen JJ, Makel I, Algra A, et al. Protection against lethal endotoxemia by anti-lipid a murine monoclonal antibodies: comparison of efficacy with that of human anti-lipid a monoclonal antibody HA-1A. *J Infect Dis* 1993;167:876–881.
213. Saravolatz LD, Wherry JC, Spooner C, et al. Clinical safety, tolerability, and pharmacokinetics of murine monoclonal antibody to human tumor necrosis factor-alpha. *J Infect Dis* 1994;169:214–217.
214. Abraham E, Wunderink R, Silverman H, et al. Efficacy and safety of monoclonal antibody to human tumor necrosis factor alpha in patients with sepsis syndrome: a randomized, controlled, double-blind, multicenter clinical trial. TNF-alpha MAb Sepsis Study Group. *JAMA* 1995;273:934–941.
215. Cronin L, Cook DJ, Carlet J, Heyland DK, Fisher CJ. Corticosteroid treatment for sepsis: a critical appraisal and meta-analysis of the literature. *Crit Care Med* 1995;23:1430–1439.
216. Palmer RM. The discovery of nitric oxide in the vessel wall: a unifying concept in the pathogenesis of sepsis. *Arch Surg* 1993;128: 396–401.
217. Minnard EA, Shou J, Naama H, Cech A, Gallagher H, Daly JM. Inhibition of nitric oxide synthesis is detrimental during endotoxemia. *Arch Surg* 1994;129:142–147.
218. Fukatsu K, Saito H, Fukushima R, et al. Detrimental effects of a nitric oxide synthase inhibitor (*n*-omega-nitro-L-arginine-methyl-ester) in a murine sepsis model. *Arch Surg* 1995;130:410–414.
219. Wang P, Ba ZF, Chaudry IH. Nitric oxide: to block or enhance its production during sepsis? *Arch Surg* 1994;129:1137–1142.
220. Jarvis WR, Martone W. Predominant pathogens in hospital infections. *J Antimicrob Chemother* 1992;29(suppl A):19–24.
221. Bross J, Talbot GH, Maislin G, Hurwits S, Strom BL. Risk factors for nosocomial candidemia: a case-control study in adults without leukemia. *Am J Med* 1989;87:614–620.
222. Wey SB, Motomi M, Pfaller MA, Woolson RF, Wenzel RP. Hospital-acquired candidemia: the attributable mortality and excess length of stay. *Arch Intern Med* 1988;148:2642–2645.
223. Anaissie E, Solomkin JS. Fungal infection: approach to the surgical patient at risk for candidiasis. In: Wilmore DW, Cheung LY, Harken AH, Holcroft JW, Meakins JL, for the American College of Surgeons, eds. *Scientific Amercan surgery*. New York: Scientific American, 1994:1–19.
224. British Society for Antimicrobial Chemotherapy. Management of deep *Candida* infection in surgical and intensive care unit patients. *Intensive Care Med* 1994;20:522–528.
225. Pittet D, Anaissie E, Solomkin JS. When to start antifungal therapy in the nonneutropenic critically ill? In: Vincent JL, ed. *Yearbook of intensive care and emergency medicine*. Berlin: Springer-Verlag, 1996: 567–577.
226. Craig CP, Connelly S. Effect of intensive care unit nosocomial pneumonia on duration of stay and mortality. *Am J Infect Control* 1984;12: 233–238.
227. Smith RL, Meixler SM, Simberkoff MS. Excess mortality in critically ill patients with nosocomial bloodstream infections. *Chest* 1991;100: 164–167.
228. Bjerke HS, Leyerle B, Shabot MM. Impact of ICU nosocomial infections on outcome from surgical care. *Am Surg* 1991;57:798–802.
229. Bueno Cavanillas A, Delgado Rodriguez M, Lopez Luque A, Schaffino

Cano S, Galvez Vargas R. Influence of nosocomial infection on mortality rate in an intensive care unit. *Crit Care Med* 1994;22:55–60.
230. Pittet D, Tarara D, Wenzel RP. Nosocomial bloodstream infection in critically ill patients: excess length of stay, extra costs, and attributable mortality. *JAMA* 1994;271:1598–1601.
231. Fagon JY, Novara A, Stephan F, Girou E, Safar M. Mortality attributable to nosocomial infections in the ICU. *Infect Control Hosp Epidemiol* 1994;15:428–434.
232. Freeman J, Goldmann DA, McGowan JE. Methodologic issues in hospital epidemiology. IV. Risk ratios, confounding, effect modification, and the analysis of multiple variables. *Rev Infect Dis* 1988;10: 1118–1141.
233. Pittet D, Thiévent B, Wenzel RP, Li N, Gurman G, Suter PM. Importance of pre-existing co-morbidities for prognosis of septicemia in critically ill patients. *Intensive Care Med* 1993;19:265–272.
234. Pittet D, Thiévent B, Wenzel RP, Li N, Auckenthaler R, Suter PM. Bedside prediction of mortality from bacteremic sepsis: a dynamic analysis of ICU patients. *Am J Respir Crit Care Med* 1996;153: 684–693.
235. Go ES, Urban C, Burns J, et al. Clinical and molecular epidemiology of *acinetobacter* infections sensitive only to polymyxin B and sulbactam. *Lancet* 1994;344:1329–1332.
236. Piedra PA, Kasel JA, Norton HJ, et al. Description of an adenovirus type 8 outbreak in hospitalized neonates born prematurely. *Pediatr Infect Dis J* 1992;11:460–465.
237. Sanchez V, Vazquez JA, Barth-Jones D, Dembry L, Sobel JD, Zervos MJ. Nosocomial acquisition of *Candida parapsilosis*: an epidemiologic study. *Am J Med* 1993;94:577–582.
238. Karanfil LV, Murphy M, Josephson A, et al. A cluster of vancomycin-resistant *Enterococcus faecium* in an intensive care unit. *Infect Control Hosp Epidemiol* 1992;13:195–200.
239. Livornese LL Jr., Dias S, Samel C, et al. Hospital-acquired infection with vancomycin-resistant *Enterococcus faecium* transmitted by electronic thermometers. *Ann Intern Med* 1992;117:112–116.
240. Watson JC, Fleming DW, Borella AJ, Olcott ES, Conrad RE, Baron R. Vertical transmission of hepatitis A resulting in an outbreak in a neonatal intensive care unit. *J Infect Dis* 1993;167:567–571.
241. De Champs C, Rouby D, Guelon D, et al. A case-control study of an outbreak of infections caused by *Klebsiella pneumoniae* strains producing CTX-1 (TEM-3) beta-lactamase. *J Hosp Infect* 1991;18:5–13.
242. Valls V, Gomez Herruz P, Gonzalez Palacios R, Cuadros JA, Romanyk JP, Ena J. Long-term efficacy of a program to control methicillin-resistant *Staphylococcus aureus*. *Eur J Clin Microbiol Infect Dis* 1994;13:90–95.
243. Guiguet M, Rekacewicz C, Leclercq B, Brun Y, Escudier B, Andremont A. Effectiveness of simple measures to control an outbreak of nosocomial methicillin-resistant *Staphylococcus aureus* infections in an intensive care unit. *Infect Control Hosp Epidemiol* 1990;11:23–26.
244. Hammami A, Arlet G, Ben Redjeb S, et al. Nosocomial outbreak of acute gastroenteritis in a neonatal intensive care unit in Tunisia caused by multiply drug resistant *Salmonella wien* producing SHV-2 beta-lactamase. *Eur J Clin Microbiol Infect Dis* 1991;10:641–646.
245. Fisher DJ, Christy C, Spafford P, Maniscalco WM, Hardy DJ, Graman P. Neonatal *Trichosporon beigelii* infection: report of a cluster of cases in a neonatal intensive care unit. *Pediatr Infect Dis J* 1993;12: 149–155.
246. Kappstein I, Schulgen G, Beyer U, Geiger K, Schumacher M, Daschner FD. Prolongation of hospital stay and extra costs due to ventilator-associated pneumonia in an intensive care unit. *Eur J Clin Microbiol Infect Dis* 1992;11:504–508.
247. Garo B, Boles JM. Le coût de l'infection nosocomiale en réanimation: une évaluation médicale et économique. *Réan Urg* 1993;2:648.

Hospital Infections, Fourth Edition,
edited by John V. Bennett and Philip S. Brachman.
Lippincott–Raven Publishers, Philadelphia © 1998

CHAPTER 26

The Newborn Nursery

Jane D. Siegel

The newborn nursery houses both healthy, full-term infants who weigh ≥ 2,000 g at birth in the normal newborn areas, as well as high-risk infants who are < 2,000 g birthweight or have complex medical problems in the high-risk nursery (HRN) area. These infants have an increased risk of acquiring infection because all components of the neonate's host defense system are deficient as compared with older infants and adults, and the severity of these deficiencies is increased as gestational age decreases [1]. Furthermore, survival of prematurely born infants has improved in recent years as a result of better supportive care, including the use of extracorporeal membrane oxygenation (ECMO) treatment of hyaline membrane disease with artificial surfactant, and improved surgical techniques. Therefore, the number of infants at risk for infection has increased. Of note, the National Nosocomial Infections Surveillance (NNIS) system of the Centers for Disease Control and Prevention (CDC) has found that the HRN in general has higher rates of nosocomial bloodstream infections, especially in very–low-birthweight infants, compared with all other intensive care units except the burn unit [2–4] (Table 26-1).

In the absence of in utero infection, the neonate is first exposed to microorganisms during passage through the birth canal. Subsequently, the normal skin and mucous membrane microflora is derived from environmental sources. Healthy term infants usually have a short hospital stay: < 72 hours, and in the managed care era, often < 24 hours. Therefore, infections are acquired infrequently in the term nursery (<1% of all admissions) and may not become manifest until after discharge, making surveillance particularly difficult. In contrast, very–low-birthweight infants may remain in the neonatal intensive care unit (NICU) for several weeks to months with continued exposure to many devices and invasive procedures, antibiotic-resistant hospital flora, and antimicrobial agents that further influence the composition of the microflora. Thus, meaningful analysis of nosocomial infection rates in the newborn nursery must use consistent definitions and risk stratification to account for the heterogeneity of its population. The HRN is the focus of nosocomial infection surveillance and prevention because of the associated increase in morbidity and mortality.

J. D Siegel: Department of Pediatrics, University of Texas Southwestern Medical Center at Dallas, Dallas, Texas 76236–9036.

DEFINITIONS

Time of Onset

Early-onset disease is defined by various investigators as positive cultures of a normally sterile body fluid obtained within the first 3, 7, or 10 days of life. For the study of nosocomial infections, 3 days is the most appropriate time interval. Infections that appear at < 48 hours of age are considered to be maternally acquired. Approximately 15% of bloodstream infections and pneumonias in the HRN are maternally acquired [5]. Outbreaks of early-onset infections are reported rarely and have remained either unexplained [6] or have been associated with fetal scalp electrode placement during labor [7] or contaminated resuscitation equipment in the delivery room [8,9].

For the purposes of tracking nosocomial infections, positive cultures obtained beyond 3 days of life are considered late-onset disease. Because clinical manifestations of infection are often delayed and it is difficult to determine if an infection was acquired from the mother or nosocomially, NNIS reports all infections except those that are transmitted transplacentally as nosocomial infections [5]. Differentiation of early- and late-onset disease is most useful when designing prophylaxis regimens. It is recommended that bacterial infections other than urinary tract infection that occur within the first month after discharge from the nursery be reported to the infant's nursery to facilitate prompt identification of an outbreak (e.g., skin infections associated with *Staphylococcus*

TABLE 26-1. *Median rates of nosocomial bloodstream infections (BSI) by intensive care unit type, National Nosocomial Infections Surveillance System (NNIS)*

	No. BSI/1,000 central-line days		No. BSI/1,000 noncentral-line days
	Oct. 1, 1986–Dec. 31, 1990	Jan. 1, 1990–Mar. 31, 1995	Jan 1, 1986–Dec. 31, 1990
Respiratory	2.1	6.1[a]	1.1
Neurosurgical	4.5	4.9	0.5
Medical/surgical	5.1	4.1	0
Trauma	5.8	6.8[a]	2.0
Surgical	5.8	3.8	0.5
Medical	6.9	5.7	0
Coronary	7.0	3.6	0
Pediatric	11.4	6.0	0.4
Burn	30.2	15.6[a]	1.2
High-risk nursery[b]			
1,000 g		12.5[c]	N/A
1,001–1,500 g	14.6[d]	5.3	N/A
1,501–2,500 g		4.7	N/A
>2,500 g	5.1[e]	3.9	N/A

N/A, not available.
[a] Pooled mean; median not available due to small number of units submitting data.
[b] Central line days includes umbilical lines.
[c] More recent period is Jan. 1, 1992–Apr. 30, 1995 for the high-risk nursery.
[d] Data pooled for birthweight groups 1,000 g and 1,001–1,500 g.
[e] Data pooled for birthweight groups 1,501–2,500 g and >2,500 g.
(Adapted from Jarvis WR, et al. Nosocomial infection rates in adult and pediatric intensive care units in the United States. *Am J Med* 1991;91:185S–191S; Gaynes RP, et al. Comparison of rates of nosocomial infections in neonatal intensive care units in the United States. *Am J Med* 192S–196S; and Hospital Infections Program, et al. NNIS semiannual report, May 1995. *Am J Infect Control* 1995; 23:377–385.)

aureus or streptococcus group A or B, omphalitis, bacterial diarrhea, especially *Salmonella* species) [8,10].

Calculation of Infection Rates in the High-Risk Nursery

Studies [3,4] have demonstrated the advantages of calculating device-associated nosocomial infection rates to control for duration of exposure to the primary risk factors. Device utilization (DU) ratios are useful for inter-hospital comparisons as long as each hospital has collected the data and calculated ratios using the same definitions and methods. The DU ratio is the measure of an intensive care unit's invasive practices that constitutes an extrinsic risk factor for nosocomial infection. The DU ratio may also serve as a marker for severity of illness or the patients' intrinsic susceptibility to infection. If the DU ratio is above the 90th percentile, a specific hospital is considered a high outlier and further investigation of that specific practice may be warranted. Device-associated infection rates and DU ratios are calculated as follows:

1. Central line-associated primary bloodstream infection (BSI) rate:

$$\frac{\text{Number of central line-associated BSIs}}{\text{Number of central line days}} \times 1{,}000$$

2. Ventilator-associated pneumonia rate:

$$\frac{\text{Number of ventilator-associated pneumonias}}{\text{Number of ventilator days}} \times 1{,}000$$

3. Device utilization (DU) ratio:

$$\frac{\text{Number of device days}}{\text{Number of patient days}}.$$

Measures of illness severity other than birthweight have been applied to the study of neonatal nosocomial infection risk only since the mid-1990s [11,12]. Using multiple regression analysis, a study [11] of coagulase-negative staphylococcal (CONS) bacteremia demonstrated a 53.9% increase in a patient's risk of experiencing at least one nosocomial bacteremia episode associated with each five-point increment in the admission day Score for Neonatal Acute Physiology (SNAP). Further analysis of the association between admission-day therapies and bacteremia attack rates among these patients using the Neonatal Therapeutic Intervention Scoring System (NTISS) demonstrated a significant positive association with phototherapy and blood pressure support with colloid or vasopressor administration.

In a study [12] of eradication of endemic methicillin-resistant *S. aureus* (MRSA) infections from our own NICU in Parkland Memorial Hospital, we used the number of patient-care hours determined for each infant by the nursing staff according to a workload quantification method called the GRASP system [13] to calculate a time-and-intensity-of-care adjusted nosocomial infection incidence density (see Chapters 15, 44). Use of the sum of all infants' daily patient-care hours as the denominator effectively controlled for the difference in risk factors between the intensive care and intermediate care areas. Further validation is required before these scoring systems can be applied routinely, but they look promising.

Distinguishing True Pathogens From Blood Culture Contaminants

Sepsis caused by pathogens that are common skin contaminants (e.g., CONS) may be associated with low colony counts [14,15] and relatively few symptoms. The following suggestions are offered to optimize the clinician's accuracy in distinguishing true sepsis from contamination (see Chapter 9):

1. Obtain at least 1 to 2 ml of blood for culture from two separate sites (preferably one peripheral site in the presence of an intravascular catheter).
2. Isolates detected within 48 to 72 hours of submission are more likely to be true pathogens.
3. A clinical course or laboratory studies compatible with sepsis are documented (e.g., absolute total neutrophil count and ratio of absolute total immature neutrophils to total neutrophils ≥ 0.2) [16].
4. The patient responds to antibiotics that are active against the isolate, usually vancomycin.

TABLE 26-2. *Risk factors for acquisition of nursery infections*

Intrinsic (host)
Decreased function of the immune system
Decreased protection from natural barriers (e.g., skin)
Developing endogenous microflora
Gestational age
Severity of illness
Underlying disease processes, e.g. congenital organ system abnormalities, chronic lung disease
Extrinsic
Use of devices
Fetal scalp electrodes
Umbilical, arterial, central venous catheters
Mechanical ventilators
Extracorporeal membrane oxygenation
Ventriculoperitoneal shunts
Fluids
Total parenteral nutrition, intralipid
Transfused blood products
Respiratory care
Breast milk
Treatments
Intravenous steroid therapy
Use of H_2 blockers
Environment
Acquisition of hospital flora
Overcrowding, understaffing
Contaminated equipment
Traffic from other sections of hospital
Radiology
Laboratory
Subspecialty consultants

RISK FACTORS

The intrinsic and extrinsic factors for nosocomial infection are summarized in Table 26-2. Birthweight and gestational age are the most important risk factors for the development of nosocomial infection. The decreased function of the immune system in the most premature infants accounts for most of the increased risk of infection. There is minimal active transport of maternal IgG antibodies across the placenta until 32 weeks' gestation, neutrophils have defective chemotaxis and phagocytosis, and the classic and alternative complement pathways have decreased activity. Attempts to improve the neonate's immune function include exchange transfusion [17], white blood cell transfusion [18], administration of intravenous immune globulin (IVIG) therapeutically [19] or prophylactically [20,21], and administration of recombinant human granulocyte colony-stimulating factor (G-CSF) [22]. Although these studies have been instructive, efficacy has not been demonstrated in adequately controlled trials and no recommendations for routine use of these products have been made. In addition to providing enhanced opsonophagocytic activity, infusions of IVIG are associated with a prompt release of neutrophils from the marrow neutrophil storage pool into the peripheral circulation and enhanced chemotaxis of neutrophils to the site of bacterial infection [19]. It does appear, however, that replacement of antibody is more effective if products containing high titers of antibody against the specific infecting agent are used, but such products are not available for routine use [23]. The neonate is particularly vulnerable to colonization with virulent and/or antibiotic-resistant bacteria because the mucosal surfaces do not have the usual protective microflora of older infants and adults [24].

Many of the extrinsic risk factors for nosocomial infection in the nursery are device and environmentally related, as observed in adult intensive care units. The use of umbilical catheters and feeding of breast milk are unique to the nursery, and specific guidelines are required for care of the umbilicus and storage of breast milk for those infants who are too sick to suckle directly from the mother's breast. For example, breast milk from a mother who was infected with group B streptococcus (GBS) or *S. aureus* has been implicated as the vehicle of transmission of these pathogens to infants [25,26]. Furthermore, viral agents that may be transmitted to infants in breast milk or in the blood contact associated with breast feeding from dry, cracked nipples include hepatitis B virus, human immunodeficiency virus (HIV), and human T-lymphotrophic virus type 1 (HTLV-1). Therefore, in countries where safe formula for bottle feeding is readily available, breast feeding is contraindicated for mothers known to be infected with HIV and HTLV-1. Hepatitis B vaccine given to neonates is protective against transmission by breast feeding. Although cytomegalovirus (CMV) is transmitted in breast milk, maternal antibody is protective against clinically significant disease. Strict guidelines developed by the CDC for banking human milk obtained from unrelated donors include screening all donors for HIV, human T-lymphotrophic virus type 1, and hepatitis B surface antigen, and pasteurization (62.5°C for 30 minutes) of all milk specimens. Bacterial counts of 10^4 colony-forming units (cfu)/ml or more of nonpathogenic organisms and the presence of gram-negative bacteria, *S. aureus*, or α- or β-hemolytic streptococci preclude use of milk specimens [27].

The use of steroids for treatment of chronic bronchopulmonary dysplasia has been associated with an increased risk of infection in two studies [28,29]. The finding of an increase in the incidence of disseminated candidal infections associated with the unique practice of single-dose steroid administration in infants with prolonged hypotension shortly after birth further supports the role of steroids as an independent risk factor [29]. The risk–benefit ratio must be carefully considered before a course of steroids is initiated in HRN infants.

SITES OF INFECTION

The sites of nosocomial infections in the HRN differ from those in adults [5]. Primary bloodstream infections account for 30% to 50% of episodes in neonates, depending on birthweight, and surgical wound infections and urinary tract infections are rare. In contrast, > 40% of hospital-acquired infections in adults are urinary tract infections and 20% are surgical wound infections (see Chapter 30). Cutaneous sites are more likely to be involved in neonates.

ETIOLOGY AND CLINICAL MANIFESTATIONS

Bacterial

A comparison of the etiologies of early- and late-onset infections in neonates born at Parkland Memorial Hospital from 1987 to 1995 is presented in Figure 26-1. This distribution is similar to the national experience [5,20,21, 28,30,31]. Since the late 1970s, GBS has been the most frequently isolated pathogen from term infants with early-onset disease, accounting for ~ 70% of cases [32]. These organisms are acquired from the mother in the peripartum period. In ~ 70% of cases, GBS infections are acquired in utero. Although the *rate* of GBS early-onset infection is inversely proportional to gestational age, 80% of cases occur in term infants.

Infections acquired in normal newborn nurseries are most frequently not invasive, usually involve the skin or mucous membranes, and result from hand carriage or contaminated equipment or medication vials. Rarely, a healthcare worker colonized with the epidemic strain has been identified and the outbreak controlled upon removal of that individual from direct patient care [33]. Impetigo (skin pustules), conjunctivitis [34], omphalitis, and soft tissue abscess are the most frequently observed clinical manifestations. *S. aureus* remains the most frequently isolated pathogen from such infants. Group A streptococcal outbreaks [35] as well as outbreaks of diarrhea caused by bacterial pathogens (e.g., *Shigella* and *Salmonella* species) may occur in both term and preterm nurseries [36,37], but have been reported less frequently in recent years (see Chapters 34, 41). CONS rarely cause early-onset disease in otherwise healthy term neonates without any devices in place.

Consistent, unexplained shifts over time in the etiology of bacterial infections in high-risk infants have been observed [38]. Invasive strains of *S. aureus* were predominant in the 1950s. For unexplained reasons, gram-negative bacilli, especially *Pseudomonas aeruginosa, Klebsiella* species, and *Escherichia coli* strains prevailed in the 1960s, to be replaced by GBS in the 1970s. GBS have

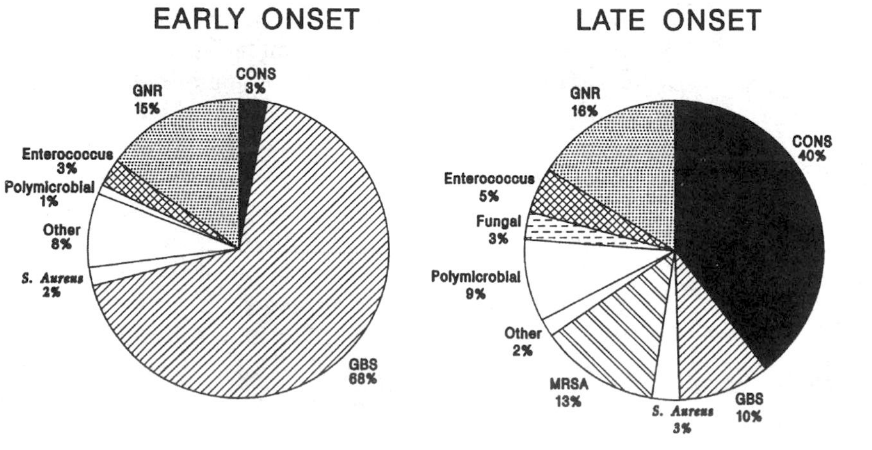

FIGURE 26-1. Invasive infections in 131,080 neonates at Parkland Memorial Hospital from January 1, 1987 through December 31, 1995. There were 347 episodes of early-onset disease (≤ 3 days of age) and 576 episodes of late-onset disease (≥ 4 days of age). Late-onset disease includes 1) infants who have been discharged and return with infection in the first 30 days of life; and 2) infants remaining in the nursery beyond 30 days of life who are monitored until discharge. GBS, group B streptococci; CONS, coagulase-negative staphylococci; GNR, gram-negative rods; MRSA, methicillin-resistant *S. aureus*.

remained the major pathogens of early-onset disease throughout the 1980s and 1990s. However, in the 1980s, MRSA and CONS emerged as prevailing pathogens of nosocomial infections in the HRN. Although CONS continue to account for 40% to 50% of hospital-acquired infections in the HRN in the 1990s, the following three pathogens associated with less than 15% to 20% of HRN infections are particularly problematic because of the difficulty in treatment: 1) enterococci, especially vancomycin-resistant strains (VRE); 2) multidrug-resistant gram-negative bacilli, especially *Enterobacter* species; and 3) fungi, predominantly *Candida* species.

Coagulase-negative staphylococci account for nearly 50% of late-onset nosocomial infections in most recent reports [5,20,21,28,31]. There are several reasons for the increased recognition of this organism as a neonatal pathogen:

1. Increased number and survival of the very–low-birthweight (< 1,500 g at birth) infants
2. Increased use of intravascular devices in the high risk neonate
3. Increased likelihood of identifying a blood culture positive for CONS as a true bacteremia with the use of more consistent definitions and methods of obtaining blood cultures (e.g., two blood cultures, preferably one from a central venous catheter and one from a peripheral site)

The epidemiology of neonatal CONS bacteremia has been studied extensively using pulsed-field gel electrophoresis, ribotyping, DNA-DNA hybridization, and restriction endonuclease analysis, in addition to the traditional methods of speciation, phage typing, and plasmid analysis. Pulsed-field gel electrophoresis is now the most reliable method to confirm identity of strains. Distinct clones of both *Staphylococcus haemolyticus* [39,40] as well as *Staphylococcus epidermidis* [40–43] may become endemic in HRNs and cause clusters of infections over periods of 6 months to as long as 10 years. At the same time, many completely unrelated strains may be isolated from infants within the same unit. Some HRNs may not have any related strains identified during a specific period of time [44–46]. Eastick et al. [47] have reported relatively stable reservoirs of CONS in the feces, around the ear, and in the axillae and nares, but small, unstable numbers of these organisms on the skin of the forearm and leg. Thus, cross-contamination among sites on the same infant as well as horizontal spread among infants are important modes of transmission. Infusion of parenteral fluids contaminated with CONS is a rare source of bacteremia in the HRN [48] (see Chapter 44).

The clinical manifestations of CONS bacteremia are most often nonspecific, and this pathogen is rarely considered a cause of death [49]. The nonspecific signs of sepsis are observed most frequently: fever, apnea and bradycardia, feeding intolerance, and lethargy. Temperature instability, thrombocytopenia, abdominal distention, and persistent bacteremia in the absence of a central venous catheter have been associated with disease caused by CONS [50]. Specific delta toxin-producing strains have been found in pure culture in the stool as well as in the blood or peritoneal fluid of patients with a mild form of necrotizing enterocolitis [51,52]. Focal infections associated with these pathogens include neck abscess, omphalitis, wound abscess, and mastitis [53]. Right-sided endocarditis caused by CONS must be considered in the presence of a central venous catheter, persistent bacteremia (> 48 hours), and thrombocytopenia during appropriate antimicrobial therapy for bacteremia [54]. There may be no other abnormal findings on physical examination, and an echocardiogram demonstrates vegetations in the right atrium or on the tricuspid valve.

After CONS, *S. aureus* was the second most frequently isolated pathogen from HRN infants in the 1986 to 1993 NNIS report [5] as well as the 1991 to 1993 report from the Neonatal Research Network [28]. Since the late 1980s, *S. aureus* outbreaks in the HRN have been associated with both methicillin-susceptible [55–58] and methicillin-resistant strains [12,59–62]. Nurseries that are situated in large general hospitals where there is a sharing of services (laboratory, radiology) as well as personnel (nurses, respiratory therapists, consulting physicians) are especially vulnerable to the acquisition of virulent strains from geographically distant foci of nosocomial MRSA infection. A single or multiple virulent strains are introduced into the nursery by a colonized infant, healthcare worker, or visiting family member [63]. Pulsed-field gel electrophoresis is the most useful method to determine if an outbreak is caused by a single or multiple different strains [64]. High rates of colonization (30% to 70%) may become established before clinical disease is recognized. The principal mode of transmission is horizontal by the transiently colonized hands of hospital personnel. Environmental sources or chronic carriers have rarely been implicated in nosocomial transmission. Unidentified virulence factors as well as environmental conditions determine the persistence of the organism in the HRN. In our own crowded HRN, MRSA persisted for a 3-year period from 1988 to 1991 [12]. Both susceptible *S. aureus* and MRSA nursery outbreaks have not been controlled until conditions of overcrowding and understaffing were corrected [12,65]. It is likely that the large number of infants who become colonized with MRSA during their stay in the HRN contributes substantially to the increased frequency of community-acquired MRSA infections observed nationwide in recent years.

Skin pustules, bullous impetigo, scalded skin syndrome [55–57], soft tissue abscesses, conjunctivitis, pneumonia with or without empyema, osteomyelitis, septic arthritis, and surgical site infections are the most frequent manifestations of both methicillin-susceptible and resistant *S. aureus* infections in neonates, and the case fatality rate associated with invasive disease may be 15% to 30%. Bacteremia with multiple foci of disease is characteristic of *S. aureus* infections.

Enterococci have been recognized as important pathogens in the HRN since 1979 [66,67], but the incidence [68–71] and number of reports of nursery outbreaks associated with *Streptococcus faecium* [72] and *Streptococcus faecalis* [73] have increased substantially since the 1980s. Outbreak strains can be distinguished from endemic strains and "background" nursery flora with the use of sensitive strain typing methods [73]. Invasion occurs most often from the infant's endogenous flora. However, in outbreaks, horizontal spread by hands of healthcare workers is an important mode of transmission. In regions of the United States where VRE have become problematic nosocomial pathogens, spread to the NICU has also occurred [71].

Most often, enterococci are isolated from the blood of low-birthweight infants with serious underlying conditions who have been in the HRN for > 30 to 60 days. Prolonged use of central venous catheters, necrotizing enterocolitis, bowel resection, and prior exposure to antibiotics are associated findings. Polymicrobial bacteremia is especially likely to occur in association with intraabdominal disease, supporting the intestine as a point of invasion of enterococci. Clinical manifestations of enterococcal infections are nonspecific. The unusual cases of meningitis [72] and endocarditis require prolonged (≥ 3 weeks and ≥ 6 weeks, respectively) treatment with combination therapy for cure.

Infections caused by gram-negative bacilli are associated with the largest case fatality rates—40% (range, 24% to 62%) in one study [28], but approaching 90–100% in earlier studies [74]. *E. coli* and *Klebsiella* and *Enterobacter* species are the most frequently isolated gram-negative rods in the absence of an outbreak [5,28,38]. Other gram-negative bacilli responsible for temporally related clusters in the HRN include *P. aeruginosa* [75–78], *Serratia* species [79,80], *Citrobacter diversus* [81–83], *Salmonella* species [10,37,84,85], *Acinetobacter* species [86], and *Flavobacterium meningosepticum* [87,88]. Nursery outbreaks of gram-negative infections have been associated with contamination of a nonchlorinated water supply [79], antiseptic solutions [80], intravenous medications and solutions [89], human breast milk [90], sinks [76], humidified ventilator circuits, suction machines [85], laryngoscopes [78], and the like. However, environmental contamination is implicated less frequently in well developed countries with clean water supplies and well defined protocols for sterilization of equipment and single use of disposable items (see Chapter 20).

In the absence of an environmental source, it is likely that a virulent epidemic strain is acquired from the infected mother or an infected healthcare worker or emerges from the infant's endogenous flora and then is transmitted horizontally on the hands of care givers. Identical strains of *C. diversus* have been identified in maternal infant pairs [82] as well as in healthcare workers and infected neonates [83]. Prolonged rectal colonization in addition to hand colonization has been implicated in outbreaks of *C. diversus* meningitis that were not controlled until colonized personnel were removed from the nursery [82,83]. Molecular fingerprinting is a valuable tool for tracing nosocomial transmission of a variety of different gram-negative bacilli in a neonatal unit [77,91–93], and should be used during outbreaks to determine if horizontal transmission or selective antibiotic pressure is the predominant mechanism of spread (see Chapter 16).

Clinical manifestations characteristic of gram-negative infections include necrotizing ophthalmitis, pneumonia, ecthyma gangrenosum, cardiovascular collapse, and meningitis. Although ecthymatous lesions are associated most frequently with *P. aeruginosa* invasive disease, they may be associated with other gram-negative pathogens as well as fungi. Biopsy and culture of such lesions are helpful for isolation of the specific pathogen. *Salmonella* species have a proclivity for causing osteomyelitis and septic arthritis, as well as a meningitis that is especially difficult to cure even with prolonged courses of antibiotics that are highly active in vitro against the infecting strain. *C. diversus* meningitis is notable for the occurrence of clusters of cases in NICUs and the association with brain abscess in 77% of cases, compared with 7% of cases of meningitis caused by other gram-negative bacilli [82). *Flavobacterium meningosepticum* is a less frequent cause of epidemic gram-negative meningitis [87,88]. This is an unusual gram-negative bacillus that is resistant to most antimicrobial agents used for empiric treatment of gram-negative meningitis in the newborn, and is treated successfully by the combination of vancomycin and rifampin [94].

The importance of antibiotic use in selection [74] of multidrug-resistant strains of gram-negative organisms has been well documented for aminoglycosides as well as third-generation cephalosporins. Carefully monitoring for development of resistance to the first-line aminoglycoside, usually gentamicin or tobramycin, is helpful. Susceptibility patterns in the HRN respond promptly to changes in antibiotic prescribing patterns. In the absence of multidrug-resistant strains, amikacin and especially third-generation cephalosporins are best reserved for rare individuals whose infections are resistant to the routine treatment regimens. The combination of an aminoglycoside and third-generation cephalosporin is recommended for treatment of gram-negative meningitis even with organisms that are fully susceptible to aminoglycosides.

Outbreaks of *Clostridium difficile*-associated colitis do not occur in the newborn nursery. In contrast to healthy adults who have an asymptomatic colonization rate of < 5%, toxin-producing strains of *C. difficile* may be recovered from the stools of as many as 50% of healthy neonates. Disease usually does not occur because the immature intestinal mucosa of the neonate lacks receptors for the *C. difficile* toxin. This organism does not play a role in the pathogenesis of necrotizing enterocolitis.

Fungal

Of the subspecialty services in NNIS hospitals conducting hospital-wide surveillance, the HRN had one of the highest nosocomial fungal infection rates for the 1986 to 1990 period: 7.6 per 1,000 discharges, after burn/trauma (16.1), cardiac surgery (11.2), and oncology (8.6) [95]. During this 5-year period, the fungal infection rate in the HRN increased from 4.7 to 9.6 per 1,000. In one study of candidemia in a pediatric population from 1988 to 1992, 25% of patients were premature infants [96]. In the 1986 to 1994 NNIS surveillance period, *Candida* species accounted for 7% of all bloodstream infections in the HRN, fourth after CONS, GBS, and *S. aureus*.

The most important risk factors for systemic fungal infections include extreme prematurity, colonization, central venous catheterization with infusion of hyperalimentation fluids containing lipid emulsions, delayed feedings, prolonged courses of broad-spectrum antibiotics, and endotracheal intubation [97–99]. In most cases, candidemia develops as a consequence of endogenous colonization rather than as a result of cross-contamination. Baley et al. [100] reported a 26.7% fungal colonization rate in infants weighing < 1,500 g at birth who were followed prospectively. Two thirds of these infants were colonized within the first week of life, reflecting maternal transmission during labor and delivery. Systemic disease developed in 7.7% of colonized infants. Once colonized, invasion arises most often from the gastrointestinal tract. Early colonization is more likely to be associated with *Candida albicans*, whereas other species, such as *Candida parapsilosis* and *Candida tropicalis* are more likely to be associated with late colonization. *C. parapsilosis* is the most commonly reported cause of epidemic candidal infections [101].

With the use of DNA fingerprinting, it has been possible to determine that several nursery outbreaks of invasive candidal infections have been associated with cross-transmission from the hands of healthcare workers [98, 99,102,103], retrograde intravenous medication administration [104], or contamination of a multidose bottle of liquid glycerin used as a suppository [101]. The presence of onychomycosis in healthcare workers has been suggested as a possible source of nosocomial candidiasis spread by hand carriage [103].

Clinical manifestations of disseminated candidiasis are nonspecific in most cases. Rarely, neonates with a maternal history of vaginal moniliasis contract congenital mucocutaneous candidiasis [105]. At birth, such infants have an intensely erythematous maculopapular eruption of the trunk and extremities that rapidly becomes vesicular and pustular and then resolves with extensive desquamation. Palms and soles are almost always affected. These infants, who are otherwise asymptomatic, do not have systemic involvement and respond well to topical antifungal therapy. In contrast, the development of a diffuse, erythematous, scaling, burnlike dermatitis in an infant of less than 1,500 g birthweight is more likely to be a manifestation of invasive disease and requires systemic therapy [106].

Candida species are recovered from blood cultures of infants with invasive candidiasis less frequently than are bacteria from infants with invasive bacterial disease. True candiduria may be a reflection of disseminated disease or localized cystitis. Candidal endocarditis associated with a central venous catheter in an infant with a structurally normal heart may be best detected by echocardiogram. Large vegetations may be present in the absence of a murmur or signs of congestive heart failure [107]. Fungal vegetations have been found at autopsy in infants with endocarditis unsuspected before death. Osteomyelitis, septic arthritis, meningitis, and brain abscess are other foci of infection that may be present with relatively few specific physical signs. The most severe cases of meningitis and endocarditis require prolonged treatment courses of amphotericin B, up to 40 to 50 mg/kg total dose or at least 6 weeks of a liposomal amphotericin preparation.

Other fungi associated with nosocomial infection in the HRN include *Aspergillus* species [108,109], *Malassezia* species [110,111], *Rhizopus* species [112], and *Trichosporon beigelii* [113]. *Aspergillus, Rhizopus*, and *Trichosporon* are acquired from the environment. Of note, infants with aspergillosis are not neutropenic, but are premature and do not have normal chemotaxis and phagocytosis. Cutaneous aspergillosis may occur as the initial manifestation of disease or as one site of involvement in disseminated disease. Because of the risk of dissemination from primary cutaneous lesions and the difficulty in distinguishing primary from secondary lesions, aggressive systemic antifungal therapy is always indicated.

Both *Malassezia furfur* [110] and *Malassezia pachydermatis* [111] have been associated with clusters of bloodstream infections in high-risk premature infants who have received intralipids through central venous catheters. *Malassezia* isolates are most frequently isolated from blood obtained through a central venous catheter and are rarely recovered from peripheral blood. *M. furfur* skin colonization rates of 25% to 84% have been reported for infants during prolonged HRN admissions, whereas no > 5% of infants hospitalized in a non-NICU setting or attending a well-baby clinic were colonized with this organism [110]. Clinical manifestations of infection are the nonspecific signs of bacterial sepsis. When temporally related cases occur, it is most likely that these organisms are carried from patient to patient on the hands of healthcare workers. Because *M. furfur* requires an exogenous source of lipids to support its growth, the clinical microbiology laboratory inoculates the specimen on a solid agar plate that is then covered with a layer of sterile olive oil. The Isolator™ blood culture system is the most convenient system available for isolation of these organisms.

Viral

Outbreaks of viral infections in the HRN have been recognized with increased frequency now that there is an awareness of the problem and techniques for isolation and identification of viruses are available in the clinical microbiology laboratory (see Chapter 9). In nursery outbreaks of viral infections, there are high rates of infection of staff members [114–116]. Because staff members have mild illness, they continue to work and continue to spread infection by direct inoculation of their infected secretions. Respiratory syncytial virus (RSV) and rotavirus are the most frequently identified viral agents associated with nosocomial spread (see Chapters 32, 34). Other respiratory viruses, notably parainfluenza, may be associated with clusters of respiratory infections having similar clinical manifestations as RSV. Manifestations of RSV infections in infants younger than 3 weeks of age are atypical and more likely to include apnea, lethargy, and poor feeding in the absence of respiratory symptoms [117]. Beyond 3 weeks of age, bronchiolitis and pneumonia are characteristic of RSV infections; apnea may precede the onset of respiratory symptoms. Infants with bronchopulmonary dysplasia requiring oxygen, congenital heart disease with pulmonary hypertension, and congenital immune deficiency syndromes are at the greatest risk for development of severe disease after infection with RSV.

Several different types of adenovirus have been associated with nursery outbreaks [116,118,119]. The most common clinical manifestations are conjunctivitis and pneumonia. Direct inoculation by ophthalmologic instruments has been documented [118]. Neonates may manifest multiorgan involvement with cardiovascular collapse and a bacterial sepsis-like clinical syndrome with a case fatality rate of 84% [119]. Nursery outbreaks of coxsackievirus and echovirus infections are well described [120]. In most outbreaks, the source cases acquired infection from their mothers and had severe disease. Case fatality rates associated with hepatitis may be as high as 83%. Those infants who acquire infection by nosocomial spread have milder disease, with case fatality rates of 12% or less. Healthcare workers may also be vectors for the spread of this group of viruses. The most common clinical manifestations of neonatal coxsackievirus and echovirus infections are hepatitis, meningoencephalitis, myocarditis, and pneumonia.

Rotavirus and hepatitis A virus are spread by the fecal–oral route. Rotavirus transmission in the nursery is well documented and infection may be asymptomatic or associated with mild to moderate or severe diarrhea. Rotavirus-associated outbreaks of necrotizing enterocolitis have been reported [115]. Nosocomial outbreaks of hepatitis A virus are extremely rare because of the relatively brief duration and low titer of viral shedding within the stool [121–123] (see Chapter 42). However, immunologically immature preterm infants may excrete hepatitis A viral antigen and RNA for as long as 4 to 5 months after the acute infection [122]. The source infants in reported outbreaks acquired hepatitis A virus either by vertical transmission from the mother before or during delivery [121], or by blood transfusion [122,123].

The following viruses are not transmitted horizontally in the nursery: HIV, hepatitis B, hepatitis C, and CMV. Observance of universal and, now, standard precautions as well as screening of blood for transfusion, and in the case of CMV, the use of filtered blood or leukocyte-poor red blood cells, has prevented transmission of infection (see Chapter 13). There is no significant increase in the excretion of CMV in infants in the nursery compared with patients in other areas of a pediatric hospital [124], nor is there a significant increase in the risk of acquisition of CMV infection among caregivers on pediatric or neonatal units compared with similar adults without hospital exposure [125]. Transmission of herpes simplex virus [126] and varicella-zoster virus [127,128] in the nursery is extremely rare. Although transmission from oral lesions of nursery personnel has been reported [129], the risk is so low that such individuals are no longer excluded from patient care. In contrast, individuals with herpetic whitlow are excluded from direct patient contact in the nursery. With more widespread use of the varicella virus vaccine licensed in 1995, the number of susceptible neonates as well as infected mothers, visitors, or healthcare workers should decrease substantially.

TREATMENT

Physicians treating specific infections may consult their local nursery guidelines or the most recent edition of the *Pocket Book of Pediatric Antimicrobial Therapy* for specific recommendations concerning choice of agent, dosing regimen, and duration of therapy [130]. Empiric therapy for early-onset disease consists of ampicillin combined with an aminoglycoside. Ampicillin provides activity against GBS, enterococci, and *Listeria monocytogenes*. If *S. aureus* is suspected, methicillin or oxacillin, or with MRSA, vancomycin, is recommended for gram-positive coverage. The choice of aminoglycoside is based on susceptibility patterns in the nursery, but amikacin is usually reserved because of its greater activity against some gram-negative bacilli that are resistant to gentamicin and tobramycin, and its increased cost. Beyond 5 days of age, vancomycin is recommended for its activity against CONS and is especially important in the presence of a central venous catheter or in a nursery with endemic or epidemic MRSA. With the exception of CONS, meningitis may be present in 10% to 20% of bacteremias. Therefore, meningitic dosages are recommended until meningitis has been ruled out.

Third-generation cephalosporins are not recommended for routine empiric use because of the rapidity of emergence of resistance in an individual patient during therapy and in microflora of the unit [74,131]. However, cefotaxime is added to the aminoglycoside if there is a strong suspicion of gram-negative meningitis. Cefatazidime is substituted for treatment of susceptible strains of *Pseudomonas* or *Stenotrophomonas* species. Ceftriaxone is not used in the neonatal period because of its displacement of bilirubin from albumin-binding sites [132] and its strong suppressive effect on the neonate's developing gastrointestinal flora [133]. There is little experience with imipenem or meropenem in neonates. However, meropenem is less toxic and maybe the only drug active against some highly resistant gram-negative bacilli. Monitoring of susceptibility patterns for gram-negative bacilli and antibiotic use is necessary to ensure that the currently recommended agents will be effective against the current pathogens (see Chapter 15).

Specific anaerobic coverage is required rarely in neonates. However, either clindamycin or metronidazole can be used; metronidazole is preferred for central nervous system infection. Chloramphenicol is not recommended for use in neonates because of its toxicity and unpredictable pharmacokinetics.

Amphotericin B remains the preferred treatment of invasive fungal disease in the neonate. Flucytosine may be added for enhanced activity in the most severe disease (e.g., meningitis, endocarditis). Fluconazole is recommended for mucocutaneous disease and isolated fungal cystitis. There is little experience with liposomal amphotericin preparations in neonates, but they may be considered in severe, life-threatening disease uncontrolled by conventional amphotericin B.

Acyclovir is the preferred treatment for herpes simplex and varicella-zoster viral infections. There is increasing experience to support the efficacy of ganciclovir for perinatally acquired CMV infection [134], and a large, multicenter trial is being conducted. Recommendations for the use of ribavirin therapy in RSV infections have been modified since the licensure of this drug in 1986 because of the continuing questions concerning efficacy. Ribavirin should be considered for use in the infected, high-risk, low-birth-weight infant with chronic bronchopulmonary dysplasia, congenital heart disease, congenital immunodeficiency syndrome, or other serious underlying conditions such as neurologic or metabolic disease, multiple congenital anomalies, and the like [135]. Ribavirin must be initiated early in the course of disease for optimum effectiveness.

PREVENTION

Nursery Design and Staffing

The American Academy of Pediatrics and the American College of Obstetrics and Gynecology have collaborated to develop guidelines for all aspects of perinatal care [136]; these guidelines are revised at regular intervals. Table 26-3 summarizes the recommended nurse/infant ratios and spatial requirements per infant based on acuity of the medical condition and the amount and type of nursing care and support equipment needed. Nurse/infant ratios below those recommended have been associated with increased rates of susceptible *S. aureus* and MRSA invasive disease in the nursery [12,65].

Isolation

The 1997 *Redbook* issued by the Committee on Infectious Diseases of the American Academy of Pediatrics has incorporated the recommendations for *standard* and *transmission*-based precautions that were published by the CDC in 1996 [137], and should be consulted for management of specific infections [138]. With the adoption of standard precautions, guidelines for isolation of neonates have been simplified. There are relatively few infections that require *contact, airborne*, or *droplet* precautions. Table 26-4 summarizes the recommended precautions for the most frequently encountered neonatal infections (see Chapter 13). It is important to note that the current category of contact precautions does not include the use of a mask within 3 feet of the patient, which was part of the former contact isolation category. Thus, if

TABLE 26-3. *Recommended staffing ratios and space according to level of care required in the newborn nursery*

Care provided	Nurse-to-infant ratio	Floor space(ft^2) per infant	Space between beds (ft)
Admissions/observation (transitional care stabilization)	1:4	40	—[a]
Newborns needing only *routine* care	1:6–8	30	3
Normal mother-newborn couplet care	1:3–4	—[a]	—[a]
Newborns requiring *continuing* care	1:3–4	40	4
Newborns requiring *intermediate* care	1:2–3	50	4
Newborns requiring *intensive* care	1:1–2	80–100	6
Newborns requiring multisystem support[b]	1:1	80–100	6
Unstable newborns requiring complex critical care[b]	>1:1	80–100	6

[a]No specific recommendation published.
[b]Increased space requirements preferred, but no specific recommendations are published.
(Adapted from American Academy of Pediatrics, American College of Obstetricians and Gynecologists. *Guidelines of perinatal care*, 3rd ed. Elk Grove Village, IL: American Academy of Pediatrics; 1992:7,23–29.)

TABLE 26-4. *Summary of 1996 isolation guidelines for infections encountered in the nursery*

Infection	Type of precautions
Abscess	
Contained by dressing	Standard
Draining, not contained by dressing	Contact
Conjunctivitis (bacterial, chlamydia, gonococcal)	Standard
Cytomegalovirus	Standard
Enteroviruses (Coxsackievirus, echovirus)	Contact
Diarrhea (bacterial or viral)	Contact
Fungal (Candidiasis, aspergillosis, *malassezia*)	Standard
Hepatitis viruses	
A	Contact
All others	Standard
Herpes simplex (maternal exposure, disease)	Contact
Human immunodeficiency virus	Standard
Listeriosis	Standard
Measles	Airborne
Meningitis	
Neisseria meningitidis, Hemophilus influenzae, type B	Droplet × 24 hr
All others	Standard
Multidrug-resistant organisms (vancomycin-resistant enterococci, methicillin-resistant *S. aureus*, resistant gram-negative bacilli)	Contact
Necrotizing enterocolitis	Standard
Respiratory viruses (respiratory syncytial, parainfluenza, adenovirus)	Contact
Rubella	Droplet
Streptococcal	Standard
Syphilis	Standard
Toxoplasmosis	Standard
Varicella	Airborne, Contact

(Adapted from Garner JS, The Hospital Infection Control Practices Advisory Committee. Guidelines for isolation precautions in hospitals. *Infect Control Hosp Epidemiol* 1996;17:54–80.)

large-particle (75μm) droplets are likely to be an important mode of transmission, droplet precautions must be added to the contact precautions (see Chapter 1). Neonates usually are unable to generate large-particle droplets. According to standard precautions, masks are indicated if splatter of respiratory secretions is anticipated (e.g., endotracheal suctioning or intubation).

It is preferable to have an isolation room with negative-pressure ventilation for isolation of neonates with perinatal exposure to maternal varicella. Most other infections require contact isolation and can be managed by cohorting and physical separation, but do not require a special room. Although enclosed isolettes provide a limited amount of barrier protection relative to open warmers or bassinets [127], they cannot be relied on to prevent spread of infections to other infants by hand carriage.

During outbreaks, cohorting infants who are colonized or infected with epidemiologically important pathogens with designated personnel who do not care for newly admitted infants or infants who are not colonized or infected is an effective method of controlling horizontal transmission [74,137,139,140]. It is very difficult to maintain strict cohorting in large, understaffed nurseries. If transmission continues in the presence of strict cohorting, continuing introduction of the epidemic organisms from a carrier or multiple different sources, or from ineffective hand antisepsis, is likely [81].

Handwashing and Gloves

As observed throughout the hospital, handwashing between patient contacts is the single most important measure for prevention of nosocomial infections in the nursery (see Chapter 13). Recommendations for the number of nursery scrub areas are as follows: 1) one scrub area at the entrance to each nursery with faucets operated by foot or knee controls; 2) scrub sinks for at least every 6 to 8 patient stations in the normal newborn nursery and for every 3 to 4 patient stations in the admission/observation, continuing care, intermediate care, or intensive care areas [136]. Antiseptic-containing foams or antiseptic-impregnated tissues must never be used as substitutes for sinks and handwashing with soap and water, but rather as adjuncts to handwashing.

Brown et al. reported the use of a video camera to record handwashing compliance and contamination episodes in the HRN [141]. The staff members were informed that the purpose of the video camera was to record traffic patterns for the optimal design of a new unit. The rates of handwashing compliance for various groups before patient contacts were nurses, 24.7%; physicians, 31.8%; respiratory therapists, 20.5%; and parents, 6.6%. Hand contamination, which may negate the effect of handwashing, occurred before 76.4% of patient contacts. The efficacy of incorporation of such a videotape into a group feedback educational program has not yet been determined. However, in a different study, Raju and Kobler [142] demonstrated an improvement of 28% to 63% in compliance with handwashing in the newborn nursery in response to intensive educational efforts using feedback of observed rates. Novel strategies to improve adherence to recommendations for handwashing are needed desperately in the nursery.

The important components of handwashing are consistency, duration of exposure, and antimicrobial content of the soap used [143] (see Chapter 13,20). Traditionally, the friction on all surfaces was believed to be sufficient to remove the transient flora, and plain soap was acceptable. However, Wade et al. demonstrated greater efficacy in removing enterococci and *Enterobacter* species using a soap that contains an antiseptic substance active against these bacteria [144]. Furthermore, the change of handwashing soap from chlorhexidine gluconate (Hibiclens) to a preparation containing 0.3% triclosan (Bacti-Stat) was associated with control of an MRSA outbreak in a newborn nursery that had continued despite the standard infection control measures [145]. The relative in vitro resistance of outbreak strains of MRSA to chlorhexidine and relative susceptibility to triclosan has been demonstrated previously.

Removal of jewelry from the hands and a 2-minute scrub from hands to forearms with an antiseptic-containing soap is recommended for nursery staff at the beginning of a work shift, and a 10- to 15-second wash between infant contacts thereafter. Plain soap that does not contain antimicrobial agents is recommended for standard precautions. However, for contact precautions and in nurseries with high rates of colonization or disease associated with epidemiologically important multidrug-resistant organisms, antimicrobial-containing soap is recommended for all handwashing. Chlorhexidine and triclosan are the most frequently used agents.

Gloves are worn whenever contact with blood or body fluids is anticipated or whenever handling anything that has come in contact with an infant in *contact* isolation. Gloves must be changed between patient contacts and are never washed. Handwashing is performed immediately upon glove removal.

Gowns, Caps, and Masks

The use of gowns on entrance into the nursery is a longstanding ritual that most nurseries are hesitant to relinquish. Studies of varying design conducted in the nursery and NICU confirm the lack of efficacy of gowns for preventing nosocomial infections [146,147]. In alternate 2-month gowning and no-gowning cycles, Pelke et al. [147] demonstrated no significant differences in the rates of bacterial colonization, nosocomial infection including RSV and necrotizing enterocolitis, and mortality. In addition, compliance with handwashing was not increased during the gowning cycles and there was no change in traffic into the unit. Thus, in a nonoutbreak setting, gowns are not required for staff or visitors upon entrance into the nursery. Gowns are indicated for the following situations: anticipated soiling with blood or body fluids, *contact* isolation, presence of clustered infections with epidemiologically important organisms that are considered to have been transmitted by contact, and parental concern for excessively soiled clothing. Some studies have continued to use gowns for handling newborn infants (e.g., cuddling, feeding).

Caps and masks are indicated for performance of sterile procedures, including central line placement. Masks also are used as part of droplet and airborne precautions or to protect an infant from personnel with respiratory tract infection who are considered indispensable and cannot be removed from the nursery.

Cord, Skin, and Eye Care

The umbilical cord may become colonized with *S. aureus* in up to 70% of infants within 48 hours after birth [148]. High colonization rates in the nursery are associated with an increased rate of postdischarge infection for term infants or later during the hospital stay for low-birthweight infants. Therefore, most nursery protocols include treatment with an antiseptic. Certainly any nursery experiencing an increased rate of *S. aureus* infections will use topical antiseptics for cord care. The delay in time to cord separation beyond 7 days in infants treated with topical antiseptics is not significant clinically. Dry cord care and isopropyl alcohol have been associated with higher colonization rates than the following antiseptic agents that may be used: 1) triple dye, a combination of brilliant green (2.29 mg/ml), proflavine hemisulfate (1.14 mg/mL), and gentian violet (2.29 mg/mL); 2) bacitracin ointment; 3) chlorhexidine; or 4) silver sulfadiazine cream (1% Silvadene™). However, greater efficacy has not been demonstrated for any one agent [136,149]. Iodine-containing agents are not recommended because of the possibility of transcutaneous absorption and suppression of neonatal thyroid function. Short-term use of mupiricin (Bactroban™) ointment for control of an outbreak associated with susceptible S. aureus or MRSA may be considered. However, mupiricin is not recommended routinely because of the emergence of resistant strains after prolonged use [150].

Traditionally, triple dye has not been used in the HRN because of theoretic concern about increased systemic absorption and rendering the umbilical stump unsuitable for vessel catheterization. However, there have been no adverse effects observed since a routine single application of triple dye to the umbilical stump was extended to infants in our intermediate care area in 1988 and then to our intensive care area infants in 1991. In the NICU, application of triple dye after umbilical vessel catheterization in the first 12 hours after birth was instrumental in controlling a prolonged MRSA outbreak [12].

Initial cleansing of the skin after birth is delayed until the neonate's temperature has stabilized. Warm water and a mild, nonmedicated soap are recommended for cleansing the skin [136]. Hexachlorophene specifically is no longer recommended for routine daily bathing of neonates because of the neurotoxicity demonstrated previously when absorbed in large concentrations. Chlorhexidine gluconate is, however, poorly absorbed through intact skin. When intramuscular injections are given in the delivery room as part of prophylaxis regimens (e.g., penicillin G for prevention of early-onset GBS disease or gonococcal ophthalmia, ceftriaxone for prevention of gonococcal ophthalmia, or vitamin K for prevention of hemorrhagic disease of the newborn), the injection site must first be cleansed well with alcohol. This prevents the introduction of microorganisms such as HIV, hepatitis B virus, and herpes simplex virus that are in maternal blood and body fluids and that may be contaminating the infant's skin.

A single application within 1 hour of delivery of topical tetracycline (1%) or erythromycin (0.5%) ophthalmic ointment is preferred for prevention of gonococcal ophthalmia. The use of 1% silver nitrate drops is discouraged because of the associated chemical irritation. The eyes should not be irrigated after instillation of any of these agents. Single-use tubes or vials must be used to prevent cross-infection. A single dose of ceftriaxone, 125 mg (25 to 50 mg/kg for low-birthweight infants) intramuscularly or intravenously, is recommended for infants born to mothers with active gonorrhea at the time of delivery.

Intravascular Catheters and Respiratory Therapy Equipment

There are few controlled investigations of care practices of intravascular catheter and respiratory therapy equipment specifically in the newborn nursery. Consequently, nurseries usually follow guidelines for care of catheters and respiratory equipment that are based on studies in older children and adults [168,169] (see Chapters). Antimicrobial- or antiseptic-impregnated catheters and cuffs are not available yet in sizes small enough for neonates. Peripherally inserted (PICC) as well as surgically placed central venous catheters are utilized in the NICU. Unique to the nursery is the use of umbilical arterial and venous catheters, for which many care issues remain unresolved. The rates of colonization and associated bacteremias are similar for umbilical artery and umbilical venous catheters. The umbilical insertion site must be cleansed with an appropriate antiseptic before catheter insertion. Tincture of iodine is not used because of the potential effect on the neonatal thyroid [168]. The chlorhexidine–gluconate-impregnated opaque foam patch (Biopatch) is not recommended for use in very–low-birthweight infants (< 1,000 g) who are younger than 7 days of chronologic age and < 27 weeks' gestation because of reports of exudative-type local reactions and pressure necrosis occurring under the patch in these very premature infants [170].

Mouth suctioning devices such as the De Lee suction trap should not be used because of the risk of exposure to potentially infectious aspirated material that could enter the mouth of the healthcare worker. When a mechanical suction apparatus is used, the negative pressure should be no greater than 100 mm Hg when the suction tubing is occluded [136].

Each nursery should develop protocols for care of the specific intravascular catheters and respiratory therapy equipment that are used in the specific unit. These protocols should be consistent with the current guidelines published by the American Academy of Pediatrics and the CDC.

Immunoprophylaxis

The presence of specific humoral antibodies to neonatal viral and bacterial pathogens is protective against infection or at least against clinically severe disease. Thus, several trials have been performed to determine the efficacy of periodic infusions of IVIG for the prevention of nosocomial infections in the HRN [20,21]. The conclusion from these studies is that, even when serum IgG levels are maintained above 400 mg/dl, there is no significant decrease in the rate of nosocomial infection or mortality associated with repeated infusions of commercially available preparations. Of note, the largest multicenter, controlled trial, which enrolled 2,416 infants, reported lot-to-lot variation in the incidence of nosocomial infection [21]. Despite the use of thousands of donors for the processing of each batch of intravenous immunoglobulin, lot-to-lot variation in antibody profile has been demonstrated [21,151]. This variation may be particularly significant for *S. epidermidis*, the most frequent pathogen associated with late-onset sepsis in the HRN. When tested in the suckling rat model, lots with ≥ 90% opsonic activity promote bacterial clearance from blood and increase survival rates, compared with lots containing ≤ 50% opsonic activity [151]. This is a plausible explanation for the failure to demonstrate efficacy in trials of IVIG.

In contrast, efficacy for prevention of RSV infection in high-risk premature infants has been demonstrated for monthly infusions of 750 mg/kg of high-titered RSV-IVIG (RespiGam™) during the RSV season [152,153]. Beneficial effects include a reduction in 1) RSV disease severity; 2) RSV-associated hospitalization and hospitalization for other respiratory viruses; and 3) the incidence of otitis media [154]; as well as reasonable cost effectiveness. Guidelines for the use of RSV-IVIG have been developed by the American Academy of Pediatrics and include the following groups: 1) infants and children younger than 2 years, with bronchopulmonary dysplasia who are or have received supplemental oxygen in the previous 6 months; 2) infants with gestational ages of < 32 weeks and chronologic ages of < 6 months at the beginning of the RSV season infants ≤ 28 weeks gestational age may benefit from prophylaxis until 12 months chronological age; and 3) RSV outbreaks in high-risk units. RSV-IVIG is not yet approved for use in infants with congenital heart disease because of concerns about a possible increase in mortality rate observed in the original study in this group of infants [152]. RSV-IVIG should be considered for high-risk infants in an HRN with one or more cases of RSV infection.

Varicella-zoster immune globulin (VZIG) is indicated for susceptible high-risk individuals exposed to varicella. After an exposure in the HRN, VZIG 125 units is administered to premature infants of > 28 weeks' gestation whose mothers have no prior history of varicella or varicella immunization, and all premature infants < 28 weeks' gestation or ≤ 1,000 g birthweight, regardless of maternal history due to lack of placental transfer of antibody in earlier stages of pregnancy [155]. Most premature infants of ≥ 28 weeks' gestation whose mothers are immune have acquired sufficient maternal antibody to protect them from severe disease and complications. However, chronologic age > 2 months and seven or more transfusions of packed red cells may be associated with increased rates of seronegativity in infants whose mothers are immune [156]. VZIG is not recommended for healthy, term infants postnatally exposed even if their mothers have a negative history of varicella. Before VZIG administration in a nursery exposure, it is helpful to obtain serum from the infants to confirm susceptibility. If antibody determinations are available within 72 hours of the exposure, VZIG administration may be delayed until results are available. If antibody is present, the infant does not require isolation during the 10 to 28 days after exposure. VZIG is not indicated if an infant has received an infusion of IVIG for other indications within the previous 3 weeks.

Chemoprophylaxis

The use of antibiotics for prevention of nosocomial infections in the HRN is strongly discouraged because of the risk of emergence of resistant microorganisms that will require more broad-spectrum and potentially more toxic antimicrobial agents for treatment (see Chapters 14, 15). Two groups of investigators have reported the efficacy of low-dose vancomycin, 25 µg/ml of total parenteral nutrition fluid, to decrease catheter colonization and bacteremia caused by CONS. In two different, prospective, randomized, controlled trials of 70 and 150 very-low-birthweight infants, respectively, CONS bacteremia was decreased in infants weighing < 1,500 g from 34% to 1.4%, and in infants weighing < 1,000 g from 26% to 2.8% [157,158]. Despite the beneficial effect, both sets of investigators as well as an accompanying editorial do *not* recommend the routine use of this regimen because of the risk of emergence of vancomycin-resistant organisms [159]. Continued exposure of the normal flora to low concentrations of vancomycin creates especially favorable conditions for resistance to occur. In addition, morbidity and mortality associated with CONS infection is not severe enough to justify the risks.

In another randomized study of 148 infants weighing < 1,500 g with percutaneous central venous catheters, the use of amoxicillin 100 mg/kg/day intravenously in three divided doses had a negligible effect on the incidence of septicemia because the rate in the control group was so low, 2.7% [160]. In conclusion, strict adherence to aseptic technique at the time of central venous catheter insertion and to protocols for catheter care remains the preferred method of prevention of intravascular catheter-related infections.

Surveillance

An active surveillance program is an essential component of prevention (see Chapter 5). In most hospitals, surveillance of positive culture results is performed by infection control personnel who are responsible for several different units in the hospital. The infection control personnel identify temporally related clusters of clinical infections and epidemiologically important pathogens, especially those that are multidrug resistant, and then collaborate with the nursery staff to develop a prevention program (see Chapter 2). On identification of an outbreak, infection control personnel notify the microbiology laboratory of the need to save strains should molecular fingerprinting studies be indicated (see Chapter 6). Designation of a nursery staff member who understands the psychology and operational logistics of the unit as the infection control liaison facilitates education and adherence to policies for cohorting, handwashing, and other aseptic practices [12,161]. Participation of nursery staff members in the design of prevention programs increases adherence and success. Most important of all is feedback to the staff of positive results when they have succeeded in controlling an outbreak.

Routine cultures of body surfaces (i.e., skin, umbilicus, mucous membranes, tracheal aspirates, rectal swabs) is not recommended in nonoutbreak settings because they do not predict which infants are at risk for sepsis and they are very costly [162,163]. In contrast, body surface cultures are helpful during an outbreak to identify infants who are colonized in addition to infants who are infected with pathogens such as MRSA, VRE, and multidrug-resistant gram-negative bacilli. Newly admitted infants must be kept in cohorts separate from colonized infants to limit horizontal transmission of the problem organism. In addition, it is now recommended that units with no clinical cases of VRE be surveyed at 6- to 12-month intervals to detect the presence of VRE before the establishment of high colonization rates and clinical disease [164].

Employee Health

All members of the nursery staff are screened by history, and serology when indicated, for susceptibility to rubella, rubeola, varicella, and hepatitis B (see Chapter 3). Appropriate immunizations are provided for those who are seronegative. Annual influenza immunizations

TABLE 26-5. *The pregnant healthcare worker: management of occupational exposures to infectious agents*

Agent	In-hospital source	Effect on fetus	Rate of perinatal transmission	Maternal screening	Prevention
Cytomegalovirus	Urine, blood; transplant patients; daycare toddlers	Hearing loss; congenital syndrome[a]	Total 40% Symptomatic 5%	Antibody protects against clinical disease; routine screening not recommended	Efficacy of cytomegalovirus-immune globulin not established; vaccine investigational.; Standard precautions
Hepatitis B	Blood, body fluids	Hepatitis; hepatocellular cancer as adult	HB_eAg positive 90% HB_eAg negative 25%	Anti-HB_sAg, HB, Ag Anti-HB_cAg	Vaccine (safe during pregnancy) Standard precautions
Hepatitis C	Blood	Hepatitis	0%–15%	Anti-HCV, HCV RNA in reference labs	ISG no longer contains anti-HCV and is not recommended Standard precautions
Herpes simplex	Vesicular fluid	Congenital malformations, sepsis, encephalitis, mucotaneous lesions	Unlikely from nosocomial exposure; maternal whitlow more likely	Not useful	Contact isolation
HIV	Blood, body fluids	No congenital malformations; AIDS by 2–3 yr of age	8%–30%	Antibody enzyme-linked immunosorbent assay, Western blot, PCR	Avoid high-risk behaviors; AZT intrapartum, post-natal for HIV pos. mothers and their babies[b] Standard precautions
Influenza	Respiratory secretions	Inconsistent	Rare	None	Vaccine (safe during pregnancy)
Parvovirus B19	Respiratory secretions, ? blood; sicklers, immunocompromised patients	Hydrops, stillbirth No congenital syndrome	Rare; 3%–9% max. adverse outcome	IgM, IgG antibody Prepregnancy antibody protective	May choose to avoid sicklers with aplastic crisis and immunocompromised patients with chronic anemia. Droplet precautions
Rubella	Respiratory secretions	Congenital syndrome[a]	45%–50% overall; 90% in first 12 wk	Antibody	Vaccine[c] Droplet precautions for acute infection Contact precautions for congenital rubella
Rubeola	Respiratory secretions	Prematurity; abortion	Rare	History, antibody	Vaccine[c]
Syphilis	Blood; vesicular fluid, amniotic fluid	Congenital syndrome[a]	10%–90% depending on stage of maternal disease	Venereal Disease Research Laboratory test	Penicillin IM after exposure Standard precautions
Toxoplasmosis	Raw meat, cat feces; no human-to-human spread	Congenital syndrome[a]	30%–50%; rate increases as pregnancy advances; previous infection protective	IgM antibody Prepregnancy antibody protective	Freeze or cook meat; avoid cat litter; wash fruit, vegetables
Tuberculosis	Sputum	Hepatomegaly, pulmonary, CNS	Rare	Skin test	Isoniazid ± ethambutol Airborne precautions
Varicella	Respiratory secretions	Malformations (skin, limb, CNS, eye); chickenpox	25%	Antibody	Vaccine;[b] varicella-zoster immune globulin within 96 hr of exposure if susceptible Airborne and central precautions

HBeAg, hepatitis B e antigen; HBsAg, hepatitis B surface antigen; HBcAg, hepatits B core antigen; HCV, hepatitis C virus; ISG, immune serum globulin; HIV, human immunodeficiency virus; CNS, central nervous system.

[a]Congenital syndrome: varying combinations of jaundice, hepatosplenomegaly, microcephaly, CNS abnormalities, thrombocytopenia, anemia, retinopathy, and skin and bone lesions

[b]Guidelines for post-exposure chemoprophylaxis in pregnant women are being developed.

[c]Live virus vaccines are given routinely prior to pregnancy.

also are administered to staff members, including pregnant women, in October and November.

Guidelines for removal of healthcare workers with highly contagious conditions from direct patient contact in the nursery should be consulted for specific recommendations [136,138]. Decisions concerning removal of personnel with respiratory, gastrointestinal, or mucocutaneous infections must be made on an individual basis. Removal of all individuals with mild illnesses may not be practical in an overcrowded, understaffed nursery. Therefore, specific instructions concerning precautions to prevent transmission of infection to patients must be given. Individuals with pertussis, active tuberculosis, varicella, exudative skin lesions, or weeping dermatitis must be removed from direct patient contact until they are no longer infectious.

Healthcare workers with herpes labialis ("cold sores") are no longer excluded from the nursery because the risk of transmission is so low. Such individuals are instructed to cover the lesions, not to touch the area surrounding the lesions, carefully observe handwashing procedures, and not to kiss or cuddle neonates under their care. The role of topical penciclovir or oral acyclovir is not established, but the quantity and duration of viral shedding is decreased in treated individuals. Personnel with herpetic whitlow must be restricted from contact with neonates until the lesions are completely crusted.

Personnel who are known to be carriers of hepatitis B surface antigen or infected with HIV are managed and counseled individually (see Chapter 42, 43). In the case of HIV, continued patient contact is determined by the stage of disease and the absence of potentially transmissible infections and is governed by state law. Percutaneous and mucocutaneous exposures to bloodborne pathogens are managed according to standard protocols, as discussed elsewhere in this text (see Chapter 44).

In the nursery, there has been much concern about the exposure of pregnant healthcare workers to neonates with congenital infections, especially CMV [165]. Frequently, the most anxiety is generated over infections that pose the least risk. Several epidemiologic studies in hospitals and day-care centers have established that the nursery staff do not have an increased risk of acquiring CMV from their patients and that exposure to toddlers in day-care centers is associated with a significantly greater risk of seroconversion [124,125,166,167]. Therefore, pregnant women are no longer restricted from caring for infants who are identified as infected with CMV. All female healthcare workers in the child-bearing age group must be taught that strict adherence to standard precautions, especially handwashing, and prepregnancy immunization against hepatitis B virus, rubella, rubeola, and varicella are the most efficacious methods of protecting themselves and their unborn children. Table 26-5 summarizes the relevant facts concerning infections that create the greatest concern among women in the child-bearing age group who are in direct contact with young infants. We have found that pregnant healthcare workers are reassured greatly by reviewing this information with them.

The only restriction that is applied to pregnant healthcare workers is avoidance of exposure to ribavirin. Although there are no data to support the theoretic risks of teratogenicity in humans, hospitals should follow the company's recommendation to restrict exposure [27].

REFERENCES

1. Lewis DB and Wilson CB. Developmental immunology and role of host defenses in neonatal susceptibility to infection. In: Remington JS, Klein JO, eds. *Infectious diseases of the fetus and newborn infant.* Philadelphia: WB Saunders, 1990:20–98.
2. Jarvis WR, Edwards JR, Culver DH, et al. Nosocomial infection rates in adult and pediatric intensive care units in the United States. *Am J Med* 1991;91(Suppl 3B):185S–191S.
3. Gaynes RP, Martone WJ, Culver DH, et al. Comparison of rates of nosocomial infections in neonatal intensive care units in the United States. *Am J Med* 1991;91(suppl 3B):192S–196S.
4. Hospital Infections Program, National Center for Infectious Disease, Centers for Disease Control and Prevention. National Nosocomial Infections Surveillance (NNIS) semiannual report, May 1995. *Am J Infect Control* 1995;23:377–385.
5. Gaynes RP, Edwards JR, Jarvis WR, et al. Nosocomial infections among neonates in high-risk nurseries in the United States. *Pediatrics* 1996;98:357–361.
6. Adams WG, Kinney JS, Schuchat A, et al. Outbreak of early onset group B streptococcal sepsis. *Pediatr Infect Dis J* 1993;12:675–670.
7. Ledger WJ. Complications associated with invasive monitoring. *Semin Perinatol* 1978;2:187–194.
8. Rubenstein AD, Fowler RN. Salmonellosis of the newborn with transmission by delivery room resuscitators. *Am J Public Health* 1955;45: 1109–1114.
9. Fierer J, Taylor PM, Gerzon HM. *Pseudomonas aeruginosa* epidemic traced to delivery-room resuscitators. *N Engl J Med* 1967;276:991–996.
10. Khan MA, Abdur-Rab M, Israr N, et al. Transmission of *Salmonella worthington* by oropharyngeal suction in hospital neonatal unit. *Pediatr Infect Dis J* 1991;10:668–672.
11. Gray JE, Richardson DK, McCormick MC, et al. Coagulase-negative staphylococcal bacteremia among very low birthweight infants: relation to admission illness severity, resource use, and outcome. *Pediatrics* 1995;95:225–230.
12. Haley RW, Cushion NB, Tenover FC, et al. Eradication of endemic methicillin-resistant *Staphylococcus aureus* infections from a neonatal intensive care unit. *J Infect Dis* 1995;171:614–624.
13. Trofino J. JCAHO nursing standards, nursing care hours and LOS per DRG: part I. *Nurse Manager* 1986;17:19–24.
14. St. Geme JW III, Bell LM, Baumgart S, et al. Distinguishing sepsis from blood culture contamination in young infants with blood cultures growing coagulase-negative staphylococci. *Pediatrics* 1990;86:157–162.
15. Schelonka RL, Chai MK, Yoder BA, et al. Volume of blood required to detect common neonatal pathogens. *J Pediatr* 1996;129:275–278.
16. Manroe BL, Weinberg AG, Rosenfeld CR, et al. The neonatal blood count in health and disease: I. reference values for neutrophilic cells. *J Pediatr* 1979;95:89–98.
17. Vain NE, Mazglumian JR, Swarner W, et al. Role of exchange transfusion in treatment of severe septicemia. *Pediatrics* 1980;66:693–697.
18. Cairo MS, Worcester CC, Rucker RW, et al. Randomized trial of granulocyte transfusions versus intravenous immune globulin therapy for neonatal neutropenia and sepsis. *J Pediatr* 1992;120:281–285.
19. Christensen RD, Brown MS, Hall DC, et al. Effect on neutrophil kinetics and serum opsonic capacity of intravenous administration of immune globulin to neonates with clinical signs of early-onset sepsis. *J Pediatr* 1991;118:606–614.
20. Baker CJ, Melish ME, Hall RT, et al. Intravenous immune globulin for the prevention of nosocomial infection in low-birth-weight neonates. *N Engl J Med* 1992;327:213–219.
21. Fanaroff AA, Korones SB, Wright LL, et al. A controlled trial of intravenous immune globulin to reduce nosocomial infections in very-low-birth-weight infants. *N Engl J Med* 1994;330:1107–1113.
22. Gillan ER, Christensen RD, Suen Y, et al. A randomized, placebo-con-

trolled trial of recombinant human granulocyte colony-stimulating factor administration in newborn infants with presumed sepsis: significant induction of peripheral and bone marrow neutrophilia. *Blood* 1994;84:1427–1433.
23. Weisman LE, Cruess DF, Fisher GW. Standard versus hyperimmune intravenous immunoglobulin in preventing or treating neonatal bacterial infections. *Clin Perinatol* 1993;20:211–224.
24. Goldmann DA. Bacterial colonization and infection in the neonate. *Am J Med* 1981;70:417–422.
25. Bingen E, Denamur E, Lambert-Zechovsky N, et al. Analysis of DNA restriction fragment length polymorphism extends the evidence for breast milk transmission in *Streptococcus agalactiae* late-onset neonatal infection. *J Infect Dis* 1992;165:569–573.
26. El-Mohandes AE, Schatz V, Keiser JF, et al. Bacterial contaminants of collected and frozen human milk used in an intensive care nursery. *Am J Infect Control* 1993;21:226–230.
27. Committee on Infectious Diseases, American Academy of Pediatrics. *1997 Redbook: report of the Committee on Infectious Diseases*. Elk Grove Village, IL: American Academy of Pediatrics, 1994:7:74–77.
28. Stoll BJ, Gordon T, Korones SB, et al. Late-onset sepsis in very low birth weight neonates: a report from the National Institute of Child Health and Human Development Neonatal Research Network. *J Pediatr* 1996;129:63–71.
29. Botas CM, Kurlat I, Young SM, et al. Disseminated candidal infections and intravenous hydrocortisone in preterm infants. *Pediatrics* 1995;95:883–887.
30. Stoll BJ, Gordon T, Korones SB, et al. Early-onset sepsis in very low birth weight neonates: a report from the National Institute of Child Health and Human Development Neonatal Research Network. *J Pediatr* 1996;129:72–80.
31. Beck-Sagué CM, Azimi P, Fonseca SN, et al. Bloodstream infections in neonatal intensive care unit patients: results of a multicenter study. *Pediatr Infect Dis J* 1994;13:1110–1116.
32. Centers for Disease Control and Prevention. Prevention of perinatal group B streptococcal disease: a public health perspective. *MMWR Morb Mortal Wkly Rep* 1996;45(RR-7):1–24.
33. Nakashima AK, Allen JR, Martone WJ, et al. Epidemic bullous impetigo in a nursery due to a nasal carrier of *Staphylococcus aureus: role of epidemiology and control measures.* Infect Control 1984;5:326–331.
34. Mooney BR, Green JA, Epstein BJ, et al. Non-gonococcal ophthalmitis associated with erythromycin ointment prophylaxis of gonococcal ophthalmia neonatorium. *Infect Control* 1984;5:138–140.
35. Campbell JR, Arango CA, Garcia-Prats JA, et al. An outbreak of M serotype 1 group A streptococcus in a neonatal intensive care unit. *J Pediatr* 1996;129:396–402.
36. Salzman TC, Scher CD, Moss R. Shigellae with transferable drug resistance: outbreak in a nursery for premature infants. *J Pediatr* 1967;71:21–26.
37. Schroeder SA, Aserkoff B, Brachman PS. Epidemic salmonellosis in hospitals and institutions: a five-year review. *N Engl J Med* 1968;279: 674–678.
38. Gladstone IM, Ehrenkranz RA, Edberg SC, et al. A ten-year review of neonatal sepsis and comparison with the previous fifty-year experience. *Pediatr Infect Dis J* 1990;9:819–825.
39. Low DE, Schmidt BK, Kirpalani HM, et al. An endemic strain of *Staphylococcus haemolyticus* colonizing and causing bacteremia in neonatal intensive care unit patients. *Pediatrics* 1992;89:696–700.
40. Patrick CJ, John JF, Levkoff AH, et al. Relatedness of strains of methicillin-resistant coagulase-negative staphylococcus colonizing hospital personnel and producing bacteremias in a neonatal intensive care unit. *Pediatr Infect Dis J* 1992;11:935–940.
41. Huebner J, Pier GB, Maslow JN, et al. Endemic nosocomial transmission of *Staphylococcus epidermidis* bacteremia isolates in a neonatal intensive care unit over 10 years. *J Infect Dis* 1994;169:526–531.
42. Lyytikäinen O, Saxén H, Rylänen R, et al. Persistence of a multiresistant clone of *Staphylococcus epidermidis* in a neonatal intensive-care unit for a four-year period. *Clin Infect Dis* 1995;20:24–29.
43. Neumeister B, Kastner S, Conrad S, et al. Characterization of coagulase-negative staphylococci causing nosocomial infections in preterm infants. *Eur J Clin Microbiol Infect Dis* 1995;14:856–863.
44. Kacia MA, Horgan MJ, Preston KE, et al. Relatedness of coagulase-negative staphylococci causing bacteremia in low-birthweight infants. *Infect Control Hosp Epidemiol* 1994;15:658–662.
45. Camargo LFA, Strabelli TMV, Ribeiro FG, et al. Epidemiologic investigation of an outbreak of coagulase-negative staphylococcus primary bacteremia in a newborn intensive care unit. *Infect Control Hosp Epidemiol* 1995;16:595–596.
46. Nesin M, Projan SJ, Kreisiverth B, et al. Molecular epidemiology of *Staphylococcus epidermidis* blood isolates from neonatal intensive care unit patients. *J Hosp Infect* 1995;31:111–121.
47. Eastick K, Leening JP, Bennet D, et al. Reservoirs of coagulase negative staphylococci in preterm infants. *Arch Dis Child* 1996;74: F99–F104.
48. Fleer A, Senders RC, Visser MR, et al. Septicemia due to coagulase-negative staphylococci in a neonatal intensive care unit: clinical and bacteriological features and contaminated parenteral fluids as a source of sepsis. *Pediatric Infectious Disease* 1983;2:428–431.
49. Hall SL. Coagulase-negative staphylococcal infections in neonates. *Pediatr Infect Dis J* 1991;10:57–67.
50. Patrick CC, Kaplan SR, Baker CJ, et al. Persistent bacteremia due to coagulase-negative staphylococci in low birth weight neonates. *Pediatrics* 1989;84:977–985.
51. Gruskay J, Abbasi S, Anday E, et al. *Staphylococcus epidermidis*-associated enterocolitis. *J Pediatr* 1986;109:520–523.
52. Scheifele DW, Bjornson GL. Delta toxin activity in coagulase-negative staphylococci from the bowels of neonates. *J Clin Microbiol* 1988;26:279–282.
53. Noel GJ, Edelson PJ. *Staphylococcus epidermidis* bacteremia in neonates: further observations and the recurrence of focal infection. *Pediatrics* 1984;74:832–837.
54. Noel GJ, O'Loughlin JE, Edelson PJ. Neonatal *Staphylococcus epidermidis* right-sided endocarditis: description of five catheterized infants. *Pediatrics* 1988;82:234–239.
55. Dancer SJ, Simmons NA, Poston SM, et al. Outbreak of staphylococcal scalded skin syndrome among neonates. *J Infect* 1988;16:87–103.
56. Dave J, Reith S, Nash JQ, et al. A double outbreak of exfoliative toxin-producing strains of *Staphylococcus aureus* in a maternity unit. *Epidemiol Infect* 1994;112:103–114.
57. Mackenzie A, Johnson W, Heyes B, et al. A prolonged outbreak of exfoliative toxin A-producing *Staphylococcus aureus* in a newborn nursery. *Diagn Microbiol Infect Dis* 1995;21:69–75.
58. Pekkala DH, Low DE, Wyper PA, et al. The utility of restriction endonuclease analysis and phage typing in the epidemiologic investigation of a *Staphylococcus aureus* outbreak in a neonatal nursery. *Diagn Microbiol Infect Dis* 1992;15:307–311.
59. Mitsuda T, Arai K, Fujita S, et al. Epidemiological analysis of strains of methicillin-resistant *Staphylococcus aureus* (MRSA) infection in the nursery: prognosis of MRSA carrier infants. *J Hosp Infect* 1995; 31:123–134.
60. Noel GJ, Kreiswirth BN, Edelson PJ, et al. Multiple methicillin-resistant *Staphylococcus aureus* strains as a cause for a single outbreak of severe disease in hospitalized neonates. *Pediatr Infect Dis J* 1992;11: 184–188.
61. Reboli AC, John JF, Levkoff AH. Epidemic methicillin-gentamicin-resistant *Staphylococcus aureus* in a neonatal intensive care unit. *American Journal of Diseases of Children* 1989;143:34–39.
62. Davies EA, Emmerson AM, Hogg GM, et al. An outbreak of infection with a methicillin resistant *Staphylococcus aureus* in a special care baby unit: value of topical mupiricin and of traditional methods of infection control. *J Hosp Infect* 1987;10:120–128.
63. Hollis RJ, Barr JL, Doebbeling BN, et al. Familial carriage of methicillin-resistant *Staphylococcus aureus* and subsequent infection in a premature neonate. *J Infect Dis* 1995;21:328–332.
64. Tenover FC, Arbeit R, Archer G, et al. Comparison of traditional and molecular methods of typing isolates of *Staphylococcus aureus. J Clin Microbiol* 1994;32:407–415.
65. Haley RA, Bregman DA. The role of understaffing and overcrowding in recurrent outbreaks of staphylococcal infection in a neonatal special-care unit. *J Infect Dis* 1982;145:875–885.
66. Buchino JJ, Ciamberella E, Light I. Systemic group D streptococcal infection in newborn infants. *Am J Dis Child* 1979;133:270–273.
67. Bavikatte K, Schreiner RL, Lemons JA, et al. Group D streptococcal septicemia in the neonate. *American Journal of Diseases of Children* 1979;133:493–496.
68. Dobson SRM, Baker CJ. Enterococcal sepsis in neonates: features by age at onset and occurrence of focal infection. *Pediatrics* 1990;85: 165–171.
69. Christie C, Hammond J, Reising S, et al. Clinical and molecular epidemiology of enterococcal bacteremia in a pediatric teaching hospital. *J Pediatr* 1994;125:392–399.

70. Rice LB, Shlaes DM. Vancomycin resistance in the enterococcus: relevance in pediatrics. *Pediatr Clin North Am* 1995;42:601–618.
71. McNeeley DF, Saint-Louis F, Noel GF. Neonatal enterococcal bacteremia: an increasingly frequent event with potentially untreatable pathogens. *Pediatr Infect Dis J* 1996;15:800–805.
72. Coudron PE, Mayhall CG, Facklam RR, et al. *Streptococcus faecium* outbreak in a neonatal intensive care unit. *J Clin Microbiol* 1984;20: 1044–1048.
73. Luginbuhl LM, Rotbart HA, Facklan RR, et al. Neonatal enterococcal sepsis: case–control study and description of an outbreak. *Pediatr Infect Dis J* 1987;6:1022–1030.
74. Toltzis P, Blumer JL. Antibiotic-resistant gram-negative bacteria in the critical care setting. *Pediatr Clin North Am* 1995;42:687–702.
75. Leigh L, Stoll BJ, Rohman M, et al. *Pseudomonas aeruginosa* infection in very low birth weight infants: a case–control study. *Pediatr Infect Dis J* 1995;14:367–371.
76. Grundmann H, Kropec A, Harting D, et al. *Pseudomonas aeruginosa* in a neonatal intensive care unit: reservoirs and etiology of the nosocomial pathogen. *J Infect Dis* 1993;168:943–947.
77. Verweij PE, Geven WB, van Belkum A, et al. Cross-infection with *Pseudomonas aeruginosa* in a neonatal intensive care unit characterized by polymerase chain reaction fingerprinting. *Pediatr Infect Dis J* 1993;12:1027–1029.
78. Neal TJ, Hughes CR, Rothburn MM, et al. The neonatal laryngoscope as a potential source of cross-infection. *J Hosp Infect* 1995;30: 315–321.
79. Pegues DA, Arathoon EG, Samayoa B, et al. Epidemic gram-negative bacteremia in a neonatal intensive care unit in Guatemala. *Am J Infect Control* 1994;22:163–171.
80. McNaughton M, Mazinke N, Thomas E. Newborn conjunctivitis associated with triclosan 0.5% antiseptic intrinsically contaminated with *Serratia marcescens. Canadian Journal of Infection Control* 1995;10:7–8.
81. Goering RV, Ehrenkranz J, Sanders CC, et al. Long term epidemiological analysis of *Citrobacter diversus* in a neonatal intensive care unit. *Pediatr Infect Dis J* 1992;11:99–104.
82. Kline MW. *Citrobacter* meningitis and brain abscess in infancy: epidemiology, pathogenesis, and treatment. *J Pediatr* 1988;113:430–434.
83. Lin FC, Devor WF, Morrison C, et al. Outbreak of neonatal *Citrobacter diversus* meningitis in a suburban hospital. *Pediatr Infect Dis J* 1987;6:50–55.
84. Kumar A, Nath G, Bhatia BD, et al. An outbreak of multidrug resistant *Salmonella typhimurium* in a nursery. *Indian Pediatr* 1995;32: 881–885.
85. Mahajan R, Mathur M, Kumar A, et al. Nosocomial outbreak of *Salmonella typhimurium* infection in a nursery intensive care unit (NICU) and pediatric ward. *J Commun Dis* 1995;27:10–14.
86. Regev R, Dolfin T, Zelig S, et al. *Acinetobacter* septicemia: a threat to neonates? Special aspects in a neonatal intensive care unit. *Infection* 1993;21:394–396.
87. Pokrywka M, Vizanko K, Mednick J, et al. *Flavobacterium meningosepticum* outbreak among intensive care patients. *Am J Infect Control* 1993;21:139–145.
88. Abrahamsen TG, Finne PH, Lingaas E. *Flavobacterium meningosepticum* infections in a neonatal intensive care unit. *Acta Paediatr Scand* 1989;78:51–55.
89. Matsaniotis NS, Syriopoulou VP, Theodoridou MC, et al. *Enterobacter* sepsis in infants and children due to contaminated intravenous fluids. *Infect Control* 1984;5:471–477.
90. Donowitz LG, Marsik FJ, Fisher KA, et al. Contaminated breast milk: a source of *Klebsiella* bacteremia in a newborn intensive care unit. *Rev Infect Dis* 1981;3:716–720.
91. Verweij PE, Van Belkum AV, Melchers WJG, et al. Interrepeat fingerprinting of third-generation cephalosporin-resistant *Enterobacter cloacae* isolated during an outbreak in a neonatal intensive care unit. *Infect Control Hosp Epidemiol* 1995;16:25–29.
92. Haertl R, Bandlow G. Epidemiological fingerprinting of *Enterobacter cloacae* by small-fragment restriction endonuclease analysis and pulsed-field gel electrophoresis of genomic restriction fragments. *J Clin Microbiol* 1993;31:128–133.
93. Alos J, Lambert T, Courvalin P. Comparison of two molecular methods for tracing nosocomial transmission of *Escherichia coli* K1 in a neonatal unit. *J Clin Microbiol* 1993;31:1704–1709.
94. Tizer KB, Cervia JS, Dunn A, et al. Successful combination vancomycin and rifampin therapy in a newborn with community-acquired *Flavobacterium meningosepticum* neonatal meningitis. *Pediatr Infect Dis J* 1995;14:916–917.
95. Beck-Sagué CM, Jarvis WR. National Nosocomial Infections Surveillance System: secular trends in the epidemiology of nosocomial fungal infections in the United States, 1980–1990. *J Infect Dis* 1993;167:1247–1251.
96. Stamos JK, Rowley AH. Candidemia in a pediatric population. *Clin Infect Dis* 1995;20:571–575.
97. Weese-Mayer DE, Fondriest DW, Brouillette RT, et al. Risk factors associated with candidemia in the neonatal intensive care unit: a case–control study. *Pediatr Infect Dis J* 1987;6:190–196.
98. Saxen H, Virtanen M, Carlson P, et al. Neonatal *Candida parapsilosis* outbreak with a high case fatality rate. *Pediatr Infect Dis J* 1995;14: 776–781.
99. El-Mohandes AE, Johnson-Robbins L, Keiser JF, et al. Incidence of *Candida parapsilosis* colonization in an intensive care nursery population and its association with invasive fungal disease. *Pediatr Infect Dis J* 1994;13:520–524.
100. Baley JE, Kliegman RM, Boxerbaum B, et al. Fungal colonization in the very low birthweight infant. *Pediatrics* 1986;78:225–232.
101. Welbel SF, McNeil MM, Kuykendall RJ, et al. *Candida parapsilosis* bloodstream infections in neonatal intensive care unit patients: epidemiologic and laboratory confirmation of a common source outbreak. *Pediatr Infect Dis J* 1996;15:998–1002.
102. Betremieux P, Chevrier S, Quindos G, et al. Use of DNA fingerprinting and biotyping methods to study a *Candida albicans* outbreak in a neonatal intensive care unit. *Pediatr Infect Dis J* 1994;13:899–905.
103. Finkelstein R, Reinhertz G, Hashman N, et al. Outbreak of *Candida tropicalis* fungemia in a neonatal intensive care unit. *Infect Control Hosp Epidemiol* 1993;14:587–590.
104. Sheretz RJ, Gledhill KS, Hampton KD, et al. Outbreak of *Candida* bloodstream infections associated with retrograde medication administration in a neonatal intensive care unit. *J Pediatr* 1992;120:455–461.
105. Santos LA, Beceiro J, Hernandez R, et al. Congenital cutaneous candidiasis: report of four cases and review of the literature. *Eur J Pediatr* 1991;150:336–338.
106. Baley JE, Silverman RA. Systemic candidiasis: cutaneous manifestations in low birth weight infants. *Pediatrics* 1988;82:211–215.
107. Mayayo E, Moralejo J, Camps J, et al. Fungal endocarditis in premature infants: case report and review. *Clin Infect Dis* 1996;22:366–368.
108. Rowen JL, Correa AG, Sokol DM, et al. Invasive aspergillosis in neonates: report of five cases and literature review. *Pediatr Infect Dis J* 1992;11:576–582.
109. Papouli M, Roilides E, Bibashi E, et al. Primary cutaneous aspergillosis in neonates: case report and review. *Clin Infect Dis* 1996;22: 1102–1104.
110. Stuart SM, Lane AT. *Candida* and *Malassezia* as nursery pathogens. *Semin Dermatol* 1992;11:19–23.
111. Welbel SF, McNeil MM, Pramanik A, et al. Nosocomial *Malassezia pachydermatis* bloodstream infections in a neonatal intensive care unit. *Pediatr Infect Dis J* 1994;13:104–108.
112. Mitchell SJ, Gray J, Morgan MEI, et al. Nosocomial infection with *Rhizopus microsporus* in preterm infants: association with wooden tongue depressors. *Lancet* 1996;348:441–443.
113. Fisher DJ, Christy C, Spafford P, et al. Neonatal *Trichosporon beigelii* infection: report of a cluster of cases in a neonatal intensive care unit. *Pediatr Infect Dis J* 1993;12:149–155.
114. Agah R, Cherry JD, Garakian AJ, et al. Respiratory syncytial virus (RSV) infection rate in personnel caring for children with RSV infections. *American Journal of Diseases of Children* 1987;141:695–697.
115. Rotbart HA, Levin MJ, Yolken RH, et al. An outbreak of rotavirus-associated neonatal necrotizing enterocolitis. *J Pediatr* 1983;103:454–459.
116. Finn A, Anday E, Talbot GH. An epidemic of adenovirus 7a infection in a neonatal nursery: course morbidity and management. *Infect Control Hosp Epidemiol* 1988;9:398–404.
117. Hall GB, Kopelman AE, Douglas RG, et al. Neonatal respiratory syncytial virus infection. *N Engl J Med* 1979;300:393–396.
118. Birenbaum E, Linder N, Varsano N, et al. Adenovirus type 8 conjunctivitis outbreak in a neonatal intensive care unit. *Arch Dis Child* 1993;68:610–611.
119. Abzug MJ, Levin MJ. Neonatal adenovirus infection: four patients and review of the literature. *Pediatrics* 1991;87:890–896.
120. Modlin JF. Perinatal echovirus infection: insights from a literature review of 61 cases of serious infection and 16 outbreaks in nurseries. *Rev Infect Dis* 1986;8:918–926.

121. Watson JC, Fleming DW, Borella AJ, et al. Vertical transmission of hepatitis A resulting in an outbreak in a neonatal intensive care unit. *J Infect Dis* 1993;167:567–571.
122. Rosenblum LS, Villarino ME, Nainan OV, et al. Hepatitis A outbreak in a neonatal intensive care unit: risk factors for transmission and evidence of prolonged viral excretion among preterm infants. *J Infect Dis* 1991;164:476–482.
123. Azimi PH, Roberto RR, Guralnik J, et al. Transfusion-acquired hepatitis A in a premature infant with secondary nosocomial spread in an intensive care nursery. *American Journal of Diseases of Children* 1986;140:23–27.
124. Brady MT, Demmler GJ, Reis S. Factors associated with cytomegalovirus excretion in hospitalized children. *Am J Infect Control* 1988; 161:41–45.
125. Balcarek KB, Bagley R, Cloud GA, et al. Cytomegalovirus infection among employees of a children's hospital: no evidence for increased risk associated with patient care. *JAMA* 1990;263:840–844.
126. Hammerberg O, Watts J, Chernesky M, et al. An outbreak of herpes simplex virus type 1 in an intensive care nursery. *Pediatric Infectious Disease* 1983;2:290–294.
127. Friedman CA, Temple DM, Robbins KK, et al. Outbreak and control of varicella in a neonatal intensive care unit. *Pediatr Infect Dis J* 1994;13:152–154.
128. Gustafson TL, Shehab Z, Brunnel PA. Outbreak of varicella in a newborn intensive care nursery. *American Journal of Diseases of Children* 1984;138:548–550.
129. Light IJ. Postnatal acquisition of herpes simplex virus by the newborn infant: a review of the literature. *Pediatrics* 1979;63:480–482.
130. Nelson JD. *1996–1997 Pocket book of pediatric antimicrobial therapy.* 12th ed. Baltimore: Williams & Wilkins, 1996.
131. Heusser, MF, Patterson JE, Kuritza AP, et al. Emergence of resistance to multiple beta-lactams in *Enterobacter cloacae* during treatment for neonatal meningitis with cefotaxime. *Pediatr Infect Dis J* 1990;9: 509–512.
132. Fink S, Karp W, Robertson A. Ceftriaxone effect on bilirubin-albumin binding. *Pediatrics* 1987;80:873–875.
133. McCracken GH, Siegel JD, Threlkeld N, et al. Pharmacokinetics of ceftriaxone in newborn infants. *Antimicrob Agents Chemother* 1983; 23:341–343.
134. Nigro G, Scholz H, Bartman U. Ganciclovir therapy for symptomatic congenital cytomegalovirus infection in infants: a two-regimen experience. *J Pediatr* 1994;124:318–322.
135. Committee on Infectious Diseases, 1995 to 1996, American Academy of Pediatrics. Reassessment of the indications for ribavirin therapy in respiratory syncytial virus infections. *Pediatrics* 1996;97:137–140.
136. American Academy of Pediatrics Committee on Fetus and Newborn, American College of Obstetrics and Gynecology Committee on Obstetrics. *Maternal and fetal medicine: guidelines for perinatal care.* 3rd ed. Elk Grove Village, IL: American Academy of Pediatrics, 1992:7, 23–29.
137. Garner JS. The Hospital Infection Control Practices Advisory Committee: guideline for isolation precautions in hospitals. *Infect Control Hosp Epidemiol* 1996;17:54–80.
138. Committee on Infectious Diseases, American Academy of Pediatrics. *1997 Redbook: report of the Committee on Infectious Diseases.* Elk Grove Village, IL: Academy of Pediatrics, 1997.
139. Jernigan JA, Titus MG, Gröschel DHM, et al. Effectiveness of contact isolation during a hospital outbreak of methicillin-resistant *Staphylococcus aureus. Am J Epidemiol* 1996;143:496–504.
140. Coovadia YM, Johnson AP, Bhana RH, et al. Multiresistant *Klebsiella pneumoniae* in a neonatal nursery: the importance of maintenance of infection control policies and procedures in the prevention of outbreaks. *J Hosp Infect* 1992;22:197–205.
141. Brown J, Froese-Fretz A, Luckey D, et al. High rate of hand contamination and low rate of handwashing before infant contact in a neonatal intensive care unit. *Pediatr Infect Dis J* 1996;15:908–910.
142. Raju TNK, Kobler C. Improving handwashing habits in the newborn nursery. *Am J Med Sci* 1991;302:355–358.
143. Larson EL, 1992, 1993 and 1994 APIC Guidelines Committee. APIC guidelines for handwashing and hand antisepsis in healthcare settings. *Am J Infect Control* 1995;23:251–269.
144. Wade JJ, Desai N, Casewell MW. Hygienic hand disinfection for the removal of epidemic vancomycin-resistant *Enterococcus faecium* and gentamicin-resistant *Enterobacter cloacae. J Hosp Infect* 1991;19:211–218.
145. Zafar AB, Butler RC, Reese DJ, et al. Use of a 0.3% triclosan (Bacti-Stat*) to eradicate an outbreak of methicillin-resistant *Staphylococcus aureus* in a neonatal nursery. *Am J Infect Control* 1995;23:200–208.
146. Cloney DL, Donowitz LG. Overgrown use for infection control in nurseries and neonatal intensive care units. *American Journal of Diseases of Children* 1986;140:680–683.
147. Pelke S, Ching D, Easa D, et al. Gowning does not affect colonization of infection rates in a neonatal intensive care unit. *Arch Pediatr Adolesc Med* 1994;148:1016–1020.
148. Verber IG, Pagan FS. What cord care—if any? *Arch Dis Child* 1993; 68:594–596.
149. Gladstone IM, Clapper L, Thorp JW, et al. Randomized study of six umbilical cord care regimens: comparing length of attachment, microbial control and satisfaction. *Clin Pediatr* 1988;27:127–129.
150. Bradley SF. Effectiveness of mupiricin in the control of methicillin-resistant *Staphylococcus aureus. Infections in Medicine* 1993;10:23–31.
151. Fisher GW, Cieslak TJ, Wilson SR, et al. Opsonic antibodies to *Staphylococcus epidermidis*: in vitro and in vivo studies using human intravenous immune globulin. *J Infect Dis* 1994;169:324–329.
152. Groothius JR, Simoes EAF, Levin MJ, et al. Prophylactic administration of respiratory syncytial virus immune globulin to high-risk infants and young children. *N Engl J Med* 1993;329:1524–1530.
153. The PREVENT Study Group. Reduction of respiratory syncytial virus hospitalization among premature infants and infants with bronchopulmonary dysplasia using respiratory syncytial virus immune globulin prophylaxis. *Pediatrics* 1997;99:93–99.
154. Simoes EAF, Groothius JR, Tristram DA, et al. Respiratory syncytial virus-enriched globulin for the prevention of acute otitis media in high-risk children. *J Pediatr* 1996;129:214–219.
155. Centers for Disease Control and Prevention. Prevention of varicella: recommendations of the Advisory Committee on Immunization Practices (ACIP). *MMWR Morb Mortal Wkly Rep* 1996;45(RR-11): 22–23.
156. Lipton SV, Brunell PA. Management of varicella exposure in a neonatal intensive care unit. *JAMA* 1989;261:1782–1784.
157. Spafford PS, Sinkin RA, Cox C, et al. Prevention of central venous catheter-related coagulase-negative staphylococcal sepsis in neonates. *J Pediatr* 1994;125:259–263.
158. Kacia MA, Horgan MJ, Ochoa L, et al. Prevention of gram-negative sepsis in neonates weighing less than 1500 grams. *J Pediatr* 1994; 125:253–258.
159. Barefield ES, Philips JB. Vancomycin prophylaxis for coagulase-negative staphylococcal bacteremia. *J Pediatr* 1994;125:230–232.
160. Harms K, Herting E, Kron M, et al. Randomized, controlled trial of amoxicillin prophylaxis for prevention of catheter-related infections in newborn infants with central venous silicone elastomer catheters. *J Pediatr* 1995;127:615–619.
161. Bradford M, Cohen SH. Critical care surveillance plan at University of California, Davis Medical Center, Sacramento, California. In: *Program and abstracts of the 3rd Decennial International Conference on Nosocomial Infections, Atlanta.* 1990:28.
162. Lee PYC, Holliman RE, Davis EG. Surveillance cultures on neonatal intensive care units. *J Hosp Infect* 1995;29:233–237.
163. Evans ME, Schaffner W, Federspiel CF, et al. Sensitivity, specificity, and predictive value of body surface cultures in a neonatal intensive care unit. *JAMA* 1988;259:248–252.
164. Hospital Infection Control Practices Advisory Committee. Recommendations for preventing the spread of vancomycin resistance. *Infect Control Hosp Epidemiol* 1995;16:105–113.
165. Valenti WM. Infection control and the pregnant healthcare worker. *Nurs Clin North Am* 1993;28:673–686.
166. Adler SP. Cytomegalovirus and child day care: risk factors for maternal infection. *Pediatr Infect Dis J* 1991;10:590–594.
167. Pass RF, Hutto C, Lyon MD, et al. Increased rate of cytomegalovirus infection among day care center workers. *Pediatr Infect Dis J* 1990; 9:465–470.
168. Pearson ML. The Hospital Infection Control Practices Advisory Committee: guideline for the prevention of intravascular-device-related infections. *Infect Control Hosp Epidemiol* 1996;17:438–473.
169. Hospital Infection Control Practices Advisory Committee. Part II: recommendations for prevention of nosocomial pneumonia. *Am J Infect Control* 1994;22:267–292.
170. Garland JS, Alex CP, Mueller CD, et al. Local reactions to a chlorhexidine gluconate-impregnated antimicrobial dressing in very low birth weight infants. *Pediatr Infect Dis J* 1996;15:912–914.

Hospital Infections, Fourth Edition,
edited by John V. Bennett and Philip S. Brachman.
Lippincott–Raven Publishers, Philadelphia © 1998

CHAPTER 27

The Operating Room

Ronald Lee Nichols

Despite the high standards set for professional performance and equipment, the controlled environment of the operating room remains potentially hostile to both the patient and the surgical team [1]. In the past, authoritative bodies have placed major emphasis on improving the operating room environment in an attempt to reduce the number of infectious complications that followed surgical procedures [2]. The national groups that have spearheaded this challenge since the early 1960s include the Committee on Operating Room Environment of the American College of Surgeons, the Association of Operating Room Nurses, the Centers for Disease Control and Prevention (CDC), the American Hospital Association, and the Medical Research Council of Great Britain. Many individuals from different disciplines have contributed valuable insights, but the names of William Altemeier, William Beck, Harvey Bernard, John Burke, Robert Condon, Harold Laufman, Joseph Moylan, Paul Nora, and Carl Walter stand out. The reduction in postoperative wound infections, in two widely quoted national studies reported in 1964 [3] and 1985 [4], appears, in part, to be due to these efforts. The 1985 study estimated that wound infections accounted for approximately 24% of the total number of nosocomial infections, which represented nearly 500,000 wound infections per year or 2.8 per 100 operations performed [4].

Many biologic, physical (electrical, radiation, laser, and new medical devices), and chemical (anesthetics and sterilization techniques) hazards are present in the modern operating room. These hazards need to be monitored, reviewed, and updated continually. Information gained from these reviews needs to be taught to all operating room personnel to provide a safe work environment [1]. This chapter concentrates on the biologic hazards, with consideration given to the patient as host and also as vector. The reader is referred to Chapter 37 for additional consideration of infections in surgical patients.

R. L. Nichols: Department of Surgery, Tulane University, New Orleans, Louisiana 70112-2699.

THE PATIENT AS A RISK FOR INFECTION

Until the late 1980s, most infection control officers, operating room nurses, and surgeons believed that the type of operative procedure performed was the most critical factor in predicting the postoperative wound infection rate [5].

Classification of Surgical Wounds

The widely accepted traditional classification of operative procedures is as follows:

Clean wounds are uninfected operative wounds in which no inflammation is encountered and the respiratory, alimentary, genital, or uninfected urinary tract is not entered.

Clean-contaminated wounds are operative wounds in which the respiratory, alimentary, genital, or urinary tract is entered under controlled conditions and without unusual contamination.

Contaminated wounds include open, fresh, accidental wounds, operations with major breaks in sterile technique or gross spillage from the gastrointestinal tract, and incisions in which acute, nonpurulent inflammation is encountered.

Dirty or infected wounds include old traumatic wounds with retained devitalized tissue and those that involve existing clinical infection or perforated viscera.

Wound infection after clean operations is usually due to exogenous microorganisms such as *Staphylococcus aureus*, whereas the usual etiologic agent or agents in the other categories of surgery generally originate from the polymicrobial aerobic–anaerobic endogenous flora. The often-quoted infection rates for the different types of operative procedures are as follows: clean, < 2%; clean-contaminated, 5% to 15%; contaminated, 15% to 30%; and dirty, more than 30% [6].

General Aspects of Risk in the Surgical Patient

The emphasis concerning the risk factors for development of postoperative infections has shifted somewhat from the type of surgical procedure to the patients themselves. Haley and colleagues [7] were the first to publish a report on the importance of identifying the individual patients who are at high risk of surgical wound infection in each category of operative procedure. To predict the likelihood of surgical wound infection from several risk factors, the authors used information collected on 58,498 patients undergoing operations in 1970 and developed a simple multivariate risk index. Analyzing 10 possible risk factors by stepwise multiple logistic regression techniques, they developed a model containing four risk factors: 1) abdominal operation, 2) operation lasting longer than 2 hours, 3) contaminated or dirty-infected operation by traditional wound classification, and 4) patient having three or more different diagnoses. They used the resultant formula to predict an individual patient's probability of contracting a postoperative wound infection. This approach was then tested on another group of 59,352 surgical patients admitted in 1975 to 1976 and was found to be a valid predictor of surgical wound infection. The authors concluded that their simplified index predicts surgical wound infection risk nearly twice as well as the traditional classification of wound contamination. Using this model, low-, medium-, and high-risk levels for contracting wound infection were identified in the traditional wound classification categories. The overall wound infection rate in this study progressively increased from clean (2.9%), to clean-contaminated (3.9%), to contaminated (8.5%), to dirty-infected (12.6%). The decrease noted from previous reports of wound infection rates in contaminated and dirty-infected procedures may relate to improved surgical techniques and more common use of proven preventive practices during the last two decades. However, a wide range of infection risk was noted among patients in each category: In clean operations, the level of risk ranged from 1.1% in the low-risk category to 15.8% in the high-risk group; in clean-contaminated operations, 0.6% were low risk and 17.7% were considered high risk; in contaminated operations, 4.5% classified as medium risk and 23.9% were high risk; and in dirty-infected operations, 6.7% were medium risk and 27.4% were high risk. No low-risk category of patients was identified in contaminated and dirty-infected operations.

Culver and other investigators from the CDC reported on a composite risk index [8]. This risk index uses the traditional wound class but attempts to improve on the previous index in several ways. First, instead of the three discharge diagnoses to identify host factors as a risk for infection, this index uses a dichotomization of the American Society of Anesthesiologists score [9]. Its ease for collecting and its objectivity seem advantageous. Second, this risk index uses a procedure-related cutoff point to indicate an extended duration of surgery for individual procedures, rather than a 2-hour cutoff point for all procedures. For some procedures (e.g., cesarean section) the cutoff point is 1 hour; for other procedures (e.g., coronary artery bypass graft operation), the cutoff point is 5 hours. This procedure-related, duration-of-surgery cutoff provides the index with additional discriminating power for specific procedures.

The widespread use of risk indexes such as the ones developed by the CDC investigators will be needed in the future. Hospitals will use the risk indexes to compare wound infection rates by risk category, either for all operations or for specific procedures. The risk indexes can provide a general guide to potential problem areas for investigation that may need further examination with procedure-specific risk factor information. The risk indexes will also help infection control programs prospectively target their surveillance and control efforts among high-risk surgical patients (see Chapter 37 for further detail).

OPERATING ROOM DESIGN AND ENVIRONMENT

More than 30 years ago, Walter and Kundsin [10] described the bacteriology of various hospital floors, including the operating room, and emphasized the relationship between the bacterial count on the floor and the airborne bacterial count. The authors recommended a standard method to attain a hygienic floor in order to make an impact on the incidence of hospital-acquired infection. Since that time, many reviews have outlined approaches that can reduce the bacterial burden within the operating room environment [6,11]. It is believed that most surgical wound infections have their origin from the bacteria that enter the operative wound at the time of operation. The causative microorganisms originate from the patient's endogenous microflora, from the operating room environment, or from bacteria shed by the operating room team. Rarely, hematogenous bacterial spread from a site of remote infection occurs during the postoperative course, resulting in wound infection.

So far, this chapter has dealt with the individual patient risk factors for infection; the remainder of the chapter emphasizes the operating room environment and personnel. A postoperative wound infection rate of zero in clean operative procedures appears to be an impossible goal even if rather dramatic techniques are used. These techniques, primarily studied in orthopedic implant surgery, include excluding the surgeon and team from the operating room environment, sealing the surrounding skin of the patient's operative site, and providing sterile operating room air [12].

Specific Microorganisms Implicated in Operating Room Infections

The microorganisms that are usually isolated from the operating room environment are the ubiquitous so-called "nonpathogens" or "commensals," which will not result in postoperative wound infection in most patients. This, however, is not true in patients undergoing implant surgery, where these low-virulence microorganisms have been shown to be commonly implicated in postoperative deep and superficial infection [13].

Staphylococcus epidermidis and other coagulase-negative staphylococci are commonly reported pathogens in implant surgery [6]. These microorganisms can be highly antibiotic resistant and frequently are associated with mucin production (slime), which acts as a virulence factor that allows for persistence of graft or implant infections [6]. *S. aureus*, a major pathogen related to the skin of the patient or a member of the operative team, is frequently implicated in postoperative wound infection.

A single outbreak of postoperative infection due to multiply β-lactam-resistant *Enterobacter cloacae*, including septicemia or mediastinitis and multiorgan failure, has been reported in five patients undergoing cardiovascular surgery. This same strain was also found in the environmental flora of the cardiovascular operating suite and in a sink reservoir in the surgery department [14]. The authors concluded that the liberal use of cephalosporins, an abundant and constant reservoir of various gram-negative bacteria within the operating room suite, and unsatisfactory infection control procedures had led to this dilemma. It should be stressed that the usual origin of gram-negative bacterial outbreaks is the intensive care unit.

Single-source outbreaks of wound or deep sternal infections due to rarely implicated pathogens have been reported after open heart surgery for coronary revascularization [15,16]. In one study, *Candida tropicalis* was isolated from sternal wounds in eight patients during a 2-month period [15]. Environmental surveillance revealed that one scrub nurse harbored the causative microorganism on the fingertips and in the nasopharynx. The removal of the suspect nurse from the cardiac team was associated with the termination of this cluster outbreak. In another single-source outbreak after open heart surgery over a 7-month period, seven patients contracted a sternal wound infection due to *Rhodococcus bronchialis* [16]. Environmental surveillance in this outbreak revealed that one circulating nurse was common to all open heart procedures that resulted in infection, and that this individual harbored *R. bronchialis* in her nose, throat, vagina, and fingers. Further investigation resulted in the culturing of this microorganism from the fur of a household pet. The spread to the patients was hypothesized to occur from the nurse's colonized hands by either droplet spread or extrinsically contaminated instruments. Since exclusion of this nurse from open heart surgery, no further cases of sternal wound infections due to *R. bronchialis* have occurred.

Wound infection outbreaks due to rapidly growing mycobacteria have also been reported after cardiac surgery [17] and augmentation mammoplasty [18]. The suggested reservoirs for these outbreaks appear to implicate the surgical environment, including the air and water. These microorganisms are the most common mycobacteria recovered from hospital dust and are known to survive in both soil and water.

An outbreak of infection due to *Serratia marcescens* was reported in eight patients who had undergone cardiovascular surgery in one hospital [19]. Two of the patients became bacteremic and one died. The epidemiologic investigation identified the cause of the outbreak to be contaminated skin cream used by a scrub nurse. This nurse also wore artificial nails, which are known to increase the carriage rate of gram-negative bacteria. The outbreak stopped after use of the cream was discontinued.

Uncommon Modes for Transmission of Infection

The usual sources for wound infections that originate in the operating room are the patient, followed by the operating room environment and healthcare workers. Wound infection may also be transmitted by some unusual vectors that are discussed here. The role that anesthesia technique and equipment play in the development of postoperative respiratory infections is beyond the general scope of this chapter. Rarely, septicemia may result from the administration of contaminated intravenous solutions [20]. An intravenous anesthetic, propofol, has been implicated in a large number of postoperative infections [21]. This drug has a unique lipid base that can support microbial growth if contaminated. Sixty-two patients at seven hospitals contracted infections after administration of propofol. These infections, at first, were attributed to the surgeon or procedure performed. Subsequently, it was found that contamination of the drug had resulted from numerous breaks in infection control technique by the anesthesia personnel [22]. Contaminated drug was then administered to the patients, resulting in the infections.

Central venous catheters placed before surgery in the operating room environment after appropriate skin cleaning and preparation rarely result in bacteremia. The use of an attachable, silver-impregnated catheter cuff may further prevent the development of these infections [23]. Suction devices used to remove blood from the operative field have been shown experimentally to have a higher degree of contamination when aspirated with operating room air [24]. This appears to correlate with a high positive suction tip culture rate when suction is used clinically with conventional operating room ventilation [25]. This finding caused the authors to recommend that suction tubes be turned off when not in use and that the tubes be changed during total hip arthroplasty.

Invasive hemodynamic monitoring in a large study of patients undergoing open heart surgery has shown differing degrees of culture-positive catheter tips after the use of central venous, intravenous, arterial, and pulmonary artery catheters [26]. However, the authors observed that no patient contracted catheter-related septicemia or endocarditis after invasive hemodynamic monitoring (see also Chapters 39, 44).

Operating Suite Design

It appears that in most operative procedures the patient and personnel are the chief problems in the control of wound infections. Nevertheless, architectural design concepts have evolved that play a role in the control of surgical infection in modern operating suites. The key features of design have been reviewed before [11] and include the isolation of the surgical suite from the mainstream of common corridor traffic and the development of the "clean central core," which serves as the supply center and supposedly offers the cleanest environment. The inner corridors that surround the clean core are designed for use by clean traffic, which includes the preoperative patient, nurses, and surgeons. The peripheral corridors are designated for traffic that includes the postoperative patient as well as surgeons and nurses after operating or between cases. Patients should be transferred before and after operation through the peripheral corridors.

The optimal size for most routine operating rooms is 20 × 20 feet with 10-foot ceilings, which allows for easy gowning, draping, and circulation of personnel and the use of equipment without the risk of contact contamination. The door of each operating room should be kept closed except for passage of equipment, personnel, and the patient. The number of personnel allowed to enter each operating room should be kept to an absolute minimum, because the origin of infecting bacteria can sometimes be traced to shedding that occurs during movement of staff within the operating room. Intraoperative surveillance of the number of people in attendance, excessive conversation, number of times the doors are opened, and the pattern of use of antibiotic prophylaxis has led to improvements regarding these factors, and was associated with a decreased postoperative infection rate in implant surgery [27]. Floors in the operating room should be nonporous and other surfaces should be as dirt resistant as possible. The use of tacky or antiseptic mats at the entrance of the operating room is contraindicated [6].

INFECTION CONTROL IN THE OPERATING ROOM ENVIRONMENT

Some of the basic operating room design aspects that appear to help in the control of infection have already been reviewed. Other important considerations are operating room cleansing and ventilation and the use of ultraviolet (UV) light.

Operating Room Cleansing

In the early morning, before people have entered, the operating room environment is nearly sterile. Wet mopping of the hard-surfaced floors with a phenolic solution between each case and wet vacuuming of the rooms and corridors at night succeeds in keeping the floors clean [11].

The practice of closing a room for 48 hours in which a "dirty" case has been treated is no longer considered necessary [11]. Appropriate clean-up techniques in these cases consist of wet mopping or flooding with a phenolic detergent followed by a wipe-down of all equipment surfaces with 70% alcohol. All rubber and plastic tubing in the room should be replaced, but the walls should be cleansed only if direct contamination has occurred. All instruments, linen, and waste should be bagged carefully in these cases, and the gowns, masks, and shoe covers used in the procedure must be left in the room in appropriate containers. Personnel must not be allowed to leave the operating room while wearing shoe covers, masks, gowns, hair covers, or gloves. If the scrub uniform is worn outside the area, it should be covered with a laboratory coat.

Sterilization of Instruments and Devices

Steam sterilization of manually cleaned instruments has remained the technique of choice since reliable control of this technique was established more than 50 years ago [28]. When performed with the correct temperature and pressure, sterilization is accomplished by the least expensive and time-consuming method. A discussion of the three major types of steam sterilizers—the gravity sterilizer, the high-speed (prevacuum) sterilizer, and the tabletop sterilizer—is beyond the scope of this chapter (see Chapter 20). Increasing the temperature in a gravity sterilizer allows for faster sterilization of unwrapped instruments or other equipment (flash sterilization). This technique should be used only in emergency situations and is not recommended by most national organizations [29].

Ethylene oxide sterilization is a technique that is more complex and expensive and can be hazardous if not handled cautiously [1,29]. This type of gas sterilization is performed only on clean and dry items and is to be used only as recommended by the manufacturers of heat-sensitive items.

Ethylene oxide sterilization requires degassing before use to avoid injuries to workers and patients. This method of sterilization is being replaced by other compounds. Peracetic acid is among the newest methods in use [30]. No matter which technique is used for sterilization, it is imperative that instruments be cleansed thoroughly before undergoing the sterilization procedures.

The sterilization processes are reviewed further in Chapter 20.

Operating Room Ventilation Systems

More than 120 years ago, Joseph Lister attempted to prevent "a floating germ" from entering during an operation by using a fine spray of dilute carbolic acid [31]. He believed that this spray would reduce the incidence of postsurgical wound infections by killing the "germs" in the air as well as on the patient's surface drapes and on the surgeon's and assistant's clothing. It appears that Lister at no time considered the use of ventilation for this purpose, and he wrote in 1890, "It seems to follow logically that the floating particles of the air may be disregarded in our surgical work" [32]. Others earlier in the same century, however, had proposed a method of ventilation to remove from the air of the hospital "pus and matters like pus floating in the air, minute hairs, epidermic scales and also living forms" [33]. Until the 1930s, the only ventilation installed in operating rooms was for removing steam produced by the sterilizers used for instrument cleansing. At this time, spurred by the inability to control the spread of respiratory diseases and childhood fevers, the possible role of airborne transmission of disease became a matter for discussion and evoked scientific interest [34]. In addition, the persistence of postoperative wound infection, despite the application of aseptic practices, resulted in Meleney's proposal [35] that organisms from the air of the operating room might play a role in its genesis. In England during the 1940s, further insights were gained when sensitive methods for the detection of airborne bacteria were developed. These techniques helped to establish that the activities of the operating room staff were the principal source for these bacteria and that the practice of extract ventilation resulted in the introduction of bacteria from the hospital corridors and wards into the operating room [33]. These observations were largely responsible for the development of the modern practice of a positive-pressure air supply for the operating room. Debate, dispute, and interest concerning the importance of airborne bacteria to postoperative wound infection, discussed first before the time of Lister, continues to the present day.

The modern conventional operating room is virtually free of bacteria or particles larger than 0.5 μm when there are no people in attendance. The source of airborne bacteria in such an operating room is largely the skin of the people present in the room, whereas the quantitative counts depend greatly on the number of people present, their level of activity, and their discipline, knowledge, and application of infection control practices. An excellent review on the subject of aerobiology in the operating room was published by Hambraeus in 1988 [36]. Despite our present knowledge, the safe level of airborne operating room environmental contamination for different surgical procedures has yet to be determined.

Today, most conventional operating rooms in America are ventilated with 20 to 25 changes per hour of high-efficiency filtered air delivered in a unidirectional vertical flow. High-efficiency particulate air (HEPA) filtration systems usually are generally used, which remove most bacteria measuring 0.5 to 5.0 μm. Therefore, the first air downstream from the HEPA filter is virtually bacteria free. Bacteria released in the operating room environment remain unaffected by the filter system. At least 20% of the air changes per hour should be with fresh air [6]. The air delivered should be at temperatures between 18° and 24°C (65° and 75°F) and with 50% to 55% humidity. Inlets should be located as high above the floor as possible and remote from the active exhaust outlets, which are located low on the walls. This arrangement allows for the unidirectionality of the ventilation system. The operating room also should be under positive pressure relative to the surrounding corridors, which minimizes the flow of air into the operating rooms when the doors are opened. Unless personnel abuses occur [11], careful maintenance of the ventilation system just described offers an environment that is virtually as clean as more costly special chambers. The use of this type of air-handling system is clearly indicated for most clean surgical procedures and for all procedures in which the patient's endogenous microflora is potentially released during the surgical procedure. The debate continues as to whether additional, highly specialized ventilation systems are advantageous when major implant surgery is to be undertaken (see Chapter 40).

The more costly specialized ventilation systems usually are referred to as *laminar flow* and comprise many types of unidirectional air-blowing systems, including those of ceiling or wall diffusers and "curtain-effect" varieties [11]. The laminar flow can be delivered in a horizontal or vertical direction, and each system has its own proponents. The principal characteristic of such a system is the delivery of air at a uniform velocity (0.5 m/second) over the whole of one wall (horizontal) or, in the case of a vertical system, from the ceiling down, at a sufficient velocity to prevent any retrograde air movements [33]. These systems also use HEPA filtration to deliver air free of particles down to 0.3 μm. The first system was devised by Whitfield in 1960 and tested by surgeons soon after [37]. Charnley [38] in 1964 reported on a prototype filtered-air enclosure that was constructed to contain the lower half of the patient's body and three surgeons of the operating team. In this system, the filtered air was forced in at the top of the enclosure and the surgeons within the enclosure wore "space suits" with respirators through which their exhaled air was extracted to prevent its mixing with the filtered air of the enclosure. The author reported preliminary results that included a reduction of airborne bacteria within the enclosure compared with outside it, and a reduction of wound infections after hip replacement from 9.5% to 1.1% when the conventional air-handling system was compared with the enclosure system. However, most of the patients did not receive prophylactic systemic antibiotics because of the author's belief that this practice was not effective and may result in increased postoperative infections [33]. In the next decade, many orthopedic surgeons performing thousands of hip replacement operations in conventional operating rooms without laminar flow chambers reported a combined 2-year infection rate of 0.45% [39].

In 1982, Lidwell and colleagues [40] reported the results of a multicenter study of infection after total hip or knee replacement in more than 8000 patients enrolled from 1974 to 1979. In patients whose implants were inserted in an operating room ventilated by an ultraclean air (laminar flow) system, the incidence of joint infection confirmed at reoperation within a 1- to 4-year period was approximately half (23 infections among 3922 patients [0.6%]) that observed in those patients whose operation was undertaken in a conventionally ventilated room at the same hospital (63 infections among 4133 patients [1.5%]). In those cases in the ultraclean group for which the surgeons wore whole-body exhaust-ventilated suits, the infection rate was noted to be approximately one fourth that found in the cases performed under conventional ventilation. However, the design of the study did not include a strictly controlled test of the effect of prophylactic antibiotics. Their use was associated with a lower incidence of sepsis (34 infections among 5,831 patients [0.6%]) compared with patients undergoing operation without antibiotic prophylaxis (52 infections among 2221 patients [2.3%]).

The results of randomized studies of arthroplasty have confirmed that a considerable reduction of sepsis can be obtained by operating in ultraclean air but that similarly low rates of infections can be achieved with normal conventional ventilation when prophylactic antibiotics are routinely given [33,41]. The question that remains is whether a combination of ultraclean air and prophylactic antibiotics can be shown in a prospective, controlled study to offer a significant reduction in infection compared with the use of either of these preventive measures alone. A review of special clean air, ultraclean air, and partial barrier systems is recommended for those interested in this subject [42].

Use of Ultraviolet Light

The bactericidal effect of UV light has long been established [42]. In a large, well-publicized, prospective, randomized study reported in 1964, it was shown that UV irradiation reduced the number of recoverable viable organisms within the operating room by more than 50% [3]. Yet, the wound infection rates observed in the same study showed no significant differences between the control operations and those done in the presence of UV irradiation. Another study reported on the value of the use of UV irradiation in preventing infection in refined clean operations at the Duke University Medical Center [43]. When used, the personnel and patients must be protected from the UV irradiation by the wearing of appropriate hoods, masks, and goggles. This approach for the prevention of operating room contamination, although used by some hospitals, has become the subject of renewed active scientific investigation [44,45]. This work has shown that UV irradiation can provide ultraclean air in the operating room. Criticism still remains regarding the need for protective clothing for exposed personnel and patients.

Scheduling of Operations

Practices aimed at scheduling "dirty" operations at the end of the day or in a specific operating room (septic room) should be discouraged [6,11]. In the modern, well managed operating suite, the chance of environmentally spread infection remains remote. This is primarily due to the high degree of efficiency in sterilizing instruments and surgical devices, efficient ventilation systems that provide clean air, and the adequacy of the techniques of operating room cleansing between cases.

Maintenance of Surveillance Records

It is recommended that all operations be classified and recorded as clean, clean-contaminated, contaminated, or dirty at the time of operation or shortly after [6]. Surgeon-specific, procedure-specific infection rates should be computed periodically and made available to the infection control committee, the department of surgery, and the individual surgeon so that interventions can be designed if increased wound infection rates are reported. All observed increases of the wound infection rates should result in the initiation of appropriate epidemiologic studies to identify possible sources for this occurrence. The hospital committee that is responsible for these functions should be designated by hospital administration.

OPERATING ROOM PERSONNEL

The importance of the conduct, personal integrity, and work ethics of operating room personnel to both the level of bacteria in the operating room and to outbreaks of wound infection has already been addressed. To understand the possible significance of the staff's actions, it is necessary to have an ongoing infection control educational and surveillance program that involves all levels of operating room employees (see Chapters 3, 5). Routine nasopharyngeal cultures of personnel who work in the operating room have been shown not to be necessary [11]. However, the practice of culturing personnel in the presence of an outbreak as part of the epidemiologic investigation, if indicated, should be carried out and is often rewarding. It is important to remember that the presence of a disseminating carrier employee, conventionally masked, gowned, and shod, in any part of the operating room is a hazard to the patient.

Surgical Gowns and Related Garb

The primary purpose of wearing a gown around the operating table is to provide a barrier to contamination that may pass from personnel to patient as well as from patient to personnel. Bernard and Beck [46] stressed in 1975 that barrier products could not be properly evaluated unless adequate tests demonstrating consistent efficacy could be established. Laufman and coworkers [47] demonstrated that the bacterial penetration of a given material used in gowns and drapes is relative, depending largely on the degree of stress placed on it, and that the materials used in surgical barriers vary greatly under the same stress. Impermeability to moisture is, of course, a basic necessity of any barrier material because the wicking effect seen in absorbent materials tends to transmit bacteria.

From the late nineteenth century until the 1950s, the standard surgical gown was reusable and constructed of 140-thread-count cotton muslin. Beck and Collette [48] questioned the suitability of this fabric in 1952 when their experiments demonstrated bacterial passage through wet, but not dry, cotton cloth. Bernard and colleagues [49] showed a reduction of bacterial transmission through gowns when a tighter weave of cotton fabric was used, whereas Moylan and colleagues [50] later demonstrated that reusable cloth gowns, even in the dry state, were ineffective bacterial barriers. Still later clinical studies by these investigators showed a significantly reduced postoperative wound infection rate when disposable, spunbonded olefin gowns and drapes were compared with either 140- or 280-thread-count cloth reusables [51]. A similar result was also reported when spun-lace disposable gowns and drapes were compared with 280-thread-count reusables [52]. We have experimentally tested the strike-through of blood in 11 types of commonly used disposable and reusable surgical gowns [53]. We observed that new cloth gowns are more resistant to strike-through than those washed 40 times and that spunbond disposable fabrics are more protective than spun lace. Most reinforced (double-layer) disposables are less vulnerable to the strike-through of blood than a single layer of the same material, and all gowns with a layer of plastic (impervious) placed between the two layers were resistant to blood strike-through.

The American Society for Testing of Materials (ASTM) has approved two emergency standards to test clothing materials. Standard F1670–97 tests fabrics for resistance to synthetic blood and Standard F1671–97a tests resistance to bloodborne pathogens using viral penetration as a test system [54]. However, much criticism has been directed at their methodology and testing standards. These standards fail to test the gown materials under normal conditions of use. Also, the results of these tests do not allow for different levels of protection (equivalent to adequate protection under varying conditions), but are simply graded as pass or fail. Consequently, it appears that only impervious materials will be able to pass these demanding tests. Finally, both test methods are time consuming and require specialized (expensive) equipment. Because conditions of use are known to vary greatly by type of procedure and task, all materials do not need to have the same level of resistance, yet the ASTM tests subject all to a single method.

Further clinical and experimental testing, with the establishment of standards, is necessary to define better the efficacy of these barrier products. The emphasis today regarding barrier efficiency mandates that healthcare workers be protected from skin contamination with their patient's blood. The Occupational Safety and Health Administration's (OSHA) *Final Rule on Occupational Exposure to Bloodborne Pathogens* addresses this by requiring that gowns be provided to protect the worker "under normal conditions of use and for the duration of time which it will be used" [55]. The materials chosen for these products should be based largely on the level of protection from blood strike-through needed in each operative procedure as well as comfort of the product. Gowns constructed with a completely impervious plastic middle layer would prevent blood strike-through but would be intolerable to wear except in the shortest operative procedures. The industry continues to develop and study new types of protective clothing for use in the operating room, as well as other areas of the hospital.

Various types of hoods, rather than caps, are being used today to cover the hair, which attracts and sheds bacterial particles. The type chosen by each operating room worker should largely be based on the amount and distribution of their scalp and facial hair. As mentioned previously, some authorities recommend the use of ventilated space suits and helmets to isolate the surgeons and assistants completely from their patients' environment during ultraclean implant surgical procedures. Closing of the trouser opening of the surgical scrubs with Velcro tape at ankle level has been shown to reduce the aerial dissemination of skin bacteria. A similar reduction of airborne bacteria did not follow Velcro closure techniques applied to the surgeon's arms or neck. The wearing of disposable shoe covers by operating room personnel, although usually recommended, has not been proved effective as an infection control measure [6,56].

The Surgical Scrub and Preoperative Skin Preparation

The surgeon and assistants who will touch the sterile surgical field or instruments are required to scrub their hands and forearms in a systematic fashion with an antimicrobial preparation before each operative procedure [6]. As late as the 1960s, the duration of this ritual was 10 minutes, with a stiff brush being used to provide friction. This technique was abandoned when it was found that bacteria from the deep dermal layers were being isolated at the surface. Today, the usual first daily surgical scrub of at least 5 minutes' duration is accomplished with a sponge impregnated with an antimicrobial-containing preparation [6]. Although the ideal duration of the scrub is not known, times as short as 5 minutes appear safe [57]. Between consecutive operations, the surgical scrub can be as short as 2 to 5 minutes. The cleansing material may be a soap or detergent containing an iodophor, hexachlorophene, or another accepted, nonirritating antimicrobial preparation that significantly reduces the number of microorganisms on the intact skin [58]. Appropriate products have been listed in categories, for choice by the hospitals, by the U.S. Food and Drug Administration [59] (see Chapter 20).

Preoperative patient skin preparation is initiated just before the time of operative incision by the limited removal of operative site hair by shaving or clipping. This is followed by the systematic washing of the operative site and surrounding areas with products similar to those used in the surgical scrub. The wash is followed by the application of an antimicrobial preparation, working from the center of the planned operative incision to the periphery [6]. Larson [58] has reviewed the agents to be considered for antimicrobial skin preparation. After the patient's skin preparation has been completed, appropriate sterile skin draping is carried out to protect the clean field from the unprepared parts of the patient. The use of plastic-impregnated drapes should not be routine, but they can be used in specific cases where isolation of an area from the operative incision is indicated (e.g., ileostomy site).

Surgical Gloves

The surgical team members, after scrubbing, should dry their hands with sterile towels and then don sterile gowns and sterile gloves. If the glove is punctured during operation, it should be promptly changed as dictated by patient safety. Some have recommended double gloving as a routine to lessen the chance of microbial contamination during total joint arthroplasty [60]. Other studies have shown that more than 12% of gloves were perforated during surgery and that this occurred in more than 30% of operations [61]. Beck [62] has stressed that traditionally gloves have been worn to protect the patient, but today, with the fear of transmission of bloodborne disease to the healthcare worker, there exists an increased level of interest concerning the efficacy of various gloves. He recommends that in the near future industry develop stronger gloves that are resistant to puncture and that, until this occurs, gloves should be changed after each hour of operative time.

Studies have shown that allergy to latex products such as surgical gloves is a growing medical problem [63,64]. It is estimated that ~ 3% of hospital physicians and nurses are affected, and higher rates have been reported in the surgical units. Allergic reactions may be delayed or immediate, and are usually local, but systemic derangements that are potentially fatal have been reported [63]. Not only are healthcare providers at risk for anaphylactic reactions, but those who have local reactions to the latex may have an increased risk of contracting a bloodborne pathogen if glove punctures occur. These local reactions include contact or atopic dermatitis that can develop into skin lesions through which contamination may enter the body. Further research is being conducted in this area.

Surgical Masks

Everyone who enters the operating room during an operation is required to wear a high-efficiency mask to cover the mouth and nose area fully [6]. If the mask becomes soiled or wet during the procedure, it should be changed. Orr [65] has argued that the efficacy of preventing wound infection with surgical masks has not been established, but that their efficiency in reducing bacterial contamination has. He noted no increase in wound infection rate in one operating room where no masks were worn during a 6-month period and concludes "that the wearing of a mask has very little relevance to the well-being of patients undergoing routine general surgery and it is a standard practice that could be abandoned" [65]. Other studies have likewise shown that contamination can be reduced with the use of the surgical mask but that the incidence of infections has not increased. Although the use of surgical masks might be considered to be a "sacred cow" to some, I believe their use should be continued in an attempt to protect both the patient from airborne contamination and the surgical team from bloodborne pathogens transmitted in any spray or splash to face, mouth, or nasal areas.

Protecting Operating Room Personnel: The Patient as Vector

A great deal of emphasis is placed on protecting the hospital employee from acquiring infectious diseases from an actively infected patient or carrier. The potential for exposure to bloodborne diseases such as human immunodeficiency virus (HIV) and hepatitis B virus is high in the operating room (see Chapters 3, 43). Because operative misadventures such as inadvertent needlestick, sharp injuries, and blood splashes to skin or mucous membranes do occur with regularity to the operative team, it has become popular to predict the probability of occupationally acquiring HIV infection during one's surgical career [66,67]. This predicted risk of acquiring infection with HIV from operative encounters appears to be primarily related to the amount of time spent in the operating room, type of operations performed, and the local seroprevalence of the patient population. The great differences in seroprevalence of HIV infection in 21 urban populations have been stressed [68]. Thirty-year career risks of HIV seroconversion, due to occupational exposure for surgeons, appear to be as high as 10% if the surgeon is actively involved in "bloody" cases in a locality that has a high seroprevalence rate [66,67]. Another risk posed by exposure to blood for the operating room staff is the acquisition of hepatitis C virus (HCV) (see Chapter 42). A documented seroconversion rate of 6% was found among healthcare workers in a study conducted by Lanphear and colleagues [69]. It is expected that the seroconversion rate after needlestick injuries with hepatitis C virus-contaminated blood will be somewhere between that seen with HIV (<1%) and hepatitis B virus (10% to 30%). The incidence of transmission of hepatitis C virus is expected to rise as a result of its unique characteristics, including the absence of a preventive vaccine, the ineffectiveness of prophylactic treatment with gamma globulin, and the unavailability of a definitive treatment. Hepatitis C has been found to be more prevalent among healthcare providers than HIV.

An observational study of more than 1300 consecutive surgical procedures at San Francisco General Hospital has shown that accidental exposure to the patient's blood occurred in 84 procedures [70]. Parenteral exposure occurred in 1.7% of cases, whereas cutaneous exposure was noted in the remainder. The risk of exposure was highest in procedures that lasted > 3 hours, when the blood loss exceeded 300 ml, and when major vascular or intraabdominal gynecologic surgery was involved. The authors concluded that surgical personnel are at risk for intraoperative exposure to blood and that preoperative testing for HIV infection did not reduce the frequency of accidental exposure to blood. Universal precautions, which include the limited and careful use of sharps, routine double gloving, use of face shields or glasses with lateral extensions, and the wearing of barrier gowns that prevent blood strike-through, appear to offer the best protection against accidental exposures to blood that may translate to seroconversion [53,70,71] (see Chapter 13).

The role that the HIV-infected surgeon or operating room employee plays in patient seroconversion and whether steps should be taken to curtail the activity of such healthcare providers remains to be determined [72]. The reader is referred to Chapter 43 for additional considerations related to HIV infections.

CONCLUSION

Risk factors related to the operating room setting include patient-associated tasks, the operating room environment, ventilation systems, cleansing and sterilization techniques and equipment, and operating room personnel. Although attempts are made to control the environment of the rooms, the operating room setting remains potentially hostile to both the patient and the surgical team. To decrease the incidence of nosocomial infections and the transmission of bloodborne pathogens, this area needs to be reviewed, monitored, and continually updated. Many new hazards and concerns are posed with new technology. Therefore, it is imperative that universal precautions are implemented and infection control measures enforced.

REFERENCES

1. LoCicero J III, Quebbeman EJ, Nichols RL. Health hazards in the operating room: an update. *Bull Am Coll Surg* 1987;72:4–9.
2. Garner JS, Emori TG, Haley RW. Operating room practices for the control of infection in U.S. hospitals, October 1976 to July 1977. *Surg Gynecol Obstet* 1982;155:873–88.
3. Ad Hoc Committee of the Committee on Trauma, Division of Medical Sciences, National Academy of Sciences National Research Council. Factors influencing the incidence of wound infection. *Ann Surg* 1964; 160(Suppl):32–81.
4. Haley RW, Culver DH, White JW, et al. The nationwide nosocomial infection rate: a new need for vital statistics. *Am J Epidemiol* 1985;121: 159–167.
5. Nichols RL. Postoperative wound infection. *N Engl J Med* 1982;307: 1701–02.
6. Nichols RL. Surgical wound infection. *Am J Med* 1991;91(Suppl 3B):54S–64S.
7. Haley RW, Culver DH, Morgan WM, et al. Identifying patients at high risk of surgical wound infection. *Am J Epidemiol* 1985;121:206–215.
8. Culver DH, Horan TC, Gaynes RP, et al. Surgical wound infection rates by wound class, operative procedure, and patient risk index. National Nosocomial Infections Surveillance System. *Am J Med* 1991;91(suppl 3B):152S–157S.
9. Keats AS. The ASA classifications of physical status a recapitulation. *Anesthesiology* 1978;49:233–236.
10. Walter CW, Kundsin RB. The floor as a reservoir of hospital infections. *Surg Gynecol Obstet* 1960;111:1–11.
11. Nichols RL. The operating room. In: Bennett JV, Brachman PS, eds. *Hospital infections.* 3rd ed. Boston: Little, Brown, 1992:461–471.
12. Wiley AM. Researches in orthopedic wound infections. *Clin Orthop* 1986;208:28.
13. Nade S. Infection after joint replacement: what would Lister think? *Med J Aust* 1990;152:394–397.
14. Andersen BM, Sorlie D, Hotvedt R, et al. Multiply beta-lactam resistant *Enterobacter cloacae* infections linked to the environmental flora in a unit for cardiothoracic and vascular surgery. *Scand J Infect Dis* 1989;21:181–191.
15. Isenberg HD, Tucci V, Cintron F, et al. Single-source outbreak of *Candida tropicalis* complicating coronary bypass surgery. *J Clin Microbiol* 1989;27:2426–2428.
16. Richet HM, Craven PC, Brown JM, et al. A cluster of *Rhodococcus (Gordana) bronchialis* sternal-wound infections after coronary-artery bypass surgery. *N Engl J Med* 1991;324:104–109.

17. Wallace RJ Jr, Musser JM, Hull SI, et al. Diversity and sources of rapidly growing mycobacteria associated with infections following cardiac surgery. *J Infect Dis* 1989;159:708–715.
18. Wallace RJ Jr, Steele LC, Labidi A, Silcox VA, et al. Heterogeneity among isolates of rapidly growing mycobacteria responsible for infections following augmentation mammoplasty despite case clustering in Texas and other southern coastal states. *J Infect Dis* 1989;160:281–288.
19. Centers for Disease Control and Prevention. Sleuths track nosocomial outbreak to skin cream. *Hosp Infect Control* 1995;22:65.
20. Duma RI, Warner JF, Dalton HP. Septicemia from intravenous infusions. *N Engl J Med* 1971;284:257–260.
21. Bennett SN, McNeil MM, Bland LA, et al. Postoperative infections traced to contamination of an intravenous anesthetic, propofol. *N Engl J Med* 1995;333:147.
22. Nichols RL, Smith JW. Bacterial contamination of an anesthetic agent. *N Engl J Med* 1995;333:184–185.
23. Maki DG, Cobb L, Garman JK, et al. An attachable silver-impregnated cuff for prevention of infection with central venous catheters: a prospective randomized multicenter trial. *Am J Med* 1988;84:307–314.
24. van Oeveren WV, Dankert J, Boonstra PW, et al. Airborne contamination during cardiopulmonary bypass: the role of cardiotomy suction. *Ann Thorac Surg* 1986;41:401–406.
25. Strange-Vognsen HH, Klareskov B. Bacteriologic contamination of suction tips during hip arthroplasty. *Acta Orthop Scand* 1988;59:410–411.
26. Damen J, Verhoef J, Bolton DT, et al. Microbiologic risk of invasive hemodynamic monitoring in patients undergoing open-heart operations. *Crit Care Med* 1985;13:548–555.
27. Borst M, Collier C, Miller D. Operating room surveillance: a new approach in reducing hip and knee prosthetic wound infections. *Am J Infect Control* 1986;14:161–166.
28. Walter CW. A reliable control for steam sterilization. *Surg Gynecol Obstet* 1938;67:526–530.
29. Crow S. *Asepsis, the right touch: something old is now new*. Bossier City, LA: Everett Publishers; 1989.
30. Crow SC. Sterilization process: meeting the demands of today's healthcare technology. *Nurse Clin N Am* 1993;28:687–695.
31. Lister J. On a case illustrating the present aspect of the antiseptic treatment in surgery. *Br Med J* 1871;1:30–32.
32. Lister J. An address on the present position of antiseptic surgery. *Br Med J* 1890;2:377–379.
33. Lidwell OM. Clean air at operation and subsequent sepsis in the joint. *Clin Orthop* 1986;211: 91–102.
34. Wells WF, Wells MW. Airborne infection. *JAMA* 1936;107:1698–1703.
35. Meleney FL: The control of wound infections. *Ann Surg* 1933;98:151.
36. Hambraeus A. Aerobiology in the operating room a review. *J Hosp Infect* 1988;11:68–76.
37. Whitcomb JC, Whitfield W, King JG, et al. Ultraclean operating rooms. *The Lovelace Clinic Review (Albuquerque, NM)* 1965;2:65–69.
38. Charnley J. A clean-air operating enclosure. *Br J Surg* 1964;51:202–205.
39. Laufman H. Current status of special air handling systems in operating rooms. *Med Instrum* 1973;7:7–15.
40. Lidwell OM, Lowbury EJL, Whyte W, et al. Effect of ultraclean air in operating rooms on deep sepsis in the joint after total hip or knee replacement: a randomised study. *Br Med J* 1982;285:10–14.
41. Hill C, Flamant R, Mazas F, Evrard J, et al. Prophylactic cefazolin versus placebo in total hip replacement. *Lancet* 1981;1:795–796.
42. Levenson SM, Trexler PC, Van der Waaij D. Nosocomial infection: prevention by special clean-air, ultraviolet light, and barrier (isolator) techniques [Review]. *Curr Probl Surg* 1986;23:453–558.
43. Hart D, Postlethwait RW, Brown IW Jr, et al. Postoperative wound infections: a further report on ultraviolet irradiation with comments on the recent (1964) National Research Council Cooperative Study report. *Ann Surg* 1968;167:728–745.
44. Berg-Perier M, Cederblad A, Persson U. Ultraviolet radiation and ultraclean air enclosures in operating rooms: UV-protection, economy, and comfort. *J Arthroplasty* 1992;7:457–463.
45. Lidwell OM. Ultraviolet radiation and the control of airborne contamination in the operating room. *J Hosp Infect* 1994;28:245–248.
46. Bernard HR, Beck WC. Operating room barriers: idealism, practicality, and the future. *Bull Am Coll Surg* 1975;60:16.
47. Laufman H, Eudy WW, Vandernoot AM, et al. Strike-through of moist contamination by woven and nonwoven surgical materials. *Ann Surg* 1975;181:857–862.
48. Beck WC, Collette TS. False faith in the surgeon's gown and surgical drape. *Am J Surg* 1952;83:125–126.
49. Bernard HR, Speers R, O'Grady F, Shooter RA, et al. Reduction of dissemination of skin bacteria by modification of operating-room clothing and by ultraviolet irradiation. *Lancet* 1965;2:458–461.
50. Moylan JA, Balish E, Chan J. Intraoperative bacterial transmission. *Surg Gynecol Obstet* 1975;141:731–733.
51. Moylan JA, Kennedy BV. The importance of gown and drape barriers in the prevention of wound infection. *Surg Gynecol Obstet* 1980;151: 465–470.
52. Moylan JA, Fitzpatrick KT, Davenport KE. Reducing wound infections: improved gown and drape barrier performance. *Arch Surg* 1987; 122:152–158.
53. Smith JW, Nichols RL. Barrier efficacy of surgical gowns: are we really protected from our patients' pathogens? *Arch Surg* 1991;126:756–763.
54. Smith JW, Nichols RL. Comment. *OR Reports* 1993;2:4–5.
55. Occupational Safety and Health Administration. *Final rule on occupational exposure to bloodborne pathogens*. 29 CFR 1910:103, 1991. 64004–64182.
56. Hambraeus A, Malmborg AS. The influence of different footwear on floor contamination. *Scand J Infect Dis* 1979;11:243–246.
57. Dineen P. An evaluation of the duration of the surgical scrub. *Surg Gynecol Obstet* 1969;129:1181–1184.
58. Larson E. APIC guidelines for infection control practice: guideline for use of topical antimicrobial agents. *Am J Infect Control* 1988;16: 253–266.
59. Zanowiak P, Jacobs MR. Topical anti-infective products. In: *Handbook of nonprescription drugs*. 7th ed. Washington, DC: American Pharmaceutical Association; 1982:525–542.
60. McCue SF, Berg EW, Saunders EA. Efficacy of double-gloving as a barrier to microbial contamination during total joint arthroplasty. *J Bone Joint Surg* (AM) 1981;63:811–813.
61. Dodds RDA, Guy PJ, Peacock AM, et al: Surgical glove perforation. *Br J Surg* 1988;75:966–968.
62. Beck WC. The hole in the surgical glove: a change in attitude. *Bull Am Coll Surg* 1989;74:15–16.
63. Masood D, Brown JE, Patterson R, et al. Recurrent anaphylaxis due to unrecognized latex hypersensitivity in two healthcare professionals. *Ann Allergy Asthma Immunol* 1995;74:311–313.
64. Mendyka BE, Clochesy JM, Workman ML. Latex hypersensitivity and occupational risk. *Am J Crit Care* 1994;3:198–201.
65. Orr NWM. Is a mask necessary in the operating theatre? *Ann R Coll Surg Engl* 1981;63:390–392.
66. Lowenfels AB, Wormser GP, Jain R. Frequency of puncture injuries in surgeons and estimated risk of HIV infection. *Arch Surg* 1989;124: 1284–1286.
67. McKinney WP, Young MJ. The cumulative probability of occupationally acquired HIV infection: the risks of repeated exposures during a surgical career. *Infect Control Hosp Epidemiol* 1990;11:243–247.
68. St. Louis ME, Rauch KJ, Petersen LR, et al. Seroprevalence rates of human immunodeficiency virus infection at sentinel Hospitals in the United States. *N Engl J Med* 1990;323:213–218.
69. Lanphear BP, Linnemann CC, Cannon CG, et al: Hepatitis C virus infection in healthcare workers: risk of exposure and infection. *Infect Control Hosp Eidemiol* 1994;15:745–50.
70. Gerberding JL, Littell C, Tarkington A, et al. Risk of exposure of surgical personnel to patients' blood during surgery at San Francisco General Hospital. *N Engl J Med* 1990;322:1788–1793.
71. Jagger J, Hunt EH, Pearson RD. Sharp object injuries in the hospital: causes and strategies for prevention. *Am J Infect Control* 1990;18: 227–231.
72. Mishu B, Schaffner W, Horan JM, et al. A surgeon with AIDS: lack of evidence of transmission to patients. *JAMA* 1990;264:467–470.

Hospital Infections, Fourth Edition,
edited by John V. Bennett and Philip S. Brachman.
Lippincott–Raven Publishers, Philadelphia © 1998

CHAPTER 28

Ambulatory Care Settings

Marguerite McMillan Jackson and Patricia Lynch

The vast majority of physician–patient contacts are in ambulatory care facilities. Statistics for 1990 indicated that ~ 77% of the population saw a physician at least once, and ~ 8% was hospitalized one or more times. Overall, each person in the United States averaged 4.8 physician visits annually, excluding telephone contacts but including inpatient care [1]. In 1995, 81% of ambulatory care visits were to physicians' offices, with an additional 8% in hospital outpatient departments. The remaining 11% were to hospital emergency departments [2].

Because of the millions of patient visits in these settings annually, questions frequently arise about the risk for nosocomial infection and about interventions to reduce these risks. Infection risk associated with care in an ambulatory setting is probably very low, although it has not been studied extensively. Most patients seen in these settings present with nonurgent problems and are not admitted to hospitals. A substantial proportion of the infections seen in ambulatory care settings (ACSs) are viral respiratory infections and probably carry with them risks of transmission similar to the risks of transmission in the community.

Nosocomial infection risk increases with the number of devices or procedures to which the patient is exposed. Except for emergent and some urgent visits to hospital emergency departments, most ambulatory care patients are not exposed to invasive devices or procedures that are known to pose significant infection risk. In addition, the duration of the patient's visit to the facility is usually limited, which is also a factor in reduced risk for nosocomial infection.

This chapter discusses the various types of ACSs, general infection risks associated with these settings, and interventions known or suspected to reduce infection risks for patients seen there. Home care is included now that an increasing number of people are being cared for in the home. As care in the home becomes more complex and includes management of devices such as intravascular catheters for administration of antibiotics and chemotherapeutic agents, device-related risks in this ACS also need careful review and evaluation.

M. M. Jackson: Epidemiology Unit, University of California at San Diego Medical Center, San Diego, California 92103.
P. Lynch: Epidemiology Associates, Seattle, Washington 98115.

AMBULATORY CARE SETTINGS

Ambulatory care may be delivered in various settings, ranging from a single physician's private office to a comprehensive emergency medical services system. The most common types of ACSs are described here.

Emergency Medical Services System

The emergency medical services system (EMSS) was developed partly in response to results from a National Academy of Sciences study of accidental death and disability, conducted in the early 1960s [3]. The Federal EMSS Act, enacted in 1973, outlined 15 separate components, defined 7 patient categories (trauma, burns, spinal cord injuries, poisoning, cardiac, neonatal, behavioral), and provided for a national EMSS framework. At the same time, communities increased emphasis on the timely delivery of care to patients with serious injuries, beginning before arrival at the hospital [4].

Prehospital Care

Prehospital care incorporates all emergency rescue, medical, and transportation services provided to ill or injured patients before they reach the hospital. The functional unit of prehospital care includes the hospital-based emergency department, personnel there who advise the field team, the field team for emergency transport, and the transport vehicle. In addition, some systems incorporate fire department personnel, community-based services, and volunteers.

Emergency Department of a Hospital

The emergency department of a hospital may provide three major services: 1) care of critically ill or injured patients, most of whom are subsequently admitted to the facility; 2) offices where physicians can examine their own patients (e.g., after office hours or when more sophisticated care is necessary than a physician's office can provide); and 3) care for people who are not critically injured or ill but who do not use any other organized ambulatory service or physician's office. Patients in the latter two categories usually are not admitted to the hospital.

Weinerman and colleagues [5] define three categories used by providers to describe requirements for emergency care that are still widely used today:

1. *Nonurgent.* Care does not require resources of an emergency service; referral for routine medical care may or may not be needed; disorder is nonacute or minor in severity. Few of these patients require hospital admission.
2. *Urgent.* Condition requires medical attention within the period of a few hours; there is possible danger to the patient if medically unattended; disorder is acute but not necessarily severe. Some of these patients require hospital admission.
3. *Emergent.* Condition requires immediate medical attention; time delay is harmful to the patient; disorder is acute and possibly threatening to life or function. Many of these patients require hospital admission and may require intensive care management.

Most visits to emergency departments are for conditions that are not considered urgent from a medical viewpoint but may be considered so by the patients presenting themselves for care. The distribution varies among hospitals according to the specific nature of the facility. In two studies of hospital emergency department visits, the two most common responses from patients regarding factors associated with their decision to visit the emergency department were expediency (e.g., available hours or comprehensive care) and immediacy [6,7]. The patient's perception of these factors may be different from that of the provider. The patient is scheduling care at his or her convenience, often because the emergency department is always open; also, third-party reimbursements may cover emergency department visits but not the same care in a physician's office.

Trauma Units

Trauma units are inpatient facilities that provide immediate and continuing care for patients with severe injuries. Some hospitals admit patients directly into the trauma unit. Infection risks associated with trauma units and the patient care provided there are discussed in Chapter 25.

Emergicenters

Emergicenters are usually freestanding facilities that care for patients with urgent or nonurgent problems. These centers are able to operate at considerably less cost than are emergency departments attached to hospitals because of the limited and exclusive nature of their function. The emergicenter functions like a physician's office with extended hours and may make referrals for more extensive care.

Outpatient Surgery

Surgicenters, or ambulatory surgery centers, are defined as centers that handle on a same-day basis those surgical procedures that cannot properly be performed in a physician's office or hospital outpatient department, but can be scheduled and performed so that the patient does not need to remain in a hospital overnight. These centers may be freestanding or part of the hospital facility. Administratively, they may be under the jurisdiction of the hospital's operating room or function independently.

In 1994, 57% of surgical operations performed in short-stay hospitals were outpatient procedures. Between 1984 and 1993, the number of freestanding ambulatory surgical centers increased from 330 to 1,862. In 1993, over 3 million procedures were performed in surgicenters, the most common of which were cataract surgery, arthroscopy, and colonoscopy [2].

Outpatient Diagnostic and Treatment Facilities

Outpatient diagnostic and treatment facilities provide care outside the usual inpatient institutional setting. This may include individual physicians' offices, clinics attached to teaching hospitals, specialty clinics, and clinics or office practices administered by groups of physicians or health maintenance organizations. Visits are usually scheduled at the request of the patient and convenience of the care provider and are usually elective in nature.

Hospital Admitting Departments

A visit to the hospital admitting department is the usual first stop for patients with scheduled elective admissions and a prehospitalization step for many patients admitted directly from clinics or emergency departments. Although emergency admissions interact with admitting departments for billing and organizational purposes, many emergency admissions go directly from the emergency department to a nursing unit or intensive care unit and do not visit the admitting department personally.

Care in the Home

Home care is a logical extension of the movement toward outpatient care, and is also viewed as a way to save money for certain conditions, although Weissert makes a convincing argument that the costs are currently about the same as existing options such as nursing homes [8]. Home healthcare was provided to almost two million people per day in 1994 by over 7,400 home health agencies. Three fourths of these people were at least 65 years of age, with almost 20% ages 85 years and older; two thirds of home care clients are women. About half of the qualifying diagnoses amounted to six types: diseases of the heart (14%), nervous system (8%), diabetes (8%), and cerebrovascular diseases, malignant neoplasms, and respiratory diseases for 6% each. Fractures, all sites, accounted for ~ 4% of qualifying diagnosis [2].

NOSOCOMIAL INFECTIONS

A nosocomial infection associated with an ACS can be defined as one that is associated temporally with the visit or with the care provided during the visit (e.g., an inadvertent exposure to a communicable disease while in the waiting room). In other words, it is an infection associated with medical intervention.

Patients seen in an ACS usually leave the facility after the visit and often are not followed up. If an infection develops associated with the visit, it may not be identified to the hospital or facility. The true incidence of these infections is not known, although several reports from ambulatory surgery settings have been published [9–15].

Risk of Nosocomial Infection in the Ambulatory Care Setting

Risk of nosocomial infection in the ACS has been demonstrated to be associated with the interaction between host defenses and exposure to potentially infectious agents in a dose sufficient to cause infection (see Chapter 1). Factors of an ACS that are different from the hospital setting include the following:

1. Large numbers of patients are seen in rapid succession in the ACS, excluding the home setting. In homes, a single patient is seen by a home care provider who may see several different patients in a day.
2. Few procedures are performed in any of the ACS settings in which access to the vascular system (e.g., intravenous therapy) or mucous membranes (e.g., intubation, laryngoscopy) is necessary.
3. A wide variety of ailments may be seen by the same care provider during a single day.
4. Most patients seen in an ACS, including emergency departments, outpatient clinics, physicians' offices, or at home, do not require admission to the hospital.

In summary, care for most patients in the ACS is for relatively minor illnesses or injuries that have not usually compromised their host defenses, or for chronic conditions that require continuing care. The duration of contact with the facility or care provider is brief, and risk for infection usually depends on instrumentation or surgical procedures. The likelihood of all three factors being sufficient to result in infection is very low.

It is widely accepted that ~ 5% of hospitalized patients contract nosocomial infections, primarily of four major types: urinary tract, surgical wound, lower respiratory, and bacteremia (see Chapter 30). Several investigators have estimated that the proportion of these infections that is potentially preventable is ~ 25% to 40% [16,17] and that most of those are related to devices and procedures. The remaining 60% to 75% are often judged unavoidable because of the patient's underlying disease combined with other factors such as the duration of hospitalization (see Chapter 30).

The incidence and preventability of nosocomial infections in the ACS have not been investigated adequately. It is reasonable to assume that most nosocomial infections in these settings are largely preventable because the duration of contact with the facility is brief, and those that do occur are usually related to medical devices and procedures.

To answer some of the questions raised about incidence of infection after ACS visits, several investigators have concentrated on patients in ambulatory surgery settings. Complications associated with ambulatory surgery were studied prospectively in 13,433 patients during a 4-year period by Natof [10]. Surgical procedures included tonsillectomy or adenoidectomy (or both), augmentation mammoplasty, submucous resection, and a variety of genitourinary procedures, primarily performed on young, healthy hosts. Only 10 of 13,433 patients contracted infections that could be associated with the ambulatory surgery procedure (3 wound infections, 3 gynecologic infections, 2 pneumonias, and 2 upper respiratory infections). The frequency of infectious complications after ambulatory surgery in this series was < 1 infection per 1,000 patients (< 0.1%).

Craig [9] summarized results of several studies of postoperative infections among ambulatory surgery patients. Despite several differences in study design, when patients and physicians responded to written questionnaires or telephone calls, the infection rate in all studies was no > 2%, and usually substantially lower.

Manion and Meyer [11] followed surgical procedures for 1 year by using a surgeon-specific, computer-generated monthly surveillance questionnaire. The response rate was 78% for outpatients and 77% for inpatients. The total wound infection rate was 0.13% (14 infections) for the 10,952 outpatients and 1.2% (116 infections) for the 9,584 inpatients. Almost 75% of the outpatient infections would have gone undetected by conventional surveillance methods; only five of them were cultured. Similar methods were used and results found by Flanders and Hinnant [12].

Zoutman et al. [13] randomly selected 25% of 2,540 day surgery procedures during a 6-month period, of which 515 were reached by telephone 1 month after their procedure by an infection control practitioner. Twenty-six (5.05%) wound infections were diagnosed, with 19 by physician diagnosis and 7 by patient description.

Infections in patients using an ambulatory podiatric surgery center were assessed by Hugar et al. [14], who found only 2 infections in 495 surgical procedures performed, for a rate of 1.35%.

Fridkin et al [15] reported four cases of *Acremonium kiliense* endophthalmitis in an ambulatory care center related to an environmental reservoir. The investigation using a case control study revealed that case patients had surgery on the first operative day of the week or had surgery significantly sooner after the operating room opened than did controls. An environmental assessment determined that the ventilation system was turned on 5–30 minutes before procedures began on the first operative day of the week, and air was filtered before but not after humidification. Cultures of the humidifier water in the ventilation system yielded isolates identical to those in case patients, suggesting the organisms were aerosolized coincident with switching on the ventilation system.

Overall, infection rates in ambulatory surgery patients appear to be lower than in patients having surgery in inpatient settings, probably largely because of the absence of most significant host risk factors that increase infection risk.

When the incidence of nosocomial infection is so low, the benefit of an intensive surveillance system is likely to be exceeded by the cost. That is, the time required to follow all patients makes the cost to identify each infection very high; however, the consequences of some nosocomial infections associated with the ACS have been serious [18,19]. In fact, Goodman and Soloman [20] characterized 53 reports of cases and clusters of infections associated with outpatient healthcare from 1961 to 1990. Twenty-three of the reports were about transmission in general medical offices, clinics, and emergency departments; 11 were in ophthalmologists' offices and clinics; 13 were in dental offices; and 6 were in alternative care settings. The modes of transmission were common source (14 injection, 15 other), 14 person-to-person, and 10 by airborne or droplet contact.

If infections in an ACS are to be monitored by surveillance, it is clear that follow-up with physicians' offices, including telephone calls to those who do not return written requests, will be required. Responsibility for this follow-up rests with various personnel, depending on the organizational structure of the agency [21,22].

Personnel Working in the Ambulatory Care Setting

The key to preventing nosocomial infections in an ACS may lie in the combination of skill in performing procedures and use of aseptic practices. As in any patient care area, personnel in the ACS should not work when they have infectious diseases and should follow the facility's program for personnel health, immunizations, and exposures to communicable diseases (see Chapter 3). Facilities that are not attached to hospitals can also use these guidelines to develop programs.

Training personnel in aseptic practices and ensuring that their skills and knowledge of invasive procedures are current is also essential in the ACS. Training patients and home caregivers is increasingly important with the trend toward managing patients with indwelling devices at home. Reports of home administration of intravenous therapy, parenteral nutrition, and dialysis were first published in the late 1970s when these practices became commonplace; few recent reports have been identified. Outpatient intravenous antibiotic therapy has been administered for a number of years [23–29], as has home parenteral nutrition [30–33], and ambulatory dialysis [33–36] (see Chapter 24). An integral component of all these programs is training for the patient or home caregiver in aseptic practices and recognition of complications. The reported incidence of infectious complications varies with the type of device, reason for and duration of therapy, host susceptibility, and many other factors.

In the home setting, some procedures likely to pose unacceptably high risks in the acute care setting can apparently be carried out acceptably. A study about aseptic technique in the use and reuse of insulin syringes by diabetic patients was conducted at an outpatient clinic of a large teaching hospital [38]. Diabetic outpatients were surveyed at the outset for compliance with recommendations for aseptic handling of syringes. The investigators then studied prospectively the effects of reusing disposable syringes in 56 diabetic patients who reused syringes a mean of 6.6 times (n=23,664 injections). Although compliance with aseptic precautions was poor, no adverse effects of syringe reuse were identified. The study reviewed other studies and case reports and then raised two important considerations. First, the initial survey established that almost half of the study subjects were reusing disposable syringes, primarily for cost reasons. Second, it found that even with poor aseptic technique associated with reuse of syringes, there were no infections. Although the authors acknowledged that the numbers of patients required to demonstrate safety statistically make it unlikely such a study will ever be done, disposable syringe reuse seems to be a fact of life for large numbers of diabetic patients and should be acknowledged by physicians providing care to diabetic patients.

THE INANIMATE ENVIRONMENT

Cleaning, Disinfection, and Sterilization

The principles of cleaning, disinfection, and sterilization of equipment and devices used in the ACS are the same as in the hospital setting (see Chapters 20, 21). However, the proportion of patients experiencing device-related procedures in the ACS is much smaller than in the inpatient setting. When a procedure involves contact with the vascular system or with mucous membranes, it is reasonable to expect risk in ambulatory patients similar to that in hospitalized patients. There may be differences, however, in the duration of exposure to the device (e.g., intravenous therapy, urinary catheterization), conditions under which the device is inserted (e.g., starting intravenous therapy without adequate preparation of the insertion site), and organisms colonizing skin and mucosal sites (see Chapters 15, 44) involved in device insertion.

Devices that are in contact with the vascular system should be sterile (e.g., instruments used to close lacerations, intravascular devices). Instruments that are in contact with mucous membranes should be sterile or receive high-level disinfection before use (e.g., vaginal specula, sigmoidoscopes, tonometers).

In general, articles and instruments that touch intact skin should be as clean as articles that are readily available in commercial establishments such as restaurants. Proper cleaning includes removal of all soil and body substances and the use of disinfectant agents appropriate to the situation. The more distant and peripheral an article is to any patient, the less infection risk there is associated with it. For example, chairs in the waiting room, cabinets in examining rooms, and curtains present virtually no infection risk.

Because of the possibility of examining tables being soiled by patient secretions, excretions, or blood, there is a common practice in the ACS to provide some barrier between the patient and the table. This is often accomplished by rolls of paper sheets or by linen sheets that are changed between patients. Unless there is soilage of the table surface, disinfection between patients is not necessary. Examination tables, countertops, floors, and other articles in the treatment areas should be cleaned on a regular schedule consistent with need in the facility.

Cleanliness of the physical facility, in general, is most easily accomplished when the number of examination rooms is sufficient and the flow of patients, personnel, and supplies can be accomplished easily.

A home care provider visiting a patient at home may not have access to amenities that are taken for granted in other ACS. It may be helpful for the home care bag to have clean barriers (e.g., a plastic-backed bedsaver pad) available to facilitate wound care or intravascular access, and foam or liquid hand disinfection agents in the event the patient's home environment makes aseptic practices and handwashing difficult or impossible.

Articles such as surgical instruments or endoscopes that are shared among a number of different facilities present a special problem. The items must be adequately cleaned, disinfected, and wrapped securely for transport before being carried back to the physicians' offices or on to the next facility. Often there is considerable pressure to accomplish these tasks more quickly than is possible. Additionally, should nosocomial infections result from inadequately disinfected material shared among different facilities, the problem is difficult to recognize because the cases are dispersed (see Chapter 20).

Ventilation Systems

Airborne transmission of potentially infectious agents by ventilation systems has been studied extensively, and data show that very few agents persist in the air for extended periods of time. The most common organism that persists in the air for extended periods is *Mycobacterium tuberculosis* (see Chapter 33). To transmit tuberculosis requires that the host be susceptible and in contact with a large enough dose of droplet nuclei for a sufficient time to become infected. Riley and colleagues [39] studied the infectiousness of a series of treated and untreated patients with tuberculosis by experiments in which air from rooms of tuberculosis patients was conducted to an exposure chamber in which guinea pigs in cages were located. Of 61 untreated patients with drug-susceptible organisms, these patients were responsible for all of the transmissions to guinea pigs; a patient with tuberculous laryngitis was the most infectious. Riley and colleagues [39] concluded that untreated patients were much more infectious than treated patients and that infectivity was also related to the number of air changes per hour in the room.

Although an ACS may provide the opportunity for the susceptible host to come in contact with a potentially infectious tuberculosis patient, the time interval of contact is usually insufficient to transmit the agent effectively. Whether an examining room in which a tuberculosis patient or multiple tuberculosis patients are seen in succession can sustain sufficient droplet nuclei to transmit tuberculosis depends on several factors: the number of infectious patients seen in a short time interval; aerosolization of droplet nuclei by the infectious patient(s) (i.e., the efficiency of dissemination); number of air changes in the examining room per unit of time, whether the air is vented directly to the outside, whether filters or ultraviolet lights are in the ventilation system and what type of filters they are; and, finally, the presence of susceptible patients or personnel in the examination room during or after the same time interval. These factors tend to have an additive effect, and risk is increased accordingly; however, the actual risk is unknown (see Chapter 33).

Many diseases that are spread by droplet contact are seen in the ACS (e.g., measles, rubella, varicella, and other childhood diseases). When a patient presents to an ACS with a fever, skin rash, or other signs characteristic of infection that may be transmitted by droplet contact, expeditious placement in a treatment room alone reduces the risk to susceptible people of contact with droplets that may be sneezed or coughed into the patient's immediate environment. In addition, many of these viral agents are transmitted most effectively by direct contact, and handwashing further reduces the risk of transmission to others [40].

Although droplets that are potentially infectious to the susceptible host do not travel more than 1 m or remain suspended in the air for extended periods of time (see Chapter 1), an outbreak of measles in a pediatric practice in 1981 [41] raised some serious questions about potential airborne transmission of the measles virus by means of droplet nuclei. Bloch and colleagues [42] investigated secondary cases of measles associated with an 11.5-month-old child who was in the office for 1 hour on the second day of rash, primarily in a single examining room, and coughing vigorously most of the time. Four of the seven children had transient contact with the source patient as he entered or exited the waiting room; only one of them had face-to-face contact within a meter. In addition, the three other children who contracted measles were never in the same room with the source patient; one arrived 1 hour after the source patient left. Airflow studies demonstrated that droplet nuclei generated in the examining room used by the source patient were dispersed throughout the entire office suite. The outbreak supports the fact that measles virus, when it becomes airborne, can survive for at least 1 hour. As a result of this outbreak, some physicians may elect not to use an examination room for at least 1 hour after it has been used by a patient diagnosed with measles, especially if the patient is coughing vigorously. This does not address the problem of air circulation throughout an office suite, particularly those in energy-efficient buildings with recirculating air.

Two other studies reported an increase in the proportion of all measles cases that were acquired in medical settings and pointed to the waiting room as a location where a reservoir of susceptible individuals may congregate, allowing for potential exposure to measles and other infectious diseases [42,43]. They also noted that the primary mode of transmission was face-to-face contact and that airborne transmission appeared to be relatively rare. In Davis and colleagues' review [42] of measles cases in 30 states from 1980 through 1984, 24% of the cases associated with medical facilities were in personnel; 76% were in patients or visitors. They concluded that more attention needs to be given to methods to prevent measles in medical facilities, including ensuring that medical personnel are immune to measles (see Chapter 3).

It is becoming increasingly common for emergency physicians to manage hospital employee health services [44] (see Chapter 3) and for the emergency department to care for employees who are exposed to airborne communicable diseases or who have these diseases but are not diagnosed until they report for work. In addition to measles, a common hospital infection control problem is varicella-zoster virus infection (chickenpox). Sayre and colleagues [44] reviewed the literature to determine a rational basis for managing the varicella-zoster virus-exposed employee and pointed out the potential for airborne transmission as an exposure route, especially if ventilation systems are defective. In the absence of immunization, attention to prompt patient placement and the use of an examination room with nonrecirculated air (if such is available) reduces the risks of transmission of varicella-zoster virus, as does assignment of care providers who are known to be immune (see Chapter 42). Farizo et al. [45] also evaluated measles transmission in Los Angeles and Houston to determine the role of pediatric emergency rooms in transmission of measles. They determined that these were common settings for transmission, and encouraged vaccination for measles in emergency rooms to provide postexposure prophylaxis and increase vaccination coverage in the community.

Potentially Infectious Body Substances

Potentially infectious agents may be present in all body substances (e.g., blood, secretions, excretions), and all body substances should be handled as if they are infectious. The implementation of these practices, in reality, is often made difficult because personnel may believe that only patients with diagnosed communicable diseases present a risk of infection. Accordingly, they may not take precautions until a diagnosis is established.

The seriousness of this problem was made clear when Dienstag and Ryan [46] published their report of prevalence of markers for hepatitis B virus (HBV) among various groups of healthcare workers (HCWs). They found that personnel with the most contact with blood (e.g., emergency room nurses) were most likely to have markers for HBV. Most such exposures resulted from contacts with patients whose HBV status was not known at the time. After this report, Jackson, Lynch, and their colleagues [47–51] began to question the efficacy of infection precautions that were initiated at the time a diagnosis was made or suspected and proposed an alternative to traditional isolation techniques that was named *body substance isolation.*

At nearly the same time, the Centers for Disease Control (now called the Centers for Disease Control and Prevention (CDC)) was also responding to increasing concerns about risks to HCWs for infection with HBV and the human immunodeficiency virus (HIV) and other bloodborne pathogens. They developed a series of recommendations intended primarily to reduce these risks to HCWs, called *universal precautions* or *universal blood and body fluid precautions* [52–55]. In 1996, the CDC established new guidelines for isolation precautions in hospitals that include standard precautions for the care of all patients, and transmission-based precautions for selected infectious agents [56] (see Chapter 13). Because these precautions are designed for acute care hospitals, some of the principles are applicable to the ACS and some are not [57–60]. The CDC and others have also addressed infection risk reduction strategies for HCWs. Additional information concerning infection risk reduction strategies for HCWs may be found in Chapters 3, 42, 43. Table 28-1 presents general precautionary measures, described according to body substance, that are applicable in the ACS.

Given the concerns of HCWs about potential risks for HIV and HBV infection, several large labor unions approached the Occupational Safety and Health Administration (OSHA) in 1986 to request that a formal rule be made to address the issue. OSHA initiated the rule-making process in 1987, and a final rule was published in December, 1991 [61]. One of the major concerns of OSHA, the CDC, and others is the lack of compliance by HCWs with obtaining the HBV vaccine, even when it is made available at no cost to the HCW [62,63] (see Chapter 42). Whether increased emphasis by OSHA about the need for HBV vaccine for HCWs will alter compliance remains to be seen.

Although many of the recommendations by OSHA emphasize the importance of having personal protective equipment (gloves, masks, gowns) readily available for the HCW, it is now well established that the greatest risk for both HIV and HBV infection is puncture injuries. Puncture injuries are often related to the design of the equipment [63], to the situation at the time [64], and to commonly used practices, such as recapping, that have long been acknowledged as risky. In fact, in a survey of needlestick injuries and needle disposal practices in Minnesota physicians' offices [65], recapping of needles was frequent (> 50% of the time) and 44% of the offices surveyed reported injuries during the past year.

To learn more about needlestick injuries sustained by care providers in the home health environment, Backinger and Koustenis [66] surveyed a random sample of 600 directors of home healthcare agencies in the United States. Almost half (46%) responded, with 102

TABLE 28-1. *General precautionary measures for handling potentially infectious body substances*

Body substance	Examples of infectious agents	Precautions for personnel in direct contact with substance	Precautions for patients or personnel in same room
Blood (e.g., uncontrolled bleeding; lacerations; GI bleed)	Hepatitis B, hepatitis C; HIV	Gloves; cover gowns for large amounts; masks and protective eyewear if splashing is likely	No direct contact, no risk
Saliva, sputum (e.g., purulent sputum, oral secretions)	Viral agents; mixed gram-positive and gram-negative bacteria	Gloves[a]	No direct contact, no risk[a]
Feces (e.g., diarrhea, fecal incontinence)	Enteric pathogens; viral agents; other gram-negative bacteria	Gloves; cover gowns for large amounts	No direct contact, no risk
Urine (e.g., incontinence)	Gram-negative bacteria	Gloves	No direct contact, no risk
Wound drainage (e.g., wound infections, abscesses, impetigo)	Gram-positive and gram-negative bacteria	Gloves; cover gowns for large amounts	No direct contact, no risk

GI, gastrointestinal; HIV, human immunodeficiency virus.

[a]For pediatric or other patients who may have a disease spread by droplet contact (e.g., chickenpox, measles, rubella, mumps), personnel with negative or unknown history of the disease or immunization should not examine the patient. Recent data suggest that some patients with measles and varicella who are coughing vigorously may produce droplet nuclei that can stay suspended in the air for up to 1 hr. Though the predominant mode of transmission of measles is by droplet spread in facilities where ventilation is poor, consideration should still be given to restricting subsequent use of such rooms to patients who are known to be immune to the disease diagnosed in the previous patient for at least an hour after the index case has vacated the room. This practice does not address problems presented by recirculated air in energy-efficient buildings that may result in airborne contamination of the entire medical office; however, transmission in such situations is rare (see text).

Note: Handwashing is usually sufficient to remove soil and potentially infectious agents from hands; however, regardless of diagnosis, when contact with these substances is anticipated, personnel should glove their hands to reduce the quantity of hand contamination and wash their hands after glove removal. Unless there is direct soilage of articles in the environment, there is no need to perform special cleaning procedures.

agencies reporting no needlestick injuries in the previous year, and 124 agencies reporting from 1 to 134 injuries, for a cumulative total of 475 injuries. There were no statistically significant differences in reported injuries between agencies using a variety of "safer" devices and those that did not use them. The authors note the limitations of these self-reported data, and call for additional research.

White and Lynch [67] evaluated the frequency of occupational blood exposures during surgical procedures performed in ambulatory care settings. They found that exposures occurred less frequently than was reported by hospital operating rooms. Reasons for this may be shorter, less complex procedures, better equipment, newer facilities, or a combination of these factors.

THE INFECTION CONTROL PRACTITIONER

Hospital-Based Settings

Infection control practitioners (ICPs) who work in hospitals usually have responsibility for infection control in the emergency department, admitting department, and ambulatory care clinics, as well as the agency's home care division (see Chapters 4, 5). These responsibilities include education of personnel about measures that reduce infection risks associated with emergency care; cleaning, disinfection, and sterilization; infection precautions; management of needlestick injuries and other exposures; and orientation for new personnel. The ICP may also act as a consultant for the development of policies and procedures. Policies and education programs should be specifically tailored for each department.

Freestanding Settings

Most freestanding settings (e.g., surgicenters, emergicenters, physicians' offices) and home care agencies not affiliated with an acute care hospital do not have a designated ICP. Consultation about infection control prevention in these settings can frequently be obtained from the local health department and ICPs in hospitals in the community.

Reportable Diseases

State and local health departments require that certain communicable (notifiable) diseases be reported to them. Designation of a person responsible for this task is essential in both the hospital-based and the freestanding ACS. In many hospitals, this is a responsibility of the ICP. In addition, local health departments may provide follow-up for contacts of patients with many infectious diseases (e.g., syphilis, gonorrhea, salmonellosis, viral hepatitis, meningococcal disease; see Chapter 2).

PATIENT AND PERSONNEL RISKS FOR NOSOCOMIAL INFECTIONS

Emergency Medical Services System

The risks to patients and personnel in the EMSS are increased by the urgency of the patient situation and the need for prompt and efficient patient management. As the urgency for intervention increases (e.g., to provide an airway, control bleeding, stabilize a fracture, provide intravenous fluids), the situation becomes less easily controlled and adherence to aseptic practices by personnel generally decreases (see Chapter 25).

Prehospital Care

Risks to patients in the prehospital care phase are usually related to aseptic practices. It is important to recognize that the need for careful aseptic practices must be balanced against the patient's need for prompt management. The duration of contact with the field situation is often brief; however, the devices inserted there and the procedures done to stabilize the patient carry with them certain infection risks. Training programs for personnel working in these situations should include information about and practice in using aseptic techniques. When the urgency of the field situation is such that aseptic practices may be difficult to use, the decision to compromise them is made for the patient and should reflect his or her best interests rather than personnel convenience. When the patient is stabilized, devices inserted under less-than-optimal conditions should be replaced aseptically and in a timely fashion. Communication among the field team, personnel in the emergency department, and, ultimately, the healthcare providers in the nursing unit where the patient is admitted helps maintain this continuity of care.

Risks to personnel depend on contact with body substances (e.g., blood, feces, saliva) that may be contaminated with an infectious agent. Infection precautions may include the use of barrier techniques (e.g., gloves) to prevent substances from soiling personnel's hands, clothing, and supplies. Personnel reduce the risk of transmitting infectious agents to patients or of acquiring infections themselves by using these barrier techniques along with handwashing (or antiseptic foams when sinks are not available).

The risks to personnel are rarely known at the onset of a transport situation, and the patient's diagnosis may never be known to the transport personnel. Accordingly, the development of standard procedures—including aseptic practices, when possible—is appropriate in any transport situation.

When communicable diseases are diagnosed, transport personnel should be included in any exposure work-ups and should receive prophylaxis when indicated. These personnel should follow the same immunization and tuberculin skin-testing routines as do hospital personnel (see Chapters 3, 33).

Fligner and associates [68] studied the prevalence of HBV serologic markers in 85 paramedics working in suburban Chicago and compared results with previously reported studies documenting rates ranging from 0.6% to 25%. In their study, 7.1% of the paramedics were found to be positive. They concluded that prehospital personnel do not constitute a homogeneous occupational category at risk for HBV infection. Using a table comparing six other studies (see Fligner et al. [68] for citations), these investigators suggested that prevalence of HBV serologic markers in paramedics is more strongly influenced by the incidence of HBV in the population of the area than by the occupational category of the HCW. They concluded that, when making decisions about the use of prophylactic vaccination versus postexposure prophylaxis and vaccination after documented exposure to blood positive for hepatitis B surface antigen, a cost-effectiveness analysis for HBV vaccine is particularly relevant for EMSSs likely to have low HBV prevalence and attack rates. The logistics of obtaining this information on patients and providing it in a timely manner to EMSS personnel was not discussed.

First responders are also concerned about the potential risk of exposure to HIV-positive blood. In a review of information known to date, Gelb [69] points out many safety issues associated with the prehospital setting when it is the scene of an accident and emphasizes the additional risk introduced by potential HIV transmission. This author concluded by supporting the need for education regarding universal precautions as well as new technologies to allow emergency HCWs to perform procedures rapidly while adequately protecting themselves from exposure. These technologic advances would involve better equipment and clothing as well as affordable disposable equipment or equipment that may be rapidly decontaminated (see Chapter 13, 43).

The transport vehicle, whether an ambulance, van, or helicopter, should be cleaned on a regular schedule; articles soiled with body substances should be cleaned and disinfected before being used for another patient. Although the patient area of the transport vehicle is a small, closed space, ventilation is easily accomplished, and it is unnecessary to provide extended ventilation times or special decontamination procedures (e.g., fumigation) before the transport of another patient.

Emergency Department of a Hospital

Risks to patients who present to an emergency department of a hospital are related to the patient's underlying condition and the procedures performed for the patient in the emergency department. In general, few procedures are performed for patients in the nonurgent category, and they are at little risk for nosocomial infection; patients in the urgent category undergo more procedures and are at somewhat greater risk; patients in the emergent category may undergo numerous procedures and are at greatest risk. In addition, it is for these patients that asepsis is most often compromised.

Respiratory infections reflect seasonal and community incidence and are usually viral. Risk to emergency department personnel of exposure to many of these infections is probably similar to that in nonhospital settings in which numbers of people are together who may be in the prodromal or acute phase of a viral illness (e.g., schools, offices, stores); however, the concentration of such people may be greater in an emergency department.

Emergency department personnel are at greater risk for exposure to HBV than are many other hospital workers because of their frequent exposure to blood. In the study by Dienstag and Ryan [46], 624 health workers were surveyed in an urban hospital in Boston. These personnel represented a spectrum of exposure to blood and to patients. Of the 30 emergency department nurses studied, 30% were positive for one or more serologic markers for HBV. Among the groups surveyed, this was the group with the highest prevalence for HBV seropositivity. Dienstag and Ryan concluded that emergency department personnel are exposed to the most severely ill patients (including those with uncontrolled bleeding), that emergency department nurses are often the first personnel to encounter such patients, and that, at the time of the study, these nurses usually did not wear gloves or protective gowns when providing such care (see Chapter 42).

Analysis of the changing epidemiology of HBV in the United States [70] points out that although the overall incidence of HBV remained relatively constant throughout the study period (January 1, 1981, through September 30, 1988), disease transmission patterns changed significantly. Of note was a 75% decline in the proportion of HBV patients reporting healthcare employment, which is primarily attributable to HBV vaccination of HCWs. New recommendations for protection against viral hepatitis, including recommendations for HCWs, were published in 1994 [71].

Hepatitis B virus and HIV infection risk for emergency department personnel has also been hypothesized from studies that have determined the prevalence of HBV and HIV antibody in serum specimens from emergency department patients [72–75]. The studies have consistently shown that patients who *are not suspected* of being HIV or HBV positive, but who *are seropositive*, are regularly seen in emergency departments. These data are used to support the need for consistent use of standard precautions when caring for all patients, although compliance with these recommendations has usually been found to be poor [76]. Similar data about unrecognized seroprevalence for HBV or HIV have also been found for patients admitted to a large teaching hospital when specimens submitted to the hospital laboratory have been tested [77].

In an editorial, Kelen [78] noted the absence of emergency specialists from studies of HCWs, and commented that data were also absent regarding the risk of seroconversion from patients with undiagnosed HIV infection. In an accompanying editorial, Baraff [79] noted concerns about cumulative risk for HCWs using a mathematical model and published data about HIV seroprevalence among emergency department patients. He suggested that if an emergency physician were to suffer one needlestick or similar exposure every year in an emergency department where 5% of the patients were HIV seropositive, and the risk of seroconversion was 0.5% per exposure, then the lifetime risk of seroconversion over a 30-year career would be approximately 0.8%, or 8 per 1,000. To put this in perspective, the risk of death from accidents, suicide, and homicide combined over a 30-year period is ~ 18 per 1,000. Baraff [79] concluded by stating that both of these figures could be modified by behavioral change and noted, "Just as most of us would not consider driving without seatbelts, we should not practice our specialty without employing universal precautions. . . ."

The advent of the HIV and acquired immunodeficiency syndrome (AIDS) epidemic has been accompanied by increasing concern about risks associated with mouth-to-mouth resuscitation. In a survey of 5,823 American Heart Association Virginia Affiliate basic cardiac life support instructors, the impact of the HIV and AIDS epidemic on attitudes, beliefs, and behaviors with regard to mouth-to-mouth resuscitation was assessed. They concluded that concern about HIV and AIDS was adversely affecting attitudes, beliefs, and self-reported behaviors of the basic cardiac life support instructors regarding mouth-to-mouth ventilation on strangers [80].

Emergicenters

Seriously injured and ill patients usually are not seen in emergicenters; most of the visits are by patients with nonurgent problems. Procedures performed in these facilities are similar to those performed in hospital emergency departments (e.g., laceration repairs, incision and drainage of abscesses, and other minor surgical procedures). The same principles of asepsis apply in this setting as in the hospital emergency department.

Outpatient Surgery

The care of instruments and the quality of aseptic practices should be the same in surgicenters as it is in hospital operating rooms. Written policies and procedures for care of instruments, cleaning of operating rooms, and personnel health practices should be developed following guidelines for hospital operating rooms (see Chapter 27). In addition, Stebben [81–82] summarized recommendations for sterile technique and prevention of wound infection in office surgery, and Drake et al. developed guidelines for office surgical facilities for the American Academy of Dermatology [83–84].

Preoperative assessment of the patient should include screening for infection and for presence of communicable diseases. Preparation and aftercare management of patients should emphasize prevention of nosocomial infection (e.g., wound care, preoperative and postoperative pulmonary management). Patients should be instructed regarding signs of infection (e.g., fever, redness, pain, swelling, drainage) and whom to contact if questions arise.

It is generally accepted that cleaning after all cases should remove all soil and body substances and that special cleaning after "dirty" cases is not necessary. Cleaning routines and preparation for subsequent cases should follow the same guidelines that are used for hospital operating rooms (see Chapter 27).

Outpatient Diagnostic and Treatment Facilities

In general, risk for nosocomial infection in outpatient diagnostic and treatment facilities is very low. In some special situations such as oncology or pediatric clinics or physicians' offices, it may be important to identify patients whose compromised immune status may place them at increased risk for infection, especially of the droplet-spread viral respiratory infections. These patients may benefit from reduced contact with other patients in the waiting room. Some pediatric clinics or physicians' offices also have separate waiting rooms for children seeking well care and for those who are ill. Some treatment rooms have doors that open directly to the outside, permitting selected patients to bypass the office waiting room entirely.

Hospital Admitting Department

In general, infection risk in the admitting department also is low. Inadvertent exposures to communicable diseases may occur there because people with unknown exposure or disease status may be together in the same waiting area for varying lengths of time. This is particularly true in pediatric facilities or hospitals with large pediatric units.

The admitting department can serve a useful role in reducing the risk of transmission of infectious agents between hospitalized patients by being attentive to the room and bed assignments for newly admitted patients and for patients who contract infections while in the hospital. In many hospitals, the ICP conveys information about potentially infectious patients to the admitting department and serves as a consultant for patient placement.

Home Care Settings

Guidelines for infection control in home health were proposed by Simmons and associates [85] in 1990 using recommendations developed for infection risk reduction in acute and long-term care settings, combined with practical suggestions for the home care environment. These are a useful starting place for a home care agency developing its own infection prevention and control standards.

Surveillance for infections and other programatic issues associated with care in the home have been described by White [86], Lorenzen and Itkin [87], and Rosenheimer [88], White and Ragland [89], and White and Smith [90].

White [86] conducted a prevalence survey of a random sample of home care clients in a home care agency in the San Francisco Bay Area. She found that 36 (20.6%) of the 175 home care clients in her study had infections but most were not associated with care in the home. In fact, only nine infections occurred during the home care period. Of the 27 infections that developed before the home care period, one third were wound infections and another one third were decubitus infections; 4 clients had chronic infections (3 with acquired immunodeficiency syndrome and 1 with hepatitis).

In the study by Lorenzen and Itkin [87], the Joint Commission on the Accreditation of Healthcare Organizations (JCAHO) requirements for home healthcare [91] is cited as a reason for developing a surveillance system. These requirements are very general and similar to expectations in the acute care setting over a decade ago, although there is an attempt to link the infection control standard to quality of care. The study site was a home care agency affiliated with an acute care hospital. Definitions of home care-related infections were linked to services performed or procedures taught in the home; however, their system was also useful for identifying hospital-associated infections with onset dates after discharge. An incident report form used by the home care nurse was completed when an infection was suspected, a culture obtained, or antibiotic prescribed. Only 16 infections were identified in 4,367 total nursing visits, of which over 75% were urinary tract infections. As a result, the agency chose to focus on risk reduction for catheter-associated urinary tract infections as a quality improvement activity.

Rosenheimer [88] also reported an approach to surveillance that addressed the problem of appropriate denominator selection. Her focus was on symptomatic urinary tract infections in patients with indwelling urinary catheters and bloodstream infections in patients receiving intravenous therapy. Only two primary bloodstream infections were identified, both in people with AIDS, during 8 months of surveillance of almost 1,500 patient intravascular therapy days (0.92%). No primary bloodstream infections were identified in patients who did not have AIDS, although the total number of patient intravascular therapy days exceeded 3,600.

White and Ragland [89] used billed supplies from a 6-month period to identify home care clients receiving intravenous care through a private visiting nurse agency in northern California. Sixty-seven individuals were identified who were having catheter care done by nurses, family care givers, or the clients themselves. Three (4.5%) of the clients had intravenous catheter-related infections identified during the 2,405 cather-days at risk for an incidence density of 12.5 infections per 10,000 catheter-days. The authors conclude that the numbers were too small to show meaningful comparisons between those with and without infections. However, the infection rates were comparable to those reported in a large study by Graham and associates [92].

White and Smith [90] described the characteristics of a sample of northern California home care agencies, including the care provided and presence of infection prevention and control standards and education. One-third (58) of the 173 agencies contacted responded to the survey, and reported a high frequency of procedures considered high risk for infection. Nearlty all had policies on universal precautions, handwashing, handling of needles and sharps, and the cleaning and disinfection of equipment. The authors point out the need to evaluate these policies and procedures for validity and reasonableness in the homecare setting, and for employee education regarding procedures that carry a high risk infection.

All of these studies show clearly that the time required to collect the data on these extremely small numbers of infections may far exceed any benefits other than to satisfy paperwork requirements. ICPs working with home care agencies should heed White's [86] suggestion that the goal of infection prevention and control in home healthcare should be prevention, early detection, and aggressive management of infections rather than focusing on calculation of home-associated infection rates.

After several years of burgeoning growth in the home care industry, the Centers for Disease Control and Prevention summarized several investigations of infections [93] associated primarily with home infusion therapy. They note that in many areas of the home care industry, technology is being introduced at a rapid pace without the benefit of either an infrastructure for infection prevention and control or, in some instances, appropriate recommendations. Several of the investigations were associated with the introduction of needleless intravascular access devices and inconsistent practices for the management of these devices [94,95,96]. In each of these outbreaks, there was a high frequency of hydrophilic gram-negative bacteria causing the bloodstream infections, suggesting that patient-catheter exposure to tap water may be an important risk factor. They urged evaluation of the CDC guideline for prevention of intravascular-device-related infections [97] to identify recommendations that could be adopted in the home care setting.

Two other articles published recently [98, 99] point out the importance of infection prevention and control education of patients and family members and the need for improved consistency in the education and training for nursing personnel providing care in the home.

Because of the large numbers of HCWs going into the homes of clients to provide care, there continues to be concern about risks to the caregiver of acquiring infections from patients, particularly AIDS. Valenti [100–101] addressed this issue from the standpoints of HIV infection risk to the patient as well as to the caregiver in the home care setting. He makes some specific recommendations for careful insertion and monitoring of vascular catheters, and for the need to use barriers appropriately when providing care in the home. In addition, training in infection control principles and practices is emphasized for caregivers and clients.

QUALITY ASSURANCE ISSUES FOR THE AMBULATORY CARE SETTING

Berman [102] presented the perspective of the JCAHO on the importance of quality assurance monitoring for ACSs. In response to increasing concerns about quality assurance, Kaplowitz [103] described a quality assurance program in a U.S. Coast Guard ambulatory care facility. A method for quality assurance monitoring for ambulatory care centers connected to hospitals was also described by Bradford and Flynn [104], who provided an outline for quality assurance rounds and clinic criteria. Emphasis was on evaluation of the structural and process elements of care. These articles stressed the challenges presented by ACSs for developing quality assurance programs that are practical and meaningful and have a significant positive impact on patient care. None of the authors specifically addressed monitoring for infections associated with care in an ACS, although some of the structural and process monitoring described by Bradford and Flynn [104] was related to infection risk. In 1993, Hurt [105] focused on the quality management issues associated with reducing exposure risks to HIV and hepatitis B for clients and staff in ambulatory care settings, and described the role of an ICP in training clinic staff members to institute safe practices within 25 clinic sites. At the end of a 30-month period, the clinic sites were in compliance with the OSHA bloodborne pathogens standard [61] and the ICP had a cadre of clinic staff members knowledgeable about infection prevention and control issues.

FUTURE TRENDS

Although ACSs are places where infection risk is usually considered to be low, the increasing use of these settings for surgical procedures, device insertions and management, and outpatient care of increasingly more immunocompromised patients will present interesting challenges for the future. Monitoring for low-frequency events such as nosocomial infections related to care in an ACS is labor intensive and costly and requires creativity to ensure efficient use of limited resources. In response to the need to use limited resources efficiently, Haim et al. [106] analyzed how the ICP assigned to a Los Angeles Veterans Affairs ambulatory healthcare center spent her time, and presented the methods used for conducting a structured work load analysis. Data revealed that about half of the ICP's time was being spent on clerical duties. The authors stressed the importance of allocating appropriate human resources to support the ICP's professional role. A model for a comprehensive infection control program in home healthcare was developed by Bellen [107] in Rochester, New York. Using traditonal quality improvement methods [108], she included activities related to direct patient care as well as activities that support the provision of such care. Some of this information may be useful to ICPs developing programs for infection prevention and control in the home care environment.

The increasing demands presented by the changes in the healthcare delivery system, by the JCAHO [92,102], and by OSHA [61] will require agencies to commit resources for ACS personnel to monitor activities and follow protocols for infection surveillance, prevention and control. For years these activities have been viewed by many ACS agencies as a low priority. Increasing awareness and commitment of resouces to meet these needs in the ACS will be one of the challenges of the next decade.

REFERENCES

1. Adams PF, Benson V. Current estimates from the National Health Interview Survey, Table 71. *Vital Health Stat 10* 1990;176.
2. National Center for Health Statistics. *Health, United States, 1994; 1996–1997*. Hyattsville, MD: Public Health Service; 1995, 1997.
3. National Academy of Sciences, National Research Council. *Accidental death and disability: the neglected disease of modern society*. Washington, DC: National Academy of Sciences; 1966.
4. Jacobs BB, Jacobs LM Jr. Prehospital emergency medical services. In: Kravis TC, Warner CG, Jacobs LM Jr, eds. *Emergency medicine*. 3rd ed. New York: Raven Press, 1993:1–29.
5. Weinerman ER, Ratner RS, Robbins A, Lavenhar MA. Yale studies in ambulatory medical care: V. determinants of use of hospital emergency services. *Am J Public Health* 1966;56:1037–1056.
6. Pisarcki G. Why patients use the emergency department. *Journal of Emergency Nursing* 1980;6(2):16–21.
7. Jacoby LE, Jones LS. Factors associated with emergency department use by repeater and nonrepeater patients. *Journal of Emergency Nursing* 1982;8:243–247.
8. Weissert WG. Home care: measuring success. In: Harrington C, Estes CL, eds. *Health policy and nursing: crisis and reform in the U.S. healthcare delivery system*. Boston: Jones and Bartlett Publishers, 1994:254–266.

9. Craig CP. Infection surveillance for ambulatory surgery patients: an overview. *Quality Review Bulletin* 1983;9:107–111.
10. Natof HE. Complications associated with ambulatory surgery. *JAMA* 1980;244:1116–1118.
11. Manion FA, Meyer L. Comprehensive surveillance of surgical wound infections in outpatient and inpatient surgery. *Infect Control Hosp Epidemiol* 1990;11:515–520.
12. Flanders E, Hinnant JR. Ambulatory surgery postoperative wound surveillance. *Am J Infect Control* 1990;18:336–339.
13. Zoutman D, Pearce P, McKenzie M, Taylor G. Surgical wound infections occurring in day surgery patients. *Am J Infect Control* 1990;18:277–282.
14. Hugar DW, Newman PS, Hugar RW. Incidence of postoperative infection in free-standing ambulatory surgery center. *J Foot Surg* 1990;29: 265–267.
15. Fridkin SK, Kremer FB, Bland LA, et al. *Acremonium kiliense* endophthalmitis that occurred after cataract extraction in an ambulatory surgical center and was traced to an environmental reservoir. *Clin Infect Dis* 1996;22:222–227.
16. Bennett JV. Human infections: economic implications and prevention. *Ann Intern Med* 1978;89(Part 2):761–763.
17. Haley RW, Culver DH, White JW, et al. The efficacy of infection surveillance and control programs in preventing nosocomial infections in U.S. hospitals. *Am J Epidemiol* 1985;121:182–205.
18. Centers for Disease Control and Prevention. Amebiasis associated with colonic irrigation: Colorado. *MMWR Morb Mortal Wkly Rep* 1981;30:101–102.
19. O'Mahoney MC, Stanwell-Smith RE, Tillett HE, et al. The Stafford outbreak of Legionnaires' disease. *Epidemiol Infect* 1990;104:361–380.
20. Goodman RA, Solomon SL. Transmission of infectious diseases in outpatient healthcare settings. *JAMA* 1991;265:2377–2381.
21. Yozzo JC. Is it feasible to track infections in an ambulatory surgery center? *Journal of Post-Anesthesia Nursing* 1989;4:255–258.
22. Redmon MC. Infection control monitoring in the ambulatory surgery unit. *Journal of Post-Anesthesia Nursing* 1993;8:28–34.
23. Antoniskis A, Anderson BC, Van Volkinburg EJ, et al. Feasibility of outpatient self-administration of parenteral antibiotics. *West J Med* 1978;128:203–206.
24. Eisenberg JM, Kitz DS. Saving from outpatient antibiotic therapy for osteomyelitis: economic analysis of a therapeutic strategy. *JAMA* 1986;255:1584–1588.
25. Kind AC, Williams DN, Persons G, Gibson JA. Intravenous antibiotic therapy at home. *Arch Intern Med* 1979;139;413–415.
26. Poretz DM, Eron LJ, Goldenberg RI, et al. Intravenous antibiotic therapy in an outpatient setting. *JAMA* 1982;248:336–339.
27. Swenson JP. Training patients to administer intravenous antibiotics at home. *Am J Hosp Pharm* 1981;38:1480–1483.
28. Graham DR, Keldermans MM, Klem LW, et al. Infectious complications among patients receiving home intravenous therapy with peripheral, central, or peripherally placed central venous catheters. *Am J Med* 1991;91(Suppl 3B):95S–100S.
29. White MC, Ragland KE. Surveillance of intravenous catheter-related infections among home care clients. *Am J Infect Control* 1993;21: 231–235.
30. Gaffron RE, Flemmong CR, Berkner S, et al. Organization and operation of a home parenteral nutrition program with emphasis on the pharmacist s role. *Mayo Clin Proc* 1980;55:94–98.
31. Jeejeebhoy KN, Langer B, Tsallas G, et al. Total parenteral nutrition at home: studies in patients surviving 4 months to 5 years. *Gastroenterology* 1976;71:943–953.
32. Miler SJ, Dickerson RN, Graziani AA, et al. Antibiotic therapy of catheter infections in patients receiving home parenteral therapy. *JPEN J Parenter Enteral Nutr* 1990;14:143–147.
33. Gouttebel MC, Saint-Aubert B, Jonquet O, et al. Ambulatory home total parenteral nutrition. *JPEN J Parenter Enteral Nutr* 1990;11:475–479.
34. Chan MK, Baillod RA, Chuah P, et al.Three years experience of continuous ambulatory peritoneal dialysis. *Lancet* 1991;1:1409–1412.
35. Harrison JT. Chronic ambulatory peritoneal dialysis [Letter]. *N Engl J Med* 1982;306:670.
36. Nolph KD, Sorkin M, Rubin J, et al. Continuous ambulatory peritoneal dialysis: three-year experience at one center. *Ann Intern Med* 1980;92;609–613.
37. Sewell CM, Clarridge J, Lacke C, et al. Staphylococcal nasal carriage and subsequent infection in peritoneal dialysis patients. *JAMA* 1982; 248:1493–1495.
38. Thomas DR, Fischer RG, Nicholas WC, et al. Disposable insulin syringe reuse and antiseptic practices in diabetic patients. *J Gen Intern Med* 1989;4:97–100.
39. Riley RL, Mills CC, O Grady F, et al. Infectiousness of air from a tuberculosis ward: ultraviolet irradiation of infected air: comparative infectiousness of different patients. *Am Rev Respir Dis* 1962;85: 511–xxx.
40. Larson E. Handwashing: it's essential: even when you use gloves. *Am J Nurs* 1989;89:934–939.
41. Bloch AB, Orenstein WA, Ewing WM, et al. Measles outbreak in a pediatric practice: airborne transmission in an office setting. *Pediatrics* 1985;75;676–683.
42. Davis RM, Orenstein WA, Frank JA, et al. Transmission of measles in medical settings: 1980–1984. *JAMA* 1986;255:1295–1298.
43. Istre GR, McKee PA, West GR, et al. Measles spread in medical settings: An important focus of disease transmission? *Pediatrics* 1987; 79:356–358.
44. Sayre MR, Lucid EJ. Management of varicella-zoster virus-exposed hospital employees. *Ann Emerg Med* 1987;16;421–424.
45. Farizo KM, Stehr-Green PA, Simpson DM, Markowitz LE. Pediatric emergency room visits: a risk factor for acquiring measles. *Pediatrics* 1991;87:74–79.
46. Dienstag JL, Ryan DM. Occupational exposure to hepatitis B virus in hospital personnel: infection or immunization? *Am J Epidemiol* 1982; 115:26–39.
47. Jackson MM. Implementing universal body substance precautions. *Occupational Medicine: State of the Art Reviews* 1989;4(Special issue):39–44.
48. Jackson MM, Lynch P, McPherson DC, et al. Clinical savvy: why not treat all body substances as infectious? *Am J Nurs* 1987;87: 1137–1139.
49 . Jackson MM, Lynch P. Infection control: too much or too little? Am J Nurs 1984;84:208–210.
50. Lynch P, Jackson MM, Cummings MJ, Stamm WE. Rethinking the role of isolation practices in the prevention of nosocomial infections. *Ann Intern Med* 1987;197:243–246.
51. Jackson MM, Lynch P. In search of a rational approach. *Am J Nurs* 1990;90:65–73.
52. Centers for Disease Control and Prevention. Recommendations for prevention of HIV transmission in health-care settings. *MMWR Morb Mortal Wkly Rep* 1987;36(Suppl 2S):1–18.
53. Centers for Disease Control and Prevention. Update: universal precautions for prevention of HIV, HBV, and other bloodborne pathogens in health-care settings. *MMWR Morb Mortal Wkly Rep* 1988;37:277–388.
54. Centers for Disease Control and Prevention. Guidelines for prevention of transmission of HIV and HBV to health-care and public-safety workers. *MMWR Morb Mortal Wkly Rep* 1989;38(Suppl S6):1–37.
55. Hughes JM. Universal precautions: CDC perspective. *Occupational Medicine: State of the Art Reviews* 1989;4(Special issue):13–20.
56. Centers for Disease Control and Prevention. Hospital Infection Control Practices Advisory Committee: Guideline for isolation precautions in hospitals. *Am J Infect Control* 1996;24:24–52.
57. Soule BM. Special Communications. The CDC and HICPAC guideline for isolation precautions in hospitals: Commentaries on an evolutionary process. *Am J Infect Control* 1996;24:199–200.
58. Jackson MM, Lynch P. Invited commentary: Guideline for isolation precautions in hospitals, 1996. *Am J Infect Control* 1996;24:203–206.
59. Stover BH. The 1996 CDC and HICPAC isolation guideline: A pediatric perspective. *Am J Infect Control* 1996;24:201–202.
60. Preston GA. HICPAC guideline for isolation precautions in hospitals: Community hospital perspective. *Am J Infect Control* 1996;24: 207–208.
61. U.S. Department of Labor and Department of Health and Human Services, Occupational Safety and Health Administration. Occupational exposure to bloodborne pathogens: final rule. *Fed Reg* 1991;56(235): 64004–64183.
62. Spence MR, Dash GP. Hepatitis B: perceptions, knowledge and vaccine acceptance among registered nurses in high-risk occupations in a university hospital. *Infect Control Hosp Epidemiol* 1990;11: 129–133.
63. Jagger J, Hunt EH, Brand-Elnagger J, Pearson RD. Rates of needlestick injury caused by various devices in a university hospital. *N Engl J Med* 1988;319:284–288.
64. Jackson MM, Lynch P. Development of a numeric Health Care Worker

Risk Assessment Scale to evaluate potential for blood-borne pathogen exposures. *Am J Infect Control* 1995;23:13–21.
65. Thurn J, Willenbring K, Crossley K. Needlestick injuries and needle disposal in Minnesota physicians offices. *Am J Med* 1989;86:575–579.
66. Backinger CL, Koiustenis GH. Analysis of needlestick injuries to healthcare workers providing home care. *Am J Infect Control* 1994;22:300–306.
67. White MC, Lynch P. Blood contact and exposures among ambulatory care personnel. *Amb Surg* 1994;2:152–155.
68. Fligner DJ, Wigder HN, Harter PM, et al. The prevalence of hepatitis B serologic markers in suburban paramedics. *J Emerg Med* 1989;7:41–45.
69. Gelb A. HIV infection control issues concerning first responders and emergency physicians. *Occupational Medicine: State of the Art Reviews* 1989;4(Special issue):61–64.
70. Alter MJ, Hadler SC, Margolis HS, et al. The changing epidemiology of hepatitis B in the United States: need for alternative vaccination strategies. *JAMA* 1990;263:1218–1222.
71. Centers for Disease Control and Prevention. Hepatitis B virus: a comprehensive strategy for eliminating transmission in the United States through universal childhood vaccination: recommendations of the Immunization Practices Advisory Committee (ACIP). *MMWR Morb Mortal Wkly Rep* 1991;40(RR-13):1–25.
72. Baker JL, Kelen GD, Sivertson KT, Quinn TC. Unsuspected human immunodeficiency virus in critically ill emergency patients. *JAMA* 1989;257:2609–2611.
73. Jui J, Mobsitt S, Fleming D, et al. Multicenter HIV and hepatitis B seroprevalence survey. *J Emerg Med* 1990;8:243–251.
74. Kelen GD, Fritz S, Qaqish B, et al. Unrecognized HIV infection in emergency department patients. *N Engl J Med* 1988;318:1645–1650.
75. Henderson DK. Risks for exposures to and infection with HIV among healthcare providers in the emergency department. *Emerg Med Clin North Am* 1995;13:199–211.
76. Baraff LJ, Talan DA. Compliance with universal precautions in a university hospital emergency department. *Ann Emerg Med* 1989;18:654–657.
77. Handsfield HH, Cummings MJ, Swenson PD. Prevalence of antibody to HIV and hepatitis B surface antigen in blood samples submitted to a hospital laboratory. *JAMA* 1987;258:3395–3397.
78. Kelen GD. Reanalysis of surveillance data regarding healthcare worker risk of nosocomial acquisition of HIV [Editorial]. *Ann Emerg Med* 1988;17:1101–1102.
79. Baraff LJ. AIDS: Implications for emergency physicians [Editorial]. *Ann Emerg Med* 1988;17:1102–1103.
80. Ornato JP, Hallagan LF, McMahan SB, et al. Attitudes of BCLS instructors about mouth-to-mouth resuscitation during the AIDS epidemic. *Ann Emerg Med* 1990;19;151–156.
81. Stebben JE. Sterile technique and the prevention of wound infection in office surgery: part I. *J Dermatol Surg Oncol* 1988;14:1364–1371.
82. Stebben JE. Sterile technique and the prevention of wound infection in office surgery: part II. *J Dermatol Surg Oncol* 1989;15:38–48.
83. Drake LA, Ceilley RI, Cornelison RL, et al. Guidelines of care for office surgical facilities: part I. *J Am Acad Dermatol* 1992;26:763–765.
84. Drake LA, Ceilley RI, Cornelison RL, et al. Guidelines for care of office surgical facilities: part II. *J Am Acad Dermatol* 1995;33:265–270.
85. Simmons B, Trusler M, Roccaforte J, et al. Infection control for home health. *Infect Control Hosp Epidemiol* 1990;11:362–370.
86. White MC. Infections and infection risks in home care settings. *Infect Control Hosp Epidemiol* 1992;13:535–539.
87. Lorenzen AN, Itkin DJ. Surveillance of infection in home care. *Am J Infect Control* 1992;20:326–329.
88. Rosenheimer L. Establishing a surveillance system for infections acquired in home healthcare. *Home Health Care Nursing* 1995;13(3):20–26.
89. White MC, Ragland KE. Surveillance of intravenous catheter-related infections among home care clients. *Am J Infect Control* 1993;21:231–235.
90. White MC, Smith, W. Infection control in home care agencies. *Am J Infect Control* 1993;21:146–150.
91. Joint Commission on Accreditation of Healthcare Organizations. *Accreditation manual for home care.* Vol. 1. Oakbrook Terrace, IL: JCAHO; 1994:353–359.
92. Graham DR, Keldermans MM, Klemm LW, et al. Infectious complications among patients receiving home intravenous therapy with peripheral, central, or peripherally placed central venous catheters. *Am J Med* 1991:91(Suppl 3B):95S-100S.
93. Garrett DO, Jarvis WR. The expanding role of healthcare epidemiology—home and long term care. *Infect Control Hosp Epidemiol* 1996;17:714–717.
94. Danzig LE, Short LJ, Collins K, et al. Bloodstream infections associated with a needleless intravenous infusion system in patients receiving home infusion therapy. *JAMA* 1995;273:1862–1864.
95. Kellerman SE, Shay DK, Howard J, et al. Bloodstream infections in home infusion patients: The influence of race and needless intravascular access devises. *J Pediatrics* 1996;129:711–717.
96. Do A, Ray B, Barnett B, et al. Evaluation of the role of needleless devices (ND) in bloodstream infections. 1996 Annual Meeting of the American Society for Microbiology, 36th Interscience Conference on Antimicrobial Agents and Chemotherapy; September 1996; New Orleans, LA. Abstract J61.
97. Centers for Disease Control and Prevention. Hospital Infection Control Practices Advisory Committee: Guideline for the prevention of intravascular-device-related infections. *Infect Control Hosp Epidemiol* 1996;17:721–725.
98. Lobato MN, Oxtoby MJ, Augustyniak L, et al. Infection control practices in the home: a survey of households of HIV-infected persons with hemophilia. *Infect Control Hosp Epidemiol* 1996;17:721–725.
99. Lobato MN, Hannan J, Simonds RJ, et al. Attitudes, practices and infections risks of hemophilia treatment center nurses who teach infection control for the home. *Infect Control Hosp Epidemiol* 1996;17:726–731.
100. Valenti WM. Infection control, human immunodeficiency virus, and home healthcare: I. infection risk to the patient. *Am J Infect Control* 1994;22:371–372.
101. Valenti WM. Infection control, human immunodeficiency virus, and home healthcare: II. risk to the caregiver. *Am J Infect Control* 1995;23:78–81.
102. Berman S. Quality assurance in ambulatory healthcare. *Quality Review Bulletin* 1988;14:18–21.
103. Kaplowitz GJ. Developing and implementing a quality assurance program in a U.S. Coast Guard ambulatory healthcare facility. *Mil Med* 1988;153:625–628.
104. Bradford M, Flynn NM. Ambulatory care infection control quality assurance monitoring. *Am J Infect Control* 1988;16:21A–24A.
105. Hurt N. The role of the infection control nurse in quality management in the ambulatory care setting. *J Healthcare Quality* 1993;15(3):43–44.
106. Haim L, Booth JH, Greaney K. Recommendations for optimizing an infection control practitioner's effectiveness in an ambulatory care setting. *J Healthcare Quality* 1994;16(2):31–34.
107. Bellen V. A model for a comprehensive infection control program in home healthcare. *J Healthcare Quality* 1996;18(3):7–17.
108. Davis ER. *Total quality management for home care.* Gaithersburg, MD: Aspen, 1994.

Hospital Infections, Fourth Edition,
edited by John V. Bennett and Philip S. Brachman.
Lippincott–Raven Publishers, Philadelphia © 1998

CHAPTER 29

Infections in Long-Term Care Facilities

Brenda A. Nurse and Richard A. Garibaldi

A wide array of healthcare settings and services fall under the designation of "long-term care facilities" (LTCF). They include, for example, chronic disease hospitals, rehabilitation centers, skilled nursing facilities, Veterans Affairs (VA) intermediate care units, nursing homes, hospice units, institutions for the mentally retarded, foster and group homes, as well as residential care facilities, adult day care facilities, and home healthcare programs. All provide care for patients who have one or more medical problems that incapacitate them for a prolonged period of time. Most patients treated in these facilities will have these problems for the remainder of their lives and will not be able to return to an independent level of care. Over two and a half million patients in this country reside in some type of LTCF. By far, the greatest number live in nursing homes. There are approximately 25,000 nursing homes that provide beds for an estimated 1.5 million residents, of whom almost 90% are elderly [1,2].

The growing number of aging Americans will likely add to the need for long-term care services in the future. People 65 years or older numbered 33.2 million in 1994. They represented 12.7% of the U.S. population, about one in every eight Americans. The number of older Americans has increased by 2.1 million or 7% since 1990, compared with an increase of 4% for the under 65 population. The older population itself is getting older. In 1994, the 65- to 74-year age group (18.7 million) was eight times larger than in 1900, but the 75- to 84-year group (10.9 million) was 14 times larger, and the 85+ group (3.5 million) was 28 times larger. In 1993, people reaching 65 years of age had an average life expectancy of an additional 17.3 years.

B. A. Nurse: University of Connecticut School of Medicine, Department of Infectious Diseases and Epidemiology, Hospital for Special Care, New Britain, Connecticut 06053.

R. A. Garibaldi: Department of Medicine, University of Connecticut School of Medicine, Farmington, Connecticut 06032.

Although a small number (1.6 million) and percentage (5%) of the 65+-year-old population lived in nursing homes in 1990, the breakdown of percentages increased dramatically with age, ranging from 1% for people 65 to 74 years to 6% for people 75 to 84 years and 24% for people 85+ years of age [3]. It is estimated that 25% of people who are now older than 65 will spend some time during their life in a nursing home [1]. As the population of elderly people continues to grow, it is anticipated that the need for temporary and permanent nursing home beds will grow as well. In addition, an increasing number of beds will be needed for patients who are not elderly but who have a variety of chronic, debilitating conditions such as acquired immunodeficiency syndrome (AIDS), severe trauma and various neuromuscular disorders such as multiple sclerosis and amyotrophic lateral sclerosis, and severe trauma, as well as patients dependent on chronic mechanical ventilation.

The 1990s are particularly challenging times to care for patients in long-term care settings. Given the continuing changes in medical insurance coverage and the managed care environment at this time, patients are spending fewer days in acute care hospitals. As a result, extended care providers, especially rehabilitation facilities, chronic disease hospitals, and home care agencies are now taking care of patients who are more acutely ill than before. They are more likely to be managed on more medications, have a central line catheter in place, and have surgical wounds or other skin care issues. They are also more likely to remain in their extended care setting if their clinical status should change and need stabilization. As a result, a more acute level of care is being provided in facilities that may lack the skilled workers and resources needed to respond to these patient care challenges.

This chapter reviews the epidemiology of infections in the long-term care setting and outlines aspects of care that lead to acquisition and transmission of these infections. Specific infections that are frequently encountered as well as common epidemiologic problems are discussed.

EPIDEMIOLOGY

The Long-Term Care Environment

Long-term care facilities vary in the level of care that they can provide. Many of them furnish a wide range of nursing, psychosocial, and rehabilitation services for patients who require different levels of medical or social supervision. Some facilities select patients according to the type of care that they require. Thus, an entire nursing home population may be comprised of patients who require close medical supervision and skilled nursing care. Others select patients who are relatively independent and require less assistance with their activities of daily living. Some facilities offer care plans that specialize in specific types of rehabilitative or recuperative services, whereas others provide supportive hospice-level care for the terminally ill. Some nursing homes have close working agreements with acute care hospitals that facilitate the exchange of patients between institutions. Hospitalized patients are transferred to long-term care facilities for less intensive, lower-cost care or specific rehabilitative services, and nursing home patients are transferred to the acute care facility for diagnostic evaluations or acute medical management. The types and frequencies of infection vary greatly according to specific referral patterns, patient population, and services provided by the facility.

Long-term care facilities are self-contained environments that provide total daily care for large numbers of needy patients. Bed capacities range from < 50 to > 300; most have between 100 to 150 beds. Patients are usually assigned to four-bed rooms or semiprivate rooms with one or two roommates. Private rooms are available for some, but are at a premium. Patients who are ambulatory usually share a common clean-up area that contains a sink, toilet, and bathing facility. Nonambulatory patients frequently require assistance with personal needs such as washing, bathing, and toileting, which are usually performed in bed or in a chair in the patient's own room or in a common area. Nursing aides or orderlies are often responsible for several patients and move from room to room to perform specified assignments. These contacts may provide opportunities for the transmission of infectious diseases.

Characteristics of Long-Term Care Facilities That Predispose to Infection

Certain activities within the LTCF are particularly conducive to the acquisition and transmission of infections. Residents are encouraged to participate in group activities. Ambulatory patients usually eat in a common area, participate in group physical and occupational therapy sessions, and are gathered together to interact with one another in recreational programs. These activities are designed to encourage social exchanges, but they may also provide opportunities for the spread of infection. Patients with mild upper respiratory illnesses, diarrhea, or conjunctivitis may participate in group activities and may serve as sources for disease transmission.

Nursing homes and chronic care facilities, like hospitals, are reservoirs for infectious agents. Patients may become colonized with pathogenic bacteria during a hospital stay and introduce them to the chronic care environment when they return. Patient-to-patient spread of bacteria in the LTCF may occur indirectly by contact with personnel whose unwashed hands may serve as vectors for transmission. The chances for this type of transmission to occur are increased when patients with indwelling catheters are placed in the same room or brought together in close proximity during group activities. Objects such as urine collection containers, bedpans, and nondisposable equipment may also become contaminated with bacteria and serve as inanimate reservoirs for common-source transmission.

The likelihood for person-to-person transmission in the long-term care environment is increased because of difficulties in identifying infected patients and diagnosing the site of their infection with accuracy. The clinical presentations of infections in elderly and chronically ill patients are frequently atypical or nonspecific. Patients are not always able to communicate changes in clinical status or accurately answer questions that would help the clinician identify or evaluate a new clinical problem. Signs and symptoms that are usually associated with infections may be absent or diminished and may result in delays in diagnosis [4]. For example, an increased respiratory rate may be the only diagnostic clue for pneumonia; urinary tract infections may present with vague, nonspecific, systemic complaints such as anorexia, nausea, confusion, or memory loss. As a result, the diagnosis and treatment of infection may be delayed, allowing transmission to occur to others. Because of the difficulties in identifying infection clinically in these patients, laboratory studies become even more critical to establish a diagnosis. However, LTCFs are often ill equipped to provide these services in a timely manner.

The lack of onsite microbiology, clinical laboratory and x-ray services may add further delay to the identification of infection. Cultures are ordered infrequently, communication to and from an outside laboratory can be slow, and quality of information may not always be consistent. The collection of specimens from possibly infected sites is often difficult because of poor patient compliance. Therefore, cultures may be unobtainable or may be contaminated with normal flora. These limitations force physicians to diagnose and treat possible infections on an empiric basis. Thus, antibiotics are prescribed more frequently than is clearly indicated, and broader-spectrum drugs are frequently chosen as initial therapy. These actions encourage the selection of antibiotic-resistant bacteria for colonization in treated patients and alter the endemic flora of bacteria found in the LTCF.

Most nursing home and LTCFs have infection control programs and designated infection control practitioners. Infection control programs are usually mandated by state law. In states where surveys have been completed, ~ 90% of nursing homes had written infection control policies and infection control committees that met at least quarterly [5,6]. In most nursing homes, however, the designated infection control practitioner has other responsibilities in addition to infection control. These responsibilities are usually administrative or supervisory in nature rather than direct nursing care. Most LTCFs do not have physicians with infectious diseases expertise to oversee their infection control activities. Although surveillance for infections is now routine in most nursing homes, it often does not directly affect patient care practices.

Certain administrative problems also contribute to the acquisition and spread of infections among LTCF patients. These include deficiencies in employee staffing and inadequate training in the basic principles of infection control. High ratios of nonprofessional staff and high rates of employee turnover may make it extremely difficult to establish and maintain efficient programs for infection control. The combination of unstructured programs and poor compliance with routine infection control practices contribute to the spread of infections in this environment.

The difficulties in maintaining effective programs for infection control are compounded by the fact that there are few published guidelines for employee health and infection prevention that focus on the unique problems of the chronic care environment. Some states have adapted infection control regulations from guidelines intended for patients in acute care hospitals. Most states mandate that patients and employees be tested for tuberculosis at the time of admission or employment and yearly thereafter. However, there are no national requirements for tuberculin skin testing or for immunizations against influenza, pneumococcal infection, or other infectious agents for either residents or nursing home staff. Most nursing homes have no formal guidelines for monitoring the health status of employees at the time of hiring or during employment. Few nursing homes have formal policies to allow absenteeism for employees with possible communicable diseases. Usually, there is no compensation for sick time; thus, employees with acute infections might choose to go to work rather than remain at home, exposing susceptible residents to infections from the community.

Nursing Home Patients

To understand the nature of infectious disease problems that occur in nursing homes and the reasons why they occur, one must be familiar with the types of patients who receive care in this setting. Most patients are elderly and functionally disabled; their average age is 80 to 85 years. As many as 20% of patients are 90 years of age or older. Most of the residents are women. Patients are usually admitted to nursing homes for functional disabilities, such as dementia, incontinence, falls, or diminished levels of self-sufficiency. More than 90% of nursing home patients require assistance in providing for their activities of daily living, such as bathing, dressing, toileting, maintaining continence, and transferring from bed or chair. In general, today's nursing home residents are more functionally disabled and dependent than ever before. In skilled nursing facilities, 35 to 50% of the population are nonambulatory and confined to bed and chair status; up to 5% are totally bedridden. As many as 50% of nursing home residents are incontinent of urine and 30% to 40% are incontinent of feces; between 5% and 10% of patients require chronic urinary drainage despite the known hazards of long-term catheterization and attempts by many nursing homes to avoid this invasive procedure.

In addition to being elderly and functionally disabled, the typical nursing home patient also has a variety of concurrent chronic conditions that may involve multiple organ systems. The average nursing home patient has more than three diagnosed conditions recorded in the medical chart. Organic brain syndrome or dementia is the most common diagnosis. Other common problems include organic heart disease, cerebrovascular accidents, hypertension, arthritis, and previous fractures, each affecting > 20% of patients [7]. Because of their long lists of underlying medical problems, most nursing home patients receive a large number of medications. Drugs are prescribed to treat underlying diseases, regulate body functions, control behavior, induce sleep, and, occasionally, prevent infections (such as suppression of urinary tract infections). Studies have shown that the average nursing home patient receives between three and seven medications per day, some of which may be unneeded or ineffective. Cathartics, analgesics, and tranquilizers are the most commonly prescribed drugs. Antibiotics account for a relatively small percentage of all prescriptions.

Host Factors That Predispose Nursing Home Patients to Infection

Many of the functional defects and underlying diseases that characterize nursing home patients are also risk factors that predispose them to infection. These factors can be classified as either normal physiologic consequences of aging or pathologic processes related to disease conditions that accelerate the aging process. Physiologic changes that occur with normal aging include declines in the functional reserve of organs such as the kidneys, lungs, and brain. Some of these changes are associated with an increased risk of infection. Poor wound healing increases the risk for decubitus ulcers. Decreased gastric acidity allows agents that cause diarrheal diseases to gain entry into the gastrointestinal tract. Diminished vital capacity, impaired gag and cough reflexes, decreased ability to clear secretions, loss of lung elastic recoil, and weakened respiratory muscles are risk factors for lower respiratory tract infections [8–10]. Incomplete bladder emptying, impaired generation of acidic urine, poor perineal hygiene, and postmenopausal estrogen deficiency predispose to urinary tract infections in the elderly.

Old age, per se, is not associated with significant physiologic deterioration or immunologic dysfunction that markedly increases susceptibility to infection. However, with aging, there is a consistent decline in T-lymphocyte function and decreased production of interleukin-2. Changes in the T-cell number and function may be important in reactivation of latent infections such as varicella-zoster (shingles) and tuberculosis. The humoral immune system remains intact; however, immune response may be quantitatively diminished. This quantitative defect results in a suboptimal responsiveness to pneumococcal and influenza vaccine in this patient population [9].

A variety of comorbidities frequently found in nursing home patients can predispose to infections. Examples of these include underlying diseases, severe levels of debility, impaired mentation, and receipt of medications that alter mental status or affect normal flora. Patients with certain chronic diseases are predisposed to infectious complications that are directly or indirectly related to their primary disease process. For instance, patients with neurologic disorders or dementia may be unable to feed themselves, communicate effectively, recognize danger, protect themselves with reflex actions, or move in bed; they are at increased risk for aspiration pneumonia and pressure sores that may become subsequently infected. In addition, they are likely to be incontinent of urine and feces and to be treated with long-term, indwelling urinary catheterization. Often, they are agitated and require sedative or tranquilizing medications that additionally diminish their physiologic responsiveness and increase their risk for infection. Similarly, patients with other underlying diseases have increased susceptibility for other infections. For instance, patients who are smokers or who have chronic pulmonary disease are at risk for respiratory infections because they are likely to have dysfunctional mucociliary clearance and depressed immunocytologic defenses. Patients with hiatal hernias, esophageal motility disorders, autonomic neuropathy involving the esophagus or stomach, or unsuspected tumors are also at increased risk for aspiration and pneumonia. Patients with obstructed urinary flow secondary to prostatic hypertrophy, calculi, or uterine prolapse have incomplete bladder emptying and urinary tract infections.

In addition to their underlying diseases, chronically ill nursing home patients have other limitations or frailties that further increase their susceptibility to infections. Systemic disorders such as glucose intolerance, osteoporosis, and degenerative arthritis are common among the elderly. Gait disturbances, difficulty with balance, impaired coordination, easy fatigue, and subtle muscle weakness increase the likelihood for falls, fractures, and subsequent immobility. Nonambulatory patients are more likely than ambulatory patients to be incontinent, require urinary catheterization, have pressure sores, and aspirate. Depression is a common problem in the elderly that may result in a loss of appetite, energy, involvement, or will to live.

Surveys have shown that between 30% to 40% of chronically ill, nursing home patients suffer from some degree of protein-calorie malnutrition. Malnourished patients frequently are unable to respond to skin test antigens, suggesting that they have significant impairments in cell-mediated immunity. Elderly patients with depressed skin test reactivity have a higher mortality (48%) during the 6-month period after testing than patients who are able to react (13%) [11]. Animal studies have shown associations between protein-calorie malnutrition and increased adherence of *Pseudomonas aeruginosa* to tracheal cells, decreased respiratory tract secretory IgA levels, and defective recruitment of macrophages into infected lungs. Deficiencies in vitamins, particularly vitamin B_6 and folate, and zinc ion may impair antibody responsiveness to antigens. Thus, malnutrition in nursing home patients may be another important factor in increasing their susceptibility to infections.

Medications and other therapies prescribed for nursing home patients may also predispose to infection. Use of sedatives and tranquilizers encourages aspiration; narcotic and atropine derivatives decrease mucociliary clearance function. Drugs that decrease lower esophageal sphincter pressure, such as beta$_2$-agonists, caffeine, benzodiazepines, and calcium channel blockers, increase the likelihood of gastric reflux and aspiration. Antacids, H_2 blockers, and drugs that interfere with gastrointestinal motility predispose to enteric infection. Antibiotics alter the indigenous flora of the gastrointestinal tract, oropharynx, vagina, and perineum, and allow colonization and infections with resistant organisms. Antacids, H_2 blockers, and drugs that interfere with gastrointestinal motility predispose to enteric infection (see Chapter 34).

ANTIMICROBIAL RESISTANCE IN LONG-TERM CARE

Since the initial development of antibiotics in the late 1940s and their successful clinical use, clinicians have assumed that effective antimicrobials would always be available. Unfortunately the ability of bacterial pathogens to adapt to their environmental milieu and continue to thrive by various mechanisms in the presence of the newest, broadest-spectrum antibiotics has been underestimated. LTCFs, like acute care hospitals, have had to face the reality of increasing problems with a growing array of antibiotic-resistant bacteria (see Chapter 14).

The appearance of various types of antibiotic-resistant bacteria has been documented in LTCFs since the 1970s. The presence of methicillin-resistant *Staphylococcus aureus* (MRSA) was first reported in 1970 when a hospital outbreak was started by an index patient referred from a nursing home. By the mid-1980s, reports of MRSA cases had increased dramatically from all types of LTCFs (see Chapter 41). In the late 1980s, quinolone resistance in MRSA strains was documented in nursing homes as well. Multiply-resistant gram-negative bacteria are found in most nursing homes in urine cultures from patients with indwelling Foley catheters. Findings of *Providencia* species and *Escherichia coli* resistant to multiple antibiotic classes are not unusual in this setting. High-level gentamicin-resistant enterococci have been reported from several nursing homes. The exact scope of the problem with vancomycin-resistant enterococci has yet to be defined (see Chapters 10, 15).

Resistant bacteria gain entry into LTCFs by a variety of routes. Newly admitted patients may be either colonized or infected with resistant bacteria that are acquired during stays in acute care hospitals, or resistant bacteria may emerge from normal flora after multiple courses of antibiotic therapy. Emergence of resistant bacteria may reflect selection or acquisition of genetic determinants that confer resistance by either spontaneous mutation or gene transfer [12]. Spontaneous mutations are thought to be rare, but have been documented in LTCFs. An outbreak of ceftazidime-resistant bacteria has been reported that arose from plasmid transmission among different Enterobacteriaceae and not from the dissemination of a single resistant bacterial isolate [13]. A similar finding has been reported from a VA home care unit in which an identical plasmid that induced gentamicin resistance was isolated from *E. coli, Citrobacter freundii*, and *Providencia stuartii* recovered from different patients [14].

Several studies have evaluated risk factors for acquiring resistant bacteria in long-term care settings. Host factors that seem most predictive include nonambulatory status, need for advanced nursing care, prior antibiotic therapy, length of stay, and presence of an indwelling urinary catheter [12]. The persistence of antimicrobial-resistant bacteria in LTCFs has been attributed to the presence of large numbers of residents with significant underlying diseases and indwelling urinary catheters, feeding tubes, or tracheostomies who frequently receive antimicrobial therapy and who stay for months to years [15].

There are many cost implications of bacterial resistance in LTCFs. True infections with resistant bacteria necessitate the use of broader-spectrum antimicrobial therapies that, without exception, are more expensive. These agents frequently are parenteral drugs that not all LTCFs are able to dispense because not all are equipped to start and maintain intravenous access. This necessitates transfers back to acute care facilities for appropriate management and increased costs of patient care. Once back in the acute care setting, the patient is at increased risk of being exposed to and acquiring infections with even more resistant organisms.

ENDEMIC INFECTIONS

General

Rates of endemic infections in LCTFs that are reported in the literature vary according to the characteristics of the patient population at the institution, the definitions that are used to identify infected patients, and the intensity of the surveillance efforts. For example, published rates from chronic disease hospitals or skilled nursing facilities that are hospital based are in general higher than those reported from residential facilities caring for patients with less specialized nursing needs. Higher rates are reported from institutions with well developed infection surveillance programs, with debilitated patient populations, and with broad definitions of infection that include asymptomatic as well as symptomatic cases. Because of the inhomogeneity of resident populations among LTCFs and a lack of standard methodologies for defining infections, it is often difficult to generalize the results of a particular study or compare rates from one LTCF to another.

In most published studies, the point-prevalence of infections in institutionalized patients is >10% [4,16–19]. Prevalence surveys tend to overestimate the presence of chronic infections such as skin or soft tissue infections, chronic bronchitis, and chronic urinary tract infection when the identification of bacteriuria is used to define the latter. It is often difficult to distinguish infection from colonization in many of the patients afflicted with chronic conditions involving these sites.

The incidence of new infections among residents of LTCFs ranges between 1.8 to 7.1 per 1,000 resident days depending on the characteristics of the patient population and intensity of surveillance methods [16,17,20–22]. The average incidence is approximately four infections per 1,000 resident days, or slightly greater than one infection per year. In most surveys, the most common sites of infections involve the urinary tract, respiratory tract, and skin. Pneumonia is most likely to be fatal.

Urinary Tract Infections

Urinary tract infections are the most common type of institutionally acquired infection among residents of LTCFs (see Chapter 31). In prevalence surveys, rates of urinary tract infection range between 1.2% and 4.7%

[17]. The incidence of new episodes of urinary tract infection for noncatheterized patients varies between 0.1 and 2.4 episodes per 1,000 resident days, depending on the criteria that are used to diagnose infection, the frequency with which urine cultures are collected, and the decision to include or not include patients with asymptomatic bacteriuria [23,24]. Rates are higher in nursing homes in which a large segment of the resident population has indwelling urinary catheters. In most facilities, between 5% and 10% of residents are catheterized; however, in institutions that provide care for more debilitated patients or patients with spinal cord injuries, as many as 50% of the resident population may be catheterized. Patients with long-term, indwelling urinary catheters are almost always bacteriuric and have a higher rate of symptomatic urinary tract infection.

The risk for development of either bacteriuria or symptomatic urinary tract infection is directly related to the degree of functional disability of the patient. Risk factors for bacteriuria in noncatheterized patients include dementia, impaired mobility, the presence of bowel or urinary incontinence, and longer durations of residence in the LTCF. Chronic diseases or therapies that impair urine flow increase bladder residual volume of urine and promote reflux. Patients with neurogenic bladders, those taking anticholinergic medicines, men with benign prostatic hypertrophy, and diabetics are at increased risk for bacteriuria and urinary tract infection. Patients who are unable to care for themselves or who have diarrhea are at increased risk of ascending infection from perineal and periurethral soilage. Patients with indwelling urinary catheters are at greatest risk for bacteriuria and infection. These patients are also prone to development of bladder calculi and nephrolithiasis that may be secondarily infected and are quite difficult to eradicate. Rates of bacteriuria and infection in incontinent patients who are managed with suprapubic catheters, intermittent catheterization, condom catheters, and diapers have not been well studied in the LTCF setting.

The specific types of bacteria and the spectrum of antibiotic resistance among urine isolates varies greatly from one LTCF to another. Most bacteriologic surveys of infections in LTCFs report results from catheterized and noncatheterized residents who have asymptomatic bacteriuria. In women without indwelling catheters, *E. coli* accounts for 50% to 60% of the isolates; other Enterobacteriaceae, including *Klebsiella, Enterobacter*, and *Proteus* species account for most of the rest [25]. In men, *Proteus* species are a more frequent cause of bacterial colonization than *E. coli*; enterococci are identified more frequently in men than in women. In catheterized patients, *Proteus* species, *P. stuartii*, and *P. aeruginosa* usually predominate as causes of bacteriuria. *P. stuartii* has a selective advantage in colonizing catheterized patients because of its unique ability to attach to catheter surfaces. Colonization in these patients is usually polymicrobial and in a constant state of flux [26]. Even MRSA have been recovered from catheterized urine in some nursing homes [27,28].

Many of the organisms that are recovered from the urinary tracts of LTCF residents are resistant to commonly prescribed antibiotics. Colonized urinary tracts are important reservoirs for resistant organisms that can be spread to other patients within the facility on the hands of caregivers. Resistance to ampicillin and cephalosporins is common among isolates of *E. coli* and other Enterobacteriaceae from these patients. *P. stuartii* are often resistant to multiple antibiotics, including the β-lactams and aminoglycosides. There are increasing numbers of reports from LTCFs of infections with *P. aeruginosa* and other gram-negative organisms that are resistant to fluoroquinolones and enterococci that are resistant to aminoglycosides. There is a growing fear that colonization or infection with vancomycin-resistant enterococci may become endemic in some LTCFs (see Chapter 15).

Respiratory Tract Infections

The epidemiology of respiratory tract infections in LTCF residents is difficult to interpret (see Chapter 32). Because of overlapping signs and symptoms and inexact case definitions, it is difficult to distinguish upper from lower respiratory tract infections. Without chest radiographs, it often is not possible to differentiate bronchitis from pneumonia. Culture surveys are often flawed because they rely on expectorated sputa to define bacteriology. Respiratory tract specimens are difficult to collect, usually contaminated with oropharyngeal flora, and often submitted for culture under suboptimal conditions.

In most surveys, respiratory tract infections are defined by clinical symptoms. In prevalence studies, they are identified in between 0.3% and 3.6% of LTCF residents [4,16–18]; the incidence of respiratory tract infections varies between 0.6 to 4.7 per 1,000 resident days [16,17,24,29]. The variability in rates reflects differences in risk factors, case definitions, methods of case identification, availability of chest radiography, seasonality, and community incidence of infection from one study to another.

It is very likely that most respiratory tract infections in LTCF patients involve only the oropharynx, sinuses, or upper airways. Little data are available from published surveys that describe the epidemiology or etiology of these infections. Most reports of upper airway infections from LTCFs describe epidemic occurrences in which an unusual incidence of infection is noted among a clustered group of residents.

Many LTCF residents are susceptible to pneumonia because of physiologic changes that occur in the aging respiratory tract and because of the frequency of preexisting, underlying chronic conditions that predispose to pulmonary infection. In addition, medications commonly prescribed for LTCF patients that dry secretions, decrease mental alertness, or alter oropharyngeal colonization also predispose patients to aspiration and infection. Studies have shown that residents of LTCFs are more likely to be colonized with gram-negative oropharyngeal flora than noninstitutionalized ambulatory patients [30]. The likelihood of oropharyngeal colonization with gram-negative organisms is greater in individuals with poor functional status, debilitating underlying diseases, nonambulatory status, and bladder incontinence. Severely debilitated patients with malnutrition who require tube feedings are at particularly high risk for aspiration pneumonia.

Bacteriologic surveys of pneumonia in LTCF residents are difficult to interpret because of the methodologic shortcomings noted previously. However, it appears that the spectrum of pathogens is quite broad and resembles infections from either a community or hospital setting [31]. Pneumococcal pneumonia remains "the old man's friend" in these patients. However, the spectrum of pathogens includes the common bacterial agents, antibiotic-resistant organisms, influenza, other viral agents and tuberculosis. It is important for physicians to be aware of the types of pathogens and their antibiotic susceptibilities that are prevalent in the LTCF setting in which they are practicing. Whenever possible, appropriate specimens should be obtained to guide treatment and identify outbreaks. When empiric therapy is prescribed, broad-spectrum antibiotics should be used; the spectrum of coverage should be narrowed once the etiologic pathogen and sensitivities are known.

Skin and Soft Tissue Infections

In general, the frequency of skin and soft tissue infections reflects the level of debility of patients within the LTCF and, to a lesser degree, the quality of nursing care. In published studies, the prevalence of skin infections ranges from 0.9% to 8.8% [16–18]. The higher rates reflect the chronic nature of these infections and difficulties in distinguishing noninfected and infected pressure ulcers. Infection rates are usually higher in surveys that use less strict clinical criteria, with or without cultures, to define an infection. Those who have the poorest levels of function and are incontinent, immobile, malnourished, and suffer sensory impairment are at greatest risk for development of skin problems.

Breakdown of the skin and secondary infection occurs when there is unrelieved pressure over prominent surfaces, shearing, friction and contamination from perspiration, urine or fecal soilage [32]. It is difficult to distinguish uninfected from infected ulcers on the basis of signs and symptoms. Wound cultures are not helpful in making the diagnosis of infection; positive cultures may reflect either colonization or infection. Cultures usually reveal polymicrobial flora with a variety of gram-positive, gram-negative, and anaerobic organisms. Studies that have identified patients with bacteremia secondary to skin infections report *S. aureus* as the most common etiologic agent; other causes include beta-hemolytic streptococci, Enterobacteriaceae, and *Pseudomonas* species.

Residents of LTCFs are at risk for cellulitis that may or may not be associated with obvious breaks in the skin or decubitus ulcers. These infections are frequently caused by group A or group B beta-hemolytic streptococci or *S. aureus* (see Chapter 41). However, the spectrum of pathogens broadens to include other gram-positive organisms, Enterobacteriaceae, and anaerobes when the cellulitis is a complication of a decubitus or chronic foot ulcer in a patient with diabetes or peripheral vascular disease.

Residents in nursing homes are susceptible to a variety of nonbacterial skin infections. Elderly patients in general are at risk for reactivation of latent herpes virus infections such as cold sores (herpes simplex virus) and shingles (herpes zoster). The incidence of these infections is no greater among residents of LTCFs than among noninstitutionalized elderly patients. On the other hand, residents in LTCFs may be at greater risk for mucocutaneous candidiasis. *Candida albicans* is responsible for a wide spectrum of clinical conditions in debilitated hosts including intertriginous infections, thrush, angular cheilosis, and vulvovaginal infections. LTCF residents who are debilitated, malnourished, incontinent, and receiving antibiotics are predisposed to candidal infections. Because of their chronic nature, some prevalence surveys report rates of candidal infections as high as 30% to 50%. One survey reported an incidence of 0.28 candidal infections per 1,000 resident days [33].

Residents of LTCFs are also at risk for conjunctival infections, although infectious causes of conjunctivitis are rarely identified by bacterial or viral cultures. In fact, most causes of chronic conjunctivitis are noninfectious in origin; they are secondary to other irritative conditions such as glaucoma, ectropion, or entropion. Reported prevalence rates of conjunctivitis range between 5% and 13% [16,20,22,34]. The most commonly identified bacterial cause of acute conjunctivitis is *S. aureus*, although other respiratory pathogens may also be responsible for some cases. Epidemic conjunctivitis secondary to bacterial or viral pathogens may occur sporadically.

Bacteremia

Bacteremia is diagnosed relatively infrequently in LTCFs. The reported incidence ranges from 0.2 to 0.4 episodes per 1,000 resident days [17,35,36]. However, this figure probably represents a gross underestimate of the true incidence of bacteremia in this setting. Blood cultures are ordered relatively infrequently to evaluate febrile episodes in LTCFs compared with acute care hospitals. In addition, in the LTCF, bacteremic patients may present with subtle, nonspecific symptoms without fever. When bacteremia is diagnosed, it is usually secondary to a focal infection at another site. Urinary tract infections are responsible for slightly more than one half of diagnosed bacteremic episodes; skin infections and pneumonia account for between 10% and 15% each. Primary bacteremia is rare given the infrequent use of central venous catheters (see Chapter 44). This may change in the future when more patients are transferred to LTCFs from acute care hospitals with intravenous lines for completion of courses of antibiotic therapy or chemotherapeutic regimens. Gram-negative organisms account for more than half the cases of bacteremia in this patient population, and gram-positive organisms account for approximately one fourth; 10% to 20% of episodes are polymicrobial. These numbers may change when intravenous therapies become more commonplace in LTCFs.

Gastrointestinal Infections

Most reports of gastrointestinal infections (see Chapter 34) in LTCFs describe epidemic occurrences of disease caused by enterotoxin-producing bacteria, invasive bacterial pathogens, or viruses. Diarrhea, however, is a common occurrence among nursing home residents; most episodes are probably noninfectious in origin. Episodes of diarrheal illness are caused by underlying medical conditions that affect digestion or absorption, as well as by high-protein dietary supplements or medications that increase intestinal motility or alter indigenous bowel flora. The true incidence of infectious diarrhea outside of the epidemic episodes is unknown.

Intestinal colonization with *Clostridium difficile* is common in many LTCFs, with a point prevalence ranging from 2% to 33%. Colonized patients are usually asymptomatic, but between 15% to 30% may have diarrhea [37,38]. Rates of colonization and infection with *C. difficile* are increased in patients who are receiving antibiotics or H_2 blockers. Once *C. difficile* is introduced into an LTCF, it is difficult to eradicate.

Human Immunodeficiency Virus Infection

Human immunodeficiency virus-infected patients are admitted to most LTCFs, but not in large numbers. Some still exclude patients with the diagnosis of AIDS. For now, AIDS patients are cared for most commonly in hospice units or chronic disease hospitals. However, this is changing as nursing home staff are becoming more familiar with and comfortable in managing patients with this diagnosis.

Human immunodeficiency virus, per se, is not a major threat to healthcare workers who adhere to universal precautions (see Chapter 13). Most of the opportunistic infections that occur in AIDS patients involve the reactivation of latent infections with pathogens that are easily controlled in people with normal immune functions. These include infections with such agents as *Toxoplasma gondii*, cytomegalovirus, or *Pneumocystis carinii*. There are, however, certain exceptions to this generalization. AIDS patients may also be infected with diarrheal pathogens such as salmonellae or *Cryptosporidia* that may be transmitted by fecal–oral spread to healthcare workers. Severe herpes virus infections with either herpes simplex virus or varicella zoster virus are also common in AIDS patients and may be transmitted through direct contact with an infected lesion. The most dangerous of the opportunistic infections that might be transmitted to healthcare workers by AIDS patients in the LTCF setting is pulmonary tuberculosis (see Chapter 33). In AIDS patients, tuberculosis may develop over a relatively short period of time, have a fulminant clinical course, and be highly infectious to staff and other patients if proper precautions are not taken. Many LTCFs do not have the appropriate administrative or environmental protections in place to adequately manage these patients.

Other Infections

A variety of other types of infections also occur in residents of LTCFs, but they are relatively uncommon and occur with a frequency that is probably no greater than that noted in noninstitutionalized populations. Individuals who are elderly, debilitated, and diseased are at risk for osteomyelitis, meningitis, infective endocarditis, diverticulitis, appendicitis, intraabdominal abscesses, and a host of other infections. Fever of unknown origin is also common among LTCF patients, particularly those with indwelling urinary catheters. This may reflect a failure to diagnose the site of primary infection or be a subtle clue to a difficult-to-diagnose inflammatory condition or malignancy.

EPIDEMIC INFECTIONS

General

The exact incidence of epidemic infections in the LTCF setting is unknown. The literature contains numerous reports of outbreaks among residents of LTCFs that document the occurrence of clustered respiratory infections, diarrheal diseases, infections with multidrug-resistant organisms, and other unusual occurrences. However, most clusters of LTCF infections go unrecognized because they are either not diagnosed in the facility in which they occur or are not thoroughly investigated.

Epidemic Respiratory Infections

There are numerous published reports of epidemic respiratory tract infections in the literature [39–46]. Among these, epidemic reports of influenza virus infection are associated with the most serious morbidity and mortality (see Chapters 30, 42). Outbreaks of influenza virus infections in LTCFs often occur concurrently with increased incidences of infection in the community. Influenza is introduced into the facility by employees or visitors who are contagious and who interact with patients. Once introduced into the LTCF, the attack rate for clinical infection among unvaccinated patients ranges between 25% to 40%; staff may also become infected. Mortality from influenza virus infection can be extremely high in patients with debilitating underlying diseases; the case fatality ratio is reported to be between 10% to 35% [42,43]. The high morbidity and mortality associated with these infections underscores the importance of aggressive annual influenza immunization programs that include both patients and employees. Although there are conflicting data on the efficacy of vaccine for preventing clinical infection among LTCF residents, immunization of both patients and staff appears to have an impact on reducing mortality of patients [47,48].

Residents of LTCFs are also at risk for a variety of other respiratory viruses such as respiratory syncytial virus, rhinovirus, or adenovirus infection that can involve either the upper or lower respiratory tract [43,45] (see Chapter 42). The number of published reports of outbreaks with these agents is relatively small and probably greatly underestimates their true occurrence. Most often, specific diagnostic tests are not performed to identify infections with these agents, outbreaks are rarely investigated epidemiologically, and reports are seldom submitted for publication.

Tuberculosis is rarely reported among residents of LTCFs (see Chapter 33). However, when it occurs in a closed setting such as this, it can have devastating consequences. Epidemics of tuberculosis in residents of LTCFs have been well documented. In one report, 47 of 102 previously uninfected residents (46%) became infected from a single index case [49]. LTCF residents with serious underlying diseases and altered immune function are at risk for reactivating latent infections. Once symptomatic, these patients may serve as index cases for primary pulmonary infection in other residents or staff through airborne transmission. It is recommended that all patients who are newly admitted to LTCFs have an initial tuberculin skin test with 5TU PPD (purified protein derivative) and undergo annual retesting thereafter. Residents who convert their skin tests from negative to positive should be considered for preventive therapy with isoniazid. Although there is a reported incidence of hepatotoxicity with the use of isoniazid that increases with increasing age, this should not prohibit the use of this drug in the elderly.

Epidemic Gastrointestinal Infections

Diarrhea is a relatively common occurrence among residents of LTCFs (see Chapter 34). Most instances are noninfectious; however, numerous reports of epidemic diarrheal illnesses have been published that include infections with a variety of bacterial and viral agents [50,51]. Epidemic salmonella infection among residents of LTCFs has been associated with both person-to-person and common-source transmission. Common source outbreaks are usually traced to contamination of tube feedings or other food items served within the facility. Sometimes a product such as raw eggs is implicated, other times a worker with asymptomatic infection is identified as the index case. Often there is significant morbidity and mortality with these infections, given the already debilitated status of many LTCF residents.

Other agents that have been incriminated as causes of epidemic foodborne gastroenteritis in LTCFs include enterotoxin-producing *S. aureus, Clostridium perfringens*, or *Bacillus cereus*. There are scattered reports of infection with other invasive pathogens such as shigellosis and enterohemorrhagic *E. coli*. Outbreaks of virus-associated diarrhea have also been reported, with rotavirus and Norwalk-like agents as the most frequently cited causes; these agents are usually spread by person-to-person transmission and have high attack rates in the LTCF setting.

Clostridium difficile is often cited as a cause of either endemic or epidemic diarrheal disease [37,38]. Some patients are asymptomatic carriers; others develop pseudomembranous colitis. Cases may be generated within the LTCF setting as a result of selective pressures from antibiotics or be secondary to the transfer of colonized patients from acute care hospitals into the LTCF. Colonized or infected patients may serve as index cases for fecal–oral spread or may contaminate objects in their environment that serve as reservoirs for common source spread. It is likely that other enteric organisms, including vancomycin-resistant enterococci, will be spread to patients and staff in similar fashion.

Epidemic Urinary Tract Infections

Outbreaks of urinary tract infections within an LTCF setting usually occur among individuals with chronic indwelling urinary catheters [12,52] (see Chapter 31). Some facilities, such as those caring for patients with spinal cord injuries, have high numbers of chronically catheterized patients who are at high risk for infection. Organisms from an infected or colonized patient can be transferred from one patient to another by passive carriage on the hands of healthcare workers. Occasionally contamination of an object or product used in the care of the catheter system is incriminated as a common source. Often, organisms such as *P. stuartii*, *Proteus* species, *Serratia marcescans*, or *P. aeuriginosa* that are resistant to multiple antibiotics are identified as the cause of urinary colonization or infection. An individual LTCF may have its own pattern of endemic flora that colonize and infect these patients.

Other Epidemic Infections

There are reports in the literature of LTCF outbreaks with a variety of pathogens. These include infections with agents as far ranging as group A streptococci, hepatitis A, and scabies. Virtually any pathogen with epidemic potential is capable of causing an outbreak in an LTCF. These facilities are also at risk for sustaining outbreaks with a variety of antibiotic-resistant organisms that may be responsible for infections or colonization at multiple sites. For instance, MRSA may be found in the nasopharynx of one resident, as the cause of a skin ulcer infection in another, and the agent responsible for a respiratory tract infection in a third. Similarly, antibiotic-resistant gram-negative bacilli may colonize the oropharynx, gastrointestinal tract, and urinary tract. Colonization in these sites is frequently cited as a reservoir for the spread of infection with these organisms throughout the LTCF.

THE INFECTION CONTROL PROGRAM

The infection control program in the LTCF setting should be designed to recognize nosocomial infection issues in a timely way as well as to prevent the transmission of these diseases to the other patients who reside there. The key to a successful program is consistent commitment to the mission of infection control.

The primary goal of any infection control program is prevention of infection and, if that is not possible, limitation of the spread of disease. Although the major objectives of infection control programs in LTCFs are similar to those in acute care hospitals (see Chapter 4), the specific issues or problems that arise may warrant different solutions based on the patient, the setting, and a reasonable assessment of patient care needs, as well as quality-of-life issues. The infection control program cannot succeed without 1) the active participation of recognized, trained personnel at the facility who have part or all of their time allotted to infection control issues; 2) a regular system of surveillance to identify problems in a timely manner (see Chapter 5); 3) a reliable mechanism to implement reasonable infection control procedures based on the setting to prevent the spread of infection; and 4) an administrative structure that is aware of, promotes, and supports the infection control staff and their program. Access to specially trained professionals such as infectious diseases physicians or certified infection control practitioners is ideal, but rarely available in the long-term care setting. Input of consultants when necessary should be part of the program.

Each institution must have clearly written policies and procedures that address infection control issues such as preadmission screening, vaccinations and tuberculosis (PPD) testing for patients and staff, food preparation, handwashing, and employee health. The staff responsible for infection control must understand the appropriate procedures for isolation and be able to communicate these directives clearly to staff both in verbal and in written form. A basic working knowledge of universal precautions is critical for all healthcare workers in all patient care settings; appropriate equipment (i.e., gloves, gowns/aprons, masks and protective eyeware/faceshields) should be available for the various tasks that staff may be called on to do in their normal work day. The importance of the different types of disease transmission (i.e., contact, droplet, airborne) should be clear to all staff members having contact with patients in the facility.

The Infection Control Committee

The core element for an effective infection control program is the infection control committee and the cooperative efforts of its members (see Chapter 4). In many LTCFs, the position of chairperson is delegated to the medical director or to an attending physician who has an interest in infectious diseases or infection control. A physician as chairperson or co-chairperson lends both credibility and authority to the committee and enables it to deal more effectively with other physicians and administrators. Critical members of the committee include an infection control practitioner, a member of administration at the decision-making level, and the director of nursing.

The role of the infection control practitioner is pivotal for program operations. Not every facility has a full-time infection control practitioner; in some institutions, the infection control practitioner is also the director of nursing. In others, the job may span two departments, incorporating employee health responsibilities with infection control. To be able to function effectively, the infection control practitioner should have a basic understanding of infectious diseases, microbiology, epidemiology, and public health, as well as an in-depth knowledge of nursing technique and aseptic practice. It is also important to have effective communication skills, the respect of the staff, and a desire to become educated in the discipline of infection control. With widespread concerns today involving work-related exposures and life-threatening infectious agents, including human immunodeficiency virus, the role of the infection control practitioner has expanded to include that of adviser and confidante as well as clinician and teacher.

The facility's administrator plays an important role on the infection control committee. At committee meetings, he or she will participate in discussions with staff about infection control issues and become informed about state or national standards that require compliance. The administrator needs to know about infectious diseases that are prevalent in the nursing home and plans for infection control. In return, the administrator can provide the committee with realistic expectations of the institution's ability to comply with the committee's recommendations. Ultimately, he or she is critical in the communication, implementation, and enforcement of facility-wide decisions.

The other members of the infection control committee should represent the interdisciplinary nature of infection control activities throughout the facility. Representatives from nursing, dietary services, pharmacy, housekeeping and building services, maintenance, and other specialty departments, if present within the facility, should be included as well. Often, a member from the local health department is invited to attend, although his or her presence is not mandatory at all meetings.

Surveillance

The optimal method for surveillance in the long-term care setting has not been defined. The system of surveillance that an institution adopts should be developed based on staffing availability, patient population, and any unique institutional issues or characteristics that exist (see Chapter 5). Rates of infection should be determined by periodic surveys of incidence or prevalence of infection. The procedures used to conduct surveillance very likely differ from institution to institution; however, the critical factor is that standardized methodology be applied consistently with the same techniques of data collection in each survey, using accepted definitions of infection, reproducible methods for case identification, and consistent data sources for the calculation of rates. By using standard techniques, individual institutions can generate data that identify background rates and monitor trends in endemic infections. With this information, the committee is able to evaluate changes in nosocomial infections and identify clusters or outbreaks. If a number of LTCFs use the same methods for data collection with similar types of patients, it may be possible to compare rates to identify problems and evaluate the effectiveness of control measures.

The surveillance program should describe institutionally acquired infections by site, etiology, nursing unit/floor, room location, date of onset, and relationship to iatrogenic manipulations. The program should highlight the occurrences of infections with resistant bacteria that are identified in the course of surveillance (i.e., MRSA, vancomycin-resistant enterococci, enterococci with high-level gentamicin resistance, and multiply resistant gram-negative bacteria). A number of approaches may be needed to identify new infections in the LTCF. Routine chart reviews do not always identify the onset of or even the presence of infections. Vital signs may not be recorded on a regular basis, making review of the vital signs sheet an incomplete source of information to screen reliably for infections. Even when the temperature is available for review, the data may be misleading because elderly patients do not always respond to infection with a febrile reaction. One of the most reliable methods for data collection is regular rounds on the nursing units, where the infection control practitioner can talk to and ask questions of the nurses and nursing assistants who provide daily direct patient care. Review of the staff nurses' notes in the medical record or bedside chart may provide helpful clues to identifying infections. Personnel should be encouraged to report significant changes in patient status and to identify newly diagnosed nosocomial infections. It can be useful to designate liaison nurses who can be trained to become infection control extenders and encouraged to participate in surveillance activities on their nursing units. Regular review of new antibiotic prescriptions can also identify newly infected patients. Routine collection of surveillance cultures from environmental sources or patients, including urine from chronically catheterized patients, is not recommended. It is the responsibility of the infection control practitioner to compile the surveillance data at regular intervals for presentation at meetings of the infection control committee.

When an unusual clustering of cases is noted, the infection control practitioner should perform an epidemiologic investigation (see Chapter 6). The investigation should include the identification of the problem, a case count, and an analysis of the cases by time, place, and person. In most instances, this type of investigation reveals the extent of the epidemic and the pattern of disease transmission; with this detailed information, the infection control practitioner can recommend appropriate control measures to be followed. In situations where the infection control problem is large or seemingly appropriate control strategies are not effective, administration or the medical director of the LTCF should be made aware of the problem and outside consultation obtained. Outside help can be solicited from certified infection control practitioners at other facilities, infectious diseases physicians in the community, the local health department, epidemiologists at a local acute care hospital, the state health department, or the Centers for Disease Control and Prevention in Atlanta.

Infection Control Procedures

Patients with active communicable diseases should be identified early and proper precautions should be undertaken to prevent the spread of infection within the institution (see Chapter 13). These patients should have their activities restricted. The type and severity of isolation precautions must be individualized according to the type of infection and the patient's total needs. When an infection control problem is identified, it is the infection control practitioner's responsibility to implement effective intervention. The problem may be an increased frequency of a specific type of infection, a breakdown in aseptic technique, failure to understand or initiate specific isolation precautions, or a possible epidemic occurrence of infection. In each of these situations, the infection control practitioner needs to intervene with an action plan to correct the problem and educate the involved staff. The practitioner should maintain contact with the staff on a regular basis to make sure that the problem is resolved.

An appropriate time to introduce the concepts and application of infection control principles to new employees is during their initial orientation to the institution. At this time, the infection control practitioner can review the risks of infections in the LTCF and the techniques of infection control. This is also a time to evaluate the new employees' knowledge and performance of infection control practices. For all employees, ongoing educational programs should be scheduled to review new techniques in infection control. These sessions should also serve as problem-solving exercises in which issues raised by employees are discussed. There are many topics on which the infection control practitioner can focus during employee updates, including review of proper techniques of indwelling urinary catheter care or decubitus ulcer prevention. Educational programs should discuss the value of handwashing and emphasize the concept of universal precautions.

Employee Health

The surveillance and control of infections in employees is critically important for the prevention of infection in patients (see Chapter 3). Nursing homes should have a system for monitoring the health status of their personnel. At the time of employment, all personnel should be evaluated to rule out the presence of acute or chronic infectious disease (e.g., PPD skin testing to rule out tuberculosis). An employee's immunization status should be questioned, checked, and updated. This information can be collected by the employee's private physician, with results sent to the LTCF, or by the employee health nurse or the infection control practitioner at the LTCF. Even though the size of the facility may preclude the feasibility of a formal employee health program, all LTCFs should maintain a file of health-related problems for each of their employees and provide a means to evaluate acutely ill staff members who might be infected. Employees who contract acute infections should be encouraged to seek early medical evaluation to determine their infectivity and be sent home, if necessary. Similarly, visitors with symptoms of acute infection should be restricted from seeing patients at the facility. Appropriate vaccinations should be offered to all employees in a timely manner. Employees who have regular exposure to blood and body fluids should receive the hepatitis B vaccine (see Chapter 3, 42). An annual influenza vaccination for employees protects not only healthcare workers but the patients with whom they work.

CONCLUSION

Long-term care facilities include a variety of different types of healthcare settings. The numbers of patients in LTCFs will continue to grow as our population ages. In the future, patients in LTCFs will have even more complicated medical conditions than today as patients get older and the trend toward shorter hospital stays in acute care continues. The patient population in LTCFs is uniquely susceptible to infection given the physiologic changes of aging, underlying chronic diseases, and the environment within which they socialize and live. LTCFs staff will need to be prepared to manage more invasive devices such as intravenous catheters and tracheostomies as well as varied diagnoses such as AIDS and ventilator-dependent lung diseases. Antibiotic resistance to a number of bacteria have been reported in LTCFs; the scope of the problem with some of these bacteria is yet to be defined.

Both endemic and epidemic infections occur relatively commonly in LTCFs. In this environment, it is important to emphasize the need for developing and supporting strong infection control programs that can initiate appropriate surveillance to monitor the rates of endemic infections and influence the prevention of epidemics. Education in infection control issues and attention to employee health is essential to enable nursing home staff to provide care safely for the current LTCF patient population, while preparing them for the more complicated patients who will be admitted in the future.

REFERENCES

1. Hing E. Nursing home utilization by current residents: United States, 1985. *Vital Health Stat* 1989;102.
2. U.S. Bureau of the Census. *The national data book.* 115th ed. Statistical abstract of the United States 1995. Washington, DC: U.S. Department of Commerce, Economics and Statistics Administration, Bureau of the Census; September, 1995.
3. American Association of Retired Persons (AARP) and the Administration on Aging (AoA), U.S. Department of Health and Human Services. *Profile of older Americans: 1995.* Washington, DC: U.S. Department of Health and Human Services, 1995.
4. Nurse BA, Garibaldi RA. Infections in the elderly. In Smith P, ed. *Infection control in long-term care facilities.* 2nd ed. Albany, NY: Delmar Publishers, 1994:25–37.
5. Khabbaz RF, Tenney JH. Infection control in Maryland nursing homes. *Infect Control Hosp Epidemiol* 1988;9:159.
6. Price LE, Sarabbi FA, Rutala WA. Infection control programs in twelve North Carolina extended care facilities. *Infect Control* 1985;6:437.
7. Garibaldi R, Brodine S, Matsumiya R. Infections among patients in nursing homes: policies, prevalence, and problems. *N Engl J Med* 1981; 305:731–735.
8. Potter J. Immunity in the elderly. In: Smith P, ed. Infection control in long-term care facilities. 2nd ed. Albany, NY: Delmar Publishers, 1994:11–23.
9. Nicolle LE, Strausbaugh LJ, Garibaldi RA. Infections and antibiotic resistance in nursing homes. *Clin Microbiol Rev* 1996:9:1–17.

10. Scherzer HH, Nurse BA. Pneumonia in the elderly stroke patient. *Physical Medicine and Rehabilitation* 1989;3:549–536.
11. Shaner HJ, Loper JA, Lutes RA. Nutritional status of nursing home patients. *J Parenter Enteral Nutr* 1980;4:367.
12. John JE, Ribner BS. Antibiotic resistance in long-term care facilities. *Infect Control Hosp Epidemiol* 1991;12:245–250.
13. Rice LB, Willey SH, Papanicolaou GA, et al. Outbreak of ceftazidime resistance caused by extended-spectrum beta-lactamases at a Massachusetts chronic care facility. *Antimicrob Agents Chemother* 1990;34: 2193–2199.
14. Shlaes DM, Lehman MH, Currie-McCumer C, et al. Prevalence of colonization with antibiotic resistant gram-negative bacilli in a nursing home care unit: the importance of cross colonization as documented by plasmid analysis. *Infect Control* 1986;7:538–545.
15. Strausbaugh LJ, Crossley KB, Nurse BA, Thrupp LD, SHEA Long-Term Care Committee. Antimicrobial resistance in long-term care facilities. *Infect Control Hosp Epidemiol* 1996;17:129–140.
16. Scheckler W, Peterson P. Infections and infection control among residents of eight rural Wisconsin nursing homes. *Arch Intern Med* 1986; 146:1981–1984.
17. Alvarez S, Shell C, Woolley T, Berk S, Smith J. Nosocomial infections in long-term facilities. *J Gerontol* 1988;43:M9–M17.
18. Setia U, Serventi I, Lorenz P. Nosocomial infections among patients in a long-term care facility: spectrum, prevalence, and risk factors. *Am J Infect Control* 1985;13:57–62.
19. Steinmiller A, Robb S, Mudler R. Prevalence of nosocomial infection in long-term-care Veterans Administration medical centers. *Am J Infect Control* 1991;19:143–146.
20. Vlahov D, Tenney J, Cervino K, Shamer D. Routine surveillance for infections in nursing homes: experience at two facilities. *Am J Infect Control* 1987;15:47–53.
21. Darnowski S, Gordon M, Simor A. Two years of infection surveillance in a geriatric long-term care facility. *Am J Infect Control* 1991;19:185–190.
22. Jackson M, Fierer J, Barrett-Connor E, et al. Intensive surveillance for infections in a three-year study of nursing home patients. *Am J Epidemiol* 1992;135:685–696.
23. Nicolle L, McIntyre M, Zacharias H, MacDonell J. Twelve-month surveillance of infections in institutionalized elderly men. *J Am Geriatr Soc* 1984;32:513–519.
24. Magnussen M, Robb S. Nosocomial infections in a long-term care facility. *Am J Infect Control* 1980;8:12–17.
25. Eberle C, Winsemius D, Garibaldi RA. Risk factors and consequences of bacteriuria in non-catheterized nursing home residents. *J Gerontol* 1993;48:66–71.
26. Warren J, Tenney J, Hoopes J, et al. A prospective microbiologic study of bacteriuria in patients with chronic indwelling urethral catheters. *J Infect Dis* 1982;146:719–723.
27. Boyd N, Gidwani R. Colonization of methicillin-resistant *Staphylococcus aureus* in southwestern Ontario. *Canadian Disease Weekly Report* 1991;17:72–74.
28. Coll PP, Nurse BA. Implications of methicillin-resistant *Staphylococcus aureus* on nursing home practice. *J Am Board Fam Pract* 1992;5: 193–200.
29. Farber B, Brennen C, Puntereri A, Brody J. A prospective study of nosocomial infections in a chronic care facility. *J Am Geriatr Soc* 1984; 32:499–502.
30. Garb J, Brown R, Garb J, Tuthill R. Differences in etiology of pneumonias in nursing home and community patients. *JAMA* 1978;240: 2169–2172.
31. McDonald A, Dietsche L, Litsche M, et al. A retrospective study of nosocomial pneumonia at a long-term care facility. *Am J Infect Control* 1992;20:234–238.
32. Nurse BA, Collins MC. Skin care and decubitus ulcer management in the elderly stroke patient. *Physical Medicine and Rehabilitation* 1989; 3:549–562.
33. Standfast S, Michelsen P, Baltch A, et al. A prevalence survey of infections in a combined acute and long-term care hospital. *Infect Control* 1984;5:177–184.
34. Boustcha E, Nicolle L. Conjunctivitis in a long-term care facility. *Infect Control Hosp Epidemiol* 1995;16:210–214.
35. Muder R, Brennen C, Wagener M, et al. Bacteremia in a long-term-care facility: a five year prospective study of 163 consecutive episodes. *Clin Infect Dis* 1992;14:647–654.
36. Setia U, Serventi I, Lorenz P. Bacteremia in a long-term care facility. *Arch Intern Med* 1984;144:1633–1635.
37. Bender B, Laughon B, Gaydos C, et al. *Clostridium difficile* endemic in chronic-care facilities? *Lancet* 1986;2:11–13.
38. Thomas D, Bennett R, Laughon B, et al. Postantibiotic colonization with *Clostridium difficile* in nursing home patients. *J Am Geriatr Soc* 1990;38:415–420.
39. Arroyo J, Postic B, Brown A, et al. Influenza A/Philippines/2/82 outbreak in a nursing home: limitations of influenza vaccination in the aged. *Am J Infect Control* 1984;12:329–334.
40. Goodman R, Orenstein W, Munro T, et al. Impact of influenza A in a nursing home. *JAMA* 1982;247:1451–1453.
41. Herman J, Stetler H, Israel E, et al. An outbreak of influenza A in a nursing home. *Am J Public Health* 1986;76:501–503.
42. Patriarca P, Arden N, Koplan J, et al. Prevention and control of type A influenza infections in nursing homes. *Ann Intern Med* 87;107:732–740.
43. Cesario T, Yousefi S. Viral infections. *Clin Geriatr Med* 1992;8:735–743.
44. Falsey A. Noninfluenza respiratory virus infection in long-term care facilities. *Infect Control Hosp Epidemiol* 1991;12:602–608.
45. Wald T, Shultz P, Krause P, et al. A rhinovirus outbreak among residents of a long-term care facility. *Ann Intern Med* 1995;123:588–593.
46. Bentley D. Tuberculosis in long-term care facilities. *Infect Control Hosp Epidemiol* 1990;11:42–46.
47. Gross P, Quinlan G, Rodstein M, et al. Association of influenza immunization with reduction in mortality in an elderly population. *Arch Intern Med* 1988;148:562–565.
48. Potter J, Stott DJ, Roberts Ag, et al. Influenza vaccination of healthcare workers in long-term-care hospitals reduces the mortality of elderly patients. *J Infect Dis* 1997;175:1–6.
49. Stead W. Tuberculosis among elderly persons: an outbreak in a nursing home. *Ann Intern Med* 1981;94:606–610.
50. Levine W, Smart J, Archer D, et al. Foodborne disease outbreaks in nursing homes, 1975 through 1987. *JAMA* 1991;266:2105–2109.
51. Jackson M, Fierer J. Infections and infection risk in residents of long-term care facilities: a review of the literature, 1970–1984. *Am J Infect Control* 1985;13:63–67.
52. Wingard E, Shlaes J, Mortimer E, et al. Colonization and cross-colonization of nursing home patients with trimethoprim-resistant gram-negative bacilli. *Clin Infect Dis* 1993;16:74–81.

PART III

Endemic and Epidemic Hospital Infections

Hospital Infections, Fourth Edition, edited by
John V. Bennett and Philip S. Brachman.
Published by Lippincott–Raven Publishers, Philadelphia, 1998

CHAPTER 30

Incidence and Nature of Endemic and Epidemic Nosocomial Infections

William J. Martone, William R. Jarvis, Jonathan R. Edwards, David H. Culver and Robert W. Haley

One of the central concepts of modern infection control is that a thorough knowledge of the occurrence of infection problems is necessary to control them most effectively. Although there is no substitute for timely information from ongoing surveillance of the current infection situation in one's own hospital, a valuable perspective can be gained from studying the incidence and nature of nosocomial infections in the nation as a whole and in hospitals similar to one's own. Such information not only points out national infection problems and trends that are likely to be mirrored in local situations but alerts infection control personnel to potentially useful concepts and techniques that can be adopted and to potential pitfalls that can be avoided.

The problem of nosocomial infections is usually discussed in two different contexts: epidemics of infections and endemic occurrences. Epidemics have been very important in the development of the modern approach to hospital infection control by presenting emergency situations that have focused concern and effort on the problem; consequently, epidemics of infections have received much attention from infection control personnel and have been the focus of much of the scientific literature on the subject. When epidemics occur, they often provoke crises that call for intensive investigation and decisive control measures. Because, however, only ~ 2% to 4% of nosocomial infections occur as part of epidemics [1,2], descriptions of nosocomial infections reflect almost entirely the nature of endemic infections and give little insight into epidemic problems.

The purpose of this chapter is, first, to describe the nationwide incidence and distribution of endemic nosocomial infections in U.S. hospitals from several studies; second, to characterize the nature of epidemics and trends in their occurrence, including the troublesome problem of pseudoepidemics; and third, to discuss methods of estimating the adverse consequences of these problems in terms of prolongation of hospital stay, extra costs, and death.

ENDEMIC NOSOCOMIAL INFECTIONS

Overall Infection Rates

The effort to estimate rates of nosocomial infections began with surveillance studies of the prevalence [3] and incidence [4,5] of infections in individual hospitals. The first effort to estimate the magnitude of the problem on a wider scale was made by the Centers for Disease Control (now the Centers for Disease Control and Prevention [CDC]) in a collaborative study of eight community hospitals known as the Comprehensive Hospital Infections Project (CHIP) [4]. Performed in the late 1960s and early 1970s, this contract-supported study involved very intensive surveillance efforts to detect both nosocomial and community-acquired infections. Validation studies were performed by CDC epidemiologists who visited the hospitals on a regular basis to estimate the percentage of infections detected by the hospitals' surveillance personnel. Based on an overall rate of 3.2 infected patients per 100 discharges and an adjustment for the percentage of true infections detected, it was estimated that in 1970

W. J. Martone: National Foundation for Infectious Diseases, Bethesda, Maryland 20814.

W. R. Jarvis, J. R. Edwards, D. H. Culver: Hospital Infections Program, National Center for Infectious Diseases, Centers for Disease Control and Prevention, Atlanta, Georgia 30333.

R. W. Haley: Department of Internal Medicine, Division of Epidemiology and Preventive Medicine, University of Texas Southwestern Medical Center, Dallas, Texas 75235–8874.

~ 5% of patients in community hospitals contracted one or more nosocomial infections (the *infection percentage*; see Chapter 5) [6], an estimate that was subsequently widely held to be the national rate of nosocomial infection.

In 1970, the CDC studies were extended to a group of approximately 80 volunteer hospitals of diverse sizes and types and called the National Nosocomial Infections Surveillance (NNIS) System. Although the same general surveillance methods were used, the quality control techniques used in CHIP were not feasible in the NNIS study; however, the advantages of the NNIS System were that the group contained a substantial number of hospitals representing the major types of hospitals in the United States, and the system could continue reporting data over a number of years. The overall infection rates reported from the NNIS hospitals, unadjusted for completeness of ascertainment, have remained relatively stable at ~ 3.2 infections per 100 discharges (the *infection ratio*; see Chapter 5) from 1970 through 1982, (although some interesting secular trends have been observed and are described in this section under the heading Secular Trends). Assuming that the completeness of ascertainment of infections in the NNIS System was similar to that in CHIP, we could derive an estimate of the nationwide infection rate in the same range as the 5% figure estimated from CHIP. Although the design of these two surveillance studies limited the precision of the estimates, they gave the first consistent estimates of the order of magnitude of the problem.

One of the objectives of the Study on the Efficacy of Nosocomial Infection Control (SENIC; see Chapter 4) was to derive a more precise estimate of the nationwide nosocomial infection rate from a statistical sample of U.S. hospitals [7]. On the basis of direct estimates made in 338 randomly selected general medical and surgical hospitals with 50 beds or more and statistically derived extrapolations to groups of small and specialty hospitals, the report from the SENIC Project estimated that ≥ 2.1 million nosocomial infections occurred among the 37.7 million admissions to the 6,449 acute care U.S. hospitals in a 12-month period in 1975 to 1976 [8]. Thus, nationwide there were 5.7 nosocomial infections per 100 admissions (the infection ratio), and ~ 4.5% of hospitalized patients experienced ~ 1 nosocomial infection (the infection percentage). Given that patients stayed a total of almost 299 million days in U.S. hospitals in 1976, the incidence-density of infections was ~ 7 infections per 1,000 patient-days (see Chapter 5).

The SENIC Project applied specifically to the 6,449 acute care U.S. hospitals and did not account for a substantial number of additional institutional infections that occur each year in chronic care hospitals, long-term care facilities (see Chapter 29), children's hospitals, and federal hospitals. On the basis of the one study from which incidence rates in nursing homes can be estimated, as many as 3.3 infections per 1,000 resident-days may be occurring, an incidence-density approaching half that in acute care hospitals [8,9]. Because there are somewhat more total institutional days spent by residents in nursing homes than by patients in hospitals (~ 451 million vs. 299 million), nursing homes may be accounting for as many as 1.5 million institutional infections per year. The total number of nosocomial and other institutional infections exceeds 4 million per year, a number substantially larger than the total number of yearly hospital admissions for all cancers, accidents, and acute myocardial infarctions combined [10].

Rates by Site of Infection

Nosocomial infections involve diverse anatomic sites, but the risks of these various types of infections, and consequently their relative frequency, appear to be very similar in most hospitals. Table 30-1 lists the estimated nationwide infection rates and the relative frequency of the most common sites found in the SENIC Project [8]. These estimates, as well as those from past studies, support the following conclusions: Nosocomial urinary tract infections make up approximately two fifths of all nosocomial infections; surgical wound infections, nearly one fourth; respiratory tract infections, approximately one eighth; bacteremia, about one sixteenth; and all other types of nosocomial infections collectively account for the remainder. Although these data are expected to vary from hospital to hospital, they have been remarkably consistent in most reported studies.

TABLE 30-1. *Rates and relative frequencies of the major types of nosocomial infections, SENIC Project 1975–1976*

	Nationwide infection rates[a]	Percentage distribution
Urinary tract infection	2.39	42
Surgical wound infection	1.39[b]	24
Lower respiratory infection	0.60	11
Bacteremia[c]	0.27	5
Other sites	1.07	18
All sites	5.72	100

[a]Ratio of number of infections to number of admissions multiplied by 100 (i.e., number of nosocomial infections per 100 admissions). (Adapted from Haley RW et al. The efficacy of infection surveillance and control programs in preventing nosocomial infections in U.S. hospitals. *Am J Epidemiol* 1985;121:159.)

[b]The ratio of surgical wound infections to total operations was 2.79 per 100 operations.

[c]Includes primary and secondary bacteremias.

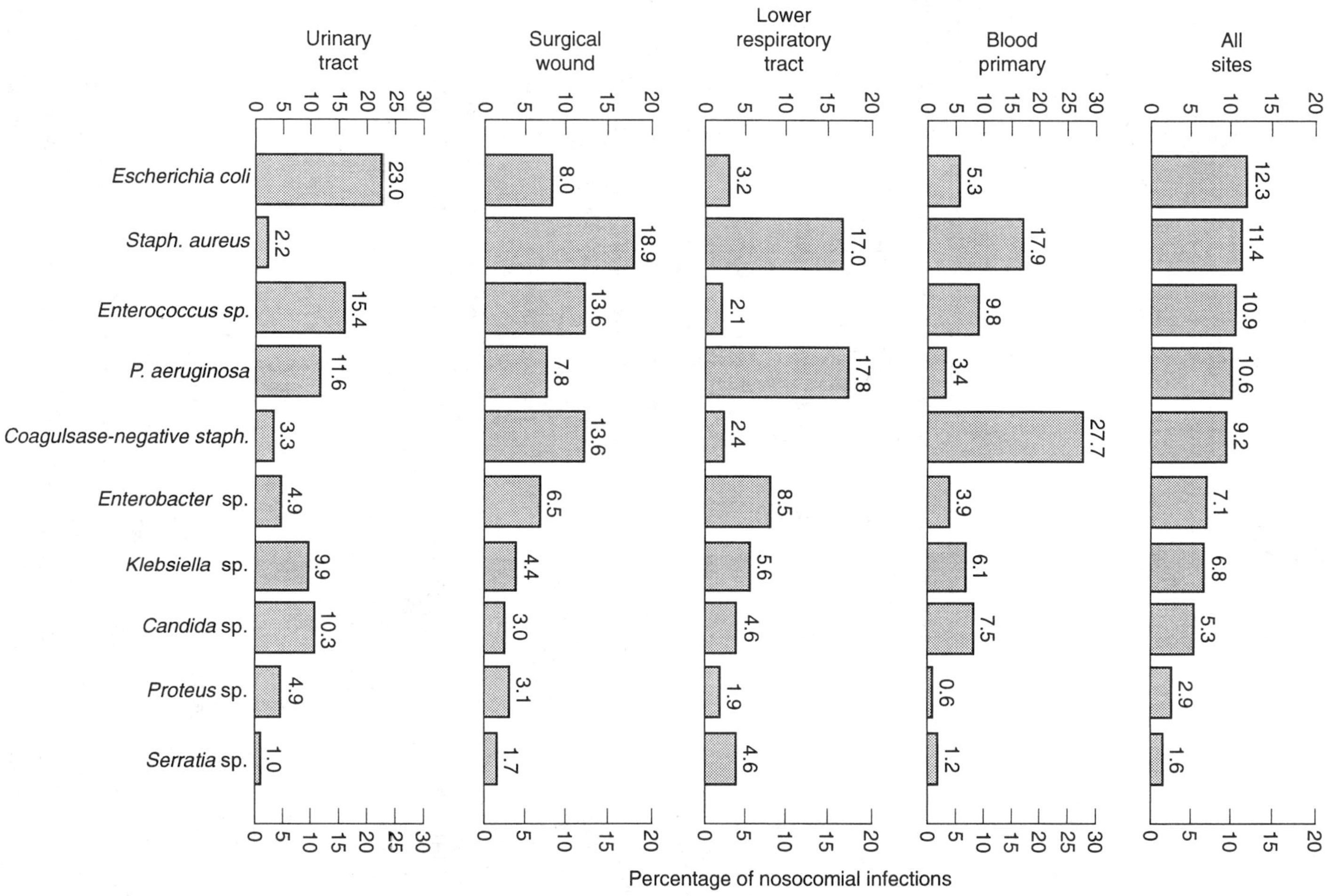

FIGURE 30-1. Percentage distribution of nosocomial infections by primary pathogen at the major sites of infection, National Nosocomial Infections Surveillance System, 1990–1994.

Rates by Pathogen

The best source of information for gaining insight into the nationwide patterns of microorganisms involved in nosocomial infections is the NNIS System. Data from the hospital-wide component of the NNIS System in the period 1990 to 1994 indicate that cultures were obtained in 84% of reported nosocomial infections, and, in 96%, at least one causative pathogen was isolated. Among these infections of known cause, 87% involved aerobic bacteria; 3%, anaerobic bacteria; 9%, fungi; and the remaining 1%, a miscellaneous group of viruses, protozoa, and parasites. On the basis of other studies [11,12], it appears that viral nosocomial infections are substantially underreported in the NNIS System, a fact that mirrors the underrecognition of viral infections in hospitals generally.

The relative frequency of the 10 most commonly isolated pathogens for each of the four major sites of infection is shown in Figure 30-1. In nosocomial urinary tract infections, *Escherichia coli* was by far the most commonly isolated pathogen, and this held true for all services except urology, where *Enterococcus* species were isolated with nearly equal frequency. The second most common urinary pathogens were *Enterococcus* species, although they were slightly exceeded by *Pseudomonas* in cardiac, orthopedic, and plastic surgery patients and by *Klebsiella* in pediatric patients. Urinary tract infections were uncommon in newborns.

In surgical wound infections, *Staphylococcus aureus* was the most common pathogen, followed by *Enterococcus* species. Enterococci were the most common pathogens in burn or trauma, general surgery, and urology patients, whereas coagulase-negative staphylococci played a predominant role in cardiac surgery and high-risk nursery patients.

In lower respiratory infections, *Pseudomonas aeruginosa* and *S. aureus* were encountered with almost equal frequency overall. *S. aureus* was the most common pathogen in burn or trauma, neurosurgery, orthopedic, pediatric, and high-risk nursery patients. *P. aeruginosa* was the most common pathogen in cardiac surgery, general surgery, plastic surgery, urology, and medical patients. Viruses were the second most common pathogen reported in pediatric and well-baby nursery patients.

Primary bacteremias are culture-documented bloodstream infections in which no other site of infection was found to be seeding the bloodstream. The microbiologic features of primary bacteremia have changed since the early 1980s, with coagulase-negative staphylococci emerging as the most significant nosocomial pathogen [13]. Coagulase-negative staphylococci made up ~ 29% of infections overall and were the most frequently reported isolate on all services except in obstetrics and well-baby nursery patients, where group B streptococci predominated. The predominance of group B streptococci in obstetrics and well-baby nursery patients may be an indication that some primary bacteremias are, in fact, secondary bacteremias in which the primary site of infection was never ascertained. *S. aureus* was the second most common cause of primary bacteremia.

On the basis of its microbiologic features, secondary bacteremia (not included in Figure 30-1) appears to be a different disease from primary bacteremia. The risk of secondary bacteremia is highest after lower respiratory infections (7.8%), surgical wound infections (6.6%), and urinary tract infections (4.4%). Complications of infection by secondary bacteremia were most common on the cardiac surgery service (9.0%), followed by general surgery service (6.5%), the high-risk nursery (6.4%), the burn or trauma service (5.6%), and the urology service (4.9%). Secondary bacteremia was least likely on the otolaryngology service (2.6%), the orthopedic service (2.5%), and the gynecology service (2.3%). Secondary bacteremia was also more likely in teaching hospitals. The organisms most commonly involved were *S. aureus* (20.9%), *E. coli* (11.3%), *P. aeruginosa* (9.6%), and *Enterococcus* species (9.2%).

Escherichia coli is the most commonly isolated pathogen from all nosocomial infections, regardless of site, because of its predominance in urinary tract infections and its substantial role in infections at all other sites. *S. aureus* is the second most commonly isolated pathogen overall, because of its frequent involvement in all types of infections except those of the urinary tract, where it is uncommonly found. The high frequency of enterococci, the third leading pathogen, has perhaps not been well enough appreciated in the past. The important role of *Pseudomonas* as the fourth most common pathogen is not surprising because of its well-known involvement in all types of nosocomial infections. More recently, coagulase-negative staphylococci have emerged as the fifth most common pathogen, largely because of their increasing importance in bloodstream infections. Improvements in surveillance and laboratory techniques are needed to clarify the roles of coagulase-negative staphylococci, anaerobic bacteria, and viruses, whose true frequencies have probably been misjudged, and perhaps more attention should be given to the endogenous mechanisms and nosocomial transmission of group B streptococci in the obstetric and newborn areas.

Patient Risk Factors

The strongest determinants of the risk of nosocomial infection are the characteristics and exposures of patients that predispose them to infection. Like the so-called chronic diseases, such as coronary heart disease and cancer, nosocomial infections arise from the complex interactions of multiple causal factors, and these factors interact differently in predisposing to the different types of infection (see Chapter 1). Much epidemiologic and clinical research has been devoted to studying the characteristics associated with the occurrence of nosocomial infection [14–25]. It has not always been clear whether the associations are truly causal, however, and these characteristics are often referred to as *risk factors*—that is, factors associated with, but not necessarily causing, infection. Undoubtedly, some of these risk factors are true causes of infection; others are only coincidentally associated with infection because they frequently follow infection or occur along with the truly causal factors. Complicating matters further is the fact that two or more risk factors often occur simultaneously in the same patient, sometimes exerting additive, or even synergistic, effects. In this respect, it is said that these risk factors are strongly intercorrelated.

To design strategies for preventing infections, it is important to try to differentiate among coincidental indicators of risk, independent causal factors, and synergistic interactions of causal factors. There have been several attempts to study multiple risk factors using modern techniques of multivariate statistical analysis. Much of this work can be illustrated by the results of analyses of risk factors performed on a group of 169,526 patients who made up a representative sample of patients admitted to acute care U.S. hospitals in 1975 to 1976 as part of the SENIC Project [19–21]. In an initial descriptive analysis, population estimates of infection rates for each of the four major types of infection were calculated within each category of exposure to between 10 and 20 separate risk factors [20]. A striking finding was that all of the risk factors were associated with infection at all four sites. At first this seems surprising, because one would not expect a direct causal association between being treated on a respirator, for example, and acquiring a urinary tract infection. The explanation, of course, is that some of the associations are indicative of direct causal relationships; others are indicative of partial causal relationships, potentiated or diminished by other concurrent influences; and others (such as that between respirators and urinary tract infection) represent largely coincidental associations (most patients on respirators also have indwelling urinary catheters that predispose them to urinary tract infection).

The two factors that appeared to exert the strongest causal influences in all four sites of infection were indicators of the degree of the patient's underlying illness: 1) in surgical patients, the duration of the patient's operation, and 2) an index of the number and type of distinct diagnoses and surgical procedures recorded (intrinsic risk index). After these, several factors were strongly associated with infections at one or two sites but not with all four. Having a combined thoracoabdominal operation was strongly associated with pneumonia and surgical wound infection; undergoing a "dirty" (or contaminated) operation was associated with surgical wound infection; having an indwelling urinary catheter was linked to urinary tract infection; being on a respirator, with pneumonia and bacteremia; previous nosocomial infection, with bacteremia; and receiving immunosuppressive therapy, with bacteremia. Examples of risk factors that had weaker associations with all four sites were age, sex, previous community-acquired infection, and length of preoperative hospitalization.

Another way of viewing these complex multivariate associations is to hypothesize that there are two general categories of causes: those that allow microorganisms access to vulnerable areas of the patient (e.g., operations, catheters, and endotracheal tubes) and those that reduce the patient's capacity for resisting the multiplication and injurious effects of the microorganisms (e.g., immunosuppressive therapy and metabolic sequelae of lengthy operations). In a later multivariate analysis of the SENIC data, this concept was tested using surgical wound infection as an example [19]. The resulting multivariate model indicated that two factors—the familiar surgical wound classification [26] and undergoing an abdominal operation—both represent the likely degree of contamination of the operative wound. These measured a portion of the risk of surgical wound infection largely separate from that measured by the other two factors—the duration of the operation and the number of diagnoses recorded. These latter two factors represent the patient's degree of susceptibility to infection. Moreover, one might infer that the degree of contamination of the wound and the patient's susceptibility were of nearly equal importance in the genesis of surgical wound infections because each of these four factors was about equally important in the multivariate model (see Chapter 7).

Multivariate modeling has demonstrated that the risk of infection is primarily determined by definable causal factors reflecting the patient's underlying susceptibility to infection or the degree to which microorganisms have access to vulnerable body sites. Modification of one or more of these factors can alter a patient's risk. Multivariate statistical models can be developed to predict accurately a patient's risk of nosocomial infection from measurable risk factors. The aggregate infection risk of a hospital, or of a subgroup of patients in a hospital—measured by its overall nosocomial infection rate—is primarily determined by the mix of patients, that is, by the causal factors present when patients are admitted and to which they are exposed in diagnosis and treatment. These conclusions form the basis for understanding much of the variation in nosocomial infection rates described in the following sections.

Rates by Service

Differences in the average risk of infection among groups have been most readily noticed in relation to the well-known differences in infection rates of different services or specialty areas. Analyses of the SENIC data showed that surgical service patients were not only at highest risk of surgical wound infections but had rates of infection for the other main sites almost three times higher than medical patients (approximately four times higher for pneumonia and approximately one and one half times higher for urinary tract infection and bacteremia). Moreover, even though surgical patients constituted only 42% of general medical and surgical patients, they accounted for 71% of nosocomial infections of the four major types (virtually all surgical wound infections, 74% of pneumonias, 56% of urinary tract infections, and 54% of bacteremias) [20]. Analysis of data collected in the NNIS System from 1990 through 1994 showed a stepwise decrease in nosocomial infection rates (calculated as the number of infections per 1,000 patient-days) by service as follows: burn or trauma service (15.0), cardiac surgery service (12.5), neurosurgery service (12.0), high-risk nursery (9.8), general surgery service (9.2), and oncology service (7.0). Lowest rates were found on the pediatric service (3.3), the well-baby nursery (1.7), and the ophthalmology service (0.6). Other investigators have quantitated the inordinately high risks of patients in special care units (see Chapters 25, 26).

Rates by Type of Hospital

It has long been apparent that overall nosocomial infection rates differ substantially from one hospital to another. In the mid-nineteenth century, Sir James Y. Simpson [27] found that the rate of death from infection of amputated extremities varied directly with the size of the hospital in which the operation was performed (with larger hospitals having higher rates), a phenomenon he called "hospitalism." The rates of surgical wound infection in the five hospitals participating in the National Research Council's prospective evaluation of ultraviolet light were found to vary from 3.2% to 11.0% [22]. The average infection rates of hospitals participating in the NNIS System were reported to vary from 1.7% in small community hospitals to more than 11% in chronic disease hospitals [6].

A multivariate analysis of the SENIC data was performed to determine what institutional characteristics of the hospitals best predicted their nosocomial infection rates. Of the many characteristics studied, those found to differentiate best were affiliation with a medical school (teaching vs. nonteaching), size of the hospital (indicated by the number of beds), type of control or ownership of the hospital (municipal, nonprofit, investor owned), and region of the country [28]. The overall nosocomial infection rates averaged 3.7% in small (< 200 beds) nonteaching hospitals, 5.1% in large (≥ 200 beds) nonteaching ones, 7.6% in nonprofit teaching hospitals, and 8.5% in the municipal teaching hospitals. These relationships tended to be consistent for each of the 4 major sites of infection. Because nonprofit teaching hospitals tend to have < 500 beds, and municipal teaching hospitals tend to have > 500, teaching hospitals could be subclassified almost as well by size as by ownership–control. In addition, within these four hospital groups, rates of urinary tract infection, surgical wound infection, and bacteremia were generally higher in the Northeast and north-central regions, whereas rates of pneumonia were higher in the West. A similar analysis of NNIS data from 1980 to 1982 found the lowest rates in nonteaching hospitals, intermediate levels in teaching hospitals with < 500 beds, and highest rates in teaching hospitals with ≥ 500 beds [7]. This relationship held consistently for infection rates at each site, on every service, and for all pathogens.

To test the hypothesis that these differences were largely due to differences in the mix of patients typically treated in the various types of hospitals, the SENIC data were additionally analyzed to try to explain the differences. Indeed, indexes of the patients' risk factors explained the greatest part of the interhospital differences and, after controlling for indexes of patients' risk factors, average length of stay, and measures of the completeness of diagnostic work-ups for infection (e.g., culturing rates), the differences in the average infection rates of the various hospital groups virtually disappeared. These findings indicate that much of the difference in observable infection rates of various types of hospitals is due to differences in the intrinsic degree of illness of their patients and related factors and, because of this, the overall infection rate per se usually gives little insight into whether the hospital's infection control efforts are effective.

Trends Over Time

The occurrence of nosocomial infections is a dynamic process. Changes are constantly occurring in the types of patients admitted to hospitals, risk factors to which they are exposed, character of the pathogens predominating in the hospital milieu, quality of patient care, thrust of infection control efforts, and other important factors. Two indicators of the dynamic nature of the problem are the seasonality of certain types of nosocomial infections and the long-term secular trends that may occur.

Seasonality

Analysis of the data from the NNIS System has repeatedly shown seasonal variations in the occurrence of nosocomial infections involving certain gram-negative rods [29–31]. The report of the 1980 to 1982 results shows clear seasonal peaks of infections in the summer and early fall with certain gram-negative bacteria, specifically *Klebsiella, Enterobacter, Serratia*, and *Acinetobacter* species as well as *P. aeruginosa*. In contrast to the seasonal occurrence of pyogenic infections in the community [32], staphylococcal and streptococcal infections show no significant seasonal variation in the hospital. There also seems to be no seasonality of infections with other common bacteria, such as *E. coli*, enterococci, *Enterobacter* species, and anaerobes. Nosocomial viral respiratory infections occur mostly during the seasons in which they occur in the community (e.g., influenza and respiratory syncytial virus infections in the winter and early spring) [11].

Secular Trends

Changes in nosocomial infection rates over time are difficult to study. In prevalence studies performed over several decades, the relatively small sample sizes have hampered the detection of secular changes. An analysis of secular trends in the NNIS System from 1970 to 1979 suggested that surgical wound infections may have decreased slightly over the decade, bacteremias may have increased, and other types of infections remained unchanged [29]. More recent analysis of hospital-wide NNIS data demonstrates a remarkable increase in nosocomial bloodstream infection rates, largely attributable to coagulase-negative staphylococci and *Candida albicans* [13]. The inability to control these analyses for other factors that could have accounted for the changes, however, rendered these findings difficult to interpret.

To address this issue, the rates from the two time periods of the SENIC Project, 1970 and 1975 to 1976, were compared after controlling for the most likely biasing factors [33]. After controlling for changes in levels of patient risk, length of stay, and completeness of ascertainment of infections, overall nosocomial infection rates in acute care hospitals were found to have increased by a statistically significant 10% over the 5-year period. Additional analysis, however, revealed three contrasting trends in different groups of hospitals. In the group that established no substantial infection surveillance and control programs, the overall infection rate increased by 18%; in the group in which moderately intensive programs were established, the rates tended to show no significant change; and in the group that established very intensive programs for preventing infections at all four of the major sites, the overall rate decreased by 36%. These findings suggest strongly that the overall nationwide trend of a 10% increase was really the result of two forces that were affecting the nationwide rate in opposite directions: 1) the continuing introduction of more invasive and immunocompromising techniques into the care of hospitalized patients, which tended to increase the infection rates; and 2) the efficacy of newly established infection surveillance and control programs, which tended to decrease them. This indicates that future secular trends in the rates of endemic nosocomial infections could be in either direction, depending strongly on the balance that hospitals achieve between technologic innovations in patient care and investments in infection surveillance and control programs.

EPIDEMIC NOSOCOMIAL INFECTIONS

Incidence, Recognition, and Control

Although many scientific articles have been written to describe individual outbreaks of nosocomial infections, very little work has been done to estimate the frequency of these epidemics. The earliest study on this subject was performed in the CDC's CHIP study in the early 1970s [1]. Among seven community hospitals participating in CHIP during 12 months in 1972 to 1973, a computerized threshold program screened the regularly reported cases of nosocomial infection for clusters of infection that might indicate an outbreak, and a CDC epidemiologist analyzed the data to eliminate purely coincidental clusters. Then CDC staff members visited the hospitals that had potential outbreaks to confirm the nature of the problem and suggest control measures, if needed. From these data it was estimated that 1 true outbreak occurred for every 10,000 hospital admissions and that outbreaks accounted for somewhere in the range of 2% of patients with nosocomial infections. Wenzel and colleagues [2] estimated that 3.7% of nosocomial infections in a large, university-affiliated referral hospital occurred in outbreaks. Although confined to a relatively small number of hospitals, these estimates appear to confirm the prevailing view that outbreaks account for a fairly small proportion of nosocomial infections.

One of the main reasons that infection control personnel are concerned about outbreaks, aside from the attention they often provoke, is that control measures can often stop outbreaks if they are recognized and investigated, thus bringing about demonstrable reductions in morbidity and mortality. In the CHIP investigations, despite the fact that the seven hospitals had very active surveillance systems, one third of the clusters had not been recognized before the CDC visit. This fact points out the difficulty of recognizing outbreaks even in the best of circumstances and suggests the usefulness of inventive computerized systems to screen surveillance data for potential epidemics (see Chapters 5, 8). It also suggests that hospitals that appear never to have outbreaks may simply be failing to recognize them.

The CHIP investigations also demonstrated that 40% of the outbreaks appeared to have resolved spontaneously, whereas the remaining 60% continued until control measures were instituted [1]. Half of the outbreaks that continued were controlled by measures taken by the hospitals' infection control staff and the other half were completely resolved only after measures suggested by the outside investigators. The rate of spontaneous resolution explains the origin of opinions against surveillance expressed by some people, but if these figures are representative of community hospitals in general—and it must be recalled that these were hospitals with very active infection surveillance systems—then a large number of outbreaks may be going unrecognized and uncontrolled, despite the advanced state of infection surveillance and control programs.

Characteristics of Epidemics

The recognition, investigation, and control of epidemics requires an understanding of the epidemiology of nosocomial outbreaks, including the most common sources, modes of transmission, and effective control measures. Each year, numerous publications describe outbreaks at individual institutions and the results of their investigation and control. From 1956 to 1995, > 445 hospital outbreak investigations were conducted by the CDC. Many factors influence the types of investigations conducted by the CDC, including which outbreaks are recognized and brought to the CDC's attention, which outbreaks are of sufficient potential public health importance (by causing significant morbidity or mortality) to warrant CDC investigation, investigator availability, and whether a CDC investigation may add to the infection control knowledge to help prevent or control similar outbreaks in the future. Thus, these outbreaks reflect problems that are unique, urgent, perplexing, or difficult to control.

The 252 hospital outbreak investigations conducted by the CDC from 1956 to 1979 have been summarized by Stamm and coworkers [34]. In the early years (1956 to 1962), the two most common problems investigated included epidemics of gastrointestinal disease, primarily due to *Salmonella* species and enteropathogenic *E. coli*, or staphylococcal infections; both types of epidemics were most frequently encountered in newborn nurseries. In the early 1960s, the investigation of staphylococcal infections abruptly decreased, which was followed in the 1970s by a decrease in the number of gastrointestinal outbreaks investigated. This probably reflects a decrease in the incidence of such outbreaks because of improved understanding of the epidemiology and control of such infections and the improved ability of hospital infection control personnel to recognize and control these outbreaks without CDC assistance. From the late 1960s until the 1980s, there was an increase in investigations of outbreaks caused by gram-negative pathogens, bacteremias, surgical wound infections, and problems related to intensive care units, newly introduced medical devices, and invasive procedures. During the 1970s, outbreaks of bacteremia were the most common problem investigated. Other problems emerging during the 1970s were outbreaks of hepatitis A and B; necrotizing enterocolitis in nurseries; sternal wound infections after open heart surgery, particularly those caused by rapidly growing mycobacteria; and nosocomial Legionnaires' disease. Also during this period, there was the emergence of the continuing problem of outbreaks due to microorganisms resistant to multiple antimicrobials, particularly aminoglycoside-resistant gram-negative bacilli and methicillin-resistant *S. aureus* (MRSA).

Outbreak investigations conducted by the CDC from 1980 to 1990 have been reviewed by Jarvis [35]. A total of 129 outbreaks were investigated; the most common sites of infection were the bloodstream or surgical wounds. Many of the bloodstream infections resulted from inadequately disinfected transducers in intensive care unit patients [36]. During this period, there were no investigations of epidemics of urinary tract infections, and < 10% of the outbreaks involved nosocomial pneumonia. From 1990 through 1994, the CDC investigated 64 outbreaks. Of these, 22 (34.3%) were bloodstream, 15 (23.4%) were respiratory, and 7 (10.9%) were surgical site infections. This probably reflects the recognition of bloodstream and surgical wound infections as serious causes of morbidity and mortality and the difficulties involved in identifying the pathogen causing nosocomial pneumonia. Furthermore, this may reflect the fact that nosocomial pneumonia most commonly results from the patient's endogenous flora or from organisms transmitted by the hands of medical personnel, whereas bloodstream or surgical wound infection clusters frequently can be traced to an invasive device, procedure, or personnel carrier (see Chapters 32, 37, 39, 44).

From 1980 to 1990, most of the investigated outbreaks were caused by bacteria. Although gram-negative organisms accounted for more than half of the outbreaks, from 1985 to 1990 outbreak investigations increasingly involved gram-positive organisms. Also during this decade, fungi, viruses, or mycobacterial outbreaks were responsible for a larger proportion of the investigations. Rapidly growing mycobacteria were recognized as causes of surgical wound infections, chronic otitis media, and infections after hemodialysis [37–39]. Outbreak investigations also implicated noninfectious causes, such as E-Ferol toxicity in neonates in intensive care units and pyrogenic reactions and chemical toxin exposures in hemodialysis centers (e.g., chloramine, hydrogen peroxide) [40–42].

From 1990 through 1994, 55 (87.6%) outbreaks were infectious in origin and 8 (12.4%) involved noninfectious complications. Of the infectious disease outbreaks, 11 (19.6%) involved nosocomial transmission of *Mycobacterium tuberculosis* [43–57], 7 (12.5%) involved fungi, and 6 (10.7%) involved viral pathogens. Sixteen (28.6%) of the infectious disease outbreaks were caused by multidrug-resistant organisms, including *M. tuberculosis*, vancomycin-resistant enterococci, and MRSA. The noninfectious disease outbreaks included aluminum toxicity in dialysis patients, carbon monoxide poisoning in surgical patients, and latex allergy [58,59].

In the 1980s, investigations probably reflected the increasing use of invasive procedures and devices and the introduction of an ever-increasing number of products. Approximately 33% of the outbreaks investigated occurred in intensive care settings, and nearly 25% of the outbreaks involved surgical patients. More than 50% of the outbreaks investigated were associated with products, procedures, or devices. For example, nine cases of *Yersinia enterocolitica* sepsis were associated with transfusion of contaminated packed red blood cells [60]. Each of these independent events was traced to mildly symptomatic or asymptomatic infection in the blood donor. Prolonged storage of the blood cells allowed proliferation of the *Y. enterocolitica*, which resulted in sepsis or endotoxin shock when the blood was transfused [61]. In another outbreak, five separate episodes of bloodstream infection or surgical wound infection were traced to extrinsic contamination of a newly introduced anesthetic agent [62,63]. The manufacturer of this soybean oil-based product, which does not contain a preservative, did not recommend refrigeration. Laboratory studies demonstrated that when contaminated with low numbers of microorganisms, rapid microbial proliferation ensued [62]. In the 1990s these trends continued, with over 30% of the outbreaks involving surgical patients and over 50% involving products, procedures, or devices. In addition, 10 (15.6%) outbreaks occurred in dialysis units, 10 (15.6%) involved human immunodeficiency virus-infected patients [58,59,64], and 8 (12.5%) involved outpatient settings, including home infusion therapy [65].

Interestingly, the sites of infection involved in epidemics investigated by the CDC differ markedly from those involved in endemic infections (Table 30-2). Of the epidemics investigated, bloodstream infections predominated, followed by surgical wounds, pneumonia, gastrointestinal infections, and meningitis. Among endemic infections, however, urinary tract infections predominate, followed by surgical wounds, pneumonia, and bloodstream infections, in that order. Similarly, the distribution of pathogens varies markedly between epidemic and endemic infections. *Pseudomonas* and *Serratia* species, *S. aureus*, and *Candida* species were the most common organisms causing epidemics, whereas *E. coli*, coagulase-negative staphylococci, and *S. aureus* predominated among endemic infections. Epidemic infections also commonly involved more unusual organisms, such as

TABLE 30-2. *Comparison of types of infections and pathogens involved in endemic and epidemic infections*

	Endemic infections[a] (%)	Epidemic investigations[b] (%)	
		January 1983–July 1990	August 1990–December 1994
Type of infection			
Urinary tract infection	37	5	<1
Surgical wound infection	17	10	10
Pneumonia	16	12	27
Cutaneous infection	2	13	2
Bacteremia	11	20	37
Meningitis	<1	5	2
Gastroenteritis	3	18	3
Hepatitis	<1	7	6
Other	12	10	13
Total	100	100	100
Pathogen			
Escherichia coli	13.8	<1	2
Enterococcus	10.7	<1	4
Staphylococcus aureus	11.2	5	9
Pseudomonas	11.2	16	<1
Proteus	3.9	<1	<1
Klebsiella	6.2	2	6
Enterobacter	6.3	4	9
Group A streptococcus	0.2	3	2
Serralia	1.7	5	<1
Salmonella	<1	2	<1
Hepatitis	<1	<1	8
Coagulase-negative staphylococci	9.7	<1	6
Candida species	7.1	5	4
Mycobacteria	<1	5	23
Other	15	48	26
Total	100	100	100

[a]National Nosocomial Infections Surveillance System, 1986–1990.

[b](Source of data for 1980–1990 adapted from Jarvis WR. Nosocomial outbreaks: The Centers for Disease Control's Hospital Infections Program experience, 1980–1990. *Am J Med* 1991;91(suppl 3B):101S.)

Ewingella americana, Tsukamurella species, *Rhodococcus bronchialis, Nocardia facinica, Ewingella hormaechei, Acremonium kiliense*, multidrug-resistant *M. tuberculosis* [44,46–49,51,54–56], mycobacteria, viruses, and fungi [35,66–69]. This probably reflects the fact that nosocomial infections vary by service or location (i.e., intensive care unit vs. nonintensive care unit) and that clusters of infections caused by unusual organisms, or usual organisms with unusual antimicrobial susceptibility patterns are more easily recognized, whereas clusters of infections caused by common organisms with unremarkable antimicrobial susceptibility patterns are probably not recognized. Also, these differences reflect the fact that unusual outbreaks are more likely to be investigated, as are outbreaks in which a common-source or personnel carrier is involved, rather than the more common problem with endemic infections whereby usual organisms are frequently transferred from patient to patient on the hands of medical personnel.

A number of selection biases influence which outbreaks are investigated by the CDC. First, a problem must be recognized at the hospital level. Once recognized, whether local expertise exists influences whether CDC assistance is requested. Second, if a problem at the hospital level is recognized and brought to the attention of the state health department, interest or expertise at the state level determines whether the state concurs with the hospital's request for CDC assistance. Because the CDC is a nonregulatory agency, any request for CDC assistance must include both an invitation by the hospital's administration and the state health department. Last, if the CDC is asked to conduct an on-site epidemiologic investigation, several factors determine the CDC's response. The likely public health importance of the problem is the most important: If an outbreak is potentially product related or is causing significant morbidity or mortality, all efforts will be made to respond. In addition, if the outbreak appears to be caused by an unusual pathogen or a common pathogen with unusual characteristics, or it involves an unusual or uncommon reservoir or mode of transmission, and if personnel are available, an on-site epidemiologic investigation by the CDC will be conducted. All investigations are conducted as collaborative efforts, and close working relationships with local, state, and federal personnel are desirable. These and other selection biases undoubtedly contribute to this profile of nosocomial epidemic problems. Of greatest value to infection control is the knowledge gained by investigation about the most common sources and modes of transmission of various pathogens in outbreaks. These data help infection control practitioners focus their preventive interventions on the areas most likely to result in containment of ongoing out-

TABLE 30-3. *Likely modes of transmission of common nosocomial outbreak pathogens*

Mode of transmission	Site or type of infection	Pathogen	Service or group
Common source	Blood	*Pseudomonas cepacia*	All
		Pseudomonas fluorescens	All
	GI	*Salmonella* species	All
	Peritonitis	*P. cepacia*	All
	Blood	*Candida parapsilosis*	All
	Blood, SWI	*Serratia marcescens*	ICU, surgical
	Blood, SWI	Mycobacteria	Hemodialysis, surgical
Human disseminator	SWI	*Staphylococcus aureus*	Surgical, obstetric
	Cutaneous	*S. aureus*	Nursery
	Hepatitis	Hepatitis A or B	All
	Pulmonary	*M. Tuberculosis*	HIV, immunocompromised
Cross-infection	SWI	*S. marcescens*	Surgical
	Pulmonary	*Xanthomonas maltophilia*	ICU
	Meningitis	*Citrobacter diversus*	Neonates
		GBS	
	Gastroenteritis	*Salmonella* species	
		Clostridium difficile	All
	Urinary tract	Gram-negative bacilli	All
	Pneumonia	Respiratory syncytial virus	Nursery
	Meningitis	Enteroviruses	Nursery
	Cutaneous	*S. aureus*	Nursery
	Hepatitis	Hepatitis A	Nursery
	SWI, pulmonary, cutaneous	MRSA	All
Airborne	Pulmonary	*Aspergillus* species	Oncology
	Pulmonary	*Mycobacterium tuberculosis*	All
	Varicella	Varicella-zoster virus	All
	Pulmonary	*Legionella*	All

GI, gastrointestinal; SWI, surgical wound infection; ICU, intensive care unit; GBS, Guillain-Barré syndrome; MRSA, methicillin-resistant *S. aureus;* HIV, human immunodeficiency virus.

breaks. In general, outbreaks can be classified into five groups according to their most likely mode of transmission: 1) common source, 2) human transmitter (carrier), 3) cross-infection (person to person), 4) airborne (microorganism traveling more than a few feet), and 5) uncertain modes of transmission. When outbreaks are classified this way, certain site–pathogen combinations, often specific to certain patient groups, become apparent (Table 30-3).

Knowledge of these site–pathogen combinations can facilitate initial investigative efforts by focusing on the most likely source or modes of transmission. For example, although nosocomial *Salmonella* infections can be transmitted from person to person, most outbreaks are traced to a common-source food (see Chapter 22). Clusters of *Pseudomonas cepacia* infections or pseudoinfections should alert infection control personnel to the possibility of contaminated solutions, including antiseptics such as povidone–iodine solution [70]. Pseudoepidemics involving endoscopy, often caused by nontuberculous mycobacteria, should lead to a review of endoscope disinfection/sterilization practices, sources of tap water, and causes of endoscope washer reservoir contamination [71]. Group A streptococcal surgical wound infections are almost always traced to a personnel carrier; carriage can involve the rectum, vagina, scalp, or other sites [72]. Intensive care unit outbreaks of gram-negative bacteremia frequently are traced to inadequately disinfected intraarterial pressure-monitoring transducers [36,73] (see Chapter 25). Clusters of *Legionella* or *Aspergillus* species pulmonary infections, particularly in the immunocompromised patient, should stimulate a search for an environmental source for airborne transmission [74] (see Chapter 32). Clusters of patients with nosocomial acquisition of *M. tuberculosis* or healthcare workers with skin test conversions should lead to an evaluation of tuberculosis patient identification and isolation practices and review of healthcare worker respiratory protective device use [44,46,48,49,51,53–55,58,59,75,76]. Recognition of patients infected or colonized with vancomycin-resistant enterococci should lead to an evaluation of isolation practices and antimicrobial use and whether current recommendations are being fully implemented [77–79].

The most common cause of both endemic and epidemic infections is cross-infection, whereby organisms are transferred from patient to patient by medical personnel. Although almost any organism can be transmitted by cross-infection, gram-negative organisms and *S. aureus* are the most commonly recognized. Nosocomial viral infections, which frequently occur in pediatric patients, also are often transmitted by cross-infection.

Multihospital Epidemics

As hospitals become more and more specialized, the possibility of multiple hospital outbreaks becomes a greater concern. This occurs most commonly by interhospital spread and less commonly through the national distribution of products that cause or predispose to infection. First, a pathogen involved in an epidemic in one hospital may be introduced into a patient population at another hospital, usually by one of three modes of transmission: 1) transfer of colonized or infected patients, particularly those with burns or decubitus ulcers [80–85]; 2) transfer of colonized or infected medical house staff [12,86]; and 3) transient colonization of hands of nurses or technicians who rotate among different hospitals [87]. Because the transfer of house staff and seriously ill patients occurs primarily among large, university-affiliated, tertiary referral hospitals, interhospital spread appears to occur most frequently in these, and less commonly among smaller community hospitals [88]; however, the increasing trend of nurses and technicians toward working in cooperatives serving several hospitals may encourage more interhospital spread. Interhospital transmission of outbreaks has been observed primarily in epidemics involving pathogens with important antimicrobial resistance patterns, such as multiply resistant *Serratia* species [87], aminoglycoside-resistant gram-negative bacilli [84], multidrug-resistant *M. tuberculosis* [44,46–49,51,52], and MRSA [85,88] (see Chapters 14–16, 41). This association could be due to the genetic colinkage of antimicrobial resistance with factors that facilitate spread. For example, strains of diverse genera that are prevalent in nosocomial infections have been shown to share the genetic information that confers resistance to important antimicrobial agents [89]. Similarly, the diversity of phage types involved in epidemiologically clear outbreaks of MRSA infections suggests the spread of genetic information among different strains that have strong predispositions to infect hospital patients. Alternatively, the association could be due merely to the fact that resistance provides a dramatic marker that increases the likelihood that an epidemic will be recognized. If so, as infection control personnel in hospitals develop more sensitive means for recognizing outbreaks and more effectively share surveillance data with their counterparts in other local hospitals (e.g., through area-wide surveillance systems supported by local health departments), interhospital transmission of infection will probably be recognized more commonly.

In the second type of multiple-hospital involvement, a widely distributed product used in patient care may cause infections in many hospitals simultaneously, because of either intrinsic contamination of the product in the factory [90] or design flaws or common usage errors that encourage in-use contamination in the hospitals [91,92] (see Chapters 39, 41). After a series of nationwide epidemics due to intrinsically contaminated products in the early 1970s, it appeared that intrinsic product contamination would become a common problem [90]. Subsequent experience has shown, however, that in-use contamination is a far more common explanation for infections related to newly introduced products and devices. Although intrinsic contamination is still recognized [60,69, 70], extrinsic contamination of products during manipulation is much more common [62,63].

In the 1980s, the widespread use of an unlicensed intravenous vitamin E preparation in neonates led to a nationwide problem of unusual illness with high fatality in neonates [41]. The recognition of this new syndrome in several neonatal intensive care units in some states led to the identification of the source and U.S. Food and Drug Administration (FDA) recall of the product. Similarly, an outbreak of bloodstream infections or surgical wound infections in five states led to the identification of a newly introduced intravenous anesthetic as the source [62,63]. Although only one species of organism was involved in each outbreak, different institutions had different pathogens, including *S. aureus, Enterobacter* species, *Moraxella* species, and *C. albicans*. On-site epidemiologic investigations at each hospital identified contamination of the product during preparation by anesthesia personnel. This led the FDA and the manufacturer to alert users of this product of the need for strict aseptic handling during preparation. The outbreaks of bloodstream infections in home infusion therapy patients demonstrate that as a new approach to patient care (i.e., home infusion) evolves, it is essential that the introduction of new techniques, such as needleless devices to reduce healthcare worker blood contacts, be evaluated for their risk of patient complications [65]. Furthermore, such studies may document the need for new infection control recommendations (e.g., more frequent end cap changes) [65]. These experiences highlight the fact that infection control personnel should remain alert to the possibility of infections or toxic reactions associated with newly introduced products or procedures. Suspicion of such problems should immediately be reported through the state health department to the CDC and the FDA.

Pseudoepidemics

Not all clusters of reported nosocomial infections constitute true epidemics of disease. In the prospective study of outbreaks in the CDC CHIP project, approximately 80% of the clusters of infection identified statistically by a computerized threshold program were judged to be coincidental, illustrating the need for epidemiologic evaluation of surveillance data to detect outbreaks [1]. More important, of those clusters that appeared to represent real outbreaks epidemiologically, approximately one third (37%) were found not to be true outbreaks after thorough investigations. Most of these pseudoepidemics were traced to systematic errors or changes in the definition of infection used, the clinical diagnosis of infection, or in reporting of infection by the infection surveillance staff. These results show the importance of using the same definitions over time, using the same surveillance methodology, and realizing that changes in the frequency of performance of various diagnostic tests will influence the detection of infections. Systematic errors in the microbiology laboratory accounted for fewer than one fourth of the pseudoepidemics. From 1959 to 1979, 11% of the CDC's hospital outbreak investigations were, in fact, pseudoepidemics. Approximately one half of these were attributed to processing errors in the microbiology laboratories [34,93]. From 1980 to 1990, 6% of outbreaks investigated were pseudoepidemics. Of these, 75% were traced to contaminated products, 12.5% were traced to environmental contamination, and 12.5% were traced to contamination of the culture during laboratory processing. From 1990 through 1994, only one (1.5%) of the epidemics investigated was a pseudoepidemic. However, this involved nontuberculous mycobacterial contamination of bronchoscopes traced to a contaminated endoscope washer reservoir [71]. Numerous similar epidemics have been published or reported to the CDC or FDA suggesting that this is a common problem.

The difference in results between the CHIP study and the CDC outbreak investigation experience is probably due to the more extensive investigation usually done by hospital personnel to rule out artifactual problems before the CDC epidemiologists undertake a formal investigation. Consequently, in the routine practice of infection control in most hospitals, most pseudoepidemics may be due to diagnostic and reporting errors, as reflected by the CHIP investigation, although truly perplexing pseudoepidemics may more often be traced to contaminated equipment or errors in the microbiology laboratory, as reflected in the CDC investigations (see Chapter 6).

ADVERSE CONSEQUENCES OF NOSOCOMIAL INFECTIONS

The reader of the scientific literature on the subject of nosocomial infections is struck by the disproportionately large number of articles on the adverse consequences—prolongation of hospital stay, extra hospital costs or charges, and deaths—of these infections. The importance of these studies stems from two factors: First, in contrast to most other hospital services, hospitals have not traditionally been able to charge patients or their insurance carriers directly for the costs of their infection surveillance and control programs; and second, it has been difficult to demonstrate how many nosocomial infections these programs prevent. Consequently, it has been necessary, or at least very helpful, in many hospitals to estimate the magnitude of adverse effects of nosocomial infections on the patients to justify the expenditures of mounting and sustaining a preventive program. The adverse outcomes most often studied are deaths and costs attributable to infection. Despite their usefulness, such estimates must be interpreted with caution because of controversies over the methods used [94–96].

Nationwide estimates of the number of deaths attributable to nosocomial infections have varied even more widely. By combining data from the SENIC Project [8] and from a concurrent assessment of mortality performed in the NNIS System [97], 19,000 deaths nationwide per year were estimated to be directly attributable to nosocomial infections and, in 58,000 more deaths, nosocomial infections contributed but were not the only cause (Table 30-4). At the other extreme, a study using multivariate logistic regression techniques, with the same drawbacks as the matched comparison approach, estimated 300,000 deaths per year nationwide attributable to nosocomial urinary tract infections alone [98]. Regardless of which estimates are used, however, the large number of deaths from nosocomial infections is a cause for concern. Counting only the 19,000 deaths directly caused by nosocomial infections—the lowest estimate derived from the NNIS System and SENIC—would place nosocomial infection just below the tenth leading cause of death in the U.S. population. These figures indicate the need for an accurate counting of nosocomial infections in our national systems for vital and health statistics [8].

Until the serious methodologic problems are solved, it seems prudent to use the more conservative estimates derived from concurrent assessments, even though they may underestimate the magnitude of the problem. Table 30-4 lists the estimates of extra days and costs derived from concurrent assessments in the SENIC pilot studies [28] and estimates of deaths derived from the NNIS System [97] and SENIC [8]. In view of the new strategies of prospective reimbursement for hospital care and the evidence for the efficacy of infection surveillance and control programs, it is likely that the direct cost reductions produced by infection control will be sufficiently obvious even if derived from the most conservative estimates (see Chapter 17).

PREVENTABILITY OF NOSOCOMIAL INFECTIONS

That large numbers of endemic as well as epidemic nosocomial infections are preventable has periodically been reaffirmed by milestone reports such as that of Semmelweis, studies on the effects of proper care of urinary catheters and respirators, and the virtual elimination of

TABLE 30-4. *Estimated extra days, extra charges, and deaths attributable to nosocomial infections annually in U.S. hospitals*

	Extra days		Extra charges			Deaths directly caused by infections		Deaths contributed by infection	
	Avg. per infection[a]	Est. U.S. total[b]	Avg. per infection (1975)[a]	Avg. per infection (1992)[c]	Est. U.S. total (1992)[b]	(%)[d]	Est. U.S. total[b]	(%)[d]	Est. U.S. total[b]
Surgical wound infection	7.3	3,726,000	$838	$3,152	$1,609,000,000	0.64	3,251	1.91	9,726
Pneumonia	5.9	1,339,000	$1,511	$5,683	$1,290,000,000	3.12	7,087	10.13	22,983
Bacteremia	7.4	762,000	$935	$3,517	$362,000,000	4.37	4,496	8.59	8,844
Urinary tract infection	1.0	903,000	$181	$680	$615,000,000	0.10	947	0.72	6,503
Other site	4.8	1,946,000	$430	$1,617	$656,000,000	0.80	3,246	2.48	10,036
All sites	4.0[e]	8,676,000	$560[e]	$2,100	$4,532,000,000	0.90[e]	19,027	2.70[e]	58,092

[a](Adapted from Haley RW, et al. Extra days and prolongation of stay attributable to nosocomial infections: A prospective interhospital comparison. *Am J Med* 1981;70:51, by pooling data from the three SENIC pilot study hospitals.)

[b]Estimated by multiplying the total number of nosocomial infections estimated in the SENIC Project (Haley RW, et al. The nation-wide nosocomial infection rate: A new need for vital statistics. *Am J Epidemiol* 1985;121:159) by the average extra days, average extra charges, or percentage of infections causing or contributing to death, respectively.

[c]Estimated from Haley RW et al. *Am J Med* 1981;70:51, by pooling data from the three hospitals and adjusting for the annual rate of inflation of hospital expenses from 1976 to 1992 (range 5.0 to 12.3%) obtained from the American Hospital Association's National Panel Survey. Estimates for inflation rates in 1991 and 1992 were projected 1987-to-1990 trend.

[d]Unpublished analyses of data reported to the National Nosocomial Infections Surveillance (NNIS) System in 1980–1982 (Hughes JM, et al. *Abstracts of the twenty-second interscience Conference on antimicrobial agents and chemotherapy,* Miami Beach, FL, October 4–6, 1982).

[e]Nationwide estimate obtained by summing the products of the site-specific estimate of the average extra days, average extra charges, or the percentage of infections causing or contributing to death, respectively, from the SENIC pilot studies (Haley RW, et al. *Am J Med* 1981;70:51), and the nationwide estimate of the proportion of nosocomial infections affecting the site from the main SENIC analysis (Haley RW, et al. *Am J Epidemiol* 1985;121:159).

epidemic bacteremia caused by intrinsic contamination of commercial intravenous solutions. Yet when a representative sample of infection control program heads were asked to estimate the percentage of nosocomial infections occurring in U.S. hospitals that are preventable, the responses varied from 1% to 100%, with a mean of approximately 50%; the program heads who had served in their positions longer and who were more knowledgeable about infection control tended to give lower estimates [99]. There are at least two reasons for this lack of agreement among those working most closely with the problem. First, it is difficult to demonstrate that infections have been prevented or to infer whether active infections were preventable [100]. Second, because new risk factors for infection are constantly appearing, necessary control measures are continually evolving, and ability to manage the patient care behavior of hospital personnel is changing, the true percentage of infections that are preventable probably changes from time to time.

Consequently, the only meaningful way of framing the preventability question is to ask what percentage of nosocomial infections can be prevented by maintaining an intensive infection surveillance and control program that continually adjusts to the new risks while attempting to manage patient care behavior. Because this was precisely the question framed in the SENIC Project, there is an approximate answer. Among U.S. hospitals in the 1970s, approximately one third of all nosocomial infections were preventable by maintaining infection surveillance and control programs with particular characteristics [33] (see Chapter 4). The fact that the approaches found to be effective were general preventive strategies aimed at managing infection control (i.e., surveillance and control programs), rather than individual preventive practices (e.g., catheter care), suggests that the SENIC estimate of preventability will remain reasonably accurate for the foreseeable future. As new infection control guidelines are published, it is important that they be implemented so that prevention efforts are maximized [79,101,102,103].

REFERENCES

1. Haley RW, et al. How frequent are outbreaks of nosocomial infection in community hospitals? *Infect Control* 1985;6:233.
2. Wenzel RP, et al. Hospital acquired infections in intensive care unit patients: an overview with emphasis on epidemics. *Infect Control* 1983;4:371.
3. Kislak JW, Eickhoff TC, Finland M. Hospital-acquired infections and antibiotic usage in the Boston City Hospital. *N Engl J Med* 1964; 271:834.
4. Eickhoff TC, Brachman PS, Bennett JV, Brown JF. Surveillance of nosocomial infections in community hospitals: I. surveillance methods, effectiveness, and initial results. *J Infect Dis* 1969;120:305.
5. Thoburn R, Fekety FR, Cluff LE, Melvin VB. Infections acquired by hospitalized patients. *Arch Intern Med* 1968;121:1.
6. Bennett JV, Scheckler WE, Maki DG, Brachman PS. Current national patterns: United States. In: *Proceedings of the International Conference on Nosocomial Infections, August 3–6, 1970*. Chicago: American Hospital Association, 1971:42–49.
7. Haley RW, Quade DH, Freeman HE, CDC SENIC Planning Committee. Study on the efficacy of nosocomial infection control (SENIC Project): summary of study design. *Am J Epidemiol* 1980;111:472.
8. Haley RW, et al. The nation-wide nosocomial infection rate: a new need for vital statistics. *Am J Epidemiol* 1985;121:159.
9. Magnussen MH, Robb SS. Nosocomial infections in a long-term care facility. *Am J Infect Control* 1980;2:12.
10. United States National Center for Health Statistics. *Utilization patterns and financial characteristics of nursing homes in the United States: 1977 National Nursing Home Survey*. (Data from the National Health Survey, Series 13, No. 53. DHHS publication no. [PHS] 81,1714). Hyattsville, MD National Center for Health Statistics, 1981.
11. Hall CB. Nosocomial viral respiratory infections: perennial weeds on pediatric wards. *Am J Med* 1981;70:670.
12. Valenti, W.M., et al. Nosocomial viral infections: epidemiology and significance. *Infect Control* 1980;1:33.
13. Banerjee SN, et al. Secular trends in nosocomial primary bloodstream infections in the United States, 1980–89. *Am J Med* 1991;91(Suppl 3B):86S.
14. Cruse PJE, Foord R. The epidemiology of wound infection: a 10-year prospective study of 62,939 wounds. *Surg Clin North Am* 1980; 60:27.
15. Dukes C. Urinary infections after excision of the rectum: their cause and prevention. *Proc R Soc Med* 1928;22:259.
16. Ehrenkrantz NJ. Surgical wound infection occurrence in clean operations: risk stratification for interhospital comparisons. *Am J Med* 1981;70:909.
17. Freeman J, McGowan JE Jr. Risk factors for nosocomial infection. *J Infect Dis* 1978;138:811.
18. Garibaldi RA, et al. Risk factors for predicting postoperative pneumonia. *Am J Med* 1981;70:677.
19. Haley RW, et al. Identifying patients at high risk of surgical wound infection: a simple multivariate index of patient susceptibility and wound contamination. *Am J Epidemiol* 1985;121:206.
20. Haley RW, et al. Nosocomial infections in U.S. hospitals, 1975–1976: estimated frequency by selected characteristics of patients. *Am J Med* 1981;70:947.
21. Hooton TM, et al. The joint associations of multiple risk factors with the occurrence of nosocomial infection. *Am J Med* 1981;70:960.
22. Howard JM, et al. Postoperative wound infections: the influence of ultraviolet irradiation of the operating room and of various other factors. *Ann Surg* 1964;160(Suppl):1.
23. Lidwell OM. Sepsis in surgical wounds: multiple regression analysis applied to records of post-operative hospital sepsis. *Journal of Hygiene (Cambridge)* 1961;59:259.
24. McCabe WR, Jackson GC. Gram-negative bacteremia: I. etiology and ecology. *Arch Intern Med* 1962;110:847.
25. Stamm WE, Martin SM, Bennett JV. Epidemiology of nosocomial infections due to gram-negative bacilli: aspects relevant to development and use of vaccines. *J Infect Dis* 1977;163(Suppl):S151.
26. Altemeir WA, et al, eds. *Manual on the control of infection in surgical patients*. Philadelphia: JB Lippincott, 1976:29–30.
27. Simpson JY. Our existing system of hospitalism and its effect: part I. *Edinburgh Medical Journal* 1869;14:816.
28. Haley RW, Morgan WM, Culver DH, Schaberg DR. *Differences in nosocomial infection rates by type of hospital: the influence of patient mix and diagnostic medical practices*. Presented at the Interscience Conference on Antimicrobial Agents and Chemotherapy, Miami, Florida, October 4, 1982.
29. Allen JR, Hightower AW, Martin SM, Dixon RE. Secular trends in nosocomial infections: 1970–79. *Am J Med* 1981;70:389.
30. Hughes JM, et al. Nosocomial infection surveillance, 1980–1982. *MMWR Morb Mortal Wkly Rep* 1983;32:1SS.
31. Retailliau HF, et al. *Acinetobacter calcoaceticus*: a nosocomial pathogen with an unusual seasonal pattern. *J Infect Dis* 1979;139:371.
32. Benenson AS. Staphylococcal disease. In: Benenson AS, ed. *Control of communicable diseases in man*. 15th ed. Washington, DC: American Public Health Association, 1990:358–366.
33. Haley RW, et al. The efficacy of infection surveillance and control programs in preventing nosocomial infections in U.S. hospitals. *Am J Epidemiol* 1985;121:182.
34. Stamm WE, Weinstein RA, Dixon RE. Comparison of endemic and epidemic nosocomial infections. *Am J Med* 1981;70:393.
35. Jarvis WR. Nosocomial outbreaks: the Centers for Disease Control's

Hospital Infections Program experience, 1980–1990. *Am J Med* 1991; 91(Suppl 3B):101S.
36. Beck-Sague CM, Jarvis WR. Epidemic bloodstream infection associated with pressure transducers: a persistent problem. *Infect Control Hosp Epidemiol* 1989;10:54.
37. Lowry PW, et al. *Mycobacterium chelonae* infection among patients receiving high-flux dialysis in a hemodialysis clinic, California. *J Infect Dis* 1990;161:85.
38. Lowry PW, et al. *Mycobacterium chelonae* causing otitis media in the ear-nose-and-throat practice. *N Engl J Med* 1988;319:978.
39. Safranek TJ, et al. *Mycobacteria chelonae* wound infections after plastic surgery employing contaminated gentian violet skin marking solution. *N Engl J Med* 1987;317:197.
40. Gordon SM, Tipple M, Bland LA, Jarvis WR. Pyrogenic reactions associated with the use of processed disposable hollow fiber hemodialyzers. *JAMA* 1988;260:2077.
41. Martone WJ, et al. Illness with fatalities in premature infants: association with an intravenous vitamin E preparation. *Pediatrics* 1986; 78:591.
42. Tipple MA, Bland LA, Favero MS, Jarvis WR. Investigation of hemolytic anemia after chloramine exposure in a dialysis center. *Trans Am Soc Artif Intern Organs* 1988;34:1060.
43. Dooley SW, Villarino ME, Lawrence M, et al. Tuberculosis in a hospital unit for patients infected with the human immunodeficiency virus (HIV): evidence of nosocomial transmission. *JAMA* 1992;267: 2632–2634.
44. Edlin BR, Tokars JI, Grieco MH, et al. An outbreak of multidrug-resistant tuberculosis among hospitalized patients with the acquired immunodeficiency syndrome: epidemiologic studies and restriction fragment length polymorphism analysis. *N Engl J Med* 1992;326: 1514–1522.
45. Tokars JI, Jarvis WR, Edlin BR, et al. Tuberculin skin testing of hospital employees during an outbreak of multidrug-resistant tuberculosis in human immunodeficiency virus (HIV)-infected patients. *Infect Control Hosp Epidemiol* 1992;13:509–510.
46. Beck-Sague CM, Dooley SW, Hutton MD, et al. Outbreak of multidrug-resistant tuberculosis among persons with HIV infection in an urban hospital: transmission to staff and patients and control measures. *JAMA* 1992;268:1280–1286.
47. Pearson ML, Jereb JA, Frieden TR, et al. Nosocomial transmission of multidrug-resistant *Mycobacterium tuberculosis*: a risk to hospitalized patients and health-care workers. *Ann Intern Med* 1992;117: 191–196.
48. Coronado VG, Valway S, Finelli L, et al. Nosocomial transmission of multidrug-resistant *Mycobacterium tuberculosis* among persons with human immunodeficiency virus infection [Abstract S50]. In: *Abstracts of the third annual meeting of the Society for Hospital Epidemiology of America*; Chicago, April 18–20, 1993.
49. Coronado VG, Beck-Sague CM, Hutton MD, et al. Transmission of multidrug-resistant *Mycobacterium tuberculosis* among persons with human immunodeficiency virus infection in an urban hospital: epidemiologic and restriction fragment length polymorphism analysis. *J Infect Dis* 1993;168:1052–1055.
50. Jarvis WR. Nosocomial transmission of multidrug-resistant *Mycobacterium tuberculosis*. *Res Microbiol* 1993;144:117–122.
51. Coronado VG, Beck-Sague CM, Pearson ML, et al. Multidrug-resistant *Mycobacterium tuberculosis* among patients with HIV infection. *Infectious Disease and Clinical Practice* 1993;2:297–302.
52. Jereb KA, Klevens RM, Privett TD, et al. Tuberculosis in healthcare workers at a hospital with an outbreak of multidrug-resistant *Mycobacterium tuberculosis*. *Arch Intern Med* 1995;155:854–859.
53. Zaza S, Blumberg HM, Beck-Sague C, et al. Nosocomial transmission of *Mycobacterium tuberculosis*: role of healthcare workers outbreak propagate. *J Infect Dis* 1995;172:1542–1549.
54. Maloney SA, Perason ML, Gordon MT, et al. Efficacy of control measures in preventing nosocomial transmission of multidrug-resistant tuberculosis to patients and healthcare workers. *Ann Intern Med* 1995;122:90–95.
55. Wenger PN, Otten J, Breeden A, et al. Control of nosocomial transmission of multidrug-resistant *Mycobacterium tuberculosis* among healthcare workers and HIV-infected patients. *Lancet* 1995;345: 235–240.
56. Stroud LA, Tokers JI, Grieco MH, et al. Evaluation of infection control measures in preventing the nosocomial transmission of multidrug-resistant *Mycobacterium tuberculosis* in a New York City hospital. *Infect Control Hosp Epidemiol* 1995;16:141–147.
57. Jarvis WR. Nosocomial transmission of multidrug-resistant *Mycobacterium tuberculosis*. *Am J Infect Control* 1995;23:146–151.
58. Kelly JK, Pearson ML, Kump VP, et al. Epidemiologic features, risk factors and latex hypersensitivity in patients with spina bifida who develop anaphylactic reactions during general anesthesia. *Am J Clin Allerg* 1994;94:53–61.
59. Burwen DR, Olsen SM, Bland LA, et al. Epidemic aluminum intoxication in hemodyalis patients traced to use of an aluminum pump. *Kidney Int* 1995;48:469–474.
60. Tipple MA, et al. Sepsis associated with transfusion of red blood cells contaminated with *Yersinia enterocolitica*. *Transfusion* 1990;30:207.
61. Arduino MJ, et al. Growth and endotoxin production of *Yersinia enterocolitica* and *Enterobacter agglomerans* in packed erythrocytes. *J Clin Microbiol* 1989;27:1483.
62. Centers for Disease Control and Prevention. Postsurgical infections associated with an extrinsically contaminated intravenous anesthetic agent. *MMWR Morb Mortal Wkly Rep* 1990;39:426.
63. Bennett SN, McNeil MM, Bland LA, et al. Multiple outbreaks of postoperative infections traced to extrinsic contamination of an intravenous anesthetic, propofol. *N Engl J Med* 1995;333:147–154.
64. Velandia M, Fridkin SK, Cardenas V, et al. Transmission of HIV in dialysis centre. *Lancet* 1995;345:1417–1422.
65. Danzig LE, Short LJ, Collins K, et al. Bloodstream infections associated with a needleless intravenous infusion. *JAMA* 1995;273: 1862–1864.
66. McNeil MM, et al. *Ewingella americana*: recurrent pseudobacteremia from a persistent environmental reservoir. *J Clin Microbiol* 1987; 25:498.
67. Richet HM, et al. A cluster of *Rhodococcus* (*Gordona*) *bronchialis* sternal wound infections after coronary-artery bypass surgery. *N Engl J Med* 1991;324:104.
68. Richet HM, McNeil MM, Edwards MC, Jarvis WR. Cluster of *Malassezia furfur* pulmonary infections in infants in a neonatal intensive care unit. *J Clin Microbiol* 1989;27:1197.
69. Tokars JI, et al. *Mycobacterium gordonae* pseudoinfection associated with a contaminated antimicrobial solution. *J Clin Microbiol* 1990;28: 2765.
70. Centers for Disease Control and Prevention. Contaminated povidone–iodine solution Texas. *MMWR Morb Mortal Wkly Rep* 1989;38:133.
71. Maloney S, Welbel S, Daves B, et al. *Mycobacterium abscessus* pseudoinfection traced to an automated endoscope washer: utility of epidemiologic and laboratory investigation. *J Infect Dis* 1994;169: 1166–1169.
72. Mastro TD, et al. An outbreak of surgical-wound infections due to group A streptococcus carried on the scalp. *N Engl J Med* 1990; 323:968.
73. Beck-Sague CM, et al. Epidemic bacteremia due to *Acinetobacter baumanni* in five intensive care units. *Am J Epidemiol* 1990;132:723.
74. Weems JJ, et al. *Candida parapsilosis* fungemia associated with parenteral nutrition and contaminated blood pressure transducers. *J Clin Microbiol* 1987;25:1029.
75. Centers for Disease Control and Prevention. Guidelines for preventing the transmission of *Mycobacterium tuberculosis* in health-care facilities, 1994. *MMWR Morb Mortal Wkly Rep* 1994;43:RR1–RR13.
76. Sinkowitz R, Fridkin S, Manangan L, et al. *Status of tuberculosis infection control programs at U.S. hospitals, 1989–1992*. Presented at the annual meeting of the Association for Professionals in Infection Control and Epidemiology, Inc., Las Vegas, Nevada, June 4–8, 1995.
77. Shay DK, Maloney SA, Montecalvo M, et al. Epidemiology and mortality risk of vancomycin-resistant enterococcal bloodstream infections. *J Infect Dis* (in press).
78. Morris G, Shay DK, Hebden JN, et al. Enterococci resistant to multiple antimicrobial agents including vancomycin. *Ann Intern Med* 1995; 123:250–259.
79. Centers for Disease Control and Prevention. Notice of a proposed report from the Hospital Infection Control Practices Advisory Committee: preventing the spread of vancomycin resistance [HICPAC-VRE]. *Federal Register* 1994;59(94):25758–25763.
80. Price EH, Brain A, Dickson JAS. An outbreak of infection with a gentamicin- and methicillin-resistant *Staphylococcus aureus* in a neonatal unit. *J Hosp Infect* 1980;1:221.
81. Sapico FL, Mongomerie JZ, Canawati HN, Aeilts G. Methicillin-

resistant *Staphylococcus aureus* bacteriuria. *Am J Med Sci* 1980;281:101.
82. Saraglou G, Cromer M, Bisno AL. Methicillin-resistant *Staphylococcus aureus*: interstate spread of nosocomial infections with emergence of gentamicin–methicillin-resistant strains. *Infect Control* 1980;1:81.
83. Shanson DC. Antibiotic-resistant *Staphylococcus aureus*. *J Hosp Infect* 1981;2:11.
84. Weinstein RA, Kabins SA. Strategies for prevention and control of multiple drug resistant nosocomial infection. *Am J Med* 1981;70:449.
85. Winn RE, et al. Epidemiological, bacteriological, and clinical observations on an interhospital outbreak of nafcillin-resistant *Staphylococcus aureus*. *Current Chemotherapy* 1979;2:1096.
86. Shanson DC, McSwiggan DA. Operating theatre-acquired infection with a gentamicin-resistant strain of *Staphylococcus aureus*: outbreaks in two hospitals attributable to one surgeon. *J Hosp Infect* 1980;1:171.
87. Schaberg DR, et al. An outbreak of nosocomial infection due to multiply resistant *Serratia marcescens*: evidence of interhospital spread. *J Infect Dis* 1976;134:181.
88. Haley RW, et al. The emergence of methicillin-resistant *Staphylococcus aureus* infections in United States hospitals: possible role of the house staff patient transfer circuit. *Ann Intern Med* 1982;97:297.
89. Schaberg DR, et al. Evolution of antimicrobial resistance and nosocomial infection: lessons from the Vanderbilt experience. *Am J Med* 1981;70:445.
90. Maki DG, Rhame FS, Mackel DC, Bennett JV. Nationwide epidemic of septicemia caused by contaminated intravenous products: I. epidemiologic and clinical features. *Am J Med* 1976;60:471.
91. Centers for Disease Control and Prevention. Nosocomial bacteremia from intravascular pressure monitoring systems. In: *National nosocomial infections study report*. Atlanta: Centers for Disease Control, 1977 (issued 1979):31–36.
92. Donowitz LG, Marsick FJ, Hoyt JW, Wenzel RP. *Serratia marcescens* bacteremia from contaminated pressure transducers. *JAMA* 1979;242:1749.
93. Weinstein RA. Pseudoepidemics in hospital. *Lancet* 1977;2:862.
94. Clark S. Sepsis in surgical wounds with particular reference to *Staphylococcus aureus*. *Br J Surg* 1957;44:592.
95. Finkler SA. The distinction between costs and charges. *Ann Intern Med* 1982;96:102.
96. Haley RW, Schaberg DR, Von Allmen SD, McGowan JE Jr. Estimating the extra charges and prolongation of hospitalization due to nosocomial infections: a comparison of methods. *J Infect Dis* 1980;141:248.
97. Hughes JM, et al. Mortality Associated with nosocomial infections in the United States, 1975–1981. In: *Abstracts of the twenty-second interscience conference on antimicrobial agents and chemotherapy,* Miami Beach, Florida, October 4–6, 1982. Washington, DC: American Society for Microbiology, 1982:189.
98. Platt R, et al. Mortality associated with nosocomial urinary tract infection. *N Engl J Med* 1982;307:637.
99. Haley RW. The "hospital epidemiologist" in U.S. hospitals, 1976–1977: a description of the head of the infection surveillance and control program. *Infect Control* 1980;1:21.
100. McGowan JE Jr, Parrott PL, Duty VP. Nosocomial bacteremia: potential for prevention of procedure-related cases. *JAMA* 1977;237:2737.
101. Centers for Disease Control and Prevention. Guideline for prevention of nosocomial pneumonia [Tablan]. *Respiratory Care* 1994;29:1191–1236.
102. Centers for Disease Control and Prevention. Management of patients with suspected viral hemorrhagic fever [Bolyard-Ebola]. *MMWR Morb Mortal Wkly Rep* 1988;37(S-3):1–16.

Hospital Infections, Fourth Edition,
edited by John V. Bennett and Philip S. Brachman.
Lippincott–Raven Publishers, Philadelphia © 1998

CHAPTER 31

Urinary Tract Infections

Walter E. Stamm

INCIDENCE

According to data from numerous hospitals [1–3] and from multihospital collaborative studies (see Chapter 5), nosocomial urinary tract infections have consistently been responsible for 35% to 45% of all hospital-acquired infections. Thus approximately 2 per 100 patients admitted to acute care hospitals in the United States, or more than 0.8 million patients per annum, acquire nosocomial bacteriuria. In the National Nosocomial Infections Surveillance (NNIS) System, urinary tract infections have consistently accounted for 40% of all hospital-acquired infections, with little change evident over the period 1970 to 1995. In this survey, the proportion of nosocomial bacteriuria cases associated with or contributing to mortality was < 3% (see Chapter 30).

ENDEMIC VERSUS EPIDEMIC INFECTIONS

Endemic acquisition accounts for most nosocomial urinary tract infections, but numerous examples of epidemic transmission have been reported [4,5]. Epidemics of nosocomial bacteriuria have resulted from inadequately disinfected cystoscopes, nonsterile irrigating solutions used on multiple patients, contaminated disinfectants in catheter insertion trays, and, most commonly, person-to-person transmission on crowded hospital wards where aseptic catheter care practices were not being used [4,5]. Frequent catheter irrigation appeared to be an important causal factor in several epidemics. Multiply drug-resistant strains of *Serratia, Proteus, Klebsiella*, and *Pseudomonas* possessing unique antimicrobial susceptibility patterns have afforded opportunities to trace the epidemiology of nosocomial urinary tract infections in the epidemic setting. Most often, epidemic investigations have demonstrated transmission of organisms from one catheterized patient to another by the hands of hospital personnel. In several epidemics, patients with unrecognized asymptomatic bacteriuria lasting for weeks or even months served as an important reservoir, with temporal and spatial clustering of subsequent cases in proximity to these source patients.

Most likely, a proportion of infections classified as endemic actually result from clusters or microepidemics of cross-infection on hospital wards. Using tertiary marker systems (e.g., pyocin typing, serotyping, and phage typing) to trace cross-infection attributable to common organisms such as *Escherichia coli*, Schaberg and coworkers [6] demonstrated that ~ 15% of endemic nosocomial infections occur in clusters suggestive of cross-infection. *Pseudomonas* and *Serratia* infections were most often clustered, and *E. coli* infections least often. Thus, attention to the same factors that prevent or terminate epidemics of nosocomial bacteriuria (see the section on Prevention) presumably would prevent some endemic infections as well.

RISK FACTORS

Nearly all nosocomial urinary tract infections occur in patients with indwelling urinary catheters (~ 80%) or after other types of transient urologic instrumentation (nearly 20%). Specific host factors associated with an increased risk of infection during or after instrumentation include female gender, older age, and an increasing degree of underlying illness (Table 31-1). The risk of development of nosocomial bacteriuria in women exceeds the risk in men by approximately twofold in each decade of life [7,8], but men more often manifest secondary bacteremia. For both men and women, the risk of catheter-associated bacteriuria increases with age [7,8]. In addi-

W. E. Stamm: Division of Allergy and Infectious Diseases, University of Washington School of Medicine, Seattle, Washington 98195.

TABLE 31-1. *Risk factors associated with infection during catheterization*

Alterable factors	Unalterable factors
Indications for catheterization	Female gender
Length of catheterization	Older age
Catheter care techniques	Severe underlying illness
Type of drainage system	Meatal colonization
Receipt of antimicrobials	

tion, 95% of deaths and 83% of bacteremic episodes occur in patients older than 50 years [8].

In addition to host factors (which, for the most part, cannot be altered), the risk of urinary infection relates directly to the type and duration of urologic instrumentation. After a single in-and-out catheterization, between 1% and 20% of patients acquire bacteriuria [9,10]; lower rates occur in healthy outpatients and higher rates in older hospitalized patients. Indwelling urethral catheters draining into an open collecting vessel result in bacteriuria in 100% of patients within 4 days [11]. With the sterile closed collecting systems used in most hospitals today, bacteriuria occurs on the average in 10% to 25% of catheterized patients [12–14]. In hospitals with active prevention programs, rates of < 10% have been reported (see Chapter 5). In prospective studies carried out in general hospital populations between 1966 and 1995 [12,15–21], there has been an apparent trend toward a reduced prevalence of catheter-associated bacteriuria (Table 31-2). Many factors may account for this decrease, including increased antimicrobial use in catheterized patients, decreasing lengths of catheterization and hospitalization, and more effective infection control efforts. The per-day risk for development of bacteriuria appears comparable throughout catheterization (3% to 6%), but the cumulative risk increases with duration of catheterization [22,23]. Thus, ~ 50% of hospitalized patients catheterized longer than 7 to 10 days contract bacteriuria [13,22] (Figure 31-1).

Bacteriuria develops more frequently in patients not receiving systemic antimicrobials and in patients in whom catheter care violations have occurred [16,24].

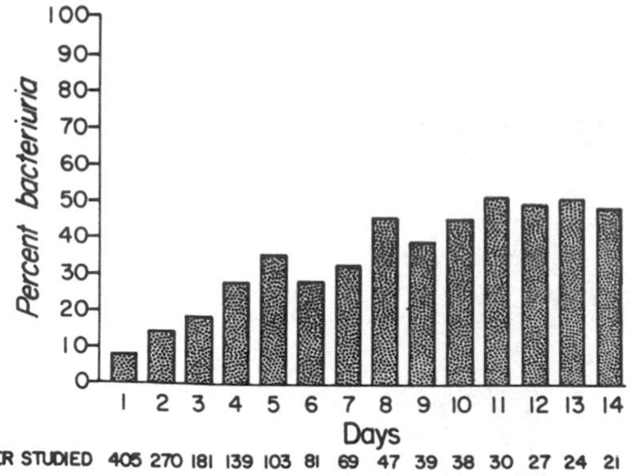

FIGURE 31-1. Percentage of catheterized patients with bacteriuria by day of catheterization. (From Garibaldi RA, et al. Factors predisposing to bacteriuria during indwelling urethral catheterization. *N Engl J Med* 1974;291:216. Reprinted by permission of *The New England Journal of Medicine.*)

ETIOLOGY

Aerobic gram-negative rods account for most catheter-associated urinary tract infections. In data collected by the NNIS System [25] (Table 31-3), Enterobacteriaceae, pseudomonads, and enterococci accounted for most of the infections, both hospital-wide and in the intensive care unit setting. Increasingly, the aerobic gram-negative rods causing nosocomial bacteriuria have been characterized by multiple antimicrobial resistance, often mediated by transmissible plasmids [26] (see Chapter 16). Candidal infections of the catheterized urinary tract appear to have increased since the early 1980s, and now predominate as the most common cause of nosocomial urinary tract infection in the intensive care unit setting.

The relative proportion of infections accounted for by an individual species, as well as their antimicrobial susceptibility patterns, vary widely from hospital to hospital and fluctuate with time in each hospital. In two studies, *E. coli* and *Proteus* species accounted for a progressively smaller percentage of nosocomial urinary tract infections as the period of hospitalization and catheterization lengthened [8,27]. Conversely, *Serratia* and *Pseudomo-*

TABLE 31-2. *Prevalence of catheter-associated urinary tract infections in prospective studies, 1966–1990*

Reference	Prevalence (%)
Kunin 1966 [17]	23
Finkelberg 1969 [12]	21
Garibaldi 1974 [15]	23
Warren 1978 [20]	17
Platt 1983 [18]	9
Thompson 1984 [19]	10
Johnson 1990 [16]	10
Riley 1995 [20a]	12

TABLE 31-3. *Pathogens causing nosocomial urinary tract infections*

Hospital-wide		Intensive care	
Pathogen	(%)	Pathogen	(%)
E. coli	26	Candida spp	25
Enterococci	16	E. coli	18
P. aeruginosa	12	Enterococci	13
Candida spp	9	P. aeruginosa	11
K. pneumoniae	7	Enterobacter spp	6

(Adapted from Jarvis WR, Martone WJ. Predominant pathogens in hospital infections. *J Antimicrob Chemother* 1992; 29:19–24.)

nas aeruginosa accounted for a progressively greater proportion of infection as hospitalization increased. These observations suggest that a proportion of catheter-associated infections are, in fact, not newly acquired but may represent recognition of previous covert bacteriuria after insertion of a urinary catheter.

PATHOGENESIS

Occasionally, nosocomial urinary tract infections result from direct introduction of urethral microorganisms at the time of catheterization, other instrumentation (usually cystoscopy), or surgery. Based on time of onset, however, most catheter-associated infections arise later in the period of catheterization. Microorganisms causing these infections enter the catheterized urinary tract either through the lumen of the catheter (intraluminal route) or along its external surface in the mucous sheath between the catheter and urethral mucosa (transurethral route; Figure 31-2). Women appear to be at greater risk than men of transurethral infection. In one study, approximately two thirds of women in whom catheter-associated bacteriuria developed were shown to have previous urethral and rectal colonization with their infecting strain, compared with only one third of men [28]. Thus, the pathogenesis of catheter-associated infections in many women resembles the pathogenesis of non–catheter-associated infections. Studies of community-acquired bacteriuria in women suggest that fecal organisms establish introital, vaginal, and urethral colonization before urinary tract infection with these strains occurs [29,30]. Because only one third of men in whom catheter-associated bacteriuria develops can be demonstrated to have antecedent urethral and rectal colonization, the urethral route of entry may be less important in men. In either sex, however, establishment of urethral colonization with a gram-negative rod apparently confers an increased risk of subsequent infection. Garibaldi and coworkers [15] showed that the increased risk of subsequent nosocomial bacteriuria associated with a positive meatal culture was approximately fourfold in women and twofold in men. However, periurethral colonization is not invariably followed by bacteriuria, and, when bacteriuria does occur, it is often > 72 hours after the establishment of periurethral colonization [31].

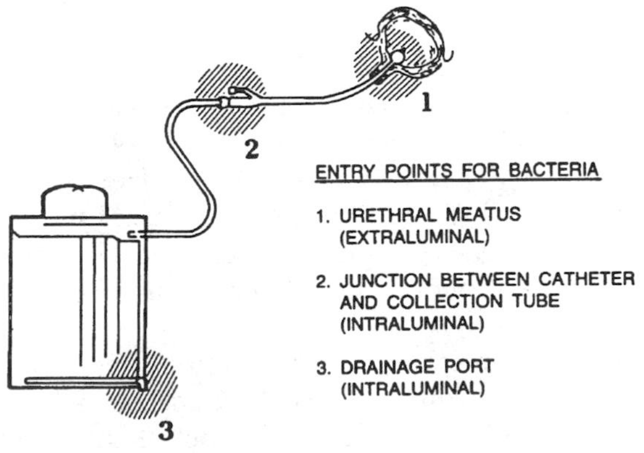

FIGURE 31-2. Entry points for bacteria causing catheter-associated urinary tract infection.

Bacteriuria may also result from microorganisms that enter the collecting system and ascend through the lumen of the urinary catheter into the bladder (intraluminal route). In studies assessing this mode of entry, ~ 15% to 20% of infected patients can be demonstrated to have their infecting organism in the collecting bag before entry into the bladder [15,31,32]. Retrograde spread of the organism from the collecting bag to the bladder occurs within 24 to 48 hours in nearly all such patients [15]. Once in the bladder, small numbers of microorganisms (e.g., 100 colony-forming units [cfu] per milliliter) increase to large numbers (> 100,000 cfu/ml) in < 24 hours [33]. Thus contamination of the collecting bag or introduction of organisms by disconnection of the distal catheter and proximal collection tube can allow entry of organisms that produce nosocomial bacteriuria. Rarely, nosocomial bacteriuria arises secondary to hematogenous seeding of the genitourinary tract or as a complication of surgical procedures involving the urinary tract or adjacent structures.

Studies since the mid-1980s have demonstrated an important role for attachment and growth of bacteria on the inner surface of the catheter in the pathogenesis of catheter-associated urinary tract infection [34–37]. Two populations of bacteria exist in the catheterized urinary tract, those growing within the urine itself (planktonic growth) and those growing on the surface of the catheter (biofilm growth). The growth of a bacterial biofilm on the urinary catheter progresses according to a well-defined sequence of events: Bacteria attach to the urinary catheter, initiate a biofilm form of growth in which sheets of organisms coat the catheter, and secrete an extracellular matrix of bacterial glycocalyces in which they become embedded. In addition, host urinary proteins such as Tamm-Horsfall protein and urinary salts are incorporated into this biofilm. Subsequently, this material leads to encrustation of the inner catheter surface. Examination of catheters by electron microscopy has demonstrated this biofilm growth on the inner surface of catheters removed from both patients and animals [34–37]. Certain genera of bacteria, particularly *Proteus* and *Pseudomonas*, are frequently associated with a propensity for biofilm growth and catheter obstruction [38].

In patients without urinary catheters who contract urinary tract infections, it has been demonstrated that a small number of "urovirulent clones" of *E. coli* produce the most serious infections [39,40]. These clones are defined on the basis of a limited number of O, K, and H serotypes and by the presence in these clones of specific virulence genes for P fimbriae, hemolysin, and siderophores. Studies to determine whether similar strains frequently infect the catheterized urinary tract have shown that the urovirulent strains seen in community-acquired urinary tract infections rarely cause bacteremic catheter-associated urinary tract infections [16,41]. The diversity of species causing catheter-associated urinary tract infections implies that compromised host defenses are probably more important than specific bacterial virulence factors in the genesis of these infections [8,42–44]. However, specific bacterial properties may be of importance in some settings. It has been demonstrated, for example, that specific strains of bacteria adhere more avidly to either catheter materials themselves or to uroepithelial cells from patients' bladders [45]. Better understanding of the interaction of bacteria and host epithelial cells could lead to novel approaches for preventing catheter-associated urinary tract infection.

Although catheter-associated bacteriuria has been clearly linked to subsequent bacteremia, the mechanism through which such bacteremia occurs has not been elucidated. Bacteremia could occur secondary to mucosal ulcerations resulting from bladder wall damage during catheterization. Cystoscopic examination of catheterized patients and animals suggests such ulcerations are common after 7 days of catheterization [3,46]. Alternatively, the well-known association of bacteremia with either insertion or withdrawal of urinary catheters or other urologic instruments suggests that bacteremia may result from the mucosal trauma associated with these events [47]. Finally, as in non–catheter-associated urinary tract infections, bacteremia may result when infection extends beyond the bladder to involve the kidney, prostate, or other portions of the upper urinary tract.

The various mechanisms through which bacteremia may develop have not been distinguished in studies of catheter-associated bacteriuria. To address this issue, localization of the site of infection in patients with catheter-associated bacteriuria and bacteremia requires additional study. Certainly, few patients with an unobstructed urinary tract contract characteristic clinical evidence of renal infection. The antibody-coated bacteria (ACB) test has been used in patients with catheter-associated bacteriuria to assess the frequency of asymptomatic renal involvement and, in some studies, has suggested the presence of clinically inapparent upper tract infection in 15% to 20% of those with bacteriuria [48,49]. However, comparison of the ACB test with other localization tests in catheterized patients has not been carried out, and thus the actual significance of a positive result has not been established.

SEQUELAE

From the short-term clinical perspective, most catheter-associated urinary tract infections appear benign. Because only 20% to 30% cause symptoms, most episodes can be classified as asymptomatic bacteriuria [50,51]. Pyuria accompanies most episodes of catheter-associated bacteriuria, however, suggesting host invasion rather than simple bladder colonization [52,53]. Not many patients with catheter-associated bacteriuria have undergone localization studies, and thus the proportion of patients with bladder, prostate, or kidney infections has not been determined. In studies using the ACB test, as many as one fourth of episodes of catheter-associated bacteriuria were positive, suggesting upper tract infection [48,49]. Clinically recognized infections, including prostatitis, epididymitis, seminal vesiculitis, and renal infection, may arise from bacteriuria originating during catheterization, but the frequency of such infections remains ill defined. In general, these complications arise primarily in patients with long-term indwelling catheters and are rare in patients whose catheterization lasts less than 10 days.

The major systemic complication of catheter-associated bacteriuria has been secondary bacteremia [54]. Although the risk of secondary bacteremia is small in any given patient, taken collectively, bacteremia arising from catheter-associated bacteriuria accounts for a large proportion of all nosocomial bacteremias. Most series of hospitalized patients with gram-negative bacteremia demonstrate that 30% to 40% of all gram-negative bacteremias acquired in the hospital originate in the urinary tract [55–58], making this the most commonly recognized source of gram-negative sepsis. Estimates of the frequency of secondary bacteremia associated with catheterization range from 1 per 50 to 150 catheterized bacteriuric patients. In one prospective study, however, 8% of patients had bacteremia after urinary catheterization [47]. Bacteremia thus may occur more often than is recognized clinically, especially on insertion, withdrawal, manipulation, or obstruction of the catheter.

Epidemiologic studies have related nosocomial bacteriuria with an increased mortality [18]. After adjustment for other factors, such as type of underlying disease, severity of illness, age, and sex, an approximately threefold relative increase in risk of death was observed by Platt and colleagues [18]. Similar studies in elderly, noncatheterized patients with asymptomatic bacteriuria have not found an association between bacteriuria and mortality [59,60]. The mechanism through which bacteriuria might produce increased mortality has not been elucidated but may relate to unrecognized septicemia or endotoxemia [18,61]. To date, catheter-associated bacteriuria has not been associated with long-term renal damage, but the natural history of this condition has not been studied prospectively.

Several authors have attempted to estimate whether increased hospital stay results from nosocomial urinary tract infection [62–64]. In a case–control study, Givens and Wenzel [62] found that urinary infections occurring in surgical patients resulted in 2.4 days of increased hospitalization and a cost of $558 per patient. Other estimates of increased hospitalization attributable to catheter-associated infection have ranged from 1 to 4 days, and estimates of increased costs have ranged from $0 to $1100 [63,64] (see Chapter 17).

CLINICAL MANIFESTATIONS

Only 20% to 30% of patients with catheter-associated bacteriuria experience symptoms attributable to infection, and thus most cases can be classified as asymptomatic bacteriuria [51]. When present, symptoms include dysuria, urgency, frequency, and hematuria. Fever, flank pain, or other clinical manifestations of pyelonephritis develop in fewer than 1% of patients with catheter-associated bacteriuria [52,53]. Despite the absence of symptoms in most patients with catheter-associated bacteriuria, the presence of pyuria suggests host invasion and actual infection rather than simple bladder colonization. Clinical findings characteristic of gram-negative bacteremia accompany bacteremia secondary to bacteriuria. Interestingly, the onset of bacteremia usually occurs within 24 hours of the onset of bacteriuria except for *Serratia marcescens* infections, in which bacteremia most commonly originates days after the onset of bacteriuria [27].

DIAGNOSIS

Most physicians diagnose catheter-associated bacteriuria by obtaining a urine specimen for culture by aspiration through a sampling port on the catheter itself. Because specimens so collected presumably represent actual bladder urine, contamination is infrequent. Catheter aspiration corresponded with cultures obtained by suprapubic aspiration in at least 90% of cases [65]. Urine cultures obtained from the catheter sampling port may not always reflect true bacteriuria in patients who have organisms growing on a biofilm on the inner surface of the catheter. Rather, bladder urine may be sterile but organisms from the catheter biofilm may contaminate the aspirated urine culture. Such contamination would be more likely to occur in patients with catheters in place for a week or more.

Quantitative culture results may demonstrate organisms ranging in quantity from 10 to $>10^5$ cfu/ml. Various authors have used quantitative bacterial counts ranging from $\geq 10^2$ to $\geq 10^5$ cfu/ml to define infection in catheterized patients. However, prospective studies to establish a specific quantitative level as more or less indicative of infection have not been carried out. For clinical purposes, bacteriuria of 10^2 cfu/ml or more, especially when associated with pyuria, can probably be taken as evidence of bladder infection [33]. Catheter-tip cultures should not be used to diagnose urinary infection [66].

TREATMENT

Because most patients with catheter-associated bacteriuria lack associated symptoms, treatment need not be undertaken unless the patient is at high risk for complications such as bacteremia or renal infection. Thus, treatment of asymptomatic bacteriuria may be useful in patients with neutropenia, obstructed urinary tracts, renal transplants, pregnancy, or other specific situations in which bacteriuria in and of itself may be of significant risk. In most patients without such complicating clinical features, however, treatment of bacteriuria should not be undertaken. In such patients, bacteriuria often resolves spontaneously with removal of the catheter; if one anticipates removal of the catheter, treatment should be postponed until that time. After catheter removal, the patient can either be observed for a period of time and subsequently treated if the bacteriuria does not resolve spontaneously, or treated empirically after the catheter has been removed. The latter may be particularly useful in elderly women in whom the risk of development of symptomatic infection is particularly high [67]. Treatment with the catheter in place often results in emergence of resistant strains, and eradication of bacteriuria in the presence of an indwelling catheter has been largely unsuccessful [68]. Because the antimicrobial susceptibility patterns of strains causing catheter-associated bacteriuria vary widely, choice of a specific antimicrobial agent should be guided by the in vitro antimicrobial sensitivities of the infecting organisms (see Chapter 14).

PREVENTION

Guidelines for prevention of catheter-associated bacteriuria have been published by the Centers for Disease Control and Prevention [69]. Until more has been learned about the pathogenesis of nosocomial bacteriuria, preventive efforts must be focused largely on aseptic care of the urinary catheter (Table 31-4). These measures are directed primarily at preventing entry of bacteria into the sterile closed drainage system and have been most effective when the period of catheterization is less than 7 days.

TABLE 31-4. *Methods for prevention of catheter-associated infections*

- Avoid catheterization
- Decrease duration of catheterization
- Use intermittent catheterization
- Insert catheters aseptically
- Use a closed sterile drainage system
- Use a condom catheter in cooperative patients
- Maintain gravity drain
- Apply topical meatal antimicrobials in women
- Give systemic antimicrobials
- Separate infected and uninfected patients

Probably the single most effective preventive measure is to avoid use of the indwelling catheter whenever possible. Indications for continued catheterization should be reviewed on a daily basis because the risk of bacteriuria associated with catheterization can be markedly reduced by removing catheters as soon as possible. Catheters should be inserted aseptically under sterile conditions. In addition, the closed drainage system should be considered a sterile site, and aseptic precautions should be observed when manipulating any portion of the system. Inadvertent or purposeful disconnection of the catheter and collecting system predisposes to bacteriuria, as does use of nonsterile technique when emptying urine from the collecting vessel. Continuous, downhill, gravity-flow drainage should be maintained at all times. Both hospital personnel and catheterized patients should be taught the importance of these principles.

Many technologic improvements in catheters and drainage systems have been proposed as means of preventing bacteriuria. These include polymeric silicone (Silastic) rather than rubber catheters; baffles, vents, or other devices for preventing reflux or retrograde infection; instillation of antimicrobial or antiseptic agents into the catheter bag; culture vents on the side of the urinary catheter; permanent junctions between the distal catheter and collecting system; and antimicrobial substances impregnated into the catheter itself. Most of these technologic improvements make sense from the standpoint of the pathogenesis of these infections, but it has been difficult in controlled trials to prove the effectiveness of most such innovations. Because opening the closed collecting system has been clearly shown to predispose to infection, sampling ports that permit cultures to be obtained without opening the system are preferred. Although sometimes inconvenient, drainage systems marketed as a single unit extending from the bladder catheter to the collecting bag prevent inadvertent disconnection of the catheter and collecting system. In a randomized, controlled trial, Platt and colleagues [70] found that sealed-junction catheters significantly reduced the risk of urinary tract infection and also reduced the risk of death in individuals not receiving systemic antimicrobials.

More controversial has been the value of using antimicrobial substances such as hydrogen peroxide or chlorhexidine in the collecting bag. In one study, Maizels and Schaeffer [71] demonstrated that hydrogen peroxide in the collecting bag successfully eradicated microorganisms introduced into the collecting system and prevented retrograde infection. In another study, use of hydrogen peroxide in the drainage spigot prevented retrograde infection [72]. On the other hand, some studies have failed to find benefit attributable to either system [19,73]. In part, the potential benefit of such a system relates to the proportion of infections acquired by the intraluminal route. In previous studies, an estimated 15% to 20% of infections occurred in this manner [28], and thus most infections may not be preventable through control measures aimed at interrupting this route of bacterial ingress. Such measures may, however, reduce reservoirs of organisms available for transfer from one catheterized patient to another on the hands of personnel. In hospitals in which technique is not optimal and intraluminal infection occurs more often, these preventive approaches may have greater benefit.

Because many infections acquired during catheterization arise after urethral meatal colonization with the infecting strain, topical application of antiseptic agents to these areas has been advocated as a preventive measure. In a large and careful study addressing this topic, Burke and coworkers [74] were unable to ascribe benefits to twice-daily application of povidone–iodine solution followed by povidone–iodine ointment. In a subsequent study, Burke and colleagues [75] demonstrated reduced infection rates using a twice-daily polyantimicrobial ointment applied at the meatal–catheter junction; however, the benefit was seen only in a specific high-risk group: women with previous meatal colonization. Therefore, although the overall efficacy of this approach remains in doubt, it is apparently effective in some patients.

Alternative means of blocking urethral colonization and ascent of organisms from the urethral meatus surface are being investigated. Many years ago, antimicrobial impregnation of catheters was assessed [76]. Although the technique was not successful in those studies, newer approaches using silver-impregnated catheters have been undertaken. This approach has an appealing logical basis in that silver ions are bactericidal, can be applied to catheters, are nontoxic, and, when used topically, have been effective in other settings such as controlling burn wound infections. Schaeffer and colleagues [77] demonstrated that silver-coated catheters (in conjunction with a silver catheter tubing junction connector and an antiseptic-filled drainage bag) reduced the incidence of catheter-associated urinary tract infections and delayed their onset in chronically catheterized patients. In a trial by Liedberg and Lundeberg [78], excellent results were also obtained in short-term catheterized patients using a silver-coated catheter. They demonstrated that 10% of the patients catheterized with the silver-coated latex catheter had urinary tract infections, vs. 37% of those receiving a Teflon control catheter [79]. However, other studies of the silver-coated catheter in general hospital populations have demonstrated less benefit [16]. Further study of these catheters and this general approach appear warranted.

Irrigation of the bladder with antimicrobial solutions is another technique that has been used to prevent catheter-associated bacteriuria [79]. Martin and Bookrajian [80] first reported prevention of infections using acetic acid or a neomycin–polymyxin B irrigant in an open collecting system. Instillation of chlorhexidine into the bladder has also been reported as efficacious [81]. However, Warren and colleagues [20], in a carefully controlled trial, were unable to ascribe any benefits to continuous irrigation with polymyxin–neomycin and found that patients on irrigation contracted infections with more resistant organisms.

Systemic antibiotic agents have been demonstrated to decrease the likelihood of bacteriuria during the first 5 to 7 days of catheterization [13,20,51,74,75]. In addition, in controlled trials, systemic antimicrobials have been associated with a decreased rate of catheter-associated bacteriuria [82–84]. Thus, systemic antimicrobial agents probably reduce the likelihood of bacteriuria developing during short-term catheterization. However, whether the risks, side effects, and costs of such antimicrobials warrant their use for this purpose requires additional study. It may be reasonable to consider systemic antimicrobials as a preventive measure in high-risk patients who have an anticipated short duration of catheterization. In patients with long-term urinary catheterization, continued antimicrobial use results in the emergence of resistant strains and probably should be avoided [85]. Antimicrobial prophylaxis has been of clear benefit in preventing postoperative urinary infection among men with sterile urine undergoing urologic surgery [55,86].

Selective decontamination of the gut (see Chapter 15) may be useful in preventing catheter-associated urinary tract infections [87]. According to Vollaard and colleagues [87], oral norfloxacin plus oral amphotericin B administered to patients with urinary catheters decreased the occurrence of catheter-associated urinary tract infections and delayed their onset.

Daily culture monitoring of catheterized patients to detect bacteriuria before onset of symptoms or bacteremia has been advocated [13]. However, Garibaldi and colleagues [23] found monitoring to be of little benefit because most symptomatic infections and bacteremias occurred within 24 hours of the onset of bacteriuria. Alternative methods of urinary drainage such as condom drainage, suprapubic catheterization, or intermittent catheterization (see next section) may be preferable in selected patients. Condom catheters have been most successfully used in alert, cooperative patients receiving meticulous skin care to prevent meatal ulceration [88,89]. In this setting, condom catheters used for 2 to 4 weeks appear to have an infection risk lower than that of indwelling catheters. In uncooperative patients who manipulate the condom catheter, however, infections occur at least as frequently as in comparable patients with indwelling catheters [88]. Suprapubic catheterization has been largely used by gynecologists and urologists for short-term catheterization after surgical procedures. Reported experience suggests that this technique may be less often associated with bacteriuria than is indwelling urethral catheterization, but a direct prospective comparison of the two techniques has not been published [90,91]. Suprapubic catheterization eliminates the urethral route of infection and thus might be expected to cause less bacteriuria than urethral catheterization.

CHRONIC CATHETERIZATION

Bacteriuria occurs in essentially all patients who require chronic catheter drainage because of spinal cord injury or other causes of neurogenic bladder [92]. Prospective evaluation of such patients has shown that they experience multiple sequential episodes of bacteriuria, usually with a different species each episode (reinfection), but occasionally with a single persisting species [93,94]. Polymicrobial infections commonly occur. Some strains, specifically Proteeae, pseudomonads, and enterococci, appear to persist in the urinary tract once present, whereas other strains frequently cycle in and out of the urinary tract [32,94]. This may be because the persisters are able to adhere more avidly to the catheter. For *Providencia stuartii*, specific fimbriae (the MR/K fimbriae) have been shown to promote adherence to the catheter and persistence in the urinary tract [95]. On the other hand, *E. coli* type 1 fimbriae have been shown to promote persistence in the urinary tract by increasing avidity of adherence to uroepithelial cells [95]. Thus there may be two populations of organisms in such patients—namely, those that attach to the catheter and those that attach to bladder uroepithelial cells. Alternatively, Proteeae have been found as persistent colonizers of the groin in nursing home patients, and such colonization may provide a reservoir from which infection originates [96].

Most bacteriuric episodes are asymptomatic, but bacteremia, pyelonephritis, epididymitis, and renal calculi occur with sufficient frequency to be of major concern [93,94,97]. These conditions probably contribute in part to deterioration in renal function, a major cause of death in this population [32].

A recurrent problem in these patients is that of catheter encrustation and eventual obstruction. The pathogenesis of catheter encrustation is similar in many ways to that of an infection stone [32]. Bacteria adhere to the catheter and produce encrustation, as described previously. The encrustation consists of bacteria, their glycocalyces, host proteins such as Tamm-Horsfall protein, and, eventually, urinary crystals such as struvite and apatite. This process is accelerated by urease-producing bacteria, especially *Proteus mirabilis*, which has a very potent urease [98,99]. The urease results in products that alkalinize the urine, promote crystallization of struvite and apatite, and promote the encrustation and obstruction process. Patient-related factors may play a role here as well in that some patients' urine leads to catheter obstruction more rapidly than others. Further study of the process of encrustation and catheter blockage would be of great interest in these patients.

Prevention of infection has been difficult in patients with chronic indwelling catheters. Aseptic techniques applied to patients with short-term catheterization have not been successful in those with longer-term catheterization. Antimicrobial treatment of asymptomatic bacteriuric episodes had no apparent impact on the frequency or natural history of infection according to one study, and instead selected for antibiotic-resistant strains [94]. Similarly, antimicrobial prophylaxis or the use of urinary antiseptics has not been successful in these patients [100–102]. Most bacteriuria in these patients is accompanied by pyuria, suggesting that more than simple bladder colonization has occurred, but studies to localize such infections to the lower or upper urinary tract have been largely unsuccessful [93,103]. Patients with chronic catheterization should probably receive antibiotic treatment only for clinically apparent pyelonephritis, epididymitis, or bacteremia—not for asymptomatic bacteriuria. Treatment should be guided by in vitro sensitivities, because infections with multiply resistant, hospital-acquired strains develop in these patients.

Experience suggests that intermittent catheterization, even if done in a nonsterile fashion, may be a significant advance over chronic indwelling catheterization. Infection reportedly can be avoided altogether in some patients and occurs periodically in others on intermittent catheterization [104,105]. In addition, low-dose, continuous antimicrobial prophylaxis may be effective in patients with intermittent catheterization [97], but it is generally not effective in patients with indwelling catheters.

REFERENCES

1. Kislak JW, Eickhoff TC, Finland M. Hospital-acquired infection and antibiotic usage in the Boston City Hospital. *N Engl J Med* 1964; 271:834.
2. McNamara MJ, et al. A study of bacteriologic patterns of hospital infections. *Ann Intern Med* 1967;66:486.
3. Moody ML, Burke JP. Infections and antibiotic use in a large private hospital. *Arch Intern Med* 1972;130:261.
4. Schaberg DR, Weinstein RA, Stamm WE. Epidemics of nosocomial urinary tract infection caused by multiply resistant gram-negative bacilli: epidemiology and control. *J Infect Dis* 1976;133:363.
5. Stamm WE, Weinstein RA, Dixon RE. Comparison of endemic and epidemic nosocomial infections. *Am J Med* 1981;70:393.
6. Schaberg DR, et al. Nosocomial bacteriuria: a prospective study of case clustering and antimicrobial resistance. *Ann Intern Med* 1980;93:420.
7. Hooton TM, et al. The joint association of multiple risk factors with the occurrence of nosocomial infections. *Am J Med* 1981;70:960.
8. Stamm WE, Martin SM, Bennett JV. Epidemiology of nosocomial infections due to gram-negative bacilli: aspects relevant to development and use of vaccines. *J Infect Dis* 1977;136S(Suppl):S151.
9. Stamm WE. Guidelines for prevention of catheter-associated urinary tract infections. *Ann Intern Med* 1975;82:386.
10. Turck M, Goffee B, Petersdorf RG. The urethral catheter and urinary tract infection. *J Urol* 1962;88:834.
11. Kass EH. Asymptomatic infections of the urinary tract. *Transactions of the Association of American Physicians* 1956;69:56.
12. Finkelberg Z, Kunin CM. Clinical evaluation of closed urinary drainage systems. *JAMA* 1969;207:1657.
13. Kunin CM. *Detection, prevention, and management of urinary tract infections*. 4th ed. Philadelphia: Lea & Febiger; 1985.
14. Thornton GF, Andriole VT. Bacteriuria during indwelling catheter drainage: II. effect of a closed sterile drainage system. *JAMA* 1970; 214:339.
15. Garibaldi RA, et al. Factors predisposing to bacteriuria during indwelling urethral catheterization. *N Engl J Med* 1974;291:215.
16. Johnson JR, et al. Prevention of catheter-associated urinary tract infections with a silver oxide coated urinary catheter: clinical and microbiological correlates. *J Infect Dis* 1990;162:1145.
17. Kunin CM, McCormack R-C. Prevention of catheter-induced urinary tract infections by sterile closed drainage. *N Engl J Med* 1966;274: 1155.
18. Platt R, Polk BF, Murdock B, Rosner B. Mortality associated with nosocomial urinary tract infection. *N Engl J Med* 1982;307:637.
19. Thompson RL, et al. Catheter-associated bacteriuria: failure to reduce attack rates using periodic instillations of a disinfectant into urinary drainage systems. *JAMA* 1984;251:747.
20. Warren JW, et al. Antibiotic irrigation and catheter-associated urinary tract infections. *N Engl J Med* 1978;299:570.
21. Riley DK, Classen DC, Stevens LE, Burke JP. A large randomized clinical trial of a silver-impregnated urinary catheter: lack of efficacy and staphylococcal superinfection. *Am J Med* 1995;98:349.
22. Garibaldi RA, et al. Meatal colonization and catheter-associated bacteriuria. *N Engl J Med* 1980;303:316.
23. Garibaldi RA, Mooney BR, Epstein BJ, Britt MR. An evaluation of daily bacteriologic monitoring to identify preventable episodes of catheter-associated urinary tract infections. *Infect Control* 1982;3:466.
24. Platt R, Polk BF, Murdock B, Rosner B. Risk factors for nosocomial urinary tract infection. *Am J Epidemiol* 1986;124:977.
25. Jarvis WR, Martone WJ. Predominant pathogens in hospital infections. *J Antimicrob Chemother* 1992;29:19.
26. Levy SB. Antibiotic resistance. *Infect Control* 1983;4:195.
27. Krieger JN, Kaiser DL, Wenzel RP. Urinary tract etiology of bloodstream infections in hospitalized patients. *J Infect Dis* 1983;148:57.
28. Daifuku R, Stamm WE. Association of rectal and urethral colonization with urinary tract infection in patients with indwelling catheters. *JAMA* 1984;252:2028.
29. Marsh FP, Murray M, Panchamia P. The relationship between bacterial cultures of the vaginal introitus and urinary infection. *Br J Urol* 1972;44:368.
30. Stamey TA, et al. Recurrent urinary infection in adult women: the role of introital enterobacteria. *Calif Med* 1971;155:1.
31. Schaeffer AJ. Catheter-associated bacteriuria. *Urol Clin North Am* 1986;4:735.
32. Warren JW. Catheter-associated urinary tract infections. *Infect Dis Clin North Am* 1987;1:823.
33. Stark RP, Maki DG. Bacteriuria in the catheterized patient: what quantitative level of bacteriuria is relevant? *N Engl J Med* 1984;311:560.
34. Cox AJ, et al. An automated technique for in vitro assessment of the susceptibility of urinary catheter materials to encrustation. *Eng Med* 1987;6:37.
35. Cox AJ, Hukins DWL, Sutton TM. Infection of catheterized patients: bacterial colonization of encrusted Foley catheters shown by scanning electron microscopy. *Urol Res* 1989;17:349.
36. Nickel JC, Grant SK, Costerton JW. Catheter-associated bacteriuria: an experimental study. *Urology* 1985;26:369.
37. Nickel JC, Gristina P, Costerton JW. Electron microscopic study of an infected Foley catheter. *Can J Surg* 1985;28:50.
38. Mobley HLT, Warren JW. Urease-positive bacteriuria and obstruction of long-term urinary catheters. *J Clin Microbiol* 1987;25:2216.
39. Johnson J. Virulence factors in *E. coli* urinary tract infections. *Clin Microbiol Rev* 1991;4:80.
40. Stamm WE, et al. Urinary tract infections: from pathogenesis to treatment. *J Infect Dis* 1989;159:400.
41. Johnson JR, Moseley SL, Roberts PL, Stamm WE. Aerobactin and other virulence factor genes among strains of *E. coli* causing urosepsis association with patients' characteristics. *Infect Immun* 1988;56:405.
42. Kennedy RP, Plorde JJ, Petersdorf RG. Studies on the epidemiology of *E. coli* infections: IV. evidence for a nosocomial flora. *J Clin Invest* 1965;44:193.
43. Sobel JD, Kaye D. Host factors in the pathogenesis of urinary tract infection. *Am J Med* 1984;76(Suppl):122.
44. Winterbauer RH, Turck M, Petersdorf RG. Studies on the epidemiology of *E. coli* infections: V. factors influencing acquisition of specific serologic groups. *J Clin Invest* 1967;46:21.
45. Daifuku R, Stamm WE. Bacterial adherence to bladder uroepithelial cells in catheter-associated urinary tract infection. *N Engl J Med* 1986; 314:1208.
46. Isaacs JH, McWhorter DM. Foley catheter drainage systems and bladder damage. *Surg Gynecol Obstet* 1971;132:889.
47. Sullivan NM, et al. Clinical aspects of bacteremia after manipulation of the genitourinary tract. *J Infect Dis* 1973;127:49.
48. Gonick P, Falkner B, Schwartz A, Pariser R. Bacteriuria in the catheterized patient: cystitis or pyelonephritis? *JAMA* 1975;233:253.

49. Thorley JD, Barbin GK, Reinarz JA. The prevalence of antibody-coated bacteria in urine. *Am J Med Sci* 1978;275:75.
50. Hartstein AI, et al. Nosocomial urinary tract infection: a prospective evaluation of 108 catheterized patients. *Infect Control* 1981;2:380.
51. Mooney BR, Garibaldi RA, Britt MR. Natural history of catheter-associated bacteriuria (colonization, infection, bacteremia): implication for prevention. In: Nelson JD, Grassi C, eds. *Current chemotherapy and infectious diseases*. Vol. 2. Washington, DC: American Society of Microbiology; 1980:1083.
52. Musher DM, Thorsteinsson SB, Airola VM. Quantitative urinalysis: diagnosing urinary tract infection in men. *JAMA* 1976;236:2069.
53. Stamm WE. Measurement of pyuria and its relationship to bacteriuria. *Am J Med* 1983;75(Suppl):53.
54. Dupont HL, Spink WW. Infections due to gram-negative organisms: an analysis of 860 patients with bacteriuria at the University of Minnesota Medical Center 1958–1966. *Medicine* 1969;48:307.
55. Falkiner FR, et al. Antimicrobial agents for the prevention of urinary tract infections in transurethral surgery. *J Urol* 1983;129:766.
56. Kreger BE, Craven DE, Carling PC, McCabe WR. Gram-negative bacteremia: III. reassessment of etiology, epidemiology, and ecology in 612 patients. *Am J Med* 1980;68:332.
57. Steere AC, Stamm WE, Martin SM, Bennett JV. Gram-negative rod bacteremia. In: Bennett JV, Brachman PS, eds. *Hospital infections.* Boston: Little, Brown; 1979:507.
58. Wenzel RP, Osterman CA, Hunting KJ. Hospital-acquired infections: I. infection rates by site, service, and common procedures in a university hospital. *Am J Epidemiol* 1976;104:645.
59. Abrutyn E, et al. Does asymptomatic bacteriuria predict mortality and does antimicrobial therapy reduce mortality in elderly ambulatory women? *Ann Intern Med* 1994;120:827.
60. Nordenstam GR, et al. Bacteriuria and mortality in an elderly population. *N Engl J Med* 1986;314:1152.
61. van Dventer SJH, et al. Endotoxemia, bacteria, and urosepsis. In: *Bacterial endotoxins: pathophysiological effects, clinical significance, and pharmacological control.* London: Alan R. Liss; 1988:213.
62. Givens CD, Wenzel RP. Catheter-associated urinary tract infections in surgical patients: a controlled study on the excess morbidity and costs. *J Urol* 1980;124:646.
63. Green MS, Rubinstein E, Amit P. Estimating the effects of nosocomial infections on the length of hospitalization. *J Infect Dis* 1982; 145:667.
64. Pinner RW, et al. High cost nosocomial infections. *Infect Control* 1982;3:143.
65. Bergquist D, Bronnestam R, Hedelin H, Stahl A. The relevance of urinary sampling methods in patients with indwelling Foley catheters. *Br J Urol* 1980;52:92.
66. Gross PA, Harlzavy LM, Barden GE, Kerstein M. Positive Foley catheter tip cultures: fact or fancy. *JAMA* 1979;228:72.
67. Harding GKM, et al. How long should catheter-acquired urinary tract infection be treated?: a randomized controlled study. *Ann Intern Med* 1991;114:713.
68. Butler HK, et al. Evaluation of specific systemic antimicrobial therapy in patients on closed catheter drainage. *J Urol* 1968;100:567.
69. Wong ES, Hooton TM. Guidelines for prevention of catheter-associated urinary tract infections. *Infect Control* 1982;2:125.
70. Platt R, Murdock B, Polk BF, Rosner B. Reduction of mortality associated with nosocomial urinary tract infection. *Lancet* 1983;1:1893.
71. Maizels M, Schaeffer AJ. Decreased incidence of bacteriuria associated with periodic instillations of hydrogen peroxide into the urethral catheter drainage bag. *J Urol* 1980;123:841.
72. Desautels RE, Chibaro EA, Lang RJ. Maintenance of sterility in urinary drainage bags. *Surg Gynecol Obstet* 1982;154:838.
73. Sarubbi FA, Rutala WA, Samsa G. Hydrogen peroxide instillations into the urinary drainage bag: should we or shouldn't we? *Am J Infect Control* 1982;10:72.
74. Burke JP, et al. Prevention of catheter-associated urinary tract infections: efficacy of daily meatal care regimens. *Am J Med* 1981;70:655.
75. Burke JP, et al. Evaluation of daily meatal care with poly-antibiotic ointment in prevention of catheter-associated bacteriuria. *J Urol* 1983; 129:331.
76. Butler HK, Kunin CM. Evaluation of polymyxin catheter lubricant and impregnated catheters. *J Urol* 1968;100:560.
77. Schaeffer AJ, Stony KO, Johnson SM. Effect of silver oxide/trichloroisocyanuric acid antimicrobial urinary drainage system on catheter-associated bacteriuria. *J Urol* 1988;139:69.
78. Liedberg H, Lundeberg T. Silver alloy coated catheters reduce catheter-associated bacteriuria. *Br J Urol* 1990;65:379.
79. Bastable JRG, Peel RN, Birch DM, Richards B. Continuous irrigation of the bladder after prostatectomy: its effect on postprostatectomy infections. *Br J Urol* 1977;49:689.
80. Martin CM, Bookrajian EN. Bacteriuria prevention after indwelling urinary catheterization. *Arch Intern Med* 1962;110:703.
81. Kirk D, Bullock DW, Mitchell JP, Hobbs SJF. Hibitane bladder irrigation in the prevention of catheter-associated urinary infections. *Br J Urol* 1979;51:528.
82. Britt MR, et al. Antimicrobial prophylaxis for catheter-associated bacteriuria. *Antimicrob Agents Chemother* 1977;11:240.
83. vanDerWall E, et al. Prophylactic ciprofloxacin for catheter-associated urinary-tract infection. *Lancet* 1992;339:946.
84. Stamm WE. Catheter-associated urinary tract infections: epidemiology, pathogenesis, and prevention. *Am J Med* 1991;91(Suppl 3B):655.
85. Warren JW, Anthony WC, Hoopes JM, Muncie HL. Cephalexin or susceptible bacteriuria in afebrile, long-term catheterized patients. *JAMA* 1982;248:454.
86. Hirschmann JV, Inui TS. Antimicrobial prophylaxis: a critique of recent trials. *Rev Infect Dis* 1980;2:1.
87. Vollaard EJ, et al. Prevention of catheter associated gram-negative bacilluria with norfloxacin by selective decontamination of the bowel and high urinary concentration. *J Antimicrob Chemother* 1989;23:915.
88. Hirch DD, Fainstein V, Musher DM. Do condom catheter collecting systems cause urinary tract infections? *JAMA* 1979;242:340.
89. Johnson ET. The condom catheter: urinary tract infection and other complications. *South Med J* 1983;76:579.
90. Hodgkinson CP, Hodrari AA. Trocar suprapubic cystostomy for postoperative bladder drainage in the female. *J Obstet Gynecol* 1966;96: 773.
91. Mattingly RF, Moore DE, Clark DO. Bacteriologic study of suprapubic bladder drainage. *Am J Obstet Gynecol* 1972;114:732.
92. Turck M, Stamm WE. Nosocomial infection of the urinary tract. *Am J Med* 1981;70:651.
93. Merritt JL, Keys TF. Limitations of the antibody-coated bacteria test in patients with neurogenic bladders. *JAMA* 1982;247:1723.
94. Warren JW, et al. A prospective microbiologic study of bacteriuria in patients with chronic indwelling urethral catheters. *J Infect Dis* 1982; 146:719.
95. Mobley HLT, et al. MR/K hemagglutination of *Providencia stuartii* correlates with catheter adherence and with persistence in catheter-associated bacteriuria. *J Infect Dis* 1988;157:264.
96. Ehrenkranz NJ, Alfonso BC, Eckert DG, Moskowitz LB. Proteeae species bacteriuria accompanying Proteeae sp. groin skin carriage in geriatric outpatients. *J Clin Microbiol* 1989;27:1988.
97. Warren JW, Muncie HL, Bergquist EJ, Hoopes JM. Sequelae and management of urinary tract infection in the patient requiring chronic catheterization. *J Urol* 1981;125:1.
98. McLean R, Nickel JC, Noakes VC, Costerton JW. An in vitro ultrastructural study of infectious kidney stone genesis. *Infect Immun* 1985;49:805.
99. Mobley HLT, Warren JW. Urease-positive bacteriuria and obstruction of long-term urinary catheters. *J Clin Microbiol* 1987;25:2216.
100. Merritt JL, Erickson RP, Opitz JL. Bacteriuria during followup in patients with spinal cord injury: II. efficacy of antimicrobial suppressants. *Arch Phys Med Rehabil* 1982;63:413.
101. Sweet DE, et al. Evaluation of H_2O_2 prophylaxis of bacteriuria in patients with long-term indwelling Foley catheters: a randomized controlled study. *Infect Control* 1985;6:263.
102. Vainrub B, Musher DM. Lack of effect of methanimine in suppression of or prophylaxis against chronic urinary infections. *Antimicrob Agents Chemother* 1977;12:625.
103. Kuhlemeier KV, Lloyd LK, Stover SL. Localization of upper and lower urinary tract infections in patients with neurogenic bladders. *Science Digest* 1982;4:29.
104. Guttman L, Frankel H. The value of intermittent catheterization in the early management of traumatic paraplegia and tetraplegia. *Paraplegia* 1966;4:63.
105. Lapides J, Diokno AC, Lowe BS, Kalish MD. Followup on unsterile, intermittent self-catheterization. *J Urol* 1974;3:184.

Hospital Infections, Fourth Edition,
edited by John V. Bennett and Philip S. Brachman.
Lippincott–Raven Publishers, Philadelphia © 1998

CHAPTER 32

Pneumonia

Donald E. Craven, Kathleen A. Steger and F. Marc LaForce

Nosocomial pneumonia, defined as an infection of lung parenchyma that was neither present nor incubating at the time of admission to the hospital, is the second most common nosocomial infection in the United States, but because of its high morbidity and mortality is considered the most serious hospital-acquired infection [1–3]. Episodes of nosocomial pneumonia are usually caused by common nosocomial bacterial pathogens, but *Legionella pneumophila, Mycobacterium tuberculosis*, viruses, or fungi are important emerging pathogens [3–6].

Accurate diagnosis is critical to understanding the epidemiology, pathogenesis, and prevention of hospital-acquired pneumonia (HAP). There is no well-accepted gold standard for diagnosis, but rather a series of definitions with variable sensitivity and specificity [7,8]. Clinical diagnosis is usually used in nonventilated patients and most ventilated patients, but invasive techniques such as bronchoalveolar lavage (BAL) or protected specimen brush (PSB) have been used more extensively since the mid-1980s [7,8]. More recently, "blind" BAL or quantitative endotracheal aspirates (QEA) have demonstrated acceptable sensitivity and specificity [7–9].

Bacteria causing nosocomial pneumonia may originate from the patient's endogenous flora, other patients, hospital staff, or environmental sources. Aspiration is the major route of bacterial entry into the lower respiratory tract, and airborne particles are the primary mode of transmission for most viruses, *M. tuberculosis*, and *Aspergillus* species.

This chapter reviews the epidemiology, pathogenesis, and treatment of nosocomial pneumonia. Prevention of nosocomial pneumonia caused by bacterial pathogens is emphasized, with an overview of lower respiratory tract infections due to viruses, fungi, and mycobacteria.

BACTERIAL PATHOGENS

Epidemiology

Etiologic agents, rates of nosocomial pneumonia and associated mortality, and costs are summarized in the following sections.

Etiologic Agents

Etiologic agents causing nosocomial pneumonia differ by hospital, patient population, and the specific diagnostic methods used [3,4,10–15]. The crude and cause-specific rates of nosocomial pneumonia are probably underestimated because of the well-known decrease in autopsy rates, the cases of pneumonia that occur after discharge, atypical presentation in immunocompromised patients, and lack of readily available diagnostic tests for patients with pneumonia due to anaerobes, *L. pneumophila*, viruses, and fungi [3,16,17] (Figure 32-1). The bacteria, viruses, and fungi causing nosocomial pneumonia may originate from several different sources, including the patient's endogenous flora, other patients, staff, contaminated devices, or the environment [18,19] (Figure 32-2). Prior hospitalization and previous antibiotic therapy are important predisposing factors.

Early-onset bacterial nosocomial pneumonia occurs during the first 4 days of the hospital stay and is more frequently caused by *Streptococcus pneumoniae, Moraxella catarrhalis, Hemophilus influenzae*, or anaerobes [11, 20–26] (Table 32-1). Conversely, late-onset bacterial pneumonia is more commonly caused by gram-negative bacilli (*Klebsiella, Acinetobacter* species, *Pseudomonas aeruginosa*) or *Staphylococcus aureus* [20,23]. Gram-negative bacilli have been implicated in > 60% of reported cases,

D. E. Craven, K. A. Steger: Department of Infectious Diseases, Clinical AIDS Program, Boston Medical Center, Boston, MA 02118-2353.

F. M. LaForce: Department of Medicine, University of Rochester School of Medicine, Rochester, New York 14642.

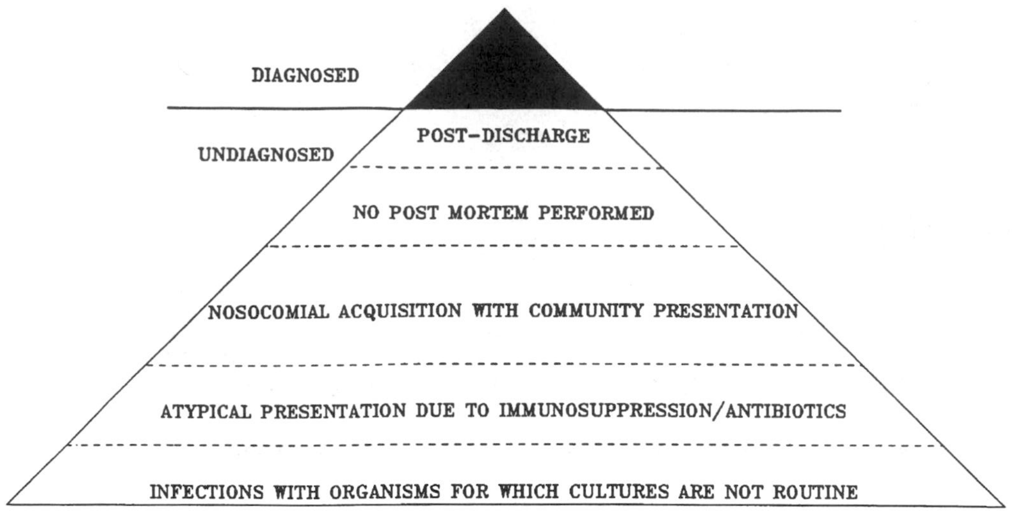

FIGURE 32-1. The pyramid of nosocomial pneumonia, indicating that many cases are not diagnosed or misclassified. Those cases that are not diagnosed may have been misclassified as community acquired, become manifest only at postmortem, or may have occurred in the outpatient setting or after discharge from the hospital. Furthermore, transmission of *Streptococcus pneumoniae*, *Hemophilus influenzae*, and *Pneumocystis carinii* pneumonia in the hospital setting is not widely appreciated. (From Craven DE, Steger KA. Hospital-acquired pneumonia: perspective for the epidemiologist. *Infect Control Hosp Epidemiol* 1997 [in press], with permission.)

and *S. aureus* between 20% and 40% of the cases in different reports. As shown in Table 32-2, isolation rates of different bacteria vary considerably depending on the population studied and the method of diagnosis [25,26].

Because critically ill patients often have severe acute and chronic underlying diseases, receive multiple antibiotics, and are exposed to numerous invasive devices, they are susceptible to multidrug-resistant (MDR) strains of gram-negative bacilli and *S. aureus* [18,19]. The virulence of different strains within the same species are variable [27–30]. Some data suggest that patients with nosocomial pneumonia caused by MDR strains of bacteria may have an increased crude mortality rate that reflects their underlying disease. In one study, patients with ventilator-associated pneumonia (VAP) due to methicillin-resistant *S. aureus* had a higher mortality, but were also more likely than patients with VAP due to methicillin-sensitive *S. aureus* to have received prior steroids and antibiotics, mechanical ventilation for more than 6 days, be older than 25 years of

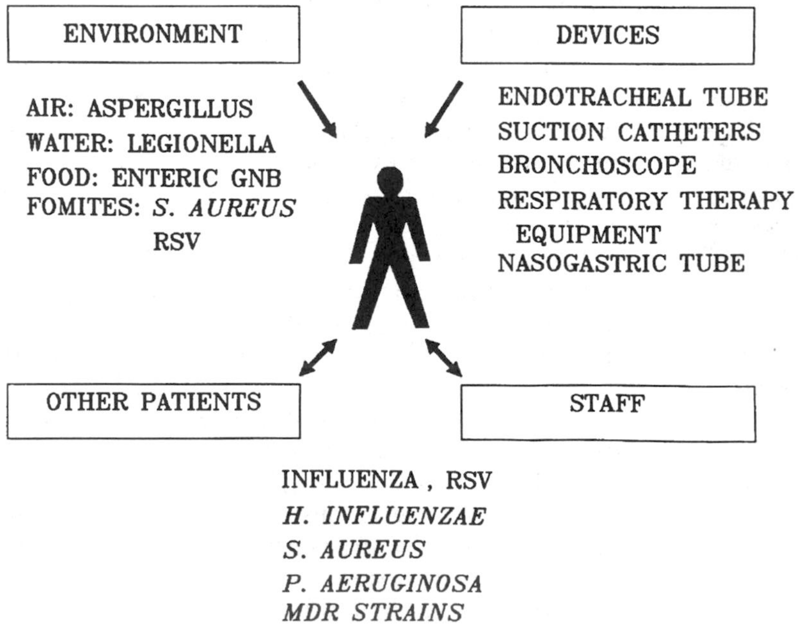

FIGURE 32-2. Sources of nosocomial respiratory tract pathogens. Microorganisms may originate from the environment, invasive devices, or other patients or hospital staff. (Adapted from Craven DE, Steger KA. Epidemiology of nosocomial pneumonia: new concepts on an old disease. *Chest* 1995;108:1S–16S, with permission.)

TABLE 32-1. *Common pathogens associated with nosocomial pneumonia*[a]

Pathogen	Onset of pneumonia	Frequency (%)	Source of organism
Bacteria			
Gram-positive cocci			
Staphylococcus aureus	Late	20%–40%	Endogenous Health care workers Environment
Streptococcus pneumoniae	Early	5%–20%	Endogenous Other patients
Aerobic gram-negative bacilli	Late	≥20%–60%	
Pseudomonas aeruginosa	Late		Endogenous
Enterobacter spp	Late		Other patients
Acinetobacter spp	Late		Environment
Klebsiella pneumoniae	Late		Enteral feeding
Serratia marcescens	Late		Health care workers
Escherichia coli	Late		Equipment/devices
Gram-negative coccobacilli			
Hemophilus influenzae	Early	<5%–15%	Respiratory droplet
Anaerobic bacteria	Early	0%–35%	Endogenous
Special pathogens			
Legionella pneumophila	Late	0%–10%	Potable water Showers, faucets Cooling towers
Mycobacterium tuberculosis	Late	<1%	Endogenous Other patients/staff
Viruses			
Influenza A and B	Early/Late	<1%	Other patients/staff
Respiratory syncytial virus	Early/Late	<1%	Other patients/staff Fomites
Fungi/Protozoa			
Aspergillus	Late	<1%	Air, construction
Candida spp	Late	<1%	Endogenous Other patients/staff
Pneumocystis carinii	Late	<1%	Endogenous Other patients

[a]Crude rates of pneumonia may vary by hospital, patient population, and method of diagnosis.

(Adapted, in part, from Horan TC, White JW, Jarvis WR, et al. Nosocomial infection surveillance, 1984. *MMWR Morb Mortal Wkly Rep* 1986;35:17SS–29SS; Tablan OC, Anderson LJ, Arden NH, et al. Guideline for prevention of nosocomial pneumonia: part I. Issues on prevention of nosocomial pneumonia, 1994. *Infect Control Hosp Epidemiol* 1994;15:588–625; and Haley RW, Hooton TM, Culver DH, et al. Nosocomial infections in US hospitals, 1975–1976: estimated frequency by selected characteristics of patients. *Am J Med* 1981;70:947–959.)

age, and have a history of preexisting chronic lung disease, bacteremia, or shock [25].

Most cases of bacterial nosocomial pneumonia are caused by more than one species of bacteria [11,14,20,23, 31–33]. As shown in Table 32-2, the specific etiology of pneumonia varies by hospital, the presence of an endotracheal tube, and the method used for diagnosis [11,13, 24,34,35]. For example, in Schleupner and Cobb's series [24], most of the medical and surgical patients in community-based teaching hospitals had pneumonia due to *S. pneumoniae* or *H. influenzae*, in contrast to reports from university hospitals in which VAP was commonly caused by gram-negative bacilli and *S. aureus* [11,24,32].

Rates of Pneumonia

Nosocomial pneumonia has accounted for 13% to 18% of all nosocomial but rates needs to be reassessed with the emergence of managed care programs and the changing healthcare delivery systems in the United States. In general, rates of HAP occur at a higher frequency in university vs. nonteaching hospitals [1,3]. Lower respiratory tract infections are diagnosed in 0.8% to 0.9% of medical and surgical patients, 17.5% of postoperative patients, and 7% of neonatal intensive care unit (ICU) patients [1,36–38]. Several studies have indicated that ~ 10% to 25% of ICU patients contract pneumonia. These rates generally reflect those of the common bacterial pathogens shown in Table 32-1.

Crude rates of VAP range from 6 to 30 cases/100 patients, depending on the population studied [11,39–41]. Several studies have demonstrated that rates of pneumonia are increased four to twenty-onefold for incubated patients [37,42,43], and range from 1% to 3% per day of intubation and mechanical ventilation [44,45]. However, because crude rates of VAP do not adjust for time or duration of mechanical ventilation, using an index of "cases/1,000 ventilator days" is recommended. Rates of

TABLE 32-2. *Microorganisms isolated from respiratory tract specimens obtained by various methods to diagnose nosocomial pneumonia*

	Schaberg [37]	Bartlett [13]	Fagon [11]	Torres [12]	Schleupner [24]
Hospital type	NNIS/UMH	Veterans	General	General	Community Teaching
Ventilated/Nonventilated	Mixed	Mixed	Ventilated	Ventilated	Mixed
Number	N/A	159	49	78	231
Specimen(s) cultured	sputum tracheal aspirate	tracheal aspirate, pleural fluid	protected specimen brush (PSB)	PSB, blood, lung aspirate, pleural fluid	sputum or tracheal aspirate
Culture results					
No organism isolated	N/A	0	0	54%[b]	11%
Polymicrobial	N/A	54%[b]	40%[b]	13%[b]	35%
Number of isolates	15499	314	111	N/A	312
Gram-negative bacilli (GNB)	50%[a]	46%[b]	75%[b]	16%[b]	9%[b]
Ps. aeruginosa	17%	9%	31%	5%	3%
Enteric GNB	27%	20%	32%	9%	6%
H. influenzae	6%	17%	10%	0%	2%
Legionella spp	N/A	N/A	2%	2%	N/A
Gram-positive cocci	17%[a]	56%[b]	52%[b]	4%[b]	27%[b]
S. aureus	16%	25%	33%	2%	4%
S. pneumoniae	1%	31%	29%	2%	23%
Anaerobes	N/A	35%	2%	0%	0
Fungi	4%	N/A	0%	1%	0
Viruses	N/A	N/A	N/A	N/A	N/A

NNIS, National Nosocomial Infection Surveillance System; UMH, University of Michigan Hospitals.
N/A, Not applicable; not tested or not reported.
[a]Percent isolates.
[b]Percent episodes (percentages not additive due to polymicrobial etiology in some episodes).
(Modified in part from Tablan OC, Anderson LJ, Arden NH, et al. Guideline for prevention of nosocomial pneumonia: part I. Issues on prevention of nosocomial pneumonia, 1994. *Infect Control Hosp Epidemiol* 1994;15:588–625.)

VAP/1,000 ventilator days range from 5/1,000 in pediatric ICU patients to 34/1,000 in patients with thermal injury [3,40,46]; rates are ~ 15 per 1,000 for medical and surgical ICU patients [40,44,45,47]. These rates of nosocomial pneumonia are probably skewed by overrepresentation of patients in university teaching hospitals [24,48].

Mortality

The crude mortality rates for nosocomial pneumonia range from 20% to 50% and reflect, in large part, the severity of underlying disease in the population studied [33,41,49–53]. In a case–control study of 200 patients who died in the hospital, nosocomial pneumonia contributed to 60% of the infection-related deaths [54]. On examination of 1,000 autopsy reports, pneumonia was not only associated with 7.5% of the deaths, but was the most common nosocomial infection contributing to death [55]. Mortality rates were usually higher in patients with pneumonia due to *P. aeruginosa*, and when secondary bacteremia was present [2,37,44,51,52,55,56].

Intensive care unit patients with nosocomial pneumonia appear to have a two- to tenfold increased risk of mortality compared to patients without pneumonia [34,44,50, 51]. Independent risk factors for mortality in nonventilated patients include "high-risk" organisms, bilateral infiltrates on chest radiography, and respiratory failure [34]. By comparison, risk factors for mortality in patients with VAP include transfer from another hospital or ward, renal failure, duration of mechanical ventilation, pneumonia on admission, coma, severe underlying disease, worsening respiratory failure, shock, inappropriate antibiotic treatment, and hospitalization in noncardiac ICUs [34,50]. VAP has been a significant risk factor for mortality in several studies [50].

In contrast to crude mortality, mortality due to the pneumonia or "attributable mortality" has been estimated to be 30% to 33% for nonventilated patients [49]. In a more recent study, the attributable mortality for patients with VAP was 27%, and increased to 43% when the etiologic agent was *P. aeruginosa* or *Acinetobacter* species [33]. Most experts believe that the attributable mortality of nosocomial pneumonia can be reduced by appropriate therapy and prevention strategies.

Cost

Nosocomial pneumonia appears to increase the duration of hospitalization two- to threefold, compared to patients without pneumonia [37,49,52,56]. In one study, the mean length of stay for patients with VAP was 34 days, compared with 21 days for matched control subjects

TABLE 32-3. Limitations and advantages of current methods used for the diagnosis of nosocomial pneumonia

Method of diagnosis	Advantages	Limitations
Clinical [3,23,24,38,48,98]	Based on widely available clinical data; fever; leukocytosis; purulent sputum by Gram stain, new & persistent pulmonary infiltrate on chest x-ray Non-invasive Relatively inexpensive Gram stain and sputum culture easy to perform Serial Gram stains in intubated patients, when correlated with clinical condition, may provide a clue for initial choice of antibiotics and aid in the interpretation of sputum culture results	Poor specificity, especially in patients with diffuse infiltrates on chest x-ray, ARDS, or CHF Poor sensitivity for immunocompromised patients or unusual organisms Poor specificity of non-quantitative sputum cultures Culture results delayed for 24–48 hr Presence of potential pathogen suggestive, *not* diagnostic Quality of specimen variable Culture for Legionella often unavailable Processing and interpretation of Gram stain varies
Clinical Pulmonary Infection Score (CPIS) [68,76]	CPIS correlates with diagnosis by bronchoscopy and PSB in ventilated patients Uses quantitative bacteriology to increase specificity	Quantitative endotracheal cultures are not widely available Results may be altered by prior antibiotic use
Bronchoscopy with (PSB) or (BAL) [7,8,10–12,33,72]	Useful for diagnosis in some mechanically ventilated and/or immunocompromised patients PSB sensitivity (≥ 10^3/mL) every 85%–90%, and specificity 95% in experienced staff BAL sensitivity (≥ 10^4/mL) every 86% to 100%, and specificity 95%–100% in experienced staff Decreases unnecessary antibiotic use and development of antibiotic-resistant organisms Useful for patient who does not respond to initial antibiotic therapy	Relies on quantitative bacteriology Prior antibiotics may decrease sensitivity May miss early cases of ventilator-associated pneumonia (VAP) Bronchoscopy is relatively costly, not always available, and invasive Delays in obtaining culture results BAL may have greater complication rate than PSB Need meticulous and prompt processing of specimens Efficacy, risk, and cost of PSB/BAL versus clinical diagnosis for various populations of patients is not well documented
Non-bronchoscopic BAL [7,8,9,73,74]	Simpler, less expensive, and appears to have comparable diagnostic yield to bronchoscopy with PSB or BAL Useful for following response to antibiotic treatment	Quantitative cultures are more costly than routine cultures Requires special skill Data on risk, benefit, and cost compared to clinical diagnosis and bronchoscopy are limited
Quantitative Endotracheal Aspirates (QEA) [76–78]	Simpler, less expensive than bronchoscopy or non-bronchoscopic BAL 65% correlation between QEA and bronchoscopy with PSB, BAL, but less specific Good negative predictive value (~70%)	Threshold for diagnosis of ventilator-associated pneumonia (VAP) varies among studies
Autopsy [223,274]	May increase diagnosis of unsuspected pathogens, such as Legionella, Aspergillus, Candida, CMV, and PCP	No clinical value for patient Not often performed

PSB, protected specimen brush; BAL, bronchoalveolar lavage; VAP, ventilator-associated pneumonia; ARDS, adult respiratory distress syndrome; CHF, congestive heart failure; CMV, cytomegalovirus; PCP, Pneumonocystis carinii pneumonia.

(Adapted in part from Craven and Steger. Hospital-acquired pneumonia: perspectives for the epidemiologist. *Infect Control Hosp Epidemiol* 1997 [in press].)

[33,57]. There is need for more current data on the cost of nosocomial pneumonia, particularly in view of the rapidly changing healthcare delivery system in the United States.

Diagnosis

Accurate data regarding etiologic agents, epidemiology, and treatment of bacterial nosocomial pneumonia are limited by the lack of a gold standard for diagnosing infection (Table 32-3). For intubated patients, there has been considerable controversy over the benefits and risk of clinical diagnosis and empiric antibiotic therapy vs. the use of more specific quantitative analysis of specimens obtained from the lower respiratory tract by bronchoscopic or blind aspirates using BAL or PSB. Clearly, randomized studies based on outcomes such as cost, duration of mechanical ventilation, hospital stay, morbidity, and mortality are needed to resolve this controversy.

Clinical Diagnosis

The clinical diagnosis of nosocomial pneumonia incorporates data on the patient's underlying disease, risk factors for infection, symptoms, and time in the hospital (early vs. late disease). Pneumonia due to *S. pneumoniae* or *H. influenzae* occurs early in the hospitalization, especially in patients with advanced age, chronic underlying disease, acquired immunodeficiency syndrome (AIDS), or head trauma. By comparison, pneumonia due to *S. aureus* usually appears later in the hospital course and should be suspected in insulin-dependent diabetics, intravenous drug users, or patients with renal failure. *Klebsiella*, *P. aeruginosa*, and other gram-negative bacillary pathogens often cause late-onset disease in mechanically ventilated patients with severe acute or chronic underlying disease.

Most patients with nosocomial pneumonia exhibit fever, malaise, dyspnea, and a productive cough. Critically ill patients are usually tachypneic, tachycardiac, and febrile, and may be agitated; some may progress to coma, hypotension, or shock. Tracheal deviation may be present if there is associated pneumothorax or empyema, with clinical evidence of consolidation, pleuritis, or pleural effusion. Information garnered from the physical examination and from laboratory data (blood leukocyte count, blood gases, chest radiographs, sputum Gram stain, and cultures) is often helpful in establishing the etiology and severity of the pneumonia. Although blood cultures are quite specific, they are uncommonly positive, and culture results are not available for 2 to 48 hours. Likewise, the Gram stain or culture of a pleural fluid may identify the specific causative agent, but is performed in only a small fraction of patients.

The chest radiograph usually shows a localized or diffuse alveolar pattern. The presence of lung abscess suggests a necrotizing infection due to anaerobes, *S. aureus*, or aerobic gram-negative bacilli. Multiple, wedge-shaped infiltrates in the periphery are suggestive of septic emboli, and pneumatoceles are associated with *S. aureus* infection. Pleural effusion occurs in > 25% of patients with pneumonia caused by pneumococci or *S. aureus*, but may occur with gram-negative bacilli as well [58]. Computed tomography scans may be helpful in the diagnosis of pneumonia or abscess in patients with adult respiratory distress syndrome (ARDS), or for the management of pneumonia complicated by empyema. Ultrasound provides similar information and may provide a portable diagnostic and therapeutic tool for patients too unstable to leave the ICU.

Atelectasis, pulmonary edema, pulmonary emboli, neoplastic processes, and some autoimmune diseases can all mimic pneumonia. Chest radiographic changes due to ARDS or congestive heart failure make the clinical diagnosis of pneumonia particularly difficult. In the intubated patient, it may be difficult to distinguish between tracheal colonization, tracheobronchitis, and early pneumonia. In critically ill patients, sputum may be produced spontaneously, induced by nebulized saline, or obtained by transtracheal aspiration or bronchoscopy.

Examination of sputum often provides ready clues to the diagnosis of pneumonia. Adequate Gram-stained sputum samples should reveal multiple inflammatory cells, a paucity of epithelial cells, and a predominant morphology of bacterial types. Highly purulent sputum usually indicates bacterial infection. Gram-positive diplococci should suggest pneumococci, whereas gram-positive cocci in clusters suggest staphylococci. Gram-negative coccobacilli (characteristic of *H. influenzae*) or diplococci (suggesting *Neisseria* species or *M. catarrhalis*) may be seen early, whereas gram-negative bacilli (*Klebsiella*, other enteric rods, or *Pseudomonas*) may occur early in chronically ill patients, those who were previously hospitalized, or patients with onset later in their hospital course.

With Gram stains demonstrating polymorphonuclear cells or macrophages, but no bacteria, legionellosis, *M. tuberculosis* infection, or partially treated bacterial infection should be considered. Because sputum is only cultured aerobically, anaerobes should be considered if there are mixed bacterial morphologies on Gram stain and the culture report reveals "normal flora." Pleural fluid, thin-needle aspirates, and blood cultures may be sent for anaerobic culture. In cases where the diagnosis remains unclear, transbronchial or open lung biopsy may be needed for diagnosis. Some investigators have looked for elastase fibers or antibody-coated bacteria in sputum and for elastolytic activity in pulmonary lavage fluid to aid in the diagnosis of pneumonia, but these methods are not widely used [59,60]. In intubated patients, serial Gram stains may be useful to monitor response to initial antibiotic therapy and culture and sensitivity testing used to adjust antimicrobial therapy. Culture data usually reflect only aerobic bacteria, and antibiotic sensitivities represent the minimum inhibitory concentrations in serum, and not those in bronchial secretions. Thus, it is prudent to make changes in antimicrobial therapy based on clinical response and the pharmacology of the agents being used.

Clinical criteria for the diagnosis of pneumonia are the standard in most hospitals, but this method lacks specificity, particularly in mechanically ventilated patients (see Table 32-3). In one study, 60 patients were suspected of having pneumonia clinically, but conclusive evidence of pneumonia was found in only 30% [61]. Similarly, only 31% of cases of clinically suspected pneumonia were correctly identified in an ICU setting, and some investigators, using vigorous chest physical therapy alone, were able to eliminate 80% of new infiltrates in ICU patients within 8 hours [10,62]. Reports of routine endotracheal aspirates, which are commonly used to diagnose pneumonia, had a sensitivity of 89% and a specificity of 14% [4]. Clearly, improved diagnostic methods are necessary for optimal management, particularly for ventilated patients [63,64].

Diagnosis of Ventilator-Associated Pneumonia by Bronchoscopy With Bronchoalveolar Lavage or Protected Specimen Brush

Because of the absence of a gold standard for diagnosis, controversy exists over the most accurate, safe, and cost-effective method of diagnosing VAP [8,65]. Bronchoscopy with PSB or BAL, coupled with quantitative bacteriology, has demonstrated greater specificity than clinical diagnosis of VAP [7,8] (see Table 32-3). Bronchoscopy with PSB ($\geq 10^3$ organisms/ml) or BAL ($\geq 10^4$ organisms/ml) has sensitivities that range from 60% to 95%, with specificities of 80% to 100% [4,7,8,10,66–69]. Early results of a meta-analysis of 15 clinical studies of PSB yielded an overall sensitivity of 91%, and specificity of 95% [70] vs. a sensitivity ranging from 86% to 100%, with 100% specificity for BAL.

Despite the seemingly encouraging results with the use of these techniques under optimal conditions, false-negative and false-positive tests are a risk, particularly when the patient has received recent antibiotic therapy [8,71]. In addition, caution is advised because of differences in study design, patient populations, definitions of pneumonia, variations in the skill of the bronchoscopist, and questions about the risk and cost–benefit ratios compared with clinical diagnosis with and without quantitative bacteriology.

Nonbronchoscopic Diagnosis of Ventilator-Associated Pneumonia

Because bronchoscopy is an invasive technique that is costly and not always available, nonbronchoscopic or blind BAL has been suggested as an effective alternative [9,68,72–76]. These methods rely on QEA, but they are simpler, less expensive, and appear to provide results similar to those obtained by bronchoscopy [77,78].

Good correlation has been observed between bronchoscopic diagnosis and the clinical pulmonary infection score (CPIS) for the clinical diagnosis of pneumonia [68]. The CPIS incorporates quantitative assessment of the patient's temperature, leukocyte count and differential, oxygenation, presence of infiltrates or ARDS on chest radiograph, and results of semiquantitative Gram stain and culture of tracheal aspirates. Serial Gram stains and quantitative cultures, when correlated with CPIS [68,76], also appear to provide a more accurate diagnosis than clinical criteria and may result in more appropriate use of antibiotics in the ICU, but further evaluation is needed. The use of blind BAL may provide another alternative to bronchoscopic diagnosis, but this technique also needs further validation. In summary, the use of quantitative tracheal aspirates and CPIS is probably superior to clinical diagnosis and similar to results obtained by bronchoscopy [79]. Understanding the risks and cost–benefit ratios of different techniques for the diagnosis of nosocomial pneumonia and their impact on clinical management, patient outcomes, and cost of care is imperative.

Pathogenesis

There are several mechanisms that contribute to the pathogenesis of pneumonia, and the relative contribution of each pathway remains controversial. Although VAP may result from bacteremia or translocation of bacteria through or between the gastrointestinal mucosal epithelial cells, aspiration of bacteria primarily from the oropharynx and sometimes of organisms refluxed from the stomach is the most important route of infection [22,43,80–88] (Figure 32-3). In the mechanically ventilated patient, leakage of bacteria around the endotracheal cuff, along with local trauma and tracheal inflammation from the endotracheal tube, increases colonization and reduces the clearance of organisms and secretions from the lower respiratory tract [22,82,83,86,89] (Figure 32-4). Tracheal colonization with bacteria and tracheobronchitis are common and may be precursors to VAP [63,64]. Bacteria may also be nebulized or inoculated directly into the lower respiratory tract.

Colonization of the Oropharynx

In contrast to healthy people, critically ill patients and patients with VAP have high rates of oropharyngeal colonization with bacterial pathogens [90,91]. Colonization with gram-negative bacilli was present in 16% of moderately ill patients vs. 57% of critically ill patients, and rates of pneumonia were increased sixfold in ICU patients who were colonized [81,92]. In another study, 36 patients with VAP had significantly higher rates of oropharyngeal colonization than the 27 mechanically ventilated patients without pneumonia [90].

The ability of gram-negative bacilli to adhere to oropharyngeal epithelial cells appears to be pivotal in establishing successful colonization. Host factors, types of bacteria colonizing the pharynx, and the use of antibiotics may alter colonization and adherence of gram-negative bacilli

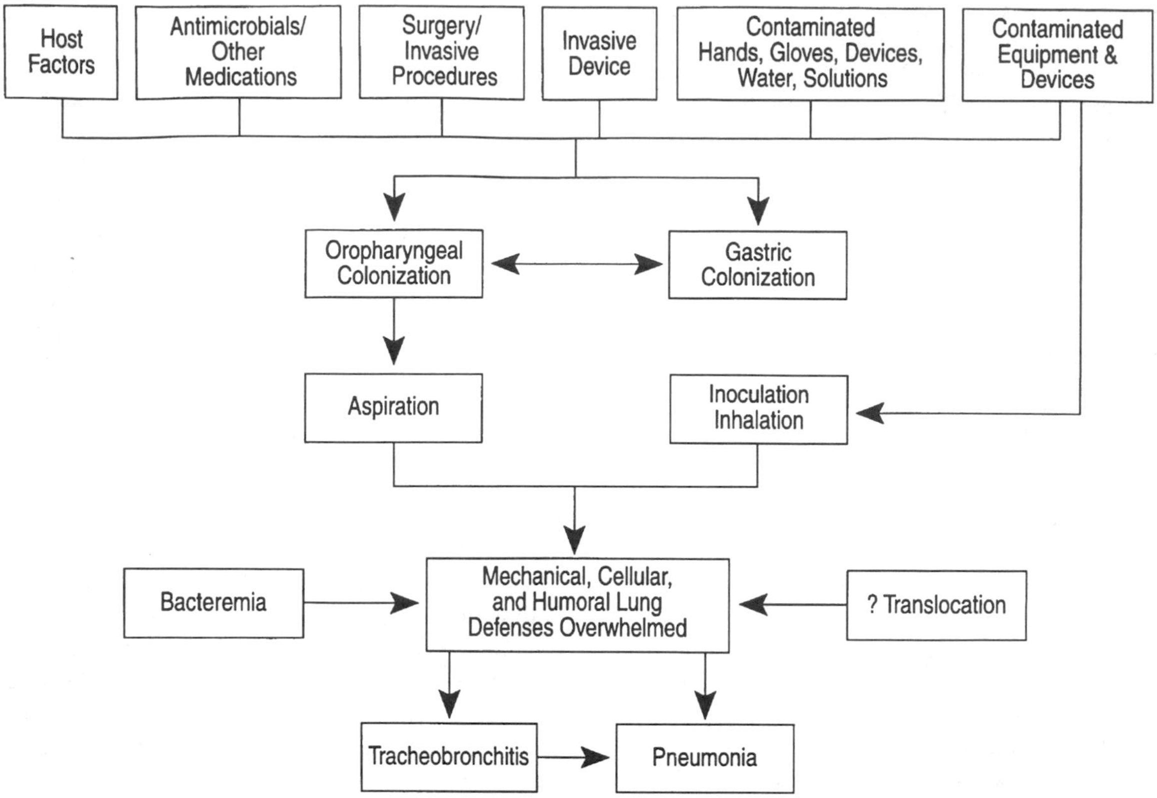

FIGURE 32-3. Summary of risk factors contributing to colonization and infection of the lower respiratory tract. Important risk factors include the inoculum and virulence of the infecting agents and response of the pulmonary host defenses in the lung. (From Craven DE, Steger KA, Fleming CA. Preventing hospital-acquired pneumonia: Current concepts and strategies. *Semin Respir* and *Crit Care Med* 1997;18:185–199, with permission.)

[47,93–95]. Oral epithelial cells rich in fibronectin bind gram-positive organisms such as streptococci and *S. aureus*, whereas those poor in fibronectin preferentially bind gram-negative bacilli such as *P. aeruginosa* [94,96,97]. High levels of elastase and small amounts of IgA in the sputum also effect bacterial adherence [94,96,97].

Gastric Colonization

In mechanically ventilated patients, the stomach and gastrointestinal tract appear to contribute to oropharyngeal and tracheal colonization with gram-negative bacilli [43,50,80,83–85,90,98–102], although some investiga-

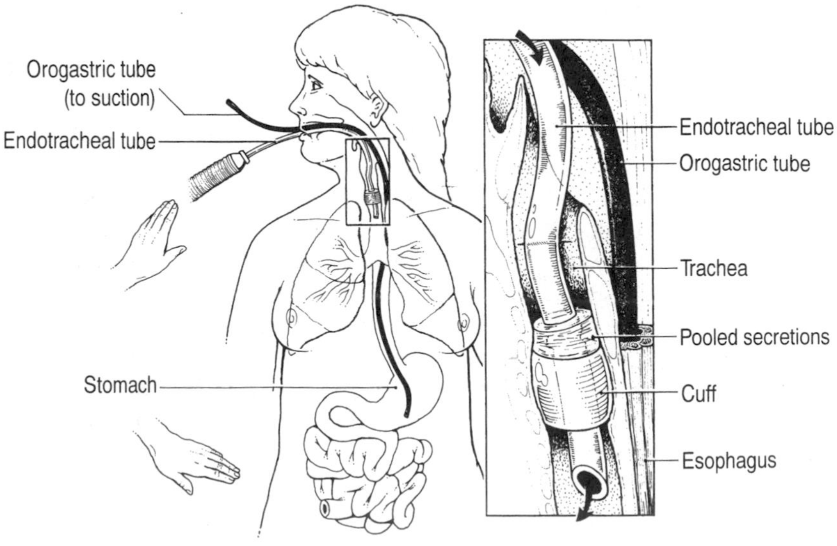

FIGURE 32-4. An intubated patient with subglottic secretions above the cuff. Removal of subglottic secretions decreases colonization of the trachea and the risk of ventilator-associated pneumonia (VAP). Note that the endotracheal and gastric tubes are also inserted through the mouth to reduce the risk of nosocomial sinusitis and VAP. (From Craven DE, Steger KA. Hospital-acquired pneumonia: perspective for the epidemiologist. *Infect Control Hosp Epidemiol* 1997 [in press], with permission.)

tors question their importance [103,104]. The stomach is often sterile when the pH is < 2 because of the potent bactericidal activity of hydrochloric acid [21,84,105]. An increase in gastric colonization occurs with achlorhydria, and in the presence of various gastrointestinal diseases, malnutrition, or use of antacids and histamine-2 (H_2) blockers [105–114]. In mechanically ventilated patients, colonization may reach 1–100 million gram-negative bacilli/ml of gastric juice when the pH is greater than 4 [21,84,99]. Retrograde colonization of the oropharynx from the stomach may increase the risk of lower respiratory tract infection, constituting the "gastropulmonary route of infection" [83,84,99–101,115].

Immune Defenses in the Lung

The response of the pulmonary host defenses to invading microorganisms plays an integral part in the pathogenesis and outcome of infection, but unfortunately progress in our understanding is limited and needs further work [116–118]. Mucociliary and mechanical clearance in the upper airway are important factors in the defense against infection. Bacterial antigens and cytokines that affect the activity and efficacy of ciliary cells in clearing bacteria from the lower airway need further study. The ability of macrophages and polymorphonuclear leukocytes to eliminate bacterial pathogens and the interaction of these cells with inflammatory cytokines probably play important roles in the pathogenesis of pneumonia [119]. Cell-mediated immune response is controlled by a complex array of lipids, peptides, and cytokines, including interleukin-1 and -2, interferons, growth factors, and chemotactic factors [59,60,116–118]. Leukotrienes, complement components, and platelet-activating factor also assist in the inflammatory response and contribute in various ways to the pathogenesis of nosocomial pneumonia [59,60,120]. Based on an improved understanding of molecular interaction between bacteria cell walls, toxins, and host defenses, strategies should be considered to enhance host defenses and supplement current antimicrobial regimens.

Risk Factors and Prevention

Risk factors for nosocomial pneumonia may be grouped into host factors, conditions that favor colonization and aspiration, cross-infection or complications from medications, invasive devices, and respiratory therapy equipment [22,23,41,43,47,50,82,83,94,98,121] (see Figure 32-3). Specific intervention strategies for intrinsic and extrinsic risk factors are shown in Figure 32-5.

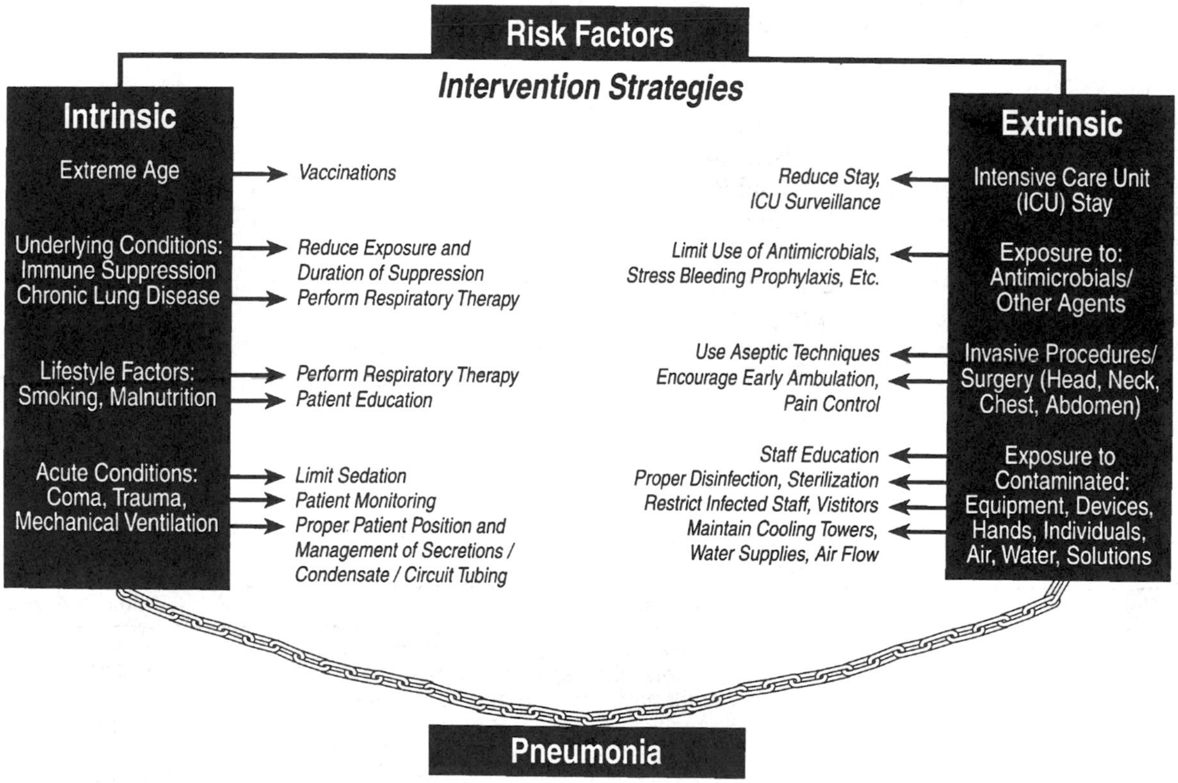

FIGURE 32-5. Intrinsic and extrinsic host factors contributing to the chain of infection for hospital-associated pneumonia caused by bacterial pathogens. Prevention efforts should emphasize interventions aimed at extrinsic risk factors. (From Craven DE, Steger KA, Fleming CA. Preventing hospital-acquired pneumonia: Current concepts and strategies. *Semin Respir* and *Crit Care Med* 1997;18:185–199, with permission.)

TABLE 32-4. *Selected risk factors and preventive measures for bacterial nosocomial pneumonia in the non-intensive care unit patient*

Risk factor	Preventative measure	CDC/HICPAC[a]
Age	Primary prevention; healthcare maintenance	NS
Underlying disease	Treat COPD; incentive spirometry	IA
	Influenza, pneumococcal vaccination	IA
Immunosuppression	Taper steroids	NS
	Minimize duration of neutropenia ±G-CSF	NS
	Avoid exposure to potential nosocomial pathogens	NS
Environmental	Awareness of seasonal pathogens (influenza, RSV)	NS
	Maintenance of cooling tower, water supply, air filter	IB[b]
Depressed consciousness	Cautious use of CNS depressants	NS
	Position patient upright at 30°–45°	NS
Antibiotic administration	Antibiotic prophylaxis for NP not recommended	IB
	Judicious administration of antibiotics	NS
Cross-infection	Educate and train personnel	IB
	Appropriate handwashing, use of gloves & gowns	IA
	Feedback surveillance data to staff	IA
	Isolation of patients with respiratory infections	NS
	Identify MDR pathogens	NS
Enteral feeding	Verify tube placement	IB
	Use sterile water	NS
	Use orogastric tube, if possible	NS
Avoid reflux	Position patient at 30°–45°; drain residual	IB
Oxygen delivery systems	Change tubing between patients	IB

NS, not specified in HICPAC guideline; COPD, chronic obstructive pulmonary disease; GCSF, granulocyte colony stimulating factor; RSV, respiratory syncitial virus; CNS, central nervous system; NP, nosocomial pneumonia; MDR, multidrug resistant

[a]Centers for Disease Control and Prevention/Hospital Infection Control Practices Advisory Committee (CDC/HICPAC) guideline categories. Specific references listed in the 1994 CDC/HICPAC guidelines. (Tablan OC, Anderson LJ, Arden NH, et al. Guideline for prevention of nosocomial pneumonia: part I. Issues on prevention of nosocomial pneumonia, 1994. *Infect Control Hosp Epidemiol* 1994;15:588–625.)

[b]Refers specifically to legionella and aspergillus infections.

Prevention measures are well summarized in the *Guideline for Prevention of Nosocomial Pneumonia* published by the Centers for Disease Control and Prevention (CDC) and the Hospital Infection Control Practices Advisory Committee (HICPAC) [3] (Table 32-4). The CDC/HICPAC guideline was reviewed and approved by a number of important infection control and pulmonary and infectious disease organizations, and is the most comprehensive document available. CDC/HICPAC Category IA is "strongly recommended for all hospitals and strongly supported by well-designed experimental or epidemiologic studies." Category IB is "strongly recommended for all hospitals and viewed as effective by experts in the field and a consensus of HICPAC based on strong rationale and suggestive evidence, even though definitive scientific studies may not have been done." Category II is "suggested for implementation in many hospitals; recommendations may be supported by suggestive clinical or epidemiologic studies, a strong theoretical rationale or definitive studies applicable to some but not all hospitals." No-recommendation categories are defined as practices for which there are insufficient data, or when there

TABLE 32-5. *Risk factors and preventive measures for bacterial nosocomial pneumonia in the nonventilated, intensive care unit patient*

Risk factor	Preventative measure	CDC/HICPAC[a]
Stress bleeding prophylaxis	Use nonalkalinizing cytoprotective agents	II
	Use only when specifically indicated	NS
Invasive equipment/devices	Appropriate cleaning and sterilization	IB
	Expeditious removal	IB
Spirometer/O_2 sensor	Clean; sterilize/disinfect between patients	IA
Resuscitation bag	Clean; sterilize/disinfect between patients	IA
Nasogastric tube	Refer to enteral feeding (Table 32-4)	IA
Cross-infection	Surveillance with feedback to staff	IA
	Infection control procedures	IA
Immobility	Lateral rotational bed	NR

NS, not specified in HICPAC guideline.

[a]CDC/HICPAC guideline criteria defined in test; specific references in text and CDC/HICPAC guidelines.

TABLE 32-6. *Risk factors and preventive measures for patients with ventilator-associated pneumonia (VAP)*

Risk factor	Preventative measure	CDC/HICPAC[a]
Gastric colonization	Selective decontamination of digestive tract	NR
Endotracheal intubation	Keep cuff inflated; aspirate subglottic secretions before deflating cuff	IB
	Continuous aspiration of subglottic secretions	NR[b]
	Oral intubation	NR
	Semi-recumbent patient positioning	NS
Ventilator circuits	Do not change more often than every 48 hours	IA
	Drain/discard condensate away from patients	IA
	Use heat-moisture exchanger (HME)	NR
In-line medication nebulizer	Disinfect between treatments	IB
	Sterilize between patients	IB
Suction catheter	Aseptic technique	IA
	Sterile single-use catheter for open system	II
	Closed circuit tracheal suction catheter	NR
	Aseptic technique when changing tubes	IB
Tracheostomy care		

[a]CDC/HICPAC guideline criteria as defined in Tables 32-4 and 32-5. Specific references in text and CDC/HICPAC guidelines (From Tablan OC, Anderson LJ, Arden NH, et al. Guideline for prevention of nosocomial pneumonia: part I: Issues on prevention on nosocomial pneumonia, 1994. *Infect Control Hosp Epidemiol* 1994;15:588–625.)

is a lack of consensus regarding efficacy. Table 32-4 provides risk factors and preventive measures for the non-ICU patient, Table 32-5 summarizes strategies for the nonventilated ICU patient, and Table 32-6 provides information on the mechanically ventilated patient.

Host Factors

Advanced age, smoking, and underlying diseases significantly increase the risk of pneumonia and colonization of the upper airway, but they may not be the best targets for prevention of the current episode of nosocomial pneumonia. These factors, however, should be targeted for prevention of future episodes of pneumonia.

Aspiration and gastric reflux are common in hospitalized patients [2,43,80,83,84,86,98,122,123]. In one study, oropharyngeal reflux was reported in ~ 70% of patients receiving tube feedings; 40% had evidence of pulmonary aspiration [122]. Maintaining the patient in an upright position appears to reduce reflux, aspiration, and VAP [41,83,123]. Because this technique is simple and has excellent risk–benefit and cost–benefit ratios, it is strongly endorsed.

The postoperative patient is at particularly high risk of nosocomial pneumonia due to a variety of pathogens that may enter the airway during intubation or be aspirated during anesthesia or into the anesthetized airway postextubation. Postoperative atelectasis, retained secretions, and pain may increase the risk of nosocomial pneumonia. CDC/HIVPAC Category IB recommendations for prevention include maintaining semiupright patient position to reduce aspiration, frequent coughing, deep breathing, incentive spirometry, and early ambulation to prevent atelectasis.

Medications

Several medications have been identified as risk factors for nosocomial pneumonia, some of which are discussed here and in review articles [121,124,125].

Sedatives and Neuromuscular Blockers

Sedatives may increase the risk aspiration and decrease cough and clearance of secretions from the lower respiratory tract. This effect is profound in elderly patients or those with impaired swallowing. Prevention strategies should include judicious use of sedation and proper positioning of patients to minimize the risk of aspiration.

Limited data are available on neuromuscular blockers as a risk factor for VAP. Prekates and coworkers studied risk factors for VAP (diagnosed by bronchoscopy with PSB and BAL) in 92 postoperative multiple trauma patients [126]. VAP occurred in 23% of these patients. Independent predictors of VAP, after stepwise logistic regression, were flail chest ($p < 0.001$) and the use of neuromuscular blockers ($p < 0.001$). The CDC/HICPAC guideline made no comment in the absence of more supporting data; clearly, further studies are needed.

Antibiotics and Selective Decontamination of the Digestive Tract

The use of antibiotics is controversial because they may either prevent or increase the patient's risk of HAP. Clearly, some antibiotics have had a role in reducing endogenous colonization with pathogens such as *S. pneumoniae* and *H. influenzae*. Thus, although broad-spectrum antibiotics such as cephalosporins may decrease the risk of early-onset

HAP, they may in turn increase the prevalence of colonization and infection due to nosocomial MDR pathogens [20,34,41,127]. We advocate the judicious use of antibiotics for early treatment of VAP. In accordance with the CDC/HICPAC guideline, we also discourage the use of prophylactic antibiotics for HAP. Finally, controlling antibiotic use in sites, such as the ICU, is frequently associated with a decrease in patient colonization and infection with MDR pathogens. With the increasing prevalence of MDR nosocomial infections, controlling antibiotic use may ultimately become necessary.

Selective decontamination of the digestive tract (SDD) uses multiple oral antibiotics (aminoglycoside, polymyxin B, and amphotericin B), with and without systemic cefotaxime, trimethoprim, or a quinolone, to prevent oropharyngeal and gastrointestinal colonization (see Chaapter 15). Several studies and review articles of SDD report dramatically reduced rates of respiratory tract colonization and infection [128–137]. However, the results of many of these studies are difficult to assess because of differences in study design, study population, and inconsistent definitions of respiratory tract infection that could include tracheobronchitis.

Two large, double-blind, placebo-controlled trials found no benefit from SDD [136,137]. In a more recent study by Ferrer et al., tracheal secretions were examined by PSB or BAL, with or without diagnosis at autopsy, and again no difference was noted in the frequency of VAP among the SDD group vs. the control subjects (18% vs. 24%) [128].

The SDD trialist group reported a 67% reduction in lower respiratory tract infection and decreased mortality in patients treated with SDD and a systemic antibiotic compared with those who received only a combination of the oral, nonabsorbable antibiotics [129]. However, the effect of SDD on the emergence of MDR strains of bacteria, coupled with the limited effect on the duration of mechanical ventilation, length of hospital stay, and overall cost effectiveness, raise concerns about its risk–benefit ratio [133,134]. The CDC/HICPAC guideline made no recommendation on the use of SDD. We, and others, do not support the routine use of SDD for all medical and surgical ICU patients [133–135]. SDD may be useful for a select population of patients, such as those with trauma, but further data are needed to delineate the most effective antibiotic regimen, issues of long-term benefit, and risk–benefit and cost–benefit ratios in an era characterized by MDR strains of bacteria.

Stress Bleeding Prophylaxis

Although antacids, H_2 blockers, and sucralfate have not been approved for stress bleeding prophylaxis by the U.S. Food and Drug Administration, they are frequently prescribed. Data have suggested that patients with prolonged mechanical ventilation are at increased risk for clinically significant gastrointestinal bleeding [138]. Although controversial, several studies have demonstrated lower rates of VAP in patients treated prophylactically with sucralfate compared to antacids and H_2 blockers [23,50,98,99,114,139,140]. Others have found no difference between these agents [21,103,104,141,142]. In meta-analyses of the efficacy of stress bleeding prophylaxis in ICU patients, respiratory tract infection was significantly less frequent ($p < 0.05$) in patients treated with sucralfate compared with patients receiving either H_2 blockers or antacids [139,143,144]. These studies have used a clinical diagnosis of pneumonia, and further studies are needed using BAL, PSB, or QEA for diagnosis.

Differences among sucralfate, antacids, and H_2 blockers may be due to gastric pH, reflux, bacterial colonization, effect on host defenses, or the bactericidal activity of sucralfate [23,80,98–100,140,145]. More recent data suggest that the differences between sucralfate and other agents primarily affect rates of late-onset bacterial pneumonia [23].

Perhaps the most important question is whether stress bleeding prophylaxis should be prescribed at all [138]. One randomized trial found no difference in rates of stress bleeding between patients receiving prophylaxis and control subjects [146]. Many of us believe that it is overprescribed.

Devices

Several devices have been identified as risk factors for HAP. Many of these devices are used in mechanically ventilated patients and are associated with VAP; intervention strategies are summarized in several review articles and in Table 32-6 [121,124,125].

Nasotracheal or Endotracheal Tubes

The endotracheal tube facilitates the entry of bacteria into the trachea, decreases clearance of bacteria and secretions from the lower airway, and significantly increases the patient's risk of VAP [22,37,42,50,80,82,86, 147–149]. Subglottic secretions and bacteria that pool above the endotracheal tube cuff may leak into the trachea and increase tracheal colonization and VAP (see Figure 32-4). Manual intermittent or continuous aspiration of subglottic secretions (CASS) decreases this risk and the incidence of VAP [82,150]. In one study, the incidence of VAP decreased from 39.6 episodes/1,000 ventilator days in control subjects to 19.6 episodes/1,000 ventilator days for the group receiving CASS [22]. Efficacy was most pronounced during the first 2 weeks after intubation. Because of the excellent risk–benefit and cost–benefit ratios, this strategy should be given serious consideration when the system becomes available in the United States.

Respiratory airway care is also important in the intubated patient [127]. In a study by Rello and coworkers, there was a significantly higher rate of VAP noted in patients who failed the CASS technique during the first eight days of mechanical ventilation, especially if the patient was not receiving antibiotics [127]. These data underscore the importance of maintaining adequate cuff pressure to reduce aspiration around the endotracheal tube cuff, and there was a trend toward a higher risk of VAP for patients with cuff pressures less than 20 cm H_2O. Clearly, maintaining cuff pressure is simple and should be routinely adapted based on its efficacy and low cost.

Over 95% of endotracheal tubes examined by scanning electron microscopy had partial bacterial colonization and 84% were completely covered by bacteria encased in a biofilm or glycocalyx [151]. Some investigators have suggested that aggregates of bacteria in biofilm, dislodged during tracheal suctioning, act as septic emboli that increase the patient's risk of VAP. Aggregates of bacteria encased in biofilm are not readily killed by antibiotics and may be more resistant to clearance by pulmonary host defenses [147,151]. Research to alter the composition of the endotracheal tube to be more resistant to biofilm is in progress.

Nasogastric Versus Orogastric Tubes and Sinusitis

A nasotracheal tube increases the patient's risk of sinusitis and VAP, and therefore should be avoided or used only when clinically indicated [149]. Most patients receiving mechanical ventilation also have a gastric tube inserted to manage secretions, prevent gastric distention, or provide nutritional support (see Figure 32-4). The nasogastric tube increases oropharyngeal colonization and gastric reflux, acts as a conduit for bacteria to migrate to the oropharynx, and causes sinusitis [42,80,149,152]. The diagnosis of sinusitis is often made clinically. The use of a computed tomography scan and needle aspiration of the sinus fluid increase the specificity of the diagnosis and identification of the specific etiologic agent. In one study, maxillary sinusitis was linked to the placement and duration of nasotracheal and gastric intubation [149]. Organisms isolated from the maxillary sinus aspirates were most commonly *P. aeruginosa*, *Acinetobacter* species, *S. aureus*, and *Candida albicans*; these isolates correlated well with organisms causing VAP. Oral gastric and endotracheal tubes significantly decreased the incidence of infectious maxillary sinusitis and VAP ($p < 0.001$) and are therefore important prevention strategies.

Enteral Feeding

Accurate assessment of the patient's nutritional status and the use of enteral feeding, rather than parenteral nutrition, appear to reduce the risk of nosocomial pneumonia [122,153,154]. Early initiation of enteral feeding may help maintain the gastrointestinal epithelium and prevent bacterial translocation, but it is not without risk (see Table 32-4). Enteral feedings may become contaminated during preparation. Therefore, we recommend the routine use of aseptic technique and sterile water for their preparation and for nasogastric tube flushes; we are concerned that tap water may be a source of legionellae and other nosocomial gram-negative bacilli (see section on *Legionella pneumophila*) [101,155].

Enteral feeding may also cause gastric distention and colonization and increase the risk of aspiration, resulting in HAP [3,154,156]. Serial monitoring and removal of the gastric residual are important strategies to decrease the risk of aspiration and HAP [3,41,83,122,157]. Aspiration or gastric reflux are common in hospitalized patients [83,84,86,98,122,123,125]. In one study, oropharyngeal reflux was reported in ~ 70% of patients receiving tube feedings; 40% had evidence of pulmonary aspiration [122]. Maintaining the patient in a semiupright position appears to reduce reflux, aspiration, and VAP (CDC/HICPAC, Category IB) [41,83,123]. Enteral feeding remains a complicated issue and controversy persists over the use of continuous vs. intermittent enteral feeding, the need to acidify enteral feedings, and the optimal site and position of the feeding tube [3,156,157]. For patients undergoing abdominal surgery, some investigators routinely insert jejunal feeding tubes in an effort to reduce aspiration and the risk of VAP.

Bronchoscopy

Mechanically ventilated patients may undergo bronchoscopy through the endotracheal tube for diagnostic purposes or removal of mucus plugs or excessive secretions. In one study, bronchoscopy was identified as a risk factor for HAP [62]. This could be related to several factors, including the use of large volumes of BAL that impede the host's removal of bacteria in the lower airway and the introduction of nosocomial pathogens into the lower airway by releasing bacteria encased in biofilm on the endotracheal tube. As discussed previously, when bacteria encased in biofilm embolize to different areas of the lung, they may be particularly difficult for host defenses to clear effectively [147,151]. Although these pathogenic mechanisms are hypothetical, they are of concern but are difficult to assess as a risk factor.

Equipment Used in Mechanically Ventilated Patients

The CDC/HICPAC guideline recommends that mechanical ventilator breathing circuits be changed no more frequently than every 48 hours, but more recent data suggest that changing ventilator circuits at intervals greater than 48 hours or not at all is both safe and cost effective [3,158–160] (Figure 32-6).

A ventilator with a humidifier may have tubing condensate containing from 10^3 to 10^6 gram-negative

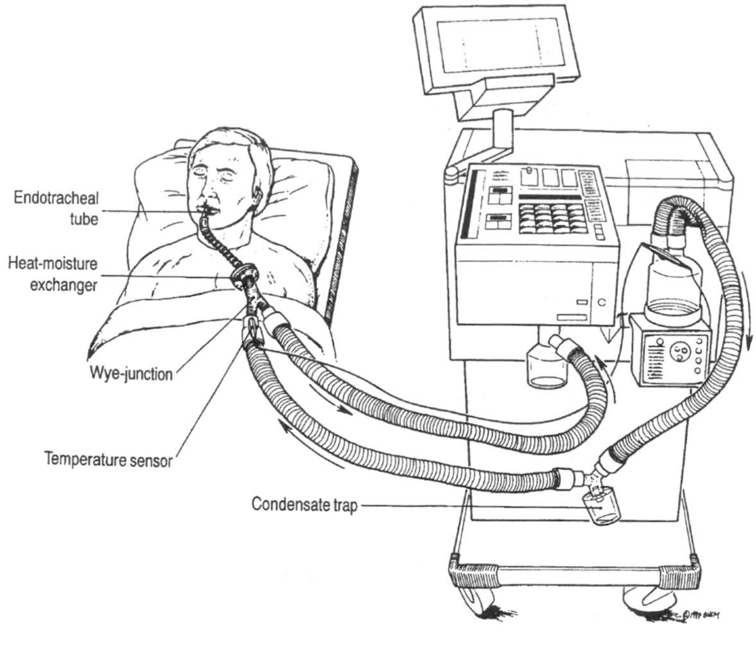

FIGURE 32-6. Mechanically ventilated patient in the upright position. The ventilator humidifies the air, which is carried through the inspiratory tubing to the Wye junction into the endotracheal tube and the patient's lower respiratory tract. The humidified air is expired out the expiratory phase tube to a "trap." If a heat–moisture exchanger (HME) is inserted between the swivel adapter and Wye junction, the humidifier can be turned off and there is no condensate in the circuit. (From Craven DE, Steger KA. Hospital-acquired pneumonia: perspective for the epidemiologist. *Infect Control Hosp Epidemiol* 1997 [in press], with permission.)

bacilli/ml, and thus reflux of condensate directly into the trachea should be avoided. Heated tubing and condensate traps reduce condensate formation and the patient's risk of pneumonia [161]. Furthermore, heat–moisture exchangers recycle exhaled moisture and eliminate circuit condensate [3,162–168]. These devices are well tolerated by most patients and are particularly useful in postoperative or lower-risk patients, but they may not provide sufficient humidity to some critically ill patients.

Tracheal suction catheters used on ventilated patients may inoculate bacteria directly into the lung or trachea. Aseptic technique with gloves is recommended during suctioning. A closed, multiuse suction system may be more convenient than a single-use catheter and causes less hypoxia for the patient, but may not reduce the risk of VAP [3,169].

Several accessory devices are also of concern. A medication nebulizer inserted into the mechanical ventilator circuit may become colonized from contaminated condensate and is of concern because aerosols are generated that have direct access to the lower airway [170]. The resuscitation bag, spirometer, temperature sensor, and oxygen analyzer are also potential sources of cross-contamination with nosocomial pathogens [2,3,171–173]. The use of molecular typing of strains may help track and identify potential sources of cross-contamination (see Chapter 16*)*.

Infection Control Measures

Intervention strategies to reduce transmission of nosocomial pathogens in the hospital are critical. Some of these targets are discussed in the following sections.

Surveillance and Infection Control

Previous studies have indicated that hospitals with effective surveillance and infection control programs have rates of pneumonia 20% lower than hospitals without such programs [3] (see Chapters 4, 5). Effective targeted surveillance for high-risk patients coupled with staff education, use of proper isolation techniques, and effective infection control practices are cornerstones for the prevention of nosocomial pneumonia [125,174]. Because of the changes in the healthcare system and the increasing impact of managed care programs, infection control staff have been decreased. We recommend that targeted surveillance of high-risk areas, such as the ICUs, should remain a priority. Also, monitoring of MDR pathogens and device-related infections should be carried out [125].

Surveillance and prevention practices vary widely among hospitals and different patient populations. We suggest that ICU staff should be involved in collection and analysis of surveillance data, and that all data should be collected and feedback provided in timely fashion. Additional infection control strategies for the prevention of nosocomial pneumonia should include identification of high-risk patients, staff education, institution of proper isolation methods, and adherence to infection control practices such as handwashing (see Chapter 5).

Cross-Infection From Patients and Staff

Cross-colonization or cross-infection is an important mechanism in the pathogenesis of nosocomial infection [24,86,174] (see Figure 32-2). Gram-negative bacilli and *S. aureus* are often present in high concentrations as indigenous flora in critically ill patients, the hospital environment, and on the hands or gloves of hospital personnel [125]. Handwashing before and after patient contact is an effective means of removing transient bacteria, but because of the vagaries of handwashing practices among hospital personnel, some investigators have advocated the use of barrier precautions (gloves and gowns) for contact with all patients. This practice has been associated with significantly decreased rates of nosocomial infections in pediatric ICUs [175]. If gloves are used, care must be taken to change them between patients [125].

Nasal carriage of *S. aureus* is common among health-care workers and outbreaks are often associated with staff with dermatitis or nasal or rectal colonization. Sherertz and coworkers emphasize the importance of viral respiratory tract infections in the transfer of airborne methicillin-resistant *S. aureus* from a physician to 8 of 43 patients in an ICU [176]. Molecular typing was performed to confirm the source of the outbreak and experimental induction of rhinovirus infection and its role in airborne dispersion of bacteria was demonstrated (the "cloud adult"). Without the use of surgical masks, the dispersal of *S. aureus* increased transmission fortyfold. These data underscore the importance of upper respiratory tract infection in the dissemination of *S. aureus* isolates and the importance of masks in preventing dissemination.

Antibiotic Treatment

Treatment of nosocomial pneumonia involves supportive care, attention to underlying disease, and appropriate antimicrobial therapy. Supportive measures include supplemental oxygen, vigorous pulmonary toilet, appropriate hydration, and careful attention to the presence and treatment of pulmonary edema.

Empiric combination therapy is often prescribed because of the polymicrobial and sometimes cryptic nature of nosocomial pneumonia. The choice of initial antibiotic therapy should be based on clinical history, severity of underlying disease, time in the hospital, previous culture data, information on indigenous nosocomial pathogens and their antimicrobial sensitivity patterns, and information gained from the Gram stain (see Chapter 14).

Empiric therapy should be broad enough to cover the suspected nosocomial pathogens [7,68,76]. Local bacterial sensitivity patterns as well as special circumstances such as focal epidemics must always be considered when deciding on empiric therapy. The American Thoracic

TABLE 32-7. *Antimicrobial therapy of nosocomial pneumonia in adults: A consensus statement of the American Thoracic Society (ATS)*[a]

Group	Pathogens	Initial Antibiotics
Mild, moderate, or severe disease[b] Early onset No risk factors.	*S. pneumoniae* *H. influenza* Enteric gram-negative bacilli *S. aureus*	Ceftriaxone (CTX) or Ampicillin/Sulbactam (Amp/Sul)
Mild or moderate disease Onset any time	*S. pneumoniae* *H. influenza* Enteric gram-negative bacilli *S. aureus*	CTX or Amp/Sul
Risk factors present:		
Aspiration	Anaerobes	CTX + Clindamycin or Amp/Sul
Coma, head trauma, diabetes, renal failure	*S. aureus* Methicillin-resistant *S. aureus* (MRSA)	Same as above CTX or Amp/Sul + Vancomycin
High-dose steroids	Legionella	Amp/Sul + Erythromycin
Intensive care unit patient (ICU), steroids, prior antibiotics, lung disease	*P. aeruginosa* Acinetobacter MRSA Legionella	Ceftazidime or Imipenem + Aminoglycoside (AG) or Ciprofloxacin Add Vancomycin Add Erythromycin
Severe disease[b] Onset any time	*S. pneumoniae* *H. influenza* Enteric gram-negative bacilli *S. aureus*	Same as ICU patient above
Risk factors present	*P. aeruginosa*, Acinetobacter MRSA Legionella	Same as ICU patient above

[a](From the American Thoracic Society (adopted by the ATS Board of Directors). Hospital-acquired pneumonia in adults: diagnosis, assessment of severity, initial antimicrobial therapy, and preventative strategies: a consensus statement. *American Journal of Respiratory Critical Care Medicine* 1996;153:1711–1725.)

[b]Severe disease = ICU admission, respiratory failure, sepsis, rapidly progressing pneumonia, organ failure, shock, > 35% 02 to maintain 02 Sat > 90%.

Society has published a consensus statement on the treatment of nosocomial pneumonia that is based on severity of disease, time of onset, and the presence of specific risk factors associated with more unusual nosocomial pathogens [177] (Table 32-7). For example, if a patient has a disease that is mild to severe but of early onset, and there are no underlying risk factors, core organisms such as *S. pneumoniae*, *H. influenzae*, nonpseudomonal gram-negative rods, and *S. aureus* should be considered, and therapy with one of the core antibiotics such as ceftriaxone or ampicillin/sulbactam is recommended. Anaerobes become more important if there is a risk of aspiration, corticosteroid therapy is associated with pneumonia due to *L. pneumophila*, and patients who have prolonged hospitalization or prior antibiotic therapy have an increased risk of colonization and infection with *P. aeruginosa* or *Acinetobacter* species. Specific therapy for these pathogens is summarized in Table 32-7.

Although combination antibiotic therapy has been prescribed traditionally, more recent data have suggested that patients treated with one drug (e.g., ceftazidime, cefoperazone, imipenem) may have similar outcomes to patients treated with combination therapy [178,179]. In general, pneumonia due to *P. aeruginosa*, *Acinetobacter* species, and Enterobacteriaceae should be treated with two drugs and physicians should monitor antimicrobial resistance and superinfection [58].

Although aminoglycosides have a wide spectrum of activity against nosocomial gram-negative bacilli, their use may be hampered by a poor toxic–therapeutic ratio, the need for antibiotic peak and trough levels to monitor toxicity, and their low penetration into bronchial secretions [58,179]. Clinical data suggest that peak levels of at least 7 μg/ml for gentamicin or tobramycin and at least 28 μg/ml for amikacin have been associated with better outcomes [180].

In patients who require prolonged therapy and have impaired renal function, aztreonam may be preferable to an aminoglycoside [179]. Quinolones, such as ciprofloxacin, are particularly useful because of their broad activity against gram-negative bacilli and excellent penetration into respiratory secretions, but additional coverage is needed for patients with pneumonia due to anaerobes or pneumococci. An adjunctive agent is recommended when treating pneumonia due to *P. aeruginosa* with ciprofloxacin.

LEGIONELLA PNEUMOPHILA

L. pneumophila is an important cause of nosocomial pneumonia [3,155,181–190]. The organism is ubiquitous in water and is regularly present in the water supply of many hospitals, particularly if there is active construction [191–194]. Because culture, serology, or urinary antigen tests for *L. pneumophila* are often not routinely performed, the incidence of legionellosis is underestimated [16].

Preventing cases of nosocomial legionellosis begins with being able to recognize disease due to *L. pneumophila* or the diagnosis of a definite case of nosocomial disease (Table 32-8). Cultures for legionellae are well within the capabilities of most hospital microbiology laboratories, and tracheal aspirates and pleural fluids should be cultured for legionellae in cases of HAP in which the microbiologic diagnosis is unclear. Such studies are particularly important in patients receiving cytotoxic chemotherapy or corticosteroids [195]. Because *L. pneumophila* is not spread person to person, the occurrence of cases in a hospital means that an environmental source is present, which, if not identified and corrected, may lead to more cases.

Nosocomial legionellosis has been traced to airborne spread of organisms from contaminated cooling towers [196]. Colony counts of *L. pneumophila* can be decreased in these units with disinfectants; however, the optimum disinfectant for contaminated systems has not yet been determined. Periodic cleaning and hyperchlorination of cooling towers are prudent measures until more specific recommendations can be offered [3]. Regardless of the maintenance schedule of these units, it is important that the location of hospital air intake vents in relation to the effluent from cooling towers be reviewed.

Contaminated potable water is probably the most important hospital reservoir of *L. pneumophila* in terms of transmission to patients, particularly those who are immunosuppressed or on corticosteroids. Inhalation of aerosols from showers, faucets, and respiratory therapy equipment and aspiration of contaminated potable water have all been proposed as methods of transmission [197]. An outbreak of nosocomial pneumonia due to *L. pneumophila* type 6 was traced to medications and enteral feedings that used potable water as a diluent [155]. Subtyping studies showed that the patient strains were remarkably similar to other *L. pneumophila* isolates from the hospital water supply and were different from other community serotype 6 strains. The outbreak was controlled by reducing the levels of legionellae in the water supply and by substituting sterile water to administer medications and dilute enteral feedings.

The CDC/HICPAC have published guidelines for prevention of legionellosis (see Table 32-8). Some investigators have recommended environmental sampling of the hospital water supply, but specific guidelines for routine environmental culturing for *L. pneumophila* have not been developed. CDC/HICPAC suggest culturing potable water if nosocomial cases are observed [3]. However, this recommendation has little meaning unless the hospital microbiology laboratory is capable of culturing *L. pneumophila* or referring to a more specialized laboratory appropriate specimens from patients with undiagnosed pneumonia. If cases of nosocomial legionellosis occur, a thorough epidemiologic investigation, including the collection and analysis of environ-

TABLE 32-8. *Issues, risk factors, and possible control measures for Legionnaire's disease*

Issues/risk factors	Control measures	CDC/HICPAC
Epidemiology		
Outbreaks documented; sporadic cases occur	Education; heightened awareness	IA
Actual rates of associated NP probably higher than 0%–14% reported	Reinforce control measures	IA
Organism common in aquatic environments; may enter hospital water supplies; colonization enhanced at 25° – 42°C	CDC/HICPAC made no recommendation for routine environmental culturing; no recommendation for maintaining certain temperature of potable H_2O or for treatments, such as chlorination	NR
Risk factors: immune suppression, chronic underlying disease & later stage acquired immunodeficiency syndrome (AIDS)	Increased awareness of risk factors	II
Moderate risk: diabetes mellitus, chronic lung disease, non-hematologic malignancy, smoking and advanced age	Establish mechanisms to provide appropriate laboratory tests for diagnosis	IA
Primary prevention		
Nebulization/Other Semicritical Devices	Proper cleaning & disinfection, use sterile H_2O to fill; avoid large-volume room-air humidifiers that create aerosols unless they can be sterilized	IA
Cooling Towers	Place so that tower drift is away from hospital's air-intake system and so that volume of aerosolized drift is minimized if possible, or install drift eliminators, use an effective biocide, & follow recommended maintenance	IB
Secondary prevention		
With single "definite" case of >2 "possible cases" within 6 mo of each other	Contact local state health department or CDC if disease is reportable in state or assistance is needed	IB
If case is identified in severely immuno-compromised patient, or if hospital houses such patients	Conduct epidemiologic/environmental investigation to determine source(s)	IB
	Otherwise conduct epidemiologic investigation via retrospective data review and initiate intensive prospective surveillance for at least two months	II
	With continued transmission, conduct epidemiologic investigation; save and subtype isolates	IB
	If source identified, continue surveillance for at least two months; defer/complete decontamination of hospital's water supply pending identification of sources	II
If heated-water system implicated	Decontaminate by superheating or hyper-chlorination and clean tanks and heaters to remove sediment/scale	IB
	Follow local regulations re: water temperature, & chlorination	II
	Treatment of water with ozone, ultra-violet light, or heavy-metal ions unresolved	NR
	Restrict immunocompromised patients from showers and use only sterile water for their consumption until organism is undetectable in water supply	II
When cooling towers/evaporative condensers are implicated	Decontaminate cooling tower system	IB
	Assess efficacy of interventions by collecting specimens for culture at 2-wk intervals for 3 mo; if negative, collect cultures monthly for 3 mo	II
	If organism detected in >1 culture(s), reassess implemented control measures, modify them as necessary, and repeat decontamination procedures	II

Adapted from the Centers for Disease Control/(CDC) Hospital Infection Control and Prevention Practices Advisory Committee's (HICPAC) Guidelines for Prevention of Nosocomial Pneumonia (NP).

(Tablan OC, Anderson LJ, Arden NH, et al. Guideline for prevention of nosocomial pneumonia: part I. Issues on prevention of nosocomial pneumonia, 1994. *Infect Control Hosp Epidemiol* 1994;15:588–625.)

mental samples, is indicated. If cases are clustered, it is prudent to substitute a new source of potable water until the results of environmental samples are known. If water samples are positive, it is very important that representative isolates be saved for subtyping studies [198,199].

There are no specific rules governing when water systems ought to be treated to eliminate or reduce contamination with legionellae. Decontamination ought to be considered when potable water cultures are positive and nosocomial infections with the same *L. pneumophila* biotype have occurred. The presence of certain at-risk

TABLE 32-9. *Issues, risk factors and control measures for viral pneumonia*

Issues/risk factors	Control measures	CDC/HICPAC
Respiratory syncytial virus (RSV)		
Most common during infancy/early childhood: uncommon in adults	Educate personnel about epidemiology, modes of transmission, & prevention	IA
Seasonal outbreaks	Alert key personnel of increased RSV activity	IB
RSV present in large numbers in respiratory secretions; transmitted directly/indirectly	Use rapid diagnostic tests for those at risk	IB
Person-to-person spread	Handwashing after contact, despite glove use; gown before anticipated soiling or when handling infants with RSV	IB
	Use gloves for handling potentially infected secretions or with contaminated fomites	IA
	Restrict staff with acute upper respiratory illness from caring for patients at risk	IB
	Limit visitors accordingly	II
	During outbreaks, use private rooms or patient/staff cohorting; defer elective admissions	II
Control of RSV outbreaks	No recommendations for using eye/nose goggles	NR
Influenza		
Associated pneumonia >in young/old, immune suppressed, or with certain chronic underlying diseases	Offer vaccine to those at high risk of complications from influenza from September until influenza activity declines	IA
	Vaccinate staff as per recommendation	IB
Outbreaks occur in winter; nosocomial outbreaks have been described	Educate staff about epidemiology	IA
	Notify staff of outbreaks	IB
	Employ prompt diagnostic techniques	IB
Person-to-person spread via droplet nuclei or small-particle aerosols,? role of fomites	Use private room/cohorting for those suspected/diagnosed	II
	Use negative air pressure in rooms for these patients or room in areas with independent air-supply-and-exhaust system	II
	Use masks for susceptibles entering room of patient with influenza	IB
	Involve employee health service in evaluating staff with suggestive symptoms	II
	During outbreaks, restrict visitors, defer elective admissions, and restrict elective pulmonary/cardiovascular surgery	IB
Control of Influenza outbreaks	Determine the outbreak strain; vaccinate susceptible patients/staff	IB
	In nosocomial outbreaks of influenza A, administer prophylaxis to all uninfected patients unless contraindicated	IB
	Administer amantadine or rimantadine as above to staff	II
	Discontinue use of these drugs if laboratory tests confirm/strongly suggest influenza type A is NOT the cause of the outbreak	IA
	If outbreak is due to influenza type A and vaccine has been administered recently to susceptibles, continue amantadine/rimantadine prophylaxis for 2 wk after vaccination	IB
	Reduce contact between those at risk of complications from influenza and those taking amantadine/rimantadine	IB

Adapted in part from the 1994 Centers for Disease Control and Prevention (CDC)/Hospital Infection Control Practices Advisory Committee's (HICPAC) Guidelines for Prevention of Nosocomial Pneumonia.
(Tablan OC, Anderson LJ, Arden NH, et al. Guideline for prevention of nosocomial pneumonia: part I. Issues on prevention of nosocomial pneumonia, 1994. *Infect Control Hosp Epidemiol* 1994;15:588–625.)

groups, such as bone marrow transplant patients, may result in a more aggressive approach to decrease levels of environmental contamination.

Methods that can be used to disinfect water distribution systems contaminated with legionellae include hyperchlorination or superheating [200,201]. Hyperchlorination, as a method of disinfection, has fallen out of favor because legionellae are relatively chlorine tolerant and the concentrations required to kill them result in significant corrosion of the plumbing system. Superheating and flushing have emerged as the most widely used method for disinfection of water distribution systems [3]. *L. pneumophila* is killed at temperatures greater than 60°C (140°F). The basic cleansing technique requires that the temperature of the water in the tank be raised to > 70°C (158°F), followed by the running of all shower heads and faucets to kill legionellae. This method provides effective short-term control but requires effective planning to ensure that it is properly done. Consultation with state, local, and federal health officials and with hospitals who have had experience dealing with environmental legionellosis is strongly recommended [3].

RESPIRATORY VIRUSES

The full extent of nosocomial viral respiratory infections is not well known. In general, respiratory viruses like influenza, parainfluenza, or respiratory syncytial virus (RSV) are introduced into the hospital environment by patients, staff, or visitors as part of the general disease burden caused by a virus circulating through a community [202,203]. Once introduced, viruses can spread nosocomially with dramatic consequences. One such example is the chaos created with the occurrence of cases of nosocomial measles that were part of the national epidemic of measles in the early 1990s [204]. However, as hospitalization stays have shortened, many of these illnesses become manifest after hospitalization.

Influenza

Nosocomial influenza usually begins dramatically when a cluster of patients or long-term care residents develop fever, myalgia, headache, coryza, and cough temporally associated with disease in the community [3,205] (see Chapter 42). Closed units such as nursing homes (see Chapter 29), chronic disease facilities (see Chapter 28), ICUs (see Chapter 25), or pediatric wards are at particular risk. Influenza is spread by droplet nuclei introduced into the respiratory tract, but direct-contact transmission may also occur. Infectivity is highest during the first 3 days of illness. The diagnosis of influenza is usually a clinical one and confirmatory cultures, if done, are performed on the first few cases. Influenza virus can be recovered from nasal or other respiratory secretions and serologic testing can also confirm influenza infection.

The control of influenza relies on prevention by immunization or chemoprophylaxis [206] (Table 32-9). Annual influenza immunization should be given to all residents of long-term care facilities such as nursing homes. Because influenza can be introduced by hospital personnel, it is prudent to emphasize their immunization as a means of decreasing risk to hospitalized patients (see Chapter 3). Unfortunately, influenza vaccine has not been well received by hospital employees even when provided conveniently and at no cost. Staff suffering from influenza-like illness should be discouraged from working because of the hazard they pose to patients.

Influenza vaccine should be given annually for all long-term care residents and offered to all hospitalized patients who are 65 years of age or younger than 65 years with cardiac, pulmonary, renal, or metabolic disease, during the influenza season. Admission to a hospital during the fall and early winter should trigger a review of influenza immunization status. Influenza vaccine is extremely effective in preventing severe influenza-related complications. Reactions to the vaccine in the elderly are infrequent and minor, consisting mainly of malaise and a sore arm, symptoms easily controlled with analgesics.

Amantadine and rimantadine are effective chemoprophylactic agents that can prevent influenza A [207]. Of importance, these antivirals do not interfere with antibody response to influenza vaccine, and a recommended approach for dealing with a high-risk, unprotected population, such as hospitalized patients during an epidemic of influenza A, is to vaccinate and treat with antivirals for 2 weeks, by which time protective antibody titers would be present [206]. Amantadine and rimantadine are not substitutes for influenza vaccine because they are effective only against strains of influenza A. Rimantadine causes fewer side effects and is the preferred agent [208].

Respiratory Syncytial Virus

Respiratory syncytial virus is a highly contagious virus that is the major cause of lower respiratory tract infection in young children and infants [3] (see Chapter 42). RSV occurs yearly, usually in the winter or spring [3]. Because of its prevalence, RSV is a common cause of nosocomial lower respiratory tract infection on pediatric units. Adults who are immunocompromised, elderly, or suffering from chronic obstructive pulmonary disease have also been shown to be at risk for severe RSV infection.

Respiratory syncytial virus is present in high concentrations in respiratory secretions and can be transmitted directly by large respiratory droplets during close contact with infected people or indirectly by contaminated hands or fomites [3]. The conjunctivae and nasal mucosa are the most important portals of entry. Culture of RSV remains the gold standard for diagnosis, but antigen detection systems are rapid and offer good sensitivity and specificity. Once a laboratory-confirmed case of RSV is identified in the hospital, subsequent cases are usually diagnosed presumptively.

Several types of RSV have been identified in nosocomial outbreaks. Prevention efforts, as outlined in the 1994 CDC/HICPAC *Guideline for Prevention of Nosocomial Pneumonia*, should be directed at containing the reservoir of virus in infected patients [3] (see Table 32-9). Emphasis should be placed on contact isolation precautions, particularly gowning and gloving [44,209]. Gloves must be changed between patients and precautions taken to avoid inoculation of eyes or noses. In controlled studies, gowning also seems to prevent transmission. Special efforts, such as private rooms or cohorting infected patients and staff, may be needed to prevent infection of high-risk patients.

FUNGI

Aspergillus

Aspergillus spores are found universally in unfiltered air [210–214]. Because of their size, *Aspergillus* spores remain suspended in air for long periods of time. When inhaled, they penetrate to the distal lung where they are inactivated by normal cellular defenses. *Aspergillus* are very hardy and once introduced into an environment persist for long periods of time. High concentrations in the hospital have been found in false ceiling dust, polystyrene linings of fireproofed doors, and fireproofing material. *Aspergillus* spores may be present in particularly high concentrations during hospital construction and renovation [212,215].

Although *Aspergillus* pneumonia is uncommon, mortality rates are high because of the necrotizing nature of the infection and its poor response to antifungal chemotherapy. Immunocompromised patients, particularly those undergoing chemotherapy resulting in prolonged neutropenia, those undergoing organ transplantation, or those with AIDS are at particular risk for aspergillosis. Diagnosis is often difficult and usually requires bronchoscopy with BAL or biopsy to discriminate between airway colonization and tissue invasion.

A single case of nosocomial *Aspergillus* pneumonia should raise suspicion and prompt a search for other cases. Prevention of nosocomial aspergillosis requires the cooperation of engineering and housekeeping services. Information for the evaluation of hospital airflow systems is contained in the 1994 CDC/HICPAC *Guideline for Prevention of Nosocomial Pneumonia* [3]. Clearly, efforts should be taken to avoid exposure of high-risk patients to environmental reservoirs. Particular attention should be paid to the risks imposed on immunosuppressed patients as a result of hospital construction in areas close to high-risk patients. If possible, fungal isolates should be type studied [210,216].

Candida albicans

C. albicans is an increasingly important nosocomial respiratory pathogen in immunosuppressed or critically ill patients [217,218]. Critically ill patients who are immunocompromised or treated with broad-spectrum antibiotics are at highest risk of infection. Molecular typing studies may help establish the mode of nosocomial transmission and locate both patient and hospital reservoirs of the organism [219].

HUMAN IMMUNODEFICIENCY VIRUS AND EMERGING PATHOGENS

Over 700,000 people in the United States are infected with human immunodeficiency virus type 1 (HIV; see Chapter 43), and more than 530,000 cases of AIDS have been reported to the CDC as of March, 1997, resulting in a steady increase in numbers of HIV-infected patients cared for in hospitals, outpatient clinics, and chronic healthcare facilities [220]. AIDS patients have a greater risk of nosocomial infection and are often exposed to invasive devices and antibiotics [221,222]. Bacterial infections are prevalent in HIV-infected patients and the lung is a common site of infection. Nichols and coworkers reported bacterial infection in 83% of 46 autopsied AIDS patients, and such infection contributed to death in 36% of these cases [223]. Pneumonia was the most common bacterial infection, occurring in more than 50% of the patients. Niedt and Schinella found bacterial infection in > 50% of 56 autopsies, and pneumonia was again the most common type of infection [224]. *S. aureus* and *P. aeruginosa* were the most common organisms isolated. There is also concern that many of the traditional "community-acquired" respiratory pathogens, such as pneumococci, *H. influenzae, M. tuberculosis*, and even *Pneumocystis carinii* may be acquired and transmitted in the hospital.

Human immunodeficiency virus-infected people have rates of pneumococcal pneumonia that are estimated to be five- to fifteenfold greater than in HIV-seronegative people, and data suggest nosocomial transmission of a type 6A MDR strain of pneumococcus between two AIDS patients who were hospitalized three rooms apart [225–228]. The isolates were unique to that hospital and had identical serotypes and unusual antibiogram resistance patterns. The second patient probably contracted pneumococcal bacteremia and pneumonia 20 days after exposure, and had been discharged from the hospital. Nosocomial transmission has been reported for outbreaks of penicillin-resistant pneumococci in Spain and South Africa [229,230], underscoring the need to reassess our current definition and emphasize the use of proper isolation until a diagnosis is established.

H. influenzae pneumonia is also increased in AIDS patients (79/100,000 vs. 2/100,000 in healthy adults) [231,232]. Published data indicate that rates of *H. influenzae* type b disease are higher in household contacts and that person-to-person spread is important in households and healthcare facilities [233–235]. Proper respiratory isolation and use of infection control techniques may be crucial in preventing the nosocomial spread of bacterial respiratory pathogens.

Mycobacterium tuberculosis

The association between HIV infection and infection due to *M. tuberculosis* (TB) in the United States has been well documented [236,237] (see Chapter 33). AIDS patients may have a negative tuberculin skin test and an atypical clinical presentation. Two epidemiologic studies using analysis of restriction fragment length polymorphisms suggested that recently transmitted TB cases accounted for two thirds of the active TB cases in HIV-infected individuals, and that HIV infection was an independent risk factor for having a "cluster isolate" [238,239].

Nosocomial outbreaks of TB involving HIV-infected people have been characterized by attack rates that range from 5% to 44%, rapid progression to active disease, evidence of significant spread in healthcare settings, and high mortality [5,240]. Several nosocomial outbreaks have been reported, many of which have strong epidemiologic data supported by a molecular analysis of the outbreak strains. Factors that contributed to the outbreaks include an increasing number of HIV-infected patients exposed to TB and delays in proper isolation, diagnosis, treatment, and drug susceptibility results. In addition, inadequate ventilation, lack of isolation rooms with positive air pressure, and inadequate precautions for cough-inducing procedures, such as administration of aerosolized pentamidine and bronchoscopy, have contributed to transmission [241].

In response to the growing number of TB outbreaks, the CDC has published a new set of guidelines for preventing TB transmission in healthcare settings [242]. These guidelines stress early identification of active disease, prompt isolation, and expeditious initiation of effective therapy. In addition, routine skin testing for TB exposure among healthcare workers is recommended (see Chapter 3), and, when appropriate, a contact investigation coupled with appropriate preventative therapy [241].

Nosocomial TB does not usually result in an acute pulmonary infection, but rather the hospital or health facility serves as a locus where patients with undiagnosed but infectious TB are bedded. If proper respiratory precautions are not taken, these patients can spread infection to other inpatients and staff. The likelihood of these events has increased with the rise in new cases of active TB and the atypical clinical presentations seen in the elderly and HIV-infected patients.

Patients with compatible roentgenographic findings or HIV-infected patients with atypical pulmonary infections should be assumed to have TB and placed in respiratory isolation until the results of Ziehl Niehlson sputum smears are known. Patients and staff who are exposed to an active case of tuberculosis should first have their tuberculin status carefully reviewed. Known tuberculin-positive individuals are not a problem because their positivity conveys protection. People who do not know their tuberculin status should have an intermediate tuberculin test done and, if negative, a second test within 2 weeks should be done to identify those in whom a booster response is needed to define positivity. People who are negative to both tuberculin tests are considered true negatives and should be retested in 6 weeks. Those who test positive at this point are classified as converters and should be offered chemoprophylaxis.

Pneumocystis carinii Pneumonia

Current epidemiologic and animal studies suggest that airborne droplets are the most likely source of *P. carinii* pneumonia (PCP) transmission. Clusters or hospital outbreaks of PCP in the United States were reported in immunosuppressed children beginning in 1968 [243]. The use of sputum induction, bronchoscopy, or aerosolized pentamidine treatment in HIV-infected patients may increase the risk of nosocomial transmission of PCP. Hoover and coworkers found temporal and geographic relationships suggesting person-to-person spread of *P. carinii* in HIV-infected men compared with HIV-seronegative control subjects [244] (see Chapter 43). Also, Haron and coworkers reported increased rates of PCP among cancer patients in their institution from 1980 to 1987, which paralleled the increasing numbers of cases of AIDS admitted to their institution [245]. Although no specific epidemiologic routes of transmission could be determined, the AIDS clinic and leukemia outpatient clinic were contiguous and the two patient populations mingled freely. In another study, PCP was diagnosed in 5 of 144 renal transplant recipients over a 22-month period [246]. All five patients attended the same outpatient facility, where they shared waiting and treatment rooms and had encounters with AIDS patients in whom PCP later developed. Although these data on nosocomial transmission are not conclusive, they are suggestive and indicate that precautions should be instituted to prevent the nosocomial spread of *P. carinii* among immunosuppressed patients.

CONCLUSION

In the 1980s, significant strides were made in our understanding of the pathogenesis of nosocomial pneumonia. Unfortunately, many of these advances have not been translated into clinically relevant decisions, and thus have not resulted in decreased incidence and mortality rates. National surveillance with better case definitions that take into account the increased number of patients with HIV infection and other causes of immunosuppression, as well as the ever-increasing pressure to discharge hospitalized patients, needs to be continued. The development of sophisticated molecular epidemiologic techniques should help better define reservoirs of specific pathogens, modes of spread, and the interactions between nosocomial pathogens and pulmonary defenses.

Diagnosis of nosocomial pneumonia remains a major problem for clinicians and hospital epidemiologists. Protocols are needed for the cost-effective use of bronchoscopy with BAL or PSB, or the use of CPIS and QEA in the diagnosis of VAP. There is a need for outcome studies comparing patients with VAP managed by clinical diagnosis vs. the use of bronchoscopy in terms of morbidity, mortality, cost, and the emergence of MDR pathogens.

There is a need for improved infection control strategies, such as maintaining the patient in a semiupright position, replacing nasotracheal tubes with oral intubation, and using orogastric rather than nasogastric tubes. In addition, the use of continuous aspiration of subglottic secretions appears to reduce early-onset VAP. Optimal management of tube feeding, coupled with the effective use of nutritional support, deserves further investigation. Well-designed clinical trials to analyze the risks, benefits, and costs of these devices should be a prerequisite to their routine use. Last, rigorous studies are needed to define the type, route, and duration of antibiotic therapy in patients with nosocomial pneumonia caused by different pathogens.

ACKNOWLEDGMENT

The authors thank Maria Tetzaguic for assistance in the preparation of the manuscript.

REFERENCES

1. Horan TC, White JW, Jarvis WR, et al. Nosocomial infection surveillance, 1984. *MMWR Morb Mortal Wkly Rep* 1986;35:17SS–29SS.
2. Craven DE, Steger KA, Barber TW. Preventing nosocomial pneumonia: state of the art and perspectives for the 1990's. *Am J Med* 1991; 91(Suppl 3B):44S–53S.
3. Tablan OC, Anderson LJ, Arden NH, et al. Guideline for prevention of nosocomial pneumonia: part I. Issues on prevention of nosocomial pneumonia, 1994. *Infect Control Hosp Epidemiol* 1994;15:588–625.
4. Torres A, De La Bellacasa JP, Xaubet A, et al. Diagnostic value of quantitative cultures of bronchoalveolar lavage and telescoping plugged catheters in mechanically ventilated patients with bacterial pneumonia. *Am Rev Respir Dis* 1989;140:306–310.
5. Fischl MA, Daikos GL, Uttamchandani RB, et al. Clinical presentation and outcome of patients with HIV infection and tuberculosis caused by multiple-drug-resistant bacilli. *Ann Intern Med* 1992;117: 184–190.
6. Arnow PM, Sadigh M, Costas C, Weil D, Chudy R. Endemic and epidemic aspergillosis associated with in-hospital replication of *Aspergillus* organisms. *J Infect Dis* 1991;164:998–1002.
7. Niederman MS, Torres A, Summer W. Invasive diagnostic testing is not needed routinely to manage suspect ventilator-associated pneumonia. *American Journal of Respiratory Critical Care Medicine* 1994;150:565–569.
8. Chastre J, Fagon JY. Invasive diagnostic testing should be routinely used to manage ventilated patients with suspected pneumonia. *American Journal of Respiratory Critical Care Medicine* 1994;150:570–574.
9. Kollef MH, Bock KR, Richards RD, Hearns ML. The safety and diagnostic accuracy of minibronchoalveolar lavage in patients with suspected ventilator-associated pneumonia. *Ann Intern Med* 1995;122: 743–748.
10. Fagon JY, Chastre J, Hance AJ, et al. Detection of nosocomial lung infection in ventilated patients: use of a protected specimen brush and quantitative culture techniques in 147 patients. *Am Rev Respir Dis* 1988;138:110–116.
11. Fagon JY, Chastre J, Domart Y, et al. Nosocomial pneumonia in patients receiving continuous mechanical ventilation: prospective analysis of 52 episodes with use of a protected specimen brush and quantitative culture techniques. *Am Rev Respir Dis* 1989;139: 877–884.
12. Torres A, Aznar R, Gatell JM, et al. Incidence, risk, and prognosis factors of nosocomial pneumonia in mechanically ventilated patients. *Am Rev Respir Dis* 1990;142:523–528.
13. Bartlett JG, O'Keefe P, Tally FP, Louie TJ, Gorbach SL. Bacteriology of hospital acquired pneumonia. *Arch Intern Med* 1986;146:868–871.
14. Rello J, Quintana E, Ausina V, et al. Incidence, etiology, and outcome of nosocomial pneumonia in mechanically ventilated patients. *Chest* 1991;100:439–444.
15. Horan T, Culver D, Jarvis W, et al. Pathogens causing nosocomial infections. *CDC: The Antimicrobic Newsletter* 1988;5:65–67.
16. Muder RR, Yu VL, McClure JK, Kroboth FJ, Kominos SD, Lumish RN. Nosocomial Legionnaires' disease uncovered in a prospective pneumonia study: implications for underdiagnosis. *JAMA* 1983;249: 3184–3188.
17. Valenti WM, Hall CB, Douglas JR, et al. Nosocomial viral infections: I. epidemiology and significance. *Infect Control* 1980;1:33–37.
18. Maki DG. Control of colonization and transmission of pathogenic bacteria in the hospital. *Ann Intern Med* 1978;89:777–780.
19. Weinstein RA. Epidemiology and control of nosocomial infections in adult intensive care units. *Am J Med* 1991;91:179S–184S.
20. Pugin J, Auckenthaler R, Mili N, Janssens JP, Lew PD, Suter PM. Diagnosis of ventilator-associated pneumonia by bacteriologic analysis of bronchoalveolar lavage fluid. *Am Rev Respir Dis* 1991;143: 1121–1129.
21. Reusser P, Zimmerli W, Scheidegger D, Marbet GA, Buser M, Gyr K. Role of gastric colonization in nosocomial infections and endotoxemia: A prospective study in neurosurgical patients on mechanical ventilation. *J Infect Dis* 1989;160:414–421.
22. Valles J, Artigas A, Rello J, et al. Continuous aspiration of subglottic secretions in the prevention of ventilator-associated pneumonia. *Ann Intern Med* 1995;122:179–186.
23. Prod'hom G, Leuenberger PH, Koerfer J, et al. Nosocomial pneumonia in mechanically ventilated patients receiving antacid, ranitidine, or sucralfate as prophylaxis for stress ulcer. *Ann Intern Med* 1994;120: 653–662.
24. Schleupner CJ, Cobb DK. A study of the etiologies and treatment of nosocomial pneumonia in a community-based teaching hospital. *Infect Control Hosp Epidemiol* 1992;13:515–525.
25. Rello J, Torres A, Ricart M, et al. Ventilator-associated pneumonia by *Staphylococcus aureus*: comparison of methicillin-resistant and methicillin-sensitive episodes. *American Journal of Respiratory Critical Care Medicine* 1994;150:1545–1549.
26. Rello J, Quintana E, Ausina V, Puzo C, Net A, Prats G. Risk factors for *Staphylococcus aureus* pneumonia in critically ill patients. *Am Rev Respir Dis* 1990;142:1320–1324.
27. Scerpella EG, Wanger AR, Armitige L, Anderlini P, Ericsson CD. Nosocomial outbreak caused by a multiresistant clone of *Acinetobacter baumannii*: results of the case-control and molecular epidemiologic investigations. *Infect Control Hosp Epidemiol* 1995;16:92–97.
28. Grattard F, Pozzetto B, Tabard L, Petit M, Ros A, Gaudin O. Characterization of nosocomial strains of *Enterobacter aerogenes* by arbitrarily primed-PCR analysis and ribotyping. *Infect Control Hosp Epidemiol* 1995;16:224–230.
29. Hearst J, Elliott K. Identifying the killer in cystic fibrosis. *Nature* 1995;1:626–627.
30. Sun L, Jiang R, Steinbach S, et al. The emergence of a highly transmissible lineage of *cbl*$^{+}$ *Pseudomonas (Burkholderia) cepacia* causing CF centre epidemics in North America and Britain. *Nature* 1995; 1:661–666.
31. Chastre J, Fagon JY, Soler P, et al. Diagnosis of nosocomial bacterial pneumonia in intubated patients undergoing ventilation: comparison of the usefulness of bronchoalveolar lavage and the protected specimen brush. *Am J Med* 1988;85:499–506.
32. Jimenez P, Torres A, Rodriguez-Roisin R, et al. Incidence and etiology of pneumonia acquired during mechanical ventilation. *Crit Care Med* 1989;17:882–885.
33. Fagon JY, Chastre J, Hance AJ, Montravers P, Nowara A, Gilbert C. Nosocomial pneumonia in ventilated patients: a cohort study evaluating attributable mortality and hospital stay. *Am J Med* 1993;94: 281–288.
34. Torres A, Aznar R, Gatell JM, et al. Incidence, risk, and prognosis factors of nosocomial pneumonia in mechanically ventilated patients. *Am Rev Respir Dis* 1990;142:523–528.
35. Schaberg DR, Culver DH, Gaynes RP. Major trends in the microbial

etiology of nosocomial infection. *Am J Med* 1991;91(Suppl 3B): 72S–75S.
36. Hemming VG, Overall JC, Britt MR. Nosocomial infections in a newborn intensive-care unit: results of forty-one months of surveillance. *N Engl J Med* 1976;294:1310–1316.
37. Haley RW, Hooton TM, Culver DH, et al. Nosocomial infections in US hospitals, 1975–1976: estimated frequency by selected characteristics of patients. *Am J Med* 1981;70:947–959.
38. Garibaldi RA, Britt MR, Coleman ML, et al.Risk factors for postoperative pneumonia. *Am J Med* 1981;70:677–680.
39. Lareau SC, Ryan KJ, Diener CF. The relationship between frequency of ventilator circuit changes and infectious hazard. *Am Rev Respir Dis* 1978;118:493–496.
40. George DL. Epidemiology of nosocomial ventilator-associated pneumonia. *Infect Control Hosp Epidemiol* 1993;14:163–169.
41. Kollef MH. Ventilator-associated pneumonia. *JAMA* 1993;270: 1965–1970.
42. Celis R, Torres A, Gatell JM, Almela M, Rodriguez-Roisin R, Augusti-Vidal A. Nosocomial pneumonia: a multivariate analysis of risk and prognosis. *Chest* 1988;93:318–324.
43. Cross AS, Roupe B. Role of respiratory assistance devices in endemic nosocomial pneumonia. *Am J Med* 1981;70:681–685.
44. Leclair JM, Freeman J, Sullivan BF, et al. Prevention of nosocomial respiratory syncytial virus infections through compliance with glove and gown isolation precautions. *N Engl J Med* 1987;317:329–334.
45. Heffner JE. Nosocomial sinusitis: den of multiresistant thieves? *American Journal of Respiratory Critical Care Medicine* 1994;150:608–609.
46. Jarvis WR, Edwards JR, Culver DH, et al. Nosocomial infection rates in adult and pediatric intensive care units in the United States. *Am J Med* 1991;91(Suppl 3B):185S–190S.
47. Niederman MS, Mantovani R, Schoch P, et al. Patterns and routes of tracheobronchial colonization in mechanically ventilated patients: the role of nutritional status in colonization of the lower airway by *Pseudomonas* species. *Chest* 1989;95:155–161.
48. Craven DE, Kunches LM, Lichtenberg DA, et al. Nosocomial infection and fatality in medical and surgical intensive care unit patients. *Arch Intern Med* 1988;148:1161–1168.
49. Leu HS, Kaiser DL, Mori M, Woolson RF, Wenzel RP. Hospital-acquired pneumonia: attributable mortality and morbidity. *Am J Epidemiol* 1989;129:1258–1267.
50. Craven DE, Kunches LM, Kilinsky V, Lichtenberg DA, Make BJ, McCabe WR. Risk factors for pneumonia and fatality in patients receiving continuous mechanical ventilation. *Am Rev Respir Dis* 1986;133:792–796.
51. Graybill JR, Marshall LW, Charache P, et al. Nosocomial pneumonia: a continuing major problem. *Am Rev Respir Dis* 1973;108:1130–1140.
52. Craig CP, Connelly S. Effect of intensive care unit nosocomial pneumonia on duration of stay and mortality. *Am J* Infect Control 1984;12:233–238.
53. Stevens RM, Teres D, Skillman JJ, et al. Pneumonia in an intensive care unit: a thirty-month experience. *Arch Intern Med* 1974;134:106–111.
54. Gross PA, Neu HC, Aswapokee P, et al. Deaths from nosocomial infection: experience in a university hospital and a community hospital. *Am J Med* 1980;68:219–223.
55. Daschner F, Nadjem H, Langmaack H, Sandritter W. Surveillance, prevention and control of hospital-acquired infections: III. nosocomial infections as cause of death: retrospective analysis of 1,000 autopsy reports. *Infection* 1978;6:261–265.
56. Freeman J, Rosner BA, McGowan JE. Adverse effects of nosocomial infection. *J Infect Dis* 1979;140:732–740.
57. Boyce JM, Potter-Bynoe G, Dziobek L, Solomon SL. Nosocomial pneumonia in Medicare patients: Hospital costs and reimbursement patterns under the prospective payment system. *Arch Intern Med* 1991;151:1109–1114.
58. Pennington JE. Nosocomial respiratory infection. In: Mandell GL, Douglas RG Jr, Bennett JE, eds. *Principles and practice of infectious diseases*. 3rd ed. New York: Churchill Livingstone; 1990:2199–2204.
59. Wunderink RG. Detection of nosocomial lung infection in ventilated patients. *Am Rev Respir Dis* 1989;139:1302–1303.
60. Wunderink RG, Russell J, Mezger E, Adams J, Popovich JC Jr. The diagnostic utility of antibody-coated bacteria test in intubated patients. *Am Rev Respir Dis* 1985;131:A81
61. Bryant LR, Mobin-Uddin K, Dillon ML, Griffen WO, Ky L. Misdiagnosis of pneumonia in patients needing mechanical respiration. *Arch Surg* 1973;106:286–288.
62. Joshi N, Localio AR, Hamory BH. A predictive risk index for nosocomial pneumonia in the intensive care unit. *Am J Med* 1992; 93:135–142.
63. Andrews CP, Coalson JJ, Smith JD, Johanson WG Jr. Diagnosis of nosocomial bacterial pneumonia in acute, diffuse lung injury. *Chest* 1981;80:254–258.
64. Bell RC, Coalson JJ, Smith JD, Johanson WG Jr. Multiple organ system failure and infection in adult respiratory distress syndrome. *Ann Intern Med* 1983;99:293–298.
65. Haley CE, McDonald RC, Rossi L, Jones WD Jr, Haley RW, Luby JP. Tuberculosis epidemic among hospital personnel. *Infect Control Hosp Epidemiol* 1989;10:204–210.
66. Chastre J, Viau F, Brun P, et al. Prospective evaluation of the protected specimen brush for the diagnosis of pulmonary infection in ventilated patients. *Am Rev Respir Dis* 1984;130:924–929.
67. Torres A, De La Bellacasa JP, Rodriguez-Roisin R, Jimenez De Anta MT, Augusti-Vidal A. Diagnostic value of telescoping plugged catheters in pneumonia using the Metras catheter. *Am Rev Respir Dis* 1988;138:117–120.
68. Pugin J, Auckenthaler R, Mili N, Janssens JP, Lew PD, Suter PM. Diagnosis of ventilator-associated pneumonia by bacteriologic analysis of bronchoscopic and nonbronchoscopic blind bronchoalveolar lavage fluid. *Am Rev Respir Dis* 1988;138:117–120.
69. Meduri GU, Beals DH, Meijub AG, Baselski V. Protected bronchoalveolar lavage: a new bronchoscopic technique to retrieve uncontaminated distal airway secretions. *Am Rev Respir Dis* 1991;143: 855–864.
70. Cook DJ, Fitzgerald JM, Guyatt GH, Walter S. Evaluation of the protected brush catheter and bronchoalveolar lavage in the diagnosis of nosocomial pneumonia. *Journal of Intensive Care Medicine* 1991;6: 196–205.
71. Warren RE, Newsom SWB, Matthews JA, Arrowsmith LWM. Medical grade compressed air. *Lancet* 1986;1:1438.
72. Rouby JJ, Rossignon MD, Nicolas MH, et al. A prospective study of protected bronchoalveolar lavage in the diagnosis of nosocomial pneumonia. *Anesthesiology* 1989;71:679–685.
73. Piperno D, Gaussorgues P, Bachmann P, Jaboulay JM, Robert D. Diagnostic value of nonbronchoscopic bronchoalveolar lavage during mechanical ventilation. *Chest* 1988;93:223
74. Gaussorgues P, Piperno D, Bachmann P, et al. Comparison of non-bronchoscopic bronchoalveolar lavage to open lung biopsy for the bacteriologic diagnosis of pulmonary infections in mechanically ventilated patients. *Intensive Care Med* 1989;15:94–98.
75. Pham LH, Brun-Buisson C, Legrand P, et al. Diagnosis of nosocomial pneumonia in mechanically ventilated patients. *Am Rev Respir Dis* 1991;143:1055–1061.
76. A'Court CHD, Garrard CS, Crook D, et al. Microbiological lung surveillance in mechanically ventilated patients, using non-directed lavage and quantitative culture. *Q J Med* 1993;86:635–648.
77. El-ebiary M, Torres A, Gonzalez J, et al. Quantitative cultures of endotracheal aspirates for the diagnosis of ventilator-associated pneumonia. *Am Rev Respir Dis* 1993;148:1552–1557.
78. Marquette CH, Georges H, Wallet F, et al. Diagnostic efficiency of endotracheal aspirates with quantitative bacterial cultures in intubated patients with suspected pneumonia. *Am Rev Respir Dis* 1993;148: 138–144.
79. Cook DJ, Brun-Buisson C, Guyatt GH, Sibbald WJ. Evaluation of new diagnostic technologies: bronchoalveolar lavage and the diagnosis of ventilator-associated pneumonia. *Crit Care Med* 1994;22: 1314–1322.
80. Craven DE, Driks MR. Pneumonia in the intubated patient. *Semin Respir Infect* 1987;2:20–33.
81. Johanson WGJ, Pierce AK, Sanford J, Thomas GD. Nosocomial respiratory infections with gram-negative bacilli: the significance of colonization of the respiratory tract. *Ann Intern Med* 1972;77: 701–706.
82. Mahul PH, Auboyer C, Jospe R, et al. Prevention of nosocomial pneumonia in intubated patients: respective role of mechanical subglottic secretions drainage and stress ulcer prophylaxis. *Intensive Care Med* 1992;18:20–25.
83. Torres A, Serra-Battles J, Ros E, et al. Pulmonary aspiration of gastric

contents in patients receiving mechanical ventilation: the effect of body position. *Ann Intern Med* 1992;116:540–542.
84. du Moulin GC, Paterson DG, Hedley-Whyte J, Lisbon A. Aspiration of gastric bacteria in antacid-treated patients: a frequent cause of postoperative colonization of the airway. *Lancet* 1982;1:242–245.
85. Atherton ST, White DJ. Stomach as a source of bacteria colonizing respiratory tract during artificial ventilation. *Lancet* 1978;2:968–969.
86. Cameron JL, Reynolds J, Zuidema GD. Aspiration in patients with tracheostomies. *Surg Gynecol Obstet* 1973;136:68–70.
87. Deitch EA, Berg R. Bacterial translocation from the gut: a mechanism of infection. *J Burn Care Rehabil* 1987;8:475.
88. Rashkin MC, Davis T. Acute complications of endotracheal intubation: relationship to reintubation, route, urgency, and duration. *Chest* 1986;89:165–167.
89. Toews GB, Gross GN, Pierce AK. The relationship of inoculum size to lung bacterial clearance and phagocytic cell response in mice. *Am Rev Respir Dis* 1979;120:559–566.
90. Torres A, El-ebiary M, Gonzalez J, et al. Gastric and pharyngeal flora in nosocomial pneumonia acquired during mechanical ventilation. *Am Rev Respir Dis* 1993;148:352–357.
91. Bryant LR, Trinkle JK, Mobin-Uddin K, Baker J, Griffen WO Jr. Bacterial colonization profile with tracheal intubation and mechanical ventilation. *Arch Surg* 1972;104:647–651.
92. Johanson WG, Pierce AK, Sanford JP. Changing pharyngeal bacterial flora of hospitalized patients: emergence of gram-negative bacilli. *N Engl J Med* 1969;281:1137–1140.
93. Reynolds HY. Bacterial adherence to respiratory tract mucosa: a dynamic interaction leading to colonization. *Semin Respir Infect* 1987; 2:8–19.
94. Niederman MS. Gram-negative colonization of the respiratory tract: pathogenesis and clinical consequences. *Semin Respir Infect* 1990;5: 173–184.
95. Valenti WM, Trudell RG, Bentley DW. Factors predisposing to oropharyngeal colonization with gram-negative bacilli in the aged. *N Engl J Med* 1978;298:1108–1111.
96. Woods DE, Straus DC, Johanson WG Jr, et al. Role of pili in adherence of *Pseudomonas aeruginosa* to mammalian buccal epithelial cells. *Infect Immun* 1980;29:1146–1151.
97. Woods DE, Straus DC, Johanson WG Jr, et al. Role of fibronectin in the prevention of adherence of *Pseudomonas aeruginosa* to buccal cells. *J Infect Dis* 1981;143:784–790.
98. Driks MR, Craven DE, Celli BR, et al. Nosocomial pneumonia in intubated patients given sucralfate as compared with antacids or histamine type 2 blockers: the role of gastric colonization. *N Engl J Med* 1987;317:1376–1382.
99. Daschner F, Kappstein I, Engels I, et al. Stress ulcer prophylaxis and ventilation pneumonia: prevention by antibacterial cytoprotective agents. *Infect Control* 1988;9:59–65.
100. Tryba M. The gastropulmonary route of infection: fact or fiction? *Am J Med* 1991;91(Suppl 2A):135S–146S.
101. File TJ, Tan J, Thomson RJ, Stephens C, Thompson P. An outbreak of *Pseudomonas aeruginosa* ventilator-associated respiratory infections due to contaminated food coloring dye: further evidence of the significance of gastric colonization preceding nosocomial pneumonia. *Infect Control Hosp Epidemiol* 1995;16:417–418.
102. Niederman MS, Craven DE. Devising strategies for nosocomial pneumonia prevention: should we ignore the stomach? *Clin Infect Dis* 1997; 24:320–323.
103. Bonten MJM, Gaillard CA, van Tiel FH, Smeets HGW, van der Geest S, Stobberingh EE. The stomach as a source for colonization of the upper respiratory tract and pneumonia in ICU patients. *Chest* 1994; 105:878–884.
104. Bonten MJM, Gaillard CA, de Leeuw PW, Stobberingh EE. The role of colonization of the upper intestinal tract in the pathogenesis of ventilator-associated pneumonia. *Clin Infect Dis* 1997;24:309–319.
105. Giannella RA, Broitman SA, Zamcheck N. Influence of gastric acidity on bacterial and parasitic enteric infections: a perspective. *Ann Intern Med* 1973;78:271–276.
106. Arnold I. The bacterial flora within the stomach and small intestine: the effect of experimental alterations of acid-base balance and the age of the subject. Am J Med Sci 1933;186:471–481.
107. Bishop RF, Anderson CM. The bacterial flora of the stomach and small intestine in children with obstruction. *Arch Dis Child* 1960; 35:487–491.
108. Drasar BS, Shiner M. Studies of the intestinal flora: II. bacteria flora of the small intestine in patients with gastrointestinal disorders. *Gut* 1969;10:812–819.
109. Hornick RB, Music SI, Wenzel R, et al. The broad street pump revisited: response of volunteers to ingested cholera vibrios. *Bull NY Acad Med* 1971;47:1181–1191.
110. Seley GP, Colp R. The bacteriology of peptic ulcers and gastric malignancies: possible bearing on complications following gastric surgery. *Surgery* 1941;10:369–380.
111. Gracey M, Suhurjano S, Stone DE. Microbial contamination of the gut: another feature of malnutrition. *Am J Clin Nutr* 1973;26:1170–1174.
112. Ruddell WSJ, Axon ATR, Findlay JM, et al. Effect of cimetidine on the gastric bacterial flora. *Lancet* 1980;1:672–674.
113. Donowitz LG, Page MC, Mileur GL, Guenthner SH. Alteration of normal gastric flora in critical care patients receiving antacid and cimetidine therapy. *Infect Control* 1986;7:23–26.
114. Kappstein I, Friedrich T, Hellinger P, et al. Incidence of pneumonia in mechanically ventilated patients treated with sucralfate or cimetidine as prophylaxis for stress bleeding: bacterial colonization of the stomach. *Am J Med* 1991;91(Suppl 2A):S125–S131.
115. Beer DJ, Matloff SM, Rocklin RE. The influence of histamine on immune and inflammatory responses. *Adv Immunol* 1984;35:209–268.
116. Toews GB. Role of the polymorphonuclear leukocyte: interaction with nosocomial pathogens. *Eur J Clin Microbiol Infect Dis* 1989;8:21–24.
117. Rose RM. Pulmonary macrophages in nosocomial pneumonia: defense function and dysfunction, and prospects for activation. *Eur J Clin Microbiol Infect Dis* 1989;8:25–28.
118. Fick RB. Lung humoral response to Pseudomonas species. *Eur J Clin Microbiol Infect Dis* 1989;8:29–34.
119. Reynolds HY. Normal and defective respiratory host defenses. In: Pennington JE, ed. *Respiratory infections: diagnosis and management.* 2nd ed. New York: Raven Press; 1989:1–33.
120. Kunkel SL, Strieter RM. Cytokine networking in lung inflammation. *Hosp Pract* 1990;25:63–76.
121. Craven DE, Steger KA, Fleming CA. Preventing hospital-acquired pneumonia: Current concepts and strategies. *Semin Respir Infect* 1997 (in press).
122. Ibanez J, Penafiel A, Raurich J, et al. Gastroesophageal reflux and aspiration of gastric contents during nasogastric feeding: the effect of posture [Abstract]. *Intensive Care Med* 1988;14(Suppl 2):296.
123. Border J, Hassett J, LaDuca J, et al. The gut origin septic states in blunt multiple trauma (ISS-40) in the ICU. *Ann Surg* 1987;206:427–448.
124. Craven DE, Steger KA. Nosocomial pneumonia in mechanically ventilated adult patients: epidemiology and prevention in 1996. *Semin Respir Infect* 1996;11:32–53.
125. Craven DE, Steger KA. Epidemiology of nosocomial pneumonia: new concepts on an old disease. *Chest* 1995;108:1S–16S.
126. Prekates A, Nanas S, Floros J, et al. Predisposing factors for ventilator-associated pneumonia in general ICU. *American Journal of Respiratory Critical Care Medicine* 1996;153:A562.
127. Rello J, Sonora R, Jubert P, Artigas A, Rue M, Valles J. Pneumonia in intubated patients: role of respiratory airway care. *American Journal of Respiratory Critical Care Medicine* 1996;154:111–115.
128. Ferrer M, Torres A, Gonzalez J, et al. Utility of selective digestive decontamination in a general population of mechanically ventilated patients. *Am Rev Respir Dis* 1992;4:A112.
129. Selective Decontamination of the Digestive Tract Trialists' Collaborative Group. Meta-analysis of randomised controlled trials of selective decontamination of the digestive tract. *Br Med J* 1993;307:525–532.
130. Stoutenbeek CP, van Saene HKF, Miranda DR, Zandstra DF. The effect of selective decontamination of the digestive tract on colonization and infection rate in multiple trauma patients. *Intensive Care Med* 1984;10:185–192.
131. Cockerill FR, Muller SM, Anhalt JP, et al. Prevention of infection in critically ill patients by selective decontamination of the digestive tract. *Ann Intern Med* 1992;117:545–553.
132. van Saene HKF, Stoutenbeek CP, Stoller JK. Selective decontamination of the digestive tract in the intensive care unit: current status and future prospects. *Crit Care Med* 1992;20:691–703.
133. Duncan RA, Steger KA, Craven DE. Selective decontamination of the digestive tract: risks outweigh benefits for intensive care unit patients. *Semin Respir Infect* 1993;8:308–324.
134. The European Society of Intensive Care Medicine, The Societe Reanimation de Langue Francaise. The first European consensus confer-

ence in intensive care medicine: selective decontamination of the digestive tract in intensive care unit patients. *Infect Control Hosp Epidemiol* 1992;13:609–611.
135. Craven DE. Use of selective decontamination of the digestive tract: is the light at the end of the tunnel red or green? *Ann Intern Med* 1992; 117:609–611.
136. Gastinne H, Wolff M, Delatour F, Faurisson F, Chevret S. A controlled trial in intensive care units of selective decontamination of the digestive tract with nonabsorbable antibiotics. *N Engl J Med* 1992;326: 594–599.
137. Hammond JMJ, Potgieter PD, Saunders GL, Forder AA. A double blind study of selective decontamination in intensive care. *Lancet* 1992;340:5–9.
138. Cook DJ, Fuller HD, Guyatt GH, et al. Risk factors for gastrointestinal bleeding in critically ill patients. *N Engl J Med* 1994;330:377–381.
139. Cook DJ, Reeve BK, Scholes LC. Histamine-2-receptor antagonists and antacids in the critically ill population: stress ulceration versus nosocomial pneumonia. *Infect Control Hosp Epidemiol* 1994;15: 437–442.
140. Tryba M. Risk of acute stress bleeding and nosocomial pneumonia in ventilated intensive care unit patients: Sucralfate versus antacids. *Am J Med* 1987;83(Suppl):117–124.
141. Gaynes R, Bizek B, Mowry-Hanley J, Kirsch M. Risk factors for nosocomial pneumonia after coronary artery bypass graft operations. *Ann Thorac Surg* 1991;51:215–218.
142. Ryan P, Dawson J, Teres D, Celoria G, Navab F. Nosocomial pneumonia during stress ulcer prophylaxis with cimetidine and sucralfate. *Arch Surg* 1993;128:1353–1357.
143. Cook DJ, Laine LA, Guyatt GH, Raffin TA. Nosocomial pneumonia and the role of gastric pH. *Chest* 1991;100:7–13.
144. Tryba M. Sucralfate versus antacids or H_2-antagonists for stress ulcer prophylaxis: a meta-analysis on efficacy and pneumonia rate. *Crit Care Med* 1991;19:942–949.
145. Mantey-Stiers F, Tryba M. Antibacterial activity of sucralfate in human gastric juice. *Am J Med* 1987;87:125–128.
146. Ben-Menachem T, Fogel R, Patel RV, et al. Prophylaxis for stressed-related gastric hemorrhage in the medical intensive care unit: a randomized, controlled, single-blind study. *Ann Intern Med* 1994;121: 568–575.
147. Inglis TJJ, Millar MR, Jones JG, Robinson DA. Tracheal tube biofilm as a source of bacterial colonization of the lung. *J Clin Microbiol* 1989;27:2014–2018.
148. Craven DE, Barber TW, Steger KA, Montecalvo MA. Nosocomial pneumonia in the 90's: update of epidemiology and risk factors. *Semin Respir Infect* 1990;5:157–172.
149. Rouby J, Laurent P, Gosnach M, et al. Risk factors and clinical relevance of nosocomial maxillary sinusitis in the critically ill. *American Journal of Respiratory Critical Care Medicine* 1994;150:776–783.
150. Ashbaugh DC. Sepsis complicating the acute respiratory distress syndrome. *Surg Gynecol Obstet* 1972;135:865–868.
151. Sottile FD, Marrie TJ, Prough DS, et al. Nosocomial pulmonary infection: possible etiologic significance of bacterial adhesion to endotracheal tubes. *Crit Care Med* 1986;14:265–270.
152. Cheadle WG, Vitale GC, Mackie CR, Cuschieri A. Prophylactic postoperative nasogastric decompression: a prospective study of its requirement and the influence of cimetidine in 200 patients. *Ann Surg* 1985;202:361–366.
153. Olivares L, Segovia A, Revuelta R. Tube feeding and lethal aspiration in neurological patients: a review of 720 autopsy cases. *Stroke* 1974;5: 654–656.
154. Pingleton SK, Hinthorn DR, Liu C. Enteral nutrition in patients receiving mechanical ventilation: multiple sources of tracheal colonization include the stomach. *Am J Med* 1986;80:827–832.
155. Venezia RA, Agresta MD, Hanley EM, Urquhart K, Schoonmaker D. Nosocomial legionellosis associated with aspiration of nasogastric feedings diluted in tap water. *Infect Control Hosp Epidemiol* 1994;15:529–533.
156. Anderson KR, Norris DJ, Godfrey LB, et al. Bacterial contamination of the tube-feeding formulas. *JPEN J Parenter Enteral Nutr* 1984;8: 673–678.
157. Montecalvo MA, Korsberg TZ, Farber HW, et al. Nosocomial pneumonia and nutritional status of critical care patients randomized to gastric versus jejunal tube feedings. *Crit Care Med* 1992;20: 1377–1387.
158. Craven DE, Connolly MGJ, Lichtenberg DA, Primeau PJ, McCabe WR. Contamination of mechanical ventilators with tubing changes every 24 or 48 hours. *N Engl J Med* 1982;306:1505–1509.
159. Dreyfuss D, Djedaini K, Weber P, et al. Prospective study of nosocomial pneumonia and of patient and circuit colonization during mechanical ventilation with circuit changes every 48 hours versus no change. *Am Rev Respir Dis* 1991;143:738–743.
160. Kollef M, Shapiro S, Fraser V, et al. Mechanical ventilation with or without 7-day circuit changes: a randomized controlled trial. *Ann Intern Med* 1995;123:168–174.
161. Craven DE, Goularte TA, Make BJ. Contaminated condensated in mechanical ventilator circuits: a risk factor for nosocomial pneumonia. *Am Rev Respir Dis* 1984;129:625–628.
162. Branson RD, Hurst JM. Laboratory evaluation of moisture output of seven airway heat and moisture exchangers. *Respiratory Care* 1987; 32:741–747.
163. Branson RD, Campbell RS, Davis KJ, Johnson DJ, Porombka D. Humidification in the intensive care unit: prospective study of a new protocol utilizing heated humidification and a hygroscopic condenser humidifier. *Chest* 1993;104:1800–1805.
164. Roustan JP, Kienlen J, Aubas P, Aubas S, du Cailar J. Comparison of hydrophobic heat and moisture exchanger with heated humidifier during prolonged mechanical ventilation. *Intensive Care Med* 1992;18:97–100.
165. Misset B, Escudier B, Rivara D, Leclercq B, Nitenberg G. Heat and moisture exchanger vs heated humidifier during long-term mechanical ventilation: a prospective randomized study. *Chest* 1991;100:160–163.
166. Martin C, Perrin G, Gevaudan MJ, Saux P, Gouin F. Heat and moisture exchangers and vaporizing humidifiers in the intensive care unit. *Chest* 1990;97:144–149.
167. Hurni J, Feihl F, Lazor R, Leutenberger P, Perret C. Safety of combined heat and moisture exchanger filters in long-term mechanical ventilation. *Chest* 1997;111:686–691.
168. Kirton OC, DeHaven B, Morgan J, Morejon O, Civetta J. A prospective, randomized comparison of an in-line heat moisture exchange filter and heated wire humidifiers: rates of ventilator-associated early onset (community-acquired) or late onset (hospital-acquired) pneumonia and incidence of endotracheal tube occlusion. *Chest* 1997; (in press).
169. Deppe SA, Kelly JW, Thoi LL, et al. Incidence of colonization, nosocomial pneumonia, and mortality in critically ill patients using a Trach Care[R] closed-suction system versus an open-suction system: a prospective, randomized study. *Crit Care Med* 1990;18:1389–1394.
170. Craven DE, Lichtenberg DA, Goularte TA, Make BJ, McCabe WR. Contaminated medication nebulizers in mechanical ventilator circuits: a source of bacterial aerosols. *Am J Med* 1984;77:834–838.
171. Craven DE, Steger KA. Nosocomial pneumonia in the intubated patient: new concepts on pathogenesis and prevention. *Infect Dis Clin North Am* 1989;3:843–866.
172. Craven DE, Steger KA, Duncan RA. Prevention and control of nosocomial pneumonia. In: Wenzel RP, ed. *Prevention and control of nosocomial infections.* 2nd ed. Baltimore: Williams & Wilkins; 1992:580–599.
173. Weems JJ Jr. Nosocomial outbreak of *Pseudomonas cepacia* associated with contamination of reusable electronic ventilator temperature probes. *Infect Control Hosp Epidemiol* 1993;14:583–586.
174. Albert RK, Condie F. Handwashing patterns in medical intensive care units. *N Engl J Med* 1981;304:1465–1466.
175. Klein BS, Perloff WH, Maki DG, et al. Reduction of nosocomial infection during pediatric intensive care by protective isolation. *N Engl J Med* 1989;320:1714–1721.
176. Sherertz RJ, Reagan DR, Hampton KD, et al. A cloud adult: the *Staphylococcus aureus*–virus interaction revisited. *Ann Intern Med* 1996;124:539–547.
177. The American Thoracic Society (adopted by the ATS Board of Directors). Hospital-acquired pneumonia in adults: diagnosis, assessment of severity, initial antimicrobial therapy, and preventative strategies: a consensus statement. *American Journal of Respiratory Critical Care Medicine* 1996;153:1711–1725.
178. Smith CR, Ambinder R, Lipsky JJ, et al. Cefotaxime compared with nafcillin plus tobramycin for serious bacterial infections: a randomized, double-blind trial. *Ann Intern Med* 1984;101:469–477.
179. LaForce FM. Systemic antimicrobial therapy of nosocomial pneumonia: monotherapy versus combination therapy. *Eur J Clin Microbiol Infect Dis* 1989;8:61–68.

180. Moore RD, Smith CR, Lietman PS. Association of aminoglycoside plasma levels with therapeutic outcome in gram-negative pneumonia. *Am J Med* 1984;77:657–662.
181. Kirby BD, Synder KM, Meyer RD, et al. Legionnaires disease: report of sixty-five nosocomially acquired cases and review of the literature. *Medicine* 1980;59:188–205.
182. Marrie TJ, MacDonald S, Clarke K, Haldane D. Nosocomial Legionnaires' disease: lessons from a four-year prospective study. *Am J* Infect Control 1991;19:79–85.
183. Hsu SC, Martin R, Wentworth BB. Isolation of *Legionella* species from drinking water. *Appl Environ Microbiol* 1984;48:830–832.
184. Haley CE, Cohen ML, Halter J, Meyer RD. Nosocomial Legionnaires' disease: a continuing common-source epidemic at Wadsworth Medical Center. *Medicine* 1979;90:583–586.
185. Brady MT. Nosocomial Legionnaires' disease in a children's hospital. *J Pediatr* 1989;115:46–50.
186. Breiman RF, Fields BS, Sanden G, Volmer L, Meier A, Spika J. An outbreak of Legionnaires' disease associated with shower use: possible role of amoebae. *JAMA* 1990;263:2924–2926.
187. Blatt SP, Parkinson MD, Pace E, et al. Nosocomial Legionnaires' disease: aspiration as a primary mode of disease acquisition. *Am J Med* 1993;95:16–22.
188. Yu VL, Beam TR Jr, Lumis RM, et al. Routine culturing for *Legionella* in the hospital environment may be a good idea: a three-hospital prospective study. *Am J Med Sci* 1987;294:97–99.
189. Giorgi JV, Detels R. T-cell subset alterations in HIV-infected homosexual men: NIAID multicenter AIDS cohort study. *Clin Immunol Immunopathol* 1989;52:10–18.
190. Archibald DW, Witt DJ, Craven DE, et al. Antibodies to HIV in cervical secretions from women at risk for AIDS [Letter]. *J Infect Dis* 1987;156:240–241.
191. Bezanson G, Burbridge S, Haldane D, Yoell C, Marrie T. Diverse populations of *Legionella pneumophila* present in the water of geographically clustered institutions served by the same water reservior. *J Clin Microbiol* 1992;30:571–576.
192. Chave J, David S, Wauters J, Van Melle G, Francioli P. Transmission of *Pneumocystis carinii* from AIDS patients to other immunosuppressed patients: a cluster of *Pneumocystis carinii* pneumonia in renal transplant recipients. *AIDS* 1991;5:927–932.
193. Marrie T, Haldane D, Bezanson G, Peppard R. Each water outlet is a unique ecologic niche for *Legionella pneumophila*. *Epidemiol Infect* 1992;108:261–270.
194. Mermel LA, Josephson SL, Giorgio CH, Dempsey J, Parenteau S. Association of Legionnaires' disease with construction: contamination of potable water? *Infect Control Hosp Epidemiol* 1995;16:76–81.
195. Carratala J, Gudiol F, Palares R, et al. Risk factors for nosocomial *Legionella pneumophila* pneumonia. *American Journal of Respiratory Critical Care Medicine* 1995.
196. Dondero TJ, Rendtorff R, Mallison GF, et al. An outbreak of Legionnaires' disease associated with contaminated air-conditioning cooling tower. *N Engl J Med* 1980;302:365–370.
197. Yu V. Could aspiration be the major mode of transmission for *Legionella*? *Am J Med* 1993;95:13–15.
198. Struelens MJ, Maes N, Rost F, et al. Genotypic and phenotypic methods for investigation of a nosocomial *Legionella pneumophila* outbreak and efficacy of control measures. *J Infect Dis* 1992;166:22–30.
199. Luck PC, Helbig JH, Gunter U, et al. Epidemiologic investigation by macrorestriction analysis and by using monoclonal antibodies of nosocomial pneumonia caused by Legionella pneumophila serogroup 1." *J Clin Microbiol* 1994;32:2692–2697.
200. Muraca PW, Yu VL, Goetz A. Disinfection of water distribution systems for *Legionella*: a review of application procedures and methodologies. *Infect Control Hosp Epidemiol* 1990;11:79–88.
201. Yu VL, Zeming L, Stout JE, Goetz A. *Legionella* disinfection of water distribution systems: principles, problems, and practice. *Infect Control Hosp Epidemiol* 1993;14:567–570.
202. Valenti WM, Hall CB, Douglas RGJ, Meneges MA, Pincus PH. Nosocomial viral infections: I. epidemiology and significance. *Infect Control* 1980;1:33–37.
203. Goldmann DA. Transmission of infectious diseases in children. *Pediatr Rev* 1992;13:283–293.
204. Rivera ME, Mason WH, Ross LA, Wright H Jr. Nosocomial measles infection in a pediatric hospital during a community-wide epidemic. *J Pediatr* 1991;119:183–186.
205. Hall CB, Douglas G, Geiman JM, et al. Nosocomial respiratory syncytial virus infections. *N Engl J Med* 1975;293:1343–1346.
206. Centers for Disease Control and Prevention. Prevention and control of influenza. *Advisory Committee Immunization Practices* 1995;44(April 21):1–38.
207. Dolin R, Reichman RC, Madore HP, Maynard R, Linton PN, Webber-Jones J. A controlled trial of amantadine and rimantadine in the prophylaxis of influenza A infection. *N Engl J Med* 1990;322:443–450.
208. Tominack RL, Hayden FG. Rimantadine hydrochloride and amantadine hydrochloride use in influenza A virus infections. *Infect Dis Clin North Am* 1987;1:459–478.
209. Valenti WM, Betts RF, Hall CB, Hruska JF, Douglas RGJ. Nosocomial viral infections: II. guidelines for prevention and control of respiratory viruses, herpes viruses, and hepatitis viruses. *Infect Control* 1981;1:165–178.
210. Denning DW, Clemons KV, Hanson LH, Stevens DA. Restriction endonuclease analysis of total cellular DNA of *Aspergillus fumigatus* isolates of geographically and epidemiologically diverse origin. *J Infect Dis* 1990;162:1151–1158.
211. Rhame FS. Prevention of nosocomial aspergillosis. *J Hosp Infect* 1991;18:466–472.
212. Arnow PM, Anderson RL, Mainous PD, et al. Pulmonary aspergillus during hospital renovation. *Am Rev Respir Dis* 1978;118:49–53.
213. Hopkins CC, Weber DJ, Rubin RH. Invasive aspergillosis infection: possible non-ward common source within the hospital environment. *J Hosp Infect* 1989;13:19–25.
214. Rhame FS. Lessons from the Roswell Park bone marrow transplant aspergillosis outbreak. *Infect Control* 1985;63:345–346.
215. Opal SM, Asp AA, Cannady F, et al. Efficacy of infection control measures during a nosocomial outbreak of disseminated aspergillosis associated with hospital construction. *J Infect Dis* 1986;153:634
216. Symoens F, Viviani MA, Nolard N. Typing by immunoblot of *Aspergillus fumigatus* from nosocomial infections. *Mycoses* 1993;36: 229–237.
217. Haron E, Vartivarian S, Anaissie E, Dekmezian R, Bodey GP. Primary *Candida* pneumonia: experience at a large cancer center and review of the literature. *Medicine* 1993;72:137–142.
218. Sanchez V, Vazquez JA, Barth-Jones D, Dembry L, Sobel JD, Zervos MJ. Epidemiology of nosocomial acquisition of *Candida lusitaniae*. *J Clin Microbiol* 1992;30:3005–3008.
219. Dembry LM, Vazquez JA, Zervos MJ. DNA analysis in the study of the epidemiology of nosocomial candidiasis. *Infect Control Hosp Epidemiol* 1994;15:48–53.
220. Craven DE, Steger KA, Hirschhorn LR. Nosocomial colonization and infection in persons infected with human immunodeficiency virus. *Infect Control Hosp Epidemiol* 1996;17:304–318.
221. Weber DJ, Becherer PR, Rutala WA, Samsa GP, Wilson MB, White GC II. Nosocomial infection rate as a function of human immunodeficiency virus type 1 status in hemophiliacs. *Am J Med* 1991;91(Suppl 3B):S206–S211.
222. Gaynes R, Martone W, Bisno A, Rimland D, Srivastara P, Culver D. Nosocomial infections among HIV-positive patients [Abstract]. In: *Second annual meeting of The Society of Health Care Epidemiology of America (Abstract M32). Chicago, Illinois,* 1992:M32.
223. Nichols L, Balogh K, Silverman M. Bacterial infections in the acquired immune deficiency syndrome: clinicopathologic correlations in a series of autopsy cases. *Am J Clin Pathol* 1989;92:787–790.
224. Niedt GW, Schinella RA. Acquired immunodeficiency syndrome: clinicopathologic study of 56 autopsies. *Arch Pathol Lab Med* 1985; 109:727–734.
225. Blumberg HM, Rimland D. Nosocomial infection with penicillin-resistant pneumococci in patients with AIDS. *J Infect Dis* 1989;160: 725–726.
226. Simberkoff MS, El Sadr W, Schiffman G, et al. *Streptococcus pneumoniae* infections and bacteremia in patients with acquired immunodeficiency syndrome with report of a pneumococcal vaccine failure. *Am Rev Respir Dis* 1984;130:1174–1176.
227. Witt DJ, Craven DE, McCabe WR. Bacterial infection in patients with acquired immunodeficiency syndrome and AIDS-related complex. *Am J Med* 1987;82:900–906.
228. Selwyn PA, Alcabes P, Hartel D, et al. Clinical manifestations and predictors of disease progression in drug users with human immunodeficiency virus infection. *N Engl J Med* 1992;327:1697–1703.
229. Pallares R, Gudiol F, Linares J, et al. Risk factors and response to

antibiotic therapy in adults with bacteremic pneumonia caused by penicillin-resistant pneumococci. *N Engl J Med* 1987;317:18–22.
230. Feldman C, Kallenbach JM, Miller SD, Thorburn JR, Koornhof HJ. Community-acquired pneumonia due to penicillin-resistant pneumococci. *N Engl J Med* 1985;313:615–617.
231. Casadevall A, Dobroszycki J, Small C, Pirofski L. *Haemophilus influenzae* type b bacteremia in adults with AIDS and at risk for AIDS. *Am J Med* 1992;92:587–590.
232. Steinhart R, Reingold AL, Taylor F, Anderson G, Wenger JD. Invasive *Haemophilus influenzae* infections in men with HIV infection. *JAMA* 1992;268:3350–3352.
233. Michaels RH, Norden CW. Pharyngeal colonization with *Hemophilus influenzae* type b: a longitudinal study of families with a child with meningitis or epiglottitis due to *Hemophilus influenzae* type b. *J Infect Dis* 1977;136:222–228.
234. Goetz MB, O'Brien H, Musser JM, Ward JI. Nosocomial transmission of disease caused by nontypeable strains of *Haemophilus influenzae. Am J Med* 1994;96:342–347.
235. Patterson JE, Madden GM, Krisiunas EP, et al. A nosocomial outbreak of ampicillin-resistant *Hemophilus influenzae* type b in a geriatric unit. *J Infect Dis* 1988;157:1002–1007.
236. Barnes PF, Bloch AB, Davidson PT, Snider DE Jr. Tuberculosis in patients with human immunodeficiency virus infection. *N Engl J Med* 1991;324:1644–1650.
237. Brudney K, Dobkin J. Resurgent tuberculosis in New York City: human immunodeficiency virus, homelessness, and the decline of tuberculosis. *Am Rev Respir Dis* 1991;144:745–749.
238. Small PM, Hopewell PC, Singh SP, et al. The epidemiology of tuberculosis in San Francisco: a population-based study using conventional and molecular methods. *N Engl J Med* 1994;330:1703–1709.
239. Alland D, Kalkut GE, Moss AR, et al. Transmission of tuberculosis in New York City: an analysis by DNA fingerprinting and conventional epidemiologic methods. *N Engl J Med* 1994;330:1710–1716.
240. Beck-Sagué C, Dooley SW, Hulton MD, et al. Hospital outbreak of multidrug-resistant *Mycobacterium tuberculosis* infections. *JAMA* 1992;268:1280–1286.
241. Blumberg HM, Watkins D, Berschling J, et al. Preventing the nosocomial transmission of tuberculosis. *Ann Intern Med* 1995;122: 658–663.
242. Centers for Disease Control and Prevention. Guidelines for preventing the transmission of *Mycobacterium tuberculosis* in health-care facilities, 1994. *MMWR Morb Mortal Wkly Rep* 1994;43.
243. Singer C, Armstrong D, Rosen PP, et al. *Pneumocystis carinii* pneumonia: a cluster of eleven cases. *Ann Intern Med* 1975;82: 772–777.
244. Hoover DR, Graham NMH, Bacellar H, et al.Epidemiologic patterns of upper respiratory illness and *Pneumocystis carinii* pneumonia in homosexual men. *Am Rev Respir Dis* 1991;144:756–759.
245. Haron E, Bodey GP, Luna MA, Dekmezian R, Elting L. Has the incidence of *Pneumocystis carinii* pneumonia in cancer patients increased with the AIDS epidemic? *Lancet* 1988;1:904–905.
246. Chave JP, Bille J, Glauser MP, Francioli P. Diagnosis of pulmonary infections in patients infected with the human immunodeficiency virus. *Eur J Clin Microbiol Infect Dis* 1989;8:123–126.

Hospital Infections, Fourth Edition,
edited by John V. Bennett and Philip S. Brachman.
Published by Lippincott–Raven Publishers, Philadelphia, 1998

CHAPTER 33

Tuberculosis

William R. Jarvis

Tuberculosis is a major cause of morbidity and mortality throughout the world, with an estimated eight million people contracting disease and three million dying annually. Worldwide, the prevalence of tuberculosis is increasing; this is in part due to the human immunodeficiency virus (HIV) epidemic. In the mid-1980s, the incidence of tuberculosis reversed its downward trend in the United States and, possibly secondary to the HIV epidemic and increased immigration from countries with a high incidence of tuberculosis, began to increase [1–6].

At about this same time, an increase in the number of outbreaks of transmission of *Mycobacterium tuberculosis*, particularly multidrug-resistant strains (MDR-TB; i.e., resistant to at least two first-line antituberculous agents), began to be reported in healthcare institutions in the United States [7].

PATHOGEN AND PATHOGENESIS

Tuberculosis is caused by bacteria in the *M. tuberculosis* complex, of which *M. tuberculosis* is the most important [2,4]. The primary mode of transmission is by airborne droplet nuclei, which may be produced when people with pulmonary or laryngeal tuberculosis cough, sneeze, speak, or sing. In addition, aerosols can be produced and transmission occur during manipulation or irrigation of tuberculosis lesions or when tissues or secretions from a person with tuberculosis are being obtained or processed. The actual sizes of the airborne droplet nuclei are not known but are estimated to be between 1 and 5 µm; such particles are light enough to be carried long distances by ambient air currents. When such airborne droplet nuclei are inhaled, they may traverse the body's defenses and become implanted in the respiratory bronchiole or alveoli. Despite capture by macrophages, the bacilli may replicate within the cell or be carried directly or by the macrophage through the lymphatics to regional lymph nodes or the bloodstream, or they may disseminate. Cell-mediated immunity usually limits further multiplication or spread, and lesions resolve. The risk of infection with *M. tuberculosis* varies depending on the concentration of droplet nuclei in the air and the duration of exposure to the contaminated air. After inhalation, the bacilli remain viable; this condition of latent *M. tuberculosis* infection is asymptomatic and is not contagious. In immunocompetent individuals, a tuberculin skin test (TST) applied 2 to 10 weeks after initial infection is positive; this is secondary to hypersensitivity to *M. tuberculosis* cell wall components. In ~ 10% of infected immunocompetent individuals, the organism begins to multiply and causes active disease in their lifetime. In ~ 5% of these individuals, this occurs within the first 1 to 2 years after infection, and in the remaining 5% disease occurs > 2 years after infection. Those with immunocompromising conditions are at a > 10% risk for development of active tuberculosis annually.

TUBERCULOSIS IN THE UNITED STATES

From 1953 through 1984, the number of people in the United States each year with active tuberculosis decreased by ~ 6% per year, from 84,304 to 22,201 [3]. However, from 1985 through 1992, the reported number of people with tuberculosis increased by ~ 20% to 26,673 [4]. Thus, from 1985 through 1992, ~ 52,000 excess episodes of tuberculosis have been reported above what would have been expected based on the 1953 to 1984 trend. In addition, the proportion of people infected with MDR-TB increased. Factors contributing to this increase in tuberculosis include the HIV epidemic, the increase in the number of people immigrating from countries with a high prevalence of tuberculosis, adverse social conditions, and inadequate infection control practices in

W. R. Jarvis: Hospital Infections Program, Centers for Disease Control and Prevention, Atlanta, Georgia 30333.

healthcare facilities, all of which facilitate transmission. The combination of an increasing prevalence of tuberculosis, HIV-infected people, and MDR-TB resulted in an increase in hospitalization of people with infectious tuberculosis and an increased risk of *M. tuberculosis* transmission in healthcare facilities to both patients (nosocomial acquisition) and healthcare workers (occupational acquisition). With increased emphasis in hospital- and community-based tuberculosis control programs, the reported incidence of tuberculosis decreased by 5.2% in 1993 and by another 3.7% in 1994 [5,6]

Of the 25,287 people reported with tuberculosis in the United States in 1993, 65% were male, 71.5% were racial and ethnic minorities, 38% were 25 to 44 years of age, and 29% were born in a country other than the United States. In 1993, 64% of the reported episodes of tuberculosis were reported from seven states—California, New York, Texas, Florida, Illinois, New Jersey, and Georgia. Factors in reversing the increasing trend in tuberculosis in the United States include the successful implementation of recommended tuberculosis control programs, including directly observed therapy and improved implementation of hospital infection control practices [8].

DIAGNOSIS OF TUBERCULOSIS

Prevention of transmission of *M. tuberculosis* depends on a high index of suspicion of tuberculosis and knowledge of the clinical signs and symptoms and the appropriate diagnostic work-up. The initial symptoms of tuberculosis may be nonspecific and insidious in onset and include fatigue, anorexia, fever, chills, myalgia, sweating, and weight loss. Pulmonary tuberculosis is the most common form and the one usually associated with transmission in healthcare facilities. In the pulmonary form of tuberculosis, the nonspecific symptoms are accompanied by an insidious cough that gradually progresses over a period of weeks to months to a productive cough with mucopurulent sputum or hemoptysis. Hoarseness or a sore throat suggests possible laryngeal involvement; laryngeal tuberculosis usually is accompanied by pulmonary disease, large numbers of acid-fast bacilli (AFB) in sputum, and a high degree of contagion. The infectivity of the patient with tuberculosis depends on the site of infection, the presence of AFB-positive sputum, the number of organisms expelled into the air, the presence of pulmonary cavitary or endobronchial lesions, the duration of effective therapy, and whether the person remains in isolation or covers his or her mouth when coughing. Extrapulmonary tuberculosis without pulmonary or laryngeal involvement usually is not contagious. However, irrigation or manipulation of tuberculosis lesions can produce infectious aerosols and transmit *M. tuberculosis*. The appropriate diagnostic work-up of a patient with signs or symptoms consistent with tuberculosis should include a chest radiograph. With initial infection, parenchymal infiltration with ipsilateral lymph node enlargement may be seen, whereas in reactivation, apical or posterior segment lesions in the upper lobes are most common. In all patients, but particularly those who are immunocompromised, such as those with HIV infection, the chest radiograph findings may range from normal to miliary in appearance [9]. In those with possible pulmonary tuberculosis, respiratory secretions should be obtained promptly for AFB smears and culture; in pediatric patients, gastric aspirates may be needed for those who do not cough. Specimens should be transported to the laboratory promptly and the most rapid laboratory diagnostic methods should be used, including fluorescent microscopy and radiometric methods for species identification and drug susceptibility testing [10]. Because the AFB smear is the most rapid presumptive diagnostic test and also provides an important assessment of the patient's infectivity, AFB smears using fluorescent microscopy should be promptly performed. The development of genetic probes facilitates the rapid identification of *M. tuberculosis* (see Chapter 9). The initial isolate from people with tuberculosis and subsequent isolates from any person not responding to appropriate treatment should be tested for antituberculous drug susceptibility. Antituberculous drug susceptibility results provide the clinician with important information for choosing an effective therapeutic regime. Furthermore, the use of genetic probes and nucleic acid amplification techniques can further shorten the time required to determine the species identification. Data show that from 1992 to 1995, the proportion of U.S. hospital laboratories in which the recommended methods were used for AFB smears, primary culture, *M. tuberculosis* identification, and antituberculous drug susceptibility testing has increased [11].

During the initial evaluation, a TST should be applied to the surface of the patient's forearm using the Mantoux method and read at 48 to 72 hours. Despite the limitations of the TST (< 100% sensitivity and specificity; positive predictive value correlates with the prevalence of tuberculosis), it remains the most practical screening method for identifying people with *M. tuberculosis* infection (i.e., latent infection). Only the presence or absence of and the extent of induration (not erythema) transverse to the long axis of the forearm should be measured.

The cutpoint used for defining a positive TST varies depending on the risk of *M. tuberculosis* exposure. For people with HIV infection, people with close contact with a person with infectious tuberculosis, or with a chest radiograph consistent with pulmonary tuberculosis, a TST reaction of 5 mm or more is considered positive [12]. For people not meeting these criteria, but who have other risk factors for tuberculosis—people born in countries with a high prevalence of tuberculosis; medically underserved populations with a high prevalence of tuberculosis; people with conditions predisposing to tuberculosis (e.g., gastrectomy, jejunoileal bypass, ≥10% below ideal body weight, chronic renal insufficiency, immunosuppressive therapy, some malignancies, diabetes mellitus, gastrectomy or silicosis); residents of long-term care facilities; or other people identified as at high risk for tuberculosis—a reaction of 10 mm or more is considered positive. For others, a reaction of 15 mm or more is considered positive.

Periodic TST is a valuable method for identifying new *M. tuberculosis* infection in those exposed to people with infectious tuberculosis. For people younger than 35 years of age and most healthcare workers, an increase in TST induration of 10 mm or more within 2 years should be considered a TST conversion. For people 35 years of age or older or healthcare workers with infrequent tuberculosis exposure, an increase in TST induration of 15 mm or more in 2 years should be considered a TST conversion. Those with TST conversions should be promptly evaluated for active tuberculosis disease and placed on preventive therapy (if active disease is ruled out).

Repeated TST of noninfected individuals does not lead to hypersensitivity to tuberculin. However, in individuals with delayed hypersensitivity to tuberculin from either past infection with mycobacteria or bacille Calmette-Guerin (BCG) vaccination, reactivity may wane over time. In these individuals, the TST may stimulate the hypersensitivity and result in an initial negative TST followed by a subsequent positive TST when tested from 1 week to a year or longer after the initial TST (i.e., the "booster phenomenon"). To avoid the booster phenomenon and reduce the likelihood of interpreting a booster reaction as representing recent infection, TSTs should be conducted periodically, with the first test being a two-step test. In the two-step test, the individual first has a TST. If negative, a second TST is performed 1 to 3 weeks later. If the second test is positive, it is probably a booster reaction. Other factors that can alter the individual's ability to react to tuberculin include 1) host factors, such as concomitant infection (e.g., viral or bacterial infections), metabolic abnormalities (e.g., chronic renal failure), nutritional factors (e.g., severe protein calorie malnutrition), lymphoid organ abnormalities (e.g., malignancy, sarcoidosis), immunosuppressive agents, age (e.g., newborns or elderly), and stress (e.g., surgery, burns); 2) factors related to the tuberculin used, such as improper storage, improper dilution, chemical degradation, or contamination; 3) factors related to the TST administration method, such as injection of too little antigen or delay in administration after drawing up the tuberculin; or 4) factors related to reading the TST, such as an inexperienced reader or misreading.

Once a presumptive diagnosis of tuberculosis is established based on clinical findings plus or minus radiologic and laboratory findings, the patient should be placed on appropriate empiric therapy that can be modified once drug susceptibility results are available [13]. If the results of antituberculous susceptibility testing indicate resistance to agents being used or the patient fails to respond to the empiric therapy, the therapeutic regime should be modified.

M. TUBERCULOSIS TRANSMISSION IN HOSPITALS

Several factors influence whether *M. tuberculosis* is transmitted to either patients or healthcare workers in a hospital or other healthcare facility. These include the likelihood that they will be exposed to *M. tuberculosis*, that they will become infected, and that the infection will progress to disease. The risk of exposure in the healthcare setting is influenced by the number of infectious tuberculosis patients admitted and the infection control practices implemented in the healthcare facility, including the methods for identifying infectious patients, the type of isolation infectious patients are placed in, the type of respiratory protection used by the healthcare worker, and the environmental and engineering controls used. Several studies have shown that if the number of tuberculosis patients admitted or cared for is low, then the risk of exposure to *M. tuberculosis* is low [14–18]. The risk that healthcare workers or patients will become infected is influenced by the concentration of airborne droplet nuclei they are exposed to, the type and duration of the exposure, and the efficacy of the infection control measures implemented; although immunocompromising conditions increase the risk of disease given infection, they do not appear to increase the risk of infection. The risk that, once infected, one will progress rapidly from infection to disease depends on the prevalence of conditions in the worker or patient populations that decrease immunity (e.g., HIV infection, malignancy, or diabetes).

Surveillance for *M. tuberculosis* Infection/Disease in Healthcare Workers

There is no national surveillance system for *M. tuberculosis* infection/disease in healthcare workers in the United States. Before 1993, the national tuberculosis surveillance system did not collect occupational data on those reported with tuberculosis. In data reported since 1993, healthcare workers accounted for 0 to 6% of those reported with tuberculosis; however, this system does not provide further investigative data to determine whether the tuberculosis was occupationally or community acquired [5]. TST conversion data (tuberculosis infection without disease) are not collected in this or any other national surveillance system. In studies conducted at individual institutions, the incidence of tuberculosis infection in healthcare workers ranged from 0.1% to 10% [17–44] (Table 33-1).

Several national surveys show that in hospitals with healthcare worker TST programs, overall TST conversion rates range from 0.33% to 5.5% [14–18] (see Table 33-1). Several studies have shown that healthcare workers originating from foreign countries or with a history of BCG have a higher prevalence of TST positivity [43,44]. Furthermore, in some regions of the country, healthcare workers have a high prevalence of TST positivity at the time of employment [14–16,42,45]. For these reasons, it has been recommended that a two-step TST be performed at the time of employment followed by periodic TST based on the risk of exposure [12,46,47].

Few studies have assessed the risk of tuberculosis disease in healthcare workers. Although healthcare workers in the United States in general are at low risk of TST conversion or tuberculosis, selected healthcare worker groups—those with the closest contact with infectious tuberculosis patients or those working in hospitals with *M. tuberculosis* outbreaks—may be at greater risk [48]. In two surveys of physicians affiliated with medical schools, active tuberculosis appeared to be more common than in the community population [28,49]. Barrett-Conner found that 3.5% of the physicians at one medical center had been treated for active tuberculosis; 75% of active disease occurred within 10 years after beginning medical school and 62% occurred after infection after the beginning of medical school [28]. In the 1938 to 1981 graduates of the University of Illinois Medical School, active tuberculosis was more common than in the general population, and > 66% of the episodes occurred ≤ 6 years after graduation [49]. Twelve studies, most based on either registries or questionnaires, have assessed the risk of tuberculosis disease in healthcare workers: in five, the risk was estimated to be greater than in the general population; in three, the risk was estimated as less than in the general population; and in four, the risk was not compared with that of the general population [18].

TABLE 33-1. *Healthcare worker (HCW) tuberculin skin test (TST) conversion rates, United States, 1960–1996*

Reference	State	Study period	Study population	Annual TST conversion rate(%)
Levine [19]	New York	1960–1967	Nursing students	1.1
Weiss [20]	Pennsylvania	1962–1971	Nursing students	4.2
Atuk & Hunt [21]	Virginia	1968–1969	HCWs	1.9
Gregg et al. [22]	South Carolina	1969–1973	HCWs	4.1
Berman et al. [23]	Maryland	1971–1976	HCWs	1.4
Craven et al. [24]	Virginia	1971–1973	HCWs	0.5
Vogeler & Burke [25]	Utah	1972–1975	HCWs	0.2
Ruben et al. [26]	Pennsylvania	1973–1975	HCWs	3.1
Ktsanes et al. [27]	Louisiana	1972–1981	HCWs	1.0
Barrett-Conner [28]	California	1974–1975	Physicians	0.4–1.8
Weinstein et al. [29]	New York	1974–1981	Medical students	0.1
Chan & Tabak [30]	Florida	1978–1981	Physicians	4.0
Bass & Serio [31]	Alabama	1979	HCWs	2.9
Thompson et al. [32]	Multiple[a,b]	1979	HCWs	2.9
Kantor et al. [33]	Illinois	1979–1986	HCWs	0.9
Price et al. [34]	North Carolina[a]	1980–1984	HCWs	1.1
Aiken et al. [35]	Washington[a]	1982–1984	HCWs	0.9
Malasky et al. [17]	Multiple[a,b]	1984–1986	Pulmonary fellow	5.7
Raad et al. [36]	Florida	1984–1987	HCWs	0.1
Raad et al. [36]	Florida	1985–1987	HCWs	0.4
Ramirez et al. [37]	Kentucky	1986–1991	HCWs	0.7
Ikeda et al. [38]	New York	1989–1990	HCWs	0.8
Condos et al. [39]	New York	1988–1992	HCWs	1.0
Redwood et al. [40]	New York	1990–1992	HCWs	10.0
Cocchiarella et al. [41]	Illinois	1991	HCWs	46.2, 4.8[c]
Adal et al. [42]	Virginia	1992	HCWs	0.2
Panlilio et al. [43], National/state survey	Multiple[a,b]	1994–1995	HCWs	1.4
Manangan et al. [44]	Texas[a] (151)[d]	1989–1991	HCWs	0.6–0.9
Sinkowitz et al. [16]	Multiple[a,b] (1,494)[d]	1989–1992	HCWs	0.4–0.5
Fridkin et al. [14,15]	Multiple[a,b] (359)[d]	1992–1993	HCWs	0.2–1.9

[a]Multiple hospitals.
[b]Multiple states.
[c]High-risk and low-risk HCWs, respectively.
[d]Number of hospitals reporting.

Nosocomial *M. tuberculosis* Transmission

Before 1989, reports of nosocomial *M. tuberculosis* outbreaks were infrequent [50–52]. The sparsity of such reports may reflect either infrequent transmission or the failure to detect such transmission. Only 5% to 10% of immunocompetent people exposed to an infectious tuberculosis patient contract tuberculosis in their lifetime, and such development would occur months to years after the exposure. Because the patient may not be readmitted to the same facility, the possibility of nosocomial acquisition might not be considered; such disease would not be linked to a prior hospitalization and nosocomial acquisition would not be documented. Thus, unless there is a large group of immunocompetent or immunocompromised patients with newly diagnosed tuberculosis, or patients infected with a strain of *M. tuberculosis* with an unusual antimicrobial susceptibility pattern, nosocomial transmission may not be suspected, detected, or reported. Hence, nosocomial patient-to-patient transmission of *M. tuberculosis* may occur more frequently than recognized or reported.

In contrast, occupational acquisition of *M. tuberculosis* infection and disease has been a well-documented risk to healthcare workers in the United States since the early 1930s. In the mid- to late 1930s, Israel et al. followed a cohort of 637 nursing students during their hospital training [53]. At study entry, 360 (57%) nurses were TST negative and 277 (43%) were TST positive. During their training, 100% of the TST-negative nursing students had TST conversions and active tuberculosis developed in 68/637 (11%). Additional studies in the 1930s and 1940s documented high (79% to 85%) TST conversion rates among nurses [54,55]. Furthermore, during this period, studies documented that the risk of active tuberculosis disease among medical school students was more than three times higher than that of the general population [56]. Risk factors for disease among the medical students included exposure to unrecognized tuberculosis patients, treating patients in the men's tuberculosis ward, or presence in the autopsy room.

Despite these studies suggesting both nosocomial and occupational transmission of *M. tuberculosis*, efforts to introduce appropriate infection control interventions were slow. Many hospitals opened wards for tuberculosis patients only, sanitaria (or entire hospitals for tuberculosis patients) were common, and, in many hospitals, obtaining routine chest radiographs at the time of patient admission to identify the previously unrecognized infectious tuberculosis patient was initiated. Concomitantly, increased suspicion of tuberculosis by clinicians, improvements in diagnostic and therapeutic modalities, and the identification of effective preventive antituberculous therapy resulted in a dramatic reduction in the incidence of tuberculosis in the United States from the mid-1940s until the mid-1980s [1].

Despite the fact that numerous studies have documented that healthcare workers are at increased risk of occupational acquisition of *M. tuberculosis*, no formal surveillance system for healthcare worker TST conversion or disease has been established. Thus, even today there are few specific data on the risk of acquisition of tuberculosis among healthcare workers in the United States and virtually no data on healthcare workers in the developing world, where the risk may be even greater because of larger numbers of patients with tuberculosis, the presence of large, open wards, and minimal or absent infection control precautions. A questionnaire administered to graduates of the University of Illinois School of Medicine from 1938 to 1981 found that in most years the incidence of tuberculosis in the graduates exceeded that in the general population [49]. In another survey of medical school-affiliated physicians in California, 3.5% of physicians had been treated for tuberculosis; 75% of active disease had occurred < 10 years after beginning medical school [28]. However, data from the North Carolina tuberculosis control program show that in 1983 and 1984 hospital personnel had similar or lower rates of tuberculosis than the general population [34]. More recently, surveys have shown that many hospitals do not have active healthcare worker TST programs, that nurses and administrative personnel are more likely to be included in the TST program than are physicians, that healthcare worker TST positivity rates at hire can be high and are related most likely to community tuberculosis prevalence, and that healthcare worker (primarily nursing staff) TST conversion rates range from 0% to 27% [14–16,48,57,58].

Nosocomial *M. tuberculosis* in Human Immunodeficiency Virus-Infected Patients

Tuberculosis is a common infection in HIV-infected patients [59,60] (see Chapter 43). Most of these episodes of tuberculosis are thought to be due to reactivation of latent *M. tuberculosis* infection. In 1985, the incidence of tuberculosis began to rise in the United States; it is unclear how much of this rise was due to HIV-infected people who are at increased risk for both reactivation of latent infection and new, primary infection [1]. Nevertheless, between 1985 and 1992, ~ 52,000 excess episodes of tuberculosis occurred above what would have been expected in the United States had the downward trend in tuberculosis been maintained; much of this increase was thought to be in HIV-infected people [1]. Thus, the interaction of the HIV and tuberculosis outbreaks has resulted in a major public health challenge. In the late 1980s, nosocomial outbreaks of drug-susceptible *M. tuberculosis* or MDR-TB began to occur in U.S. hospitals [7]. In 1989, Dooley et al. investigated an outbreak of tuberculosis among patients on an HIV ward of a hospital in

Puerto Rico [61]. They found that HIV ward patients with exposure to an infectious tuberculosis patient were 11 times more likely to contract tuberculosis than were HIV ward patients without such an exposure. In addition, nurses (i.e., those with patient care responsibilities) working on the HIV or internal medicine wards were significantly more likely to have a positive TST than were clerical staff (i.e., those without direct patient care responsibilities) working on other wards at that hospital. This investigation documented that HIV-infected patients sharing a room with an HIV-infected patient with infectious tuberculosis were at increased risk of nosocomial acquisition of *M. tuberculosis*, that the incubation period was most consistent with primary infection, that the risk for development of active disease given exposure to an infectious tuberculosis patient was high, and that the duration from *M. tuberculosis* infection to disease (i.e., incubation period) was shortened in HIV-infected patients. These findings were consistent with those from another outbreak investigation that documented increased risk of nosocomial transmission of *M. tuberculosis* among hospitalized, HIV-infected patients [62].

Nosocomial *M. tuberculosis* Outbreaks

As with healthcare worker tuberculosis infection or disease, there is no national surveillance or reporting system specifically for nosocomial *M. tuberculosis* outbreaks. Thus, our knowledge of such outbreaks is based on published reports. From 1960 through 1996, over 20 nosocomial outbreaks in the United States were reported [2,33,38,51,52,61,63–77]. All the reported outbreaks involved adults and airborne transmission. These outbreaks primarily occurred at acute care, general medical–surgical facilities, but outbreaks at a hospice and a health department clinic also have been reported [65,66]. In the healthcare facility, outbreaks have involved the emergency department, inpatient medical wards, inpatient HIV wards, inpatient renal transplant ward, inpatient prison ward, intensive care units, surgical or radiology suites, the outpatient HIV clinic, and an autopsy suite. Most of the reports in the 1960s to 1980s involved patient-to-healthcare worker *M. tuberculosis* transmission, and patient-to-patient transmission was infrequently detected or reported. In contrast, most of the reports in the 1980s and 1990s involved immunocompromised patients and have included both patient-to-patient and patient-to-healthcare worker *M. tuberculosis* transmission.

Nosocomial Multidrug-Resistant *M. tuberculosis* Outbreaks

In the late 1980s and early 1990s, numerous nosocomial tuberculosis outbreaks occurred in the United States, caused by strains of *M. tuberculosis* resistant to two or more antituberculous agents, most commonly isoniazid and rifampin. In 1990, Edlin et al. investigated an outbreak of MDR-TB among acquired immunodeficiency syndrome (AIDS) patients at a New York City hospital [69]. From 1989 through 1990, 18 AIDS patients had acquired infections with *M. tuberculosis* strains resistant to isoniazid and streptomycin; in contrast, only 3 patients had had such infections in the preceding 3 years. Compared with 30 AIDS patients with tuberculosis caused by drug-susceptible strains of *M. tuberculosis*, the 18 MDR-TB AIDS patients were significantly more likely to be homosexual men, to have had AIDS for a longer period, or to have been hospitalized at the outbreak hospital within the 6 months preceding diagnosis of their tuberculosis. Furthermore, the MDR-TB patients were significantly more likely than AIDS patients infected with drug-susceptible strains of *M. tuberculosis* to have been hospitalized during their exposure period on the same ward at the same time as another patient with infectious MDR-TB. Compared with a group of AIDS patients infected with drug-susceptible strains of *M. tuberculosis* and similar durations of hospitalization, the MDR-TB AIDS patients were more likely to have occupied rooms closer to the room of an infectious MDR-TB patient. Restriction fragment length polymorphism (RFLP) analysis of the strains of 16 MDR-TB AIDS patients showed that 13 had an identical pattern. Thus, this investigation provided both epidemiologic and laboratory data supporting nosocomial acquisition of *M. tuberculosis* by these MDR-TB AIDS patients. The attack rate was 21/346 (6.1%) among all AIDS patients and 18/189 (9.5%) among AIDS patients hospitalized no more than two rooms away from an infectious MDR-TB AIDS patient's room. The estimated period from exposure to the development of active disease (i.e., incubation period) was estimated at 1.5 to 6 months. An environmental evaluation showed that only 1 of 16 patients' rooms had negative pressure. A TST survey conducted at the time of the investigation identified TST conversions (from documented negative to positive) in 11/60 (18.3%) healthcare workers; those with a follow-up TST more than 2 years before their baseline negative TST had a TST conversion rate of 9/31 (29%), whereas those with a follow-up TST of 2 years or less after their negative baseline had a TST conversion rate of 2/29 (6.9%) [79]. The *M. tuberculosis* strain from the one healthcare worker with active MDR-TB had an identical RFLP pattern to that of the MDR-TB AIDS patient's strain.

At about the same time as the aforementioned outbreak, another MDR-TB outbreak, caused by a strain of *M. tuberculosis* resistant to isoniazid and rifampin, was occurring at a hospital in Florida [70,71,77]. From 1988 through 1990, 25 MDR-TB patients were identified among HIV-infected patients admitted to the hospital's HIV ward. Compared with HIV ward patients with tuberculosis caused by drug-susceptible strains, the MDR-TB

TABLE 33-2. *Characteristics of Centers for Disease Control and Prevention-investigated nosocomial multidrug-resistant* Mycobacterium tuberculosis *outbreaks, 1988–1992*

Hospital	Outbreak period	Number of case-patients	Number HIV-positive case-patients (%)	Outbreak ward	Mortality number (%)	Infecting strain: Resistance pattern[a]	Infecting strain: RFLP type	Number healthcare worker TST conversions (%)	Number isolation rooms negative pressure (%)	References
1	1988–1989	25	25 (100)	HIV	21 (84)	INH, RIF	Two strains	13/39 (33)	17/23 (74)	[70,71]
2	1988–1990	18	18 (100)	Medicine	10 (56)	INH, SM	One strain	11/60 (18)	1/16 (6)	[69,78]
3	1989–1991	17	16 (94)	Medicine	14 (82)	INH, RIF, SM	One strain	88/352 (25)[a]	None	[48]
4	1990–1991	23	21 (91)	HIV	19 (83)	INH, RIF	One strain	6/12 (50)	None	[72]
5	1991–1991	8	1 (12.5)	Medicine	1 (12.5)	INH, RIF, EMB, ETA, KM, SM, RTB	One strain	46/696 (6.6)	None	[38]
6	1990–1991	16	14 (88)	Medicine	14 (88)	INH, RIF, SM	One strain	Unknown	None	[74]
7	1990–1992	13	13 (100)	Infectious disease	11 (85)	INH, RIF	One strain	5/10 (50)	None	[73]
8	1991–1992	37	35 (96)	HIV	34 (93)	INH, RIF	One strain	Unknown	None	[77]
9	1990–1992	42	41 (98)	Prison	32 (79)	INH, RIF	One strain	N/A	None	[79]

HIV, human immunodeficiency virus; RFLP, restriction fragment length polymorphism; TST, tuberculin skin test; INH, isoniazid; RIF, rifampin; EMB, ethambutol; ETA, ethionamide; KM, kanamycin; SM, streptomycin; RBT, rifabutin; N/A, not applicable.

[a] Eleven healthcare workers with active tuberculosis.

patients were more likely to have had an opportunistic infection before being diagnosed with tuberculosis, to have been exposed to an AFB sputum smear-positive MDR-TB patient during their hospitalization preceding the diagnosis of tuberculosis, to have failed to respond to antituberculous therapy, or to have died. MDR-TB patients remained AFB sputum smear positive for a significantly greater proportion of their hospitalization than did HIV-infected patients with tuberculosis caused by drug-susceptible strains 375/860 (44%) vs. 197/1445 (14%) person-days). Exposure to AFB sputum smear-positive, culture-positive patients was significantly more likely to result in transmission of *M. tuberculosis* than was exposure to AFB sputum smear-negative, culture-positive patients. Exposures to infectious MDR-TB patients occurred both on the HIV ward and the HIV outpatient clinic. Patients who attended the HIV clinic to receive aerosolized pentamidine were at greater risk for development of MDR-TB than were those attending the clinic but not receiving aerosolized pentamidine. All of the available 13 MDR-TB patient *M. tuberculosis* isolates had one of two RFLP patterns. Healthcare workers on the HIV ward and clinic were significantly more likely than healthcare workers on a comparison ward to have a TST conversion during the study period (13/39 vs. 0/15). There was a strong correlation between risk for healthcare worker *M. tuberculosis* infection and the number of days that an AFB sputum smear-positive MDR-TB patient was hospitalized on the HIV ward. Six of the 23 AFB isolation rooms were found to have positive pressure. In the HIV clinic, the aerosolized pentamidine administration rooms had positive pressure compared with the treatment room, which was positive pressure relative to the discharge waiting room; also, air from the patient treatment rooms was recirculated back into the clinic.

From 1990 through 1992, the Centers for Disease Control and Prevention (CDC) conducted nine nosocomial MDR-TB outbreak investigations [7,38,48,69–75,77–79] (Table 33-2). These outbreaks all occurred between 1988 and 1992 and involved 8 to 42 (median, 18) patients at each facility. Seven of nine outbreaks occurred in New York State, with six of these in New York City hospitals. In all the outbreaks, the *M. tuberculosis* strain transmitted was resistant to isoniazid; in eight outbreaks the strain also was resistant to rifampin. Depending on the outbreak, the strains were also resistant to streptomycin, ethambutol, ethionamide, kanamycin, or rifabutin. In two outbreaks, some of the infecting strains were resistant to seven antituberculous agents [38,48]. The proportion of patients in these outbreaks who had HIV infections ranged from 12.5% to 100%; most of these outbreaks occurred either on HIV wards or on wards where most of the patients admitted had HIV infection. Mortality ranged from 12.5% to 93% (median, 83%). The interval from diagnosis of tuberculosis until death ranged from 4 to 16 (median, 4) weeks.

Risk Factors for Nosocomial Transmission of Drug-Susceptible or Multidrug-Resistant *M. tuberculosis*

A wide variety of factors were responsible for patient-to-patient or patient-to-healthcare worker *M. tuberculosis* transmission in these outbreaks (Table 33-3). These included factors affecting the likelihood of exposure, the likelihood of infection given exposure, and the likelihood

TABLE 33-3. *Risk factors for nosocomial transmission of drug-susceptible and multidrug-resistant* M. tuberculosis

- Patient risk factors
  - Human immunodeficiency virus infection
  - Acquired immunodeficiency syndrome
  - Low CD4 T-lymphocyte count
  - Prior hospital admission
    - Admission to a room near (< 3 rooms) an infectious MDR-TB patient
    - Exposure to an AFB sputum smear-positive MDR-TB patient
- Clinical risk factors
  - Delayed diagnosis
    - Nonclassic signs/symptoms
    - Nonclassic chest radiograph
    - Low index of suspicion of tuberculosis by physicians
    - Delays in laboratory results (identification and susceptibility)
  - Delayed patient isolation
    - Low index of suspicion of tuberculosis
    - Delayed recognition of MDR-TB
    - Inadequate number of isolation rooms
  - Delayed institution of effective therapy
    - Delayed recognition of MDR-TB
    - Delayed laboratory susceptibility data
- Infection control factors
  - Inadequate isolation
    - Isolation rooms
      - Positive pressure
      - < 6 Air changes per hr
      - Air recirculated
      - Doors open
    - Infectious patients leave rooms
      - For nonmedical reasons (social, smoking, TV)
      - Premature discontinuation of isolation
  - Inadequate precautions during aerosol generating procedures
  - Inadequate microbiologic methods
    - AFB smears not done
    - Slow turnaround of identification and susceptibility testing
    - Rapid methods not performed for:
      - Culture
      - Identification
      - Antimicrobial susceptibility testing
    - Delayed communication of results from referral laboratories
    - Delayed communication of results to clinicians
    - Failure to monitor *M. tuberculosis* antimicrobial susceptibility results
    - Failure to maintain or analyze results/records of *M. tuberculosis* identification or susceptibility testing

MDR-TB, multidrug-resistant tuberculosis; AFB, acid-fast bacilli.

of active disease given infection. Patient risk factors included having HIV or AIDS, prior hospitalization at the outbreak hospital, the close proximity of AFB sputum smear-positive (i.e., infectious) tuberculosis patients and patients with HIV infection or AIDS, or exposure to an infectious tuberculosis patient either because of close proximity of the rooms or exposures outside of the patient's room. Other risk factors included delayed recognition of tuberculosis in the patient because of nonclassic signs, symptoms, or chest radiograph; low index of suspicion by physicians; delayed recognition of infecting MDR-TB strains because of delayed laboratory identification or communication to the clinicians; and delayed institution of effective antituberculosis therapy. In addition, a number of inadequate infection control practices were identified, including delayed initiation of appropriate AFB isolation; isolation rooms without at least six air changes per hour, negative pressure, or air exhausted to the outside; failure to isolate tuberculosis patients until they were no longer infectious, lapses in AFB isolation such as allowing infectious patients in isolation to leave their rooms without wearing a mask or for nonmedical reasons (e.g., to attend group social events, to walk the halls, go to common bathrooms, or visit the lounge or television areas); leaving AFB isolation room doors open; inadequate duration of AFB isolation; and inadequate precautions during aerosol-generating procedures such as sputum induction or aerosolization of pentamidine. Last, delay in institution of effective therapy contributed to prolonged infectiousness and increased the risk of transmission of MDR-TB strains.

In these MDR-TB outbreaks, the failure rapidly to identify and appropriately isolate infectious patients, combined with the prolonged infectiousness of these patients secondary to delays in diagnosis and treatment, led to exposure of other patients and healthcare workers. In each outbreak, the major risk factor for MDR-TB or for a TST conversion was exposure to an infectious MDR-TB patient. Delayed identification of infectious MDR-TB patients may have been contributed to by a low index of suspicion for tuberculosis in HIV-infected patients with pulmonary symptoms and the fact that many of the MDR-TB patients did not present with classic signs, symptoms, or chest radiographs (i.e., cavitary or miliary patterns) for tuberculosis [9,75]. In some instances, neither TSTs nor AFB sputum smears were performed on potentially infectious patients. Most MDR-TB patients had abnormal chest radiographs; however, they usually had interstitial patterns rather than classic miliary or cavitary patterns. When cultures were obtained, the results of cultures or antituberculosis susceptibility testing were not available for a median of 7 weeks because the most rapid methods were not used; in some instances, the results were not available for 6 months. These delays in diagnosis resulted in delays in recognition of MDR-TB, in instituting effective antituberculosis therapy, and in appropriate patient isolation; in turn, these lapses resulted in prolonged periods of exposure of infectious tuberculosis patients to other patients and healthcare workers. Although in most of the outbreaks infectious tuberculosis patients were the source, outbreaks have been associated with a healthcare worker with infectious tuberculosis and with irrigation or manipulation of an undiagnosed tuberculous skin abscess or ulcer [67,68,76].

Molecular Typing of Multidrug-Resistant *M. tuberculosis* Outbreak Isolates

A critical element in confirming the epidemiologic evidence of nosocomial *M. tuberculosis* transmission in each of the MDR-TB outbreak investigations was the molecular typing of the infecting strains (see Chapter 9). In the early 1990s, a new method to type *M. tuberculosis* isolates, RFLP, was developed [80]. Thus, in each MDR-TB outbreak, available isolates from patients and healthcare workers with active tuberculosis disease were obtained and RFLP typed. Although occasionally a similar strain was identified at more than one facility, particularly in New York City, where patients may have either had contact in or outside of the hospital, in most instances, one or more unique strains was documented to have been transmitted within each facility (see Table 33-2). In one instance, use of a newly developed polymerase chain reaction-based RFLP method was necessary because the source-case isolate was no longer viable [76,81]. The combination of epidemiologic and molecular typing data conclusively proved that MDR-TB strains were being transmitted within these facilities. Future application of RFLP and other molecular typing techniques should facilitate further elucidation of nosocomial and community transmission of *M. tuberculosis*.

Risk for Tuberculosis Infection in Healthcare Workers

In each outbreak, occupational acquisition of tuberculosis was suspected. However, conclusive documentation was difficult because in most instances the healthcare workers had infection but not disease. Furthermore, at a number of the outbreak hospitals, the healthcare worker TST program was inadequate; often, the healthcare workers had not had either a baseline two-step TST or a routine TST within the past 1 to 2 years [69,78]. At one MDR-TB outbreak hospital, 18% of healthcare workers in whom a TST was applied during the investigation had a positive TST; MDR-TB developed in one healthcare worker, and the infecting isolate had the same RFLP pattern as that recovered from MDR-TB outbreak patients [69,78]. In one investigation, the outbreak ward healthcare workers with or without TST conversions were similar in age, race, sex, duration of employment on the outbreak ward, occupation, and shift worked [70]. However, compared with healthcare workers on control wards where tuberculosis patients were not admitted, outbreak ward and clinic healthcare workers were at significantly greater risk for TST conversion. Risk for TST conversion was associated with exposure to MDR-TB patients who were AFB sputum smear positive rather than to drug-susceptible tuberculosis patients; healthcare worker infection risk was significantly lower (although not zero) when they had exposure to AFB sputum smear-negative, culture-positive patients. In three MDR-TB outbreak hospitals, adequate TST data were available to assess healthcare worker TST conversion risk; at these institutions, 22% to 50% of healthcare workers had TST conversions during the outbreak periods [69,70,72–75]. At the time of these investigations, at least 16 healthcare workers had contracted active MDR-TB; 7 were HIV positive, 7 were HIV negative, and 2 were of unknown HIV status [75]. Five of the 16 (31.2%) healthcare workers died; 4 of these 5 were known to be HIV infected. In many if not most instances, healthcare workers were not wearing the 1990 CDC tuberculosis guidelines-recommended respiratory protection (i.e., particulate [dust-mist, dust-fume-mist, or high-efficiency particulate air filter [HEPA] respirators); often, the healthcare workers either wore no or improperly wore respiratory protection [46].

TUBERCULOSIS INFECTION CONTROL PROGRAMS IN THE UNITED STATES

The aforementioned nosocomial MDR-TB outbreaks raised considerable concern about the status of tuberculosis infection control programs at U.S. hospitals. Several surveys have been conducted to assess these programs. In 1992, the American Hospital Association (AHA) in collaboration with the CDC conducted a survey of all U.S. municipal, Veterans Administration, and university hospitals, and a 20% random sample of private hospitals [57]. Responses were received from 763 (71%) of the 1076 surveyed hospitals; of the 763 respondents, 178 (25%) hospitals in 39 states admitted MDR-TB patients. Among the 763 hospitals, the number of AFB isolation rooms meeting 1990 CDC tuberculosis guidelines recommendations ranged from 0 to 60 (median, 7); 219 (29%) hospitals had no AFB isolation rooms meeting the CDC criteria. Healthcare worker TST programs varied widely. Fifteen (2%) reported nosocomial transmission of *M. tuberculosis* to patients and 91 (13%) reported tuberculosis transmission to healthcare workers.

In 1993, the Society of Healthcare Epidemiology of America (SHEA) in collaboration with the CDC, conducted a survey of the SHEA membership, most of whom are at medical school-affiliated teaching hospitals [14,15]. From 1989 through 1992, the number of SHEA member hospitals admitting MDR-TB patients increased from 10/166 (10%) to 49/166 (30%). During this period, the median healthcare worker TST positivity rate at the time of hire increased from 0.54% to 0.81%; in contrast, the median healthcare worker TST conversion rate remained stable at ~ 0.34% during the period (range, 0.35% to 0.33%). AFB isolation rooms meeting CDC 1990 tuberculosis guidelines recommendations were reported at 113/181 (62%) hospitals responding to the question. During the study period, the proportion of 191 respondent hospitals in which surgical submicron masks or dust-mist or dust-fume-mist respirators were used increased from 9 (5%) to 85 (43%).

In another survey, conducted in 1993 by the Association for Professionals in Infection Control and Epidemiology (APIC), in collaboration with the CDC and covering the same period, most of the 1494 respondents were smaller community hospitals and the proportion of hospitals admitting drug-susceptible tuberculosis or MDR-TB patients increased from 46.4% to 56.6% and 0.8% to 4.5%, respectively [16]. From 1989 through 1992, the healthcare worker pooled mean TST positivity rate at hire rose from 0.95% to 1.14% and the TST conversion rate increased from 0.4% to 0.5%. In 1992, rooms compliant with the CDC 1990 tuberculosis guidelines recommendations for AFB isolation were reported at 66% of the hospitals, and at 64% of the hospitals healthcare workers still used surgical masks for respiratory protection; from 1989 through 1992, the number of hospitals in which particulate respirators were used increased from 0.4% to 13.8%.

Nosocomial transmission of *M. tuberculosis* is a particular concern in emergency departments where a wide variety of patients, many of whom have fever and cough, seek care. Moran et al. found that among patients with active pulmonary tuberculosis at an urban emergency department, tuberculosis was often not suspected and isolation of these infectious patients was delayed [82]. In 1993, Moran et al. conducted a survey of infection control practices in emergency departments at a sample of the hospitals responding to the AHA/CDC survey [83]. Of the 446 emergency departments surveyed, 298 returned completed questionnaires. The proportion of emergency departments in which tuberculosis patients were seen daily, weekly, monthly, or less frequently was 12.6%, 17.2%, 23.3%, and 46.9%, respectively. The proportion in which tuberculosis isolation rooms meeting CDC 1990 tuberculosis guidelines recommendations were available in triage or waiting rooms or in the emergency department itself was 1.7% and 19.6%, respectively. One or more healthcare workers had TST conversions in 16.1% of the surveyed emergency departments in 1991 and 26.9% in 1992. Prevention and control of *M. tuberculosis* in emergency departments depends on 1) education of the staff about the high-risk groups for and signs and symptoms of tuberculosis so that they will suspect and promptly identify infectious patients; 2) ensur-

TABLE 33-4. *Evaluation of preventive interventions on patient-to-patient MDR-TB transmission at three MDR-TB outbreak hospitals*

			Number of case-patients			Proportion of patients with MDR-TB[a]		Mortality		Nosocomial MDR-TB exposure	
Hospital	Initial period	Intervention period	Outbreak period	Intervention period	Total	Outbreak period	Intervention period[a]	Outbreak period	Intervention period	Outbreak period	Intervention period
1	Jan. 90–May 90	Jun. 90–Jun. 92	15	11	26	26/180	28/498[b] (TB)	—	—	12	0
2	Jan. 89–Mar. 90	Apr. 90–Sep. 92	16	22	38	19/216	9/277 (A)	6	8	11	5[c]
4	Jan. 90–Jun. 91	Jul. 91–Aug. 92	30	10	40	30/95	10/70[c] (O)	25	4	20	1[d]

MDR-TB, multidrug-resistant tuberculosis
[a]All tuberculosis patients (TB), all outbreak ward patients (O), or all AIDS patients (A)
[b]$p<0.01$
[c]Four patients were exposed on HIV ward in initial period, $p=002$
[d]$p=0.003$

ing that emergency departments have adequate isolation facilities for infectious tuberculosis patients; 3) rapid isolation of screened patients who may have infectious tuberculosis; and 4) a comprehensive healthcare worker TST program.

The microbiology laboratory plays a critical role in the rapid identification of infectious tuberculosis patients (see Chapter 9). However, the microbiologic methods used in many laboratories are not the most rapid, and communication between the laboratories and the clinicians often is inadequate [11,14–16,57,84]. In one survey of hospital-based laboratories in the United States, rapid methods were used for AFB microscopy in 47%, primary culture in 72%, *M. tuberculosis* identification in 38%, and drug susceptibility testing in 13% of the laboratories surveyed [57]. Approximately 46% of hospitals surveyed, and an estimated 30% of laboratories at all U.S. hospitals with 100 beds or more, performed the minimal number of mycobacterial cultures deemed necessary to maintain competence [10,11]. Fortunately, since 1992, there has been a significant improvement in compliance with recommended methods for AFB smear, culture, and antimicrobial susceptibility testing [11].

These outbreak and survey data show that the emergence of MDR-TB as a major public health problem was associated with the incomplete implementation of the CDC tuberculosis guidelines recommendations [46,47]. Many hospitals do not have the recommended patient isolation facilities, healthcare worker TST or respiratory protection programs, or laboratory processing practices. Although the APIC/CDC survey shows that as many as 50% of community hospitals do not admit tuberculosis patients routinely and few admit MDR-TB patients, the SHEA/CDC and AHA/CDC surveys show that urban, larger hospitals and those with a medical school affiliation routinely admit tuberculosis or MDR-TB patients [14–16,57]. Data from the SHEA/CDC and APIC/CDC surveys show that there continues to be improvement in the degree of implementation of CDC tuberculosis guidelines recommendations since the initial AHA/CDC survey.

Efficacy of the CDC Tuberculosis Guidelines Recommendations

The nosocomial tuberculosis and especially the MDR-TB outbreaks raised concern in the infectious disease, infection control, occupational medicine, and industrial hygiene communities about the effectiveness of the CDC tuberculosis guidelines recommendations [46,47]. To assess the efficacy of these control measures, follow-up investigations were conducted at three of the hospitals where MDR-TB outbreaks had occurred and at one where a drug-susceptible *M. tuberculosis* outbreak occurred. In each MDR-TB hospital, a wide variety of infection control measures, similar to those in the CDC 1990 and 1994 tuberculosis guidelines, were implemented (Tables 33-4 and 33-5). Because same-ward exposure to an infectious MDR-TB patient was identified as the most significant risk factor in the initial MDR-TB outbreak investigations, this was assessed as a measure of nosocomial or occupational acquisition of tuberculosis in the follow-up studies. In the first follow-up investigation at an MDR-TB outbreak hospital in New York City, Maloney et al. documented that the proportion of patients with MDR-TB strains decreased, the proportion of MDR-TB patients with same-ward exposures decreased, and the TST conversion rates of healthcare workers assigned to the outbreak wards were lower in the follow-up or intervention period than in the outbreak period [85]. In the second follow-up investigation, Wenger et al. showed that, after implementation of control measures on the MDR-TB outbreak HIV ward, no episodes of MDR-TB could be traced

TABLE 33-5. *Evaluation of preventive interventions on patient to healthcare worker MDR-TB transmission at three MDR-TB outbreak hospitals*

			Susceptible HCWs		Number of HCWs with tuberculin skin test conversion		Number of HCWs with active TB		
Hospital	Initial period	Intervention period	Initial period	Intervention period	Initial period	Intervention period	Initial period	Intervention period	Total
1	Jan. 90–May 90	Jun. 90–Jun. 92	25	27	7	3[a,b]	1	0	1
2	Jan. 89–Mar. 90	Apr. 90–Sep. 92	60	29	11	5	4	0	4
4	Jan. 89–Jun. 91	Jul. 91–Aug. 92	90	78	15	4[c]	1	1	2

MDR-TB, multidrug-resistant tuberculosis; HCW, healthcare worker.
[a]All had been exposed to unknown infectious MDR-TB patient.
[b]$p<0.01$
[c]$p<0.02$

to contact with infectious MDR-TB patients and that healthcare worker TST conversions were terminated [86]. In the third follow-up study, Stroud et al. documented that, after implementation of recommended CDC tuberculosis infection control measures, the MDR-TB attack rate for AIDS patients decreased from 19/216 (8.8%) to 5/193 (2.6%) [87]. Blumberg et al. conducted a fourth follow-up investigation, at a hospital in which a drug-susceptible *M. tuberculosis* outbreak had occurred [76,88]. Their study documented that, after the hospital introduced mostly administrative controls—more rapid identification of infectious tuberculosis patients, isolation of infectious patients in rooms with increased air exhaust, and improved healthcare worker respiratory protection—a decrease occurred in the number of exposures to infectious tuberculosis patients (4.4 to 0.6 per month), cumulative number of days per month that infectious tuberculosis patients were not in isolation (35.4 to 3.3), and healthcare worker TST conversions (3.3% to 0.4%) [88].

Each of these studies shows that with more complete implementation of administrative and engineering/environmental controls and use of respiratory protective devices for healthcare workers, *M. tuberculosis* outbreaks can be terminated and further *M. tuberculosis* transmission from patient to patient or patient to healthcare worker can be either terminated or reduced to background tuberculosis rates seen on wards where tuberculosis patients are not admitted routinely [89]. These data document that the CDC tuberculosis guidelines work if they are fully implemented.

CDC Tuberculosis Guidelines

In 1990, the CDC published *Guidelines for Preventing the Transmission of Tuberculosis in Health Care Settings, with Special Focus on HIV-Related Issues* [46]. These guidelines provided the recommended elements of an infection control program to prevent the transmission of *M. tuberculosis* in healthcare facilities. Emphasis was placed on methods to prevent the generation of infectious airborne droplet nuclei, early identification of infectious tuberculosis patients, preventing the spread of *M. tuberculosis* through source controls, air disinfection to reduce microbial contamination of the air, disinfection and sterilization, and surveillance for tuberculosis infection or disease in healthcare workers. Recommendations for patient AFB isolation rooms included having six or more air changes per hour, negative pressure in relation to other rooms or corridors, and exhausting the air from the room directly to the outside. The guidelines also recommended the use of particulate respirators as respiratory protection for healthcare workers.

As a result of the nosocomial tuberculosis outbreaks and in response to requests for changes or clarifications in the CDC 1990 tuberculosis guidelines, the CDC revised these guidelines, and published the *Guidelines for Preventing the Transmission of* Mycobacterium tuberculosis *in Health-Care Facilities, 1994* [47] (Table 33-6). The 1994 CDC tuberculosis guidelines include a recommendations section followed by four extensive supplements. The recommendations include sections on assignment of responsibility, risk assessment, development of the tuberculosis infection control program, and periodic risk assessment; identifying, evaluating, and initiating treatment for patients who may have active tuberculosis; management of patients in ambulatory care settings or emergency departments who may have active tuberculosis; management of hospitalized patients who have confirmed or suspected tuberculosis; engineering control recommendations; healthcare worker respiratory protection; cough-inducing and aerosol-generating procedures; education and training of healthcare workers; healthcare worker counseling, screening, and evaluation; problem evaluation; coordination with the Public Health Department; and additional considerations for selected areas in healthcare facilities and other healthcare settings. The supplements include discussion of determining the infectiousness of a tuberculosis patient; diagnosis and treatment of both latent infection and active tuberculosis disease; engineering controls (i.e., ventilation and ultraviolet germicidal irradiation); respiratory protection; and decontamination (i.e., cleaning, disinfecting, and sterilizing of patient care equipment).

Hierarchy of Controls

The 1994 CDC tuberculosis guidelines emphasize the importance of understanding the hierarchy of tuberculosis control measures; these include administrative controls to identify infectious tuberculosis patients promptly and reduce healthcare worker and patient exposure to such patients, engineering controls to reduce the generation and spread of airborne droplet nuclei, and respiratory protective devices to protect healthcare workers from inhalation of infectious airborne droplet nuclei. Although each of these measures was discussed in the 1990 CDC tuberculosis guidelines, the 1994 CDC tuberculosis guidelines highlight the importance of these measures. The first and most critical tuberculosis control measure is the use of administrative controls to reduce the risk of patient or healthcare worker exposure to people with infectious tuberculosis. Compliance with this recommendation requires the development of effective written policies and protocols and implementation of these into practice to ensure that clinicians maintain a high index of suspicion for tuberculosis in patients with respiratory symptoms and conduct an appropriate diagnostic work-up of patients suspected of having tuberculosis; that rapid laboratory techniques (fluorescence stains for AFB smears, radiometric methods for species identification and susceptibil-

TABLE 33-6. *Basic elements of an effective tuberculosis (TB) infection control program*[a]

I. Assignment of responsibility
  A. Assign responsibility for the TB infection control program to qualified people.
  B. Ensure that people with expertise in infection control, occupational health, administration, and engineering are identified and included.

II. Risk assessment, TB infection control plan, and periodic reassessment
  A. Initial risk assessments
    1. Obtain information concerning TB in the community.
    2. Evaluate data concerning TB patients in the facility.
    3. Evaluate data concerning PPD tuberculin skin test conversions among HCWs in the facility.
    4. Rule out evidence of person-to-person transmission.
  B. Develop written TB infection-control program
    1. Select initial risk protocol(s).
    2. Develop written TB infection control protocols.
  C. Repeat risk assessment at appropriate intervals.
    1. Review current community and facility surveillance data and PPD tuberculin skin test results.
    2. Review records of TB patients.
    3. Observe HCW infection control practices.
    4. Evaluate maintenance of engineering controls.

III. Identification, evaluation, and treatment of TB patients
  A. Screen patients for signs and symptoms of active TB
    1. On initial encounter in emergency department or ambulatory care setting.
    2. Before or at the time of admission.
  B. Perform radiologic and bacteriologic evaluation of patients who have signs and symptoms suggestive of TB.
  C. Promptly initiate treatment.
  D. Periodically reevaluate response to therapy; modify regimen if no improvement.

IV. Managing outpatients who have possible infectious TB
  A. Promptly initiate TB precautions.
  B. Place patients in separate waiting areas or TB isolation rooms.
  C. Give patients a surgical mask or box of tissues, and instructions regarding the use of these items.
  D. Instruct patients to cover their mouth and nose with tissue when coughing or sneezing.

V. Managing inpatients who have possible infectious TB
  A. Promptly isolate patients who have suspected or known infectious TB.
  B. Monitor the response to treatment.
  C. Follow appropriate criteria for discontinuing isolation.

VI. Engineering recommendations
  A. Design local exhaust and general ventilation in collaboration with people who have expertise in ventilation engineering.
  B. Use a single-pass air system or air recirculation after HEPA filtration in areas where infectious TB patients receive care.
  C. Use additional measures, if needed, in areas where TB patients may receive care.
  D. Design TB isolation rooms in health care facilities to achieve at least 6 air changes per hr for existing facilities and at least 12 air changes per hr for new or renovated facilities.
  E. Regularly monitor and maintain engineering controls.
  F. TB isolation rooms that are being used should be monitored daily to ensure they maintain negative pressure relative to the hallway and all surrounding area.
  G. Exhaust TB isolation room air to outside or, if absolutely unavoidable, recirculate after HEPA filtration.

VII. Respiratory protection
  A. Respiratory protective devices should meet recommended performance criteria.
  B. Respiratory protection should be used by people entering rooms in which patients with known or suspected infectious TB are being isolated, by HCWs when performing cough-inducing or aerosol-generating procedures on such patients, and by people in other settings where administrative and engineering controls are not likely to protect them from inhaling infectious airborne droplet nuclei.
  C. A respiratory protection program is required in all facilities in which respiratory protection is used to protect health care workers.

VIII. Cough-inducing procedures
  A. Do not perform such procedures on TB patients unless absolutely necessary.
  B. Perform such procedures in areas that have local exhaust ventilation devices (e.g., booths or special enclosures) or, if this is not feasible, in a room that meets the ventilation requirements for TB isolation.
  C. After completion of procedures, TB patients should remain in the booth or special enclosure until their coughing subsides.

IX. HCW TB training and education
  A. All HCWs should receive periodic TB education appropriate for their work responsibilities and duties.
  B. Training should include the epidemiology of TB in the facility.
  C. TB education should emphasize concepts of the pathogenesis of and occupational risk for TB.
  D. Training should describe work practices that reduce the likelihood of transmitting *M. tuberculosis.*

X. HCW counseling and screening
  A. Counsel all HCWs regarding TB and TB infection.
  B. Counsel all HCWs about the increased risk to immunocompromised people for development of active TB.
  C. Perform PPD skin tests on HCWs at the beginning of their employment, and repeat PPD tests at periodic intervals.
  D. Evaluate symptomatic HCWs for active TB.

XI. Evaluate HCW PPD test conversions and possible nosocomial transmission of *M. tuberculosis.*

XII. Coordinate efforts with public health department.

PPD, purified protein derivative; HCW, healthcare worker; HEPA, high-efficiency particulate air.

[a]A program such as this is appropriate for healthcare facilities in which there is a high risk for transmission of *M. tuberculosis.*

(Adapted from Centers for Disease Control and Prevention. Guidelines for preventing the transmission of *Mycobacterium tuberculosis* in health-care facilities, 1994. *MMWR Morb Mortal Wkly Rep* 1994;43(RR1–13))

ity testing, or genetic probes for species identification) are used; that laboratory results are rapidly communicated to clinicians; and that infectious tuberculosis patients are promptly isolated to minimize exposure to other patients or unprotected healthcare workers [46,47].

Administrative source controls are essential for preventing *M. tuberculosis* transmission. A critical element of any tuberculosis control program is education of healthcare workers about the epidemiology of tuberculosis, the importance of suspecting tuberculosis particularly in patients with HIV infection, the importance of healthcare worker TST and respiratory protection programs, the need for clinicians to know the susceptibility of prevalent *M. tuberculosis* strains in the hospital and community, the importance of rapidly and appropriately isolating tuberculosis patients, and the importance of initiating an effective treatment regimen in infectious tuberculosis patients.

The next level of the hierarchy is the use of engineering/environmental controls to prevent the generation and spread of airborne droplet nuclei and to reduce the concentration of these infectious particles. These include 1) direct source control using local exhaust ventilation, 2) controlling the direction of air flow to prevent contamination of air in adjacent areas, 3) dilution and removal of contaminated air by general ventilation, and 4) air disinfection by air filtration or ultraviolet germicidal irradiation.

The third and last level of the hierarchy is the use of personal respiratory protective devices by healthcare workers in areas where the risk of exposure to infectious droplet nuclei and resultant occupational acquisition of *M. tuberculosis* is suspected to be higher than normal (e.g., AFB isolation rooms and where cough-inducing or aerosol-producing procedures are performed).

The outbreak investigations, the follow-up studies at outbreak hospitals, and the surveys have not documented the independent importance of these different measures. Furthermore, because the control measures recommended in the CDC tuberculosis guidelines are intended to be implemented as a group, neglecting any one measure could lead to the failure of the others to eliminate or reduce nosocomial transmission of *M. tuberculosis*. Most of the nosocomial or occupational acquisition of tuberculosis results from exposure to an unsuspected or undetected infectious tuberculosis patient.

Risk Assessment

Another important addition in the 1994 CDC tuberculosis guidelines is the introduction of the concept of conducting a risk assessment. The purpose of the risk assessment is to identify healthcare facilities or areas within those facilities in which the risk of exposure to infectious tuberculosis patients and subsequent patient-to-patient or patient-to-healthcare worker *M. tuberculosis* transmission is minimal, very low, low, intermediate, or high. In this way, the tuberculosis control program can be individualized for a specific area or hospital so that high- or low-risk facilities would not need to comply with the same recommendations; greater flexibility could be given both between and within institutions. This risk assessment is used to determine the frequency of healthcare worker TST, repeat risk assessment and ventilation evaluation and to suggest supplemental engineering/environmental interventions.

Tuberculosis Control Program

The basic elements of the tuberculosis control program are applicable to all types of healthcare facilities (see Table 33-6). These elements emphasize the following:

1. Use of rapid laboratory methods to facilitate rapid diagnosis of tuberculosis patients
2. The recommendation that smear results be available within 24 hours of specimen collection
3. The importance of considering tuberculosis in HIV-infected patients even if another pathogen is identified
4. The importance of rapid evaluation and triage of infectious patients in outpatient settings
5. The importance of directly observed therapy
6. That patient tuberculosis isolation rooms (i.e., private room, negative pressure, six or more air changes per hour, air exhausted directly outside) can have recirculation of air to the same patient's room or general ventilation if the air is passed through a HEPA filter in the ventilation system
7. That all infectious tuberculosis patients (drug-susceptible or MDR-TB strains) remain in isolation until clinically improved *and* they have negative AFB sputum smears on 3 consecutive days (because the decision to remove from isolation is usually made before susceptibility results are available)
8. That consideration should be given to keeping MDR-TB patients in AFB isolation for their entire hospitalization
9. That discharge should be coordinated with the community's public health department and private clinicians so that compliance with therapy is ensured, and to avoid exposure of individuals to an infectious tuberculosis patient outside of the healthcare setting.

Respiratory Protection

The 1990 CDC tuberculosis guidelines recommended particulate respirators, which include dust-mist, dust-fume-mist, or HEPA filter respirators, for use as respiratory protection against tuberculosis. However, the 1994 CDC tuberculosis guidelines established new criteria for respiratory protection: 1) the ability to filter particles 1 μm in size (in the unloaded state) with a filter efficiency of 95% or better (i.e., filter leakage < 5%), given flow rates of up to 50 liters/minute; 2) the ability to be qualitatively or quantitatively fit tested in a reliable way; 3) the ability to be adequately fit checked before each use in a reliable way; and 4) the ability to fit healthcare workers with different facial sizes and characteristics, which can usually be met by the availability of at least three sizes of respirator. The criteria were based on the characteristics thought to be most desirable in a respirator and on the in-use experience at drug-susceptible or MDR-TB outbreak hospitals where patient-to-healthcare worker *M. tuberculosis* transmission was terminated by using submicron masks or dust-mist respirators together with implementation of the 1990 CDC tuberculosis guidelines recommendations [85–89].

When the 1990 CDC tuberculosis guidelines first recommended particulate respirators to protect healthcare workers from occupational acquisition of *M. tuberculosis*, it became clear that the use of respirators was for protection of healthcare workers from patient infections, and not vice versa. This area then came under the jurisdiction of the U.S. Occupational Safety and Health Administration (OSHA) [90,91]. Thereafter, no matter which respirator was recommended, the law required a healthcare worker respirator training, education, and fit testing program. OSHA requires that when healthcare workers wear a respiratory protective device to protect them from disease, they must use a National Institute for Occupational Safety and Health (NIOSH)-certified respirator. Therefore, in 1992, OSHA asked NIOSH to assess and recommend which respirator would be required to protect healthcare workers from occupational *M. tuberculosis* acquisition. Because of a lack of data about the concentration of *M. tuberculosis* in airborne droplet nuclei, what the minimal infectious dose is, the exact size and size distribution of airborne droplet nuclei particles, the potential of mortality given infection, the risk of toxic reaction from antituberculous prophylactic or therapeutic agents, and the NIOSH/OSHA interest in providing a zero-risk environment, NIOSH recommended a powered air-purifying respirator (PAPR) with a HEPA filter for moderate exposures and a positive-pressure, air-line respirator with a tight-fitting half-mask respirator for high-risk exposures [92]. By law, NIOSH may not consider either cost or practicality in making its recommendation. During 1992 and 1993, various OSHA regions made respirator recommendations ranging from dust-mist respirators to PAPRs.

To understand the complexity involved in arriving at an appropriate respirator recommendation for healthcare workers to prevent occupational acquisition of *M. tuberculosis*, it is important to understand the relationship between OSHA and NIOSH [90]. OSHA requires that any respiratory protective device used to protect healthcare workers must be NIOSH certified [92]. Before 1995, the existing NIOSH respirator certification process did not adequately test the efficacy of dust-mist or dust-fume-mist respirators against low-concentration aerosols in the size range of *M. tuberculosis* droplet nuclei (best estimated at 1 to 5 μm). Subsequently, studies documented that there was wide variability in penetration of dust-mist or dust-fume-mist respirators when challenged by either 1-μm particles or *M. chelonae* aerosols [93]. Although some manufacturers' dust-mist or dust-fume-mist respirators prevented 95% or more of these particles from penetrating, other manufacturers' respirators allowed up to 40% penetration. Thus, in contrast to HEPA filter respirators, all of which are certified to prevent penetration of less than 0.03% of 0.3-μm particles, the efficacy of dust-mist and dust-fume-mist respirators varied widely and could not be ensured. For this reason, the 1994 CDC tuberculosis guidelines indicated that although some dust-mist or dust-fume-mist respirators would meet the new guidelines criteria, only HEPA-filtered respirators always meet these criteria and were certified by NIOSH to do so [47,90,94].

In 1996, NIOSH implemented a new respirator certification process that tests respirators with a 0.3-μm test particle and designates them into different classes of respirator based on 99.95%, 99%, or 95% filtration efficacy [95]. All three classes of respirators surpass the minimum filter criteria recommended in the 1994 CDC tuberculosis guidelines (i.e., the ability to filter 95% of 1-μm particles). These 95% filtration efficiency respirators, designated N-, P-, or R-95s, are available for use to protect healthcare workers from occupational exposure to *M. tuberculosis*. Because of the 1994 tuberculosis guidelines recommendations and this new NIOSH respirator certification process, a greater variety of respirators and respirator sizes have become available at lower cost to protect healthcare workers from *M. tuberculosis*. Follow-up data at several of the MDR-TB outbreak hospitals show that use of submicron surgical masks or dust-mist respirators by healthcare workers together with implementation of recommendations similar to those in the 1990 CDC tuberculosis guidelines terminated patient-to-healthcare worker *M. tuberculosis* transmission on outbreak wards [85–89]. Furthermore, survey data have shown that at healthcare facilities with > 6 tuberculosis patients or with > 200 beds, respirators with submicron filter capability reduce the risk of healthcare worker TST conversion [14,15]. In addition, studies show that some dust-mist or dust-fume-mist respirators filter more than 95% of particles with a mean size of 0.8 μm, smaller than the estimated particle size of *M. tuberculosis* droplet nuclei [93]. The new NIOSH respirator certification process permits the use of respirators similar to those shown to be effective in outbreak settings and reduces the controversy surrounding the use of respirators in healthcare facilities to protect workers from *M. tuberculosis*.

Respirator education and fit-test programs are integral parts of any healthcare worker respiratory protection program. These are mandated by OSHA for any healthcare worker potentially exposed to *M. tuberculosis*. Factors to consider when selecting a respirator include face-seal leakage and the ability to fit test and fit check the respirator. healthcare workers with facial hair (e.g., beards) will not be able to get an adequate face seal with the new N-95 or older particulate respirators. For these healthcare workers, particularly those performing very–high-risk procedures on infectious tuberculosis patients, PARPs may be an alternative.

Healthcare Worker Education/Problem Evaluation

Another new section in the 1994 CDC tuberculosis guidelines is on education and training of healthcare workers. All healthcare workers with possible *M. tuberculosis* exposure should be taught the epidemiology of tuberculosis; the potential for occupational exposure; the principles of tuberculosis infection control; the importance of routine and periodic healthcare worker TST; the principles of preventive therapy; the importance of seeking evaluation if the healthcare worker has symptoms of tuberculosis; and the higher risk of disease given infection in those who are immunocompromised, particularly those infected with HIV. In addition, counseling of healthcare workers and options for voluntary work reassignment should be provided. The guidelines also emphasize the importance of the two-step Mantoux TST for all healthcare workers at the time of hire and that periodic TST should be performed based on the healthcare worker's risk assessment. Furthermore, a section on evaluating problems provides guidance on investigation of TST conversions or active disease in healthcare workers or possible patient-to-patient tuberculosis transmission. In one nosocomial tuberculosis outbreak, a healthcare worker was the source. Both the healthcare worker's lack of recognition of symptoms as consistent with tuberculosis and the occupational health department's delay in recognition of tuberculosis in other healthcare workers with TST conversions and abnormal chest radiographs contributed to the outbreak [88].

Guideline Supplements

In the five supplements, extensive details are provided on the rationale, methods, and guidance for implementation of various elements of the tuberculosis control program. For example, the supplement on diagnosis and treatment provides a table on TST interpretation, treatment options, and drug dosages. The supplement on engineering controls discusses the basis for current science on ventilation and use of ultraviolet germicidal irradiation; and the supplement on respiratory protection discusses the factors to consider when choosing a respirator, including the key components of a respirator training program and the advantages and disadvantages of the various respirator types.

Cost of Tuberculosis Control Measures

Much of the debate about recommendations for the control of *M. tuberculosis* transmission in healthcare facilities has involved concerns about the cost of these measures. To facilitate identification of the extent of the infection control program that would be necessary at low-risk versus high-risk hospitals, the 1994 tuberculosis guidelines recommend conducting a risk assessment. Restricting admission of infectious tuberculosis patients to selected areas of the facility may significantly reduce the cost of the control program by limiting the area requiring environmental/engineering modifications and the number of healthcare workers requiring respirator education and fit testing and frequent TST monitoring. The major tuberculosis infection control measure costs are related to environmental/engineering modifications of existing older facilities to improve the number of air exchanges or to make the room negative pressure. Although these costs can be substantial, the modifications are long-term and the costs can be amortized over the life of the equipment. Recent estimates of the cost of such environmental changes at MDR-TB outbreak hospitals varied widely (median, $229,000; range, $70,000–$559,000) depending on the extent and type of modifications required [96].

Most of the concerns about costs of the tuberculosis control program have centered around the cost of the respirators and respirator education and fit testing program. Several authors have estimated the cost of respirators or respirator education and fit testing programs based on the number of healthcare workers at the facility. Nettleman et al. have estimated that the use of HEPA-filtered respirators would cost $7 million per case of tuberculosis prevented and $100 million per life saved [97]. Adal et al. estimated that at $7.51 to $9.08 per HEPA-filtered respirator, it would cost $1.3 to $18.5 million to prevent one episode of occupational acquisition of *M. tuberculosis* [98]. Both of these estimates come from institutions with a very low incidence of tuberculosis. Furthermore, a number of assumptions were made, such as single rather than repeated use of the respirator, admission of tuberculosis patients throughout the facility, and inclusion of all healthcare workers at the institution in the respiratory protection program, which may have artificially inflated the estimates. Kellerman et al. found that actual costs of respirators and respiratory education and fit testing programs were substantially less than these estimates at several of the MDR-TB hospitals; the median annual cost of respirators at four MDR-TB outbreak hospitals was $109,000 (range, $70,000–$223,000) and the median annual cost of respirator education and fit testing programs was $10,000 (range, $3700 to $19,700) [96].

Bacille Calmette-Guerin Vaccination

Because of concern about occupational acquisition of *M. tuberculosis* by healthcare workers, use of BCG vaccination as a protective measure has been raised. Although in many other countries BCG has been given routinely to all infants for more than 60 years, routine BCG administration in any age group has never been implemented in the United States. In 1988, the U.S. Advisory Committee on Immunization Practices (ACIP) removed the healthcare worker category from the list of people for whom BCG vaccination should be considered. The MDR-TB outbreaks in the late 1980s and 1990s resulted in a revisiting of this issue. Meta-analyses of the efficacy of BCG found that the data were inadequate (methodologic flaws) to evaluate the effectiveness of BCG in protecting healthcare workers [99,100]. Furthermore, the situation in the United States would be different from countries in which BCG is given in infancy. In the United States, if protecting healthcare workers were the goal, such vaccination would have to be given to adults. No data are available on how effective BCG administered only in adulthood would be. Furthermore, BCG is unlikely to provide protection for immunocompromised healthcare workers and might lead to disseminated BCG disease. Many of the countries in which BCG is routinely administered have a very high prevalence of tuberculosis in their populations, suggesting that BCG does not prevent pulmonary disease, although it may decrease the risk of disseminated disease. In such countries with HIV and tuberculosis outbreaks, the healthcare workers still may be at risk for occupational acquisition of *M. tuberculosis*. Few of these countries have either healthcare worker tuberculosis infection or disease surveillance programs; thus, there are few data on current rates of tuberculosis in BCG-vaccinated healthcare worker populations in areas with high prevalence of HIV or tuberculosis, or both. As a result of these and other factors, the ACIP and the American Committee for the Elimination of Tuberculosis decided to maintain their recommendation that use of BCG should be made on an individual basis but that it is not recommended in low-risk areas and in healthcare facilities with effective infection control programs [101].

Pediatric Settings

There has been similar controversy about the need for the CDC tuberculosis guidelines recommendations in pediatric settings. Many believe that because most pediatric patients have primary disease, poor or absent cough, and infrequent bronchial and laryngeal tuberculosis, transmission is unlikely. Although the risk for such transmission may be less, it is not zero. Furthermore, there are few data to document the lack of risk to healthcare workers in these settings. One survey of pediatric facilities showed that of 158 hospital respondents, 62 (40%) had a tuberculosis infection control policy specific for children, 147 (93%) reported admitting less than 6 tuberculosis patients, and 104 (66%) reported admitting no tuberculosis patients [102]. At 141/154 (92%) hospitals, a tuberculosis isolation policy existed; most isolated pediatric patients with positive AFB smears (139/143; 97%), evidence of cavitary tuberculosis on chest radiograph (141/145; 97%), or an AFB-positive gastric aspirate (107/140; 76%). At 10/154 (6.5%) facilities, clusters of more than two healthcare workers with similar occupational exposures had TST conversions in the preceding 5 years. Thus, like adults, pediatric patients should be evaluated at the time of admission for possible tuberculosis. Those with possible tuberculosis should be evaluated for potential infectiousness (i.e., positive sputum AFB smears). Those considered infectious should be placed in appropriate tuberculosis isolation.

Nosocomial Transmission of *M. tuberculosis* in International Settings

With the worldwide epidemics of HIV and tuberculosis, many countries throughout the world are admitting large numbers of patients with HIV infection, tuberculosis, or HIV infection and tuberculosis to their healthcare facilities. In many of these countries, overall infection control programs are minimal and tuberculosis infection control programs are nonexistent; such facilities often have no healthcare worker TST programs, no tuberculosis isolation rooms meeting the CDC-recommended criteria, and minimal laboratory diagnostics for tuberculosis (i.e., no rapid AFB smear, culture, or susceptibility capability). In such facilities, *M. tuberculosis* transmission from patient to patient and patient to healthcare worker undoubtedly occurs. It is incumbent on such facilities to conduct a risk assessment and determine the risk of such transmission to both their healthcare workers and patients. In these situations, simple control measures, such as enhanced administrative controls, healthcare worker respiratory protection, separation of infectious patients, and improved ventilation or ultraviolet germicidal irradiation may be useful in reducing the risk of *M. tuberculosis* transmission.

REFERENCES

1. Centers for Disease Control and Prevention. Expanded tuberculosis surveillance and tuberculosis morbidity: United States, 1993. *MMWR Morb Mortal Wkly Rep* 1994;43:361–366.
2. Kochi A. The global tuberculosis situation and the new controls strategy of the World Health Organization. *Tubercle* 1991;72:1–6.
3. Centers for Disease Control and Prevention. Tuberculosis, final data:

United States, 1986. *MMWR Morb Mortal Wkly Rep* 1988;36: 387–389, 395.
4. Cantwell MF, Snider DE Jr, Cauthen GM, Onorato IM. Epidemiology of tuberculosis in the United States, 1985 through 1992. *JAMA* 1994; 272:535–539.
5. Centers for Disease Control and Prevention. Expanded tuberculosis surveillance and tuberculosis morbidity: United States, 1993. *MMWR Morb Mortal Wkly Rep* 1994;43:361–366.
6. Centers for Disease Control and Prevention. Tuberculosis morbidity: United States, 1994. *MMWR Morb Mortal Wkly Rep* 1995;44: 387–389, 395.
7. Centers for Disease Control and Prevention. Nosocomial transmission of multidrug-resistant tuberculosis among HIV-infected person: Florida and New York, 1988–1991. *MMWR Morb Mortal Wkly Rep* 1991;40:585–591.
8. Frieden TR, Fujiwara PI, Washko RM, Hamburg MA. Tuberculosis in New York City: turning the tide. *N Engl J Med* 1995;333:229–233.
9. Coronado VG, Beck-Sague CM, Pearson ML, et al. Clinical and epidemiologic characteristics of multidrug-resistant *Mycobacterium tuberculosis* among patients with human immunodeficiency virus (HIV) infection. *Infect Dis Clin Pract* 1993;2:297–302.
10. Tenover FC, Crawford JT, Huebner RE, Geiter LJ, Horsburgh CR, Good RC. Guest commentary. The resurgence of tuberculosis: is your laboratory ready? *J Clin Microbiol* 1993;31:767–770.
11. Tokars JI, Rudnick JR, Kroc K, et al. U.S. hospital mycobacteriology laboratories: status and comparison with state public health department laboratories. *J Clin Microbiol* 1996;34:680–685.
12. Centers for Disease Control and Prevention. Screening for tuberculosis and tuberculosis infection in high-risk populations, and the use of preventive therapy for tuberculosis infection in the United States: recommendations of the Advisory Committee for Elimination of Tuberculosis. *MMWR Morb Mortal Wkly Rep* 1990;39(RR-8):1–7.
13. Centers for Disease Control and Prevention. Management of persons exposed to multidrug-resistant tuberculosis. *MMWR Morb Mortal Wkly Rep* 1992;41(RR-11):59–71.
14. Fridkin SK, Manangan L, Bolyard E, SHEA, Jarvis WR. SHEA-CDC TB survey: part I. status of TB infection control programs at member hospitals, 1989–1992. *Infect Control Hosp Epidemiol* 1995;16: 129–134.
15. Fridkin SK, Manangan L, Bolyard E, SHEA, Jarvis WR. SHEA-CDC survey: part II. efficacy of TB infection control programs at member hospitals, 1992. *Infect Control Hosp Epidemiol* 1995;16:135–140.
16. Sinkowitz R, Fridkin S, Manangan L, Wenger P, APIC, Jarvis WR. Status of tuberculosis infection control programs at U.S.hospitals, 1989–1992. *Am J Infect Control* 1996;24:226–234.
17. Malasky C, Jordan T, Potulski F, Reichman LB. Occupational tuberculosis infections among pulmonary physicians in training. *Am Rev Respir Dis* 1990;142:505–507.
18. Menzies D, Fanning A, Yuan L, Fitzgerald M. Tuberculosis among healthcare workers. *N Engl J Med* 1995;332:92–98.
19. Levine I. Tuberculosis risk in students of nursing. *Arch Intern Med* 1968;121:545–548.
20. Weiss W. Tuberculosis in student nurses at Philadelphia General Hospital. *Am Rev Respir Dis* 1973;107:136–139.
21. Atuk NO, Hunt EH. Serial tuberculin testing and isoniazid therapy in general hospital employees. *JAMA* 1971;218:1795–1798.
22. Gregg D, Gibson M. Employee TB control in a predominantly tuberculosis hospital. *J S C Med Assoc* 1975;71:160–165.
23. Berman J, Levine ML, Orr ST, Desi L. Tuberculosis risk for hospital employees: analysis of a five-year tuberculin skin testing program. *Am J Public Health* 1981;71:1217–1222.
24. Craven RB, Wenzel RP, Atuk NO. Minimizing tuberculosis risk to hospital personnel and students exposed to unsuspected disease. *Ann Intern Med* 1975;82:628–632.
25. Vogeler DM, Burke JP. Tuberculosis screening for hospital employees: a five year experience in a large community hospital. *Am Rev Respir Dis* 1978;117:227–232.
26. Ruben FL, Norden CW, Schuster N. Analysis of a community hospital employee tuberculosis screening program 31 months after its inception. *Am Rev Respir Dis* 1977;115:23–28.
27. Ktsanes VK, Williams WL, Boudreaux VV. The cumulative risk of tuberculin skin test conversion for five years of hospital employment. *Am J Public Health* 1986;76:65–67.
28. Barrett-Conner E. The epidemiology of tuberculosis in physicians. *JAMA* 1979;241:133–138.
29. Weinstein RS, Oshins J, Sacks HS. Tuberculosis infection in Mount Sinai medical students: 1974–1982. *Mt Sinai J Med* 1984;51:283–286.
30. Chan JC, Tabak JI. Risk of tuberculous infection among house staff in an urban teaching hospital. *South Med J* 1985;78:1061–1064.
31. Bass JB, Serio RA. The use of repeat skin tests to eliminate the booster phenomenon in serial tuberculin testing. *Am Rev Respir Dis* 1981;123:394–396.
32. Thompson NJ, Glassroth JL, Snider DE Jr, Farer LS. The booster phenomenon in serial tuberculin testing. *Am Rev Respir Dis* 1979;119: 587–597.
33. Kantor HS, Poblete R, Pusateri SL. Nosocomial transmission of tuberculosis from unsuspected disease. *Am J Med* 1988;84:833–838.
34. Price LE, Rutala WQ, Samsa GP: Tuberculosis in hospital personnel. *Infect Control* 1987;8:97–101.
35. Aitken ML, Anderson KM, Albert RK. Is the tuberculosis screening program of hospital employees still required? *Am Rev Respir Dis* 1987;136:805–807.
36. Raad I, Cusick J, Sheretz RJ, Sabbagh M, Howell N. Annual tuberculin skin testing of employees at a university hospital: a cost–benefit analysis. *Infect Control Hosp Epidemiol* 1989;10:465–469.
37. Ramirez JA, Anderson P, Herp S, Raff MJ. Increased rate of tuberculin skin test conversion among workers at a university hospital. *Infect Control Hosp Epidemiol* 1992;13:579–581.
38. Ikeda RM, Birkhead GS, DiFerdinando GT Jr, et al. Nosocomial tuberculosis: an outbreak of a strain resistant to seven drugs. *Infect Contr Hosp Epidemiol* 1995;16:152–159.
39. Condos R, Scluger N, Lacouture R, Rom W. Tuberculosis infections among housestaff at Bellevue Hospital in an epidemic period [Abstract]. *Am Rev Respir Dis* 1993;147(Suppl):A124.
40. Redwood E, Anderson V, Felton CP, Findley S, Ford JG. Tuberculin conversions in hospital employees in a high tuberculosis prevalence area [Abstract]. *Am Rev Respir Dis* 1993;147(Suppl):A119.
41. Cocchiarella LA, Cohen RAC, Conroy L, Wurtz R. Positive tuberculin skin testing reactions among house staff at a public hospital in the era of resurgent tuberculosis. *Am J Infect Control* 1996;24:7–12.
42. Adal KA, Anglim AM, Palumbo CL, Titus MG, Coyner BJ, Farr BM. The use of high-efficiency particulate air-filter respirators to protect hospital workers from tuberculosis: a cost-effectiveness analysis. *N Engl J Med* 1994;331:169–173.
43. Panlilio AL, Burwen DR, the TB Infection Surveillance Project. Tuberculosis skin testing surveillance of healthcare workers [Abstract]. *Infect Control Hosp Epidemiol* 1996;17:P17.
44. Manangan LP, Perrotta DM, Banerjee SN, Hack D, Simonds D, Jarvis WR. Status of tuberculosis infection control programs at Texas hospitals, 1989–1991. *Am J Infect Control* 1997;25:229–235.
45. Sepkowitz KA, Fella P, Rivera P, Villa N, DeHovitz J. Prevalence of PPD positivity among new employees at a hospital in New York City. *Infect Control Hosp Epidemiol* 1995;16:334–337.
46. Centers for Disease Control and Prevention. Guidelines for preventing the transmission of tuberculosis in health-care settings, with special focus on HIV-related issues. *MMWR Morb Mortal Wkly Rep* 1990;39 (RR-17).
47. Centers for Disease Control and Prevention. Guidelines for preventing the transmission of *Mycobacterium tuberculosis* in health-care facilities, 1994. *MMWR Morb Mortal Wkly Rep* 1994;43(RR1-13).
48. Jereb JA, Klevens RM, Privett TD, Smith PJ, et al. Tuberculosis in healthcare workers at a hospital with an outbreak of multidrug-resistant *Mycobacterium tuberculosis*. *Arch Intern Med* 1995;155: 854–859.
49. Geisler PJ, Nelson KE, Crispin RJ, Moses VK. Tuberculosis in physicians: a continuing problem. *Am Rev Respir Dis* 1986;133:773–778.
50. Pope AS: An outbreak of tuberculosis in infants due to hospital infection. *J Pediatr* 1942;40:297–300.
51. Ehrenkranz JN, Kicklighter LJ. Tuberculosis outbreak in a general hospital: evidence for airborne spread of infection. *Ann Intern Med* 1972;77:377–382.
52. Alpert ME, Levison ME. An epidemic of tuberculosis in a medical school. *N Engl J Med* 1965;272:718–721.
53. Israel HL, Hetherington HW, Ord JG. A study of tuberculosis among students of nursing. *JAMA* 1941;117:839–844.
54. Brahdy L. Immunity and positive tuberculin reaction. *Am J Public Health* 1941;31:1040–1043.
55. Badger TL, Ayvazian LF. Tuberculosis in nurses: clinical observations on its pathogenesis as seen in a fifteen year follow-up of 745 nurses. *Am Rev Tubercule* 1949;60:305–327.

56. Abruzzi WA, Hummel RJ. Tuberculosis: incidence among American medical students, prevention and the use of BCG. *N Engl J Med* 1953; 248:722–729.
57. Rudnick JR, Kroc K, Manangan L, Banerjee S, Pugliese G, Jarvis W. *Are U.S. hospitals prepared to control nosocomial transmission of tuberculosis?* Presented at the First World Congress on Tuberculosis, Rockville, Maryland, November 15–18, 1992.
58. Ramaswamy R, Corpuz M, Hewlett D. Tuberculosis surveillance of community hospital employees: a recommended strategy. *Arch Intern Med* 1995;155:1637–1639.
59. Barnes PF, Bloch AB, Davidson PT, Snider DE Jr. Tuberculosis in patients with human immunodeficiency virus infection. *N Engl J Med* 1991;324:1644–1650.
60. Selwyn PA, Hartel D, Lewis VA, et al. A prospective study of the risk of tuberculosis among intravenous drug users with human immunodeficiency virus infection. *N Engl J Med* 1989;320:545–550.
61. Dooley SW, Villarino ME, Lawrence M, et al. Tuberculosis in a hospital unit for patients infected with the human immunodeficiency virus (HIV): evidence of nosocomial transmission. *JAMA* 1992;267: 2632–2634.
62. Di Perri G, Cruciani M, Danzi MC, et al. Nosocomial epidemic of active tuberculosis among HIV-infected patients. *Lancet* 1989;2: 1502–1504.
63. Cantanzaro A. Nosocomial tuberculosis. *Am Rev Respir Dis* 1982; 125:559–562.
64. Haley CE, McDonald RC, Rossi L, Jones D Jr, Haley RW, Luby P. Tuberculosis epidemic among hospital personnel. *Infect Control Hosp Epidemiol* 1989;10:204–210.
65. Hutton MD, Stead WS, Cauthen GM, Bloch AB, Ewing WM. Nosocomial transmission of tuberculosis associated with a draining abscess. *J Infect Dis* 1990;161:286–295.
66. Calder RA, Duclos P, Wilder MH, et al. *Mycobacterium tuberculosis* transmission in a health clinic. *Bulletin of the International Union for Tuberculosis and Lung Disease* 1991;66:103–106.
67. Pierce JR Jr, Sims SL, Holman GH. Transmission of tuberculosis to hospital workers by a patient with AIDS. *Chest* 1992;101:581–582.
68. Frampton MW: An outbreak of tuberculosis among hospital personnel caring for a patient with a skin ulcer. *Ann Intern Med* 1992;117: 312–313.
69. Edlin BR, Tokars JI, Grieco MH, et al. An outbreak of multidrug-resistant tuberculosis among hospitalized patients with the acquired immunodeficiency syndrome: epidemiologic studies and restriction fragment length polymorphism analysis. *N Engl J Med* 1992;326: 1514–1522.
70. Beck-Sague CM, Dooley SW, Hutton MD, et al. Outbreak of multidrug-resistant tuberculosis among persons with HIV infection in an urban hospital: transmission to staff and patients and control measures. *JAMA* 1992;268:1280–1286.
71. Fischl MA, Uttamchandani RB, Daikos GL, et al. An outbreak of tuberculosis caused by multiple-drug-resistant tubercle bacilli among patients with HIV infection. *Ann Intern Med* 1992;117:177–183.
72. Pearson ML, Jereb JA, Frieden TR, et al. Nosocomial transmission of multidrug-resistant *Mycobacterium* tuberculosis: a risk to hospitalized patients and health-care workers. *Ann Intern Med* 1992;117: 191–196.
73. Coronado VG, Valway S, Finelli L, et al. Nosocomial transmission of multidrug-resistant *Mycobacterium tuberculosis* among intravenous drug users with human immunodeficiency virus infection. In: *Abstracts of the third annual meeting of the Society for Hospital Epidemiology of America;* Chicago, April 18–20, 1993. *Infect Control and Hosp Epidemiol.*
74. Coronado VG, Beck-Sague CM, Hutton MD, et al. Transmission of multidrug-resistant *Mycobacterium tuberculosis* among persons with human immunodeficiency virus infection in an urban hospital: epidemiologic and restriction fragment length polymorphism analysis. *J Infect Dis* 1993;168:1052–1055.
75. Jarvis WR. Nosocomial transmission of multidrug-resistant *Mycobacterium tuberculosis*. *Res Microbiol* 1993;144:117–122.
76. Zaza S, Blumberg HM, Beck-Sague C, et al. Occupational risk of infection with *Mycobacterium tuberculosis*: patients and healthcare workers as a source of infection. *J Infect Dis* 1995;172:1542–1549.
77. Centers for Disease Control and Prevention. Outbreak of multidrug-resistant tuberculosis at a hospital: New York City, 1991. *MMWR Morb Mortal Wkly Rep* 1993;42:427–434.
78. Tokars JI, Jarvis WR, Edlin BR, et al. Tuberculin skin testing of hospital employees during an outbreak of multidrug-resistant tuberculosis in human immunodeficiency virus (HIV)-infected patients. *Infect Control Hosp Epidemiol* 1992;13:509–510.
79. Valway SE, Greifinger RB, Papania M, et al. Multidrug-resistant tuberculosis in the New York State prison system, 1990–1991. *J Infect Dis* 1994;170:151–156.
80. Cave MD, Eisenbach KD, McDernott PF, Bates JH, Crawford JT: IS6110. conservation of sequence in the *Mycobacterium tuberculosis* complex and its utilization in DNA finger printing. *Mol Cell Probes* 1991;5:73–80.
81. Haas WH, Butler WR, Woodley CL, Crawford JT. Mixed-linker polymerase chain reaction: a new method for rapid fingerprinting of the *Mycobacterium tuberculosis* complex. *J Clin Microbiol* 1993;31: 1293–1298.
82. Moran GJ, McCabe F, Morgan MT, Talan DA. Delayed recognition and infection control for tuberculosis patients in the emergency department. *Ann Emerg Med* 1995;26:290–295.
83. Moran GJ, Fuchs MA, Jarvis WR, Talan DA. Tuberculosis infection control practices at emergency departments in the United States, 1993–1994. *Ann Emerg Med* 1995;26:283–289.
84. Huebner RE, Good RC, Tokars JI. Current practices in mycobacteriology: results of a survey of state public health laboratories. *J Clin Microbiol* 1993;31:771–775.
85. Maloney SA, Pearson ML, Gordon MT, et al. Efficacy of control measures in preventing nosocomial transmission of multidrug-resistant tuberculosis to patients and healthcare workers. *Ann Intern Med* 1995; 122:90–95.
86. Wenger PN, Otten J, Breeden A, et al. Control of nosocomial transmission of multidrug-resistant *Mycobacterium tuberculosis* among healthcare workers and HIV-infected patients. *Lancet* 1995;345: 235–240.
87. Stroud LA, Tokars JI, Grieco MH, et al. Evaluation of infection control measures in preventing the nosocomial transmission of multidrug-resistant *Mycobacterium tuberculosis* in a New York City hospital. *Infect Control Hosp Epidemiol* 1995;16:141–147.
88. Blumberg HM, Watkins DL, Berschling JD, et al. Preventing the nosocomial transmission of tuberculosis. *Ann Intern Med* 1995;122: 658–663.
89. Jarvis WR. Nosocomial transmission of multidrug-resistant *Mycobacterium tuberculosis*. *Am J Infect Control* 1995;23:146–151.
90. Jarvis WR, Bolyard EA, Bozzi CJ, et al. Respirators, recommendations, and regulations: the controversy surrounding protection of healthcare workers from tuberculosis. *Ann Intern Med* 1995;122:142–146.
91. Occupational Safety and Health Administration. OSHA 29DFR-OSH. 29 CFR 1910.134—*Occupational safety and health standards, personal protective equipment, respiratory protection.* Code of Federal Regulation. Washington, DC: U.S. Government Printing Office, Office of the Federal Register 1972;37:1910–1934.
92. Leidel NA, Mullan RJ. NIOSH recommended guidelines for personal respiratory protection of workers in health-care facilities potentially exposed to tuberculosis. Atlanta: U.S. Department of Health and Human Services, Public health Service, Centers for Disease Control and Prevention, National Institute for Occupational Safety and Health; 1992.
93. Chen SK, Vesley D, Brosseau LM, et al. Evaluation of single-use masks and respirators for protection of healthcare workers against mycobacterial aerosols. *Am J Infect Control* 1994;22:65–74.
94. National Institute for Occupational Safety and Health. NIOSH 30CFR-NIOSH. 30 CFR Part II—*Respiratory protective devices; tests for permissibility, fees.* Code of Federal Regulations. Washington, DC; U.S. Government Printing Office, Office of the Federal Register. 1972;37:6243–71.
95. U.S. Department of Health and Human Services. 42 CFR Part 84: Respiratory protective devices; proposed rule. *Federal Register* 1994; 59:26849–26889.
96. Kellerman S, Tokars JT, Jarvis WR. The costs of complying with CDC tuberculosis guidelines at hospitals with a history of multidrug-resistant *Mycobacterium* tuberculosis outbreaks [Abstract]. *Infect Control Hosp Epidemiol* 1996;17:17.
97. Nettleman MD, Fredriskson M, Good NL, Hunter SA. Tuberculosis control strategies: the cost of particulate respirators. *Ann Intern Med* 1994;121:37–40.
98. Adal KA, Anglim AM, Palumbo CL, Titus MG, Coyner BJ, Farr BM. The use of high-efficiency particulate air-filter respirators to protect

hospital workers from tuberculosis: a cost-effectiveness analysis. *N Engl J Med* 1994;331:169–173.

99. Brewer TF, Colditz GA. Bacille Calmette-Guerin vaccination for the prevention of tuberculosis in healthcare workers. *Clin Infect Dis* 1995; 20:136–142.
100. Brewer TF, Colditz GA. Relationship between bacille Calmette-Guerin (BCG) strains and the efficacy of BCG vaccine in the prevention of tuberculosis. *Clin Infect Dis* 1995;20:126–135.
101. Centers for Disease Control and Prevention. The role of BCG vaccine in the prevention and control of tuberculosis in the United States. *MMWR Morb Mortal Wkly Rep* 1996;45(RR-4):1–18.
102. Kellerman S, Simonds D, Jarvis W, Lee T. Tuberculosis infection control policies and procedures at hospitals caring for children: the APIC-CDC survey. In: *Twenty-third annual meeting of the Association for Professions in Infection Control and Epidemiology, Inc.;* Atlanta, Georgia, June 2–6, 1996. *Am J Infect Control* 1996;24:93.

Hospital Infections, Fourth Edition,
edited by John V. Bennett and Philip S. Brachman.
Lippincott–Raven Publishers, Philadelphia © 1998

CHAPTER 34

Infectious Gastroenteritis

Herbert L. DuPont and Bruce S. Ribner

Microorganisms that cause outbreaks of foodborne illness in the community also have the potential for causing similar events in hospitalized patients. However, certain forms of gastroenteritis—such as that caused by foodborne toxins of *Clostridium perfringens, Clostridium botulinum, Staphylococcus aureus*, and *Bacillus cereus*, as well as that produced by the ingestion of food contaminated with group A streptococci and *Vibrio parahaemolyticus*—have not been recognized to be transmissible from person to person within the hospital. The control of these diseases in the hospital depends on safe food-handling practices, as discussed in Chapter 22, and such forms of gastroenteritis are not considered additionally in this chapter.

Infectious or communicable gastroenteritis caused by *Salmonella* other than *Salmonella typhi, Escherichia coli, Shigella*, and rotavirus receive primary attention in this chapter. In addition, the chapter separately addresses *Clostridium difficile* (an agent with a high degree of communicability that causes antibiotic-associated diarrhea and colitis), *Yersinia enterocolitica* (an agent that has produced communicable nosocomial infections involving the gastrointestinal tract), staphylococcal enterocolitis (a noncommunicable form of nosocomial gastroenteritis), and necrotizing enterocolitis (a disease of uncertain, possibly infectious cause). Nosocomial transmission of *Vibrio cholerae* has produced nosocomial infectious gastroenteritis in areas endemic for this disease, but the agent is not discussed here because of the rarity of endemic cases in the United States.

Infectious gastroenteritis differs from most other hospital-associated infections, which characteristically result from endogenous organisms in people with markedly altered resistance. Enteric infections caused by the agents just mentioned are nearly always exogenously acquired, often occur in clusters or epidemics, and are usually due to the introduction of a virulent organism through the ingestion of contaminated foods or medications, through short-term carriers among patients and hospital staff, or through patient-to-patient transmission on the hands of personnel. Although host factors such as age and debility are important, healthy patients and hospital personnel also are frequently involved in outbreaks of these infections.

INCIDENCE

Although the true incidence of nosocomial infectious gastroenteritis is not known, it is evident that its occurrence is greatly underestimated. The common occurrence of noninfectious diarrhea among patients and personnel, the lack of standard criteria for the diagnosis of nosocomial infectious gastroenteritis, and the limited ability of many hospital laboratories to identify the most common agents responsible for infectious gastroenteritis have all contributed to the underreporting of this condition. These factors have also contributed to the great differences in rates of nosocomial infectious gastroenteritis reported by investigators in the literature.

It is important to distinguish between nosocomial diarrhea and nosocomial infectious gastroenteritis. Nosocomial diarrhea has been reported to occur in 7.7% to 41% of the patients admitted to adult intensive care units [1,2], 1.2% to 2.1% of all patients admitted to pediatric teaching hospitals [3], and 1.5% of children admitted to two pediatric wards [2]. When compared with nosocomial infections occurring at other body sites in the same populations, nosocomial diarrhea represented either the first or second most common nosocomial illness. However, most studies do not require the isolation of a pathogen for the diagnosis of nosocomial diarrhea. Where sought, pathogens are found in slightly more than half of the

H. L. DuPont: Baylor College of Medicine, University of Texas at Houston, St. Luke's Episcopal Hospital, Houston, Texas 77030.
B. S. Ribner: Ralph H. Johnson DVA Medical Center, Medical University of South Carolina, Charleston, South Carolina 28401.

affected patients in unselected populations [4] and in as few as 17% of the patients who contract nosocomial diarrhea while receiving tube feedings [5]. Thus, nosocomial infectious gastroenteritis accounts for only a portion of those patients who experience nosocomial diarrhea.

The National Nosocomial Infections Surveillance (NNIS) System (see Chapter 30) for the period January, 1990 through December, 1994 found that, for hospitals reporting all nosocomial infections, 2.27 per 1,000 patients discharged experienced a nosocomial gastrointestinal infection. There were marked differences among services. The highest rates were found in high-risk nurseries (9.58 per 1,000), reflecting the underlying susceptibility of the hosts and the ease of transmission of the pathogens responsible for infectious gastroenteritis in this age group. Surgical services had the next highest rate (3.21 per 1,000), followed by medicine and pediatrics (2.82 and 2.04 per 1,000, respectively). Obstetric services had the lowest rates of enteric nosocomial infection (0.14 per 1,000 discharges).

Causative pathogens also tended to differ substantially by service. On pediatric services and in high-risk nurseries, rotaviruses were responsible for 72% and 38%, respectively, of all instances of nosocomial infectious gastroenteritis. In contrast, *C. difficile* accounted for 94% of such disease on general surgery services and 96% on medical services.

DIAGNOSTIC CRITERIA

Clinical and Microbiologic Criteria

There is wide variation in the clinical symptoms experienced by patients with these enteric infections. Some patients become asymptomatic excreters of a potential pathogen, whereas others show varying forms of diarrheal disease. Organisms that invade the intestinal epithelial lining often elicit a febrile response in addition to causing diarrhea. In infections with pathogens that invade the colonic mucosa primarily, symptoms of colitis occur, including urgency, tenesmus, and passage of bloody, mucoid stools (dysentery). Diarrhea or loose stools in a patient with unexplained fever should be diagnosed as infectious gastroenteritis, regardless of culture results for bacterial pathogens. When diarrhea or loose stools occur in an afebrile patient or in a febrile patient whose fever has other likely causes, the identification of a recognized pathogen in stools or by serologic testing is necessary for this diagnosis.

Diarrhea of noninfectious origin—such as that caused by cathartics, inflammatory diseases of the gastrointestinal tract, and surgical resections and anastomoses—should be carefully differentiated from the diarrhea of infectious gastroenteritis. Alterations in the gastrointestinal flora because of antibiotic administration are commonly associated with diarrhea; such cases of diarrhea should not be reported as gastroenteritis unless enterocolitis occurs, in which event they should be reported as noninfectious gastroenteritis.

Classification of Infections

Diarrhea with onset after admission that is associated with a positive culture for organisms recognized as causative of infectious gastroenteritis should be regarded as a nosocomial infection. The interval between the time of admission and the onset of clinical symptoms must be greater than the known minimum incubation period for that agent (see subsequent sections). Alternatively, nosocomial infections may be diagnosed if a stool culture obtained shortly before or just after admission is negative for the pathogen in question and the pathogen is subsequently cultured from the patient.

PREDISPOSING HOST FACTORS

Defective Gastric Defenses

There is evidence to indicate that gastric acid plays an important role in the defense against ingested organisms. The bactericidal action of stomach acid greatly reduces or eradicates ingested organisms and thus reduces the inoculum of organisms that subsequently reaches the intestine. Physiologic or pathologic achlorhydria, which is most common in premature infants and elderly patients, may underlie the increased risks of certain enteric bacterial infections seen in these groups. Although unstudied, variations in gastric acidity may also partly determine which person becomes ill after the ingestion of a contaminated common vehicle. Antacid use has been shown greatly to facilitate colonization of the intestine with vaccine strains of *Shigella* and to increase the frequency of gastrointestinal acquisition of nosocomial strains of aerobic gram-negative rods. Similar effects are produced by agents such as cimetidine. It is probable that anticholinergic medications act similarly. People with histories of gastric resection and vagotomy are known to be at higher risk of acquiring cholera than otherwise healthy people.

The time during which ingested substances are in contact with gastric acid may be important. Water without food tends to traverse the stomach more rapidly than solid food, reaching the neutralizing secretions of the duodenum more rapidly. The inoculum of organisms required to produce infection is probably reduced when transmitted by water. Waterborne outbreaks of salmonellosis have occurred when low concentrations of the organism are present, whereas large numbers are usually required for foodborne transmission of these organisms.

Antibiotic Therapy

The oral or systemic administration of antibiotics to which an epidemic strain is resistant greatly facilitates cross-colonization and infection (see Chapter 14). These effects presumably occur because of a reduction in the competitive interference of normal, sensitive flora against the ingested strains, which in effect reduces the inoculum required for establishment of the pathogen. The continued administration of the drug after acquisition of the pathogen may permit the selective outgrowth of the pathogen and result in much greater concentrations of the organism in the feces than might otherwise occur. The chances of transmission and risk of disease are thereby increased.

Antibiotic administration may also predispose certain patients to diarrhea caused by enteric pathogens resistant to the antibiotic. This may occur during therapy or shortly after termination of the antibiotic. In such cases, the pathogen is able to replicate more rapidly than the suppressed normal flora, reaching concentrations not normally achievable when the normal flora is at pretherapy levels. These elevated concentrations may lead to enteritis and increase the risk of cross-infection in a manner similar to that of resistant pathogens.

Although almost all antibiotics have been associated with infectious diarrhea, agents active against anaerobic bacteria, such as clindamycin and the β-lactam antibiotics, seem to present the greatest risk.

Crowding and Staffing Factors

A ratio of staff to patients that is insufficient encourages infractions in handwashing and isolation techniques, especially in critical care areas. Even careful handwashing, however, is sometimes ineffective in removing gram-negative rods from the hands, and a slight but definite risk of transmitting organisms by direct contact with successive patients exists even after handwashing. Thus inordinately low staff-to-patient ratios may lead to increased risk of cross-colonization and infection. Crowding of patients also increases the risk of cross-infection. Although crowding of patients is often accompanied by insufficiencies in staff, it may be independently important in that it increases the risk of indirect contact spread through environmental sources, especially in nurseries.

Gastrointestinal Endoscopy

Gastrointestinal endoscopy has become an important diagnostic and therapeutic procedure. It is estimated that over eight million such procedures are performed annually in the United States. Although nosocomial infectious gastroenteritis after endoscopy is uncommon, the large number of endoscopies performed has resulted in an increasing number of recognized nosocomial gastrointestinal infections after these procedures. Gastrointestinal infections caused by *Salmonella* species, *C. difficile*, and *Campylobacter* species have all been reported after gastrointestinal endoscopy.

It is inherently difficult to remove pathogenic organisms from gastrointestinal endoscopes because the instruments have a complex structure and are difficult to clean, the materials used in their construction are fragile and usually do not tolerate sterilization procedures or total immersion in disinfectants, and the instruments tend to become heavily soiled during use. Because of these difficulties, it is often possible to detect the presence of large numbers of bacteria in the channels of these instruments after disinfection has been completed. Preventing transmission of pathogenic organisms by contaminated gastrointestinal endoscopes requires policies that ensure adequate training of personnel responsible for cleaning and disinfecting the endoscopes, stress meticulous cleaning, ensure adequate contact time of parts with an Environmental Protection Agency-registered disinfectant, and include steps to dry thoroughly all channels before storage [6–8].

GENERAL CONTROL MEASURES

In controlling the spread of enteric infections in the hospital environment, a number of general measures can be taken regardless of the specific pathogen responsible. The most important mode of cross-infection for enteric bacterial pathogens in the hospital is usually the fecal–oral route, by which indirect contact spread of organisms occurs from patient to patient on the hands of personnel. Outbreaks may also result from the ingestion of contaminated food, medication, or test materials.

Handwashing

Because the most important means of spread of enteric bacterial pathogens is by hand transfer, effective handwashing is among the most important measures to prevent disease transmission. Although it is unlikely that all potentially pathogenic microorganisms can be removed by handwashing, the level of contamination can be reduced, in most cases, below that necessary for disease transmission among healthy children and adults. At least one study has demonstrated that a handwashing agent containing an antiseptic is more effective in removing enteric pathogens from the hands of healthcare workers than an agent that does not contain an antiseptic. This observation may be especially important when caring for debilitated patients or newborn infants, because the dose of enteropathogens needed to produce disease in these patients probably is substantially lower. In areas housing such patients, additional measures for the prevention of cross-infection may be required.

Surveillance

It is necessary to have an alert hospital surveillance program that continually reviews clinical patterns of infection in the hospital and evaluates bacteriologic reports from the diagnostic microbiology laboratory. Such a program is often instrumental in defining the extent of an outbreak before it has reached serious proportions and represents the foundation of an effective infection control program (see Chapter 5).

Surveillance must include hospital personnel, particularly food handlers, as well as patients. One important means of minimizing nosocomial diarrheal disease is to establish an effective personnel health service. Food handlers, nurses, and ancillary staff having direct contact with patients should be encouraged to communicate with the personnel health service when an episode of acute gastroenteritis occurs among themselves. Stool cultures should be performed and the ill person removed from work until culture results and the clinical course of the disease can be evaluated (see Chapter 3).

All personnel with an acute diarrheal illness should be removed from food handling and direct patient contact until the diarrhea has resolved. If stool cultures reveal the presence of an infectious pathogen, the employees should not return to food handling and should not care for patients in high-risk areas (e.g., intensive care units, newborn nurseries, transplant services) until two stool specimens obtained a minimum of 24 hours apart are negative for the pathogen. Employees from whom an enteric pathogen is isolated may care for patients in low-risk areas on resolution of diarrhea and before elimination of the infectious pathogen from the stool. However, such employees must be instructed to pay careful attention to thorough handwashing after use of toilet facilities.

No infant born of a mother with diarrhea or with stool cultures positive for an enteric pathogen should be admitted to the nursery ward. Any infant with loose, watery, or bloody diarrhea should be handled with enteric precautions until a noninfectious cause for the diarrhea has been identified.

Similarly, patients of all ages admitted to the hospital with unexplained diarrhea, or in whom diarrhea develops while in the hospital, should be placed in enteric isolation until an infectious etiology has been ruled out. Historically, such patients have led to well-documented outbreaks of nosocomial gastroenteritis due to both bacterial and viral agents.

Use of Antimotility Drugs

Treatment of acute gastroenteritis with drugs to decrease the motility of the gut and produce symptomatic relief of diarrhea may have undesirable side effects in select patients. In people with severe illness due to invasive pathogens (*Shigella, Salmonella*, and *Campylobacter*), worsening of clinical illness may result. Drugs such as diphenoxylate hydrochloride and atropine (Lomotil) or loperamide (Imodium) should be avoided in the treatment of nosocomial gastroenteritis when patients have significant fever or are passing bloody mucoid stools.

Prompt Investigation of Cases

The occurrence of two or more cases of nosocomial infectious gastroenteritis caused by the same organism within a few weeks should prompt a review of the exposures common to these cases (see Chapter 6). Case–control investigations are less likely to establish the source of infections conclusively when the number of cases is small, and microbiologic sampling of foods, medications, or equipment common to cases may be of special value in this circumstance. Culture surveys of other patients hospitalized in the same patient care areas as those with cases of disease and of employees working in these areas may identify asymptomatically infected people, and such people should be included with symptomatic patients for purposes of epidemiologically establishing possible sources.

Hospital outbreaks of enteric disease may be caused by patients or hospital personnel who are short-term carriers of a specific pathogen. Comparison of the exposures of cases and control subjects to specific personnel (see Chapter 6) and culture surveys of hospital personnel and asymptomatic patients may help to identify the carriers responsible for such outbreaks. Occasionally, environmental factors such as air, dust, bedside tables, thermometers, and mattresses are important in contact spread. If a common vehicle such as food, contaminated equipment, or contaminated oral medication or test solution can be identified, its removal or disinfection may assist in terminating the outbreak.

Secondary cases often occur after disease outbreaks caused by contaminated vehicles, and the chance of epidemiologically identifying responsible sources may be improved in such situations by focusing attention on early cases and on patients whose illnesses seem unlikely to have derived from person-to-person spread.

On occasion, epidemiologic studies may indicate that the central kitchen is responsible for the dissemination of a bacterial pathogen. Removal of food handlers with recent diarrheal disease or kitchen personnel with positive cultures on culture surveys may result in termination of the epidemic. In most instances, however, foodborne outbreaks of nosocomial gastroenteritis derive from inadequate handling of products from food-producing animals rather than from contamination of the food by food handlers.

Outbreak Management

During an epidemic, it is usually helpful to isolate patients with asymptomatic as well as symptomatic infections in separate rooms with separate lavatory facilities. Enteric precautions are necessary, of which glove-gown-stool precautions should be a part.

In nurseries in which enteric isolation of individual cases is not possible, cohort systems (see Chapter 26) should be used during an epidemic to minimize the risk of cross-infection. Successful control of outbreaks sometimes requires repeated culture surveys coupled with a special type of cohorting. Infants who are ill or colonized with the epidemic organism can sometimes be grouped together into a cohort that is physically separated from noninfected infants. Personnel caring for these infants must not care for noninfected infants, and no equipment should be shared between the two groups. Only milk packaged in sterile containers should be used, common equipment shared among babies should be removed, and infants should be confined to their own bassinets or Isolettes. To prevent additional spread of infection, infants born outside the hospital should not enter the nursery during an epidemic of diarrhea. Unnecessary contact with babies by hospital personnel or contact between infants should be eliminated during epidemics. An adequate-sized nursing and hospital staff is especially important in the management of nursery epidemics.

Not only is it important to isolate patients with active disease as long as indicated (see Chapter 13), but infected patients should be discharged from the hospital as soon as their condition allows them to be managed at home. Uninfected patients should also be discharged as soon as possible from hospital areas experiencing an outbreak of nosocomial gastroenteritis.

SALMONELLA INFECTIONS

General Aspects

Clinical and Microbiologic Features

In salmonellosis, fever, nausea, and vomiting develop and are followed shortly by abdominal pain and watery diarrhea. Frequently, mucous strands can be found in stool specimens, whereas gross blood is found in slightly < 10% of cases. In shigellosis and *Campylobacter* enteritis, stools are bloody in approximately 50% of cases.

Newborns have a predisposition to disease. Approximately 50% of exposed infants become ill once a case is introduced into a nursery. *Salmonella* infections in infants may result in septicemia or disseminated focal disease such as meningitis, abscesses, or osteomyelitis. They may also result in asymptomatic intestinal colonization. Some neonates become persistent intestinal carriers of salmonellae, and their cultures may remain positive for more than a year.

Others who are at high risk are the aged, individuals with the acquired immunodeficiency syndrome, and the debilitated. Patients with malignant disease have an unexplained predisposition to the development of salmonellosis, and the frequency of bloodstream invasion in such patients is quite high. People housed in nursing homes represent another segment of hospitalized patients in whom explosive outbreaks may occur with high fatality rates [9].

In a patient with acute gastroenteritis, the isolation of *Salmonella* from a stool culture usually is sufficient to establish the cause of the disease. This is true because of the relatively high degree of pathogenicity of these enteric bacteria, plus the fact that long-term carriers are unusual.

Therapy

Antimicrobial therapy has been shown in numerous studies to prolong the intestinal excretion of salmonellae. Mild, uncomplicated *Salmonella* gastroenteritis should not be treated. However, in patients in whom bloodstream invasion occurs—most commonly newborns, the immunocompromised, or extremely debilitated patients, particularly those with malignant disease—antimicrobials often are instrumental in recovery from infection and may be lifesaving. In general, trimethoprim–sulfamethoxazole, a fluoroquinolone (adults), and ceftriaxone provide the most effective therapy.

In addition to prolonging the period of excretion of the infecting strains, the administration of antimicrobial agents may, on occasion, make the clinical infection more severe or cause clinical relapse of infection when the drug administered is one to which the infecting strain is resistant. Antimicrobial therapy also increases the chance of the infecting organism acquiring additional resistances (see Chapter 14).

Epidemiologic Considerations

Classification of Infections

Incubation periods for salmonellosis vary from 6 to 72 hours. The incubation period varies inversely with the size of the infecting dose. Patients with positive cultures and an onset of gastroenteritis 72 hours or more after admission should be considered to have nosocomial infections. People with onsets within 6 to 72 hours of admission should be considered to have nosocomial infections only when epidemiologic evidence makes nosocomial acquisition likely. Isolation of salmonellae from a patient's stool in the absence of clinical symptoms of gastroenteritis should be reported as a nosocomial infection only if previous stool cultures during hospitalization were negative.

Transmissibility

Whereas person-to-person transmission of *Salmonella* strains is unusual among healthy people outside of the hospital environment, these organisms can be transmitted on the hands of healthcare workers or by person-to-person spread among the aged, debilitated, or newborn patients in the hospital setting. Communicability of this organism from patients to hospital personnel or to community contacts is uncommon because larger doses are necessary to infect healthy people and the precautions routinely used by hospitals in managing patients with gastroenteritis usually are effective.

Incidence

Approximately 50% of infections occur on the newborn service or pediatric floor. The remaining cases occur mainly among patients on the surgical or medical services.

Since 1963, the Centers for Disease Control and Prevention (CDC) has maintained nationwide surveillance of salmonellosis. Between 1963 and 1972, 112 (or 28%) of the total reported outbreaks occurred in institutions (hospitals, nursing homes, and custodial institutions) [10]. Approximately 3,500 cases were reported in these outbreaks among institutionalized populations, which represented 13% of the total reported cases. In 1979, 13% of reported outbreaks in the United States occurred in institutions. These outbreaks accounted for only 1.4% of all the cases occurring in outbreaks that year. The average institutional outbreak involved 6 patients, contrasting with the average noninstitutional outbreak, which involved 69 patients.

Sources and Modes of Acquisition

The nosocomial salmonellosis that occurs in the pediatric population, especially in newborns, is characteristically spread from person to person. The organism is typically introduced into the nursery by an infant who acquired the infection from its mother at delivery, but it can also be introduced by a carrier among the personnel or, more rarely, through foods and medications. Spread from infant to infant within the nursery then occurs on the hands of personnel. Fomites may be important in cross-infections, and persistence of the organism in dust and other environmental sites is sometimes responsible for perpetuating an outbreak. Epidemics have been traced to contaminated delivery room resuscitation equipment and the water baths used for heating infant formula [11]. A commercially distributed, special nutritional formula that contains contaminated egg albumin has caused *Salmonella* Infantis outbreaks when administered orally or by tube feeding. Outbreaks of *Salmonella* Kottbus, a serotype that has a tendency to be excreted from infected bovine mammary glands, have been traced to contamination of human breast milk collected to feed premature infants. Although it is unclear whether the breast milk was primarily or secondarily contaminated, inadequate storage and handling of the milk after collection allowed the organisms to proliferate to significant levels.

Outbreaks in nurseries usually are smaller than those commonly seen in nosocomial *Salmonella* infections in adults [10]. In adult infections, a common source can usually be incriminated. The common source may be previously contaminated, raw, or undercooked meats or other products of food-producing animals (e.g., eggs or milk products), or food that has become contaminated after cooking because of organisms on equipment or surfaces in the kitchen [12,13]. Food contaminated by a short-term *Salmonella* carrier working in the kitchen is much less commonly responsible. On occasion, a medication contaminated by *Salmonella* serves as a vehicle, especially medications containing enzymes and hormones of animal origin (e.g., pepsin, bile salts, vitamins, and endocrine gland extracts). Sporadic cases caused by intermittent exposure to infrequently used medications can produce a puzzling epidemiologic problem that requires a careful case–control approach for its solution (see Chapter 6).

In homes for the aged, epidemics often are initiated by the ingestion of contaminated food, and the epidemic may be perpetuated by cross-infection among debilitated patients by means of healthcare workers (see Chapter 29).

Less frequent sources of *Salmonella* infections include yeast, dried coconut, carmine dye, and inadequately disinfected equipment used on successive patients (e.g., Gomco suction and endoscopy equipment).

The specific serotype of *Salmonella* may provide a clue to the source. Some serotypes commonly infecting humans, such as *Salmonella* Typhimurium, derive from a variety of sources, but some have strong associations with particular sources that may be likely in human infection: *Salmonella* Choleraesuis is associated with porcine sources; *Salmonella* Cubana, with cochineal insects used to prepare carmine dye; *Salmonella* Dublin, with bovines; *Salmonella* Pullorum, with poultry sources; and so on. Many additional correlations exist between serotypes and sources among the > 2,000 serotypes of *Salmonella*. Establishing that several different cases were caused by the same serotype may also be of value in suggesting a common source of infection. This is especially true when cases have occurred sporadically in different hospital areas. For this reason, all *Salmonella* isolated from nosocomial infections should be serotyped.

Control

Safe food-handling practices, as outlined in Chapter 22, are especially important in the prevention of nosocomial salmonellosis. In addition to the prompt epidemiologic identification and removal of common sources and implementation of the measures mentioned earlier in this chapter concerning outbreak management, thorough cleaning and disinfection of fomites and environmental surfaces in a nursery after discharge of infected infants is also important (see Chapter 26). Prophylactic antibiotics are contraindicated as a control measure.

ESCHERICHIA COLI INFECTIONS

General Aspects

Clinical and Microbiologic Features

E. coli can produce gastroenteritis in children and adults by several different mechanisms. Strains that produce keratoconjunctivitis in the guinea pig eye (the Sereny test) tend to produce an invasive, *Shigella*-like illness. Disease caused by such strains appears rare in the United States, although large foodborne outbreaks have been documented. Loose, watery diarrhea, usually mild but sometimes severe and resembling that of cholera, is associated with certain strains of *E. coli* that produce enterotoxins. Both heat-labile and heat-stable toxins have been identified. Disease can be produced by either type of enterotoxin, although both are frequently produced by the same strain. Enterotoxin-producing strains appear to be major causes of travelers' diarrhea and are frequent causes of gastroenteritis in infants living in developing countries. Enterotoxigenic *E. coli* occasionally causes outbreaks of diarrhea in the United States, characteristically traced to contaminated food or water. One large hospital nursery outbreak has been reported [14].

E. coli belonging to the classic enteropathogenic serotypes (EPEC) appears to produce disease by mechanisms not yet fully understood, because disease caused by such strains cannot be explained on the basis of the previously described mechanisms [15]. A high percentage of EPEC strains have been enteroadherent, as seen in HEp-2 tissue culture cells [16]. EPEC has previously been considered a common cause of nursery outbreaks, which sometimes were explosive, with high attack rates and fulminating clinical courses [17]. Reports of such outbreaks are not common in the United States in recent years. Undoubtedly, this relates at least in part to the decreasing availability of serotyping procedures in hospital diagnostic laboratories. During any hospital outbreak of diarrhea, particularly when it has occurred in the newborn nursery, EPEC should be considered in the differential diagnosis.

The clinical expression of EPEC infections varies considerably—probably as a result of differences in pathogenic mechanisms—from minimal, watery diarrhea to fulminating disease with septicemia. There appears to be a great deal of unexplained variability even among strains with the same serotype, and occasional outbreaks occur in newborn nurseries in which attack rates exceed 50% and mortality is high. EPEC outbreaks are almost totally confined to newborn nurseries, and infants and young children, especially those younger than 2 years, appear to be primarily at risk. The association of EPEC disease with the very young may not be totally correct, because infection with such strains is usually considered to occur only in children younger than 4 years of age with diarrhea, and appropriate laboratory tests are performed only in this age group.

Clinicians should be aware that the laboratory procedures used to determine the serogroup of isolates have certain deficiencies. Non-EPEC serotypes that cross-react with EPEC serotypes can agglutinate in pooled test sera to give a false-positive test result that can be identified only by complete serotyping. Also, *E. coli* implicated in cases of diarrhea not belonging to EPEC serotypes and not producing the conventional heat-labile or heat-stable toxins of enterotoxigenic *E. coli* may be *E. coli* that show EPEC-like adherence in HEp-2 cells.

Shigatoxin-producing *E. coli* 0157:H7 is an important cause of acute hemorrhagic colitis. Patients are typically present with bloody diarrhea and severe cramps without important fever. Hemolytic uremic syndrome (HUS) may complicate the illness.

Therapy

Disease caused by enterotoxin-producing strains of *E. coli* was shown to respond favorably to antibiotics to which the organisms are susceptible in studies conducted in Mexico, an area where such disease has a high endemic frequency [18]. The duration and severity of diarrhea are reduced by such therapy. Although controlled trials have not been conducted, antibiotic therapy would appear to be indicated on clinical grounds for *Shigella*-like disease caused by invasive strains, and responses comparable to those seen in treatment of shigellosis (see the section on *Shigella* Infections) might be anticipated.

The value of antimicrobial therapy for EPEC disease is controversial, part of this controversy doubtlessly deriving from the difficulty in ensuring that EPEC was the cause of the gastroenteritis. In some instances, a lack of response to antibiotics may have occurred because EPEC isolated from cases was an incidental finding in disease caused by other agents, especially rotaviruses. When gastroenteritis occurs in a premature or full-term nursery and a causative role can be ascribed to EPEC, uncontrolled trials suggest that orally administered gentamicin, colistin, or neomycin for a 1-week course of treatment may be of value [19]. Systemic antibiotics should also be given to all such patients if sepsis occurs in one or more affected infants. Because the isolation of EPEC in a sporadic case of gastroenteritis is of uncertain value in establishing the cause, such laboratory findings offer little or no guidance for the clinician; the clinical severity of the illness is the only factor useful in deciding whether to institute treatment.

Antimicrobial therapy is not recommended for diarrhea due to *E. coli* 0157:H7 since therapy may predispose to the development of HUS.

Epidemiologic Considerations

Classification of Infections

Incubation periods for EPEC disease are commonly 24 to 48 hours, but they may occasionally be much longer. Children with onset of gastroenteritis 48 hours or longer after admission should be considered to have nosocomial infections, as well as all infants in whom EPEC disease develops at any time during hospitalization after birth in the hospital. Isolation of an enteropathogenic serotype of *E. coli* from a stool culture in the absence of clinical symptoms of gastroenteritis should not be reported as an infection. For consistency in surveillance, an infection should be reported when an EPEC strain is isolated from a patient with gastroenteritis in whom no other recognized pathogen is identified.

Transmissibility

The only known populations at risk for development of nosocomial enteric infections due to *E. coli* strains are newborn infants and young children. When an enteropathogenic *E. coli* strain is introduced into a nursery, hospital personnel and community contacts may become asymptomatic carriers of the organism, especially during an episode of infantile diarrhea, and may serve as an important epidemiologic link in the transmission of the disease to the newborns [20]. Enteric disease caused by enterotoxigenic *E. coli* is only very rarely transmitted from person to person.

Incidence

Enteropathogenic *E. coli* are an unusual cause of infectious nosocomial diarrheal disease caused by bacteria in the NNIS data (see Chapter 30). These organisms are identified by serotype analysis. Outbreaks ascribed to EPEC have become much less common since the mid-1980s. Only a few outbreaks of nosocomial disease caused by enterotoxin-producing *E. coli* have been reported [14].

Sources and Modes of Acquisition

The most common source of EPEC infections is an infected child admitted to a newborn nursery or readmitted to a pediatric ward. The infant may have acquired the infection at the time of delivery or may have acquired the organism during hospitalization and had an onset of enteric disease in the early days after discharge from the hospital. Secondary spread of the infecting strain to other infants occurs on the hands of hospital personnel or from articles in the nursery that have been contaminated with the strain during an epidemic. Pharyngeal colonization of infants is common during epidemics and, although unproved, may be an important intermediate step in producing disease in some cases. Proliferation of organisms at this site might produce an inoculum that is capable of establishing infection in the lower gastrointestinal tract.

Epidemics of infantile EPEC diarrhea have occurred at times when the organism can be detected in the dust and fomites in the hospital environment. Asymptomatic carriers are probably important as a cause of epidemics among susceptible infants and include antepartum mothers, hospital staff, or other children without disease. During periods of infantile diarrhea outbreaks, ~ 5% of pediatric patients without intestinal infection and up to one third of antepartum women have been shown to harbor EPEC organisms in their stool. Outbreaks in the nursery usually follow the introduction of a new serotype of EPEC by a newly admitted, infected child or by colonized hospital personnel. The infecting strain is transmitted among children, usually on the hands of attendants or through articles and equipment in communal use.

A single, large, protracted nosocomial outbreak caused by a strain of *E. coli* that produced heat-stable enterotoxin and did not belong to a recognized enteropathogenic serotype has been reported [14]. The disease appears to have been transmitted by means of cross-contamination of oral feedings. The epidemic strain did not colonize or produce disease in adults despite its presence in multiple environmental sites. Illness was mild and characterized by 3 to 5 days of watery diarrhea without pus or blood in the stools. Prophylactic oral colistin, to which the multiply drug-resistant strain was sensitive, was ineffective in preventing acquisition. Antibiotic resistance and enterotoxin production were colinked on a transmissible plasmid of the epidemic strain [21].

Control

Control measures mentioned earlier in this chapter and elsewhere [22] can be helpful in curtailing an EPEC outbreak. Such measures are not indicated, however, unless a causative role can be ascribed to an EPEC strain on the basis of the previously outlined criteria. Colonization of infants with an EPEC strain in the absence of enteric disease attributable to the strain is not an indication for control measures.

Enterotoxigenic *E. coli* strains are believed to be transmitted mainly by food and water, and prevention of disease from these sources can be accomplished by proper food handling and chlorination of water supplies

SHIGELLA INFECTIONS

General Aspects

Clinical and Microbiologic Features

Shigellosis, or bacillary dysentery, often represents a distinct clinical entity. Fever develops in 50% of the patients, and mucus with or without blood can be documented in the stool within 1 or 2 days after the onset of diarrhea. Patients are usually more toxic and symptoms more severe with this form of enteric infection than with others.

When newborns are infected by a *Shigella* strain, the mortality is higher, and complications (e.g., intestinal perforation and septicemia) develop with a higher frequency than in other common bacterial causes of gastroenteritis [23,24]. Although there is some evidence that breast-fed infants show an increased resistance to *Shigella*, nearly all hosts are extremely susceptible to these organisms.

Shigella sonnei and *Shigella flexneri* are the species principally responsible for disease in the United States. *S. sonnei* strains can be differentiated from one another by colicin typing, and *S. flexneri* strains by serotyping. Clinicians should be aware that *Salmonella–Shigella* agar, a popular medium for stool cultures in many clinical laboratories, is toxic to many *S. flexneri* strains. For optimal recovery of strains, specimens should not be placed in holding or transport media but should be plated directly onto blood or xylose, lysine, and deoxycholate agar as soon as possible after collection.

Therapy

In bacillary dysentery, appropriate antimicrobial agents are clearly beneficial in decreasing the excretion of the pathogenic shigellae and improving clinical symptoms. A fluoroquinolone is the treatment of choice in adults when susceptibility data are not available. Because of the potential toxicity of quinolones, trimethoprim–sulfamethoxazole is the treatment of choice for empiric therapy in children and pregnant women. A 3- to 5-day course usually is adequate. For children infected by trimethoprim-resistant shigellae, nalidixic acid 55 mg/kg/day in four equally divided doses or, for mild to moderately severe cases, furazolidone 7.5 mg/kg/day in four equally divided doses for 5 days is recommended. Antibiotic therapy is associated with the emergence of multiple drug resistance in originally sensitive strains, which is presumably caused by R-factor transfer from endogenous gastrointestinal flora. Thus, patients should remain in enteric isolation until posttreatment cultures are negative.

Epidemiologic Considerations

Classification of Infections

Incubation periods for shigellosis vary from 1 to 6 days. Patients with positive cultures and an onset of gastroenteritis 24 hours or more after admission should be considered to have nosocomial infections unless epidemiologic evidence of community-acquired infection is found (e.g., occurrence of shigellosis in family contacts before the onset of the patient's illness). Isolation of shigellae from a patient's stool in the absence of clinical symptoms of gastroenteritis should be reported as a nosocomial infection only if previous stool cultures during hospitalization were negative, or isolation occurs during a documented hospital outbreak due to the recovered strain.

Transmissibility

Although *Shigella* strains represent the most potentially communicable of the bacterial pathogens, the striking clinical disease often helps the physician spot the illness early and promptly institute effective therapy and control measures. Such early detection partly explains the usual, surprising lack of spread in the normal hospital environment. Other patients, hospital personnel, and community contacts appear to be at risk for development of bacillary dysentery when exposed to an infected patient because of the very low dose of organisms (less than 10^2) necessary to produce disease.

Incidence

Although any hospitalized patient is at risk for development of nosocomial shigellosis when a case is admitted, only rarely do outbreaks occur [25]. The only population at high risk is that of people housed in residential institutions for the mentally retarded, where crowded living conditions, poor personal hygiene, and overworked nursing personnel all appear to be important causes of serious outbreaks.

Shigellosis was reported in only 1 of the 3,363 patients with nosocomial enteric infections during the 1986 to 1989 period in NNIS data [26]. How many of the 10,000 to 13,000 cases of shigellosis reported each year in the

United States come from hospitals is unknown. Between 10% and 20% of the cases of shigellosis reported each year, however, originate in residential institutions for the retarded.

Sources and Modes of Acquisition

The usual sources are short-term carriers of the organism who are either ill or in the convalescent stages of their disease. In custodial institutions, a few long-term carriers may be present and may serve as an important reservoir. Long-term carriage, however, is rare. On occasion, shigellosis develops when contaminated food is ingested that was prepared by a person carrying the organism after an episode of disease. Most cases, however, are secondary to person-to-person spread of infection. Infections are rarely acquired by indirect contact spread from inanimate environmental sources because these organisms are able to survive only for short periods in the environment.

Control

Antibiotics are effective in eradicating sensitive strains of *Shigella* from the gastrointestinal tract, but, as noted earlier, infecting strains have a propensity to develop multiple drug resistance in response to therapy. Thus, treatment of culture-positive patients should be coupled with individual enteric isolation procedures for each patient to prevent the potential emergence and continued spread of a strain that has acquired additional antibiotic resistances (see Chapter 14).

Living, orally administered vaccine strains of *Shigella* have been tested as potential immunoprophylactic agents in several studies. The duration of protection is short. Furthermore, multiple oral doses of vaccine must be given, vaccine strains can be transmitted to nonimmunized patients, and there is a potential risk of reversion of some of these strains to virulent organisms.

VIRAL GASTROENTERITIS

Rotaviruses have been shown to be important causes of nosocomial gastroenteritis [27–29]. Nosocomial transmission of rotavirus [28–31], hepatitis A virus [32], and adenoviruses [31] has been documented. Nosocomial adenoviral gastroenteritis, which appears to be much less frequent than rotaviral infections and produces milder clinical illness, is not discussed in this section.

Although the transmission of hepatitis A infection is rare in the hospital setting, it is mentioned here briefly because of the occasional presentation of patients with unexplained diarrhea caused by hepatitis A (see Chapter 42). The diarrhea may antedate the onset of clinical jaundice by several days, or jaundice may not occur. The high titers of infectious virus in the stool during the preicteric phase make these patients excellent sources of hepatitis A nosocomial infection in settings in which good handwashing practices are not followed.

Incidence of Rotavirus Infections

Rotaviruses are the most frequent enteric pathogens found in people younger than 5 years in the United States (see Chapter 42). They have also been established as the leading cause of nosocomial infectious gastroenteritis in pediatric patients. Prospective studies in hospital nurseries have shown 33% to 70% of the infants may shed rotavirus in the stool by the fifth day of life, with 8% to 28% of those shedding the virus demonstrating clinical symptoms [3,33,34]. Similar studies in pediatric patients have shown rotaviruses to account for nearly one half of all nosocomial infectious gastroenteritis [3,4,28]. Data from the NNIS System for 1986 to 1989 recorded rotavirus as the causative agent in 75% of pediatric patients with nosocomial infectious gastroenteritis and in 51% of such patients in high-risk nurseries [26]. When patients are stratified by age, rotavirus is far more likely to cause nosocomial infectious gastroenteritis in patients younger than 2 years [3]. Infection rates tend to follow the seasonal pattern observed in the general community, with peak incidence in the winter and spring and lowest incidence in the summer [3].

Although less common in adults, rotaviruses may be responsible for nosocomial infectious gastroenteritis in this age group. Yolken and colleagues [35] found rotaviruses to be the causative agent in 9 of 31 patients who experienced infectious diarrhea on a bone marrow transplant unit. Outbreaks of rotavirus infection have also been reported in hospitalized geriatric patients [1] and in elderly patients on a long-stay ward [36]. For the period 1986 to 1989, the NNIS System found rotavirus to account for 4% and 2% of the nosocomial infectious gastroenteritis on oncology services and general surgical services, respectively, but for less than 1% of such disease on other adult services.

Clinical Aspects

Illness begins with the sudden onset of fever, abdominal pain, and vomiting and continues with moderate or severe watery diarrhea that usually lasts ~ 3 to 8 days. Rotavirus disease severe enough to require hospitalization occurs in 2% of all children during their lifetime [37]. Rotavirus can be identified in the stool or heavily inoculated rectal swab specimens from infected patients through direct or immune electron microscopy. Commercially available kits for the accurate and rapid identification of rotavirus are available. These kits make use of either a modified enzyme-linked immunosorbent assay or latex agglutination. Because of the high incidence of asymptomatic shedding of rotavirus in children younger than 2 years of age, positive assays in isolated cases must be interpreted with caution.

Sources and Modes of Acquisition

Rotavirus disease appears to be highly infectious, and it can be spread from patients with disease to susceptible people by direct contact. The peak incidence in winter suggests that droplet spread from the upper respiratory tract may play a role in transmission, because respiratory spread is a common feature of most illnesses with seasonal peaks in the winter. Infants admitted to the hospital shedding rotavirus are the major sources of nosocomial outbreaks [38]. Nosocomial transmission probably occurs indirectly from patient to patient on the hands of hospital personnel as well as by person-to-person spread from patients with disease to susceptible people when such patients are inadequately isolated. Hospital personnel usually are immune and do not carry the virus.

Prevention and Control

Rotaviruses are highly immunogenic, and serologic studies indicate a high level of acquired immunity in people older than 5 years of age. These findings raise the possibility of ultimate control of the disease by vaccine. Vaccine candidates are being tested for safety and efficacy [39,40]. Children with nosocomial nonbacterial gastroenteritis should be placed on enteric precautions; although not currently recommended in CDC guidelines, consideration should be given to the use of masks on older children to prevent potential droplet transmission when they are transported out of the isolation area.

CLOSTRIDIUM DIFFICILE INFECTION

General Aspects

Clinical and Microbiologic Features

C. difficile produces a spectrum of clinical illness ranging from mild diarrhea to fulminant pseudomembranous colitis. Characteristically, *C. difficile* disease causes profuse diarrhea and fever that are temporally related to having received antimicrobial therapy in an institutional setting. Stools often contain mucus and blood.

It is generally believed that the administration of antimicrobials disrupts the normal flora of the bowel. This, in turn, allows the proliferation of *C. difficile*, with a resulting release of toxins that cause mucosal injury, inflammation, and fluid secretion [41].

Therapy

In patients with mild disease, the initial management should consist of discontinuing antimicrobial therapy or switching to an antimicrobial that is less predisposing to *C. difficile* disease (see section on Sources and Modes of Acquisition) whenever possible. Many patients respond to this approach alone. In patients who require continuation of their antimicrobial therapy, who do not respond to discontinuation or change in antimicrobials, or who have more severe disease, both oral metronidazole and oral vancomycin have proven effective. Because of increasing vancomycin resistance among the gram-positive cocci, CDC guidelines have encouraged the use of metronidazole as the agent of choice for the treatment of *C. difficile* infection.

Epidemiologic Considerations

Classification of Infections

The diagnosis of *C. difficile* infection in most cases depends on the demonstration of *C. difficile* toxin in the stool.

Transmissibility

Although direct patient-to-patient spread is uncommon, *C. difficile* is easily spread in the hospital setting from infected and colonized patients to their environment. Most transmission is thought to occur through hand carriage by healthcare workers.

Incidence

Prospective studies have documented that ~ 1% of healthy adults and 7% of patients being admitted to the hospital are colonized with *C. difficile*. One fifth of all adults admitted to general hospital units become colonized with *C. difficile*, with colonization becoming more prevalent with increasing length of stay. Of those patients who become colonized, diarrhea develops in approximately one third. Approximately 20% to 30% of pseudomembranous colitis is caused by *C. difficile*.

C. difficile outbreaks may occur among geriatric populations in general hospitals or among the elderly residents of long-term care facilities [42]. In the pediatric population, over half of all healthy neonates are asymptomatic carriers of *C. difficile*. However, disease in this population is rare.

Sources and Modes of Acquisition

The major reservoir for *C. difficile* in the hospital setting is patients who are colonized or infected with *C. dif-*

ficile. A relatively high prevalence of culture positivity for *C. difficile* at admission to tertiary care hospitals helps to explain the high rates of infection in these settings [43]. Patients with symptomatic disease heavily contaminate their immediate hospital environment, and this contamination can be demonstrated to persist for months. The hands of healthcare workers who care for these patients also become contaminated with the organism, and routine handwashing with non–antiseptic-containing soaps frequently does not remove these bacteria.

The major risk factors for *C. difficile* acquisition are hospitalization and antimicrobial administration. Antimicrobials active against anaerobic bacteria, such as clindamycin and the β-lactam antimicrobials, are most frequently associated with *C. difficile* colonization and disease. Although less important, gastrointestinal surgery and impaired host defense also appear to be associated with *C. difficile* acquisition.

Control

The most important measure for prevention of *C. difficile* transmission is good handwashing practices. Although there are data to support the use of antiseptic-containing handwashing agents, this issue remains unsettled. Patients identified with *C. difficile* disease should be placed in enteric precautions (see Chapter 13). The role of isolation in managing patients with asymptomatic carriage has not been determined. Nosocomial epidemics of *C. difficile* may be controlled by restricting use of antimicrobials, particularly clindamycin [44].

OTHER GASTROINTESTINAL DISEASES

Staphylococcal Enterocolitis

In contrast to *C. difficile* colitis, staphylococcal enterocolitis is not transmissible from person to person; however, the disease may be an important source from which nosocomial strains of *S. aureus* can be transmitted.

Incidence

The true incidence of such infections is unknown. Since the appreciation of *C. difficile* as the common cause of pseudomembranous colitis, the reported incidence of staphylococcal enterocolitis has dropped sharply. No cases were reported in the NNIS reporting period of 1986 to 1989 [26]. Staphylococcal enterocolitis occurs sporadically, and epidemics have not been reported.

Clinical Aspects

In certain hosts in whom there is impaired resistance due to surgery, antimicrobial therapy, alcoholism, or diabetes mellitus, staphylococci may grow to large numbers in the intestinal tract and be responsible for morphologic damage to the intestinal mucosa that results in diarrhea and fever of varying severity. Intestinal involvement varies widely from minimal and self-limiting enteritis to fulminating pseudomembranous enterocolitis [45]. Patients with enteritis have diarrhea of a variable nature, often mild and watery, and may have low-grade fever, but they are not extremely toxic. Pseudomembranous enterocolitis frequently presents with fulminating and dehydrating diarrhea; bloody, mucoid stools; fever; leukocytosis; and toxemia. The entire colon may be involved with the disease, and there may be some involvement of the small intestine. Mortality in such patients is high and ranges from 10% to 50%.

The diagnosis is established by documenting abundant polymorphonuclear leukocytes and sheets of gram-positive cocci in stool specimens, which on subsequent culture grow large numbers of *S. aureus*. Proctologic examination shows a white membrane that reflects areas of mucosal necrosis in those with pseudomembranous enterocolitis.

Patients should receive replacement fluid and electrolytes. Both oral vancomycin [46] and fecal retention enemas containing stool flora from a healthy person (the latter may have only historical significance) have been shown to be of value in treating patients with serious forms of the disease. Parenteral semisynthetic penicillinase-resistant penicillin treatment is advised for very toxic patients.

Sources and Modes of Acquisition

S. aureus can be cultured from the stool of ~ 10% of normal adults, but it is usually present in small numbers. Intestinal carriage of these organisms is twice as common in hospitalized patients as in people outside the hospital environment. Most strains that cause staphylococcal enterocolitis are multiply drug resistant, and some have been shown to produce an enterotoxin in laboratory tests. Pathogenic strains are probably acquired mainly from nosocomial sources, and they proliferate to displace normal flora when antibiotics to which they are resistant are administered. Staphylococcal enterotoxin is probably not important in the pathogenesis of the disease, because otherwise clinically identical pseudomembranous enterocolitis occurs after infection with nonenterotoxigenic strains. Destruction or replacement of normal endogenous flora is probably the principal inciting factor.

Prevention and Control

Prompt cessation of previously administered antibiotics and administration of oral vancomycin to patients with more serious staphylococcal enteritis may prevent the disease from progressing to pseudomembranous enterocolitis. Large numbers of *S. aureus* are often disseminated from patients with these diseases, and strict, rather than enteric, isolation procedures should be considered (see Chapter 13).

Neonatal Necrotizing Enterocolitis

Neonatal necrotizing enterocolitis (NEC) is a frequently fatal disease that usually affects low-birthweight infants with preexistent perinatal complications. The disease is characterized by ischemic necrosis of the gastrointestinal tract and intramural gas (pneumatosis intestinalis), and it frequently results in intestinal perforation, peritonitis, and septicemia. NEC often occurs in epidemics in nurseries, which suggests an infectious cause. Three pathogenetic factors underlie the occurrence of disease: injury to the intestinal mucosa, due to relative ischemia from stress in newborns or other causes; the presence of intraluminal enteric bacteria; and enteral feedings that provide a metabolic substrate for the bacteria.

Most reports of NEC have not incriminated a particular bacterium as a cause of the disease, perhaps indicating that many strains of gram-negative bacteria or viruses may be involved in its pathogenesis. However, a particular strain of bacteria prevalent in the nursery has occasionally been linked with an epidemic of NEC [47]. The prophylactic use of systemic antibiotics does not prevent colonization of an infant's gastrointestinal tract with gram-negative bacteria, and most studies have shown no efficacy of such drugs in preventing NEC. The prophylactic use of oral kanamycin, however, appeared effective in one study [48], as did oral administration of IgA-IgG given to low-birthweight infants [49].

Additional studies of sporadic and epidemic NEC cases, including careful aerobic and anaerobic culture studies of cases and control subjects, should assist in determining the role of microorganisms in this disease.

Yersinia enterocolitica Infections

Nosocomial transmission of infections caused by *Y. enterocolitica* has rarely been reported, but it probably occurs far more commonly than reports indicate. The organism, a gram-negative rod, can easily be misidentified, and sometimes prolonged cold enrichment is required for its optimal recovery from stool specimens. Early symptoms are usually those of fever and acute enterocolitis, and the abdominal pains are frequently so similar to those of appendicitis that appendectomies are performed. Mesenteric adenitis or ileitis usually is discovered. A wide variety of other features can be seen, including arthritis and erythema nodosum. Although the reservoir of the organism is in animals, person-to-person transmission also occurs, and nosocomial transmission has sometimes involved personnel [50].

A more deliberate search for this organism in otherwise unexplained nosocomial gastroenteritis outbreaks should be encouraged when clinical features suggest it is a possible causative agent. In addition to culture studies, serologic tests may be helpful in establishing the diagnosis of infection with this organism.

Other Pathogens

In addition to the enteropathogens discussed, outbreaks of nosocomial gastroenteritis have been caused by *Citrobacter freundii* [51], *Listeria monocytogenes* [34], and a variety of other agents. Although *Campylobacter jejuni* was encountered only rarely in the NNIS survey, it will undoubtedly prove to be an important cause of nosocomial gastroenteritis now that the organism can be readily identified in hospital laboratories. The ability of pathogens other than those normally associated with gastrointestinal disease to produce gastroenteritis must be remembered when evaluating an outbreak. The clinician should be cautious not to dismiss lightly unusual pathogens recovered from stool cultures during the investigation of nosocomial enterocolitis.

REFERENCES

1. Kelly TWJ, Patrick MR, Hillman KM. Study of diarrhea in critically ill patients. *Crit Care Med* 1983;11:7.
2. Lima N, Searcy M, Guerrant R. Nosocomial diarrhea rates exceed those of other nosocomial infections on ICU and pediatric wards [Abstract 1050]. In: *Proceedings of the Interscience Conference on Antimicrobial Agents and Chemotherapy*. Washington, DC: American Society of Microbiology; 1986.
3. Brady MT, Pacini DL, Budde CT, Connell MJ. Diagnostic studies of nosocomial diarrhea in children: assessing their use and value. *Am J Infect Control* 1989;17:77.
4. Welliver RC, McLaughlin S. Unique epidemiology of nosocomial infections in a children's hospital. *American Journal of Diseases of Children* 1984;138:131.
5. Edes TE, Walk BE, Austin JL. Diarrhea in tube-fed patients: feeding formula not necessarily the cause. *Am J Med* 1990;88:91.
6. Kaczmarek RG, Moore RM, McCrohan J, et al. Multi-state investigation of the actual disinfection/sterilization of endoscopes in healthcare facilities. *Am J Med* 1992;92:257.
7. Martin MA, Reichelderfer M. APIC guideline for infection prevention and control in flexible endoscopy. *Am J Infect Control* 1994;22:19.
8. Spach DH, Silverstein FE, Stamm WE. Transmission of infection by gastrointestinal endoscopy and bronchoscopy. *Ann Intern Med* 1993; 118:117.
9. Taylor JL, et al. Simultaneous outbreak of *Salmonella enteriditis* and *Salmonella schwarzengrund* in a nursing home: association of *S. enteriditis* with bacteremia and hospitalization. *J Infect Dis* 1993;167: 781.
10. Baine WB, Gangarosa EJ, Bennett JV, Barker WH, Jr. Institutional salmonellosis. *J Infect Dis* 1973;128:357.
11. Schroeder SA, Aserkoff R, Brachman PS. Epidemic salmonellosis in hospitals and institutions: a five-year review. *N Engl J Med* 1968;279: 674.
12. Hirsch W, et al. *Salmonella edinburg* infection in children: a protracted hospital epidemic due to a multiple drug resistant strain. Lancet 1965; 2:828.
13. Mackerras IM, Mackerras MJ. An epidemic of infantile gastro-enteritis in Queensland caused by *Salmonella bovis-morbificans* (Basenau). *Journal of Hygiene (Cambridge)* 1949;47:166.

14. Ryder RW, et al. Infantile diarrhea produced by heat-stable enterotoxigenic *Escherichia coli. N Engl J Med* 1976;295:849.
15. Goldschmidt MC, DuPont HL. Enteropathogenic *Escherichia coli*: lack of correlation of serotype with pathogenicity. *J Infect Dis* 1976;133: 153.
16. Cravioto A, Gross RJ, Scotland SM, Rowe B. An adhesive factor found in strains of *Escherichia coli* belonging to the traditional infantile enteropathogenic serotypes. *Curr Microbiol* 1979;3:95.
17. Taylor J. Infectious infantile enteritis, yesterday and today. *Proc R Soc Med* 1970;63:1297.
18. Oberhelman RH, et al. Efficacy of trimethoprim-sulfamethoxazole in treatment of acute diarrhea in a Mexican pediatric population. *J Pediatr* 1987;110:960.
19. DuPont HL, Pickering LK. *Infections of the gastrointestinal tract: microbiology, pathophysiology, and clinical features*. New York: Plenum; 1980.
20. Rogers KB. The spread of infantile gastroenteritis in a cubicled ward. *Journal of Hygiene (London)* 1951;49:40.
21. Wachsmuth IK, Falkow S, Ryder RW. Plasmid-mediated properties of a heat-stable enterotoxin-producing *Escherichia coli* associated with infantile diarrhea. *Infect Immun* 1976;14:403.
22. Harris AH, et al. Control of epidemic diarrhea of the newborn in hospital nurseries and pediatric wards. *Ann NY Acad Sci* 1956;66:118.
23. Haltalin KC. Neonatal shigellosis: report of 16 cases and review of the literature. *American Journal of Diseases of Children* 1967;114:603.
24. Whitfield C, Humphries JM. Meningitis and septicemia due to *Shigellae* in a newborn infant. *J Pediatr* 1967;70:805.
25. Salzman TC, Scher CD, Moss R. Shigellae with transferable drug resistance: outbreak in a nursery for premature infants. *J Pediatr* 1967; 71:21.
26. Centers for Disease Control and Prevention, National Nosocomial Infections Surveillance (NNIS) System, Hospital Infections Program, Atlanta, GA, Robert Gaynes, M.D., personal communication.
27. Echeverria P, Blacklow NR, Smith DH. Role of heat-labile toxigenic *Escherichia coli* and reovirus-like agent in diarrhea in Boston children. *Lancet* 1975;2:1113.
28. Ford-Jones EL, Mindorff CM, Gold R, Petric M. The incidence of viral-associated diarrhea after admission to a pediatric hospital. *Am J Epidemiol* 1990;131:711.
29. Ryder RW, McGowan JE, Hatch MH, Palmer EL. Reovirus-like agent as a cause of nosocomial diarrhea in infants. *J Pediatr* 1977;90:698.
30. Davidson GP, et al. Importance of a new virus in acute sporadic enteritis in children. *Lancet* 1975;1:242.
31. Flewett TH, Boyden AS, Davies H. Epidemic viral enteritis in a long-stay children's ward. *Lancet* 1975;1:4.
32. Goodman RA, et al. Nosocomial hepatitis A transmission by an adult patient with diarrhea. *Am J Med* 1982;73:220.
33. Jayashree S, Bhan MK, Raj P, et al. Neonatal rotavirus infection and its relation to cord blood antibodies. *Scand J Infect Dis* 1988;20:249.
34. Larsson S, et al. *Listeria monocytogenes* causing hospital-acquired enterocolitis and meningitis in newborn infants. *Br Med J* 1978;2:473.
35. Yolken RH, et al. Infectious gastroenteritis in bone marrow transplant recipients. *N Engl J Med* 1982;306:1009.
36. Cubitt WD, Holzel H. An outbreak of rotavirus infection in a long-stay ward of a geriatric hospital. *J Clin Pathol* 1980;33:306.
37. Centers for Disease Control and Prevention. Viral agents of gastroenteritis: public health importance and outbreak management. *MMWR Morb Mortal Wkly Rep* 1990;39(RR-5):1.
38. Gaggero A, Avendaño LF, Fernández J, Spencer E. Nosocomial transmission of rotavirus from patients admitted with diarrhea. *J Clin Microbiol* 1992;30:3294.
39. Flores J, et al. Reactions to and antigenicity of two human–rhesus rotavirus reassortant vaccine candidates of serotype 1 and serotype 2 in Venezuelan infants. *J Clin Microbiol* 1989;27:512.
40. Bernstein DI, et al. Evaluation of rhesus rotavirus monovalent and tetravalent reassortant vaccines in U.S, children. *JAMA* 1995;273:1191.
41. Bartlett JC. Antibiotic-associated diarrhea. *Clin Infect Dis* 1992;15:573.
42. Simor AE, Yake SL, Tsimidis K. Infection due to *Clostridium difficile* among elderly residents of a long-term-care facility. *Clin Infect Dis* 1993;17:672.
43. Samore MH, et al. *Clostridium difficile* colonization and diarrhea at a tertiary care hospital. *Clin Infect Dis* 1994;18:181.
44. Pear SM, et al. Diarrhea in nosocomial *Clostridium difficile*-associated diarrhea by restricting clindamycin use. *Ann Intern Med* 1994;120:272.
45. Dearing WH, Baggenstoss AH, Weed LA. Studies on the relationship of *Staphylococcus aureus* to pseudomembranous enterocolitis and to postantibiotic enteritis. *Gastroenterology* 1960;38:441.
46. Khan MY, Hall WH. Staphylococcal enterocolitis: treatment with oral vancomycin. *Ann Intern Med* 1966;65:1.
47. Hill HR, Hunt CE, Matsen JM. Nosocomial colonization with *Klebsiella*, type 26, in a neonatal intensive care unit associated with an outbreak of sepsis, meningitis, and necrotizing enterocolitis. *J Pediatr* 1974;85:415.
48. Egan EA, Mantilla G, Nelson RM, Eitzman DV. A prospective controlled trial of oral kanamycin in the prevention of neonatal necrotizing enterocolitis. *J Pediatr* 1976;89:467.
49. Eibl MM, Wolf HM, Fürnkranz H, Rosenkranz A. Prevention of necrotizing enterocolitis in low-birth-weight infants by IgA-IgG feeding. *N Engl J Med* 1988;319:1.
50. Toivanen P, Toivanen A, Olkkonen L, Aantaa S. Hospital outbreak of *Yersinia enterocolitica* infection. *Lancet* 1973;1:801.
51. Parida SN, Verma IC, Deb M, Bhujwala RA. An outbreak of diarrhea due to *Citrobacter freundii* in a neonatal special care nursery. *Indian J Pediatr* 1980;47:81.

Hospital Infections, Fourth Edition,
edited by John V. Bennett and Philip S. Brachman.
Lippincott–Raven Publishers, Philadelphia © 1998

CHAPTER 35

Puerperal Endometritis

William J. Ledger

NATURE OF INFECTIONS

Incidence

There is good evidence that the incidence of puerperal endometritis reported from individual hospitals with active surveillance of these infections (1% to 4%) is probably unchanged from the most accurate figures available from the preantibiotic decade of the 1920s. This statement is not an apology for modern obstetrics, for the status of puerperal endometritis and sepsis has dramatically changed in that same time interval. The incidence of cesarean sections has increased from < 5% to >20%, and these have a higher risk of infection, whereas the most severe infections—those resulting in maternal death from sepsis—have virtually been eliminated from modern obstetrics.

The actual incidence of puerperal endometritis is higher than that noted in the National Nosocomial Infections Study (NNIS; see Chapter 30), in which an incidence of <1% was found. Possible reasons for this lower incidence are noted in the following sections.

Deficiencies in Reporting Infections

Obstetricians tend to underestimate the incidence of nosocomial infections, including postpartum endometritis. This phenomenon of individual physician inaccuracy in assessing the frequency of infections reflects commonly observed patterns of clinical practice. Most patients with the early symptoms of a postpartum endometritis, such as temperature elevation, are first discovered at night and not during the traditional early-morning rounds of physicians [1] (Figure 35-1). In most occasions, these patients are placed on systemic antibiotics without prior culture studies. A nationwide evaluation of over 12,000 women undergoing hysterectomy who were cared for by obstetrician–gynecologists revealed that > 50% had received systemic antibiotics without prior culture tests [2]. A rapid response of the patient to the administered antibiotics with a quick return of temperature levels to normal may cause the attending physician to disregard the case as "true" morbidity. In addition, early discharge of patients from the hospital under the Diagnosis-Related Groups system or because of pressures for early discharge from Health Maintenance Organizations or other insurance organizations means that many infections will be diagnosed outside of the hospital. Thus, any nationwide survey will detect only a portion of all cases of endometritis during any study interval. Despite the fact that some cases are inevitably missed by surveillance systems such as that of the NNIS, pooled microbiologic data from cases that are reported do provide an assessment of the pathogens involved in postpartum endometritis. The failure of many hospitals to provide adequate anaerobic microbiology means that the importance of anaerobes in these mixed bacterial infections is often overlooked.

Underestimates of the incidence of endometritis in modern obstetrics are also based on continued dependence on a preantibiotic-era definition of morbidity based on temperature elevations. This definition was established by American obstetrician–gynecologists between the First and Second World Wars, and it is based on four separate oral temperature recordings each postpartum day; *morbidity* is defined as an oral temperature of 38°C (100.4°F) or greater on any 2 of the first 10 postpartum days, excluding the first 24 hours after delivery. This is in contrast to the early discharge system now in place, which precluded these observations for 10 days. Modern obstetrics has in-house observation for 1 day after vaginal delivery and 2 days after cesarean section. The old definition excluded from consideration patients with one temperature elevation shortly after delivery as well as those who had a single temperature elevation later but no evidence

W. J. Ledger: Department of Obstetrics and Gynecology, The New York Hospital–Cornell Medical Center, New York, New York 10021.

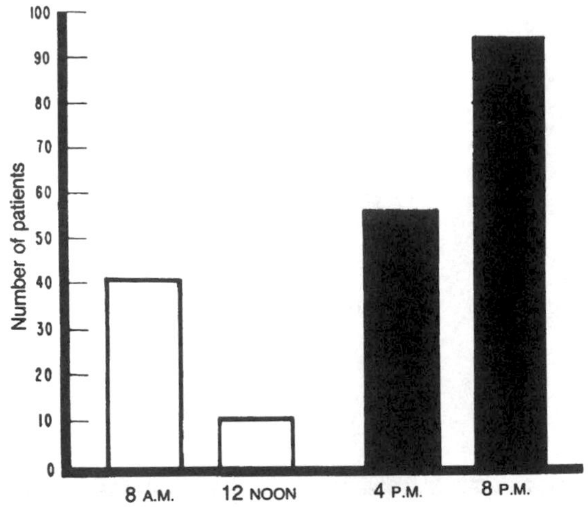

FIGURE 35-1. The first temperature elevation of obstetric patients with postpartum morbidity. Most patients had initial rises in the late afternoon or evening hours.

of a postpartum pelvic infection. On a statistical basis, nearly all the women from the preantibiotic era who met these temperature criteria for morbidity had a pelvic infection, whether uterine or urinary tract. Appropriate microbiologic studies could be performed, and such patients could be isolated from other obstetric patients. Most of these patients now are being treated at home.

Another great setback for a clear understanding of infectious disease in antibiotic-era obstetrics has been adherence to this old standard in the face of antibiotic use. Use of powerful systemic antibiotics in postpartum patients with the first elevation of temperature may yield an immediate clinical response with rapid and persistent defervescence of fever. If the obstetric service adheres to traditional temperature-defined morbidity standards, the patient is not counted in morbidity statistics. This accounts in part for the frequent discrepancy between the low recorded morbidity figures and the high systemic antibiotic use in obstetric units.

Community-Acquired Versus Nosocomial Infections

All postpartum endometritis should be considered a nosocomial infection, unless the amniotic fluid is infected at the time of admission or the patient was admitted 24 hours or more after rupture of the membranes. Some infections in the latter group are nosocomial, however, and available microbiologic, clinical, and epidemiologic data should be carefully reviewed to determine whether the infection is community acquired or nosocomial.

Mechanisms of Infection

The uterus has excellent local defense mechanisms to protect itself against invasion by contaminating organisms from the lower genital tract. These defenses are present in the nonpregnant state, as is demonstrated by the rapid clearance of the lower genital tract bacteria that are carried into the endometrial cavity during the insertion of an intrauterine device [3]. During pregnancy, Galask and associates [4] have demonstrated inhibition of bacterial growth by the amniotic fluid. The labor and delivery results in uterine acquisition of organisms from the varied flora of the lower genital tract, but most postpartum patients remain free of symptoms because the uterus rapidly clears itself of the potentially pathogenic bacteria introduced from the vagina. This upward passage of bacteria occurs with labor, but is enhanced by vaginal examination during labor. In women with premature rupture of membranes, vaginal examination increases the risk of infection and hastens the onset of labor [5].

Postpartum endometritis occurs when these efficient uterine defense mechanisms are overcome by a combination of too many bacteria, the introduction of especially virulent bacterial strains, or local alterations (e.g., soft tissue damage or the incomplete removal of the placenta) that provide a nidus for a postpartum infection. The virulence of organisms is probably a more important factor than was realized in the past. The increased risk for infection in women with bacterial vaginosis reflects the greater risks with an overgrowth of many different strains of bacteria, particularly anaerobes [6].

Postpartum pelvic infection follows a pattern of progression (Figure 35-2), with ascension of the organisms into the endometrial cavity, invasion of the myometrium, extension into parametrial areas beyond the uterus, and bloodstream invasion in some instances [7]. If this progression is unchecked by the appropriate use of systemic antibiotics, then myometrial, parametrial, or adnexal abscesses can occur with suppurative involvement of the pelvic veins, septic pelvic thrombophlebitis, and even distant septic metastases to the liver and lung. In addition to the appropriate use of systemic medical agents, adequate uterine drainage must be ensured, and intervention for the drainage or removal of a pelvic abscess may be necessary for cure. This can occur even when what seem to be appropriate antibiotics are used. A subhepatic abscess has been reported after cesarean sections [8] and necrotizing fasciitis have been seen in postpartum patients [9]. These serious infections still occur.

PREDISPOSING HOST FACTORS

Host Susceptibility

The better-nourished pregnant patient with a middle-class background is far less likely to have infectious problems than her poorly nourished, anemic, lower-class counterpart, a victim of her social class. The latter class increased in numbers since 1980, as did the abuse of drugs in this population. Drug abuse had an impact on

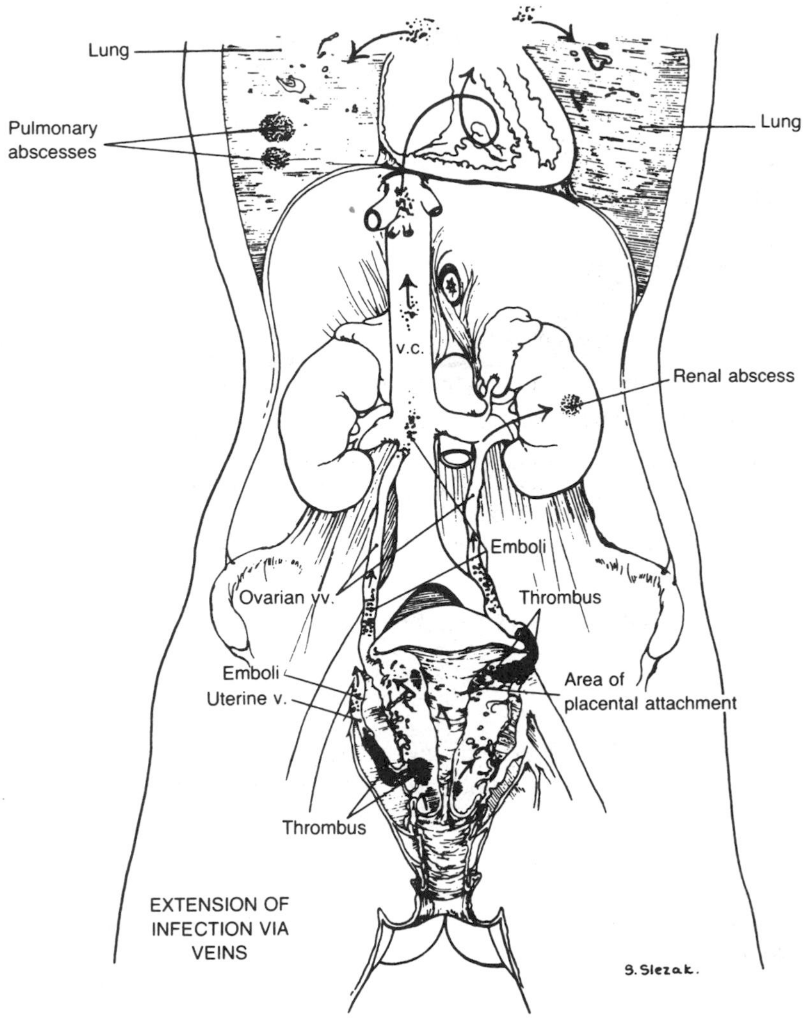

FIGURE 35-2. Potential spread of untreated postpartum endometritis.

maternal nutrition as well as exposing these women to potentially dangerous pathogens through prostitution and shared intravenous needles. Both human immunodeficiency virus infection [10] and syphilis [11] are increasing in frequency in this population. In addition, risk of infection increases with prolonged rupture of the fetal membranes before delivery, with increasing length of labor, and with retention of fetal membranes or placental fragments after delivery.

Transvaginal Monitoring

In addition to reducing mortality rates, the availability of antibiotics has dramatically changed the practice of obstetrics–gynecology. Prolonged transvaginal monitoring of maternal intraamniotic pressures and transvaginal attachment of a fetal scalp electrode for electrocardiograph reading could not have been considered if antibiotics were not available for postpartum use by obstetricians and neonatologists. These invasive procedures have been accompanied by enhanced infection risks. Among obstetric patients, the incidence of endometritis is higher in monitored patients compared with unmonitored patients [12]. In a clinic population, where there is a moderately high level of background infection, this difference is less apparent [13] (Figures 35-3 and 35-4).

Cesarean Section

Advances in the science of neonatology have increased fetal survival and increased the incidence of cesarean section for fetal indications in situations in which maternal risk of postpartum infection is increased. The frequency of infection after a cesarean section is 10 times greater than that after vaginal delivery. The obstetric service at the New York Hospital–Cornell Medical Center is now doing cesarean sections for infants estimated to weigh 500 g. One result of this new criterion has been a reduction in perinatal mortality [14], but these results have been achieved by judgments that increase the maternal risk of infection. Cesarean sections are performed at the first instance of fetal distress in these small infants. At

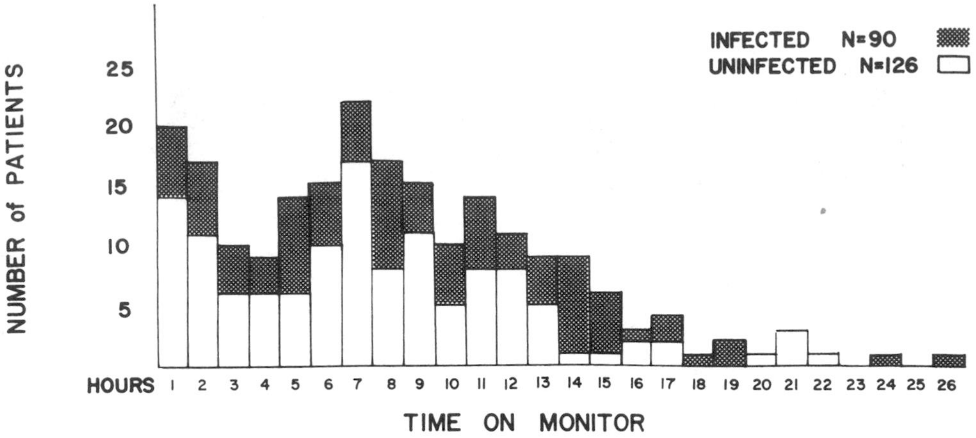

FIGURE 35-3. The length of time of internal monitoring and the number of women with and without infection who delivered vaginally. Each bar represents the total number of women monitored for that time interval. (Reprinted with permission from Gassner CB, Ledger WJ. The relationship of hospital-acquired maternal infection to invasive intrapartum monitoring techniques. *Am J Obstet Gynecol* 1976;126:33.)

least one study showed an increase in central nervous system damage among premature newborns whose distress was observed for 30 minutes or more before delivery was done [15]. Our own assessment would be that the benefits to the fetus of this new obstetric philosophy outweigh the risks to the mother.

DIAGNOSTIC CRITERIA

Clinical

The clinical diagnosis of postpartum endometritis is based on a number of findings, but the most significant

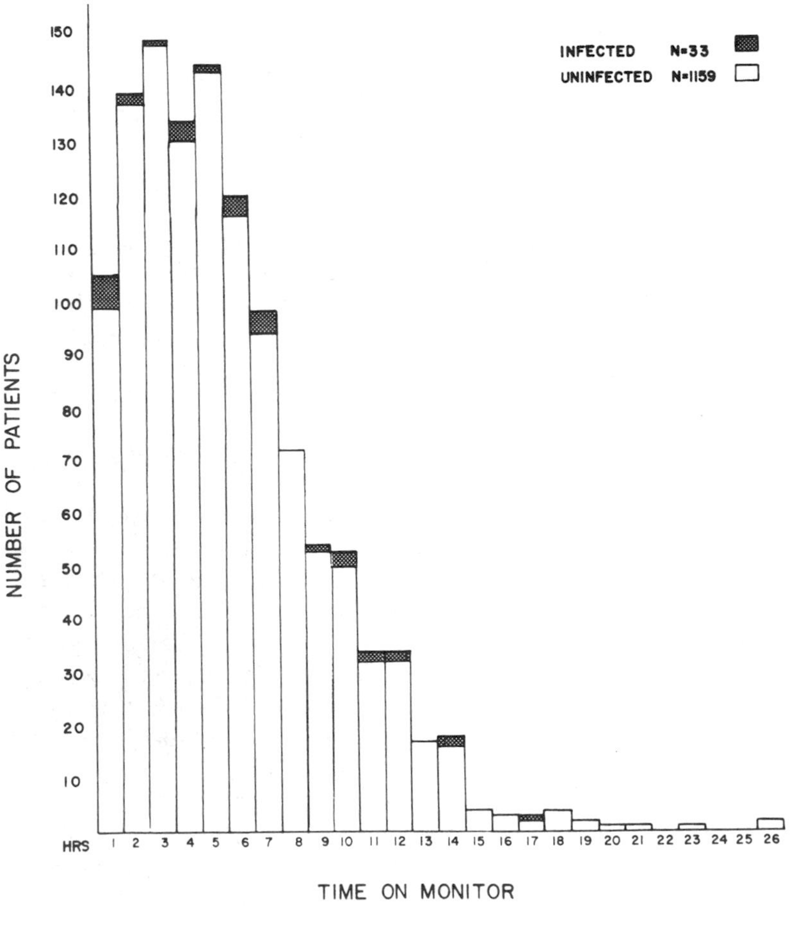

FIGURE 35-4. The length of time of internal monitoring and the number of women with and without infection who delivered by cesarean section. Each bar represents the total number of women monitored for that time interval. (Reprinted with permission from Gassner CB, Ledger WJ. The relationship of hospital-acquired maternal infection to invasive intrapartum monitoring techniques. *Am J Obstet Gynecol* 1976;126:33.)

factor is fever. In general, these women have an oral temperature elevation to about 38°C (100.4°F) and a tachycardia consistent with this rise. Patients usually have uterine tenderness and sometimes have tenderness beyond the uterus in the parametrial and adnexal regions. A decrease in the normal postpartum uterine lochial flow is often noted 6 to 12 hours preceding the temperature elevation, and the lochial flow may be foul smelling. If the physician makes a clinical diagnosis of endometritis and begins administration of systemic antibiotics with or without positive culture results, the patient should be included in all infection surveillance and postpartum morbidity statistics.

Attempts to assess the presence of a postpartum endometritis through evaluation of commonly used, indirect hematologic measures of infection have not been successful. The phenomena of labor and delivery are accompanied by changes in the commonly used parameters to measure the presence or absence of a bacterial infection. Thus, a normal patient in labor or postpartum who has no evidence of an active bacterial infection may have an elevated white blood cell count (even above 20,000) with an increase in the percentage of immature leukocytes, and an elevated sedimentation rate. In addition, the amniotic fluid of a patient in labor has white blood cells present even when there is no clinical evidence of infection [16]. Bearing these facts in mind, there should be no enthusiasm for dependence on such laboratory tests to determine the diagnosis of infection.

Microbiologic

Isolations of bacteria in the clinical microbiology laboratory from endometrial cultures does not establish the diagnosis of a postpartum endometritis. Exceptions are the discovery of a group-A β-hemolytic streptococci, *Neisseria gonorrhoeae,* or *Chlamydia trachomatis*, which should trigger specific physician responses for treatment. The reasons for the usual lack of useful diagnostic, but not therapeutic, information from the microbiologic laboratory are manifold. Most culture techniques for sampling the postpartum endometrial cavity include a transcervical approach, which of necessity involves contamination by the abundant bacterial flora normally present in the endocervical canal of asymptomatic women. There have been a number of sheathed culture apparatuses that have been developed, but there has been no widespread physician acceptance of these methods. Also, the organisms recovered from the endometrial cavity of patients with endometritis are usually the same as those normally inhabiting the vagina and endocervix of sexually active women.

The preceding considerations do not mean that the laboratory will not be helpful, for it may indirectly contribute to the diagnosis or lack of diagnosis and give therapeutic guidance for treating postpartum endometritis. Assistance in excluding the diagnosis of postpartum endometritis may be provided, for example, in the febrile postpartum patient with no localizing uterine signs of infection when a significant bacterial colony count is obtained from a properly collected urine sample, and the fever resolves successfully after therapy with an antibacterial agent (e.g., a nitrofurantoin) with limited action outside of the urinary tract.

SPECIMEN COLLECTION AND TRANSPORT

Transvaginal Specimens

The greatest difficulty facing clinicians in their attempts to sample the postpartum endometrial cavity microbiologically is in obtaining specimens that are free of vaginal and cervical contamination. To date, most techniques have stressed the transvaginal and transcervical approach to the endometrial cavity. Various techniques have been tried to decrease contamination from endocervical canal organisms, including the use of plastic or metal tubing through which specimens can be collected. There has been little physician enthusiasm for these more complicated diagnostic procedures. Also, there have been no reports of attempts to quantitate the recovery of bacteria, similar to the methods of the colony counts of urine specimens, that might separate vaginal and endocervical contaminants from the more numerous pathogens from the site of infection.

Use of Blood Cultures

The most useful microbiologic technique, when it is positive, is the blood culture. A positive result focuses the clinician's attention on the most significant microorganisms in the infectious process. Those that invade the bloodstream are critical for the physician's therapeutic consideration. Despite some enthusiasm for this diagnostic intervention, one study could not support this as a routine procedure in patients with chorioamnionitis when costs were analyzed [17].

Transport

Significant changes in microbiologic sampling and the transportation of specimens have been brought about by physician awareness of the importance of anaerobic microorganisms in postpartum infections. The recovery of anaerobes is crucially dependent on the clinician's efforts to reduce exposure of the specimens to atmospheric oxygen. Time is a critical factor, because exposure of a swab of the infection site to atmospheric oxygen for a few minutes or less reduces or eliminates certain anaerobic organisms. A number of alternative laboratory systems have been proposed to eliminate such exposure. Transport media have been used, either liquid for primary culture or semisolid for transport to the laboratory and primary plating there. Alternatively, gassed tubes, free of oxygen, have been used for transport to a laboratory where primary plating and anaerobic incubation can be performed (see Chapter 9).

There are major weaknesses in all these clinical schemes for the obstetrician–gynecologist. Figure 35-1 documents the first temperature elevation of obstetric patients with postpartum morbidity, which is the logical time for initial patient evaluation [18]. It is clear that most microbiologic samples are obtained late in the afternoon or in the early evening, when laboratory coverage, particularly by technicians with familiarity in anaerobic methods, is usually inadequate. In addition, with early discharge, most of the temperature elevations occur at home where cultures before treatment are less likely to be done.

GENERAL CONTROL MEASURES

Patient Care Practices

Prenatal Care

The emphasis on the preventive aspects in patient care has been heavily weighted toward patient management during pregnancy, labor, and delivery. For the patient in labor, most obstetricians believe that the results of prenatal care culminating in delivery largely determine the frequency and severity of postpartum endometritis.

Rectal and Vaginal Examinations

One of the great changes in practice patterns in obstetrics since the 1960s has been the abandonment of the rectal examination during labor. Rectal examination was firmly established in the preantibiotic era and was predicated on the belief that it would avoid the introduction of exogenous organisms into the vagina. Because the most feared bacterial pathogens—the group-A β-hemolytic streptococci and the pneumococci—were often introduced into the vagina from personnel sources, prohibition of vaginal examination was undoubtedly beneficial. A number of studies demonstrated no differences in the postpartum endometritis rate when patients undergoing vaginal examination during labor were compared with those having rectal examination. These results probably reflect the low frequency of involvement of exogenous organisms in postpartum endometritis. Both rectal and vaginal examinations, however, can result in the displacement of organisms from the lower genital tract to the uterus, and these manipulations, as well as other manipulations with similar risks (e.g., intrauterine placement of forceps or the physician's hand at delivery), should be limited to as few as necessary for good management of the patient.

Prophylactic Antibiotics

Prophylactic antibiotics for the patient in labor who needs a cesarean section (see Chapter 14) is the standard of care in the United States. Studies have shown diminished postpartum morbidity with their use [19]. The timing of the dosage for prophylaxis varies. Preoperative administration delivers a therapeutic level of antibiotic to the fetus, which can make evaluation for neonatal sepsis more difficult. The standard of care is administration after clamping of the cord. The use of antibiotic solution lavage in the operating room has had a variety of outcomes. In some studies, the results are not as good as with intravenous antibiotics [20].

Handwashing and Gloves

In the nineteenth century, Semmelweis recognized the importance of hand transfer of organisms from the postmortem room and the autopsy in the production of endometritis; physicians carried the bacterial pathogens from the autopsy room on their hands and clothing to the vagina and endocervix of the patient in labor, which led to the subsequent development of infection. Semmelweis's great achievement was to require hand-bathing in an antiseptic solution by physicians before the next patient was seen to break the chain of bacterial contamination and infection. Handwashing and the use of sterile gloves for vaginal examinations remain important general control measures.

Environmental Factors

Environmental factors are infrequently involved in the development of postpartum endometritis. Indeed, studies of the effect of ultraviolet irradiation on the rate of all postoperative wound infections [21] suggest that this would be the case in the delivery room, because the studies showed that there was little impact on clinical results despite reductions in the bacterial contamination of air (see Chapter 37). The lack of importance of the environment would be especially anticipated in the case of endometritis, because most of these infections derive from the patients' endogenous bacterial flora.

Therapy

The cornerstones of therapy in patients with a postpartum endometritis are adequate uterine drainage and the use of appropriate antimicrobials. Uterine drainage must be ensured, and the maneuver of removing membranes at the time of pelvic examination provides the patient undergoing clinical examination the added benefit of an assessment of the extent of infection; a microbiologic specimen may also be obtained at this time.

Antibiotics are usually required for cure. They are prescribed before the results of culture susceptibility tests are known, and the initial choices reflect the individual physician's philosophy of antibiotic use, which should be based on past experiences with similar patients. At the New York Hospital–Cornell Medical Center, physicians frequently use a single antibiotic like ampicillin or a cephalosporin to treat the patient who is not allergic to penicillin and who has had a vaginal delivery. This course usually results in cure, even in the patient with a concomitant bacteremia, because these agents provide coverage against most of the commonly recovered organisms. In patients who have had a cesarean section, there are a number of antibiotic choices available. Standard therapy has been a combination of clindamycin and an aminoglycoside, usually gentamicin [22]. This combination of antibiotics provides coverage against most of the commonly recovered aerobes and anaerobes and has shown superior results to the previously used combination of penicillin and an aminoglycoside. A concern has been the maintenance of adequate levels of gentamicin on standard doses, based on body weights [23]. I have favored obtaining serum levels to correct low levels found in 40%, but one study suggests that this is infrequently necessary [24]. Alternatively, a second cephalosporin such as cefoxitin or cefotetan, one of the newer broad-spectrum penicillins such as mezlocillin, or penicillins with a β-lactamase inhibitor can be used alone. A number of studies indicate the standard 10-day length of treatment is not needed in these patients [25]. These women can be treated until they have been afebrile 48 hours.

ENDOGENOUS INFECTIONS FROM LOWER GENITAL TRACT FLORA

The microorganisms mainly responsible for postpartum endometritis are nearly always endogenous to the patient; that is, they normally reside in the gastrointestinal and lower genital tracts (vagina and endocervix) of asymptomatic, pregnant women. Bacterial vaginosis, which is associated with a manyfold increase in the number of vaginal bacteria, increases the risk of infection [6]. The stress of labor and delivery, rupture of the membranes, frequent vaginal examinations by the medical team caring for the patient, use of invasive monitoring devices in the vagina, and delivery by the intrauterine placement of forceps or physicians' hands all introduce opportunities for uterine acquisition of lower genital tract flora. After introduction, they may find a suitable uterine environment where they can survive and invade.

The endogenous organisms that most frequently become pathogenic and result in an endometritis include certain aerobic streptococci (α-hemolytic streptococci, the group-B β-hemolytic streptococci, and the enterococci); anaerobic cocci (*Peptostreptococcus*); gram-negative aerobes (*Escherichia coil, Klebsiella* species, and *Hemophilus influenzae*); and, finally, gram-negative anaerobic rods, *Bacteroides fragilis, Bacteroides bivius,* and *Bacteroides disiens.* There is evidence that nearly all of the patients with endometritis, particularly those with severe infections, have a mixed infection with more than one organism involved.

Epidemics of endometritis caused by these organisms have not been recognized, and their control depends on avoiding predisposing factors, when possible, and adherence to general control measures.

Gram-Negative Aerobic Infections

Gram-negative aerobes are less frequently recovered from these women today than they were in the 1970s. The most frequently isolated organisms are *E. coli, Klebsiella,* and *H. influenzae*, with an associated bacteremia. There are no distinctive clinical signs, however, to alert the clinician to the possibility that an associated bacteremia is present.

The low frequency of antimicrobial-resistant organisms is a major advantage to the clinician treating women with endometritis in which gram-negative aerobes are involved. Most postpartum obstetric patients have intact host defense mechanisms and usually have not had prolonged exposure to systemic antimicrobial therapy before labor and delivery or prolonged hospitalization before delivery. Effective first-line drugs include the aminoglycosides, gentamicin and tobramycin. Because there are a few resistant gram-negative aerobic organisms seen in these patients, we usually rely on gentamicin as our most frequently used aminoglycoside, with amikacin reserved for the patient who is suspected of having gram-negative aerobic bacterial sepsis or who had repeated exposure to antibiotics for urinary tract infections during pregnancy. The cephalosporins and broad-spectrum penicillins are highly effective against such gram-negative aerobes, and these are an acceptable alternative to aminoglycosides, as is azithromycin.

Gram-Negative Anaerobic Infections

Incidence

Studies show that *Bacteroides* species were frequently isolated from patients with postpartum endometritis [26]. Most of these isolates are *B. bivius* or *B. disiens,* but *B. fragilis* has been isolated in patients with serious infection.

Clinical Features

Patients with postpartum endometritis due to *B. fragilis, B. bivius,* or *B. disiens* can be seriously ill, and they frequently have lochia with a fecal odor. Although most patients respond to antibiotics, pelvic abscess formation can occur and operative drainage or removal may be necessary for cure, despite the use of appropriate antibiotics in adequate dosages. Septic thrombophlebitis can follow infections with those organisms, but this is a much less frequently seen entity since physicians have used antibiotics effective against gram-negative anaerobes from the beginning of therapy.

Therapy

Postpartum endometritis due to *B. fragilis, B. bivius,* or *B. disiens* requires specific antibiotic strategies. The first-line drugs of choice are clindamycin and metronidazole. Clindamycin has been associated with pseudomembranous enterocolitis, a serious clinical entity that affects about 1 in 25,000 treated patients (see Chapters 14, 34). Alternative drugs include cephalosporins and broad-spectrum penicillins.

Operative removal and drainage of pelvic abscesses, treatment of septic pelvic thrombophlebitis with intravenous heparin therapy, and continued use of appropriate antibiotics may result in a rapid defervescence of fever in a patient with previously persisting temperature spikes.

Gram-Positive Anaerobic Infections

Incidence

There is a consistency in the bacterial causes of endometritis. Microbiologic studies of patients with postpartum endometritis in the preantibiotic era showed *Peptostreptococcus* to be the most commonly isolated organism [27], and it is a common isolate today [20]. In surveillance studies of obstetric infections with proper anaerobic culture techniques, *Peptostreptococcus* and *Peptococcus* are each frequently recovered from the endometrium [26] and bloodstream [28] of patients with endometritis.

Clinical Features

A postpartum endometritis due to gram-positive anaerobic cocci can be suspected in a patient whose lochia has a putrid, fecal odor. Pelvic abscess formation rarely occurs, but when it does, operative drainage or removal may be necessary for cure, despite the use of appropriate antibiotics as judged by in vitro antibiotic susceptibility testing. The postpartum retention of fetal membranes or placental fragments has frequently been observed with these infections.

Therapy

Peptostreptococcus is quite susceptible to clindamycin in dosage levels that are easily exceeded in the serum by frequently administered therapeutic doses of this agent. Other alternative antibiotics include the newer cephalosporins and penicillins.

Aerobic Infections

Incidence

There was an increasing evidence of group-B β-hemolytic streptococcal maternal infections in the late 1980s [26]. The enterococci are also frequently encountered. Group-A infections are rare, but serious.

Clinical Features

Postpartum endometritis due to aerobic streptococci has no characteristic clinical findings that distinguish it from endometritis due to other organisms.

Therapy

The group-B β-hemolytic streptococci and α-hemolytic streptococci are susceptible to penicillin and clindamycin. The group-D streptococci have unique antibiotic susceptibility patterns. In the laboratory, the organism is frequently not susceptible to penicillin or an aminoglycoside alone, but when both antibiotics are used together or when ampicillin is substituted for penicillin, there is both laboratory and clinical evidence of a response. In the penicillin-allergic patient with enterococcal endometritis, vancomycin is the antibiotic of choice, because the cephalosporins and clindamycin have little effectiveness against this group of organisms. A new hospital problem has been the emergence of vancomycin resistant enterococci [29] (see Chapter 14). Fortunately, this still is an uncommon problem in postpartum units.

GROUP-A B-HEMOLYTIC STREPTOCOCCAL INFECTIONS

In contrast to the preceding category of infections, endometritis caused by group-A streptococci commonly derives from exogenous sources, is highly invasive and transmissible, and has produced outbreaks requiring special measures for control.

General Aspects

Transmissibility

The group-A β-hemolytic streptococci are highly contagious agents (see Chapter 41). For this reason, obstetricians justifiably fear the introduction of this organism into the labor room environment lest it be transmitted to patients in labor and result in serious cases of postpartum endometritis. A patient with an active *Streptococcus pyogenes* infection can transmit these organisms to patients or medical personnel, resulting in colonization. Hospital personnel can be asymptomatic carriers of group-A streptococci and transmit the organisms to patients in labor. Community contacts may be important in the transmission of this organism to patients in labor, particularly in the modern obstetric setting that allows husband and wife to be together during all of labor and delivery. This practice can be a problem if the husband is a carrier of group-A streptococci.

Incidence

The importance of group-A β-hemolytic streptococcal infections infections is not based on a high frequency of infections but rather on the clinical invasiveness and epidemiologic virulence of such strains. The low frequency of isolation matches our surveillance experience with endometritis and the bacteremia associated with it.

Sources and Modes of Acquisition

Endogenous sources are probably mainly responsible for specific cases. The vagina of such patients is often asymptomatically colonized with group-A streptococci when the patient is admitted to the delivery room, but patients may also have an upper respiratory tract infection or skin lesion that harbors such organisms.

The most common method of spread of exogenous organisms involves direct transmissions of the organism from personnel who are asymptomatic carriers to the patients. Clinically infected personnel may also be responsible (see Chapters 37, 41). Personnel may become colonized after providing care to a patient with postpartum endometritis; they may then transmit these organisms to patients in labor.

Clinical Considerations

Manifestations

There are a number of distinctive clinical features seen in the patient with group-A β-hemolytic streptococcal endometritis. Historically, this entity has been called "puerperal fever," "puerperal sepsis," and "childbed fever." The most striking feature is the early onset of high, spiking fevers (Figure 35-5) in the postpartum patient [30]. Patients appear critically ill, but abdominal and pelvic examinations reveal diffuse tenderness with no localizing signs. The cervical discharge is usually clear and watery, is not purulent, and contains many gram-positive cocci when the exudate is Gram stained. Although this organism is very susceptible to penicillin and clindamycin, patients with endometritis frequently do not become afebrile for 48 hours or more (see Figure 35-4).

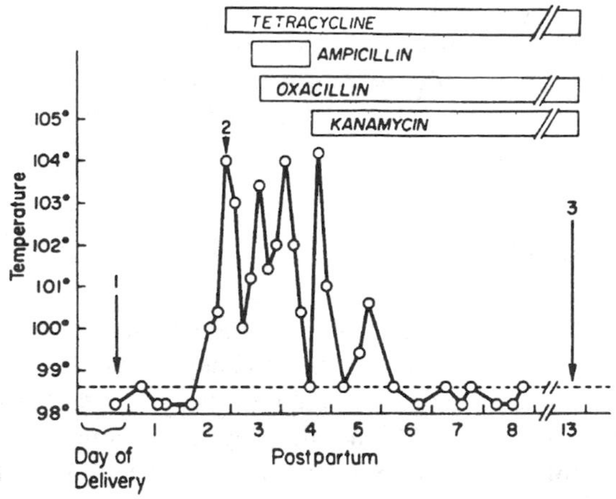

FIGURE 35-5. The early onset of a high, spiking temperature pattern in a postpartum patient with group-A β-hemolytic streptococcal endometritis. Despite the use of penicillin analogs (ampicillin and oxacillin), the patient required several days to become completely afebrile. The patient delivered at point 1 on the chart was started on antibiotic treatment at point 2 and was discharged at point 3.

Therapy

The drug of choice for treating group-A β-hemolytic streptococcal endometritis remains penicillin G; clindamycin is also effective against this organism. Tetracycline is not an acceptable alternative for treating patients with this infection because of the frequency of resistant strains.

Epidemic Infections

Reported Outbreaks

Since the introduction of antibiotics, sporadic outbreaks of group-A β-hemolytic streptococcal endometritis epidemics have been reported in New York City [31] and Boston [1]. In the New York City outbreak, there were 9 confirmed cases, whereas in Boston there were 20 women with this diagnosis.

Sources

In the New York City outbreak, the sources of the bacteria that were disseminated around the hospital were colonized, asymptomatic newborns [31]. In Boston, a common source was the cutaneous lesions of an anesthesiologist [1]. A preantibiotic-era study of this problem found many personnel colonized with such streptococci [32]. Colonization of medical personnel and subsequent transmission to patients in labor seem to be the crucial ingredients in the maintenance of an epidemic. Another outbreak of group-A streptococcal infections affecting obstetric–gynecologic patients was ultimately traced to an anesthesiologist who was an asymptomatic rectal carrier of the organism [33]. Thus, operating room sources of this type should be suspected in endometritis outbreaks that exclusively or primarily involve patients with cesarean sections.

Prevention and Control

Infections due to this organism are so serious that the discovery of one case of puerperal sepsis should be considered an epidemic. The patient needs to be placed in wound and skin isolation, and hospital personnel should gown and glove before providing personal care (see Chapter 13). All labor and delivery room personnel on duty during this patient's labor and delivery should be screened for possible infections by history and physical examination, and cultures should be obtained on their nose, throat, any suspected skin lesion, and rectum. Lochial culture specimens should be obtained from postpartum patients who had been in the delivery room at the same time as the infected patient, and appropriate antibiotics should be given to those whose cultures are positive for the same strain as the one isolated from the infected patient (which is established by M and T typing). Such personnel should be relieved of patient care responsibilities until appropriate antibiotic therapy has resulted in negative cultures. All culture-positive personnel should be treated if the typing of strains cannot be done expeditiously.

There were a number of significant differences between the preantibiotic-era epidemics and those more recently reported. The preantibiotic-era study reported maternal deaths, and the outbreak was controlled only by closing the maternity service of the hospital until all infected patients had been discharged [32]. The more recent epidemics have been controlled by the use of the appropriate antibiotics, isolation of infected patients, epidemiologic identification of disseminating carriers, and eradication of carried strains by proper treatment of colonized or infected hospital personnel. If initial nose and throat cultures of personnel epidemiologically associated with the outbreak are negative, multiple culture specimens should be obtained, including ones from rectal and vaginal sites. In Boston, all admissions to the service in the midst of the epidemic were treated with penicillin or penicillin-like antibiotics [1]. Such broad-scale prophylaxis may be especially indicated at the time an outbreak is first recognized, because it may permit a maternity unit to remain open while epidemiologic and microbiologic investigations are undertaken. If such investigations are successful in identifying the sources and modes of spread, then attention focused on these areas should obviate the need for continued chemoprophylaxis of patients. Outbreaks should be promptly reported to local health authorities.

Coagulase-Positive *Staphylococcus*

Maternal infections due to these organisms occur. They most frequently involve the breast and are discovered after patients have been discharged from the hospital. If these organisms are found in women with an endometritis, the same control measures as the group-A β-hemolytic streptococcus should be used.

REFERENCES

1. Jewett JF, Reid DE, Safon LE, Easterday CL. Childbed fever: a continuing entity. *JAMA* 1968;206:344.
2. Ledger WJ, Child M. The hospital care of patients undergoing hysterectomy. *Am J Obstet Gynecol* 1973;117:423.
3. Mishell DR, Bell JH, Good RG, Moyer DL. The intrauterine device: a bacteriologic study of the endometrial cavity. *Am J Obstet Gynecol* 1966;96:119.
4. Larsen B, Snyder IS, Galask RP. Bacterial growth inhibition by amniotic fluid. *Am J Obstet Gynecol* 1974;119:492.
5. Wagner MV, Chin VP, Peters CJ, Drexler B, Newman LA. A comparison of early and delayed induction of labor with spontaneous rupture of membranes at term. *Obstet Gynecol* 1989;74:93.
6. Watts DH, Krohn MA, Hillier SL, Eschenbach D. Bacterial vaginosis as a risk factor for post-cesarean endometritis. *Obstet Gynecol* 1990;75:52.
7. Eastman NJ, Hellman LM. In: Williams LW, ed. *Obstetrics.* 20th ed. New York: Appleton-Century-Crofts; 1966 Chapter 24.
8. Harper AK, Slocumb JT. Right subhepatic abscess for cesarean section: a case report. *J Reprod Med* 1989;34:376.
9. Golde S, Ledger WJ. Necrotizing fasciitis in postpartum patients: a report of four cases. *Obstet Gynecol* 1977;50:670.
10. Ellerbrock T, Bush T, Chamberland M, Oxtoby M. Epidemiology of women with AIDS in the United States, 1981 through 1990. *JAMA* 1991;265:2971.
11. Reyes MP, Hunt N, Ostrea EM Jr, George D. Maternal/congenital syphilis in a large tertiary-care urban hospital. *Clin Infect Dis* 1993; 17:1041.
12. Larsen JW, Goldkrand JW, Hanson TM, Miller CR. Intrauterine infection on an obstetric service. *Obstet Gynecol* 1974;43:838.
13. Gassner CB, Ledger WJ. The relationship of hospital-acquired maternal infections to invasive intrapartum monitoring techniques. *Am J Obstet Gynecol* 1976;126:33.
14. Paul RH, Hon EH. Clinical fetal monitoring: V. effect on perinatal outcome. *Am J Obstet Gynecol* 1974;118:529.
15. Shy KK, Lathy DA, Bennett FC. Effects of electronic fetal heart rate monitoring, as compared with periodic auscultation on the neurologic development of premature infants. *N Engl J Med* 1990;322:588.
16. Bobitt JR, Ledger WJ. Amniotic fluid analysis. *Obstet Gynecol* 1978; 51:56.
17. Locksmith GJ, Duff P. Assessment of the value of routine blood cultures in the evaluation and treatment of patients with chorioamnionitis. *Infectious Disease in Obstetrics and Gynecology* 1994;2:111.
18. Ledger WJ, Reite AM, Headington JT. A system for infectious disease surveillance on an obstetric service. *Obstet Gynecol* 1971;37:769.
19. Wong R, Gee CL, Ledger WJ. Prophylactic use of cefazolin in monitored obstetric patients undergoing cesarean section. *Obstet Gynecol* 1978;51:407.
20. Conover WB, Moore TR. Comparison of irrigation and intravenous antibiotic prophylaxis at cesarean section. *Obstet Gynecol* 1984;63: 787.
21. Howard JM, Barker WF, Culberson WR, et al. Postoperative wound infections: the influence of ultraviolet irradiation of the operating room and of various other factors. *Ann Surg* 1964;160(Suppl):1.
22. DiZerega G, Yonekura L, Roy S, Nakamura RM, Ledger WJ. A comparison of clindamycin–gentamicin and penicillin–gentamicin in the treatment of post-cesarean section endomyometritis. *Am J Obstet Gynecol* 1979;134:238.
23. Zaske DE, Cipolle RJ, Strate RG, Malo JW, Koszalka MF Jr. Rapid gentamicin elimination in obstetric patients. *Obstet Gynecol* 1980; 56:559.

24. Briggs GG, Ambrose P, Nageotte MP. Gentamicin dosing in postpartum women with endometritis. *Am J Obstet Gynecol* 1988;160:309
25. Gall SA, Addison WA, Hill GB. Moxalactam therapy for obstetric and gynecologic infections. *Rev Infect Dis* 1982;4:S701.
26. Newton ER, Prihoda TJ, Gibbs R. A clinical and microbiologic analysis of risk factors for puerperal endometritis. *Obstet Gynecol* 1990; 75:402.
27. Schwarz OH, Dieckman WJ. Puerperal infection due to anaerobic streptococci. *Am J Obstet Gynecol* 1927;13:467.
28. Ledger WJ, Norman M, Gee C, Lewis W. Bacteremia on an obstetric gynecologic service. *Am J Obstet Gynecol* 1975;121:205.
29. Eliopoulos GM. The ten most common questions about resistant enterococcal infections. *Infectious Disease in Clinical Practice* 1994;3:125.
30. Ledger WJ, Headington JT. The group A beta-hemolytic streptococcus. *Obstet Gynecol* 1972;39:474.
31. Mead PB, Ribble JC, Dillon TF. Group A streptococcal puerperal infection. *Obstet Gynecol* 1968;32:460.
32. Watson BP. An outbreak of puerperal sepsis in New York City. *Am J Obstet Gynecol* 1928;16:157.
33. McIntyre DM. An epidemic of *Streptococcus pyogenes* puerperal and postoperative sepsis with an unusual carrier site—the anus. *Am J Obstet Gynecol* 1968;101:308.

Hospital Infections, Fourth Edition,
edited by John V. Bennett and Philip S. Brachman.
Lippincott–Raven Publishers, Philadelphia © 1998

CHAPTER 36

Central Nervous System Infections

W. Michael Scheld and Barry M. Farr

Nosocomial infection of the central nervous system (CNS) is a rare but serious occurrence in the modern hospital. As with other types of nosocomial infections, infection of the CNS most often follows a procedure, which provides access for microbes to bypass normal host barriers. While a majority of cases follow neurosurgery, other neuroinvasive procedures, such as lumbar puncture or placement of an epidural catheter, can occasionally infect the CNS [1,2]. Nosocomial CNS infections that are not due to microbial contamination during procedures generally affect neonates, who possess an immature blood-brain barrier that may be more easily crossed during bacteremia, and the immunosuppressed. Nosocomial CNS infections range from superficial surgical site infections as the result of neurosurgery to meningitis, meningoencephalitis, and focal suppurations, including brain abscess, subdural empyema, and epidural abscess.

INCIDENCE

Data from the National Nosocomial Infection Surveillance (NNIS) program, which were collected in 163 U.S. hospitals between 1986 and 1993, document 5.6 nonsurgical nosocomial CNS infections for every 100,000 patients discharged [3]. This rate is approximately half of what it was a quarter of a century ago (1/10,000 discharges) [4]. Meningitis is the most common CNS infection, accounting for 91% of the total, followed by intracranial abscesses in 8% and spinal abscesses in only 1%.

Somewhat higher rates of CNS infection have been observed among the immunosuppressed, ranging from 20 per 100,000 discharges for cancer patients [5] to 5 to 12 per 100 discharges among transplant patients [6]. Meningitis has constituted 71% of CNS infections among cancer patients, followed by brain abscess and encephalitis (making up 27% and 2% of cases, respectively) [5]. Brain abscess appears to be more common among transplant patients (see Chapter 45), accounting for ~40% of CNS infections after heart and heart-lung transplants [7]. The highest rate of infection for a hospital service has been 45 per 100,000 discharges for the newborn nursery, according to NNIS data collected between 1986 and 1990 [8].

The incidence of CNS infection is relatively high among neurosurgical patients, compared with other groups of patients. Among patients with American Society of Anesthesiology (ASA) scores below 3, an operative duration less than the 75th percentile, and a wound classification of "clean" or "clean contaminated," infection rates in the NNIS program have been 0.56/100 craniotomies, 0.70/100 spinal fusions, and 3.85/100 ventricular shunts [9]. Among patients with higher ASA scores (i.e., greater severity of underlying illnesses), longer durations of the procedure, and/or contamination of the wound, higher rates were observed [9]. The most common infection following neurosurgical procedures has been superficial surgical site infection, accounting for 60% of surgical site infections after craniotomy and 75% after laminectomy, according to NNIS data [3]. Meningitis is the second most common CNS infection after craniotomy, accounting for 22% of cases, and it is the most common form of CNS infection after ventricular shunt placement, accounting for 76% of cases.

RISK FACTORS

The most obvious risk factor for nosocomial CNS infection has been neurosurgery. Skin flora, which usually cannot be cultured from the operative site immediately after antiseptic preparation, regrow during the operation and can be cultured from a majority of operative sites just before closure [10]. As with other types of surgery, it is thus likely that most infections occur during

W.M. Scheld, B.M. Farr: Department of Internal Medicine, University of Virginia Health Sciences Center, Charlottesville, Virginia 22908.

the procedure while the wound is open, becoming contaminated from regrowth of the patient's own skin flora at the margins of the wound or occasionally by organisms from the operative team introduced on contaminated gloves or instruments or settling from the air into the wound. Infection at another body site is also a risk factor for infection of the neurosurgical wound. In an outbreak of meningitis due to *Klebsiella* spp, for example, colonization and/or infection of the respiratory or urinary tracts appeared to precede CNS infection [11]. Another study found that in 70% of neurosurgery patients with meningitis, there was antecedent or simultaneous isolation of the same organism from another body site [12].

Factors that amplify the risk of postcraniotomy infection have included duration of the operation, external drainage, reexploration, and operation through a paranasal sinus [13]. The risk factors contributing to the development of meningitis/ventriculitis after placement of a ventriculostomy have included intracerebral hemorrhage, other neurosurgical operations, drainage for > 5 days, an air-vented system, irrigation of the system, and intracranial pressure > 20 mm Hg [13,14]. The risk for infection of cerebrospinal fluid (CSF) shunts has increased with duration of the procedure, thrombosis of the catheter, externalization of the shunt, inexperience on the part of the surgeon, and type of shunt (ventriculoatrial carrying a higher risk than ventriculoperitoneal shunting) [13]. A persistent CSF leak after surgery heightened the risk of infection thirteen-fold in one study [15]; concurrent infection at a remote site increased the risk of CNS infection sixfold.

Placement of an intracranial pressure monitor is associated with different rates of infection, depending on where the monitor is positioned. One study found a 7.5% infection rate with a subarachnoid screw, a 14.9% rate with a subdural cup catheter, and a 21.9% rate for a ventriculostomy catheter [16]. Another study found a 0.6% rate for epidural monitors, a 3% rate for a subdural bolt, and a 4% rate for intraventricular or parenchymal brain monitors [17].

Patients with head trauma are at increased risk of CNS infection, especially meningitis. Cerebrospinal fluid fistula raises the risk of infection in this population. A CSF leak was found to be present in 13% of cases of nosocomial meningitis after head trauma in one case series [18]. Infection of the paranasal sinuses may be followed by CNS infection in these patients [19].

Premature birth also appears to be an important risk factor, as neonates cared for in neonatal intensive care units have had the highest rates of CNS infection according to NNIS data [8]. This finding seems to be related to the high risk of bacteremia from critical care instrumentation coupled with an increased risk of secondary meningitis from bacteremia stemming from the neonate's immature blood-brain barrier. Immunosuppression is another important risk factor for nonsurgical CNS infection, usually due to hematogenous spread.

ETIOLOGIC AGENTS

Staphylococci and gram-negative bacilli accounted for almost 70% of CNS infections documented in the NNIS hospitals between 1986 and 1992 [3]. During this time *Staphylococcus aureus* was the most common pathogen after both craniotomy and laminectomy, followed by coagulase-negative staphylococci. These organisms were followed by enterococci, *Streptococcus* spp, *Pseudomonas aeruginosa*, *Acinetobacter* spp, *Citrobacter* spp, *Enterobacter* spp, *Klebsiella pneumoniae*, *Escherichia coli*, miscellaneous other gram-negative bacilli, and yeast, which each accounted for < 10% of cases. After shunt procedures, *S. aureus* remained the most common pathogen causing superficial site infections, but coagulase-negative staphylococci were more typical causes of deeper infections; gram-negative bacilli were responsible for 19% of deeper infections related to shunts [3].

If all CNS infections are considered, coagulase-negative staphylococci were the most frequent pathogens, making up 31% of cases, compared with 27% for gram-negative bacilli, 11% for *S. aureus*, 18% for streptococcal species, 4% for yeast, and 9% for others [3]. For meningitis, the most frequently encountered CNS infection, coagulase-negative staphylococci accounted for 32%, followed by gram-negative bacilli (29%), *Streptococcus* spp (18%), *S. aureus* (10%), yeast (4%), and others (9%) [3]. For intracranial infections, gram-negative bacilli were the cause of 23% of cases, followed by *S. aureus* (19%), coagulase-negative staphylococci (17%), anaerobes (11%), fungi (8%), *Streptococcus* spp (8%), viruses (4%), yeast (3%), and others (8%). Spinal abscess displayed a dramatically different distribution of etiologic agents—67% were due to *S. aureus*, and 33% were due to coagulase-negative staphylococci [3].

The largest study of nosocomial meningitis from a single hospital was conducted by Durand and colleagues, who reviewed 197 cases among 151 adult patients at Massachusetts General Hospital during a 27-year period [18]. These nosocomial cases accounted for 40% of the total of 493 episodes of bacterial meningitis observed during the study period. The proportion of cases that were nosocomial increased during the 27-year period. In this study, gram-negative bacilli were most common, accounting for 38% of cases, followed by *S. aureus* (9%), coagulase-negative staphylococci (9%), *Streptococcus* spp (9%), *Hemophilus influenzae* (4%), *Listeria monocytogenes* (3%), and *Enterococcus* spp (3%) [18]. The microbes responsible for nosocomial gram-negative meningitis in this study were *E. coli* (30%), *Klebsiella* (23%), *Pseudomonas* (11%), *Acinetobacter* (11%), *Enterobacter* (9%), *Serratia* (9%), *Citrobacter* (4%), *Pro-*

teus (2%), coliform types (2%), and nonenteric types (2%) [18]. The higher proportion of gram-negative and lower proportion of staphylococcal isolates in this study than in the more recent NNIS data could be due to the fact that there were only two years of overlap between the 27-year study and the NNIS data.

Pathogens most frequently isolated from brain abscesses have been streptococci, *Enterobacteriaceae*, and anaerobes, together constituting ≤ 70% of cases. Among immunocompromised patients, the frequency distribution of etiologic agents is somewhat different; *Toxoplasma gondii* and *Cryptococcus neoformans* are most frequent in patients with the acquired immunodeficiency syndrome, *Aspergillus* and *T. gondii* are the most common after heart and heart-lung transplants, and *Aspergillus* and *C. neoformans* are the most typical after kidney and liver transplants [20]. Among marrow transplant recipients, fungi accounted for 92% of cases in a recent study—*Aspergillus* in 58% of cases and *Candida* in 33% of cases [20].

Outbreaks of CNS infection among neonates or in neurosurgical patients have most often involved aerobic gram-negative bacilli [10, 21–25]. Such outbreaks have sometimes been linked to a healthcare provider carrying the organism [26] and at other times to contaminated equipment, such as respirators [27] or a shaving brush used for preoperative hair removal [25]. Outbreaks due to gram-positive bacteria, such as *Streptococcus* spp (both groups A and B), *S. aureus*, and *L. monocytogenes*, have also been reported [28–34]. Secondary spread of *Neisseria meningitidis* and *H. influenzae* within the hospital setting appears to be rare [35–37].

CLINICAL MANIFESTATIONS AND DIAGNOSIS

Meningitis

The typical manifestations of meningitis—fever, headache, neck stiffness, and depressed level of consciousness—are usually present with nosocomial CNS infection, but the last three of these symptoms and signs are also frequently present in postneurosurgical patients who don't have meningitis. These findings may stem from the underlying disease or the surgery. For this reason, changes in the degree of these symptoms and signs over time may be more important indications than their mere presence. Meningitis usually begins within 10 days of neurosurgery and almost always within a month. Fever is the most reliable single sign because it is not usually seen in postsurgical patients and because it is a component of almost all cases of nosocomial meningitis; 94% of patients with meningitis after neurosurgery had fever within the first day of illness in one study [12]. These usual clinical manifestations are more diagnostically useful indicators in nonsurgical patients, with some exceptions, such as neonates and the immunosuppressed. Neonates with meningitis usually have fever but may fail to manifest other classic findings of meningitis, such as nuchal rigidity or a bulging fontanelle. Instead there may be a weak cry, decreased muscle tone, lack of movement, poor sucking, diarrhea, vomiting, dyspnea, or apnea [38]. Likewise, the geriatric patient may not show classic symptoms or signs. High-dose corticosteroid therapy or severe neutropenia may significantly alter the clinical presentation of meningitis [6,39].

Because the clinical picture is often more difficult to interpret for nosocomial than for community-acquired meningitis, CSF analysis is correspondingly more important for confirming the diagnosis. Unfortunately, CSF abnormalities due to underlying disease and/or aseptic inflammation after neurosurgery can result in confusion, especially very early after surgery [40]. Administration of OKT3 has been associated with development of aseptic meningitis in transplant patients with negative results of cultures for bacteria, fungi, and viruses [41]. The CSF findings most predictive of nosocomial bacterial meningitis have been neutrophilic pleocytosis, with most who are affected having a CSF white blood cell count > 1,000/mm^3 (and almost all having a CSF white blood cell count > 100/mm^3), > 50% neutrophils, and hypoglycorrachia (usually < 40 mg/dl). Hypoglycorrachia appears to be the most reliable indicator of infection in the absence of positive results on Gram's stain or culture [12].

Gram's stain confirmed the presence of a pathogen in ~ 50% and culture in 83% of nosocomial cases in one large study [18]. After neurosurgery, Gram's stain proved *Candida* to be the causative agent in 36% of 18 reported cases; it is worth noting that *Candida* meningitis resulted in neutrophilic pleocytosis in 62%, with CSF white counts ranging from 13 to 8,000/mm^3 and a CSF glucose level of < 40 mg/dl in only 12% [42]. False-positive results of Gram's stains reportedly have been due to organisms in stain reagents, on glass slides, in media used for swabs, and in tubes used to centrifuge the CSF [43–47]. Culture results will often be rendered negative within 24 hours of starting antibiotic therapy, but changes in glucose, protein, and white cells usually take days to detect [48]. Antigen detection testing is seldom helpful in nosocomial meningitis but may be useful for detecting *C. neoformans* in immunosuppressed patients [39].

CSF Shunt Infection

Infection of a shunt is classified by the Centers for Disease Control and Prevention as nosocomial if it occurs within 1 year of placement, although most cases occur within the first 2 months. Pathogens such as *S. aureus* are associated with early-onset infections, while coagulase-negative staphylococci are associated with a later onset

[49]. Fever is the most reliable symptom [50]. Infection of the proximal end of a ventricular shunt often results in symptoms of shunt obstruction as well, such as nausea, vomiting, and headache. Nuchal rigidity is present in one third [49] of cases. Symptoms and signs of distal infection of a shunt depend upon the location of the tip. With ventriculoperitoneal shunts, peritonitis is the usual manifestation, but intestinal obstruction, intestinal perforation, and intrabdominal abscess have each been reported. Aseptic inflammation about the distal end has resulted in development of a peritoneal pseudocyst [51]. A tunnel infection with inflammation along the catheter may be seen.

Ventriculopleural shunts result in empyema with distal infection, while ventriculoatrial catheters are characterized by symptoms of endocarditis, such as lethargy and fever of several weeks' duration. Blood cultures usually show positive results, and nephritis may be detected by urinalysis and serum creatinine measurement. Whenever a shunt infection is suspected, aspiration of shunt fluid is indicated for cytology, Gram's stain, and culture. The sensitivity of the Gram's stain is ~50% and of culture ~80% [3]. Nine of 10 patients with shunt infection will have > 100 white cells per mm^3. Glucose and protein determinations on CSF from a shunt have not proved useful [52].

Brain Abscess

Brain abscess can occur after neurosurgery, sinus infection, sinus surgery, bloodstream infection, and penetrating head trauma, such as gunshot wounds [53–57]. Headache, fever, and focal neurologic abnormalities are the most typical findings, while seizures, nuchal rigidity, nausea, vomiting, and papilledema can each be seen up to half the time. Computed tomography scanning or magnetic resonance imaging may be useful in confirming the anatomic location and size of lesions. Stereotactic aspiration with computed tomography guidance can be used for therapeutic drainage as well as for obtaining fluid for cytologic and microbiologic stains and cultures to guide therapy.

Meningoencephalitis

Meningoencephalitis involves inflammation of brain parenchyma as well as the meninges. Meningoencephalitis has occurred in rare cases as a nosocomial infection after corneal or dural transplants taken from cadavers and after neurosurgery using contaminated instruments or electrodes. Both rabies virus and the agent of Creutzfeldt-Jakob disease have been transmitted in this manner. The incubation period for rabies following transplantation was 1 month, while for Creutzfeldt-Jakob disease it was about 18 months [13].

Creutzfeldt-Jakob disease is a rapidly dementing illness with prominent myoclonus. Hypokinesia, rigidity, nystagmus, tremor, and ataxia may each be present in more than half of cases. Seizures occur in 10% to 20%. The disease generally ends with coma and death after 7 to 9 months. Rabies begins with a prodrome of nonspecific symptoms, such as fever, headache, malaise, anorexia, nausea, vomiting, and diarrhea. The prodrome is followed after 2 to 20 days by an acute neurologic phase, which may be characterized by hyperactivity and disorientation (furious rabies) or by paralysis. Coma usually supervenes within 10 days of the onset of neurologic symptoms and may last for hours in untreated patients to months in treated patients. The average duration of coma is 7 days in untreated patients and 13 days in patients receiving intensive care. Only three recoveries from rabies have been reported.

Spinal Epidural Abscess

The classic stages of an epidural abscess are back pain, radicular pain, radicular weakness, and then paralysis. Other symptoms may include bowel and/or bladder dysfunction, sensory deficits, stiff neck, and altered mental status. Fever is usually present at the time of diagnosis. Laboratory evaluation of peripheral blood usually demonstrates leukocytosis and an elevated erythrocyte sedimentation rate. Magnetic resonance with gadolinium-DTPA contrast allows the best delineation of an abscess in preparation for surgery, which is done rapidly to preserve or salvage cord function.

Subdural Empyema

Cranial subdural empyema can follow paranasal sinusitis, otitis media, penetrating trauma, or a neurosurgical procedure. Symptoms generally begin with fever and headache followed by seizures, altered mental status, focal neurologic symptoms, nausea, and vomiting. Computed tomography scan or magnetic resonance imaging can be used to differentiate empyema from brain abscess. Spinal subdural empyemas have occurred very rarely and show symptoms similar to spinal epidural abscess, but tenderness may be absent on physical exam [3].

PROGNOSIS

Infections of the CNS are regarded as being among the most serious because of the potentially disabling morbidity and mortality. Of 53 deaths among patients with CNS infection in NNIS hospitals between 1988 and 1993, 49 (92%) were believed to have been precipitated by the infection rather than a preexisting illness [3]. The case fatality rate for nosocomial bacterial meningitis in the study by Durand et al. was 35%, compared with 25% for cases of community-acquired bacterial meningitis in adults [18].

Cerebrospinal fluid shunt infections were associated with an attributable mortality rate of 23% in a study by Schoenbaum et al. [49]. Walters et al. confirmed the mortality associated with shunt infections, finding a doubling of the case fatality rate as well as a tripling of the number of additional surgical procedures and significant prolongation of hospital stay among survivors [58]. The type of therapy appears to have an important effect on outcome. Antimicrobial therapy alone had a 36% success rate in treating shunt infections in one study, compared with 65% for antimicrobial therapy and immediate shunt removal and 96% for shunt removal, antibiotic therapy, and ventricular aspirates or external drainage [59]. Mayhall et al. found a case fatality rate of 100% among untreated patients with ventriculostomy infection [14]. Decline in cognitive ability has been documented following shunt infections [60].

Brain abscess is associated with a case fatality rate of ~10% [53,55] and permanent neurologic side effects in almost half of the survivors [54,56]. Adverse prognostic factors include very young or very old age, ventricular rupture, delay of antimicrobial therapy, altered mental status at diagnosis, larger size and greater number of abscesses, and fungal or gram-negative bacillary pathogens [54,56,57]. Spinal epidural abscess was associated with a case fatality rate of 13% in a review of seven case series including 188 patients [61], but a more recent study of 43 patients reported only two deaths (5%) [62]. Paralysis was observed in 22% of cases in the review [61] and 20% of patients in the more recent series [62]. Intracranial subdural empyema is associated with a case fatality rate of 20% to 30% and a high incidence of seizures and other side effects in survivors [63]. The most common CNS infection after neurosurgery—superficial surgical site infection—has little effect on mortality but does prolong hospital stay [3].

Prognosis is often related to the specific cause of the CNS infection. In the study by Durand et al., case fatality rates for the three most common nosocomial pathogen groups were 36% for gram-negative bacilli, 39% for *S. aureus*, and 0% (0 of 16) for coagulase-negative staphylococci [18]. The etiologic agent has an important effect upon prognosis among the immunosuppressed, with case fatality rates of 84% for gram-negative bacilli, 24% for *S. aureus*, and 37% for *L. monocytogenes* [6,64]. Patients with cerebral aspergillosis rarely survive [65]. The type of underlying illness also affects prognosis in immunosuppressed patients with CNS infection. Case fatality rates of 90% have been observed among patients with leukemia, compared with 77% for lymphoma and 59% for solid tumors of the head or spine [5,64].

PREVENTION

Since most CNS infections acquired in the hospital are related to surgery, efforts to prevent these infections will prominently include general measures for prevention of surgical wound infection, which is discussed in detail in Chapter 37. Such measures include strict attention to antiseptic preparation of the skin and aseptic technique, hair removal by depilatory or clipping rather than shaving, and minimizing the duration of operation while avoiding hemorrhage or creation of a CSF fistula, both of which can promote infection. Prophylactic antibiotics reduce the risk of infection with craniotomy at least threefold. Either cefazolin or vancomycin is acceptable, since most infections are caused by staphylococci [66]. Cefazolin would be preferred for hospitals with low rates of infection by methicillin-resistant staphylococci (see Chapter 41) because high usage of vancomycin appears to select for vancomycin-resistant enterococci (see Chapter 15) within an institution [67]. In hospitals with high rates of infection due to methicillin-resistant staphylococci, however, vancomycin would be the preferred agent.

For spinal surgery, antibiotic prophylaxis has not been standard because of the perception that infection rates are low without antibiotic prophylaxis. While some studies have documented rates < 1% [68–71], others have observed rates from 2.3% to 5.0% [72–75]. One study has shown significant prevention with antibiotic prophylaxis for patients undergoing lumbar laminectomy [76]. It is likely that large randomized trials with adequate statistical power would document benefit, as has been demonstrated recently for two other clean surgical procedures with generally low infection rates, herniorrhaphy and breast surgery [77]. Gantz and Godofsky suggested that prophylactic antibiotics are already being used routinely for high-risk situations, such as for spinal procedures involving fusion or prolonged operations, immunosuppressed patients, and implantation of hardware [3].

Prevention of infection of a CSF shunt using antibiotic prophylaxis has been difficult to confirm despite 12 randomized trials of this question. Only one of the 12 trials showed significant prevention, but there was very low statistical power in each trial. All but one of the 12 trials showed a trend toward benefit from prophylaxis, which was continued for 24 or 48 hours in 10 of the 12 trials. To have 80% power to show a statistically significant benefit in the mean reduction of infection in these 12 trials would require a sample size of 790, but the average sample size in the 12 trials was only 113. A meta-analysis of these trials verified a 48% relative reduction in the rate of infection and suggested that this reduction might be beneficial [78]. The infection rate in the treatment group in these trials averaged 6.8%, however, which led the authors of the meta-analysis to suggest that a different strategy, such as use of a catheter with antimicrobial or anti-adherence qualities, may be needed for more effective prevention.

Respiratory isolation of patients with suspected meningococcal meningitis in a private room (with clinicians wearing masks) until 24 hours after the start of effective therapy has been associated with only very rare cases of transmission to other patients [37] or to health-care personnel; usually the latter form of transmission has been due to exceptional exposure to the patient's respiratory secretions, such as mouth to mouth resuscitation [79–81]. Chemoprophylaxis of household or other very close contacts of patients with meningitis due to *N. meningitidis* or *H. influenzae* is indicated and may be arranged by the local public health department, which should be contacted promptly after admission of a patient with this disease. Eradication of the organism from the index patient before discharge may require additional therapy with rifampin, since many regimens used for therapy of meningitis do not eliminate carriage [8].

REFERENCES

1. Teele DW, Dashefsky B, Rakusan T, Klein JO. Meningitis after lumbar puncture in children with bacteremia. *N Engl J Med* 1981;305: 1079–1081.
2. Watanakunakorn C. *Escherichia coli* meningitis and septicemia associated with an epidural catheter. *Clin Infect Dis* 1995;21:713–714.
3. Gantz NM, Godofsky EW. Nosocomial central nervous system infections. In: Mayhall CG, eds. *Hospital epidemiology and infection control*. Baltimore: Williams & Wilkins, 1996: 246–269.
4. Bennett J. Incidence and nature of endemic and epidemic nosocomial infection. In: Bennett J, Brachman P, eds. *Hospital infections*. Boston: Little, Brown, 1979:233–238.
5. Chernik N, Armstrong D, Posner J. Central nervous system infections in patients with cancer. *Medicine* 1973;52:563–581.
6. Hooper D, Pruitt A, Rubin R. Central nervous system infection in the chronically immunosuppressed. *Medicine* 1985;61:166–188.
7. Hall W, Martinez A, Dummer S, et al. Central nervous system infections in heart and heart-lung transplant recipients. *Arch Neurol* 1989;46:173–177.
8. Reingold AL, Broome CV. Nosocomial central nervous system infections. In: Bennett JV, Brachman PS, eds. *Hospital infections*, 3rd ed. Boston: Little, Brown, 1992:673–683.
9. Culver D, Horan T, Gaynes R, et al. Surgical wound infection rates by wound class, operative procedure, and patient risk index. *Am J Med* 1991;91(suppl 3B):152S–157S.
10. Bayston R, Lari J. A study of the sources of infection in colonized shunts. *Dev Med Child Neurol* 1974;16(suppl 32):16.
11. Price DJE, Sliehg JD. *Klebsiella meningitis*: report of nine cases. *J Neurol Neurosurg Psychiatry* 1972;35:903.
12. Mangi RJ, Quintiliani R, Andriole VT. Gram-negative bacillary meningitis. *Am J Med* 1975;59:829–836.
13. Stephens JL, Peacock JE. Uncommon infections: eye and central nervous system. In: Wenzel RP, eds. *Prevention and control of nosocomial infections*, 2nd ed. Baltimore: Williams & Wilkins, 1993:746–775.
14. Mayhall CG, Archer N, Lamb VA, et al. Ventriculostomy-related infections: a prospective epidemiologic study. *N Engl J Med* 1984;310: 553–559.
15. Mollman HD, Haines SJ. Risk factors for postoperative neurosurgical wound infection. *J Neurosurg* 1986;64:902–906.
16. Aucoin P, Lotilainen H, Gantz N, Davidson R, Kellogg P, Stone B. Intracranial pressure monitors: epidemiologic study of risk factors and infections. *Am J Med* 1988;80:369–376.
17. Blei A, Olafsson S, Webster S, Levy R. Complications of intracranial pressure monitoring in fulminant hepatic failure. *Lancet* 1993;341: 157–158.
18. Durand ML, Calderwood SB, Weber DJ, et al. Acute bacterial meningitis in adults: a review of 493 episodes. *N Engl J Med* 1993;328:21–28.
19. Humphrey MA, Simpson GT, Grindlinger GA. Clinical characteristics of nosocomial sinusitis. *Ann Otol Rhinol Laryngol* 1987;96:687.
20. Hagensee ME, Bauwens JE, Kjos B, Bowden RA. Brain abscess following marrow transplantation: experience at the Fred Hutchinson Cancer Research Center, 1984–1992. *Clin Infect Dis* 1994;19:402–408.
21. Sautter RL, Mattman LH, Legaspi RC. *Serratia marcescens* meningitis associated with a contaminated benzalkonium chloride solution. *Infect Control Hosp Epidemiol* 1984;5:223.
22. Parry MF, Hutchinson JH, Brown NA, et al. Gram-negative sepsis in neonates: a nursery outbreak due to hand carriage of *Citrobacter diversus*. *Pediatrics* 1980;65:1105–1109.
23. Goossens H, Henocque G, Kremp L, et al. Nosocomial outbreak of *Hemophilus influenzae* type b meningitis in an enclosed hospital population. *Lancet* 1986;2:146–149.
24. Abrahamsen TG, Finne PH, Lingaas E. *Flavobacterium meningosepticum* infections in a neonatal intensive care unit. *Acta Paediatr Scand* 1989;78:51.
25. Ayliffe GAJ, Lowbury EJL, Hamilton JG, et al. Hospital infections with *Pseudomonas aeruginosa* in neurosurgery. *Lancet* 1965;2:365–369.
26. Burke JP, Ingall D, Klein JO, et al. *Proteus mirabilis* infections in a hospital nursery traced to a human carrier. *N Engl J Med* 1971;284: 115–121.
27. Berkowitz FE. *Acinetobacter* meningitis: a diagnostic pitfall. A report of three cases. *S Afr Med J* 1982;61:448.
28. Aber RC, Allen N, Howell JT, et al. Nosocomial transmission of group-B streptococci. *Pediatrics* 1976;58:346–353.
29. Campbell AN, Sill PR, Wardle JK. *Listeria* meningitis acquired by cross-infection in a delivery suite. *Lancet* 1981;2:752.
30. Ho JL, Shands KN, Friedland G, et al. An outbreak of type 4b *Listeria monocytogenes* infection involving patients from eight Boston hospitals. *Arch Intern Med* 1986;146:520–524.
31. Larsson S, et al. *Listeria monocytogenes* causing hospital-acquired enterocolitis and meningitis in newborn infants. *Br Med J* 1978;2: 473–474.
32. Nelson KE, et al. Transmission of neonatal listeriosis in a delivery room. *Am J Dis Child* 1985;139:903–905.
33. Schuchat A, et al. Outbreak of neonatal listeriosis associated with mineral oil. *Pediatr Infect Dis J* 1991;10:183–189.
34. Schlech WF, et al. Epidemic listeriosis: evidence for transmission by food. *N Engl J Med* 1983;308:203–206.
35. Glode MP, et al. An outbreak of *Hemophilus influenzae* type b meningitis in an enclosed hospital population. *J Pediatr* 1976;88:36–40.
36. Barton LL, Granoff DM, Barenkamp SJ. Nosocomial spread of *Haemophilus influenzae* type b infection documented by outer membrane protein subtype analysis. *J Pediatr* 1983;102:820.
37. Cohen MS, Steere AC, Baltimore R, et al. Possible nosocomial transmission of group Y *Neisseria meningitidis* among oncology patients. *Ann Intern Med* 1979;91:7–12.
38. Overall JC. Neonatal bacterial meningitis: analysis of predisposing factors and outcome compared with matched control subjects. *J Pediatr* 1970;76:499.
39. Tunkel AR, Scheld M. Central nervous system infection in the immunocompromised host. In: Rubin RH, Young LS, eds. *Clinical approach to infection in the compromised host*, 3rd ed. New York: Plenum Medical Book Company, 1994:163–210.
40. Rahal LJ. Diagnosis and management of meningitis due to gram-negative bacilli in adults. In: Remington JS, Swartz MN, eds. *Current clinical topics in infectious diseases*. New York: McGraw-Hill, 1980:68–84.
41. Martin MA, Massanari RM, Nghiem DD, Smith JL, Corry RJ. Nosocomial aseptic meningitis associated with administration of OKT3. *JAMA* 1988;259:2002–2004.
42. Nguyen MH, Yu VL. Meningitis caused by *Candida* species: an emerging problem in neurosurgical patients. *Clin Infect Dis* 1995;21: 323–327.
43. Ericsson CD, Carmichael M, Pickering LK, et al. Erroneous diagnosis of meningitis due to false-positive Gram stains. *South Med J* 1978;71: 1524.
44. Hoke CH, Batt JM, Mirrett S, et al. False-positive Gram-stained smears. *JAMA* 1979;241:478–480.
45. Musher DM, Schell RF. False-positive Gram stains of cerebrospinal fluid. *Ann Intern Med* 1976;79:603.
46. Peterson E, Thrupp L, Uchiyama N, et al. Factitious bacterial meningitis revisited. *J Clin Microbiol* 1982;16:758.
47. Weinstein RA, Bauer FW, Hoffman RD, et al. Factitious meningitis: diagnostic error due to nonviable bacteria in commercial lumbar puncture trays. *JAMA* 1975;233:878–879.
48. Roos KL, Tunkel AR, Scheld MR. Acute bacterial meningitis in children and adults. In: Scheld MR, Whitely RJ, Durack DT, eds. *Infections of the central nervous system*. New York: Raven Press, 1991:335–409.
49. Schoenbaum SC, Gardner P, Shilito J. Infections of cerebrospinal fluid

shunts: epidemiology, clinical manifestations, and therapy. *J Infect Dis* 1975;131:543–552.
50. Gardner P, Leipzig T, Phillips P. Infections of central nervous system shunts: symposium on infections of the central nervous system. *Med Clin North Am* 1985;69:297–314.
51. Parry SW, Schumacher JF, Llwellyn RC. Abdominal pseudocysts and ascites formation after ventriculoperitoneal shunt procedures. *J Neurosurg* 1975;43:476–480.
52. Noetzel MJ, Baker RP. Shunt fluid examination: risks and benefits in the evaluation of shunt malfunction and infection. *J Neurosurg* 1984; 61:328–332.
53. Mampalam T, Rosenblum M. Trends in the management of bacterial brain abscesses: a review of 102 cases over 17 years. *Neurosurgery* 1988;23:451–458.
54. Wispelwey B, Dacey R, Scheld W. Brain abscess. In: Scheld W, Whitely R, Durack D, eds. *Infections of the central nervous system*. New York: Raven Press, 1991:457–486.
55. Alderson D, Strong A, Ingham H, et al. Fifteen-year review of the mortality of brain abscess. *Neurosurgery* 1981;8:1–86.
56. Carey ME, Chou SN, French LA. Long-term neurologic residua in patients surviving brain abscess with surgery. *J Neurosurg* 1971;34: 652–656.
57. Carey ME, Chou SN, French LA. Experience with brain abscesses. *J Neurosurg* 1972;36:1–9.
58. Walters BC, Hoffman JH, Hendrick EB, Humphreys RP. Cerebrospinal fluid shunt infection: influences on initial management and subsequent outcome. *J Neurosurg* 1984;60:1014–1021.
59. Yogev R. Cerebrospinal fluid shunt infections: a personal view. *Pediatr Infect Dis J* 1985;4:113–118.
60. McLone D, Cryzewski D, Raimondi A, et al. Central nervous system infections as a limiting factor in the intelligence of children with myelomeningocele. *Pediatrics* 1982;70:338–342.
61. Danner RL, Hartman BJ. Update on spinal epidural abscess: 35 cases and review of the literature. *Rev Infect Dis* 1987;9:265–274.
62. Darouiche RO, Hamil RJ, Greenberg SB, Weathers SW, Musher DM. Bacterial spinal epidural abscess: review of 43 cases and literature survey. *Medicine* 1992;71:369–385.
63. Mauser HW, Tulleken CA. Subdural empyema: a review of 48 patients. *Clin Neurol Neurosurg* 1984;86:255–263.
64. Chernik N, Armstrong D, Posner J. Central nervous system infections in patients with cancer: changing patterns. *Cancer* 1977;40:268–274.
65. Weiland D, Ferguson R, Peteron P, et al. Aspergillosis in 25 renal transplant patients: epidemiology, clinical presentation, diagnosis, and management. *Ann Surg* 1983;198:622–629.
66. Anonymous. Antimicrobial prophylaxis in surgery. *Med Lett* 1993; 35:91–94.
67. Anonymous. Recommendations for preventing the spread of vancomycin resistance: Hospital Infection Control Practices Advisory Committee (HICPAC) [Review]. *Infect Control Hosp Epidemiol* 1995; 16:105–113.
68. Lindholm TS, Pylkkanen P. Discitis following removal of intervertebral disc. *Spine* 1982;7:618–622.
69. El-Gindi S, Aref S, Salama M, Andrew J. Infections of intervertebral discs after operation. *J Bone Joint Surg Br* 1965;58:114–116.
70. Odum G, Hart D, Johnson Smith W, Brown I. A seventeen-year survey of the use of ultraviolet radiation. Presented at the *Proceedings of the 24th Meeting of the American Academy of Neurologic Surgery*. New Orleans, 1962.
71. Puranen J, Makela J, Lahde S. Postoperative intervertebral discitis. *Acta Orthop Scand* 1984;56:461–465.
72. Savitz MH, Katz SS. Prevention of primary wound infection in neurosurgical patients: a 10-year study. *Neurosurgery* 1986;18:685–688.
73. Green JR, Kanshepolsky J, Turkian B. Incidence and significance of central nervous system infection in neurosurgical patients. *Adv Neurol* 1974;6:223–228.
74. Quadery LA, Medlery AV, Miles J. Factors affecting the incidence of wound infection in neurosurgery. *Acta Neurochir (Wien)* 1977;39: 133–141.
75. Wright RL. *Craniotomy infections*. Springfield, Ill.: Charles C Thomas, 1966.
76. Horowitz NH, Curtin JA. Prophylactic antibiotics and wound infections following laminectomy for lumbar disc herniation. *J Neurosurg* 1975;43:727–731.
77. Platt R, Zaleznik DF, Hopkins CC, et al. Perioperative antibiotic prophylaxis for herniorrhaphy and breast surgery. *N Engl J Med* 1990; 322:153–160.
78. Langley J, LeBland J, Drake J, Milner R. Efficacy of antimicrobial prophylaxis in placement of cerebrospinal fluid shunts: meta-analysis. *Clin Infect Dis* 1993;17:98–103.
79. Feldman HA. Recent developments in the therapy and control of meningococcal infections. *Dis Mon* 1966;(Feb):1–30.
80. Centers for Disease Control. Nosocomial meningococcemia—Wisconsin. *MMWR* 1978;27:358.
81. Artenstein MD, Ellis RE. The risk of exposure–avea patient with meningococcal meningitis. *Mil Med* 1968;133:474.

Hospital Infections, Fourth Edition,
edited by John V. Bennett and Philip S. Brachman.
Lippincott–Raven Publishers, Philadelphia © 1998

CHAPTER 37

Surgical Infections

E. Patchen Dellinger and N. Joel Ehrenkranz

HISTORICAL BACKGROUND

Up to the end of the nineteenth century, infection was the greatest risk associated with any surgical procedure. Although the practice of surgery had spread rapidly following the introduction of ether at the Massachusetts General Hospital in 1846, even relatively minor procedures could be complicated by severe systemic infection and death, while for major procedures this was the expected outcome. Increasing knowledge regarding the relationship between bacteria and infection, advanced at the end of the century by such legendary figures as Pasteur, Lister, and Koch, led to a series of discoveries and the development of techniques that ultimately paved the way for modern surgery. Pasteur studied the relationship between bacteria and putrefaction. Lister recognized the role of bacteria in surgical wound infections and in 1867 introduced the practice of spraying antiseptics into wounds to combat bacteria. He gave scant attention, however, to the role of hands in introducing bacteria into surgical wounds. In an early application of his own postulates concerning microbial pathogens, Koch produced, in 1878, experimental wound infections by the injection of bacteria. Subsequently, in 1881, he verified the superiority of heat over antiseptics for killing bacteria and preventing access of bacteria to wounds [1].

The role of the surgeon's hands in introducing bacteria into wounds was slow to be recognized despite the work of Semmelweis in 1847. In 1882, when Ernst Bergmann arrived at the Ziegelstrasse Clinic in Berlin and was asked what was new in surgery, he replied, "Today we wash our hands *before* operation" [1]. Although rubber gloves were first developed for the use of Halsted's scrub nurse in 1889, to protect her hands from harsh antiseptics, widespread use of rubber gloves in surgical procedures did not become established until well into the twentieth century.

In the twentieth century, the standardization of aseptic practices in the operating room has greatly improved the safety of clean operative procedures, but operations involving anatomic structures with a dense endogenous flora that cannot be eliminated before operation, such as the colon and rectum, continue to carry a very high risk of infection. A major collaborative study organized by the National Research Council (NRC) documented the rate of surgical wound infection following 15,613 operations carried out over 27 months from 1959 to 1962 in 16 operating rooms of five university hospitals [2]. The study was designed to investigate whether the reduction of airborne bacteria in the operating room, accomplished with ultraviolet light irradiation, could achieve a reduction in surgical wound infections. The study found that ultraviolet light produced a significant reduction in airborne bacteria, but this reduction had no effect on wound infections except in the class of "refined clean" wounds, those wounds with the lowest probability for contamination by endogenous bacteria. The infection rates in all other classes of wounds—other (clean), clean-contaminated, contaminated, and dirty—were unaffected by ultraviolet irradiation.

This study was one of the earliest and certainly one of the most convincing studies to document the importance of endogenous bacteria as the primary etiologic agent of surgical wound infections. This report also introduced a system for classifying wounds according to the risk of endogenous contamination (and thus of postoperative wound infection), which provided a basis for comparing wound infection statistics. Although more sensitive and specific wound classification systems employing additional risk factors for wound infection have been developed since then [3,4], they all continue to incorporate elements of this original scheme. This report was also the largest and most carefully conducted study in its day to examine a host of other factors related to the patient and

E. P. Dellinger: Department of Surgery, University of Washington School of Medicine, Division of General Surgery, University of Washington Medical Center, Seattle, Washington 98195-6410.

N. J. Ehrenkranz: Florida Consortium for Infection Control, South Miami, Florida 33143-5163.

the environment that influenced the risk of postoperative wound infections. Multivariate analysis of this large body of data provided convincing evidence of changes in the risk of developing postoperative infections influenced by the patient's age, obesity, steroid administration, malnutrition, presence of remote infection, use of drains, duration of operation, and duration of preoperative hospitalization. It is interesting to note that although diabetic patients had a higher infection rate than nondiabetics, this apparent difference disappeared after correction for the influence of age.

Although antibiotics were introduced near the end of the Second World War, their use did not appear to result in a lower infection rate despite early optimism. In fact, some careful observers of surgical practice published articles citing a higher rate of surgical site infection with the use of antibiotics than without. This paradox was undoubtedly due to the ineffective (usually postsurgery) use of antibiotics in patients recognized by their surgeons to be at high risk of infection. The effective use of antibiotics for prevention of postoperative infection was ultimately made possible by the pioneering studies of John Burke, who used an animal model to demonstrate the critical importance of the timing of prophylactic antibiotic administration [5]. He showed, in a guinea pig model, that the appropriate antibiotics, given before bacterial contamination, could cause a significant reduction in the risk of infection, while the same antibiotic, given after bacterial contamination, was much less effective. This information was translated into trials demonstrating clinically and statistically significant effects in human patients undergoing scheduled operative procedures, first by Bernard and Cole [6] and then by Polk and Lopez-Mayor [7] in the 1960s. Work on prophylactic antibiotics since that time has focused on defining those procedures and circumstances most likely to benefit from the use of prophylactic antibiotics and on examining the relative efficacy of different drugs and different routes and regimens of administration (see Chapter 14).

As improvements in anesthetic care and understanding of surgical physiology permitted more aggressive and widespread surgical intervention during the second half of this century, the importance of surveillance for infectious complications became more evident. One result of the NRC study cited earlier was the observation of widespread differences in infection rates between the participating hospitals for similar classes of wounds. This was probably one of the inspirations for the careful analysis of additional factors influencing infection risk that was carried out with that study. Data of this sort encouraged the systematic collection of information regarding postoperative infection rates and factors known to influence these rates.

In the 1970s the Centers for Disease Control and Prevention (CDC) began the National Nosocomial Infections Study (NNIS), later renamed the National Nosocomial Infections Surveillance system [8]. From the beginning, although it included all nosocomial infections, this project emphasized the collection of data on postoperative infections. Data from the NNIS project provide a rich source of information about the relative occurrence of infections at all sites in hospitalized surgical patients [9]. Also in the 1970s, reports of surveillance by surgical groups of large numbers of incisions validated the relationship between wound class and differing risks of infection as well as the beneficial effect of reporting wound infection data to the operating surgeons [10].

BIOLOGY OF SURGICAL WOUND INFECTIONS

Surgical wound infections are caused by bacteria, and in the absence of bacteria they do not occur. However, surgeons have known for years that many other factors also influence the risk of infection. Burke demonstrated in 1963 that all (50 of 50) clean surgical incisions contain bacteria at the end of an operation, but only a small number (4% in that report) become infected [11]. An animal study of the relationship between bacterial inoculum and infection risk showed an increasing risk of infection with increasing numbers of bacteria. This was described by a typical sigmoid, biologic curve when inoculum size was graphed against infection incidence. However, there was no inoculum in that study of 1,028 incisions that resulted either in a zero or in a 100% risk of infection [12]. The authors concluded that the development of infection in a surgical incision is "dependent on many factors other than the presence of bacteria." They further predicted that reductions in the incidence of postoperative infection could be achieved by techniques both to reduce the numbers of bacteria that gain access to surgical wounds and by focusing on methods to increase the efficiency of host defenses in resisting those bacteria that do gain access to the wound. Modern surgical surveillance and surgical infection control must acknowledge both of these areas to achieve its goals of minimum postoperative infection rates.

SURGICAL SURVEILLANCE AND CLASSIFICATION OF SURGICAL WOUNDS

As indicated earlier, the oldest and best-established definitions of surgical wound classes originated with the NRC study of the efficacy of ultraviolet light for reducing wound infections. In this study, all wounds were placed into one of five classes [2]:

1. Refined-clean: Clean elective operations, not drained, and primarily closed.
2. Other (clean): Operations that encountered no inflammation and experienced no lapse in technique. In addition, there was no entry into the gastrointestinal or respiratory tract except for incidental appen-

TABLE 37-1. *Infection rate by wound class, historical series*

Years	1960–1962	1967–1977	1975–1976	1977–1986	1987–1990
No. of patients	15,613	62,939	59,352	25,919	84,691
[Reference]	Howard, 1964 [2]	Cruse, 1980 [10]	Haley, 1985 [3]	Olson, 1990 [13]	Culver, 1991 [4]
Wound class					
Clean	5.1	1.5	2.9	1.4	2.1
Clean-contaminated	10.8	7.7	3.9	2.8	3.3
Contaminated	16.3	15.2	8.5	8.4	6.4
Dirty	28.0	40.0	12.6	—	7.1

dectomy or transection of the cystic duct in the absence of signs of inflammation. Entrance into the genitourinary tract or biliary tract was considered clean if the urine and/or bile were sterile.

3. Clean-contaminated: Gastrointestinal tract or respiratory tract entered without significant spill. Minor lapse in technique. Entry into the genitourinary tract or biliary tract in the presence of infected urine or bile.
4. Contaminated: Major lapse in technique (such as emergency open cardiac massage), acute bacterial inflammation without pus, spillage from the gastrointestinal tract, or fresh traumatic wound from relatively clean source.
5. Dirty: Presence of pus, perforated viscus, or traumatic wound that is old or from a dirty source.

All reports since the original NRC report have condensed this system into four groups, combining refined-clean and other (clean) into the one category of clean. Subsequent reports indicate a general consistency of the trends, with a tendency toward decreased overall infection rates that is most marked in the contaminated and dirty classes of wounds (Table 37-1) [2–4,10,13]. These rates may have been influenced by a variety of factors, including a better understanding of the effective use of prophylactic antibiotics and of the bacteriology of dirty operative cases as well as a reduction in the practice of closing the skin in dirty cases.

Since the NRC study, much effort has been put into understanding which factors other than wound class affect the risk of infection. This trend was actually begun with the original analysis of additional risk factors performed with the original NRC study. The earliest efforts at control of surgical infection focused on lessening infection rates for clean wounds since these wounds should theoretically have a zero infection rate if all bacteria could be eliminated from the wound. Efforts thus focused on aseptic technique for prevention of infection. Subsequent work found that even clean wounds become contaminated with some bacteria, and evaluation of historical data (Table 37-1) discovered a potential for reducing infection rates even in high-risk wounds. This provided an incentive to understanding the underlying risk of infection in order to be able to compare, in a sensible manner, wound infection rates from time to time in the same institution and from institution to institution at any time.

Another major effort in this area came from the Study of Efficacy of Nosocomial Infection Control (SENIC) project initiated by the CDC in 1974. The SENIC project collected data on surgical site infections and potential risk factors from 59,352 surgical patients admitted and operated on in 388 representative U.S. hospitals during 1975 and 1976 [3]. Multivariate analysis uncovered four risk factors with roughly equal weight in predicting wound infection. These were having an abdominal operation, having an operation that lasted > 2 hours, having a contaminated or dirty operation by the traditional NRC definitions, and having three or more discharge diagnoses. A comparison of the predictive accuracy of the SENIC system compared with the NRC classification system is given in Table 37-2. This system is clearly more discriminating than the old NRC classification of wounds. The range of relative risks of infection among clean wounds with different SENIC risk indexes is 1:14, and that of clean-contaminated wounds is 1:30; within the SENIC risk index the range is 1:2.4 among wounds with

TABLE 37-2. *Comparison of SENIC and NRC risk predictions for surgical wound infection*

	SENIC risk index						
NRC class	0	1	2	3	4	All	Maximum ratio[a]
Clean	1.1	3.9	8.4	15.8	—	2.9	14.4
Clean-contaminated	0.6	2.8	8.4	17.7	—	3.9	29.5
Contaminated	—	4.5	8.3	11.0	23.9	8.5	5.3
Dirty	—	6.7	10.9	18.8	27.4	12.6	4.1
All	1.0	3.6	8.9	17.2	27.0	4.1	—
Maximum ratio[a]	1.8	2.4	1.3	1.7	1.1	—	—

[a]Ratio of the lowest to the highest infection rate in wound class or in risk index.

TABLE 37-3. *Comparison of NNIS and NRC risk predictions for surgical wound infection*

NRC class	NNIS risk index 0	1	2	3	All	Maximum ratio[a]
Clean	1.0	2.3	5.4	—	2.1	5.4
Clean-contaminated	2.1	4.0	9.5	—	3.3	4.5
Contaminated	—	3.4	6.8	13.2	6.4	3.9
Dirty	—	3.1	8.1	12.8	7.1	4.1
All	1.5	2.9	6.8	13.0	2.8	—
Maximum ratio[a]	2.1	1.7	1.8	1.0	—	—

[a]Ratio of the lowest to the highest infection rate in wound class or in risk index.

one risk factor and < 1:2 for all other risks. One weakness of the SENIC index is the employment of the number of discharge diagnoses as a factor, since this number can be determined accurately only at the time of discharge.

The CDC has subsequently produced a new and simplified risk index in connection with the NNIS project previously described [4]. In the NNIS risk system, the preoperative assessment by the anesthesiologist according to the physical status index of the American Society of Anesthesiologists [14] is used, instead of the number of discharge diagnoses. One point is assigned for a preoperative assessment (ASA) score of 3, 4, or 5. Instead of counting any operation lasting > 2 hours, a table was developed that indicated the 75th percentile for operative duration for most operative procedures. A point is assigned for operative duration above the 75th percentile. The wound classification of contaminated or dirty is retained as in the SENIC risk index and adds one point to the risk score. The risk factor for abdominal operation is dropped. Thus, the NNIS index has a possible score of 0 to 3.

A comparison of the predictive accuracy of the NNIS index with the old NRC classification can be seen in Table 37-3. This simpler index retains the increased accuracy and consistency within risk strata of the SENIC index while being easier to apply. One can see that the ratio of risks within single NRC wound classes ranges between 3.9 and 5.4, while the ratio of risks within single NNIS risk strata all fall between 1.0 and 2.1. The NNIS program continues to gather data using this index, and it is hoped that further data regarding its accuracy will be forthcoming. For surveillance programs with limited resources, it can be seen that surveillance of the 53% of patients with one or more risk factors would yield data on 75% of all wound infections, thus increasing the efficiency of surveillance efforts [4].

Despite its advantages over the NRC wound classification system as a sole method of estimating infection risk, the NNIS index, as is the case with all indexes, cannot predict the outcomes for individual patients. In addition, it lacks predictive power for certain highly standardized procedures, such as coronary artery bypass grafting [15], cesarean section [16], or craniotomy [17]. While the NNIS index may accurately distinguish the risk of procedures from different categories of operative procedures, it does a poor job of distinguishing higher- and lower-risk procedures among all patients undergoing the same procedure. In this case, different risk factors specific to the procedure and to the population become more important. Another potential problem with this system is inconsistency in assignment of ASA scores [18]. A comparison of the sensitivity and specificity of ASA scores compared with the presence of three or more discharge diagnoses would be of interest. This comparison could probably be carried out on the original data sets used in the studies by Haley et al. [3] and Culver et al. [4].

HOST FACTORS THAT INFLUENCE INFECTION RISK

Many individual host factors influence infection risk. Several have been listed in the discussion of the NRC study earlier in this chapter. Most have been determined in studies like the NRC study, where patients undergoing one procedure or a variety of procedures and stratified by other known risk factors and/or by multivariate analysis have been followed to determine outcomes and the association of postulated risk factors with those outcomes. In most cases, the precise mechanism of action that links the risk factor and the infectious outcome are not known, although plausible explanations have often been provided based on logical reasoning but not on proof. Thus, the increased infection rates observed with advanced age, extreme obesity, weight loss, hypoalbuminemia, and, possibly, diabetes mellitus have been attributed to nonspecific defects in host defenses. The increased risk of infection observed in patients with anergy is not easily related to other measurable immune functions.

Patients who have an active infection at another site in the body are at increased risk of postoperative surgical site infection [2]. This finding may relate to the increased risk that significant numbers of bacteria will gain access to the wound during the procedure or to inoculation of the surgical wound by bacteremia [19]. Data from human wounds suggests that the risk of postoperative infection is very great whenever the wound inoculum exceeds 10^5 bacteria [20]. Although lymphatics have been suspected as a route of infection in patients with distal infections, evidence is lacking [21]. Patients who have been shaved at the surgical site before the time of operation have a higher risk of infection, and this is thought to be due to the tiny nicks and cuts that are caused by the razor and subsequent bacterial proliferation and inflammation in those injuries [22]. In vascular surgery, similar operations have a higher risk of postoperative infection in the groin region than in the arm or neck [23]. This may stem from local vascularity, local differences in bacterial number and type, or both.

INTRAOPERATIVE EVENTS THAT INFLUENCE INFECTION RISK

Infection risk is correlated with several factors that can be measured in the operating room. Other than wound class, one of the most consistently reported factors is the duration of the operative procedure. The precise connection between duration and infection risk is not known. It is plausible that a prolonged operation results in more desiccation of tissues, potential for hypothermia [24] of the patient, and increased exposure of the wound to bacteria. It is also possible, however, that a longer operative duration is a marker for other, unmeasured factors, such as the underlying difficulty of the procedure, more scarring, larger tumor, obesity of the patient, or difficulty in exposure. No trial has been, or will be, conducted in which the same surgeon, in cases of equal severity, deliberately varies the duration of the procedure. An operation that is rushed may heighten the risk of intraoperative contamination or of imperfect hemostasis, with subsequent increased risk of infection. Operations should not be prolonged unnecessarily, but emphasis on the speed of operation may be misleading.

Operative technique and skill are widely believed to influence the risk of infection and of other operative complications, but direct evidence is wanting. However, it can be shown that gross contamination of the operative field [25], poor hemostasis in the wound [7], and the need for homologous blood transfusions [26] are all associated with a higher incidence of postoperative infection. Surgeons commonly believe that leaving "dead space" or fluid in a wound increases the risk of infection. However, animal models of infection demonstrate that placing sutures to eliminate dead space [27] or placing drains to close wounds and evacuate fluid [28] actually amplifies the risk of infection. Few prospective, controlled trials of this type are available for clinical surgery [29]; however, most observational studies also demonstrate a greatly increased risk of infection with the use of drains [30,31].

Any event that supports the access of bacteria to the operative wound will increase the risk of infection. As discussed earlier, in intestinal operations gross spill is associated with a higher rate of infection. In clean operations, a lapse in technique or in the usual protective devices is associated with increased infection risk. In particular, glove punctures [32,33] or other episodes of contamination of the sterile field [33] raise the rate of infection. While few data directly confirm the value of hand scrubbing by the surgical team, the practice is firmly entrenched and presumably provides some protection against serious bacterial contamination when glove punctures occur. One recent observational study provides support for the importance of good hand preparation techniques [34]. The efficiency of the surgical drapes and gowns in preventing bacterial access to the surgical field also influences surgical risk. Impervious synthetic drapes result in a lower rate of infection in clean wounds when compared with more loosely woven materials [35]. While most bacteria that cause wound infections come from the endogenous flora of the patient, and a smaller number come by direct contact from the hands and torn gloves of the operating team, occasional wound infection epidemics can be traced to a member of the operating team, including a circulating nurse or anesthesiologist who does not appear to have direct contact with the wound [36,37]. Such infections can occur without observed breaches of aseptic practice.

Preparation of the Patient and Operative Site

Despite much study, some common practices are of unknown efficacy for preventing wound infection. Different reports indicate reduction in infection or no effect from preoperative bathing of the patient with antiseptic soaps [38]. If practical, the lowest wound infection rate for clean wounds is associated with no hair removal at the operative site. If hair removal is necessary, depilatory is preferable to clipping, which is preferable to shaving. Any hair removal should be done as close to the time of incision as possible [22]. Several agents are suitable for antiseptic preparation of the operative site. They include chlorhexidine preparations, various iodophor compounds, and tincture of iodine. Most operative sites are prepared first by the use of an antiseptic soap, followed by an antiseptic preparation without detergent. Various commercial systems that employ foam or adherent plastic drapes with an antiseptic contained within the adhesive also seem to produce acceptable reduction in resident bacteria at the operative site while enhancing convenience or saving time in the operating room.

ANTIMICROBIAL PROPHYLAXIS

Since the first articles [6,7] were published that cited the effectiveness of perioperative prophylactic antimicrobial administration, literally thousands of articles covering this topic have come out (see Chapter 14). The recommendations from a recent review sponsored by the Infectious Diseases Society of America and endorsed by it and by the Surgical Infection Society are summarized in Tables 37-4,

TABLE 37-4. *Recommendations for procedures that should receive prophylactic antimicrobial agents*[a]

Procedure	Strength of recommendation	Quality of evidence
Surgical procedures that enter the gastrointestinal tract	A	I
Esophageal		
Gastric[b]		
Small intestinal		
Biliary[c]		
Colonic[d]		
Appendiceal[e]		
Head and neck procedures that enter the oropharynx	A	I
Abdominal and lower-extremity vascular procedures	A	I
Craniotomy	A	I
Orthopedic procedures with hardware insertion	A	I
Cardiac procedures with median sternotomy	A	I
Hysterectomy	A	I
Primary cesarean section or other cesarean sections involving prolonged rupture of membranes[f]	A	I
Procedures that include the implantation of permanent prosthetic materials[g]	B	III
Optional		
Breast and hernia procedures[h]	B	I
Other "clean" procedures where the clinical setting indicates an increased infection risk[h]	B	III
Initially clean procedures that become contaminated during the conduct of the procedure	C	III
Low-risk gastric and biliary procedures[h]	B	III
There are not currently available data to apply these recommendations to so-called minimally invasive procedures, such as laparoscopic cholecystectomy or laparoscopically assisted bowel resections. Pending further data, it seems safest to apply the same standards as would be used for the same procedure done through a traditional incision.	C	III
Open gynecologic and urologic procedures that involve bowel are covered by the same guidelines that have been developed for general surgical procedures. The literature for transurethral procedures is large and controversial. It seems prudent to clear bacteriuria before any urinary tract procedure when clinical circumstances permit. Beyond that, local guidelines for implementation of the standard should reflect local practice.	B	III
It is common practice among pediatric surgeons to employ broad-spectrum antimicrobial prophylaxis for most operative procedures on newborn infants < 30 days old. There are no specific data regarding the necessity or effectiveness of this practice.	C	III

A, strongly recommended; B, recommended; C, optional; I, evidence from at least one properly randomized, controlled trial; II, evidence from at least one well-designed clinical trial without randomization, from cohort or case-controlled analytic studies (preferably from more than one center), from multiple time series studies, or from dramatic results in uncontrolled experiments; III, evidence from opinions of respected authorities, based on clinical experience, descriptive studies, or reports of expert committees.

[a]Specific recommendations are not referenced to the original source(s).

[b]"High risk" patients are those undergoing gastric procedures for cancer, gastric ulcer, bleeding, or obstruction or morbidly obese patients or those with iatrogenic or natural suppression of gastric acid secretion.

[c]"High risk" patients are those over the age of 60 with recent symptoms of acute inflammation, common duct stones, or jaundice or those who have previously had biliary operation.

[d]Oral prophylaxis with neomycin and erythromycin or another proven regimen for 18 hr before surgery is sufficient for scheduled colon operations where effective cleansing of the bowel can be achieved. Where cleansing cannot be achieved owing to obstruction or other emergency conditions, or where the surgeon desires additional prophylactic protection for a high-risk patient, parenteral antimicrobials may also be administered. An agent effective against *Enterobacteriaceae* and *Bacteroides fragilis* group organisms should be used (see Table 37-5).

[e]If the appendix is freely perforated or associated with an abscess, antimicrobial administration is considered therapeutic for the abdominal cavity, not prophylactic, and should be continued until an appropriate clinical response is obtained. The preoperative dose may function in a prophylactic manner for the incision, but treatment of established infection in the abdominal cavity requires continuation of the antimicrobial regimen after surgery. An agent effective against Enterobacteriaceae and *B. fragilis* group organisms should be included in regimens both for prophylaxis and for therapy.

[f]For cesarean section, standard practice is to administer the prophylactic antimicrobial immediately after the cord is clamped.

[g]This standard is widely recommended and practiced, although specific data for the wide range of prosthetic devices in common use are not available. These devices would include various central nervous system shunts, vascular access devices, prosthetic mesh for hernia repair, and many others in addition to specific devices, such as orthopedic hardware and cardiac valves, covered under other standards.

[h]Many authorities believe that these patients do not require antimicrobial prophylaxis. Certain clinical contexts increase the risk of postoperative infection and might strengthen the motivation to use prophylactic antimicrobials. These factors include American Society of Anesthesiologists (ASA) preoperative assessments of 3, 4, or 5; three or more major preoperative diagnoses; an operation expected to last > 2 hr; and an operation that lasts longer than the 75th percentile for that procedure. An undesirable local rate of wound infection may also heighten the benefit achieved from prophylactic antimicrobials, but the underlying cause of such a rate should be sought and corrected.

(The entire table is modified from Dellinger EP, Gross PA, Barrett TL, et al. Quality standard for antimicrobial prophylaxis in surgical procedures. *Clin Infect Dis* 1994;18:422–427.)

TABLE 37-5. *Choice of antimicrobial agents*[a]

Choice of agent	Strength of recommendation	Quality of evidence
Many antimicrobials have been demonstrated to be effective for perioperative prophylaxis. The drug chosen should have activity against the pathogens most commonly associated with wound infections that occur after the type of procedure being performed and against the pathogens endogenous to the body region being operated upon. For procedures on the distal ileum, colon, or appendix, the antimicrobial(s) used should always have activity against both *Enterobacteriaceae* and the common enteric anaerobic species, especially the *Bacteroides fragilis* group. Although infections that occur after gynecologic operations, especially hysterectomy, often involve anaerobic organisms, there has not been a demonstration of superiority by adding specific anti-anaerobic antibiotics compared with cefazolin alone. A very acceptable choice is to use cefotetan or cefoxitin for operations on the distal ileum, appendix, or colon and to use cefazolin for all other procedures.	A	I
Vancomycin can be given instead of cefazolin for patients who are allergic to cephalosporins or in conditions where methicillin-resistant *S. aureus* (MRSA) infections are determined by the infection control committee to be prevalent. Since vancomycin does not provide any activity against facultative gram-negative rods that may be present in the context of upper-gastrointestinal surgery, lower-extremity vascular surgery, or hysterectomies, another agent with gram-negative activity should be added in these cases. If vancomycin is being given because of concern over MRSA, cefazolin can also be given. If cephalosporin allergy is the concern, one can include aztreonam or an aminoglycoside with vancomycin. An aminoglycoside combined with clindamycin or metronidazole, or aztreonam combined with clindamycin, can be substituted for cefoxitin or cefotetan in allergic patients who are scheduled to undergo a colonic procedure. Aztreonam should not be used alone in combination with metronidazole because this combination lacks activity against gram-positive cocci and may lead to an increase in infections caused by *S. aureus.* If this combination is used, an agent with activity against gram-positive cocci must also be included. Unfortunately, data regarding the efficacy of these alternative recommendations are not available.	C	III

A, strongly recommended; B, recommended; C, optional; I, evidence from at least one properly randomized, controlled trial; II, evidence from at least one well-designed clinical trial without randomization, from cohort or case-controlled analytic studies (preferably from more than one center), from multiple time series studies, or from dramatic results in uncontrolled experiments; III, evidence from opinions of respected authorities, based on clinical experience, descriptive studies, or reports of expert committees.

[a]Specific recommendations are not referenced to the original source(s).

(The entire table is modified from Dellinger EP, Gross PA, Barrett TL, et al. Quality standard for antimicrobial prophylaxis in surgical procedures. *Clin Infect Dis* 1994;18:422–427. Detailed reference sources can be found there.)

37-5, and 37-6 [39]. Each recommendation given in these tables is classified by us according to the strength of the recommendation for or against a particular use and according to the quality of the evidence on which the recommendation is based. These categories are adapted from those published in an article by McGowan et al. and Gross et al. [40,41].

For most questions there is a consensus about general principles. The most contentious areas remaining for antimicrobial prophylaxis relate to the use of prophylaxis for some clean operative procedures, the specific agent used in some contexts, the duration of antimicrobial administration, and the relative merits of oral antimicrobial agents, parenteral antimicrobial agents, or both for prophylaxis in colorectal procedures. Most practitioners agree that antimicrobial prophylaxis is beneficial for procedures that involve entry into the gastrointestinal tract with resulting exposure of the surgical site to endogenous intestinal bacteria.

In the case of gastric operations, the highly acid gastric contents keep endogenous bacterial numbers very low in patients undergoing elective peptic ulcer operations, and antimicrobial prophylaxis is not considered necessary. With the recent understanding of the role of *Helicobacter pylori* in the pathogenesis of peptic ulcer disease, elective operations for this condition have essentially ceased. Procedures on the stomach for cancer, gastric ulcer, bleeding, obstruction, and perforation are considered high risk because of the greater bacterial densities encountered and the increased risk of postoperative infection; prophylaxis is thus recommended for these types of surgery. Prophylaxis is also recommended for gastric operations on morbidly obese patients [42–47].

The biliary tract is sterile in healthy persons, and colonization rates are low during elective operations for symptomatic stone disease. Higher rates of colonization and of postoperative infection are encountered in patients who are > 60 years old or who have common duct stones, bile duct obstruction, recent episodes of acute cholecystitis, or previous operations on the biliary tract. Antimicrobial prophylaxis is recommended for patients in these high-risk categories [39,42–47].

TABLE 37-6. *Dose, timing, and duration of antimicrobial administration for prophylaxis*[a]

Antimicrobial administration	Strength of recommendation	Quality of evidence
Dose: Very few reports have ever focused on the appropriate dose to use when administering a prophylactic antimicrobial. The dose used should never be less than the standard therapeutic dose for that drug. Considering the very short duration of administration recommended for prophylaxis and the safety profile of most prophylactic antimicrobial agents, it is reasonable to use a dose on the high side of the usual therapeutic range (1–2 g of cefazolin, cefoxitin, or cefotetan for adults and 30–40 mg/kg for children).	C	III
Timing: The goal should be to achieve inhibitory antimicrobial levels at the time of incision and to maintain adequate levels for the duration of the procedure. Parenteral perioperative prophylactic antimicrobials should be administered intravenously during the interval beginning 60 minutes before the incision is made. A time of administration as close as possible to the time of incision is preferred.	A	I
For cesarean section, the antimicrobial should be delayed until the umbilical cord is clamped and then should be administered immediately. Cefazolin, 2 g, is recommended.	A	I
Duration: The optimal duration of antimicrobial administration for perioperative prophylaxis is not known. Many reports document effective prophylaxis when a single dose of drug has been administered. It is likely that no further benefit is obtained by administering additional doses after the patient has left the operating room. Thus, pending further data, postoperative dosing is not recommended. Antimicrobials for prophylaxis should be discontinued within 24 hr of the operative procedure.	B	II
The optimal duration of prophylaxis for cardiac operations is still the subject of debate, and many believe longer durations are needed. However, continuing prophylaxis until all catheters and drains have been removed is not appropriate.	C	III
Repeat doses during the surgical procedure: The necessity of administering additional doses of a prophylactic antimicrobial during an operative procedure of long duration has not been clearly defined. A number of reports, however, cite a reduced effectiveness of prophylactic antimicrobials for prevention of infection, either for long-duration procedures or in cases where measurement of serum or tissue levels show low levels of drug during the procedure. Based on current information, additional intraoperative doses of antimicrobial agents should be given at intervals of one or two times the half-life of the drug so that adequate levels are maintained during the entire operation.[b]	C	III

[a]Specific recommendations are not referenced to the original source(s).

[b]Representative half-lives (with normal renal function) of the usually recommended prophylactic antimicrobial agents are cefazolin, 1.8 hr; vancomycin, 3–9 hr; cefoxitin, 40–60 min; cefotetan, 3–4.6 hr; aztreonam, 1.6–2.1 hr; aminoglycosides, 2 hr; clindamycin, 2.4–3 hr; and metronidazole, 8 hr.

(The entire table is modified from Dellinger EP, Gross PA, Barrett TL, et al. Quality standard for antimicrobial prophylaxis in surgical procedures. *Clin Infect Dis* 1994;18:422–427. Detailed reference sources can be found there.)

Elective colon and rectal procedures are followed by very high infection rates in the absence of antimicrobial prophylaxis, and such prophylaxis is widely practiced [46,48]. For procedures other than colorectal operations, parenteral administration of the antimicrobial agent is standard. For colorectal procedures the opportunity exists to use oral (luminal) agents to lower the endogenous bacterial load before operation. Both routes of antimicrobial administration have been found to cut down infections when compared with placebo, but the additional benefit of using both together has not been firmly established [48]. Nevertheless, the most common practice in the United States is to achieve mechanical cleansing of the bowel combined with oral administration of antimicrobial agents designed to reduce the luminal bacterial load on the day before the scheduled procedure and to administer parenteral agents in the operating room immediately before the operation [48,49]. The oral regimen that has the best support is the administration of 1 g each of neomycin and erythromycin base at 19, 18, and 9 hours before the scheduled time for the colon procedure [50].

Some procedures do not enter the gastrointestinal tract but nevertheless have a high rate of postoperative infection without prophylaxis. They include lower-extremity vascular procedures, hysterectomy, primary cesarean section, and craniotomy. Some other procedures do not have excessive infection rates, but any infections that do occur have devastating consequences. These operations include joint replacement and placement of other prosthetic devices, cardiac procedures, and aortic graft placements (see Chapters 39, 40). These procedures are widely regarded as benefiting from prophylactic antimicrobial administration [39, 42–47].

The use of prophylactic antimicrobial agents for clean operations in which the risk of infection is relatively low and the consequences of infection are considered mild is controversial [43,51,52]. When infection rates are low and the consequences small, use of antimicrobial agents may expose many patients to drug to prevent a single infection, which may predispose to the development of bacterial resistance and/or to an increase in adverse drug reactions in the population being treated. One proposal has been to limit the use of prophylactic antimicrobial agents to those clean procedures that can be demonstrated to carry a high risk of surgical site infection using one of the risk indexes we have discussed [46].

Many agents have been found to be effective for perioperative prophylaxis. In recent years most new antimicrobial agents with any potential for surgical use have been licensed with one or more prophylaxis indications. The primary requirement for a prophylactic antimicrobial agent is that it be active against the pathogens known to be present at the operative site and those typically recovered from surgical site infections. The agent most commonly recommended for procedures that do not involve the distal ileum, colon, rectum, or appendix, and that therefore do not entail much risk of exposure to colonic anaerobes, is cefazolin [39,42–47]. Procedures that do involve these sites require an antimicrobial agent with activity against *Bacteroides fragilis* and other colonic anaerobes as well as the *Enterobacteriaceae* [48]. Cefoxitin or cefotetan are the two most commonly recommended agents. Newer, so-called advanced-generation agents have not been confirmed to be superior to cefazolin, cefoxitin, or cefotetan for the prophylactic indications for which these three drugs have been recommended [47]. Regimens with specific activity against *Enterococcus* species have not been shown to achieve superior results in colorectal procedures. Such regimens (ampicillin, amoxicillin, or vancomycin combined with gentamicin) are recommended for prophylaxis against bacterial endocarditis when gastrointestinal or genitourinary procedures are performed on patients with high-risk cardiac conditions [53].

The timing of antimicrobial administration for prophylaxis is important (see Chapter 14). For maximum effectiveness the agent must be present in blood and body fluids before an incision is made. The original successful reports of prophylaxis specified that drugs were administered to patients “on call” to the operating room [7]. Before then, the practice had been to begin antibiotic therapy in the recovery room after the completion of the procedure. This was ineffective. Recent reports have confirmed the importance of administering prophylactic agents in the immediate preoperative period, usually within 120 minutes or less of the incision [54,55]. Unfortunately, postoperative initiation of “prophylaxis” is still relatively common [54,56,57].

The necessary duration of antimicrobial prophylaxis is not established, although analysis of data from some published reports suggests that antimicrobial activity should be present in blood and wound fluids at the time of closure for maximal effectiveness. Most early trials employed administration on a schedule that gave the third and last dose 12 hours after the first, preoperative dose. Some trials report longer durations, and prolonged administration of prophylactic agents is common in clinical practice [54,56,57]. Although a single report suggests better results with longer use of prophylactic therapy in certain high-risk patients undergoing peripheral vascular procedures [58], most published articles support a short duration of antimicrobial prophylaxis [47,59,60]. Another area of controversy is the prevention of infection after traumatic injuries that expose the patient to bacterial contamination before antimicrobial treatment can be initiated. Because prophylactic agents cannot be administered before contamination, some have termed their use therapeutic rather than prophylactic. However, prophylaxis can be achieved for the operative wounds created in treating the injuries. A number of recent studies have established that even in this context, a short duration of antibiotic treatment is as effective as a prolonged one, and probably preferable [60,61].

SELECTIVE DIGESTIVE DECONTAMINATION

More than 10 years ago, Stoutenbeek and co-authors proposed a method of selective digestive decontamination (SDD) to lower the infection rate in post-traumatic surgical patients in the intensive care unit (ICU) [62]. The concept holds that potentially pathogenic bacilli reside in an intestinal reservoir and serve as the source for many nosocomial infections. The proposed regimen—tobramycin, polymyxin B, and amphotericin B by nasogastric tube and oral paste for the duration of ICU stay and parenteral cefotaxime for the first 5 days—is supposed to suppress potentially pathogenic microorganisms in the gastrointestinal tract while preserving the useful anaerobic flora that promote colonization resistance. Despite 10 years of study and numerous publications, the concept is still the subject of much controversy. It has many proponents in Europe but has failed to garner much enthusiasm or be put into wide practice in the United States except among some solid-organ transplant groups [63]. While many articles report a reduction in nosocomial lower respiratory tract infections, few cite any important differences in mortality rates or duration of ICU stay, and the suspicion arises that what has changed is the diagnosis of pneumonia, a notoriously difficult task in ICU patients. A number of the articles written about SDD report the early emergence of resistant gram-positive cocci [64,65]. Some recent reviews make clear that the role of SDD is still very unsettled [65,67]. At present SDD remains a program in search of a role.

SYSTEMIC SURVEILLANCE OF POSTOPERATIVE INFECTION

The basic elements of a successful infection surveillance program include a definition of specific types of postoperative infections, a method for screening patients at risk, and a reliable means of recording and retrieving information (see Chapter 5). The observer who records the presence or absence of infection (infection control practitioner or hospital epidemiologist) should have no conflict of interest in performing these duties. The surgical staff should be aware of methodology for screening and recording infection and should accept the criteria to define infections. It is useful for the observer to make rounds with several surgeons to ensure agreement on the use of definitions. The general criteria put forth by the CDC [68] have recently been updated (Table 37-7). A common definition error is to equate infection with recovery of a certain bacterial species from the wound site. Bacteriologic findings do not distinguish between colonization and infection.

Surveillance objectives should be defined. All surgical infections are not necessarily equally important to identify. Highest priority is given to detecting infections that lead to death, reoperation, increased intensity of services, and special diagnostic or therapeutic measures (including parenteral administration of antimicrobials, prolongation of hospital stay, or hospital readmission). Lower priority is assigned to finding superficial infections that do not lead to the outcomes just cited and that are readily treated on an ambulatory basis, without a major increase in therapeutic costs or delay in the patient's return to regular activities. Infections, especially deep ones, complicating operations involving cardiac, vascular, and neurologic structures; bones; joints; stomach; bowel; or rectum are more likely to compromise a patient's well-being than are similar infections complicating hernia repair, uterus, gallbladder, or thyroid operations.

Postoperative infections beyond the operative site may bring about considerable morbidity and should be included in routine systematic surveillance. This is particularly true for pneumonia (see Chapter 32). In special-care surgical units, surveillance of various infections caused by multiply drug-resistant bacteria may be especially useful in providing information to surgeons about possible inappropriate antibiotic usage and may serve as an indicator of personnel or environmental transmission of bacteria. Hospital-wide outbreaks of infections due to methicillin-resistant *S. aureus* or vancomycin-resistant enterococci and clusters of diarrhea or colitis due to *Clostridium difficile* toxin may manifest first among postoperative patients (see Chapter 34). Surveillance activities should be geared to identify them.

Hospital episodes of surgical site infections and postoperative episodes of bacteremia, pneumonia, and symptomatic urinary tract infection should be identified for the three categories of elective clean, clean-contaminated, and contaminated operations. Whereas patients having dirty operations may acquire a new infection as a complication of the operative procedure, it is often difficult to separate this event from extension of the infection already present at the time of operation. As the surveillance findings from patients undergoing specific types or groups of operations become large enough for meaningful interpretation, infection rates for various procedures may be established as a baseline and to reflect the specific populations of patients being treated. After a database has been collected, cluster definitions and threshold levels for outbreak investigation may be defined.

The relative sensitivities of various methods for finding nosocomial infection have been reported [69] (see Chapter 5). It may not be possible, because of methodologic and interobserver differences as well as differences in groups of patients, to directly compare infection rates complicating specific operations done at different hospitals. At the Florida Consortium for Infection Control, an organization of nonteaching community hospitals, a retrospective medical audit has been found useful in assessing the accuracy of infection control personnel (ICP) in reporting all categories of postoperative infections. The expected ICP sensitivity for detecting infections at the operative site is ≥ 80%; the specificity is ≥ 97%. At the Minneapolis VA Medical Center, the infection control nurse uses the floor nurses who see patients' wounds as part of daily care as sensitive indicators [70]. They have been trained to recognize and to report to the nurse epidemiologist all clinically suspicious wounds. Such wounds are personally examined by the nurse epidemiologist, who makes a determination of the wound status. In addition, every nurse on a surgical ward is authorized to send wound fluid for culture without a specific order.

A positive culture is not, by itself, a sign of infection. Instead, the fact that a culture was sent alerts the nurse epidemiologist that the wound was regarded as suspicious and prompts the nurse to inspect the wound personally. This system allows the nurse epidemiologist to focus his or her efforts on only the most suspicious wounds and also provides a complete microbiologic record for those wounds that are determined to be infected [70]. Cardo et al. have reported on the accuracy of a similar system and found that sensitivity varied between 80% to 90%, depending on the degree of experience of the nurse epidemiologist, and that specificity was in excess of 99% [71].

The surveillance methods described here are all highly labor intensive. Moreover, the learning period for the ICP may vary from several months to several years [71,72], depending on the intensity of training. Once a satisfactory level of surveillance sensitivity is achieved, it can be maintained only in direct proportion to the time available for ICP to conduct surveillance. Yokoe and Platt have outlined a novel screening method in which antibiotic treat-

TABLE 37-7. *CDC definitions of nosocomial surgical site infections (SSIs), 1992*

Superficial incisional SSIs: Infection occurs within 30 days after the operative procedure **and** involves only skin or subcutaneous tissue of the incision **and** at least **one** of the following signs or symptoms is present:

- Purulent drainage from the superficial incision
- Organisms isolated from an aseptically obtained culture of fluid or tissue from the superficial incision
- At least one of the following signs or symptoms of infection: pain or tenderness, localized swelling, redness, or heat; **and** superficial incision is deliberately opened by the surgeon or attending physician
- Diagnosis of superficial incisional SSI by the surgeon or attending physician
  - The following are not reported as superficial incisional SSIs: stitch abscess (minimal inflammation and discharge confined to the points of suture penetration), infection of an episiotomy or a neonate's circumcision site[a], infected burn wound[a], and incisional SSI that extends into the fascial and muscle layers (see *Deep incisional SSI*).

Deep incisional SSIs: Infection occurs within 30 days after the operative procedure if no implant[b] is left in place or within 1 yr if implant is in place and the infection appears to be related to the operative procedure **and** involves deep soft tissues (e.g., fascial and muscle layers) of the incision **and** at least **one** of the following signs or symptoms is present.

- Purulent drainage from the deep incision but not from the organ/space component of the surgical site
- A deep incision spontaneously dehisces or is deliberately opened by a surgeon when the patient has at least one of the following signs or symptoms: fever (> 38°C), localized pain, or tenderness, unless culture of the incision gives negative results
- An abscess or other evidence of infection involving the deep incision found on direct examination, during reoperation, or by histopathologic or radiologic examination
- Diagnosis of a deep incisional SSI by a surgeon or attending physician

Organ/space SSIs: An organ/space SSI involves any part of the anatomy (e.g., organs or spaces), other than the incision, opened or manipulated during the operative procedure. Specific sites are assigned to organ/space SSIs to identify the location of the infection. The specific sites that must be used to differentiate organ/space SSIs are listed here. An example is appendectomy with subsequent subdiaphragmatic abscess, which would be reported as an organ/space SSI at the intraabdominal site. Organ/space SSIs must meet the following criteria. Infection occurs within 30 days after the operative procedure if no implant is in place and the infection appears to be related to the operative procedure **and** infection involves any part of the anatomy (e.g., organs or space) other than the incision opened or manipulated during the operative procedure **and** at least **one** of the following is present:

- Purulent drainage from a drain that is placed through a stab wound[c] into the organ/space
- Organisms isolated from an aseptically obtained culture of fluid or tissue in the organ/space
- An abscess or other evidence of infection involving the organ/space on direct examination, during reoperation, or by histopathologic or radiologic examination

SSIs involving more than one site:

- Infection that involves **both** superficial and deep incision sites is classified as deep incisional SSI
- Occasionally an organ/space infection drains through the incision. Such infection generally does not require reoperation and is considered a complication of the incision. It is therefore classified as a deep incisional SSI

Specific sites of organ/space SSI:

Arterial or venous infection	Meningitis or ventriculitis
Breast abscess or mastitis	Myocarditis or pericarditis
Disc space	Oral cavity (mouth, tongue, or gums)
Ear, mastoid	Osteomyelitis
Endocarditis	Other infections of the lower respiratory tract
Endometritis	Other infections of the urinary tract
Eye, other than conjunctivitis	Other male or female reproductive tract
Gastrointestinal tract	Spinal abscess without meningitis
Intraabdominal, not specified elsewhere	Sinusitis
Intracranial, brain, or dural infections abscess	Upper respiratory tract, pharyngitis
Joint or bursa	Vaginal cuff
Mediastinitis	

[a]Specific criteria are used for infected episiotomy and circumcision sites and for burn wounds.

[b]An implant is defined as a nonhuman-derived implantable foreign body (e.g., prosthetic heart valve, nonhuman vascular graft, mechanical heart, or hip prosthesis) that is permanently placed in a patient during an operation.

[c]If the area around a stab wound becomes infected, it is not an SSI. It is considered a skin or soft-tissue infection, depending on its depth.

(Modified from Horan TC, Gaynes RP, Martone WJ, et al. CDC definitions of nosocomial surgical infection, 1992: a modification of CDC definitions of surgical wound infections. *Am J Infect Control* 1992;20:271–274.)

ment of patients serves as a marker of those with possible operative site infection [73]. This method has some promise to be labor efficient.

Any wound infection rate determined in such a system is, of course, a minimum estimate of the infection rate, since wounds that escape surveillance or that manifest only after discharge will not be counted. A recent consensus paper by a joint Surgical Wound Infection Task Force representing the Society for Hospital Epidemiology of America, the Association for Practitioners in Infection Control, the CDC, and the Surgical Infection Society has recommended that some form of postdischarge surveillance should be undertaken [74]. Tools to identify postdischarge infections include questionnaires sent to surgeons or to patients, telephone follow-up with surgeons or patients, and systems to detect readmission of patients to hospitals and postoperative antibiotic prescriptions. The best method for accomplishing such surveillance is not known, and some systems appear to be both expensive and insensitive [75].

Another area that has received very little attention to date is the surveillance of outpatient operative procedures. The NNIS system specifically tracks only patients who have been admitted to the hospital on one day and discharged on another [8,68]. An increasing number of operative procedures are being performed on patients who are not admitted to a hospital, 50% or even more in many hospitals (see Chapter 28). Preliminary information suggests that infections in these patients are less common than in patients having similar procedures as inpatients [76,77]. However, very little systematic information is available.

A surveillance worksheet, indicating the criteria used for definition, is useful to record important details about an infected patient. Only the minimum information necessary for further tabulation to identify clusters or outbreaks should be included. Patients' demographic characteristics and details of operations are generally readily available in the medical record and need not be routinely recorded. On infrequent occasions, when clusters of infection are found, additional information about host risk factors, technical aspects of surgical procedures, or environmental details concerning the patients' care may be important in terms of stratification for analysis. Computer analysis of surveillance data is helpful only to the extent that the data output is consonant with the previously determined objectives (see Chapter 8).

ANALYSES OF CRUDE DATA: INVESTIGATIONS OF OUTBREAKS AND CLUSTERS

In the workup of an apparent excess frequency of infection at the operative site, acquisition of infection may be evaluated in relation to the sequence of surgical care: preoperative (therapeutic and host factors), intraoperative, and postoperative. By identifying a specific operation as the point of selection, rather than an operator, a wide range of possible contributions to individual infection risks is more likely to be fully explored. Operations should be surveyed for postoperative infections at operative and nonoperative sites.

It is especially important to recognize the potentially pejorative implications of incorrectly interpreting crude data sets of postoperative infections. Dissemination of crude data to an uncritical audience has the power to cause damage to a surgeon or an institution. The limitations of crude findings of postoperative infections should be identified for those who review them. Access to crude data sets should be restricted to those who have an actual need to know about interval findings of work in progress. There should also be constant concern about disseminating interpretations of a single set of data indicating highly unusual findings, because of possible sampling bias or other biases and for type 1 error due to inadequate sample size (see Chapter 7). Failure to identify potential limitations in interpreting crude data and possible sampling errors in small clusters may result in a loss of credibility of the surveillance program, may create a climate of suspicion and animosity among the surgical staff, and may jeopardize the success of any future efforts. Thus, sound epidemiologic methods and strict confidentiality of records are central to an effective program.

Clusters of infections may be sought by grouping infected patients according to characteristics such as time, place, person, infecting organisms, surgeons, types of operations, preoperative host and surgical risk factors, use of various devices, characteristics of critical care, preoperative duration of hospitalization, and postoperative intervals to onset of infection (see Chapter 6). In stratification, the analyst seeks to identify possible commonality in sources of infection. For example, a lengthy preoperative period of hospitalization may be an indicator of patients with unusual or complex manifestations of disease. Relatively long periods from operation to onset of infection may suggest that a postoperative event has played a role in infection. In the latter instance, time periods in excess of 10 to 12 days raise the possibility of that postoperative factors (including hematoma, seroma, remote site infection, prolonged or unnecessary use of surgical drains, or postoperative manipulation of the wound) aided in the initiation of infection. An open conduit at the surgical site (e.g., Penrose drain) may also be a factor in permitting infection to take hold after operation.

An increase in the incidence postoperative infection may be due to a change in risk characteristics of the patients with the introduction of a population having an increased susceptibility to infection. In small clusters of surgical infections, chance alone may bring about a concatenation of unrelated events, giving the false appearance of a group of infections linked by common causation. Alternatively, a small cluster of serious postoperative infections in high-risk patients may be an indicator of a much larger outbreak with a wide array of disease manifestations (see Chapter 6). A systematic search for unreported infections, including those arising after hospital discharge, is usually necessary to determine the actual size of such clusters. Case-control analysis, stratified as necessary, is useful when new equipment, procedures, or processes have been introduced.

SURGEON-SPECIFIC SURVEILLANCE

Following the outline of the 1964 NRC study [2], Cruse and Foord [10] devised a program of concurrent observation of surgical wounds in patients undergoing clean operations to provide individual surgeons with infection rates. This study and others [13] have demonstrated that providing infection rates to the surgical staff results in a decrease in wound infections. These findings are consonant with the results of a large SENIC study [69], in which reduction of surgical infections was found to be associated with a strong infection control program that included an effective hospital epidemiologist and a system for reporting specific surgical wound infection rates to the specific surgeon. Surgeon-specific infection rates may be readily determined. Aggregated infection rates for different classes of operations may be calculated for individual surgeons from NNIS surgical site risk index data and compared with a standardized infection ratio [78].

The goal of surgeon-specific surveillance is to lower the rate of wound infection by making individual surgeons aware of excesses in infection rates and thereby promote adherence to accepted principles of operative care. Implicit in this approach is the assumption that surgical infections may be entirely attributed to flaws in surgical techniques or judgment (including incorrect use of antibiotic prophylaxis). Also implicit is the assumption that any reduction in surgical wound infection rates following the provision of information regarding excess rates to an individual surgeon results from improvement in faulty surgical technique, protocols, or judgment. Massanari has pointed out some concerns for small sample sizes, validity of methods for risk adjustment, and reliability of data collection methods in this context [79].

Nonetheless, an actual problem in surgical technique may exist for one or several surgeons. This is a thorny issue. There is no methodology to evaluate operative technique as a surveillance activity. Moreover, providing some surgeons with surgeon-specific data may not bring about the desired results. In some instances in community hospitals, surgeons with a high rate of postoperative infection have simply moved their practices to other hospitals in which surveillance is less intense.

Lee has suggested that rather than focusing too much attention on absolute rates of infection, the hospital epidemiologist and surgeon should concentrate on classifying each surgical site infection into the dichotomous classes of *potentially avoidable* and *apparently unavoidable infections* [70]. A potentially avoidable infection is an infection that occurs under circumstances where any indicated infection-reducing adjuncts were omitted. Such adjuncts would include use of prophylactic antibiotics when indicated; avoidance of razor shaving on the day before operation; appropriate skin preparation at the operative site; avoiding elective operations in the presence of distant site, active infections; and so on. An apparently unavoidable infection is one that occurs despite the application of all known appropriate infection-reducing measures. The goal of a surgical infection surveillance program should be *zero avoidable wound infections* [70]. Where a particular infection-reducing strategy is well accepted but not always reliably applied, such as the indicated use of perioperative prophylactic antibiotics, a quality assurance program designed to ensure the reliable application of this method may have a greater effect on wound infection rates than feedback on wound infection rates alone [39].

VIRAL INFECTIONS

Studies of patients receiving transplants have confirmed that viral infection is a surgical complication in this context [80] (see Chapter 45). The principal agents are transferred by human tissue organs and blood. Cytomegalovirus, herpesvirus, hepatitis B, hepatitis C, and varicella zoster are the viruses most frequently identified (see Chapter 42). Human immunodeficiency virus is the one most feared (see Chapter 43). Routine methods for surveillance of viral postoperative infections need to be developed.

FUNGAL INFECTIONS

Candida species are gaining prominence as causes of operative site infection. This is particularly true in the surgical treatment of transplant patients, burned patients, and patients with prosthetic devices (see Chapters 38–40, 45,46). Intravenous catheters and urine cultures may yield fungi on culture before systemic involvement, and it is likely that patients are infected from such sources by hematogenous spread. Improved methods to identify and control such infections will become more important as technical advances in surgery lead to treatment of more immunocompromised subjects.

THE COSTS OF SURGICAL INFECTIONS

Postoperative infections in surgical patients may prolong the length of hospitalization for substantial periods, depending on the type of operation, and thereby greatly increase the cost of their care. Cardiothoracic, orthopedic, and gastrointestinal operations are likely to be especially costly in this regard, as a result of both pulmonary and operative site infections [81,82]. In addition to the higher direct costs of care, indirect costs are a consideration in calculating the consequences of postoperative infection. These costs include the time lost by the patient from gainful employment and the possible medicolegal actions that may be taken against a hospital or the surgical staff (see Chapters 17,18).

NEW DIRECTIONS IN PREVENTION OF POSTOPERATIVE INFECTION

As the incidence of wound infection progressively declines, new thinking is required to define the next step in improving the care of patients in relation to controlling postoperative infection. Perioperative colonization with virulent bacteria may serve as a source of both endogenous infection and cross-infection. The association between nasal carriage of *S. aureus* and postoperative infection is well known [83]. Some evidence exists that topical nasal treatment with mupirocin may serve to reduce endogenous surgical wound infection with *S. aureus* [84,85] as well as to minimize *S. aureus* cross-infection in a surgical intensive care unit (see Chapter 41). Additional studies are in progress to confirm these findings. Both nasal colonization with *S. aureus* [85] and lower respiratory tract colonization with *Haemophilus* species [86] appear to be sources of postoperative pulmonary infection. How to identify and reduce the latter, especially in the preoperative treatment of the patient with traumatic injury, remains to be established. After surgery, there are a number of additional potential measures for control of surgical infections [87], such as intravenous administration of immunoglobulins, that may lessen the frequency of postoperative acquisition of bloodstream infection and pneumonia. Aggressive and consistent infection control activities will be important in further reducing the incidence of postoperative infections.

REFERENCES

1. Wangensteen OH, Wangensteen SD. *The rise of surgery: from empiric craft to scientific discipline*. Minneapolis: University of Minnesota Press, 1978:785.
2. Howard JM, Barker WF, Culbertson W, et al. Postoperative wound infections: the influence of ultraviolet irradiation on the operating room and of various other factors. *Ann Surg* 1964;160(suppl 2):1–196.
3. Haley RW, Culver DH, Morgan WM, et al. Identifying patients at high risk of surgical wound infection: a simple multivariate index of patient susceptibility and wound contamination. *Am J Epidemiol* 1985;121: 206–215.
4. Culver DH, Horan TC, Gaynes RP, et al. Surgical wound infection rates by wound class, operative procedure, and patient risk index: National Nosocomial Infections Surveillance System. *Am J Med* 1991;91(3B): 152S–157S.
5. Burke J. The effective period of preventive antibiotic action in experimental incisions and dermal lesions. *Surgery* 1961;50:161–168.
6. Bernard H, Cole W. The prophylaxis of surgical infection: the effect of prophylactic antimicrobial drugs on the incidence of infection following potentially contaminated operations. *Surgery* 1964;56:151–157.
7. Polk HC Jr, Lopez-Mayor JF. Postoperative wound infection: a prospective study of determinant factors and prevention. *Surgery* 1969;66(1): 97–103.
8. Emori TG, Culver DH, Horan TC, et al. National Nosocomial Infections Surveillance System (NNIS): description of surveillance methods. *Am J Infect Control* 1991;19(1):19–35.
9. Horan TC, Culver DH, Gaynes RP, et al. Nosocomial infections in surgical patients in the United States, January 1986–June 1992. *Infect Control Hosp Epidemiol* 1993;14:73–80.
10. Cruse PJ, Foord R. The epidemiology of wound infection: a 10-year prospective study of 62,939 wounds. *Surg Clin North Am* 1980;60(1): 27–40.
11. Burke JF. Identification of the source of staphylococci contaminating the surgical wound during operation. *Ann Surg* 1963;158(5):898–904.
12. Morris PJ, Barnes BA, Burke JF. The nature of the "irreducible minimum" rate of incisional sepsis. *Arch Surg* 1966;92(3):367–370.
13. Olson MM, Lee JT Jr. Continuous, 10-year wound infection surveillance: results, advantages, and unanswered questions. *Arch Surg* 1990; 125(6):794–803.
14. Anonymous. New classification of physical status. *Anesthesiology* 1963;24:111.
15. Morales EA, Embrey RP, Herwaldt LA, et al. A new severity of underlying illness scale to predict postoperative wound infections following coronary artery bypass surgery [Abstract]. *Infect Control Hosp Epidemiol* 1995;16 (suppl 4, part 2):43.
16. Horan TC, Culver DH, Gaynes RP. Risk factors for surgical site infections following C-section: preliminary results of a multicenter study [Abstract]. *Infect Control Hosp Epidemiol* 1995;16 (suppl 4, part 2):22.
17. The Neurosurgical Infections Study Group, France. Risk factors for surgical wound infections in craniotomy: a multicenter study in 2,944 patients [Abstract]. Presented at the 35th Interscience Conference on Antimicrobial Agents and Chemotherapy of the American Society for Microbiology, San Francisco, September 17–20, 1995:J161.
18. Salemi CS, Anderson D, Flores D. Surgical site infection NNIS risk indexing: a problem with anesthesia department ASA scoring [Abstract]. *Infect Control Hosp Epidemiol* 1995;16(suppl 4, part 2):21.
19. Howe CW. Experimental wound sepsis from transient *Escherichia coli* bacteremia. *Surgery* 1969;66(3):570–574.
20. Robson M, Krizek T, Heggers J. Biology of surgical infection. *Curr Probl Surg* 1973;3:2–62.
21. Josephs LG, Cordts PR, DiEdwardo CL, et al. Do infected inguinal lymph nodes increase the incidence of postoperative groin wound infection? *J Vasc Surg* 1993;17(6):1077–1080.
22. Alexander JW, Fischer JE, Boyajian M, et al. Influence of hair-removal methods on wound infections. *Arch Surg* 1983;118:347–352.
23. Kaiser AB, Clayson KR, Mulherin JL Jr., et al. Antibiotic prophylaxis in vascular surgery. *Ann Surg* 1978;188(3):283–289.
24. Kurz A, Sessler DI, Lenhardt R. Perioperative normothermia to reduce the incidence of surgical-would infection and shorten hospitalization. Study of wound infection and temperature group. *N Engl J Med* 1996;334(19):P1209–1215.
25. Hojer H, Wetterfors J. Systemic prophylaxis with doxycycline in surgery of the colon and rectum. *Ann Surg* 1978;187:362–368.
26. Ford CD, VanMoorleghem G, Menlove RL. Blood transfusions and postoperative wound infection. *Surgery* 1993;113(6):603–607.
27. DeHoll D, Rodeheaver G, Edgerton MT, et al. Potentiation of infection by suture closure of dead space. *Am J Surg* 1974;127(6):716–720.
28. Magee C, Rodeheaver G, Golden G, et al. Potentiation of wound infection by surgical drains. *Am J Surg* 1976;131:547–549.
29. Monson JR, Guillou PJ, Keane FB, et al. Cholecystectomy is safer without drainage: the results of a prospective, randomized clinical trial. *Surgery* 1991;109(6):740–746.
30. Cerise E, Pierce W, Diamond D. Abdominal drains: their role as a source of infection following splenectomy. *Ann Surg* 1970;171: 764–769.
31. Simchen E, Rozin R, Wax Y. The Israeli study of surgical infection of wound infection in operations for hernia. *Surg Gynecol Obstet* 1990; 170(4):331–337.
32. Le Gallou F, Fleury M, Baranger F, et al. Could surgical gloves play a role in the peroperative transmission of methicillin-resistant *Staphylococcus aureus*? Presented at the 35th Interscience Conference on Antimicrobial Agents and Chemotherapy of the American Society for Microbiology. San Francisco, September 17–20, 1995:J156.
33. Roy M-C, Stephens D, Herwaldt LA, et al. Risk factors for surgical site infections [Abstract]. Presented at the 35th Interscience Conference on Antimicrobial Agents and Chemotherapy of the American Society for Microbiology. San Francisco, September 17–20, 1995:J157.
34. Grinbaum RS, de Mendonca JS, Cardo DM. An outbreak of hand-scrubbing-related surgical site infections in vascular surgical procedures. *Infect Control Hosp Epidemiol* 1995;16:198–202.
35. Moylan JA, Kennedy BV. The importance of gown and drape barriers in the prevention of wound infection. *Surg Gynecol Obstet* 1980;151(4):465–470.
36. Berkelman RL, Martin D, Graham DR, et al. Streptococcal wound infections caused by a vaginal carrier. *JAMA* 1982;247(19): 2680–2682.
37. Beck-Sague CM, Chong WH, Roy C, et al. Outbreak of surgical wound infections associated with total hip arthroplasty. *Infect Control Hosp Epidemiol* 1992;13(9):526–534.
38. Lynch W, Davey PG, Malek M, et al. Cost-effectiveness analysis of the use of chlorhexidine detergent in preoperative whole-body disinfection in wound infection prophylaxis. *J Hosp Infect* 1992;21(3): 179–191.
39. Dellinger EP, Gross PA, Barrett TL, et al. Quality standard for antimi-

crobial prophylaxis in surgical procedures. *Clin Infect Dis* 1994;18: 422–427.
40. McGowan JE Jr, Chesney PJ, Crossley KB, et al. Guidelines for the use of systemic glucocorticoids in the management of selected infections. *J Infect Dis* 1992;165:1–13.
41. Gross PA, Barrett TL, Dellinger EP, et al. Purpose of quality standards for infectious diseases. *Clin Infect Dis* 1994;18:421.
42. Kaiser AB. Antimicrobial prophylaxis in surgery. *N Engl J Med* 1986;315:1129–1138.
43. Meakins JL. Prophylactic antibiotics. In: Wilmore DW, Brennan MF, Harken AH, Holcroft JW, Meakins JL, eds. *American College of Surgeons: care of the surgical patient*, vol. 2. New York: Scientific American Medicine, 1991 (section 6):1–10.
44. Nichols RL. Postoperative infections and antimicrobial prophylaxis. In: Mandell GL, Douglas RG Jr, Bennett JE, eds. *Principles and practice of infectious diseases*, 2nd ed. New York: John Wiley & Sons, 1985: 1637–1644.
45. Polk HC Jr, Malangoni MA. Chemoprophylaxis of wound infections. In: Howard RJ, Simmons RL, eds. *Surgical infectious diseases*, 2nd ed. Norwalk: Appleton & Lange, 1988:351–361.
46. Page CP, Bohnen JMA, Fletcher JR, et al. Antimicrobial prophylaxis for surgical wounds: guidelines for clinical care. *Arch Surg* 1993;128: 79–88.
47. ASHP Commission on Therapeutics. ASHP therapeutic guidelines on antimicrobial prophylaxis for surgery. *Clin Pharm* 1992;11:483–513.
48. Gorbach SL. Antimicrobial prophylaxis for appendectomy and colorectal surgery. *Rev Infect Dis* 1991;13(suppl 10):S815–S820.
49. Solla JA, Rothenberger DA. Preoperative bowel preparation: a survey of colon and rectal surgeons. *Dis Colon Rectum* 1990;33:154–159.
50. Clarke JS, Condon RE, Bartlett JG, et al. Preoperative oral antibiotics reduce septic complications of colon operations: results of prospective, randomized, double-blind clinical study. *Ann Surg* 1977;186(3): 251–259.
51. Platt R, Zaleznik DF, Hopkins CC, et al. Perioperative antibiotic prophylaxis for herniorrhaphy and breast surgery. *N Engl J Med* 1990;322: 253–260.
52. Hopkins CC. Antibiotic prophylaxis in clean surgery: peripheral vascular surgery, noncardiovascular thoracic surgery, herniorrhaphy, and mastectomy. *Rev Infect Dis* 1991;13(suppl 10):S869–S873.
53. Dajani AS, Bisno AL, Chung KJ, et al. Prevention of bacterial endocarditis: recommendation by the American Heart Association. *JAMA* 1990;264:2919–2992.
54. Classen DC, Evans RS, Pestotnik SL, et al. The timing of prophylactic administration of antibiotics and the risk of surgical-wound infection [Comments]. *N Engl J Med* 1992;326(5):281–286.
55. DiPiro JT, Vallner JJ, Bowden TA, et al. Intraoperative serum and tissue activity of cefazolin and cefoxitin. *Arch Surg* 1985;120:829–832.
56. Crossley K, Gardner LC, Task Force on Prophylactic Antibiotics in Surgery. Antimicrobial prophylaxis in surgical patients. *JAMA* 1985; 245:722–726.
57. Currier JS, Campbell H, Platt R, et al. Perioperative antimicrobial prophylaxis in middle Tennessee, 1989–1990. *Rev Infect Dis* 1991; 12(suppl 10):S874–S878.
58. Richet HM, Chidiac C, Prat A, et al. Analysis of risk factors for surgical wound infections following vascular surgery. *Am J Med* 1991; 91(suppl 3B):170s–172s.
59. DiPiro J, Cheung R, Bowden T Jr. Single dose systemic antibiotic prophylaxis of surgical wound infections. *Am J Surg* 1986;152: 552–559.
60. Dellinger EP. Antibiotic prophylaxis in trauma: penetrating abdominal injuries and open fractures. *Rev Infect Dis* 1991;13(suppl 10): S847–S857.
61. Fabian TC, Croce MA, Payne LW, et al. Duration of antibiotic therapy for penetrating abdominal trauma: a prospective trial. *Surgery* 1992; 112:788–795.
62. Stoutenbeek CP, van-Saene HK, Miranda DR, et al. The effect of selective decontamination of the digestive tract on colonisation and infection rate in multiple trauma patients. *Intensive Care Med* 1984;10(4): 185–192.
63. Wiesner RH, Hermans P, Rakela J, et al. Selective bowel decontamination to prevent gram-negative bacterial and fungal infection following orthotopic liver transplantation. *Transplant Proc* 1987;19(1): 2420–2423.
64. Blair P, Rowlands BJ, Lowry K, et al. Selective decontamination of the digestive tract: a stratified, randomized, prospective study in a mixed intensive care unit. *Surgery* 1991;110(2):303–309.
65. Kollef MH. The role of selective digestive tract decontamination on mortality and respiratory tract infections: a meta-analysis. *Chest* 1994; 105(4):1101–1108.
66. Brun-Buisson C. Selective decontamination in critical care: interpreting the synthesized evidence [Editorial, Comment]. *Chest* 1994;105(4): 978–980.
67. Heyland DK, Cook DJ, Jaeschke R, et al. Selective decontamination of the digestive tract: an overview [Comments]. *Chest* 1994;105(4): 1221–1229.
68. Horan TC, Gaynes RP, Martone WJ, et al. CDC definitions of nosocomial surgical site infections, 1992: a modification of CDC definitions of surgical wound infections. *Am J Infect Control* 1992;20: 271–274.
69. Haley RW, Culver DH, White JW, et al. The efficacy of infection surveillance and control programs in preventing nosocomial infections in U.S. hospitals. *Am J Epidemiol* 1985;121(2):182–205.
70. Lee JT. Wound infection surveillance. *Infect Dis Clin North Am* 1992; 6(3):643–656.
71. Cardo DM, Falk PS, Mayhall CG. Validation of surgical wound surveillance. *Infect Control Hosp Epidemiol* 1993;14(4):211–215.
72. Ehrenkranz NJ, Sultz JM, Richter E. Recorded criteria as a "gold standard" for sensitivity and specificity estimates of surveillance of nosocomial infection: a novel method to measure job performance. *Infect Control Hosp Epidemiol* 1995;16:697–702.
73. Yokoe DS, Platt R. Surveillance for surgical site infections: the uses of antibiotic exposure. *Infect Control Hosp Epidemiol* 1994;15(11): 717–723.
74. Sherertz RJ, Garibaldi RA, Marosok RD, et al. Consensus paper on the surveillance of surgical wound infections. *Am J Infect Control* 1992;20: 263–270.
75. Manian FA, Meyer L. Comparison of patient telephone survey with traditional surveillance and monthly physician questionnaires in monitoring surgical wound infections. *Infect Control Hosp Epidemiol* 1993; 14:216–218.
76. Audry G, Johanet S, Achrafi H, et al. The risk of wound infection after inguinal incision in pediatric outpatient surgery. *Eur J Pediatr Surg* 1994;4(2):87–89.
77. Zoutman D, Pearce P, McKenzie M, et al. Surgical wound infections occurring in day surgery patients. *Am J Infect Control* 1990;18(4): 277–282.
78. Culver D, Horan T, Gaynes R. Comparing surgical site infection (SSI) rates using the NNIS SSI index and the standardized infection ratio. *Am J Infect Control* 1994;22:102.
79. Massanari RM. Profiling physician practice: a potential for misuse. *Infect Control Hosp Epidemiol* 1994;15(6):394–396.
80. Lubbers MJ. Infection in organ transplant recipients: problems and solutions. *Curr Opin Surg Infect* 1993;1:53–56.
81. Wenzel RP, Osterman CA, Hunting KJ. Hospital-acquired infections. II. Infection rates by site, service and common procedures in a university hospital. *Am J Epidemiol* 1976;104(6):645–651.
82. Penin GB, Ehrenkranz NJ. Priorities for surveillance and cost-effective control of postoperative infection. *Arch Surg* 1988;123(11):1305–1308.
83. Wenzel RP, Perl TM. The significance of nasal carriage of *Staphylococcus aureus* and the incidence of postoperative wound infection. *J Hosp Infect* 1995;31:13–24.
84. Kluytmans JA, Mouton JW, Ijzerman EP, et al. Nasal carriage of *Staphylococcus aureus* as a major risk factor for wound infections after cardiac surgery. *J Infect Dis* 1995;171(1):216–219.
85. Talon D, Rouget C, Cailleaux V, et al. Nasal carriage of *Staphylococcus aureus* and cross-contamination in a surgical intensive care unit: efficacy of mupirocin ointment. *J Hosp Infect* 1995;30(1):39–49.
86. Morran GG, McNaught W, McArdle CS. The relationship between intraoperative contamination of the lower respiratory tract and postoperative chest infection. *J Hosp Infect* 1995;30(1):31–37.
87. Ehrenkranz NJ. Control of surgical infections. *Curr Opin Surg Infect* 1994;2:103–109.

Hospital Infections, Fourth Edition,
edited by John V. Bennett and Philip S. Brachman.
Published by Lippincott–Raven Publishers, Philadelphia, 1998

CHAPTER 38

Infections of Burn Wounds

David W. Mozingo, Albert T. McManus, and Basil A. Pruitt, Jr.[1]

Infection, the risk of which is proportional to the extent of injury, continues to be the predominant determinant of outcome in thermally injured patients despite improvements in overall care in general and wound care in particular. The control of invasive burn wound infection through the use of effective topical chemotherapy, prompt surgical excision, and timely closure of the burn wound has resulted in unsurpassed survival rates. Even so, infection remains the most common cause of death in these severely injured patients.

ETIOLOGY OF BURN INJURY

Burns are estimated to affect > 1.4 million people in the United States annually [1]. Of this number, 54,000 patients require hospital admission, 16,000 of whom have injuries of such significance that care is best undertaken in a burn center. House and structure fires are responsible for > 70% of the yearly 5,400 burn-related deaths, of which three fourths result from smoke inhalation or asphyxiation and one fourth are due to burns. However, these fires are responsible for only 4% of burn admissions. Injuries due to contact with flame or ignition of clothing are the most common cause of burn in adults, whereas scald burns are most common in children. The majority of patients sustain burns of such limited severity and extent (> 80% of burns involve < 20% of the body surface) that they can be treated on an outpatient basis. There are 250 to 275 patients per million population per year who require hospital admission owing to the extent of their burns or to other complicating factors. Approximately one third of patients who require in-hospital care have a major burn injury—as defined by the American Burn Association on the basis of burn size, causative agent, preexisting disease, and associated injuries—and should be treated in a tertiary care burn center [2].

Changes in wound care over the past thirty years, including the use of effective topical antimicrobial chemotherapy and excision of the burned tissue to achieve timely closure of the burn wound, have significantly reduced the occurrence of invasive burn wound infection and its related morbidity and mortality. Regular collection of cultures from patients permits early identification of the causative pathogens of those infections that do arise. Moreover, infection control procedures, including strict enforcement of patient and staff hygiene and use of patient isolation methods, have been effective in controlling the spread of resistant organisms and eliminating them from the burn center. These advances and the improvements in the general care of critically ill burn patients have resulted in markedly improved survival rates. However, as a manifestation of the systemic immunosuppressive effects of burn injury, infection at other sites, predominantly in the lungs, remains the most typical cause of morbidity and death in these severely injured patients (Figure 38-1).

HOST IMMUNE FUNCTION

Thermal injury initiates a deleterious pathophysiologic response in every organ system, with the extent and duration of organ dysfunction proportionate to the size of the burn. Direct cellular damage is manifested by coagula-

D. W. Mozingo: Department of Surgery, Shands Burn Center, University of Florida College of Medicine, Gainesville, Florida 32610-0286.

A. T. McManus: Microbiology Branch, U.S. Army Institute of Surgical Research, Fort Sam Houston, Texas 78234-6315.

B. A. Pruitt, Jr.: Department of Surgery, University of Texas Health Science Center at San Antonio, San Antonio, Texas 78284-7842.

[1]The views of the authors contained herein do not purport to reflect the positions of the Department of the Army or the Department of Defense.

FREQUENCY OF INFECTION IN BURN PATIENTS

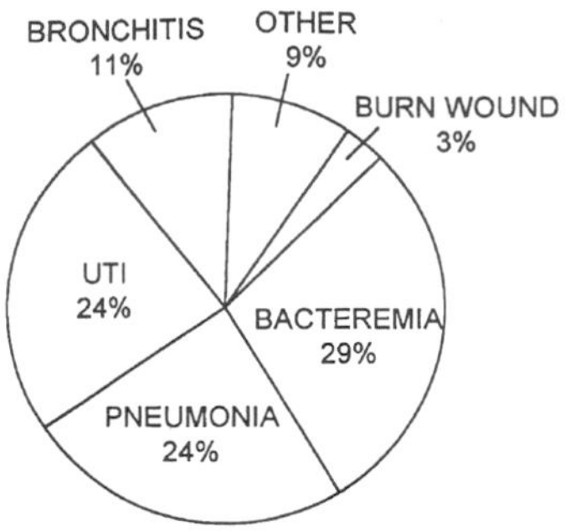

FIGURE 38-1. The frequency of infection by site expressed as a percentage of all infections complicating thermal injury. (From United States Army Institute of Surgical Research, 1991–1995.)

tion necrosis, with the depth of tissue destruction determined by the duration of contact and the temperature to which the tissue is exposed. Following burn, the normal skin barrier to microbial penetration is lost, and the moist, protein-rich avascular eschar of the burn wound provides an excellent culture medium for microorganisms. While destruction of the mechanical barrier of the skin contributes to the increased susceptibility to infection, postburn alterations in immune function may also be of significant importance. Every component of the humoral and cellular limbs of the immune system appears to be affected after thermal injury; the magnitude and duration of dysfunction are proportional to the extent of injury.

During the first weeks after injury, the total white blood cell count is elevated, but peripheral blood lymphocyte counts decrease. Alterations in lymphocyte subpopulations, including reversal of the normal ratio of T-helper cells to T-suppressor cells, have been described [3,4]. Delayed hypersensitivity reactions and peripheral blood lymphocyte proliferation in the mixed lymphocyte reaction are both inhibited following burns. Alterations in interleukin-2 (IL-2) production and IL-2 receptor expression by lymphocytes have been observed with burn injury; a direct correlation has been established between the extent of the burn and the decline of IL-2 production by peripheral lymphocytes [5].

Increased numbers of circulating B lymphocytes are evident early in the postburn course; however, serum immunoglobulin G (IgG) levels decline after burn injury and gradually return to normal over the succeeding 2 to 4 weeks. The association of higher numbers of circulating B cells but reduced serum levels of IgG suggests a defect in the ability of B cells to generate a normal response after burn injury [6]. Similar findings have been observed in IgM producing cells isolated from murine mesenteric lymph nodes and spleens following burns [7]. Exogenous administration of IgG to burn patients has been shown to promptly restore IgG levels to normal but exerts no demonstrable effect on the incidence or outcome of infections [8].

Burn injury induces a severity-related shift in the maturity of circulating granulocytes that continues for several weeks after injury. Alterations in granulocyte function, including those of chemotaxis, adherence, degranulation, oxygen radical production, and complement receptor expression, have been identified [9]. Granulocytes isolated from burn patients exhibit increased cytosolic oxidase activity and greater than normal oxidase activity after in vitro stimulation, suggesting that these neutrophils are primed and capable of producing more tissue and organ injury [10]. Recent investigations have verified significant elevations of F-actin content and impaired ability to polymerize F-actin in the granulocytes of burn patients when compared with those of controls [11]. These alterations may in part be responsible for the observed changes in chemotaxis and migration after thermal injury.

ETIOLOGY OF BURN WOUND INFECTION

Both the nature of the burn wound and microorganism-specific factors influence the rate of microbial proliferation in and penetration of the burn eschar. Burn tissue, rich in coagulated protein and well hydrated by the trans-eschar movement of fluid and serum, creates an excellent microbial culture medium. The eschar is avascular owing to thermal thrombosis of nutrient vessels, limiting both the delivery of systemically administered antibiotics and the migration of phagocytic cells into the burned tissue. Bacterial proliferation in the wound may also be enhanced by such factors as wound maceration, pressure necrosis, and wound desiccation with neo-eschar formation. In addition, secondary impairment of blood flow to the wound may further predispose the patient to invasive infection by curtailing the delivery of oxygen, nutrients, and phagocytic cells to the viable subeschar tissue.

The character of the microbial flora of the burn wound changes with time. The gram-positive organisms that predominate in the early postburn period are replaced by gram-negative organisms by the second week. Without the application of topical antimicrobial agents, the density of bacteria grows progressively, and the microorganisms penetrate the eschar by migration along sweat glands and hair follicles until the eschar/nonviable tissue interface is reached. Further microbial proliferation occurs in the subeschar space, enhancing the lysis of denatured collagen and sloughing of the eschar. If the density and invasiveness of the microorganisms exceed the defense capacity of the host, proliferating organisms in the subeschar space may invade the underlining viable tissue, leading to invasive burn wound infection and even systemic spread to remote tissues and organs. Bacterial invasion is uncommon unless the number of microorganisms exceeds 10^5/g of biopsy tissue.

Certain strain-specific factors also appear to be important in the pathogenesis of invasive burn wound infection. The production of enzymes, such as collagenase, elastase, protease, and lipase, may enhance the organisms' ability to penetrate the eschar. Moreover, bacterial motility and antibiotic resistance appear to be important in the development of invasive infection. Effective topical antimicrobial chemotherapy limits intraeschar bacterial proliferation and the attendant risk of invasive infection.

HISTOLOGIC STAGING OF BURN WOUND COLONIZATION AND INFECTION

The presence of microorganisms in the nonviable burned tissue, termed colonization, is a distinctly different entity from the presence of microorganisms in viable tissue beneath the burn eschar, termed invasive burn wound infection. Histologic examination of a biopsy of the burn wound and underlying viable tissue is the most rapid and reliable method for differentiating microbial colonization from invasive infection [12]. Burn wound biopsy is performed as an intensive care unit or ward procedure. An elliptical biopsy (0.5 × 1.0 cm), which includes the subjacent unburned viable tissue, is obtained by scalpel dissection from an area of burn wound suspected of being infected. Hemostasis is easily achieved by the application of direct pressure or by electrocoagulation. One half of the specimen is cultured for identification of microorganisms and their antibiotic sensitivities. The remaining half is submitted to the pathology laboratory for histologic examination. Using the rapid section technique, results are available in 3 to 4 hours, whereas a frozen-section technique may yield a diagnosis in 30 minutes, albeit with an attendant 4% falsely negative diagnosis rate [13]. The presence of microorganisms in viable tissue confirms the diagnosis of invasive burn wound infection (Figure 38-2). When the organisms are confined to the necrotic eschar or there is suppuration in the subeschar space separating nonviable from viable tissue, the wound is considered to be colonized and not infected (Figure 38-3). A histologic staging scheme for burn wound colonization and infection is presented in Table 38-1.

Surface cultures of the burn eschar cannot distinguish colonization from invasive infection. Quantitative bacteriologic cultures of the burn wound, although commonly used in clinical practice, correlate poorly with the presence of invasive burn wound infection. When bacteriologic counts are < 10^5/g of biopsy tissue, invasive burn wound infection is rarely present; however, even when

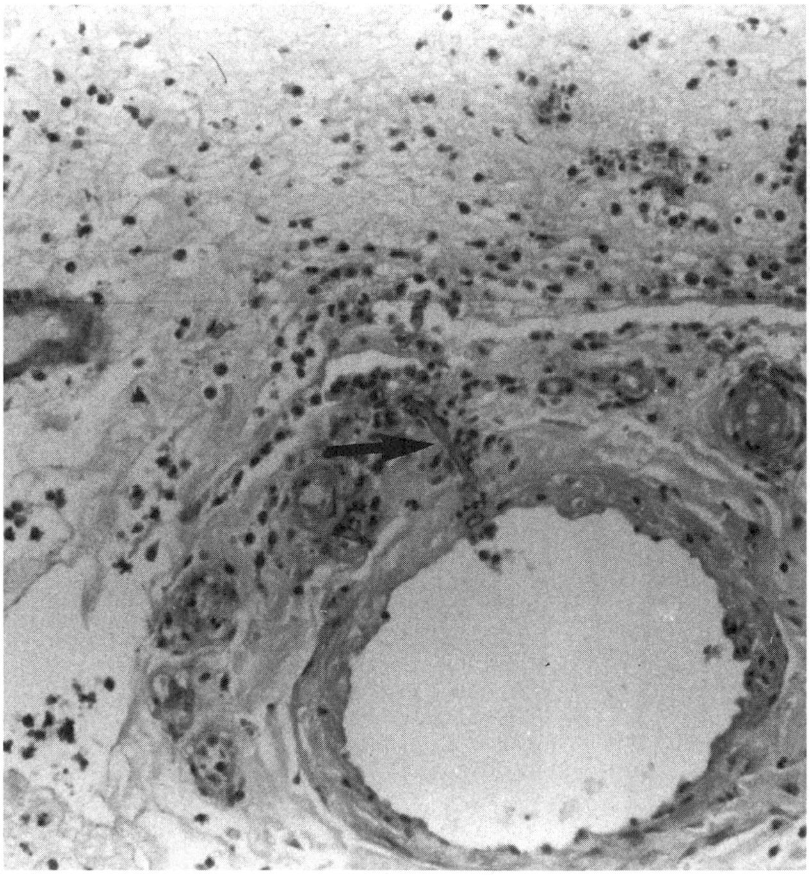

FIGURE 38-2. Photomicrograph of a burn wound biopsy specimen showing hyphae typical of *Aspergillus* species present in unburned tissue. The perivascular location of the hyphal element indicates stage IIC invasion.

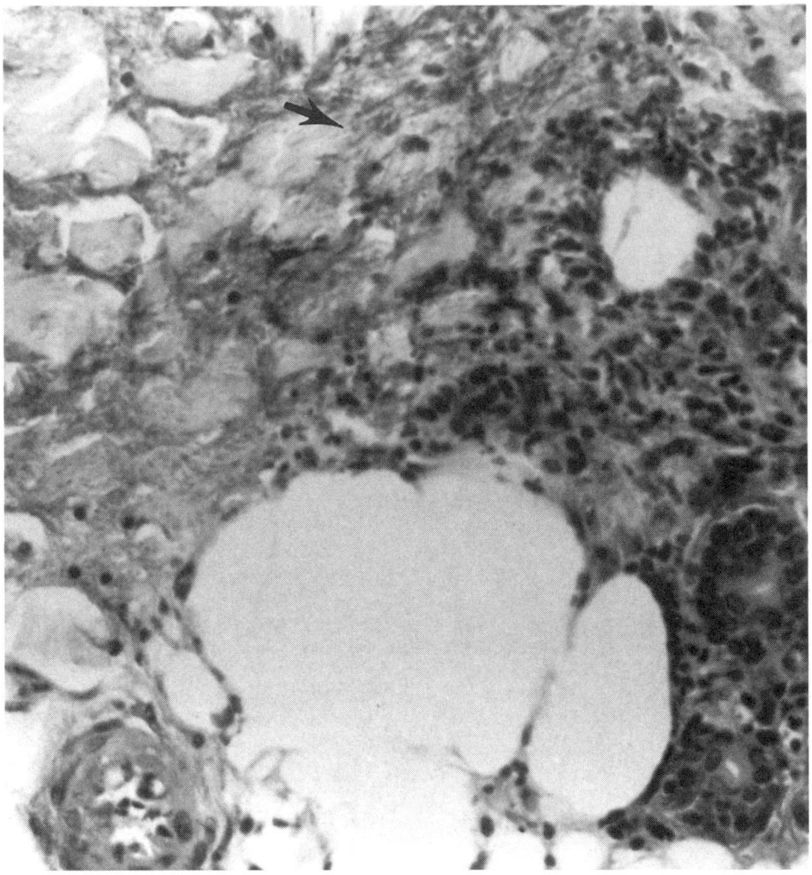

FIGURE 38-3. Photomicrograph of a burn wound biopsy specimen shows dense inflammatory cell accumulation at the interface of the viable tissue to the right and the nonviable tissue to the left. Branched hyphal elements are localized in this area, indicating stage IC colonization (*arrow*).

quantitative counts exceed 10^5 organisms per gram of biopsy tissue, histologic examination confirms the presence of invasive infection in less than half of such specimens. Burn wound biopsies may, at times, yield misleading results, but less commonly than wound cultures. Failing to include viable subeschar tissue in the biopsy specimen or sampling of a noninfected area may limit the usefulness of this technique. Negative biopsy results in the presence of clinical deterioration necessitate reexamination of the burn wound and procurement of biopsy material from other areas when other sources of systemic infection have been discounted.

TABLE 38-1. *Histologic staging of burn wound colonization and invasion*

Stage I: colonization
Superficial: sparse microbial population on surface of burn wound
Penetration: microorganisms present in variable thickness of eschar
Proliferation: dense population of microorganism at the interface of viable and nonviable tissue
Stage II: invasion
Microinvasion: microscopic foci of organisms in viable tissue immediately subjacent to subeschar space
Generalized: widespread penetration of microorganisms deep into viable subcutaneous tissues
Microvascular: involvement of lymphatics and microvasculature

BURN WOUND MICROBIAL FLORA

Over the past twenty years, significant changes in the microbial ecology of the burn wound have been noted. The recovery of *Pseudomonas* and other gram-negative species, which were once the most common organisms causing burn wound infection, has markedly declined with improvements in the isolation of patients [14]. Consequently, invasive *Pseudomonas* burn wound infection has essentially disappeared as a complication of burn

TABLE 38-2. *Microorganisms causing burn wound infection*—From U.S. Army Institute of Surgical Research, 1991–1995

Type	No.
Aspergillus species	12
Mucor species	3
Enterobacter cloacae	1
Aeromonas hydrophila	1
Enterococcus faecalis	1
Total	18

TABLE 38-3. *Organisms isolated from burn wound biopsy specimens*—From U.S. Army Institute of Surgical Research, 1991–1995

Gram-negative species		
Pseudomonas aeruginosa	174	
Other species	270	
Total	444	(29.1%)
Gram-positive species		
Staphylococcus aureus	157	
Other species	271	
Total	428	(28.0%)
Nonbacterial pathogens		
Mold species (principally *Aspergillus* species)	557	
Candida albicans	71	
Other yeasts	26	
Total	654	(42.9%)
Total	1,526	

patients treated in tertiary burn centers [15]. Tables 38-2 and 38-3, respectively, review all burn wound biopsy results in general and those demonstrating invasive burn wound infection in particular during a recent 5-year period at the U.S. Army Institute of Surgical Research and confirm this fact. Patients who have received broad-spectrum antibiotics for perioperative coverage or treatment of septic complications and whose wounds remain open for many days owing to the extent of the burn are at increased risk of burn wound colonization and infection by yeasts, fungi, or multiple antibiotic-resistant bacteria. The true fungi have replaced bacteria as the most common microbes causing burn wound infection in recent years [16]. This predominance of fungal wound infections must be viewed in the context of the marked overall decline in wound infections that has taken place. Moreover, improperly cared for or neglected burn wounds have the same high risk of bacterial infection as was common in this country several decades ago.

Viral burn wound infections are relatively uncommon and are usually caused by herpes simplex virus type 1 (see Chapter 42) [17]. Recently healed or healing partial-thickness burns, particularly those in the nasolabial area, are most frequently affected. The appearance of serrated crusted lesions, particularly on the lips, is characteristic of viral infection. Diagnosis is made by histologic examination of biopsy material or scrapings from the cutaneous lesions. Applications of topical 5% acyclovir ointment every 3 hours for 1 week has been reported to shorten the time to healing of these lesions, the duration of associated pain, and the duration of viral shedding. Even without treatment, these infections usually are self-limited and of little or no systemic consequence. However, if systemic signs and symptoms of disseminated infection are present, such as unexplained sepsis or unrelenting fever, the diagnosis of disseminated viral infection should be entertained.

PREVENTION OF BURN WOUND INFECTION

Progress in the general care of the critically burned patient has included a significant emphasis on the prevention of infectious complications. These efforts have focused mainly on the areas of environmental control (through single-bed rooms and other forms of isolation) and topical antimicrobial prophylaxis of the burn wound. Effective infection control programs are essential to reducing the exposure of patients in critical care units to nosocomial pathogens. Such control includes strictly enforced hand washing, gowning, and gloving policies. When new endemic microbial strains are identified, increased efforts to prevent patient-to-patient spread and unit environmental contamination may be accomplished using cohort patient care techniques (see Chapters 13, 26). Cohort care, which entails the assignment of patient care personnel in teams to provide care for only a specific patient or only patients colonized or infected with a targeted organism limits the spread of, and can even eliminate, antibiotic-resistant endemic organisms [18].

Effective infection control programs for burn centers should include scheduled microbial surveillance of colonization of patients, environmental hygiene monitoring procedures (see Chapter 20), biopsy assessment of the microbial status of the burn wound as necessary, monitoring of the incidence and causes of infection, and timely review of culture and clinical data by an infection control committee (see Chapter 5). The patient colonization surveillance program typically includes thrice weekly cultures of sputum and the burn wound surface and twice weekly cultures of urine and stool. The determination of a panel of antibiotic sensitivities for the predominant isolated organisms or targeted organisms aids in the recognition of problems with cross-contamination or introduction of multiply resistant bacterial strains into the unit's usual flora. Strict criteria for the definition and identification of infections that occur in burn patients are necessary, to avoid non-essential and inappropriate antibiotic use. To minimize the emergence of microbial resistance, antibiotics are used in general only for specific indications. Effective infection control policies require continual reevaluation of surveillance culture results and correlation with the sites and treatment of infections. Prompt institution of effective infection control practices is required when cross-contamination or other breaches in infection control are identified through these surveillance programs.

Patient isolation in single-bed rooms has been shown to lower the incidence of cross-contamination and subsequent infections complicating the hospital course of burn patients [19]. In general, the air flow patterns of the isolation rooms are probably not as important as the prevention of patient-to-patient contact. However, positive air flow design may delay colonization by nosocomial flora. Negative air flow rooms in burn centers are generally reserved for patients with infections spread by the airborne route (such as those caused by *Mycobacterium tuberculosis*), which may be hazardous to other patients or hospital staff members (see Chapter 33).

BURN WOUND HYGIENE AND TOPICAL ANTIMICROBIAL THERAPY

Care of the burn wound begins at the accident scene by covering the wounds with clean sheets or blankets to preserve body temperature and prevent continued environmental exposure. In the absence of gross contamination, burn wounds may be safely treated without topical antimicrobial agents for the first 24 to 48 hours. When the patient arrives at the definitive care facility, initial burn wound debridement should be performed. General anesthesia is not necessary; intravenous analgesia is sufficient for pain control during this procedure. The burns are gently cleansed with a surgical detergent disinfectant, and nonviable epidermis is debrided. Bullae should be excised and body hair shaved from the area of thermal injury beyond the margin of normal skin. The patient is placed in a clean bed, and bulky dressings may be positioned beneath the burned parts to absorb the often copious serous exudate. These dressings should be changed when they become saturated or soiled and patients should be turned frequently to prevent maceration of burned and unburned skin. The initial debridement and daily cleansing with an antimicrobial-containing surgical scrub is best performed in a shower area using a hand-held shower head, with the patient lying on a disposable plastic sheet–covered litter or specially designed shower cart. Alternatively, the patient may be placed on a slanted plinth suspended over a physical therapy tank. Immersion hydrotherapy is not necessary and may only serve to disseminate the fecal flora or other contaminating organisms over the entirety of the burn wound. For patients whose general condition is too critical to permit movement to a shower area, daily wound care may be carried out at the bedside. Following cleansing and debridement, the topical antimicrobial agent of choice is applied.

Mafenide acetate (Sulfamylon), silver sulfadiazine (Silvadene), and silver nitrate are the three most commonly employed topical antimicrobial agents for burn wound care. Each agent has specific limitations and advantages with which the physician must be familiar to ensure the patient's safety and optimal benefit. Mafenide acetate and silver sulfadiazine are available as topical creams to be applied directly to the burn wound, whereas silver nitrate is applied as a 0.5% solution in occlusive dressings. Either cream is applied in a ⅛-inch layer to the entire burn wound in an aseptic manner after initial debridement and reapplied at 12-hour intervals or as required to maintain continuous topical coverage. Once daily, all of the topical agents should be cleansed from the patient using a surgical detergent disinfectant solution and the burn wounds examined by the attending physician. Silver nitrate is applied as a 0.5% solution in multi-layered occlusive dressings that are changed two times each day.

Mafenide acetate burn cream is an 11.1% suspension in a water-soluble base. This compound diffuses freely into the eschar owing to its high degree of water solubility. Sulfamylon is the preferred agent if the patient has heavily contaminated burn wounds or has had burn wound care delayed by several days. Sulfamylon has the added advantage of being highly effective against gram-negative organisms, including most *Pseudomonas* species. Physicians using this agent must be aware of several potential clinical limitations associated with its use. Hypersensitivity reactions occur in 7% of patients, and pain or discomfort of 20 to 30 minutes' duration is common when it is applied to partial-thickness burn wounds. This agent is also an inhibitor of carbonic anhydrase, and a diuresis of bicarbonate is often observed after its use. The resultant metabolic acidosis may accentuate postburn hyperventilation, and significant acidemia may develop if compensatory hyperventilation is impaired. Inhibition of this enzyme rarely persists for > 7 to 10 days, and the severity of the acidosis may be minimized by alternating applications of Sulfamylon with silver sulfadiazine cream every 12 hours.

Silver sulfadiazine burn cream is a 1% suspension in a water-miscible base. Unlike Sulfamylon, Silvadene has limited solubility in water and, therefore, limited ability to penetrate into the eschar. The agent is most effective when applied to burns soon after injury to minimize bacterial proliferation on the wound's surface. This agent is painless upon application, and serum electrolytes and acid-base balance are not affected by its use. Hypersensitivity reactions are uncommon; an erythematous maculopapular rash subsides upon discontinuation of the agent. Silver sulfadiazine occasionally induces neutropenia by a mechanism thought to involve direct bone marrow suppression; white blood cell counts usually return to normal following discontinuation [20]. With continual use, resistance to the sulfonamide component of silver sulfadiazine is common, particularly in certain strains of *Pseudomonas* and many *Enterobacter* species. However, the continued sensitivity of microorganisms to the silver ion of this compound has maintained its effectiveness as a topical antimicrobial agent.

A silver nitrate solution, 0.5%, has a broad spectrum of antibacterial activity imparted by the silver ion. This agent does not penetrate the eschar, since the silver ions are rapidly precipitated upon contact with any protein or cationic material. Use of this agent is not associated with more intense wound pain except from the mechanical action required for dressing changes. The dressings, which are changed twice daily, are moistened every 2 hours with the silver nitrate solution to prevent evaporation from increasing the silver nitrate concentration to cytotoxic levels within the dressings. Transeschar leaching of sodium, potassium, chloride, and calcium should be anticipated, and these chemical constituents should be appropriately replaced. Hypersensitivity to silver nitrate has not been described. Mafenide acetate, silver sulfadiazine, and 0.5% silver nitrate are effective in the prevention of invasive burn wound infection; however, because of their lack of eschar penetration, silver nitrate soaks and silver sulfadiazine burn cream are most effective when applied soon after burn injury.

The acceptance and widespread appliance of prompt burn wound excision in the early care of burn patients has also contributed to the decreased incidence of bacterial burn wound infection. Surgical excision and split-thickness skin grafting of burns diminish the time during which the wound is at risk of invasive infection. In patients with burns of < 40% of the total body surface, excision is associated with shorter hospital stays, and the burn wounds may be definitively grafted in one or two surgical procedures [21]. In patients with burns over ≥ 40% of the total body surface, burn wound excision may shorten the duration and magnitude of injury-related physiologic stress and the subsequent degree of immunologic impairment. As soon as the initial burn resuscitation is complete, and the patient is physiologically stable, burn wound excision may be initiated in staged procedures such that the entirety of the full-thickness or deep partial-thickness wounds can be removed within several weeks. When skin donor sites are not available for complete grafting of these wounds, a variety of skin substitutes or biologic dressings may be used as a bridge to complete wound coverage. The exact contribution of surgical treatment to the decline in incidence of invasive bacterial burn wound infection has not been well documented; however, the temporal relationship cannot be ignored.

CLINICAL DIAGNOSIS OF BURN WOUND INFECTION

Burn wound infection occurs most commonly in patients in whom the extent of burn exceeds 30% of the body surface or in those who have suffered skin graft failure, leaving an open wound. Successful treatment of burn wound infection requires early detection; it is therefore mandatory that the entire wound be examined daily to detect changes in wound appearance. The clinical signs of invasive burn wound infection are often indistinguishable from those observed in uninfected hypermetabolic burn patients or in burn patients with other forms of sepsis. These findings may include hyper-or hypothermia, tachycardia, tachypnea, ileus, glucose intolerance, and disorientation. Physical and tinctorial changes in the appearance of the burn wounds are more reliable signs of invasive burn wound infection (Table 38-4). Conversion of an area of partial-thickness burn to full-thickness necrosis or the appearance of focal areas of dark hemorrhagic or black discoloration are the most commonly noted changes indicative of burn wound infection (Figure 38-4). The development of clinical signs and symptoms of sepsis in the thermally injured patient should prompt a thorough examination of the burn wound to identify areas suspected of harboring invasive infection. Confirmation of the diagnosis of burn wound infection is made by histologic examination of a biopsy specimen, as previously described.

TABLE 38-4. *Clinical signs of burn wound infection*

- Focal dark brown or black discoloration of wound
- Conversion of second-degree burn to full-thickness necrosis
- Degeneration of wound with neo-eschar formation
- Unexpectedly rapid eschar separation
- Hemorrhagic discoloration of subeschar fat
- Violaceous or erythematous edematous wound margin
- Metastatic septic lesions in unburned skin or distant organs

The emergence of nonbacterial opportunists as the major pathogens invading the burn wound has resulted in changes in the classic clinical presentation of burn wound infection. *Candida* species rarely invade the wound to cause systemic infection. However, *Candida* infection may arise in the interstices of a meshed skin graft or in an excised burn wound that remains unclosed as a consequence of the loss of a skin graft or a biologic dressing. Filamentous fungi are more aggressive invaders of the burn wound and may cause severe infection. These fungi rarely traverse fascial planes and remain confined to the subcutaneous tissues. *Aspergillus* species may be detected as colonizers or occasionally as invaders of the burn eschar by histopathologic examination of burn wounds at the time of excision and skin grafting. But the clinically relevant infections occur relatively late in the hospital course of patients with extensive burns who have already undergone multiple operative procedures (for which they have received perioperative broad-spectrum antibiotics) and still have unexcised eschar or previously excised, ungrafted open wounds. These infections often resemble a colony of mold with a somewhat fuzzy texture, appearing in a skin graft interstice or an area of open wound. This surface appearance is often accompanied by subcutaneous burrowing tunnels filled with the invading fungus, which are detected at the time of surgical debridement.

The phycomycetes are typically more aggressive, spreading rapidly along tissue plains, traversing fascia, and invading blood vessels and lymphatics [22]. Infections caused by these organisms are characterized by expanding soft-tissue ischemic necrosis with a peripheral edematous rim and, frequently, hematogenous dissemination to remote sites. The diagnosis is confirmed, as with bacterial burn

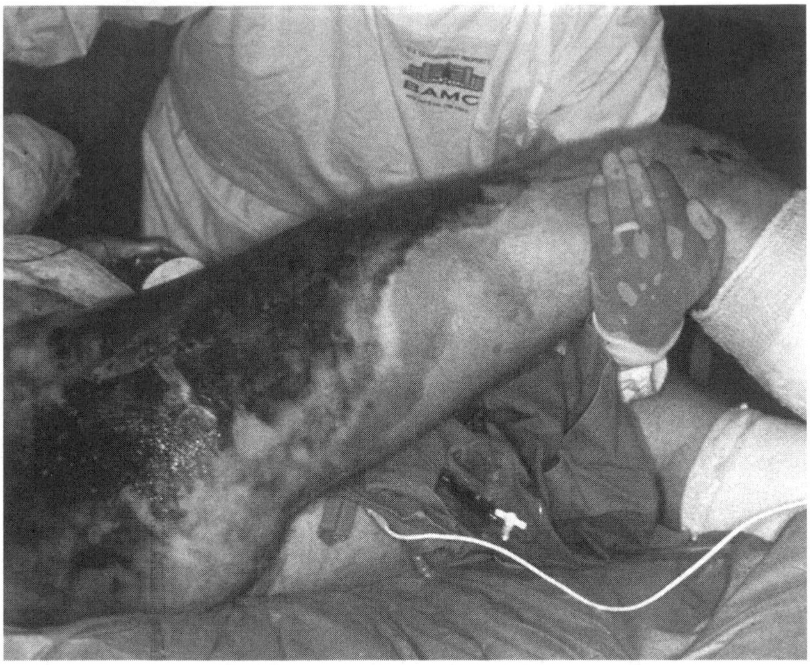

FIGURE 38-4. Multiple areas of dark discoloration on the thigh and buttocks of this patient, accompanied by unexpectedly rapid eschar separation, are characteristic of burn wound infection.

wound infection, by histologic examination of a biopsy specimen.

TREATMENT OF BURN WOUND INFECTION

The treatment of burn wound infection is initiated upon histologic confirmation of the presence of microorganisms in viable tissue. If only colonization is present (stage 1A to stage 1C), no specific change in antimicrobial therapy is indicated unless serially obtained biopsy specimens document progression of the colonization stage. If stage 2 (invasion) is observed, prompt treatment for invasive burn wound infection should begin. In the case of bacterial burn wound invasion, topical twice-daily applications of mafenide acetate should be used. The eschar-penetrating ability of this agent extends the antimicrobial activity throughout the depth of the burn eschar. Systemic antibiotic therapy is initiated based on previous burn wound surveillance cultures or burn center organism prevalence. Further refinements in antibiotic treatment are based on the individual patient's wound culture and sensitivity results. Supportive critical care is employed to maintain hemodynamic and respiratory stability, as for other severely ill patients.

Injection of an antibiotic solution into the subcutaneous tissue beneath the eschar (subeschar clysis) is recommended before surgical excision of an infected burn wound, to minimize the risk of hematogenous seeding and precipitation of florid septic shock [23]. Half of the daily dose of a broad-spectrum antipseudomonal penicillin, such as piperacillin or ticarcillin, delivered in 1 L of normal saline is infused into the subeschar tissues using a no. 20 spinal needle to minimize the number of injection sites. The patient is prepared and scheduled for surgical excision of the infected tissue within the next 6 to 12 hours, and the subeschar clysis is repeated immediately before surgery.

Excision of the burn wound to the level of the investing muscle fascia ensures complete removal of all nonviable infected tissue. After excision of the burn, the wound is treated with moist dressings containing an antimicrobial agent, such as 0.5% silver nitrate solution (the authors use a 5% mafenide acetate solution, which is not generally available). Alternatively, a biologic dressing may be applied if all nonviable tissue has been removed and the exposed tissue appears to be uninfected. The patient is returned to the operating room in 24 to 48 hours; at that time the wound is inspected, and redebridement or split-thickness skin grafting can be performed as needed.

The treatment for candidal or fungal burn wound infection is similar to that of invasive bacterial infection. Infection or neocolonization of previously excised or grafted wounds requires treatment by twice-daily application of a topical antifungal agent, such as clotrimazole cream or ciclopiroxolamine cream. Such treatment usually controls surface colonization. However, if the superficial infection continues to extend or the fungal infection is shown to involve deep tissue such as fascia or muscle, if it has invaded the microvasculature of underlying viable tissue, or if it is associated with systemic signs of sepsis, parenteral administration of amphotericin B should be initiated. The infected tissue must be widely debrided and treated with a topical antifungal agent applied beneath occlusive dressings, which should be changed two to three times daily. The patient is returned to the operating room 24 to 48 hours later for further debridement and closure of the burn wound by autografting or application of a biologic dressing as dictated by the adequacy of the initial debridement.

INFECTIONS OF SPECIAL CONCERN

Clostridium Tetani

Tetanus, caused by the neurotoxin of *Clostridium tetani*, an anaerobic, gram-positive, spore-forming rod ubiquitous in soil and the gastrointestinal tracts of humans and animals, has been reported as a rare complication of thermal injury. This organism thrives in hypoxic wounds and necrotic tissue, both of which exist in the full-thickness burn. The diagnosis of tetanus is based on characteristic physical findings because wound cultures often fail to detect the causative organism. The usual initial signs and symptoms are severe trismus with stiffness of the paraspinous and abdominal musculature. Localized or generalized muscle spasm, dysphagia, and laryngospasm may develop; the disease may progress to involve more muscle groups, causing generalized rigidity. Ventilation may be impaired by involvement of the diaphragm, chest, and abdominal musculature. In severe cases, endotracheal intubation and mechanical ventilation are required. Treatment is mainly supportive and involves aggressive critical care management of the hemodynamic and respiratory systems.

When the diagnosis is made, tetanus immune globulin should be administered immediately to neutralize any circulating free exotoxin. The usual dose is 3,000 to 6,000 u given intramuscularly. Intravenous penicillin G (10 to 40 million u per day) should be given to eradicate the clostridial organisms. Muscle spasms, when uncontrolled, may lead to rhabdomyolysis and skeletal fractures. Morphine, magnesium sulfate, and epidural anesthesia have all been used to reduce muscle spasticity. Sedation with benzodiazepines or barbiturates may be necessary, and, in severe cases, neuromuscular blockade may be required.

Fortunately, tetanus is readily prevented. During the initial care of the burn patient, the tetanus immunization status should be determined. The burn patient who has been immunized against tetanus should be given a booster dose of tetanus toxoid if the last dose was administered > 5 years earlier. Patients with no history or an uncertain history of active immunization should receive tetanus immune globulin in addition to the initial dose of tetanus toxoid. Active immunization is subsequently completed according to the routine dosage schedule.

Staphylococcus Aureus

Toxin-producing staphylococcal species have been isolated from both colonized and infected burn wounds as well as other sites of infection [24,25] (see Chapter 41). The emergence of gram-positive organisms as the predominant flora in burn patients has contributed to a lessening in the impact of infection; the virulence of Staphylococcus aureus may be strain specific, and bacteremia resulting from strains possessing the gene for the production of toxic shock syndrome toxin has been associated with episodes of unexplained profound hemodynamic instability. This gene, however, has been identified in staphylococcal strains recovered from patients with wound colonization, bacteremia, and other infections without evidence of profound physiologic disturbance.

In thermally injured patients with staphylococcal infections who manifest hemodynamic instability that responds poorly to treatment and that is out of proportion to what is usually encountered in gram-positive infections, the diagnosis of a variant of the toxic shock syndrome should be considered. Initial treatment requires aggressive intravenous fluid resuscitation to restore hemodynamic stability. Vancomycin should be administered intravenously unless the organism is known to be sensitive to methicillin, in which case a β-lactamase-resistant antistaphylococcal antibiotic, such as nafcillin, may be given.

At present, an antitoxin to the toxic shock syndrome toxin 1 is not available. Approximately 90% of the general population have antibodies against the toxin, but nearly all patients with toxic shock syndrome related to menstruation have had undetectable antibodies at the onset of the disease. Although this relationship has not been confirmed in thermally injured patients thought to have the variant toxic shock syndrome, the isolation of a strain of *S. aureus* producing the toxic shock syndrome toxin 1 and the absence of circulating antibodies to the toxin may help establish the definitive diagnosis.

Antibiotic-resistant bacteria of special note and the subject of much controversy are the methicillin-resistant strains of *S. aureus* (see Chapters 15, 41). Since the 1960s, these strains have been reported and treated as if they were distinct pathogens with more virulence than other methicillin-sensitive strains. Undoubtedly, the emergence of antibiotic-resistant organisms is of concern, and efforts should be made to limit their inroads. However, the unique concern about methicillin-resistant strains, in particular, has resulted in temporary closure of burn and other intensive care facilities and restriction of patients' movements among levels of care. The benefits of these practices must always be weighed against their clinical, epidemiologic, and economic value.

The virulence and pathologic significance of methicillin-resistant *S. aureus* (MRSA) strains compared with methicillin-sensitive strains causing infections in burn wound patients were evaluated in a recent study [26]. Colonization with any strain of staphylococcus was identified in 658 burn patients treated during a 6-year period; of this total, 319 (or nearly half) of these patients were colonized by MRSA. In this group, a total of 253 staphylococcal infections occurred in 178 patients—58% of infections were pulmonary, and 38% were bacteremic. In 58 of the 178 patients, infections were caused by the methicillin-resistant strains. The outcomes of patients infected by MRSA and methicillin-sensitive strains of *Staphylococcus aureus* were compared using a multiple logistic regression analysis of mortality. In both groups, all patients were treated with vancomycin, and no differences in the observed and predicted mortality were found between groups. We believe these findings seriously question the need for unique precautions, isolation, or treatment in patients with MRSA infections, as is often proposed by other researchers. The main concern related to frequent use of vancomycin is the possible development of vancomycin and MRSA resistance, prompted by the recent recognition of vancomycin-resistant strains of enterococci (see Chapter 15). The clinical development of vancomycin-resistant staphylococcal species has not yet been reported. Even so, strict criteria for diagnosing specific infections in burn patients and specific indications for antibiotic use based on the prevalence of resistant organisms should be adopted at individual centers to avoid inappropriate prescription of vancomycin and other antibiotics.

Aeromonas Species

Human infection with Aeromonas species is most often associated with either traumatic injuries, contaminated with water or soil, or with immunosuppression. Infections in burn patients caused by Aeromonas species are rare—there are < 20 cases reported in the English language literature. A recent report by Barillo et al. describes a series of eight thermally injured patients treated over a 35-year period in whom Aeromonas hydrophila bacteremia developed during their hospital stays [27]. In six of these eight patients, the organism was isolated from wound cultures as well. Aquatic exposure was known or suspected in only three of the patients, and five of the eight patients died. In general, soft-tissue infection with Aeromonas species has a rapid onset, usually within 48 hours of injury. Subcutaneous abscess formation is common but may not be clinically apparent on initial examination. Infections are usually polymicrobial and accompanied by a foul odor. Aeromonas is particularly destructive of muscle, and necrotizing myonecrosis, resulting in amputation or death, may develop from local infections or hematogenous spread in otherwise healthy individuals. Aeromonas infection may mimic Pseudomonas infection in the formation of ecthyma gangrenosum or may produce gas in soft-tissue planes similar to that seen with clostridial infection.

The treatment of Aeromonas burn wound infection includes systematic antibiotic administration and surgical intervention. Aeromonas species produce β-lactamase and are resistant to penicillins and first-generation cephalosporins. Aminoglycosides, aztreonam, ciprofloxacin, and third-generation cephalosporins are usually effective against this organism. Surgical debridement should be accomplished expeditiously, as outlined previously for the management of burn wound infection.

SUMMARY

Despite significant improvements in the survival of burn patients, infectious complications continue to be the major cause of morbidity and mortality. Control of invasive bacterial burn wound infection by effective topical antimicrobial agents and prompt excision and split-thickness skin grafting of the burn wound is clearly possible with modern burn care. In addition, strict isolation techniques and infection control policies have significantly minimized the occurrence of burn wound infections in general and those caused by gram-negative organisms in particular. In those patients in whom a burn wound infection develops, bacterial infection has been largely supplanted by infection caused by nonbacterial opportunists, namely, fungi and yeasts. Scheduled wound surveillance and microbiologic monitoring, with the use of wound biopsies to provide histologic confirmation of burn wound infection, permits prompt diagnosis of microbial invasion at a stage when timely institution of antibiotic therapy and surgical intervention can save the patient.

REFERENCES

1. Pruitt BA Jr, Mason AD Jr. Epidemiological, demographic and outcome characteristics of burn injury. In: Heradon DN, ed. *Total burn care*, London: WB Saunders, 1996.
2. Resources for optional care of patients with burn injury. In: *Resources for optimal care of the injured patient.* Chicago: Committee on Trauma, American College of Surgeons, 1993:63.
3. Zapata-Sirvent RL, Hansbrough JF. Temporal analysis of human leucocyte surface antigen expression and neutrophil respiratory burst activity after thermal injury. *Burns* 1993;19:5–11.
4. Burleson DG, Vaughn GK, Mason AD Jr, et al. Flow cytometric measurement of rat lymphocyte subpopulations after burn injury and burn injury with infection. *Arch Surg* 1987;122(2):216–220.
5. Wood JJ, Rodrick ML, O'Mahony JB, et al. Inadequate interleukin-2 production: a fundamental immunological deficiency in patients with major burns. *Ann Surg* 1984;200:311–320.
6. Molloy RG, Nestor M, Collins KH. The humoral immune response after thermal injury: an experimental model. *Surgery* 1994;115(3): 341–348.
7. Tabata T, Meyer AA. Effects of burn injury on class-specific B-cell population and immunoglobulin synthesis in mice. *J Trauma* 1993; 35(5):750–755.
8. Shirani KZ, Vaughn GM, McManus AT, et al. Replacement therapy with modified immunoglobulin G in burn patients: preliminary kinetic studies. *Am J Med* 1984;76(3A):175–180.
9. Cioffi WG, Burleson DG, Pruitt BA Jr. Leukocyte responses to injury. *Arch Surg* 1993;128:1260–1267.
10. Cioffi WG Jr, Burleson DG, Jordan BS, et al. Granulocyte oxidase activity after thermal injury. *Surgery* 1992;112:860–865.
11. Drost AC, Cioffi WG Jr, Carrougher GJ, et al. The relationship of gran-

ulocyte F-actin levels and infection following thermal injury Presented at *The Third International Congress on the Immune Consequences of Trauma, Shock and Sepsis*. Munich, Mar 2–5, 1994.
12. Kim SH, Hubbard GB, Wurley BL, et al. A rapid section technique for burn wound biopsy. *J Burn Care Rehabil* 1985;6:433–435.
13. Kim SH, Hubbard GB, Wurley BL, et al. Frozen section technique to evaluate early burn wound biopsy: a comparison with the rapid section technique. *J Trauma* 1985;25:1134–1137.
14. McManus AT, McManus WF, Mason AD Jr, et al. Microbial colonization in a new intensive care burn unit. *Arch Surg* 1985;120:217–223.
15. Pruitt BA Jr, McManus AT. The changing epidemiology of infection in burn patients. *World J Surg* 1992;16:57–67.
16. Mozingo DW, Pruitt BA Jr. Infectious complications after burn injury. *Curr Opin Surg Infect* 1994;2:69–75.
17. Kagan RJ, Maraquis, Matsuda T, et al. Herpes simplex virus and cytomegalovirus infections in burn patients. *J Trauma* 1985;25:40–45.
18. Shirani KZ, McManus AT, Vaughn GM, et al. Effects of environment on infection in burn patients. *Arch Surg* 1986;121:31–36.
19. McManus AT, Mason AD Jr, McManus WF, et al. A decade of reduced gram negative infections on mortality associated with improved isolation of burn patients. *Arch Surg* 1994;129:1306–1309.
20. Gamelli RL, Paxton TP, O'Reilly M. Bone marrow toxicity by silver sulfadiazine. *Surg Gynecol Obstet* 1993;177:115–120.
21. Muller MJ, Herndon DN. The challenge of burns. *Lancet* 1994;343: 216–220.
22. Pruitt BA Jr. Phycomycotic infections. In: Alexander SW, ed. *Problems in general surgery*. Philadelphia: Lippincott, 1984.
23. McManus WF, Goodwin CW Jr, Pruitt BA Jr. Subeschar treatment of burn-wound infection. *Arch Surg* 1983;118:291–294.
24. Egan WC, Clark WR. The toxic shock syndrome in a burned victim. *Burns* 1988;14:135.
25. Frame JD, Eve MD, Hackett MEJ, et al. The toxic shock syndrome in burned children. *Burns* 1986;11:234–241.
26. McManus AT, Mason AD Jr, McManus WF, et al. What's in a name? Is methicillin-resistant *Staphylococcus aureus* just another *S. aureus* when treated with vancomycin? *Arch Surg* 1989;124:1456–1459.
27. Barillo DJ, McManus AT, Cioffi WG, et al. *Aeromonas* bacteraemia in burn patients. *Burns* 1996;22(1):48–52.

Hospital Infections, Fourth Edition,
edited by John V. Bennett and Philip S. Brachman.
Lippincott–Raven Publishers, Philadelphia © 1998

CHAPTER 39

Infections of Cardiac and Vascular Prostheses

John P. Burke

The development of synthetic materials that are chemically inert and durable enough to retain their geometric and other physical properties over many years has made possible the wide application of reconstructive operations on the heart and blood vessels. Devices that are commonly implanted in the cardiovascular system include cardiac valve prostheses, patches for repairing congenital heart defects, arterial grafts, permanent cardiac pacemakers and implantable defibrillators, and arteriovenous shunts for performing hemodialysis. Ventriculoatrial shunts for treating hydrocephalus are discussed in Chapter 36 and will not be specifically addressed in this chapter.

All prosthetic devices have the propensity to fail because of mechanical, thromboembolic, or infectious complications. The risk of these complications continues throughout the life of the prosthesis. Operations to implant prostheses, therefore, should be viewed as palliative rather than curative. Fortunately, failure of the prosthesis need not be catastrophic because replacement is often feasible. In 1988, the Medical Device Implant Survey estimated that in the United States, 279,000 artificial heart valves were in use and that pacemakers were implanted in 460,000 persons [1]. Although there were complications associated with one of five artificial heart valves and one of four pacemakers, nearly 95% of heart valves and 84% of pacemakers are never replaced. More than one half of the heart valves had been implanted ≥ 5 years earlier.

At present, > 60,000 valve implantations are performed annually in the United States [2]. Although many varieties of cardiac valve substitutes have been developed, only a few have achieved widespread use [2,3]. Heart valve prostheses may be classified as either mechanical or bioprosthetic. The caged-ball, single-tilting-disk, and bileaflet-tilting-disk valves are the principal types of mechanical prostheses and are composed of metal or carbon alloys. Bioprosthetic valves may be of either human or animal origin. In recent years, the use of cryopreserved human aortic valve homografts has increased. The various types of porcine xenografts that have been widely implanted in the past two decades are constructed of an aortic valve removed from a pig, treated with glutaraldehyde for sterilization and tanning, and mounted on a metal support. Bovine pericardial xenografts are similar to the porcine valves but are no longer marketed in the United States. All heart valve prostheses have similar and persistent risks of infection—so-called prosthetic valve endocarditis (PVE), in contrast to native valve endocarditis (NVE)—but late structural failure is more common with bioprosthetic than with mechanical valves [4].

J. P. Burke: Department of Clinical Epidemiology and Infectious Diseases, LDS Hospital, Salt Lake City, Utah 8418-1827.

NATURE OF INFECTIONS

Incidence

Patients who receive cardiovascular implants are predisposed to a variety of nosocomial infections. The overall incidence of infections following open-heart operations, for example, has ranged from 8% to 44% [5,6]. The highest rates of infection have been found when special efforts have been made to identify minor and asymptomatic infections. The most common infections are of the respiratory tract, the sternal wound and mediastinum, and the bloodstream [7–10].

The risk of prosthesis infection (PVE) is greater after valve replacement than the risk of NVE after other types of open-heart surgery. The incidence of PVE is now lower than it was in patients operated on in the 1960s, a decrease that has been attributed to antimicrobial prophylaxis; in recent studies 1% to 4% of prostheses eventually become infected [11]. Nonetheless, PVE appears to be on the increase because of surgical advances that permit more patients to undergo replacement of native valves.

TABLE 39-1. *Incidence of cardiovascular prosthesis–associated infections*

Type of prosthesis [reference]	Percentage of patients with infections
Cardiac valve [12]	
1 yr after surgery	1.5[a]
5 yr after surgery	3.0[a]
10 yr after surgery	5.0[a]
Vascular graft [13]	0.77–7
Permanent pacemaker [13]	1–6
Implantable defibrillator [13]	1–6
Hemodialysis fistula/graft [14]	1.3[b]

[a]Cumulative rates.
[b]Rate per 100 patient-months.

Table 39-1 shows representative rates of infection according to actuarial methods of data analysis, if available, for each of the major groups of cardiac and vascular prostheses. The highest rates of infection are associated with such devices as external arteriovenous cannulas that are continuously exposed to skin flora and with vascular grafts that require incision of the groin. The incidence of PVE is unrelated to the valve make, position (aortic or mitral), or to model or the number of valves implanted [12,15]. The risk of PVE is greatest after valve replacement for active endocarditis (either NVE or PVE) with cumulative rates of recurrent infection as high as 20% at 10 years [16].

Infections at the site of a prosthetic implant account for a miniscule proportion of the entire spectrum of nosocomial infections. Nonetheless, the morbidity and mortality rates and the costs of these infections are high compared with those of many other types of nosocomial infection [17,18]. Indeed, one third of all deaths after open-heart surgery are caused by infection [19], and the case-fatality rate of PVE continues to be 30%–35% [18].

The small numbers of reported cases, the anecdotal nature of many reports, and the lack of a centrally coordinated national surveillance of patients who receive prosthetic implants are each responsible for important gaps in epidemiologic information. Case-report information is not reliably returned to the hospital or physician responsible for the implantation of the device, and surveillance of in-hospital events will miss prosthetic device–related infections that often appear at a distance both in time and place. It has been proposed that existing infection control units develop a system to return case data to the hospital of origin [20]. The intense focus on outcomes measurement in cardiac surgery in recent years has led to the development of new criteria for risk adjustment and improved guidelines for reporting morbidity and mortality after cardiac operations [21,22]. Differences in prosthetic device–associated infections that may occur across institutions or individual surgeons may eventually be examined as an indicator of the quality of care.

Epidemics in cardiac surgery units have generally been recognized by the occurrence of infections due to an unusual pathogen rather than from an analysis of the overall infection rate. Several outbreaks of PVE caused by filamentous fungi (*Aspergillus* species and *Penicillium* species) have been traced to environmental contamination in the operating room [23,24]. Organisms of the *Mycobacterium fortuitum* complex, including *Mycobacterium chelonei*, have been recognized as an intrinsic contaminant of porcine valve prostheses, a cause of epidemic sternal wound infections after cardiac surgery, and a cause of PVE. While modifications of the glutaraldehyde disinfection regimen used by a company to prepare porcine bioprostheses appear to have reduced the risk of such intrinsic contamination, the usual source of contamination in most outbreaks has been the local environment rather than contaminated commercial materials or devices [25]. Nonsterile ice water used for cooling the cardioplegic solution was the possible environmental source in one outbreak.

Outbreaks due to common organisms may not be immediately recognized and thus may be insidious and protracted, both because the overall infection rate may not be above control limits and because the incubation period for PVE originating during surgery may be prolonged—as long as 12 months after implantation [26]. Clustering of cases of PVE caused by *Staphylococcus epidermidis* has been observed. Methicillin-resistant *S. epidermidis* sternal wound infections and PVE have been linked to a surgeon who carried the epidemic strain on his hands [27], but the reservoir for most outbreaks appears to be the patients themselves [28].

Other investigations have identified continuing, though unusual, problems with contamination of surgical materials, such as cardioplegic solution that is prepared locally and not considered suitable for autoclave sterilization because it is heat-labile, pressure transducers, and even tap water used in the intensive care unit [29–31]. Gram-negative pathogens, such as *Serratia marcescens*, *Enterobacter cloacae*, *Stenotrophomonas maltophilia*, and *Legionella* spp, have been recognized in these circumstances. More recently, advances in molecular typing methods have enabled investigators to link clusters of sternal wound infections due to *Candida albicans*, *Can-*

dida tropicalis, and *Rhodococcus bronchialis* to transmission by scrub nurses [32–34] and of PVE due to *Candida parapsilosis* to contaminated cardiac bypass equipment [35].

Finally, outbreaks associated with the injudicious use of quaternary ammonium compounds as disinfectants have been a recurring problem in cardiovascular surgery units (see Chapter 20). In the early years of open-heart surgery, improper cleaning of cardiopulmonary bypass equipment with these agents was responsible for bacteremic infections. Contaminated disinfectants used on various surfaces in the operating room have also been associated with contamination of blood in extracorporeal circulators and with subsequent cases of sternal wound infection and endocarditis due to *S. marcescens* [36].

Pathogens

A wide variety of bacterial, mycobacterial, fungal, and rickettsial species have been identified from infections associated with cardiovascular prostheses, with many unusual infecting species described in individual case reports. Although gram-negative bacilli are the most common isolates in many nosocomial infections, this has not been true of cardiac and vascular prosthesis–associated infections (Table 39-2). Gram-negative bacilli are especially common in retroperitoneal vascular prostheses contaminated from the gastrointestinal or genitourinary tract, and several organisms can often be isolated in mixed culture from infections associated with arterial grafts of the groin and abdomen [37] and with cardiac pacemakers, especially from pulse-generator pocket abscesses [13,38,39]. *Staphylococcus aureus* is the pathogen most frequently responsible for infections of implantable cardiac defibrillators and of vascular access sites for hemodialysis [14]; however, an appreciable number of cases are due to enteric gram-negative bacilli and *Pseudomonas* species. Recent reports have documented hemodialysis fistula infections due to unusual organisms, such as *Legionella pneumophila* and *Cephalosporium* species [40,41] (see Chapter 24).

Organisms that have been judged to be of low virulence are often recovered from these infections and cannot be easily dismissed as contaminants in blood cultures. Staphylococci, especially *S. epidermidis*, are involved most often in PVE [42] and have also been recognized to have increasing importance in late arterial graft infection [43]. Streptococci, enterococci, a variety of enteric gram-negative bacilli, diphtheroids, fastidious gram-negative coccobacilli (the so-called HACEK group), *Candida*, and *Aspergillus* are also commonly found in PVE. The patterns of microbial species reported from infections associated with patch repairs for congenital heart defects are similar to those from PVE, although staphylococci may be more typical with PVE.

Classification of Infections

The revised surveillance definitions for nosocomial infections from the Centers for Disease Control and Prevention (CDC) are formulated as algorithms and now include criteria for cardiovascular system infection that can be applied to PVE and mediastinitis after open-heart surgery [44,45]. Infections of an arteriovenous graft, shunt, or fistula are grouped as vascular infections under the heading of organ/space surgical site infection. A physician's diagnosis of infection derived from direct observation during surgery or other diagnostic study, or

TABLE 39-2. *Causative agents of infections associated with cardiac valve and aortofemoral vascular prostheses*

	No. (%) of cases							
	Cardiac valve prosthesis[a]				Aortofemoral prosthesis[b]			
Organism	≤ 12 mo[c]		> 12 mo		≤ 4 mo		> 4 mo	
Coagulase-negative staphylococci	41	(56.9)	10	(22.7)	—	—	15	(48.4)
Staphylococcus aureus	5	(6.9)	5	(11.4)	1	(25)	2	(6.5)
Gram-negative bacilli	3	(4.2)	1	(2.3)	3	(75)	8	(25.8)
Streptococci (nonenterococcal)	1	(1.4)	12	(27.2)	—	—	2	(6.5)
Enterococci	2	(2.8)	4	(9.1)	1	(25)	—	—
Diphtheroids	4	(5.6)	1	(2.3)	—	—	—	—
Fungi	4	(5.6)	1	(2.3)	—	—	—	—
Fastidious gram-negative coccobacilli	1	(1.4)	7	(15.9)	—	—	—	—
Other	5	(6.9)	1	(2.3)	—	—	1	(3.2)
Culture negative	6	(8.3)	2	(4.5)	—	—	3	(9.7)
Total	72	(100.0)	44	(100.0)	4	(100)	31	(100.1)

[a]Multiple organisms reported in two cases (other). (From Calderwood SB, Swinski LA, Waternaux CM, Karchmer AW, Buckley MJ. Risk factors for the development of prosthetic valve endocarditis. *Circulation* 1985;72:31.)

[b]Multiple organisms reported in five cases. (From Bandyk DF, Berni GA, Thiele BL, Towne JB. Aortofemoral graft infection due to *Staphylococcus epidermidis*. *Arch Surg* 1984;119:102.)

[c]Time of onset after surgery.

based on clinical judgment, is recognized as an acceptable criterion unless there is compelling evidence to the contrary. Positive blood cultures alone are insufficient evidence of prosthesis-associated infection because patients may have bacteremia or fungemia from a focal infection without involvement of the prosthesis. In contrast, others with prosthesis-associated infection may not have positive results on blood culture, as when subvalvular ring abscesses are present and direct communication with the bloodstream is absent [46].

The clinical onset of infection related to a cardiovascular prosthesis may be delayed until weeks or months after the operative procedure and discharge from the hospital. The incubation period of postoperative infections related to prosthetic materials is often uncertain and probably varies within broad limits, perhaps depending on such factors as the virulence of the organism, size of the inoculum, prophylactic use of antibiotics, and host resistance. Infections related to prosthetic cardiac valves have been classified according to the time of onset of symptoms as either early (< 60 days after the operation) or late (> 60 days after). In recent studies the similarities in the patterns of organisms causing PVE throughout the initial 12 months after surgery [42] (Table 39-2) and the association of these organisms with nosocomial acquisition have suggested that 12 months may be a better breakpoint for defining nosocomial infection than the 60-day period [11,18]. For example, nearly all *S. epidermidis* infections in the first 12 months are methicillin resistant, whereas only ~30% of those occurring later are methicillin resistant. Infections throughout the initial 12-month period are considered to arise most commonly either from intraoperative contamination or from perioperative invasive devices and catheters, while the late-onset cases arise from bacteremias, such as those associated with dental, urinary, or other medical procedures (see Chapter 46).

Infections associated with vascular prostheses may also be classified as either early or late in onset, although a 4-month breakpoint is commonly suggested (Table 39-2). Vascular grafts may be more susceptible to infection from bacteremias during the first 4 months after surgery, but the majority of infections in both early and late groups are thought to arise from contamination at the time of implantation. Therefore, infections that become apparent within 12 months after placement of a cardiovascular prosthesis should be classified as nosocomial even though some patients with community-acquired infections will be incorrectly classified. In addition, intravascular infections that stem from nosocomial infections at other sites, such as the urinary or respiratory tract, should be considered separate nosocomial infections even though their onset may occur after hospital discharge. A patient who enters the hospital with an intravascular infection for which he or she receives a vascular graft or prosthesis and in whom a postoperative infection with a new and different organism involving the implanted material later develops should also be considered to have a nosocomial infection.

Diagnostic Criteria

The sudden appearance of a regurgitant murmur or cardiac failure or an abnormal tilting motion of the valve, dehiscence of the valve, or evidence of a new vegetation or periannular abscess seen on echocardiogram are each virtually diagnostic of endocarditis in patients with prosthetic cardiac valves and sustained bacteremia. Furthermore, bacteremia that is persistent after extracardiac sources of infection have been eliminated strongly supports a diagnosis of endocarditis.

Criteria have been defined to categorize the diagnosis of endocarditis as "definite," "probable," or "possible" [47]. Recently, new diagnostic criteria have been proposed (the Duke criteria) that use echocardiographic as well as clinical and microbiologic evidence and that are modeled after the Jones criteria for the diagnosis of acute rheumatic fever [48]. These criteria recognize the improved diagnostic sensitivity of transesophageal echocardiography compared with transthoracic echocardiography. Transesophageal echocardiography is especially valuable in patients with prosthetic valves, although it is not as sensitive in endocarditis involving mechanical valves as in NVE. The Duke criteria require that bacteremia with coagulase-negative staphylococci be persistent to be considered a major criterion for endocarditis. Persistence is further defined as positive results on blood cultures drawn >12 hours apart or on all of three or a majority of four or more separate blood cultures, with the first and last drawn >1 hour apart. Serologic evidence of recent infection with known valvular pathogens, such as *Brucella* spp, *Legionella* spp, *Chlamydia* spp, or *Coxiella burnetii*, is considered only a minor criterion. The Duke criteria appear to be superior to previously published guidelines and have been evaluated for NVE and, less adequately, for PVE [49].

Varying combinations of findings that support a diagnosis of endocarditis in the context of an intracardiac prosthesis are listed in the CDC's definitions for nosocomial infection [44]. This surveillance definition requires that in the absence of isolation of the organism from direct culture of the valve itself or a vegetation, the physician must have instituted appropriate antimicrobial therapy if the diagnosis was made antemortem. Positive blood culture results are not as common in patients with vascular graft infections as in those with PVE. Bleeding, clotting, or other evidence of malfunction of the graft are diagnostic of infection in the context of purulent wound drainage, exteriorization of the graft, or systemic sepsis.

If there is clinical evidence of infection, the discovery of microorganisms by microscopy or culture in vegetations or pus removed from completely intravascular prostheses at either re-operation or autopsy is confirmation of active infection. A positive culture from a removed arteriovenous cannula or an extruded cardiac pacemaker in conjunction with the recovery of the same organism from a blood culture obtained from a different site is also evidence of prosthesis infection. In most other instances, the diagnosis of infection at the site of a cardiovascular prosthesis is indirect and is based on the presence of typical clinical findings or repeated positive results on blood cultures or both.

Predisposing Factors

Postoperative endocarditis occurs more often after open-heart surgery that requires the implantation of foreign material than with other open-heart procedures. Foreign bodies may potentiate infection both by reducing the inoculum of bacteria required to induce inflammation and by promoting sequestration of bacteria in areas inaccessible to host defenses [50] (see Chapter 41). Bacterial adherence to the prosthetic device, conditioned by a layer of host substances known as biofilm, is also important in the genesis of foreign-body-associated infections. Adherence to these host proteins appears to be responsible for the ability of *S. aureus* to cause device-related infections, whereas *S. epidermidis* commonly produces a slime layer that facilitates colonization of the device [51].

The risk of infection has generally been thought to be greater in procedures involving the placement of a prosthesis in a high pressure system with turbulent blood flow, which might explain, in part, the higher infection rates with prosthetic valve implantations than with patch repairs of congenital heart defects. The risks of infection are similar for all available cardiac valve prostheses. However, two reports document a significantly higher risk in the early months after valve replacement with mechanical prostheses than with bioprostheses [42,52]. However, based upon 5 years of follow-up there appears to be no significant difference in the cumulative risk between mechanical and porcine valve recipients [42].

Cardiopulmonary bypass itself seems to reduce the defense mechanisms of patients as well as to increase the opportunities for operative contamination, and the deleterious hematologic consequences may be greater with bubble than with membrane oxygenators [53–55]. Concomitant or early postoperative infection at other sites, such as the urinary or lower respiratory tract, the surgical wound, venous and arterial catheters, and pacing wires, provides a source for direct contamination or may predispose to bacteremia with seeding of the prosthetic device in the immediate postoperative period, when the risk of infection is greatest [8]. The conclusion of earlier studies that PVE would be unlikely if bacteremia were due to a gram-negative enteric bacillus or if a portal of entry could be established has not been supported by a recent multisite study [56,57]. Indeed, 74 (43%) of 171 bacteremic patients with prosthetic heart valves either had PVE or went on to show signs of it.

The most important single factor shaping the character of postoperative endocarditis and other infections related to cardiovascular prostheses is the use of antimicrobial agents before, during, and after operative procedures. Extensive preoperative use of antibiotics may increase the risk of postoperative endocarditis when an intracardiac prosthesis is implanted [58]. The reasons for this risk are not clear, but they may be related to the replacement of normal flora by antibiotic-resistant species and the overgrowth of certain microbial flora of the skin, mucous membranes, or gastrointestinal tract. The use of prophylactic antimicrobial agents during and after operations has been responsible for shifting the patterns of infecting agents to a more antibiotic-resistant group of pathogens, including *S. epidermidis*, the diphtheroids, and various fungi [59].

Certain patients have other risk factors that are commonly associated with nosocomial infections. Serious underlying illnesses (e.g., congestive heart failure, rheumatoid arthritis, and diabetes mellitus) and the use of medications (e.g., steroids and nonsteroidal anti-inflammatory drugs) are associated with impaired host resistance and often with defective inflammatory or immune responses, which thereby increase the risks of both prosthesis-associated infection and other focal infections. A high carriage rate of *S. aureus* in asymptomatic patients receiving hemodialysis has been suggested to be related to a higher incidence of shunt infections and bacteremia [60]. This finding is in agreement with the observation that the risk of staphylococcal infections of incisional wounds in general is increased in patients who carry *S. aureus* in the anterior nares (see Chapter 41).

SPECIMENS

Collection

Isolation of the pathogen from blood cultures is the essential laboratory procedure for the diagnosis and effective treatment of intravascular infections. The techniques for obtaining specimens are far more important than the use of special media or the ability of the laboratory to isolate unusual microbial species (see Chapter 9). The bacteremias accompanying PVE have not been studied with quantitative blood cultures during the untreated course of the disease, as were those of NVE in the preantibiotic era. Patients with PVE appear to have a lower incidence of positive blood culture results than do patients with NVE, and positive rates as low as 68% have been reported [47]. Nonetheless, when bacteremia occurs, it is probably continuous, and timing of blood cultures should not be critical. Blood cultures should be obtained at various intervals to document the persistence as well as the presence of bacteremia. Continuous bacteremia can be documented by requiring that two or more culture sets show positive results for the same organism.

The blood obtained from one venipuncture site defines a single blood culture, even though the blood is distributed between aerobic and anaerobic culture bottles at the time of collection. The volume of blood sampled is critically important because there is a direct relationship between the volume and culture yield. In adults, a total blood sample of 50 to 60 ml should be sufficient to allow detection of low-density bacteremia. Therefore, 4 to 6 blood culture sets are usually recommended when endocarditis is suspected, with each set containing ≥ 10 ml of blood; 1- to 2-ml samples are often taken from neonates, 2 to 3 ml in infants ≤ 2 years old, and 3 to 5 ml in children [61]. However, some automated detection systems supply culture bottles that accommodate volumes of blood that are < 10 ml, and additional blood culture sets may be needed. The use of antimicrobials within the previous two weeks appears to lower the rate of blood culture positivity and may justify the collection of > six blood culture sets as well as incubation longer than the usual 7 days [62].

The microorganisms that are the most common contaminants in blood cultures (e.g., *S. epidermidis* and diphtheroids) are also often responsible for infections associated with cardiac and vascular prostheses. Strict adherence to aseptic technique and avoidance of sampling from indwelling catheters can reduce the chance of contaminants introduced during blood collection being assigned clinical importance. Between 1% and 5% of blood cultures have been reported to be falsely positive [62], and the rate of false-positive cultures depends on the aseptic precautions used in obtaining specimens.

Use of alcohol (70 to 95% isopropanol or 70% ethanol) for skin cleansing followed by tincture of iodine (2%) is preferred for preparing the skin for venipuncture to collect blood for culture. Solutions of benzalkonium chloride and other quaternary ammonium compounds should not be used for skin disinfection because these agents are relatively inactive against gram-negative bacilli and may become contaminated with such organisms. Outbreaks of pseudobacteremia caused by contaminated blood-drawing equipment, collection tubes, benzalkonium chloride, and povidone-iodine have been reported [63].

The disinfecting agent should be allowed to act for ~1 minute, and the venipuncture site should not be probed with a finger unless it has been decontaminated or surgical gloves are worn. The diaphragm top of the culture bottle should be wiped with alcohol or tincture of iodine before the needle is inserted. Even though the results of a recent meta-analysis have suggested that changing the needle before inoculating the culture bottle may reduce contamination rates slightly, the single-needle method should continue to be the standard because of the risk of needle-stick injury [64].

Evaluation and Special Procedures

Direct communication between the physician and laboratory personnel is necessary for evaluating these serious infections. The physician should be responsible for ensuring that a colony of any microorganism recovered is placed in a holding medium and not discarded by the laboratory as a "contaminant." A separate colony from each positive culture should be preserved for later typing by biochemical reactions, antibiotic susceptibility patterns (antibiograms), phage typing, or serologic methods when these results may be useful for determining whether the organisms are pathogens or contaminants (see Chapter 9). If the isolates are clearly different, their probable clinical significance is diminished. Specimens of the isolated microorganism will also be necessary for tests to estimate the effectiveness of antibiotic treatment.

When the clinical findings suggest intravascular infection and the conventional blood culture results are negative, special procedures should be employed to recover potential pathogens. In patients receiving antimicrobials, the optimal blood-to-broth ratio of 1:5 to 1:10 dilutes out most antimicrobial agents to noninhibitory concentrations and also neutralizes the bactericidal effects of whole blood. Because of these antibacterial properties, blood for culture must be inoculated into the medium at the bedside or into collection tubes containing the anticoagulant sodium polyanetholsulfonate. This substance inhibits phagocytosis, lysozyme, and complement as well as aminoglycoside antibiotics and is included in many commercially available media. Various other antimicrobial inactivating agents and resins have been marketed, but whether they improve microbial recovery or are cost-effective is the subject of controversy.

No one medium or culture system is capable of detecting all microorganisms. The lysis-centrifugation system continues to be the best method for detecting filamentous fungi [64]. In special instances, incubation of routine cultures should be continued for 2 to 3 weeks when fungemia or bacteremia due to fastidious gram-negative coccobacilli (*Hemophilus* species, *Actinobacillus actinomycetemcomitans*, *Cardiobacterium hominis*, *Eikenella corrodens*, and *Kingella kingae*), *Legionella*, or *Brucella* is suspected.

Negative blood culture results may be found in patients with intravascular infections due to *Legionella*, *Chlamydia*, *Rickettsia*, *Aspergillus*, *Candida*, and certain other fungi. If embolism to a major artery occurs, the embolus should be removed and later examined and cultured to detect the presence of fungi. *Candida* and *Aspergillus* may be isolated more often from arterial blood than from venous blood. Blood cultures are also occasionally negative when bacterial infection involves the right side of the heart. When tissue from a removed prosthesis is examined by histology and culture, grinding of the tissue may be indispensable for cultivating the agent [65].

CLINICAL ASPECTS OF INTRAVASCULAR INFECTIONS

Manifestations

General Features

The symptoms and signs of intravascular infection related to prosthetic materials are similar to those of NVE, with some important differences in PVE, such as more frequent signs of valve dysfunction, myocardial invasion, and congestive heart failure. Prosthetic valve endocarditis is often difficult to diagnose, and its presentation is frequently more subtle than NVE, for example, fewer days of fever and fewer clinical criteria [66]. The intravascular location is the feature that all these infections have in common and that is responsible for their protean manifestations. The specific clinical features are determined by the type and location of the prosthesis, the nature of the responsible microbial agent, and the presence of underlying chronic illness, especially uremia. The most common symptoms are nonspecific, such as fever, malaise, and weakness. Fever and other signs of infection may be suppressed by injudicious antibiotic treatment before the true nature of the infection is recognized, or they may not occur in the presence of chronic illness, such as uremia. In patients whose illness begins early in the postoperative period, the dominant symptoms may be of associated infection, such as pneumonia and surgical site infection.

Valvular Prostheses

In patients with prosthetic cardiac valves, regurgitant murmurs and severe cardiac failure as a result of dehiscence of the prosthesis are highly suggestive of endocarditis, but valve dysfunction may be due to technical or mechanical problems rather than to endocarditis. Prosthetic valve endocarditis is frequently accompanied by embolic phenomena and paravalvular myocardial abscesses. The valve itself may become occluded by a thrombus. Other findings usually associated with endocarditis—such as anemia, hematuria (macroscopic or microscopic), Roth's spots, subungual hemorrhages, conjunctival petechiae, and enlargement of the spleen—help direct attention to the possibility of intravascular infection but are less common in PVE than in NVE. Acute fulminant symptoms with hypotension may occur, especially with infections caused by *S. aureus* or *Streptococcus pyogenes* [18]. Fungal endocarditis with unusually large and friable vegetations is often complicated by embolic occlusion of the large arteries, especially those in the lower extremities. The complications of uveitis or endophthalmitis are especially suggestive of infection due to *Candida* species.

Other Vascular Prostheses

In endocarditis that follows repair of a congenital heart defect (e.g., ventricular septal defect), the only evidence of infection may be fever, either low grade or spiking. Separation of the patch with or without subsequent embolism may occur. Inflammation at the operation site may be found in patients with infected arterial grafts, subcutaneous cardiac pacemakers, and arteriovenous shunts. Common signs of infections related to arterial grafts are bleeding, clotting of the prosthesis, localized abscess, chronic draining sinus, and peripheral septic emboli with secondary abscesses. Arteriovenous shunts may also show instability of the cannula, oozing of blood, repeated clotting, or local abscess.

Management

Initial Treatment

The management of bacterial infections associated with intravascular prostheses requires the use of high doses of bactericidal antimicrobial agents intravenously and, possibly, the removal and replacement of the prosthesis. The principles of antimicrobial therapy are similar to those for the treatment of NVE [67]. Full bacteriologic study of the susceptibility of the pathogen is necessary for optimal treatment of these intravascular infections. Nonetheless, chemotherapy is often begun before the results of the susceptibility tests are available. The selection of antimicrobial agents at that time is based on consideration of the usual sensitivities of the specific pathogen and the antimicrobial agents previously used for that patient. The pathogen should be assumed to be resistant to the prophylactic antibiotics used for open-heart surgery. Postoperative infections with organisms that are susceptible to prophylactic antibiotics commonly develop, however, as determined by conventional laboratory tests, especially in infections due to *S. aureus* [68].

In fulminant PVE, especially when it is complicated by hemodynamic instability due to prosthetic valve dysfunction, it is necessary to begin treatment promptly. Even in urgent circumstances, it is possible to obtain several blood cultures before treatment is begun. Initial treatment before culture results are available commonly includes vancomycin and gentamicin. Some experts also recommend that ampicillin or an expanded-spectrum cephalosporin be used as well to treat possible fastidious gram-negative coccobacilli when the onset of infection is ≥ 6 months after surgery [18].

Treatment for Specific Pathogens

The details of antimicrobial therapy for the various pathogens reflect an evolving science that is beyond the scope of this discussion, but some general guidelines and comments are warranted. Antimicrobial treatment regimens for intravascular infection in the presence of prosthetic devices differ from those required for treatment of infections not associated with foreign bodies. The treatment of PVE nearly always requires the use of a combination of two or more antibiotic agents, and treatment is generally continued for longer periods of time, usually 6 weeks. A penicillinase-resistant penicillin is used for infections due to *S. aureus*, although penicillin G can be used if the minimum inhibitory concentration (MIC) of the organism is < 0.1 μg/ml. The addition of an aminoglycoside for the initial 2 weeks of therapy has been advocated for more rapid killing of *S. aureus*, provided that the isolate is susceptible. Use of rifampin as part of a combination regimen has been advocated based on animal studies [67].

The majority of strains of coagulase-negative staphylococci are resistant to methicillin. Special care is required when disk susceptibility or microbroth dilution tests are used to detect resistance to penicillinase-resistant penicillins because the resistance is heterogeneic, that is, only a small subpopulation of organisms is highly resistant while the bulk of the population is susceptible. Apparent susceptibility should be confirmed using higher inocula on agar containing the antibiotic or other special tests (see Chapter 15). Unless susceptibility to methicillin can be confirmed, coagulase-negative staphylococci should be assumed to be resistant to all β-lactam antibiotics, including cephalosporins. Optimal therapy for methicillin-resistant staphylococci (*S. epidermidis*) is provided by vancomycin combined with gentamicin (for the initial 2 weeks of therapy) and rifampin. Rifampin therapy should be delayed until the organism can be shown to be susceptible to gentamicin in order to prevent the development of resistance to rifampin. If the organism is resistant to gentamicin, another aminoglycoside or a quinolone to which it is susceptible should be used.

Intravascular prosthesis–associated infections due to viridans streptococci, enterococci, or diphtheroids may usually be treated with combined penicillin G and gentamicin. The American Heart Association recommends at present that gentamicin be given for at least the first 2 weeks of therapy even for highly penicillin-susceptible viridans streptococci [67]. Nutritionally variant streptococci should be treated with this combination therapy for the full duration of treatment. The increasing frequency of highly resistant enterococci among clinical isolates means that all enterococcal strains causing PVE must be screened to define antimicrobial resistance patterns and that routine use of previously standard recommendations may not provide optimal treatment. Some strains of diphtheroids are resistant to the combination of penicillin and gentamicin, and other strains may be difficult to test for susceptibility because of their slow growth. Vancomycin with or without gentamicin appears to be an effective alternative.

Most patients with infections due to nonenterococcal streptococci or methicillin-sensitive staphylococci who are allergic to penicillin can be safely treated with first-generation cephalosporins. A cephalosporin can be used if the reaction to penicillin is mild or the history is vague. Vancomycin is a suitable alternative for patients with a history of an immediate or life-threatening reaction to either penicillin or a cephalosporin and should be used in most instances when there is a history of an anaphylactic reaction to penicillin therapy. In rare instances, the physician may wish to consult detailed protocols for penicillin desensitization.

Selection of antibiotics for treating infections due to gram-negative bacilli is based on in vitro susceptibility testing and, when available, studies of antibiotic synergy. Initial therapy must always include at least two antimicrobial agents that are likely to be effective against recent nosocomial isolates of that species in the hospital in which the patient was most likely infected. The newer expanded-spectrum cephalosporins and carbapenem antibiotics and the monobactam aztreonam are useful additions to the aminoglycosides and ureidopenicillins that have been mainstays in the treatment of serious gram-negative bacillary infections. Nonetheless, these infections nearly always require early operative intervention, and removal and replacement of the prosthesis may be lifesaving.

Fungal infections, which are usually due to *Candida* or *Aspergillus* species, require removal of the prosthesis and systemic treatment with amphotericin B. The value of combining amphotericin B with either 5-fluorocytosine or rifampin is unclear. The newer imidazoles, fluconazole and itraconazole, may be useful in the context of *Candida* and *Aspergillus* PVE, respectively, but they may antagonize amphotericin B.

The effectiveness of chemotherapy in bacterial infections is commonly monitored by determining the antibacterial activity of the patient's serum against the organism recovered from the blood (or from the prosthesis itself) with a serial, twofold dilution test. Numerous problems have been associated with such tests, including determining the most appropriate time for collection of the blood specimen (peak versus trough antibiotic levels), lack of standardized methods for performing the tests, and lack of evidence that the results are of prognostic value. The test is especially likely to result in misleading information in assessing regimens that rely on combinations of antibiotics to produce bactericidal synergy. Antibiotic assays are a suitable substitute for serial, twofold dilution tests of the patient's serum when the infecting organism is known to be susceptible, and such assays can assist in preventing toxicity from excessive drug levels. Assays are also preferable in monitoring therapy with antibiotics that are highly protein-bound or sensitive to pH changes, since erratic results are sometimes seen with the serum dilution method.

Removal of Prostheses

Vigorous antibiotic therapy will cure some intravascular prosthesis infections; in others, antibiotics may suppress the systemic signs and symptoms while the infection persists at the site of the prosthesis. Antibiotic therapy of PVE fails more often in cases with an early postoperative onset than in those with a late onset. To detect antibiotic failure at the earliest possible time, it is useful to obtain blood for culture periodically during treatment and once or twice in the 8 weeks after the completion of treatment.

Removal of an intracardiac prosthesis is necessary when antibiotic therapy has failed to clear the bacteremia or if fever persists for ≥ 10 days during appropriate antibiotic therapy. Other indications for the removal of a prosthetic valve, in addition to uncontrolled infection or resistance of the organism to available bactericidal chemotherapeutic agents, include moderate to severe heart failure due to prosthesis dysfunction; invasive and destructive paravalvular infection manifest by partial valve dehiscence, new or progressive conduction system disturbances, or purulent pericarditis; and recurrent arterial embolism.

Furthermore, it seems advisable to recommend removal of the prosthesis early in the course of PVE complicated by other factors associated with an unfavorable outcome [69]. Such factors include infection caused by organisms not easily treated by antibiotics (e.g., fungi, gram-negative bacilli, *S. aureus*, and coagulase-negative staphylococci). When there are indications for the removal of the prosthesis, temporizing for >10 to 14 days with antibiotic therapy does not reduce the risk of relapse, and longer periods of antibiotic therapy before surgery do not correlate with the inability to recover bacteria from intraoperative cultures or with a more favorable outcome [70]. The most important consideration in determining the time of cardiac surgery is the hemodynamic status of the patient. Patients with culture-negative endocarditis and continued fever during empiric antibiotic therapy will often be found to have fungal endocarditis, and removal of the prosthesis is necessary for cure.

EPIDEMIOLOGIC CONSIDERATIONS

Sources and Prevention

In general, nosocomial infections at the site of a prosthetic implant may arise either from direct contamination at the time of operation or from bacteremic seeding of the tissues adjacent to the prosthesis stemming from another focal infection. Appropriate preoperative care and aseptic surgical technique may lessen the risk of the former circumstance; practices described elsewhere in this book related to prevention of urinary, respiratory, surgical site, and vascular access device–related infections will assist in the control of the latter situation (see Chapters 31, 32, 37, 44). In the past two decades striking increases have been noted in the incidence of nosocomial endocarditis in patients with preexisting prosthetic cardiac valves. Three separate studies have also reported that nearly one half of the cases were the result of infected intravascular devices and were judged to be preventable by the application of currently accepted infection control procedures and practices, including the optimal insertion and care of invasive devices, aggressive early treatment of bacterial infections, and proper use of prophylaxis [71–73]. An important preventive measure is routine surveillance of patients after surgery. Surveillance should be maintained not only during hospitalization but also after discharge and for the period during which nosocomial infection remains a potential threat (see Chapter 5).

Patient Care Practices

Many operative procedures to implant cardiac or vascular prostheses are semi-elective, allowing for meticulous preoperative care. Special attention should be given to the preoperative diagnosis and treatment of focal infections, especially periodontal, prostate, and urinary infections. Some surgeons recommend washing the patient's skin daily with hexachlorophene- or chlorhexidine-containing soaps for 1 to 2 days before operation. Preoperative shaving is associated with increased infection rates; clipping immediately before the operation is the preferred method for hair removal [74].

Many procedures to implant a cardiovascular prosthesis are so complex and lengthy that eventual breaks in aseptic technique are almost inevitable. Gloves, for example, are punctured with nearly every sternotomy. Considering the many opportunities for contamination of the operative field, the low infection rates observed suggest that infections may be caused by either uncommonly massive contamination, unusually virulent microorganisms, or especially dangerous personnel shedders. Nonetheless, firm discipline in the operating room, avoidance of unnecessary traffic and talking, and exclusion of personnel with overt skin infections should assist in the control of infection.

The prompt recognition and treatment of other postoperative infections, especially those related to intravascular lines and catheters, could also have a role in preventing late-stage prosthesis-associated infection. For example, from 31% to 92% of patients with early-onset PVE have been found to have predisposing postoperative infections at other sites with the same bacterial species [18]. Measures for the prevention of arteriovenous shunt–associated infections are similar to those for the prevention of intravenous catheter–associated infections (see Chapters 24 and 44). Because the cannula is exposed on the surface of an extremity, the site is continually subject to microbial contamination from the patient's own flora as well as from external sources, including dialysis fluid and equipment. The surgically created subcutaneous arteriovenous fistula or graft is used more often than external cannulas in most hemodialysis centers, in part because there is a lower risk of infection with the internal fistula.

All access site punctures should be performed with meticulous aseptic technique. Disinfection of the site with a povidone-iodine solution appears to be satisfactory, and gloves (either sterile or nonsterile) as well as a face mask should be worn. A recent randomized study found no difference in infection rates between the use of sterile gloves and drapes and the use of so-called clean technique for skin preparation [14]. Efforts to further limit the risk of infection in hemodialysis patients have focused on the use of newer topical and oral antimicrobial agents (such as mupirocin and rifampin) for the prophylactic eradication of *S. aureus* from the nose [75].

Environmental Factors

The majority of infections associated with cardiovascular prostheses that occur in the initial 12 months after cardiac surgery are thought to be nosocomial in origin. Some of these infections, including those with a prolonged latent period, may occur as a consequence of operative field and bypass equipment contamination, whereas others may result from postoperative infections. Conflicting data exist as to the relative importance of operative field versus bypass equipment contamination. In one study, the most common site of microbial contamination was the repaired area of the myocardium and the prosthesis just before wound closure, and the bypass equipment was infrequently contaminated [76]. In other reports, positive cultures of the pump-oxygenator blood have been associated with a higher risk of later infection. Contamination of the extracorporeal circuit has been found in 3% to 75% of patients after bypass, and persistence of a single strain of coagulase-negative staphylococcus for as long as 1 year has been confirmed in one center [77].

An additional potential source for contamination during cardiopulmonary bypass is the "cell saver apparatus," a centrifuge for intraoperative autotransfusion that has been widely used. However, positive cultures from the apparatus have not been linked to postoperative infections [78]. The instruments and equipment for bypass procedures should be thoroughly cleaned of debris, autoclaved, and assembled under aseptic conditions. The use of disposable membrane and bubble oxygenators has simplified the problems of sterilization. Many centers use a bacterial filter in the oxygen supply line because the oxygen itself and the junction between the nonsterile oxygen tank and the oxygenator may be sources of potential contamination.

The operating room air should have a slight positive pressure in relation to surrounding areas, and the doors must be kept closed (see Chapter 27). The American Institute of Architects Committee on Architecture for Health has published guidelines that require at least 15 complete changes of operating room air per hour and that describe other architectural requirements for rooms for cardiovascular surgery [79]. The development of clean-room technology and laminar (or unidirectional) airflow systems that are capable of reducing the microbial concentration to fewer than one organism per cubic foot has provided a research tool for the investigation of the relationship of airborne microbes to wound infection (see Chapters 20, 40). Conventional air-conditioning systems with HEPA filtration, however, are capable of lowering the microbial concentration in operating room air to between 1 to 3 organisms per cubic foot. Nonetheless, it seems advisable to protect prostheses from prolonged exposure to operating room air before their insertion in the patient.

A variety of other unproven measures has been recommended to reduce environmental contamination in the operating room. A few, such as regular cleaning of the operating room floor with a phenolic disinfectant and using disposable, waterproof, paper draping materials and surgical gowns, are reasonable and in widespread use; others, such as changing shoe covers at the entrance to the operating room and passing all traffic over disinfectant-soaked blankets, seem irrational and useless. All such measures should be secondary to proper aseptic techniques, hand-scrubbing, and limiting personnel and traffic in the operating room (see Chapter 27).

Inadequate sterilization of the prosthesis before insertion has also been suspected as a cause of subsequent infection (see Chapter 20). Prosthetic materials that cannot be autoclaved are frequently sterilized by ethylene oxide. Intrinsic contamination is more likely for materials treated with ethylene oxide. Neither of these techniques is used for porcine valves, which are treated with glutaraldehyde. When sterilization is undertaken by a hospital, the process should be monitored with bacterial spore strips. Some surgeons have resorted to soaking the device in an antibiotic-containing solution just before insertion, with the hope of killing any surviving organisms in the interstices of the fabric of the prosthesis. This practice has been discouraged because contamination of the prosthesis could occur from soaking in a nonsterile antibiotic solution and patients allergic to the antibiotics used may be inadvertently exposed to serious reactions. Rifampin and gentamicin/clindamycin impregnation of the sewing rings of prostheses has been reported as a promising approach to prevention of infection in high-risk valve replacement for active endocarditis, but prospective clinical trials have not yet been done [80,81].

Prophylactic Antibiotics

The use of antibiotic prophylaxis has become standard practice during surgery involving the implantation of prosthetic devices and vascular grafts [82]. However, the benefits of such prophylaxis remain uncertain because placebo-controlled studies have ended prematurely, owing to the devastating consequences of implant infections among placebo recipients, or have yielded inconclusive results. No placebo-controlled study of antibiotic prophylaxis in cardiac valve replacement surgery has been performed in the past two decades, and there is no available information on infection rates in patients not receiving antibiotics. On the other hand, antibiotic prophylaxis was significantly associated with lower wound infection rates in at least six placebo-controlled trials involving placement of vascular grafts. However, important caveats include the facts that infection of the prosthetic material itself was not shown to be significantly limited in any of these studies and that the predominant pathogens causing infections in the prosthetic devices often differ substantially from those causing wound infections.

Antibiotic prophylaxis directed at specific pathogens known to be susceptible to the drug will probably be effective. Thus prophylactic use of penicillinase-resistant penicillins or first- and second-generation cephalosporins probably reduces the incidence of postoperative infection with *S. aureus* and other susceptible pyogenic cocci. The selection of optimal regimens, however, remains challenging. Controlled studies in cardiac surgery have yielded conflicting results on the relative efficacy of the various cephalosporins in preventing sternal infections due to methicillin-susceptible staphylococci. In centers where methicillin-resistant staphylococci are frequently encountered, surgeons have often substituted vancomycin for cephalosporins.

The optimal timing of prophylaxis is more important than the choice of agent used. In ordinary clinical practice there is considerable variation in the time of administration [83]. Prophylactic antibiotics should be started no earlier than 2 hours before the operation, and intraoperative dosing should be used for a drug with a short half-life and in the circumstance of prolonged operative durations. Several studies have shown no benefit in their postoperative use beyond 2 days. Many surgeons insist on continuing them, however, until all possible sources of contamination, such as arterial catheters, have been removed.

Management of Outbreaks

Methods of Investigation

The identification of the source and mode of spread of the pathogen is the first goal of the epidemiologist and is a necessary basis for applying control measures for an outbreak (see Chapter 6). The first step is to prepare a line listing of the cases. Although there may be only a few cases, a detailed list of the clinical and epidemiologic circumstances of each case is made, and each feature shared by two or more patients is expressed as a ratio. The list should include the nature of the operative procedures; other concurrent procedures, such as coronary artery bypass grafts and the use of the internal mammary artery as a graft; and the dates of onset and the outcomes of infections. Additional factors might include the age and gender of each patient, underlying diseases that predispose to such infections, durations of preoperative hospitalization, dates of operations, types and suppliers of the prostheses, methods of sterilization and handling of prostheses before insertion, locations of the operating rooms, names of surgeons and other members of the surgical teams, results of cultures and antibiograms of isolates, prophylactic antimicrobial agents used, durations of anesthesia and pump time, proportions of emergency and nighttime procedures and of emergency reoperations, proportions of patients who experienced such intraoperative problems as bleeding and difficulty in weaning from the pump, and the presence of other focal infections. These data should also be collected from a group of patients who underwent comparable surgical procedures during the same time period but who did not show signs of infection associated with their prostheses. Analysis of these data might suggest factors associated with the cases that will determine directions for the investigation.

Recent operating room records should be reviewed to determine the total number of operative procedures of a similar nature that have been performed. These procedures should be tabulated separately for periods before and during the epidemic, for use in determining changes in the infection rate. At the same time that these data are being collected and analyzed, a review of aseptic techniques, methods for disinfecting equipment, and the mechanics of the ventilating system in the operating room may reveal a productive area for special bacteriologic study (see Chapter 20).

The pathogen recovered from each case should be saved whenever possible, both for serum inhibition tests to be used in evaluating treatment and for later laboratory study to characterize the epidemic strain. Review of the susceptibilities to antimicrobial agents of the pathogens will help determine whether a single strain or several strains are involved, and such susceptibility data may lead the epidemiologist to recommend changes in prophylactic antibiotic use (see Chapters 9, 14).

While the investigation is proceeding, the epidemiologist should recommend a protocol for collecting prospective data from new patients. For example, culture of blood from the bypass machine after each operation will help establish the incidence of contamination from this source. If such cultures have been routinely performed, an immediate review of the results from pre-epidemic and epidemic periods may be useful. Prospective cultures of prostheses just before insertion might also be undertaken, especially when the epidemic strain is an organism that is more likely than others to resist sterilization or the prostheses are subjected to disinfecting rather than sterilizing procedures. Diphtheroids, staphylococci, and spore-forming bacilli, for example, are more difficult to kill than gram-negative bacilli, and mycobacterial species appear to be relatively resistant to certain disinfectants. The temptation to obtain nasopharyngeal or other swabs for culture from personnel and environmental cultures from the operating room should be resisted until the foregoing tasks have been completed. Because the pathogens from these infections are ubiquitous, positive cultures from such human and environmental sites have limited meaning and may be misleading. Cultures from these sites should be obtained only when epidemiologic data suggest that one of these sites may be relevant to the outbreak, and isolates of appropriate identity should then be fully characterized and compared with isolates of the epidemic strain.

Control

The measures taken to control an epidemic are determined by the epidemiologic findings and the urgency of the problem. In an outbreak with a high attack rate that is recognized as a grave threat to the safe conduct of such operations, it may be necessary to close the operating room temporarily and suspend procedures. In less urgent circumstances—usually when the outbreak is insidious and protracted—thoughtful investigation may precede the application of control measures. Appropriate control measures should not be withheld pending completion of the investigation if there is a reasonable chance that additional cases will be prevented by their institution (see Chapters 6, 9). Available data should be reported to local and federal health authorities. Pooled data from many institutions may be necessary to establish conclusively the presence of low-frequency, intrinsic contamination of commercially distributed prosthetic materials.

If the investigation fails to uncover the source of the outbreak, the operating room should be temporarily closed and thoroughly cleaned. The importance of hand washing and aseptic technique should be stressed to personnel. In some circumstances, discontinuation of the use of ineffective prophylactic antibiotics may alone control the outbreak, even if the source is not found. Prompt removal or elimination of a possible source suggested by the epidemiologic investigation, even when the data are inconclusive, will allow the epidemiologist to evaluate a hypothesis through well-planned, continuing surveillance. Regardless of the solution to the problem, surveillance of patients on the involved services should continue, with the purpose of either evaluating the control and prevention measures or providing additional data that might help define the cause (see Chapter 6).

REFERENCES

1. Moss AJ, Hamburger S, Moore RM Jr., Jeng LL, Howie LJ. *Use of selected medical device implants in the United States, 1988.* Hyattsville, Md.: National Center for Health Statistics. 1990. (Advance data from vital and health statistics, no. 191.)
2. Vongpatanasin W, Hillis LD, Lange RA. Prosthetic heart valves. *N Engl J Med* 1996;335:407–416.
3. Collins JJ Jr. The evolution of artificial heart valves. *N Engl J Med* 1991;324:624–626.
4. Schoen FJ, Levy RJ. Pathology of substitute heart valves: new concepts and developments. *J Card Surg* 1994;9(suppl):222–227.
5. Rosendorf LJ, Daicoff G, Baer H. Sources of gram-negative infection after open-heart surgery. *J Thorac Cardiovasc Surg* 1974;67:195–201.
6. Conte JE Jr., Cohen SN, Roe BB, Elashoff RM. Antibiotic prophylaxis and cardiac surgery: a prospective double-blind comparison of single-dose versus multiple-dose regimens. *Ann Intern Med* 1972;76:943–949.
7. L'Ecuyer PB, Murphy D, Little JR, Fraser VJ. The epidemiology of chest and leg wound infections following cardiothoracic surgery. *Clin Infect Dis* 1996;22:424–429.
8. Ehrenkranz NJ, Pfaff SJ. Mediastinitis complicating cardiac operations: evidence of postoperative causation. *Rev Infect Dis* 1991;13:803–814.
9. Fariñas MC, Peralta FG, Bernal JM, Rabasa JM, Revuelta JM, González-Macías J. Suppurative mediastinitis after open-heart surgery: a case-control study covering a seven-year period in Santander, Spain. *Clin Infect Dis* 1995;20:272–279.
10. Gaynes R, Marosok R, Mowry-Hanley J, et al. Mediastinitis following coronary artery bypass surgery: a 3-year review. *J Infect Dis* 1991; 163:117–121.
11. Weinstein L, Brusch JL. *Infective Endocarditis*. New York: Oxford University Press, 1996:210–228.
12. Rutledge R, Kim BJ, Applebaum RE. Actuarial analysis of the risk of prosthetic valve endocarditis in 1,598 patients with mechanical and bioprosthetic valves. *Arch Surg* 1985;120:469–472.
13. Kearney RA, Eisen HJ, Wolf JE. Nonvalvular infections of the cardiovascular system. *Ann Intern Med* 1994;121:219–230.
14. Kaplowitz LG, Comstock JA, Landwehr DM, Dalton HP, Mayhall CG. A prospective study of infections in hemodialysis patients: patient hygiene and other risk factors for infection. *Infect Control Hosp Epidemiol* 1988;9:534–541.
15. Hammermeister KE, Sethi GK, Henderson WG, Oprian C, Kim T, Rahimtoola S, for the Veterans Affairs Cooperative Study on Valvular Heart Disease. A comparison of outcomes in men 11 years after heart-valve replacement with a mechanical valve or bioprosthesis. *N Engl J Med* 1993;328:1289–1296.
16. Haydock D, Barratt-Boyes B, Macedo T, Kirklin JW, Blackstone E. Aortic valve replacement for active infectious endocarditis in 108 patients: a comparison of freehand allograft valves with mechanical prostheses and bioprostheses. *J Thorac Cardiovasc Surg* 1992;103:130–139.
17. Boyce JM, Potter-Bynoe G, Dziobek L. Hospital reimbursement patterns among patients with surgical wound infections following open heart surgery. *Infect Control Hosp Epidemiol* 1990;11:89–93.
18. Karchmer AW, Gibbons GW. Infections of prosthetic heart valves and vascular grafts. In: Bisno AL, Waldvogel FA, eds. *Infections associated with indwelling medical devices*, 2nd ed. Washington, D.C.: American Society for Microbiology, 1994:213–249.
19. Asensio A, Torres J. Proportion of mortality caused by severe hospital-acquired infection in open-heart surgery. *Clin Perform Qual Health Care* 1996;4:67–73.
20. Hopkins CC. Recognition of endemic and epidemic prosthetic device infections: the role of surveillance, the hospital infection control practitioner, and the hospital epidemiologist. *Infect Dis Clin North Am* 1989; 3:211–220.
21. Daley J. Criteria by which to evaluate risk-adjusted outcomes programs in cardiac surgery. *Ann Thorac Surg* 1994;58:1827–1835.
22. Edmunds LH Jr., Clark RE, Cohn LH, Grunkenmeier GL, Miller DC, Weisel RD. Guidelines for reporting morbidity and mortality after cardiac valvular operations. *J Thorac Cardiovasc Surg* 1996;112:708–711.
23. Mehta G. *Aspergillus* endocarditis after open heart surgery: an epidemiological investigation. *J Hosp Infect* 1990;15:245–253.
24. Fox BC, Chamberlin L, Kulich P, Rae EJ, Webster LR. Heavy contamination of operating room air by *Penicillium* species: identification of the source and attempts at decontamination. *Am J Infect Control* 1990; 18:300–306.

25. Wallace RJ Jr., Musser JM, Hull SI, et al. Diversity and sources of rapidly growing mycobacteria associated with infections following cardiac surgery. *J Infect Dis* 1989;159:708–716.
26. Archer GL, Vishniavsky N, Stiver HG. Plasmid pattern analysis of *Staphylococcus epidermidis* isolates from patients with prosthetic valve endocarditis. *Infect Immun* 1982;35:627–632.
27. Boyce JM, Potter-Bynoe G, Opal SM, Dziobek L, Medeiros AA. A common-source outbreak of *Staphylococcus epidermidis* infections among patients undergoing cardiac surgery. *J Infect Dis* 1990;161:493–499.
28. Menzies R, MacCulloch D, Cornere B. Investigation of nosocomial prosthetic valve endocarditis due to antibiotic-resistant *Staphylococcus epidermidis*. *J Hosp Infect* 1991;19:107–114.
29. Hughes CF, Grant AF, Leckie BD, Baird DK. Cardioplegic solution: a contamination crisis. *J Thorac Cardiovasc Surg* 1986;91:296–302.
30. Villarino ME, Jarvis WR, O'Hara C, Bresnahan J, Clark N. Epidemic of *Serratia marcescens* bacteremia in a cardiac intensive care unit. *J Clin Microbiol* 1989;27:2433–2436.
31. Lowry PW, Blankenship RJ, Gridley W, Troup NJ, Tompkins LS. A cluster of *Legionella* sternal-wound infections due to postoperative topical exposure to contaminated tap water. *N Engl J Med* 1991;324:109–113.
32. Pertowski CA, Baron RC, Lasker BA, Werner SB, Jarvis WR. Nosocomial outbreak of *Candida albicans* sternal wound infections following cardiac surgery traced to a scrub nurse. *J Infect Dis* 1995;172:817–822.
33. Doebbeling BN, Hollis RJ, Isenberg HD, Wenzel RP, Pfaller MA. Restriction fragment analysis of a *Candida tropicalis* outbreak of sternal wound infections. *J Clin Microbiol* 1991;29:1268–1270.
34. Richet HM, Craven PC, Brown JM, et al. A cluster of *Rhodococcus* (*Gordona*) *bronchialis* sternal-wound infections after coronary-artery bypass surgery. *N Engl J Med* 1991;324:104–109.
35. Johnston BL, Schlech WF III, Marrie TJ. An outbreak of *Candida parapsilosis* prosthetic valve endocarditis following cardiac surgery. *J Hosp Infect* 1994;28:103–112.
36. Ehrenkranz NJ, Bolyard EA, Wiener M, Cleary TJ. Antibiotic-sensitive *Serratia marcescens* infections complicating cardiopulmonary operations: contaminated disinfectant as a reservoir. *Lancet* 1980;2:1289–1292.
37. Bandyk DF, Berni GA, Thiele BL, Towne JB. Aortofemoral graft infection due to *Staphylococcus epidermidis*. *Arch Surg* 1984;119:102–108.
38. Choo MH, Holmes DR Jr., Gersh BJ, et al. Permanent pacemaker infections: characterization and management. *Am J Cardiol* 1981;48:559–564.
39. Wade JS, Cobbs CG. Infections in cardiac pacemakers. In: Remington JS, Swartz MN, eds. *Current clinical topics in infectious diseases*, vol. 9. New York: McGraw-Hill, 1988:44–61.
40. Kalweit WH, Winn WC Jr., Rocco TA Jr., Girod JC. Hemodialysis fistula infections caused by *Legionella pneumophila*. *Ann Intern Med* 1982;96:173–175.
41. Onorato IM, Axelrod JL, Lorch JA, Brensilver JM, Bokkenheuser V. Fungal infections of dialysis fistulae. *Ann Intern Med* 1979;91:50–52.
42. Calderwood SB, Swinski LA, Waternaux CM, Karchmer AW, Buckley MJ. Risk factors for the development of prosthetic valve endocarditis. *Circulation* 1985;72:31–37.
43. Golan JF. Vascular graft infection. *Infect Dis Clin North Am* 1989;3:247–258.
44. Garner JS, Jarvis WR, Emori TG, Horan TC, Hughes JM. CDC definitions for nosocomial infections, 1988. *Am J Infect Control* 1988;16:128–140.
45. Horan TC, Gaynes RP, Martone WJ, Jarvis WR, Emori TG. CDC definitions of nosocomial surgical site infections, 1992: a modification of the CDC definitions of surgical wound infections. *Am J Infect Control* 1992;20:271–274.
46. Heimberger TS, Duma RJ. Infections of prosthetic heart valves and cardiac pacemakers. *Infect Dis Clin North Am* 1989;3:221–245.
47. von Reyn CF, Levy BS, Arbeit RD, Friedland G, Crumpacker CS. Infective endocarditis: an analysis based on strict case definitions. *Ann Intern Med* 1981;94(part I):505–518.
48. Durack DT, Lukes AS, Bright DK, and the Duke Endocarditis Service. New criteria for diagnosis of infective endocarditis: utilization of specific echocardiographic findings. *Am J Med* 1994;96:200–209.
49. Bayer AS, Ward JI, Ginzton LE, Shapiro SM. Evaluation of new clinical criteria for the diagnosis of infective endocarditis. *Am J Med* 1994;96:211–219.
50. Vaudaux PE, Lew DP, Waldvogel FA. Host factors predisposing to and influencing therapy of foreign body infections. In: Bisno AL, Waldvogel FA, eds. *Infections associated with indwelling medical devices*, 2nd ed. Washington, D.C.: American Society for Microbiology, 1994:1–29.
51. Christensen GD, Baldassarri L, Simpson WA. Colonization of medical devices by coagulase-negative staphylococci. In: Bisno AL, Waldvogel FA, eds. *Infections associated with indwelling medical devices*, 2nd ed. Washington, D.C.: American Society for Microbiology, 1994:45–78.
52. Ivert TSÅ, Dismukes WE, Cobbs CG, Blackstone EH, Kirklin JW, Bergdahl LAL. Prosthetic valve endocarditis. *Circulation* 1984;69:223–232.
53. Ide H, Kakiuchi T, Furuta N, et al. The effect of cardiopulmonary bypass on T cells and their subpopulations. *Ann Thorac Surg* 1987;44:277–282.
54. van Oeveren W, Dankert J, Waldevuur CRH. Bubble oxygenation and cardiotomy suction impair the host defense during cardiopulmonary bypass: a study in dogs. *Ann Thorac Surg* 1987;44:523–528.
55. van Oeveren W, Kazatchkine MD, Descamps-Latscha B, et al. Deleterious effects of cardiopulmonary bypass: a prospective study of bubble versus membrane oxygenation. *J Thorac Cardiovasc Surg* 1985;89:888–899.
56. Gordon SM, Keys TF. Bloodstream infections in patients with implanted prosthetic cardiac valves. *Semin Thorac Cardiovasc Surg* 1995;7:2–6.
57. Fang G, Keys TF, Gentry LO, et al. Prosthetic valve endocarditis resulting from nosocomial bacteremia: a prospective, multicenter study. *Ann Intern Med* 1993;119:560–567.
58. Lord JW Jr., Imperato AM, Hackel A, Doyle EF. Endocarditis complicating open-heart surgery. *Circulation* 1961;23:489–497.
59. Archer GL, Armstrong BC. Alteration of staphylococcal flora in cardiac surgery patients receiving antibiotic prophylaxis. *J Infect Dis* 1983;147:642–649.
60. Kirmani N, Tuazon CU, Murray HW, Parrish AE, Sheagren JN. *Staphylococcus aureus* carriage rate of patients receiving long-term hemodialysis. *Arch Intern Med* 1978;138:1657–1659.
61. Paisley JW, Lauer BA. Pediatric blood cultures. *Clin Lab Med* 1994;14:17–30.
62. Wilson ML, Weinstein MP. General principles in the laboratory detection of bacteremia and fungemia. *Clin Lab Med* 1994;14:69–82.
63. Washington JA. Collection, transport, and processing of blood cultures. *Clin Lab Med* 1994;14:59–68.
64. Weinstein MP. Current blood culture methods and systems: clinical concepts, technology, and interpretation of results. *Clin Infect Dis* 1996;23:40–46.
65. Gunthard H, Hany A, Turina M, Wust J. *Proprionibacterium acnes* as a cause of aggressive aortic valve endocarditis and importance of tissue grinding: case report and review. *J Clin Microbiol* 1994;32:3043–3045.
66. Sanabria TJ, Alpert JS, Goldberg R, Pape LA, Cheeseman SH. Increasing frequency of staphylococcal infective endocarditis: experience at a university hospital, 1981 through 1988. *Arch Intern Med* 1990;150:1305–1309.
67. Wilson WR, Karchmer AW, Dajani AS, et al. Antibiotic treatment of adults with infective endocarditis due to streptococci, enterococci, staphylococci, and HACEK microorganisms. *JAMA* 1995;274:1706–1713.
68. Kernodle DS, Classen DC, Burke JP, Kaiser AB. Failure of cephalosporins to prevent *Staphylococcus aureus* surgical wound infections. *JAMA* 1990;263:961–966.
69. Calderwood SB, Swinski LA, Karchmer AW, Waternaux CM, Buckley MJ. Prosthetic valve endocarditis: analysis of factors affecting outcome of therapy. *J Thorac Cardiovasc Surg* 1986;92:776–783.
70. Baumgartner WA, Miller DC, Reitz BA, et al. Surgical treatment of prosthetic valve endocarditis. *Ann Thorac Surg* 1983;35:87–102.
71. Terpenning MS, Buggy BP, Kauffman CA. Hospital-acquired infective endocarditis. *Arch Intern Med* 1988;148:1601–1603.
72. Friedland G, von Reyn CF, Levy B, Arbeit R, Dasse P, Crumpacker C. Nosocomial endocarditis. *Infect Control Hosp Epidemiol* 1984;5:284–288.
73. Chen SCA, Dwyer DE, Sorrell TC. A comparison of hospital and community-acquired infective endocarditis. *Am J Cardiol* 1992;70:1449–1452.
74. Ko W, Lazenby WD, Zelano JA, Isom OW, Krieger KH. Effects of shaving methods and intraoperative irrigation on suppurative mediastinitis after bypass operations. *Ann Thorac Surg* 1992;53:301–305.
75. Chow JW, Yu VL. *Staphylococcus aureus* nasal carriage in hemodialy-

sis patients: its role in infection and approaches to prophylaxis. *Arch Intern Med* 1989;149:1258–1262.

76. Kluge RM, Calia FM, McLaughlin JS, Hornick RB. Sources of contamination in open heart surgery. *JAMA* 1974;230:1415–1418.
77. van Belkum A, Kluijtmans J, van Leeuwen W, Goessens W, ter Averst E, Verbrugh H. Investigation into the repeated recovery of coagulase-negative staphylococci from blood taken at the end of cardiopulmonary by-pass. *J Hosp Infect* 1995;31:285–293.
78. Schwieger IM, Gallagher CJ, Finlayson DC, Daly WL, Maher KL. Incidence of cell-saver contamination during cardiopulmonary bypass. *Ann Thorac Surg* 1989;48:51–53.
79. American Institute of Architects Committee on Architecture for Health. *Guidelines for construction and equipment of hospital and medical facilities*. Washington, D.C.: American Institute of Architects Press, 1987:25–26,47–52.
80. French BG, Wilson K, Wong M, Smith S, O'Brien MF. Rifampicin antibiotic impregnation of the St. Jude Medical mechanical valve sewing ring: a weapon against endocarditis. *J Thorac Cardiovasc Surg* 1996;112:248–252.
81. Cimbollek M, Nies B, Wenz R, Kreuter J. Antibiotic-impregnated heart valve sewing rings for treatment and prophylaxis of bacterial endocarditis. *Antimicrob Agents Chemother* 1996;40:1432–1437.
82. Haas D, Kaiser AB. Antimicrobial prophylaxis of infections associated with foreign bodies. In: Bisno AL, Waldvogel FA, eds. *Infections associated with indwelling medical devices*, 2nd ed. Washington, D.C.: American Society for Microbiology, 1994:375–388.
83. Classen DC, Evans RS, Pestotnik SL, Horn SD, Menlove RL, Burke JP. The timing of prophylactic administration of antibiotics and the risk of surgical-wound infection. *N Engl J Med* 1992;326:281–286.

Hospital Infections, Fourth Edition,
edited by John V. Bennett and Philip S. Brachman.
Lippincott–Raven Publishers, Philadelphia © 1998

CHAPTER 40

Infections of Skeletal Prostheses

Daniel P. Lew and Francis A. Waldvogel[1]

INFECTED ORTHOPEDIC PROSTHESES

Over the past decades, joint replacement has become one of the most common types of prosthetic surgery because of its success in restoring function to disabled arthritic persons [1–4]. The initial procedure, total prosthetic hip implantation, was soon followed by total knee replacement, total shoulder replacement, total elbow replacement, and then ankle, wrist, and other replacements. The prevalence of total hip replacement varies according to the country studied. In data obtained in Western Europe for the year 1988, this rate varied between 54 (the U.K.) and 104 (Sweden and France) per 100,000 habitants, whereas it was between 64 and 80 in the United States [5]. It is estimated that between 500,000 and 1,000,000 total hip replacements per year were performed worldwide during the late 1980s, and the numbers are probably higher now. Data on surgery of other joints are not available, but in the United States it is estimated that total knee replacement is performed as frequently as total hip replacement [5].

Second to loosening of the prosthesis, infection is the most common complication of orthopedic implant surgery. In a Swedish study collecting follow-up information on 92,675 primary total hip replacements, 4,828 required an at least first-time revision. The causes for revision were aseptic loosening (79%), infection (10%), technical error (6%), and dislocation (2%) [5]. It is agreed that for hip surgery, the infection rate should be < 1.0%, but for other joints it may be higher because of their proximity to the skin surface and less experience in joint design. An infection rate of 0.5%, when universally attained, will still represent several thousand new cases of infection each year. The economic burden to health care associated with septic prosthetic joints is very high. The cost to treat patients with hip or knee prosthetic osteomyelitis, respectively, has been calculated to be 5.3- and 7.2-fold higher than the primary operations [6]. Prosthesis removal, which usually is necessary to treat these infections, produces large skeletal defects, shortening of the extremity, and severe functional impairment. Therefore, the patient faces protracted hospitalization, sizable financial expense, and, most distressing, renewed disability and sometimes death.

Incidence and Risk Factors

Prosthetic joints become infected by three different pathogenic mechanisms. One is introduction of microorganisms during the operative procedure, the second is contiguous spread of postoperative wound infection, and the third is colonization by hematogenous seeding. The freshly implanted biomaterial is highly susceptible to infection. Thus, during operation, colonization by even small numbers of bacteria (which, under other circumstances, might not produce infections) can lead to joint sepsis. During the early postimplantation period, when superficial infections can develop, the fascial layers have not healed, and the deep, periprosthetic tissue is not protected by the usual physical barriers. Any factor or event that delays wound healing increases the risk of infection: ischemic necrosis, hematomas, and, more directly, wound sepsis (with or without identifiable cellulitis) or suture abscesses [7–9].

Any bacteremia can induce prosthetic joint infection by hematogenous seeding. Dentogingival infections and manipulations, although exceptional, have been described as causes of viridans group streptococcal and anaerobic (peptococci and peptostreptococci) infections of prostheses. Pyogenic skin processes can cause staphylococcal (*Staphylococcus aureus* and *S. epidermidis*) and streptococcal (group A, B, C, and G streptococci) infec-

D.P. Lew, F.A. Waldvogel: Department of Internal Medicine, Geneva University Hospital, Geneva, CH-1211 Geneva 14, Switzerland.

[1]Research was supported by a grant (no. 3245810.95) from the Swiss National Foundation.

tions of replaced joints (see Chapter 41). Genitourinary and gastrointestinal tract surgeries or infections are associated with gram-negative bacillary, enterococcal, and anaerobic infections of prostheses.

Incidence of Infection After Hip or Knee Replacement

Infections have been categorized by the postoperative period in which they occur. By this classification, acute infection (stage 1) is defined as occurring within six months of surgery (≤ 40% of total infections); they are often evident within the first few weeks. These infections stem from operative contamination or from infected skin, subcutaneous tissue, and/or operative hematoma. Subacute infection (stage 2) develops within two years of operation (≤ 45% of total infections). Late infections (stage 3) emerge after two years of pain-free mobility (≥ 15% of total infections) and are mostly attributed to late-stage transient bacteremia with selective persistence of the microorganisms in the joint. This classification is, however, artificial and flawed, since a number of factors can influence the timing of symptom appearance. Smoldering infection with low-grade pathogenic microorganisms may be attributed to postoperative pain, and diagnosis may be delayed as a result. Many patients with late-stage infection probably harbor microorganisms for prolonged periods before the diagnosis is established.

The rate of infection after total hip arthroplasty in early surgical series was initially unacceptably high [10]. Wilson and colleagues reported an infection rate of > 11%, whereas in Charnley's early series, the infection rate was 7%. None of these patients was given antibiotic prophylaxis, and standard operating rooms and attire (no air filtration or body exhaust suits) were used. As a result, the source of infection in these early series was thought to be primarily local contamination. This high incidence of sepsis declined after the introduction of new operative and prophylactic measures. Air filtration and prophylactic antibiotics reduced the rate of infection to 0.6% in Charnley's later series [11]. At present, the rate of infection after total hip arthroplasty is thought to be ~1% over the entire lifetime of the prosthesis.

More precise data are now available from large series. Among 39,013 total hip or knee prostheses implanted over 23 years (1969 to 1991) at the Mayo Clinic [12], the infection rate per 1,000 joint-years was 1.32 for total hip prostheses and 2.29 for total knee prostheses. The incidence rates of prosthetic joint infection at 0 to 3 months after surgery fell from six and 12 per 1,000 joint-years (for total hip prostheses and total knee prostheses, respectively), to < 2 infections per 1,000 joint-years 24 to 48 months after implantation. These results demonstrate that the risk of infection depends on the joint replaced and that it declines with time. Late-stage infections represent the combination of smoldering infection and secondary seeding of bacteremia from another source.

Specific Risk Factors

Conditions favoring total hip arthroplasty infection include concomitant autoimmune diseases. The infection rate for patients with rheumatoid arthritis or systemic lupus erythematosus is twice as high as that for patients undergoing the same operation but without the same underlying disease. In general, the incidence of infection appears to be higher among corticosteroid-dependent patients. Another risk factor is reintervention. The rate of infection after revision hip surgery is at least twice as high as that for primary total hip arthroplasty. There are several reasons for this increased infection rate, among them, longer operating times and larger surgical exposures, resulting in the potential for increased direct contamination. Infection in an artificial joint is a risk factor for infection in the same individual with another prosthesis. Such joint infections are often due to the same causative organism and occur within the first year after the index infection [13].

Infecting Microorganisms

The data from several series indicate that a single pathogen can be identified in only about two thirds of cases; the remaining cases are equally divided between polymicrobial and sterile cultures [14]. The predominant microorganisms are staphylococcal species (~50% in several series), evenly divided between *S. epidermidis* and *S. aureus*. Aerobic streptococci are responsible for a significant group of infections (between 10% and 20% in different series). Gram-negative aerobic bacilli have been identified in some series in ≤ 25% of cases, and anaerobes usually do not account for > 10% of all pathogens. The full spectrum of microbial agents capable of causing prosthetic joint infections is very large and includes organisms ordinarily considered "contaminants" of cultures, such as *Corynebacteria* spp, *Propionibacteria* spp, and *Bacillus* spp. Primary infections with fungi (particularly *Candida* spp) and mycobacteria have been rarely described.

DIAGNOSIS

Clinical Presentation

Most patients experience a long, indolent course of infection, characterized by steadily increasing joint pain and the occasional formation of cutaneous draining sinuses. A minority of patients have an acute fulminant illness associated with high fever, severe joint pain, local swelling, and erythema. In a large series of infected hip prostheses, the rates of presenting symptoms were as follows: joint pain, 95%; fever, 43%; periarticular swelling, 38%; and wound or cutaneous sinus drainage, 32%.

Patients with persistent pain six months after total knee arthroplasty must be considered infected until proved otherwise. In a study of 52 patients with knee replacements who had been treated for infection, the workups were evaluated for accuracy in determining infection. Considerable pain was present in 96% of the patients, 77% had swelling of the knee, 27% were febrile, and 27% showed signs of active drainage. Thus, pain is the overriding complaint in patients with such infection [15]. The pattern of clinical presentation is determined largely by the nature of the infecting microorganism (i.e., the symptoms are more prominent in *S. aureus* infections compared with *S. epidermidis*). Infection must be differentiated from aseptic mechanical problems, which are the most common cause of pain and inflammatory symptoms in these patients [16]. Constant joint pain suggests infection, whereas mechanical loosening commonly causes pain only with motion and weight-bearing.

Erythrocyte Sedimentation Rate and C-Reactive Protein Levels

Persistent elevation of the erythrocyte sedimentation rate suggests infection but is neither very sensitive nor very specific, since it may be due to many other causes [17]. The combined measurement of C-reactive protein levels and the erythrocyte sedimentation rate seems to be more accurate. These two parameters are more appropriate to measure as follow-up during therapy than for diagnosis.

Radiology

A plain radiograph can display abnormal lucencies (> 2 mm in width) at the bone-cement interface, changes in the position of prosthetic components, cement fractures, periosteal reaction, or motion of components on stress views. Intraarticular injection of dye (arthrography) may show abnormal communications between the joint space and multiple defects in the bone-cement interface [1,18]. These radiologic abnormalities are found in 50% of septic prostheses. They are related to the duration of infection, since such changes may not become evident before several months. These radiographic changes are not specific to infection because they are also seen frequently with aseptic processes. When both the distal and proximal components of a prosthetic joint demonstrate radiographic abnormalities, infection is more likely than simple mechanical loosening. The presence of fistula (detected by arthrography) between the joint and soft tissue is a very significant finding in favor of infection.

Magnetic resonance or computed tomography techniques for evaluating prosthetic joints for infection are of little help because metal present in prostheses interferes with these images. Radionuclide imaging techniques have been extensively used for diagnosing prosthetic joint infection [18]. Radioisotopic scans with technetium diphosphonate demonstrate increased uptake in areas of bone with enhanced blood supply or increased metabolic activity. Increased technetium uptake is seen routinely around normal prostheses for six months after arthroplasty. After this time, interpretation of a positive scan is difficult. Persistent periprosthetic activity on bone scintigrams has been described even several years after implantation, but without evidence of clinical significance [19]. Some authors claim it reflects inflammation and possible loosening, but not specifically infection, of the implant. Abnormal gallium scans may be associated with "abundant granulation tissue" related to chronic loosening, rather than infection. In conclusion, a normal bone scan is often considered to exclude the need for surgical intervention aimed at correcting loosening or infection of the joint. Abnormal bone and gallium scans do not appear to reliably distinguish between infection and loosening.

Joint Aspiration

Aspiration of fluid associated with arthrography from a painful total joint prosthesis has been described as a highly accurate method of identifying infected joints [4,17,20]. Hip aspiration arthrography had a sensitivity of 79% for diagnosing the infection and a specificity of 100% [1]. The sensitivity rose to 91% when any one of the following features was observed: leukocytosis of the joint fluid of >10,000 white cells/mm^3, the presence of a fistula on arthrography, or isolation of a microorganism from the joint fluid or the rinsing liquid.

Ultrasonography has virtually replaced fluoroscopic techniques. There are some patients with no fluid at initial tap in whom ultrasound examination of the joint disclose the presence of loculated fluid (usually posterior to the greater trochanter) that can be aspirated under ultrasonic guidance. Arthrocentesis demonstrates the causative pathogen in 85% to 98% of cases. When intraarticular fluid is difficult to obtain, irrigation with sterile normal saline (without antiseptic preservative additives) can provide the necessary fluid for culture. When initial cultures indicate a relatively avirulent microorganism (*S. epidermidis,* corynebacteria, propionibacteria, and *Bacillus* spp), a second aspiration should be considered in order to confirm the bacteriologic diagnosis and to eliminate the possibility of contamination. Quantitative bacterial cultures are extremely useful in such situations. Quantitative measurement should be done by direct culture on a plate agar of a known amount of fluid. Culture of joint fluid in broth may be misleading, since a positive result can result from contamination. Cultures obtained at operation are diagnostic if the patient has not received antimicrobial therapy for several weeks before the procedure. Several specimens of tissue and fluid should be submitted for culture. Since fastidious microorganisms, including anaerobes, may be responsible for prosthetic arthroplasty infections, specimens should be cultured immediately in appropriate media. Tissue specimens should also be submitted for histopathologic study—special staining techniques may reflect unusual or slowly growing microorganisms.

In the study by Levitsky and colleagues [21], the sensitivities of different techniques to diagnose infection were as follows: arthrocentesis fluid Gram's stain, 32%; histopathology (leukocytic infiltrate in osseous and nonosseous periprosthetic tissue), 55%; fluid culture, 85% to 98%; and operative culture, 100% [21]. The identification of an infected implant before a revision operation is important because it will determine the extent of the surgery required [17]. In the presence of infection, cement removal must be complete, and radical excision of infected soft tissue and bone is required. The use of bone grafts is probably contraindicated. Preoperative knowledge of the antibiotic sensitivity of the infecting organism will aid in making the appropriate choice of antibiotics to administer both parenterally and in and around the cement. As with hip prostheses, the workup of an infected total knee arthroplasty should include preoperative aspiration under sterile conditions. Superficial sinus cultures poorly predict the causative pathogen.

PREVENTION

Prevention of infection is a key element in the success of joint replacement procedures. It is efficacious, has few side effects, and is certainly more cost-effective than therapy.

Benefits of Antibiotic Prophylaxis and Ultraclean Air Systems

Various reviews [3,22] have dealt with the subject of antibiotic prophylaxis subsequent to total joint replacement (see Chapter 14) [10]. Between 1970 and 1980, several studies suggested that antimicrobial prophylaxis reduces the incidence of deep incisional surgical site infection after total joint replacement [23]. Hill and coworkers reported that prophylaxis with cefazolin significantly lowered the incidence of wound infections compared with placebo [24]. However, when the results were examined according to the type of operating theater used, differences were found to be significant only among patients whose surgery was performed in a conventional setting. In a "hypersterile" environment, the rates of infection were the same for cefazolin-treated and placebo-treated groups. Thus, antibiotic prophylaxis and ultraclean air systems appear to be independent factors in limiting the rate of foreign body infection.

A recently published cost-benefit analysis concluded that for departments performing ≥ 100 total joint replacement procedures per year, a combination of parenteral antibiotic administration and use of an ultraclean air system would be "the most attractive means of prophylaxis." This also appeared to be the most cost-effective system. For departments performing < 100 arthroplasties each year, the authors argued that a combination of parenteral and local antibiotics (the latter delivered in antibiotic-impregnated cement) would be the most cost-effective means of limiting infection. In view of the economic costs and the high morbidity rates associated with infection of prosthetic joints, adherence to these recommendations seems worthwhile until other techniques for the prevention of deep infection are shown to be effective and cost-efficient.

Optimal Agents and Duration of Prophylaxis

Cefazolin has generally been used for prophylaxis in total joint replacement, but many reports in the surgical literature also evaluate the newer cephalosporins. Relatively few reported studies have compared various cephalosporins for prophylaxis in total joint replacement. Given the low incidence of deep incisional surgical site infection, a comparative trial large enough to show a difference between agents is obviously impractical. Despite the lack of such comparisons, both first-generation (cefazolin) and second-generation cephalosporins (cefamandole, cefuroxime) appear to be appropriate for this type of use [22].

Several studies have also found that administration of antibiotics for 12 to 24 hours is as effective as prolonging antibiotic therapy for several days. Therefore, administration of parenteral antibiotics just before surgery (about 30 to 90 minutes before incision), with discontinuation within 24 hours, is the optimal timing for prophylaxis [25].

Antibiotic-containing Cement in Total Joint Replacement

Antibiotic-containing cement is widely used for prophylaxis and therapy of implant surgery infections. However, the subject of antibiotic-impregnated cement in total joint replacement remains controversial [26–28]. Many antibiotics appear to be released from the cement in potentially efficacious amounts, but the duration of time over which these antibiotics continue to be released is less certain. Even for specific combinations of antibiotic and cement, different investigators have derived markedly different data. For example, the period of release of gentamicin from cement has been reported to range from 13 days to 5 years. Moreover, the use of antibiotic-impregnated cement is usually only one of a series of determining variables in clinical studies. Thus, a lowering of the infection rate is often difficult to attribute to the use of antibiotic-impregnated cement alone. It is worth noting that gentamicin, the most widely used compound, is not the agent of choice to prevent or treat staphylococcal infections.

McQueen and colleagues [29] performed a well-controlled, prospective, randomized trial including 295 arthroplasties of the hip and knee, using a second-generation cephalosporin-impregnated cement. The impact of systemic cefuroxime on the development of early infection was compared with that of cefuroxime-impregnated bone cement. The cement group received 1.5 g of cefuroxime in 40 g of cement powder; the parenteral antibiotic group received 1.5 g of cefuroxime intravenously at the induction of anesthesia and two additional doses of 750 mg each, 6 and 12 hours later. The follow-up period was only three months. The observed rate of deep infection was 0.7% in the cement group and 1.3% in the parenteral antibiotic group. The authors found at least equal efficacy of the cefuroxime-impregnated bone cement and parenterally administered cefuroxime in the prevention of early infection in total joint replacement [29].

Prophylaxis Against Hematogenous Seeding

Some experimental evidence suggests that there is a high risk of infection of joint implants in the context of bacteremia, especially in the early postoperative period. There is also clear evidence that hematogenous infection of prosthetic joints sometimes stems from overt infections elsewhere in the body, particularly those of the urinary tract or the skin. Thus, vigorous treatment of infection elsewhere in the body is required before total joint replacement. The situation with regard to dental procedures is less clear. Analysis of large series of patients indicates that the incidence of late-stage prosthetic joint infections associated with dental treatment is low.

Jacobson and co-workers created a computer simulation model to assess the risks and efficacy of no prophylaxis, orally administered penicillin prophylaxis, and orally administered cephalexin prophylaxis among dental patients at risk of late-stage prosthetic joint infection [30]. In the framework of the assumptions made by the authors, the analysis suggested that there was a very small risk of infection (29 to 68 cases per 10^6 dental visits); this risk was lower than that of death from a reaction to an antibiotic. The authors concluded from their model that routine antibiotic prophylaxis for all dental patients with prosthetic joints is not indicated but that prophylaxis might be appropriate in high-risk patients. The clinical profile of high risk patients remains to be fully elucidated. Treatment of severe periodontal disease and abscess of the teeth and gums, in the presence of foreign body, certainly requires administration of systemic antibiotics [14].

TABLE 1. *Antibiotic treatment of prosthetic joint infection*

Microorganisms isolated	Parenteral therapy: Treatment of choice	Parenteral therapy: Alternatives	Oral therapy[a]
S. aureus or coagulase negative			
Penicillin sensitive	Penicillin G (4 million u every 6 hr)	A cephalosporin II[b], clindamycin (600 mg every 6 hr), or vancomycin	Amoxicillin (750 mg every 8 hr)
Penicillin resistant	Nafcillin[c] (2 g every 6 hr)	A cephalosporin II[b], clindamycin (600 mg every 6 hr), or vancomycin	Quinolone[d]-rifampin (600 mg every 24 hr) or flucloxacillin-rifampin
Methicillin resistant	Vancomycin (1 g every 12 hr)	Teicoplanin[e] (400 mg every 24 hr, first day every 12 hr)	Not recommended
Various streptococci (group A or B β-hemolytic, *S. pneumoniae*)	Penicillin G (3 million u every 4 to 6 hr)	Clindamycin (600 mg every 6 hr), erythromycin (500 mg every 6 hr), or vancomycin	Amoxicillin (750 mg every 8 hr)
Enteric gram-negative rods	Quinolone[d] (initially i.v., followed by early oral switch)	A cephalosporin III[f]	Quinolone[d]
Serratia spp, *P. aeruginosa*	Piperacillin[g] (4 g every 6 hr) and gentamicin (5 mg/kg/day)	A cephalosporin III[f,g] or quinolone quinolone (with aminoglycosides)	Quinolone[d]
Anaerobes	Clindamycin (600 mg every 6 hr)	Amoxicillin-clavulanic acid (2.2 mg every 8 hr) or metronidazole for gram-negative anaerobes (500 mg every 8 hr)	Clindamycin (600 mg every 6 hr)
Mixed infection (aerobic and anaerobic microorganisms)	Amoxicillin-clavulanic acid (2.2 mg every 8 hr)	Imipenem[h] (500 mg every 6 hr)	Amoxicillin-clavulanic acid (750 mg every 8 hr)

[a]Oral therapy is usually given after 4 to 6 wk of parenteral therapy with the exception of quinolones.
[b]Second generation, such as cefuroxime (1.5 g every 6 hr).
[c]Flucloxacillin in Europe.
[d]Quinolone, such as ofloxacin (200 mg every 8 hr), ciprofloxacin (500–750 mg every 12 hr), or fleroxacin (400 mg every 24 hr).
[e]Teicoplanin is presently available only in Europe; it may be given by the intramuscular route.
[f]Third generation, such as ceftazidime (2 g every 8 hr).
[g]Depends on sensitivities; piperacillin/tazobactam and imipenem are useful alternatives.
[h]In cases of aerobic gram-negative microorganisms resistant to amoxicillin-clavulanic acid.

TREATMENT

The optimal treatment of a prosthetic joint infection requires a well-balanced and timed approach of antibiotic therapy (parenteral and oral) associated with a variety of surgical procedures.

Choice of an Optimal Antibiotic Regimen

Single-agent chemotherapy is usually adequate for the treatment of prosthetic joint infection. The conventional choices of antimicrobial agents for the most commonly encountered microorganisms in infections of skeletal prostheses are given in Table 1. Antibiotics should be chosen based on the antimicrobial susceptibility of the isolated microorganism. As a general principle, these antibiotics should be given parenterally for 4 to 6 weeks, which may be followed by several weeks to months of oral therapy.

Antibiotic Therapy Without Prosthesis Removal

Antibiotic treatment without the removal of the prosthesis is not considered standard therapy for prosthetic joint infection and has been associated with a failure rate of > 90% [6]. However, in selected patients, initial parenteral antibiotic therapy (for several weeks) followed by oral antibiotic therapy (for several months) may be contemplated. While there are no comparative studies for these indications, this treatment has a greater chance of success (a) when microorganisms are of low virulence and highly susceptible to orally administered antibiotics, such as streptococci (of nonenterococcal origin); (b) early in the course of infection and if the prosthesis is not loose (this approach may be successful in the context of an early aggressive debridement); (c) when a total hip prosthesis is infected by staphylococci. A small series of patients in a nonrandomized trial were treated with the combination of quinolone-rifampin for 6 months with success. This treatment requires, however, that the prosthesis not loosen; if it does, prosthesis removal is indicated [31]. In addition, in cases where removal of the prosthesis is not feasible (owing to medical and surgical contraindication or the patient's refusal to undergo surgery) and the patient tolerates an active drug for prolonged periods, suppressive antimicrobial therapy may be attempted. Careful monitoring is important because of the danger of extension of the septic process or progressive bone resorption.

Prosthesis Removal

In order to achieve a microbiologic cure, it is almost always necessary to remove the prosthesis and all associated cement and completely debride devitalized tissue and bone. Antibiotics should be given concurrently as soon as sufficient material is obtained for culture or the microorganisms are isolated. Upon removal of the prosthesis, there are several options; they include resection arthroplasty without reimplantation, arthrodesis, and one-stage or two-stage reimplantation of a new prosthesis. The decision concerning the best approach depends on careful assessment of the patient's general status, the condition of the specific site, the type of prosthesis, and the experience of the surgical team.

Resection Arthroplasty

Resection arthroplasty involves complete removal of the infected prosthesis, any associated cement, and additional infected tissue, followed by prolonged parenteral therapy. If debridement is performed very carefully and extensively and the microorganism is sensitive to currently used antimicrobials, the chance of cure is high. However, without additional surgery, joint function is lost. This approach is recommended for patients who are unable to walk or when the condition of the specific site does not allow further surgery.

Arthrodesis

Surgical fixation by fusion of the joint surfaces is the treatment of choice for infection of the total knee joint when the patient's mobility is important and reimplantation of a prosthesis is not feasible for technical reasons. In addition to prolonged parenteral and oral therapy, fixation (either external or intramedullary) is necessary for prolonged periods until bone union is achieved. This may also require bone graft and prolonged immobility. However, infection may recur.

Reimplantation

Reimplantation of a new prosthesis will result in the best functional outcome.

Reimplantation in Total Hip Arthroplasty

Two surgical approaches to treatment exist. With one-stage exchange arthroplasty, the infected components are excised, surgical debridement is performed, and a new prosthesis is immediately put in place under antibiotic coverage. Buchholz and colleagues [32], the chief proponents of this technique, use cement containing an antimicrobial drug. Analysis of published series does not show any advantage of one-stage exchange arthroplasty with or without antibiotic cement.

A second approach, described by investigators at the Mayo Clinic and elsewhere, requires careful surgical removal of all foreign body material and infected tissue followed by prolonged parenteral and oral therapy [33,34]. Reconstruction is performed ≥ 3 months after the end of therapy for less virulent infection but is delayed for ≥ 1 year for more virulent infection. The advantages of two-stage reimplantation are that it allows for additional debridement and optimization of the choice of antibiotic and duration of therapy for more virulent microorganisms. The disadvantage is that, as a result of scarring, the second intervention is more difficult to perform. In patients who have experienced extensive bone loss, a third stage, consisting of bone grafting, is required between resection and reimplantation.

In a recent review by Steckelberg and Osmon, data were collected from articles on the subject of one-step or two-stage exchange arthroplasty for total hip arthroplasty infection [35]. Among a total of 1,143 infections treated with one-stage exchange arthroplasty and with antibiotic-impregnated cement, 915 did not recur (80% success rate). The success rate of two-stage arthroplasty (with or without antibiotic-impregnated cement) is slightly higher (85%) among a total of 262 patients analyzed.

In the absence of a prospective randomized study with prolonged follow-up comparing these two different surgical approaches, it is difficult at present to recommend one- over two-stage arthroplasty [36]. Most centers in the United States and Europe use two-stage arthroplasty, with a variable intermediate period between excision and reimplantation, because it appears to give the best chance of curing infection. In selected patients (such as elderly patients in whom prolonged immobility might lead to greater rates of morbidity) and in the presence of easy-to-treat microorganisms, a one-stage procedure might be a reasonable alternative.

Total Knee Arthroplasty

The experience with one-stage arthroplasty has been disappointing in terms of the high rates of recurrence of infection in the knee joint, and only small series of patients have been treated with this procedure. Most surgeons have favored delayed two-stage exchange arthroplasty. Among a total of 197 published and reviewed cases, the success rate was 88%. However, with the two-stage procedure, patients are at risk of scarring, with resultant loss of range of motion after resection, and, thus, the period of parenteral antimicrobial therapy is not prolonged beyond 6 weeks to preserve joint function. During this intermediate period, polymethylmethacrylate antibiotic-containing cement and spacers are often used. Additional debridement is performed before secondary reimplantation.

Other Prostheses

Well-documented cases of infection have been reported for different joint replacements. Although there is not much clinical experience, the general principles described earlier are usually applicable to any other joint infection.

Concluding Remarks

With modern medical surgery and adequate prophylaxis, the incidence of prosthetic joint infection has declined over the past 20 years, but it remains a regular and dreadful complication. It is associated with serious morbidity and some mortality as well as additional costs. Researchers and clinicians have provided the means to understand better the pathophysiology of foreign body infections as well as their prevention. Improved diagnostic tools and optimal medical and surgical means to treat infections of skeletal prostheses have also been developed. In order to allow more elderly and joint-disabled individuals to optimally benefit from orthopedic bioprosthesis, new biomaterials and novel preventive strategies are necessary. Such strategies will have considerable impact on this difficult clinical problem.

REFERENCES

1. Brause BD. Infected orthopedic prostheses. In: Bisno AL, Waldvogel FA, eds. *Infections associated with indwelling medical devices*. Washington, D.C.: American Society for Microbiology, 1989.
2. Salvati EA, Small RD, Brause BD, et al. Infections associated with orthopedic devices. In: Sugarman B, Young EJ, eds. *Infections associated with prosthetic devices*. Boca Raton, Fla.: CRC Press, 1984.
3. Fitzgerald RH Jr. Total hip arthroplasty: sepsis, prevention, and diagnosis. *Orthop Clin North Am* 1992;23:259–264.
4. Cuckler JM, Star AM, Alavi A, et al. Diagnosis and management of the infected total joint arthroplasty. *Orthop Clin North Am* 1992;22: 523–530.
5. Malchau H, Herberts P, Ahnfelt L. Prognosis of total hip replacement in Sweden: follow-up of 92,675 operations performed 1978–1990. *Acta Orthop Scand* 1993;64:497–506.
6. Bengtson S. Prosthetic osteomyelitis with special reference to the knee: risks, treatment and costs. *Ann Med* 1993;25:523–529.
7. Rasul AT Jr., Tsukayama D, Gustilo RB. Effect of time of onset and depth of infection on the outcome of total knee arthroplasty infections. *Clin Orthop* 1991:x:98–104.
8. Sanderson PJ. Infection in orthopaedic implants. *J Hosp Infect* 1991;18[suppl A]:367–375.
9. Gordon SM, Culver DH, Simmons BP, et al. Risk factors for wound infections after total knee arthroplasty. *Am J Epidemiol* 1990;131: 905–916.
10. Nasser S. Prevention and treatment of sepsis in total hip replacement surgery. *Orthop Clin North Am* 1992;23:265–277.
11. Charnley J. Postoperative infection after total hip replacement with special reference to air contamination in the operating room. *Clin Orthop* 1972;87:167–187.
12. Vaudaux P. Host factors influencing staphylococcal foreign body infections. In: Philipps I, ed. *Focus on coagulase-negative staphylococci*. Royal Society of Medical Services, 1989 [International Congress and Symposium Series].
13. Murray RP, Bourne MH, Fitzgerald RH Jr. Metachronous infections in patients who have had more than one total joint arthroplasty. *J Bone Joint Surg* 1991;73-A:1469–1474.

14. Gillespie WJ. Infection in total joint replacement. *Infect Dis Clin North Am* 1990;4:465–484.
15. Windsor RE. Management of total knee arthroplasty infection. *Orthop Clin North Am* 1992;22:531–538.
16. Whyte W, Hodgson R, Tinkler J, et al. The isolation of bacteria of low pathogenicity from faulty orthopaedic implants. *J Hosp Infect* 1981;2:219–230.
17. Roberts P, Walters AJ, McMinn DJW. Diagnosing infection in hip replacements: the use of fine-needle aspiration and radiometric culture. *J Bone Joint Surg* 1992;74B:265–269.
18. Alazraki NP. Diagnosing prosthetic joint infection [Editorial; Comment]. *J Nucl Med* 1990;31:1955–1957.
19. Palestro CJ, Swyer AJ, Kim CK, et al. Infected knee prosthesis: diagnosis with In-111 leukocyte, Tc-99m sulfur colloid, and Tc-99m MDP imaging. *Radiology* 1991;179:645–648.
20. Lopitaux R, Levai JP, Raux P, et al. Value of puncture-arthrography in the diagnosis of infection of total hip arthroplasty [In French]. *Rev Chir Orthop Reparatrice Appar Mot* 1992;78:34–37.
21. Levitsky KA, Hozack WJ, Balderston RA, et al. Evaluation of the painful prosthetic joint: relative value of bone scan, sedimentation rate, and joint aspiration. *J Arthroplasty* 1991;6:237–244.
22. Norden CW. Antibiotic prophylaxis in orthopedic surgery. *Rev Infect Dis* 1991;13:S842–S846.
23. Hirschmann JV. Antibiotics in the prevention of infection associated with prosthetic devices. In: Sugarman B, Young EJ, eds. *Infections associated with prosthetic devices*. Boca Raton, Fla.: CRC Press, 1984.
24. Hill C, Flamant R, Mazas F, et al. Prophylactic cefazolin versus placebo in total hip replacement: report of a multicentre double-blind randomised trial. *Lancet* 1981;1:795–796.
25. Classen DC, Evans RS, Pestotnik SL, et al. The timing of prophylactic administration of antibiotics and the risk of surgical-wound infection [Comments]. *N Engl J Med* 1992;326:281–286.
26. Bucholz HW, Elson RA, Heinert K. Antibiotic-loaded acrylic cement: current concepts. *Clin Orthop* 1984;19:96–108.
27. Hope PG, Kristinsson KG, Norman P, et al. Deep infection of cemented total hip arthroplasties caused by coagulase negative staphylococci. *J Bone Joint Surg Br* 1989;71:851–855.
28. Duncan CP, Masri BA. The role of antibiotic-loaded cement in the treatment of an infection after a hip replacement. *J Bone Joint Surg Am* 1994;76A:1742–1751.
29. McQueen MM, Hughes SP, May P, et al. Cefuroxime in total joint arthroplasty: intravenous or in bone cement. *J Arthroplasty* 1990;5:169–172.
30. Jacobson JJ, Schweitzer SO, Kowalski CJ. Chemoprophylaxis of prosthetic joint patients during dental treatment: a decision-utility analysis. *Oral Surg Oral Med Oral Pathol* 1991;72:167–177.
31. Drancourt M, Stein A, Argenson JN, et al. Oral rifampin plus ofloxacin for treatment of *Staphylococcus*-infected orthopedic implants. *Antimicrob Agents Chemother* 1993;37:1214–1218.
32. Buchholz HW, Elson RA, Engelbrecht E, et al. Management of deep infection of total hip replacement. *J Bone Joint Surg Br* 1981;63-B:342–353.
33. McDonald DJ, Fitzgerald RH, Ilstrup DM. Two-stage reconstruction of a total hip arthroplasty because of infection. *J Bone Joint Surg Am* 1989;71:828–832.
34. Windsor RE, Insall JN, Urs WK, et al. Two-stage reimplantation for the salvage of total knee arthroplasty complicated by infection. *J Bone Joint Surg Am* 1990;72:272–278.
35. Steckelberg JM, Osmon DR. Prosthetic joint infections. In: Bisno AL, Waldvogel FA, eds. *Infections associated with indwelling medical devices*. Washington, D.C.: American Society for Microbiology, 1994.
36. Britt MW, Calhoun JH, Mader JT. Principles of current management of prosthetic joint infections. In: Jauregui LE, ed. *Diagnosis and management of bone infections*. New York: Marcel Dekker, 1995.

Hospital Infections, Fourth Edition,
edited by John V. Bennett and Philip S. Brachman.
Lippincott–Raven Publishers, Philadelphia © 1998

CHAPTER 41

Epidemiology of Staphylococcus and Group A Streptococci

Kenneth E. F. Sands and Donald A. Goldmann

HISTORICAL CONTEXT

A review of staphylococcal and streptococcal epidemiology leads directly to the historical roots of infection control. Epidemics of puerperal sepsis first suggested that hospital-acquired infections could be a major cause of morbidity and mortality and might require an organized approach to control. Modern-day hospital infection control programs have developed largely in response to outbreaks of staphylococcal disease in the 1950s and 1960s. Thus, it is not surprising that the early infection control literature was dominated by studies concerning the epidemiology of streptococcal and staphylococcal infection, and a rich and varied literature it is. In the following decades other pathogens, particularly gram-negative bacilli, appeared to be supplanting gram-positive cocci on hospital wards, and the emphasis of the infection control literature changed accordingly. More recently, the field has come full circle as the emergence of methicillin-resistant *Staphylococcus aureus* (MRSA) and *Staphylococcus epidermidis* (see Chapters 15, 30), the increasing incidence of gram-positive nosocomial infections, and evidence of the growing incidence and pathogenicity of group A streptococcal infections have rekindled interest in the epidemiology of these organisms.

K. E.F. Sands: Department of Medicine, Beth Israel Deaconness Medical Center, Boston, Massachusetts 02215.

D. A. Goldmann: Children's Hospital, Harvard Medical School, Boston, Massachusetts 02115.

EPIDEMIOLOGY OF GROUP A STREPTOCOCCAL INFECTIONS

Transmission

Although streptococci have been a scourge of obstetric wards and surgical services for centuries, group A streptococcal nosocomial infection is relatively rare today. Group A streptococci are recovered from < 1% of all surgical wound infections in hospitals participating in the National Nosocomial Infections Surveillance (NNIS) System. Thus, the occurrence of even one group A streptococcal infection is reason for concern, and two or more cases in a short period of time should alert the infection control team that a full-scale epidemic investigation is warranted, to determine the source of the outbreak.

Perhaps because streptococcal epidemics occur sporadically and unpredictably in hospitals, much of what we know about the transmission of group A streptococci comes from a series of remarkably careful studies in military populations performed by Rammelkamp and Wannamaker and their colleagues [1–3]. It had already been demonstrated that streptococcal infections could be spread by direct contact with either infected cutaneous lesions or secretions inoculated into the pharynx. The military studies were designed to answer two pivotal questions. (a) Can streptococci be transmitted by droplet nuclei generated from the respiratory tract of infected or colonized persons, and (b) can dust and other environmental fomites serve as reservoirs for the airborne spread of streptococci? These studies therefore addressed one of the fundamental issues in infection control—the relative importance of airborne and contact transmission of infection.

To obtain a rough assessment of the relative significance of airborne transmission via dust or droplet nuclei versus direct contact spread via large droplets or respira-

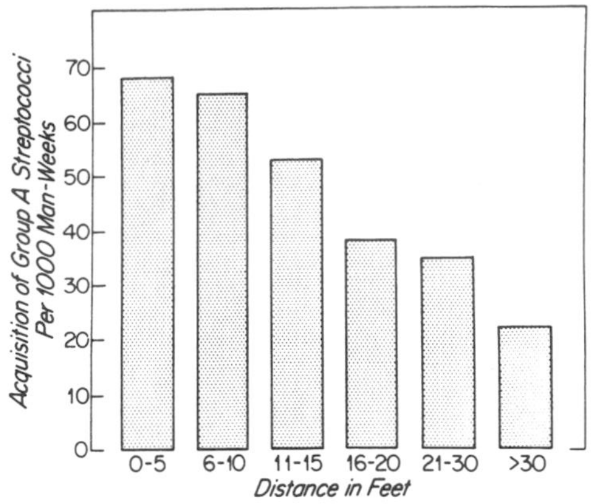

FIGURE 41-1. Acquisition rates for group A streptococci according to bed distance from the nearest carrier. (Reprinted with permission from Rammelkamp CH Jr., Mortimer EA Jr., Wolinsky E, et al. Transmission of streptococcal and staphylococcal infections. *Ann Intern Med* 1964; 60:753.)

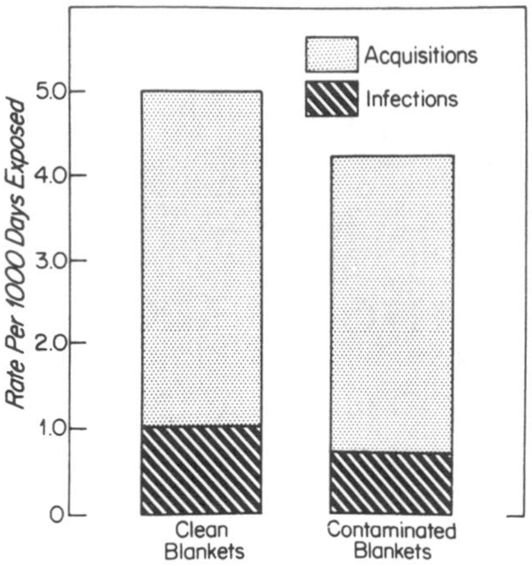

FIGURE 41-2. Acquisition and infection rates with eight types of streptococci of men with clean or contaminated blankets. (Reprinted with permission from Perry WD, Siegel AC, Rammelkamp CH Jr, et al. Transmission of group-A streptococci. I. The role of contaminated bedding. *Am J Hyg* 1957;66:85–95.)

tory secretions, Rammelkamp's group studied the incidence of streptococcal disease among susceptible soldiers as a function of the distance of their bunks from the beds of colonized or infected recruits [4]. If the risk of infection turned out to be higher only among soldiers whose bunks were very close to those of the index cases, the direct contact theory would be supported. On the other hand, if the incidence of infection turned out to be independent of location in the barracks, airborne spread would be the most likely explanation. In fact, the risk of a recruit acquiring group A streptococci was found to be inversely proportional to the distance between his bunk and that of a carrier (Figure 41-1). At a distance of 30 feet, the acquisition rate was no higher than the background incidence of streptococcal acquisition among recruits in a control population. If the beds were located right next to each other, the risk more than tripled.

Although this study suggested that most streptococcal disease is transmitted by direct contact with large droplets, the possibility remained that some infections could be spread by contaminated dust or other environmental reservoirs. It seemed particularly important to rule out airborne transmission, since it was known that soldiers who carry streptococci in their throats or noses expel a prodigious number of bacteria onto their clothes, blankets, and other personal articles. Moreover, dust collected from barracks housing colonized or infected soldiers routinely yields enormous numbers of streptococci, and streptococci can remain viable in the environment for days. To find out whether contaminated dust or blankets could spread group A streptococcal infections among susceptible persons, the following experiments were performed.

The initial studies were made possible by a bizarre but routine military procedure. Each new recruit was issued a set of wool blankets that he used until he was transferred to another unit or was admitted to a hospital. Unless these blankets were grossly soiled, they were reissued to a new recruit without cleaning. Thus, it was common practice to issue blankets heavily contaminated with streptococci to susceptible soldiers. In the clinical study, blankets were donated by 83 colonized soldiers, including 15 who had just been hospitalized because of streptococcal disease. The blankets were stored for either 24 hours or 6 days and then reissued. Recipients were followed closely for acquisition of streptococci and clinical disease. A control group received laundered blankets that were shown not to harbor streptococci. Acquisition rates turned out to be slightly lower in soldiers issued the contaminated blankets (Figure 41-2), although this difference was not statistically significant. Six recruits who received contaminated blankets did develop streptococcal disease, but in only two cases did the serotype isolated from the throat of the soldier match the serotype from the contaminated blanket.

In the next experiment, five volunteers were placed in a small enclosure while ~50 g to 100 g of contaminated dust was blown in. The soldiers were asked to sweep the floor for 10 minutes and to rest in a chair for 10 additional minutes. Air samples taken during the study period contained 100 to 1,600 streptococci per cubic foot. It was obvious that the volunteers had inhaled a considerable amount of contaminated dust, since dust could be seen easily in mucus expelled by coughing or nose blowing for as long as 6 hours after exposure. No volunteer became infected, even though none had antibody to the streptococcal serotypes found in the dust. To further document the inability of contaminated dust to transmit streptococcal infections, dust was sprinkled on the pharynx of 13 volunteers. Six other volunteers had dust containing 1,800 to 42,000 streptococci blown into the mouth. Streptococci could be recovered from the pharynx only transiently, and there were no infections. Finally, 37 airmen were placed in a barracks while 50 g to 150 g of contaminated dust were blown into the room. The airmen lived in the barracks for 18 to 24 hours before sweeping it clean. No infections occurred.

These experiments suggest that airborne streptococci are not very infectious and rarely, if ever, produce pharyngitis in susceptible persons. Instead, it appears that close contact with respiratory secretions or droplets from colonized or infected patients is critical for transmission to occur. Although airborne streptococci seem to be virtually incapable of producing pharyngitis, it does not necessarily follow that streptococci falling into a wound from contaminated air would be unable to initiate a streptococcal wound infection. Only a few streptococcal surgical wound infection outbreaks have been reported in the modern nosocomial infection literature, making data concerning the transmission of these infections scarce.

It is worth noting that the literature is virtually devoid of descriptions of outbreaks traced to a nasopharyngeal carrier on the medical or nursing staff, and outbreaks involving personnel with streptococcal skin lesions or attributed to extensive patient-to-patient transmission via hands (or, in a recent case, forearms) of personnel have been reported rarely in the past few decades [5]. Several epidemics have been attributed to vaginal or anal carriers among operating personnel [6]. It is possible that this finding reflects a reporting bias; anal or vaginal carriers may be perceived as unusual and therefore worthy of documentation [7], whereas epidemics caused by nasopharyngeal carriers may be seen as too mundane to warrant publication. Regardless, the reported outbreaks provide reasonably strong evidence that streptococci may reach operative wounds via the air [6,8–13].

Streptococci have been recovered from settling plates placed in operating rooms occupied by carriers who were linked epidemiologically to the surgical wound infections, and it has been suggested that streptococci are aerosolized by flatus or shed during exercise. As emphasized previously, mere dissemination of bacteria into the environment does not prove that these organisms actually were responsible for the observed infections. However, the carriers in some of the reported outbreaks had no direct contact with the infected patients. It is not known why airborne streptococci disseminated by carriers apparently can cause wound infections but not pharyngitis. Perhaps the open surgical wound is much more susceptible than the pharynx to airborne streptococci.

Increased Virulence of Group A Streptococci

An apparent increase in the occurrence of severe group A streptococcal infections has captured the attention of both the medical community and the general public [14]. Conclusive epidemiologic data are not available because continuous population-based surveillance for these infections has been initiated only recently. However, reports from North America, Australia, Asia, and Europe all suggest an increased incidence of invasive group A streptococcal infections [15–24]. These outbreaks have been largely community-based, but 22% of cases were hospital-acquired in one report [15], and a rise in nosocomial group A streptococcal bacteremia was noted during a community epidemic in another [25]. Public anxiety has been so great that hospital epidemiologists can expect publicity and scrutiny whenever group A streptococcal infections develop in their institutions.

In adults, the most common presentations are aggressive soft-tissue infections (necrotizing fasciitis) and/or bacteremia. In children, primary bacteremia is also common, and varicella infection, immunosuppression, and neoplasms have been identified as risk factors [19,26,27]. Infection may be accompanied by a syndrome of fulminant shock with multi-organ failure, now defined as streptococcal toxic shock syndrome [28,29] and associated with a mortality rate of 30% to 50% [24,30].

The full pathogenesis of invasive group A streptococcal disease remains to be elucidated, but most studies have focused on the roles of exotoxin (specifically pyrogenic exotoxins A and B), and specific M proteins. Isolates that produce exotoxin A or contain the gene (*speA*) for its production are greatly over-represented among patients with streptococcal toxic shock syndrome [15,24,31–34]. Exotoxin A functions as a superantigen; it can stimulate T cells in a nonspecific fashion and trigger massive release of immunologic modulators [35]. However, streptococcal toxic shock has been reported in strains that produce only exotoxin B [30]. Exotoxin B may play a role in localized soft-tissue destruction [19]. Specific M types, especially M1 and M3, have also been linked to invasive infection, perhaps because the capsules of these serotypes provide better protection for the organism from phagocytosis [36]. Variable presentations of infection may relate to the presence of the specific M-proteins and exotoxins mentioned, plus the level of immunity to these antigens present in the individual host [37].

In addition to the reported increase in invasive group A streptococcal infections, there have been reports of nonsuppurative complications. A resurgence in rheumatic fever was described in the 1980s from several regions of the United States [16,38–41], and while the incidence may have declined, cases continue to occur with greater frequency than was seen in the 1970s [42,43]. Rheumatic fever has been associated with specific mucoid M types of streptococci [44,45]. The virulence of these strains may be mediated by the capsular hyaluronic acid that these mucoid strains produce in abundance, as demonstrated by loss of virulence in acapsular mutant strains [46,47].

Epidemic Investigation

As soon as an outbreak of group A streptococcal nosocomial infection is recognized, the infection control team should immediately initiate a search for a carrier on the hospital staff (see Chapter 6). Of course, the possibility of person-to-person transmission via the hands of personnel cannot be ignored, particularly in the newborn nursery and on other nonsurgical services, but streptococcal operative wound infections are generally inoculated in the operating room and can virtually always be traced to a carrier. As noted earlier, the recent literature suggests that the carrier is more likely to be colonized with streptococci in the anus or vagina than in the throat, but the prudent epidemiologist will not begin an investigation by indiscriminately culturing a particular anatomic site. A formal epidemiologic investigation should be undertaken to ascertain whether infected patients had a significantly greater exposure to individual members of the staff. Personnel identified by the epidemiologic investigation should be questioned closely about recent sore throats, skin infections, or vaginal or anal symptoms. Although perineal disseminators may be totally asymptomatic, most of the carriers reported in the literature have had mild symptoms that could easily be missed by a casual investigation. For example, the surgeon responsible for the outbreak reported by Richman and colleagues [11] suffered from external hemorrhoids to which he applied corticosteroid ointment daily. The circulating nurse implicated in the epidemic described by Berkelman and associates [8] had chronic bouts of diarrhea complicated by shallow perineal ulcers.

Isolation of streptococci from anal or vaginal cultures taken from someone who has been linked epidemiologically to an outbreak is strong evidence pointing to the source of the problem, particularly since group A streptococci are rarely found at these sites in healthy adults. Occasionally, the symptom complex caused by the streptococci is so distinctive that it is clear that all the cases are associated with the same strain. For example, Richman and co-workers [11] recognized their outbreak when two cases of scarlet fever occurred on the orthopedic service within a short period of time. However, it is usually desirable to obtain additional laboratory data to prove that the carrier is colonized or infected with the same strain of group A streptococci that was recovered from the nosocomial infections. First, serogrouping should be performed to confirm that the organism is indeed group A, since streptococci of groups B, C, and G can also be both α-hemolytic and bacitracin-susceptible.

If additional microbiologic confirmation is required, group A streptococci can be classified by reference laboratories according to their M- and T-antigens and by their serum opacity reaction [48]. More recently, molecular epidemiologic techniques have been applied to investigate streptococcal outbreaks, including DNA sequencing [49] and restriction endonuclease analysis [50]. Even the most basic strain analysis occasionally yields surprises. Goldmann and Breton [51] found that the α-hemolytic streptococci recovered from a small cluster of orthopedic infections were of group C, and group C streptococci were subsequently isolated from the anus of a member of the surgical staff. On the other hand, there are examples where sophisticated techniques demonstrated that an outbreak actually represented clusters of infections due to multiple strains [50,52].

Nasopharyngeal carriers of group A streptococci can usually be treated successfully with penicillin or erythromycin. If streptococci are not eradicated by these regimens, amoxicillin-clavulanic acid or a penicillinase-resistant cephalosporin may be effective. The addition of a 4-day course of rifampicin to the standard penicillin regimen may be advisable [53,54]. Vaginal and anal carriers pose a greater challenge. Oral penicillin may fail to eradicate anal carriage. Oral vancomycin, which is not absorbed from the bowel, has been advocated as a supplement to penicillin therapy. Other regimens may have to be tried empirically. Even if it appears that anal or vaginal carriage has been eliminated, vigilance should be maintained. In one outbreak [8], vaginal carriage recurred with a different strain of *Streptococcus*, leading to a renewed outbreak of streptococcal disease that received considerable attention in the national press. In another outbreak [6], a persistent anal carrier was associated with widely separated cases of endometritis and bacteremia over the course of more than a year, despite treatment with various regimens of penicillin, rifampicin, and oral vancomycin. When a specific carrier cannot be identified, or when analysis suggests that the outbreak is not of clonal origin, rigorous adherence to infection control practices should be observed and usually are successful [55].

EPIDEMIOLOGY OF *STAPHYLOCOCCUS AUREUS* NOSOCOMIAL INFECTIONS

Transmission

Group A streptococcal nosocomial infections gave the advocates of airborne and direct contact theories of transmission an excuse to have a skirmish; the epidemics of *S. aureus* infection in the 1950s and 1960s provided an opportunity to start a war. British investigators performed a vast number of detailed microbiologic studies to demonstrate how carriers of staphylococci could heavily contaminate the air. This extensive literature is not well known in the United States, and Americans with an interest in staphylococcal epidemiology have largely ignored the careful work of Hare, Ridley, Shooter, Nobel, Davies, Blowers, Lidwell, and many other of their British colleagues. Indeed, with the exception of Walter and Kundsin [56], who elaborated on the principles developed by Wells [57], the concept of airborne transmission of staphylococci has had few advocates in the United States. Among the many investigators who have sought to put airborne spread in perspective are Rammelkamp in the United States [4] and Williams in Great Britain [58]. The issues have been summarized succinctly by Williams, who wrote in 1966: "It is a characteristic of the airborne route of infection . . . that whenever there is the possibility of aerial transfer there is almost always the possibility of transfer by other routes. This is perhaps especially true of the forms of staphylococcal infection that have been most extensively studied, namely, those occurring in hospitals" [58]. This debate between proponents of airborne and contact spread is of more than historical interest; those who enthusiastically promote the performance of surgery in laminar airflow operating rooms [59] or under ultraviolet lights [60] are merely reflecting their continued belief in the importance of airborne spread of staphylococci and other bacteria.

Since most of the outbreaks of staphylococcal disease in the 1950s and 1960s were caused by a single phage type (often referred to as 80/81, although these strains were generally also lysed by other phages), early British investigators naturally concentrated on identifying carriers who might be disseminating the epidemic strain on wards and in the operating room. Had they been faced with the kinds of outbreaks that we tend to see today, which generally are caused by more than one clonal strain, it is possible that their research would have focused on the role of the patient's endogenous staphylococcal flora and the importance of transmission of staphylococci on the hands of personnel. Instead, they doggedly pursued staphylococcal carriers and shedders.

The principal site of staphylococcal colonization is the anterior nares. If repeated cultures are performed, ≤80% of adults are found to harbor *S. aureus* in the nose at one time or another [61]. In most persons, the carrier state is transient, but 20% to 40% of adults remain colonized for months or even years. Often the same strain remains in residence for prolonged periods of time and, if it is eradicated, a new strain of *Staphylococcus* tends to take its place. The factors that predispose to stable colonization are unknown. Hospital personnel and patients tend to have higher colonization rates than persons outside the hospital environment, particularly during nosocomial staphylococcal outbreaks.

Increased nasal colonization rates have also been noted in insulin-dependent diabetics [62], persons on hemodialysis [63] and continuous ambulatory peritoneal dialysis [64], intravenous drug abusers [65], and even in patients receiving routine allergy injections [66]. Thus, percutaneous injections or catheterization may predispose to colonization, although the pathogenesis of this phenomenon is unclear. It has also been suggested that patients with symptomatic human immunodeficiency virus infection have a higher than normal colonization risk [67].

When it was recognized that hospital personnel could be carriers of staphylococci, some hospitals required routine nasal cultures of personnel so that they could be treated before they transmitted their staphylococci to patients. This practice never gained widespread acceptance for a number of reasons.

1. Many carriers do not disseminate staphylococci during normal breathing [68].
2. Staphylococci are most efficiently liberated directly from the nose of a healthy carrier when air is forcefully expelled, creating a loud snorting sound [69].
3. Many carriers may be present on hospital wards without any infections occurring in patients.
4. Even if there is an outbreak of staphylococcal infection on a ward, personnel who become nasal carriers may be innocent bystanders rather than the cause of the problem.
5. Routine nasal cultures are expensive, and the resulting reams of data are generally uninterpretable.
6. Some carriers may be culture-positive at the perineum while being culture-negative in the nose [70].
7. Eradication of the nasal carrier state may be difficult.

Shedding is more likely to occur in nasal carriers who have a heavy growth of staphylococci on nasal swab cultures [71] and in those with upper respiratory infections [72,73]. Moreover, the nose is the site that supports colonization of the entire skin surface of most carriers. Eradication of staphylococci from the nose is generally accompanied by elimination of *S. aureus* from the entire body. In some staphylococcal carriers, however, the perineum is the primary site of colonization, and staphylococci may not be found on repeated cultures of the nose [74].

Both nasal and perineal carriers continually shed staphylococci on skin squamae—aptly called rafts by British investigators. Because of their size, shape, and weight, these contaminated squamae may be carried along on currents of air in the hospital, resulting in airborne dispersal of staphylococci (see Chapter 1). Fortunately, most colonized hospital personnel shed modest numbers of squamae, and the relatively small number of staphylococci dispersed into the environment are quickly diluted by conventional air-handling systems and washed away by standard housekeeping practices. A small percentage of colonized persons disperse much larger numbers of staphylococci into their immediate environment, however, and are referred to as heavy shedders. High concentrations of airborne staphylococci may result, and staphylococci contaminating the environment may remain viable for long periods of time. Dermatologic disorders, such as eczema and psoriasis, clearly predispose to skin scaling and shedding, but, in most cases, the reason for heavy shedding is not readily apparent. Carriers who have a heavy growth of staphylococci on culture of

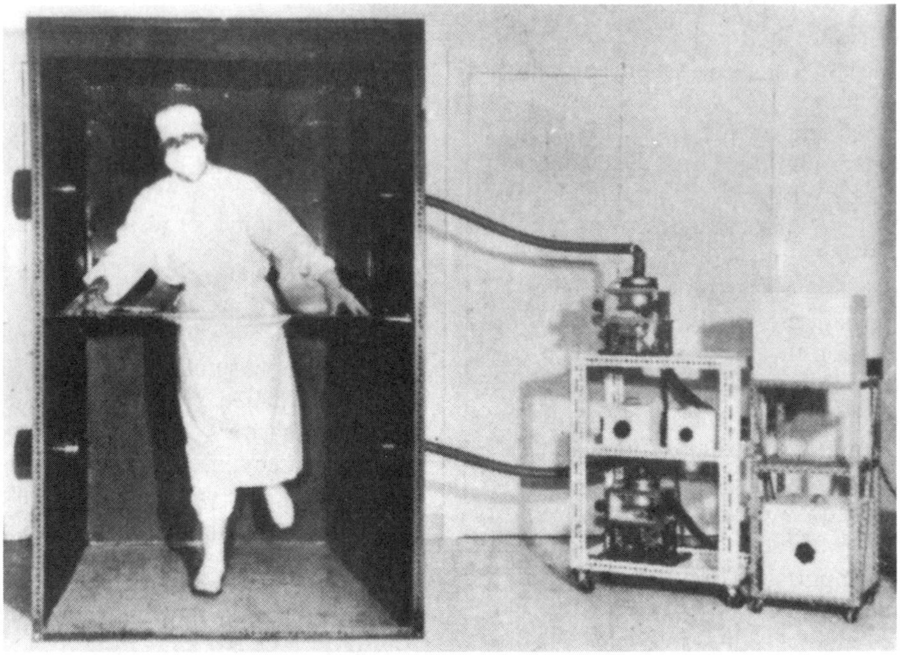

FIGURE 41-3. Test chamber with door removed showing waistline division, air-inlet filters, and air-sampling equipment. (Reprinted with permission from Bethune DW, Blowers R, Parker M, et al. Dispersal of *Staphylococcus aureus* by patients and surgical staff. *Lancet* 1965;27:4.

the anterior nares tend to colonize body sites more readily than carriers with scant nasal colonization [75], but this observation does not explain the phenomenon of heavy shedding per se.

Some insight into staphylococcal shedding patterns has been gained by studying the dispersion of staphylococci from volunteers confined to a small enclosure. The test chamber may be either rudimentary or very elaborate (Figure 41-3), but the basic principle involves collecting and quantitatively culturing the air in the chamber for staphylococci while the subject wears various types of clothing and moves about as instructed. Using this experimental technique, it has been repeatedly shown that men are more likely than women to be heavy shedders [68,76]. If a male heavy shedder is placed in a chamber clothed only in polyethylene or tightly woven cloth underpants, dispersal of staphylococci is practically eliminated, suggesting that most bacteria are shed from the perineum of carriers [68]. However, in a recent impressive recreation of these shedding experiments, Sherertz and associates found that staphylococcal dispersal dramatically increased in a colonized physician with symptomatic rhinovirus infection and that wearing a mask substantially decreased, but did not eliminate, staphylococcal dispersal [77].

Taken to the extreme, efforts to eliminate shedding in the operating room have led to the development of total body suits with individual ventilation and exhaust systems. Although these suits are a logical extension of the staphylococcal shedding experiments just mentioned, it is important to emphasize that such radical and costly measures should rarely be necessary, since very few hospital personnel actually shed significant numbers of staphylococci. Nosocomial outbreaks of staphylococcal infection, whether in the operating room or on the wards, have seldom been traced to a shedder on the hospital staff or to environmental contamination. For this reason, most hospital epidemiologists discourage extreme measures to eliminate shedding and concentrate instead on good aseptic surgical technique, careful hand washing, and other measures designed to minimize direct contact transmission.

Epidemic Investigation

The key to detecting the presence of a staphylococcal shedder lies not in surveillance cultures but in careful surveillance for nosocomial staphylococcal infections (see Chapter 5). If an increasing incidence of infection is noted, phage typing may help determine whether a single epidemic strain is responsible (see Chapter 9). However, many strains cannot be typed with routine phage panels, and even strains with similar phage patterns may be unrelated epidemiologically. Recently, the Centers for Disease Control and Prevention (CDC) abandoned the routine use of phage typing for outbreak investigation in favor of molecular-based techniques. However, other public health laboratories, such as the Colindale Public Health Laboratory in England, continue to offer phage typing. Capsular serotyping is of limited practical utility because most clinical strains fall within the same few serotypes

[78,79]. Occasionally, antibiotic resistance profiles may be helpful, particularly if the isolates are resistant to methicillin or specific aminoglycosides. However, multiply resistant strains may be epidemiologically distinct, and plasmid-mediated resistance patterns (see Chapters 14,16) may change in the course of an outbreak owing to selective antibiotic pressure and the gain or loss of plasmids [80].

More stable phenotypic profiles may be obtained from techniques such as immunoblotting and multilocus enzyme electrophoresis, which characterize bacterial protein expression [81–83]. Molecular genetic epidemiologic techniques, including both chromosomal and plasmid analysis, offer the greatest ability to characterize the relatedness of staphylococcal strains and are becoming more generally available. Chromosomal DNA may be characterized by pulsed-field gel electrophoresis, restriction endonuclease digestion, DNA-specific probes, and the polymerase chain reaction. All are highly reliable and discriminatory techniques that have proved useful in the investigation of staphylococcal outbreaks [84–87]. For example, a cluster of *S. aureus* postoperative wound infections was linked to a neurosurgeon by DNA blot hybridization using DNA probes specific for chromosomal determinants of β-lactamase production and erythromycin and spectinomycin resistance [88]. Since the affected patients had manifestations of the toxic shock syndrome, the outbreak strains were also examined with a toxic shock toxin gene probe and were found to have identical hybridization patterns. When plasmids are present, electrophoretic analysis of whole-plasmid DNA and restriction endonuclease digests of plasmid DNA can provide information about the common origin of plasmids and their acquisition or loss [80,87,89–93]. However, plasmid data must be interpreted with caution because of the instability of plasmids in bacterial populations. Excellent reviews of the methodologies, advantages, and disadvantages of this expanding spectrum of molecular techniques are available [85].

When an epidemic strain is identified, personnel should not be cultured indiscriminately. The microbiologic investigation should focus on persons who appear to be associated epidemiologically with infected patients (see Chapter 6). These persons should be examined carefully for signs of infection and questioned regarding recent infections or skin problems. Cultures of the nose, perineum, and sites of possible skin infection or dermatitis should be obtained, and any resulting *S. aureus* isolates should be characterized by one of the molecular techniques described earlier. Of course, it is difficult to know whether a staff member is colonized because of his or her contact with infected patients or vice versa. Formal shedding studies are cumbersome, but a rough measure of the intensity of shedding can be obtained by quantitatively culturing the carrier's clothing or by asking the carrier to exercise in a small, poorly ventilated room in which settling plates have been placed.

Staphylococcal epidemics caused by heavy shedders definitely are the exception rather than the rule, and most hospital epidemiologists probably will never be confronted by such an outbreak. At some point in the workup of almost all staphylococcal outbreaks, however, the infection control team will be forced at least to consider the possibility that a carrier is at the heart of the problem. Understandably, staff members tend to become apprehensive as the investigation proceeds, particularly if the investigators seem to be interested in their contact with the infected patients. It is extremely important to proceed in a frank and forthright manner, to eschew premature conclusions based on incomplete data, and to avoid capricious culturing forays. If the epidemiologic study clearly implicates one person, the infection control team must expect to encounter guilt and fear. A surgeon, for example, may have justifiable anxiety about possible litigation and damage to his or her career. Depending on the tact and skill of the investigators, the implicated staff member may be fully cooperative or may display the hostility and defensiveness of someone accused. It is essential for the infection control team to speak with one voice and to follow a rational plan of action that has been discussed fully with the directors of the appropriate services.

If the epidemiologic evidence is very strong, it is prudent to remove the presumed carrier from activities related to the care of patients while cultures are obtained. If staphylococci are recovered on culture, treatment is generally begun before molecular typing information becomes available. Because the carrier will usually want to return to work as soon as possible, the infection control team will be under considerable pressure to expedite treatment and issue work clearance. Unfortunately, there are no universally accepted criteria for determining when it is safe to send a carrier back to the wards. Certainly the carrier should not be permitted to work until cultures of at least the nose and perineum show negative results, although it must be realized that negative results of cultures taken while therapy is still under way may indicate that the carrier state is suppressed but not eradicated. When treatment is concluded, therefore, the carrier should again be removed from work until follow-up cultures are performed and the results are available. A more conservative approach would be to suspend the staff member from engaging in patient care for the entire period of treatment until follow-up culture results are negative, but the efficacy of topical mupirocin (see later discussion) probably makes this step unnecessary. In either case, careful surveillance should be carried out after the carrier returns to work, since the carrier state and shedding may recur. Some authorities advocate placing settling plates in the immediate work environment for a period of several months as an additional, as yet untested, security measure.

A staggering array of systemic and topical antimicrobial regimens has been used in an effort to eradicate nasal carriage of staphylococci [94–96]. Systemic agents have included cephalosporins, semi-synthetic penicillins, erythromycin, tetracycline, fusidic acid, and ciprofloxacin. All these agents temporarily suppress the carrier state during therapy, but when adequate follow-up cultures are performed, staphylococci reappear in the majority of persons. Ciprofloxacin is effective, but resistance tends to emerge rapidly [96]. Rifampicin can be given in combination with another systemic agent, such as trimethoprim-sulfamethoxazole or ciprofloxacin, to retard emergence of rifampicin resistance [74,94,97–100]. Alternatively, some investigators have attempted to prevent resistance by combining rifampicin with an intranasal topical agent, such as bacitracin [70,74,100], but this strategy may fail if there are extranasal sites of colonization [97].

If the staphylococci acquire resistance to the antibiotic being administered, shedding may actually increase, perhaps reflecting suppression of competing nasal flora. Most topical antimicrobials, including lysostaphin, gentamicin, neomycin, chlorhexidine, vancomycin, and bacitracin, have been equally unsuccessful in eradicating the carrier state [101]. However, topical mupirocin (pseudomonic acid), an inhibitor of protein biosynthesis, has shown considerable promise when applied intranasally two to three times daily for 5 to 7 days [76,102–105]. Recent reports have suggested that eight doses given over 48 hours is sufficient to eliminate carriage, that carriers may return to work within 24 hours of commencing therapy, and that for the majority of persons carriage is eliminated for ≥ 4 weeks [106]. Mupirocin has been used primarily in the treatment of carriers of MRSA (see the section "Methicillin-Resistant *S. Aureus*"), but its effectiveness against methicillin-susceptible strains has been confirmed [106]. Predictably, mupirocin-resistant staphylococci are now well described, both in individual cases and in outbreaks [107–109]. Resistance has been seen primarily in the context of intensive use [107,110–112], so this agent remains an appropriate option for the selected situations when elimination of carriage of staphylococci is deemed appropriate [105]. Mupirocin is available in a propylene glycol base for dermatologic use and in a paraffin base that is less irritating to mucous membranes.

Other strategies for eliminating staphylococcal carriage have a theoretical rationale but have not been evaluated systematically. Although suppression of nasal staphylococci eventually leads to elimination of staphylococci from other sites, it seems logical to try to hasten this process along by prescribing a daily hexachlorophene shower and shampoo during the treatment period. This approach is especially appealing for carriers who are colonized at the perineum or other sites in the absence of nasal colonization. Since other members of the carrier's family may also be colonized with the outbreak strain, thus providing a reservoir for recolonization of the shedder, it seems reasonable to treat them if nasal cultures yield staphylococci. In refractory cases, it may be advisable to recommend laundering of clothing and bedding, as well as a thorough house cleaning, to reduce the burden of staphylococci in the household.

Rarely, persistent or recurrent shedding of staphylococci may jeopardize a health professional's career. When all else fails, it is reasonable to consider trying bacterial interference. In the 1960s, Shinefield and co-workers [113] discovered that implantation of *S. aureus* strain 502A in the umbilicus and nose of neonates could prevent—or interfere with—colonization and infection with more virulent staphylococcal strains, such as phage type 80/81. Bacterial interference with strain 502A was subsequently tried in adults suffering from recurrent furunculosis; it showed considerable success provided the carrier state was first suppressed with antibiotics [114]. Although the implantation of strain 502A in neonates occasionally resulted in 502A infections, this complication has not been noted in adults and presumably would not cause problems for otherwise healthy carriers. Of course, it is unknown whether successfully recolonized carriers would become heavy shedders of 502A, which might then produce infections in susceptible patients.

The vast literature concerning staphylococcal carriers and shedders tends to obscure the fact that the patients themselves frequently serve as reservoirs for staphylococci and that staphylococci are transmitted from patient to patient on the hands of personnel. Thus, prompt isolation of patients with documented staphylococcal infections is extremely important. When drainage is slight or easily contained by a dressing, it is sufficient to wear gloves when touching infectious material (see Chapter 13). For patients with more extensive infections, such as a major wound or burn, full contact precautions are indicated. These precautions call for placing the patient in a private room, dedicating equipment and items to that patient, and donning both gown and gloves upon entering the room if substantial contact with the patient or environmental surfaces is expected. A private room increases the likelihood of appropriate hand washing between contacts with patients [115] and lessens the possibility of spread by fomites or skin squamae. Most authorities do not recommend special respiratory precautions for patients with staphylococcal pneumonia, although there may be a slight potential for airborne dissemination via droplet nuclei. These recommendations are consistent with CDC guidelines for isolation precautions [116].

The effectiveness of mupirocin has rekindled interest in prophylactic treatment of colonized patients at high risk of *S. aureus* infection. Recent studies confirm the reports in older literature [117–119] that nasal carriage of *S. aureus* is associated with increased risk of certain infections, namely, sternal wound infection [120], saphenous vein harvest site infection [121], bacteremia in hemodialysis patients [63], and catheter-related infections and peritonitis in peritoneal dialysis patients [122]. Nasal mupirocin therapy has been associated with a lower rate of surgical site infections in cardiothoracic surgery patients [123], *S. aureus* bacteremias in hemodialysis patients [124,125], and *S. aureus* peritonitis in peritoneal dialysis patients [126]. These data are intriguing but still preliminary; larger, controlled studies are needed to guide therapy so as to maximize benefit while minimizing the indiscriminate use that is clearly associated with resistance [127].

Staphylococcal Disease in the Nursery

Over the years, the nursery has provided numerous opportunities to study the acquisition and transmission of *S. aureus*. Newborns seldom acquire staphylococci from their mothers at the time of birth, but in a matter of days colonization may reach 40% to 90% if these newborns are admitted to a nursery where many babies are already colonized [84,128]. The umbilicus is usually the initial site of colonization [129], but staphylococci quickly spread to the nose and other skin sites. Spread from infant to infant undoubtedly occurs via the hands of the doctors and nurses who care for colonized babies; airborne transmission almost never takes place. These principles, which are widely accepted today, were hotly disputed before Rammelkamp and colleagues [4] performed their classic studies of nursery staphylococcal epidemiology in the 1950s.

Rammelkamp's studies were carried out in a small ward containing seven bassinets (Figure 41-4). A baby known to be colonized with staphylococci was placed in

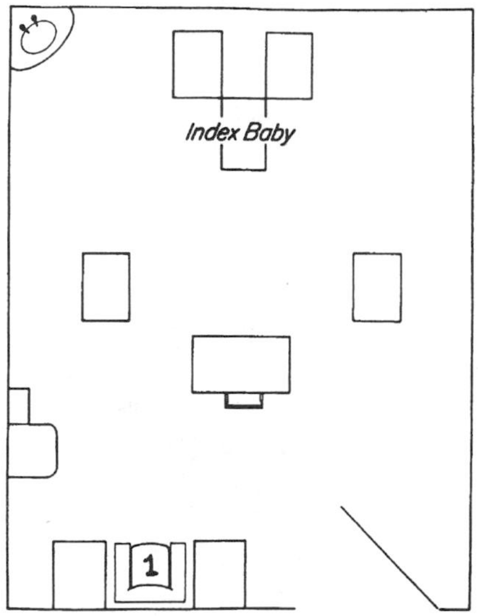

FIGURE 41-4. Results of exposure of infants to carriers of staphylococci. (Reprinted with permission from Rammelkamp CH Jr., Mortimer EA Jr., Wolinsky E, et al. Transmission of streptococcal and staphylococcal infections. *Ann Intern Med* 1964;60:753.)

one of these beds. Newborns were then admitted directly to the ward and placed either right next to the index baby or 4.5 or 11 feet away. The three nurses who cared for the noncolonized newborns wore double masks and washed their hands with hexachlorophene after each contact with patients; the index patient was cared for by separate personnel. Nasal cultures were obtained from the babies every other day. Of the 91 newborns brought onto this special ward, only three became colonized with the index baby's staphylococcal strain. During two weeks of this study, one of the nurses, who was colonized with *S. aureus*, sat for 8 hours per day in the chair between the two bassinets in position 1 of Figure 41-4. Although she did not wear a mask, none of the babies in the room acquired her strain of *Staphylococcus*. This is hardly surprising, since the probability that she was a heavy shedder was very small. More interesting results were obtained by allowing this nurse and another colonized nurse to handle the noncolonized babies in a routine fashion. Approximately 20% of the babies cared for by these nurses acquired their caretakers' staphylococcal strains.

A subsequent study showed that these staphylococci were transferred to the babies by direct contact with organisms on the nurses' hands. In this study, the same two nurses and a third carrier handled 37 infants for 10 minutes each through the ports of an Isolette incubator. Fifty-four percent of these babies acquired staphylococci from their nurses, as determined by phage typing of organisms recovered from cultures of the nose and umbilicus. This study demonstrated that so-called Isolettes do not effectively shield newborns from the most important route of staphylococcal cross-infection in the nursery—transmission via the hands.

Even in spacious, well-staffed nurseries, spread of staphylococci may be difficult to control (see Chapter 26). Transmission occurs much more readily in crowded, hectic nurseries. Staffing appears to be a particularly critical factor. Haley and Bregman [130] were able to verify that clusters of staphylococcal infections occur significantly more frequently when patient-staff ratios are highest. Control of nursery staphylococcal outbreaks is facilitated by prompt recognition, but detection is not always easy. Most well babies spend only 1 or 2 days in the nursery, so hospital-acquired staphylococcal infections may not manifest clinically until the baby is at home. Moreover, the majority of infections are mild and do not require readmission to the hospital. Therefore, community pediatricians must be encouraged to report all staphylococcal infections to the infection control office. Seemingly trivial infections, such as pustulosis, omphalitis, circumcision wound infection, and conjunctivitis, have just as much epidemiologic significance as infant mastitis, septic arthritis, or osteomyelitis. Community obstetricians should also participate in the reporting process, since a single case of maternal mastitis may be the initial sign of a nursery problem.

In an effort to predict when a staphylococcal outbreak is imminent, some nurseries routinely monitor staphylococcal colonization rates by culturing the umbilicus and nose when babies are discharged. Such surveillance cultures are expensive and rarely helpful. Although there is a rough correlation between the number of babies colonized with staphylococci and the incidence of staphylococcal infections [131], many nurseries routinely find high colonization rates without experiencing an outbreak [84,132,133]. Surveillance cultures may be more informative when performed to determine the impact of specific control measures on transmission of staphylococci in the nursery or to verify that a particular epidemic strain has been eradicated.

The severe outbreaks of staphylococcal disease that struck nurseries in the 1950s and 1960s led to the introduction of a variety of infection control measures. Perhaps the simplest and most effective was routine bathing of neonates with 3% hexachlorophene [134]. Hexachlorophene, with its excellent and persistent activity against gram-positive bacteria, drastically reduced staphylococcal colonization and subsequent infection. By eliminating the normal gram-positive cutaneous flora along with the *S. aureus*, hexachlorophene paved the way for colonization by nosocomial gram-negative bacilli such as *Pseudomonas* [132]. But this appeared to be a minor disadvantage at the time, since neonatal gram-negative infections seemed to be a much less severe problem. Of greater concern were reports of hexachlorophene toxicity. In patients with burns or extensive dermatitis who were bathed with large amounts of hexachlorophene, a convulsive disorder developed that was associated with cystic degenerative changes in the white matter.

Similar neuropathologic changes were seen in infant animals treated with topical hexachlorophene [135] as well as in human neonates, particularly premature infants [136,137]. The human studies were retrospective, and there has been no convincing evidence that bathing full-term infants with hexachlorophene is hazardous. Nonetheless, in 1972 the Food and Drug Administration recommended against the routine use of hexachlorophene in nurseries. This recommendation resulted in a sharp decline in hexachlorophene bathing and a significant increase in the number of outbreaks of nursery staphylococcal disease in the United States [138]. Balancing the potential risks and benefits of hexachlorophene, it seems reasonable to avoid its use in the routine bathing of newborns. However, hexachlorophene may be a valuable adjunct to other control measures during a staphylococcal outbreak. As an added measure of safety, some investigators suggest diluting the hexachlorophene 1:4 or 1:5 and omitting baths for premature infants, although it is possible that these compromises could reduce efficacy. Chlorhexidine (0.5% in 70% alcohol) has been used as an alternative; it appears to be safe and effective [139] and is deserving of further study.

Since the umbilicus is one of the initial sites of staphylococcal colonization in the neonate, a variety of topical antiseptics have been applied to it in an effort to abort colonization without washing the entire body surface. The basic validity of this approach has been demonstrated by studies using triple dye, an aqueous mixture of brilliant green, proflavine hemisulfate, and crystal violet [140,141], but the safety of this agent has not been evaluated extensively. Other topical antiseptics, such as bacitracin, alcohol, chlorhexidine gluconate, and iodophors, may be as effective as triple dye and more acceptable aesthetically, but none has been studied adequately. The little information about the use of mupirocin in the newborn population is equivocal. One group has reported that an outbreak of MRSA was controlled in part by applying mupirocin to the umbilicus and nose twice daily for 7 days, coupled with a dusting of 0.3% hexachlorophene powder over the umbilicus, axillae, and perineum [142]. In a different neonatal unit, mupirocin therapy failed to eradicate MRSA colonization in one outbreak [143].

When topical antiseptics and conventional infection control measures failed to halt epidemics of severe staphylococcal disease in the 1960s, Shinefield and colleagues [113] tried the more radical approach of bacterial interference (see previous discussion). In general, implantation of *S. aureus* 502A in the nose and umbilicus was highly successful in preventing colonization by nosocomial staphylococcal strains. Although this strategy fell into disfavor when epidemics of staphylococcal disease abated and reports of occasional serious disease due to 502A appeared, bacterial interference remains a possible approach in difficult-to-control nursery epidemics.

The emphasis in the medical literature on topical antiseptics and bacterial interference tends to obscure the fact that adherence to standard infection control routines is of primary importance in limiting the transmission of staphylococci in the nursery. Thorough hand washing after contact with infants is imperative (see Chapters 13, 26). Hexachlorophene may be used for routine hand washing when a staphylococcal problem is recognized in the nursery, but it probably should be avoided at other times because its use may encourage transmission of gram-negative bacilli on the hands. Chlorhexidine gluconate and triclosan, both of which have broad-spectrum antimicrobial activity, are reasonable alternatives. The use of triclosan for hand washing as well as infant bathing may have been instrumental in the control of an MRSA outbreak in one nursery [144].

Infants with staphylococcal infections should be placed on contact precautions (see Chapter 13). Consideration should be given to placing babies with intercurrent viral respiratory infections on more stringent precautions (masking when close to the patient and single room required), because such babies tend to aerosolize large numbers of staphylococci into the environment—the so-called cloud baby phenomenon described by Eichenwald and colleagues [145]. Colonized babies may be segregated, with infected babies in a separate part of the nursery, and, if possible, assigned separate nursing staff (see Chapter 26). Some nursery staffs have elected to use a cohort admissions system to reduce the opportunity for person-to-person spread. In a typical system, all infants admitted in a 48-hour period are placed in a single room, and traffic of personnel from this room to other rooms is minimized or avoided altogether. After 48 hours, the room is closed to additional admissions and not reopened until the entire cohort has been discharged and the room cleaned thoroughly. Clearly, the success of cohorting depends on the availability of separate nursery areas and sufficient personnel. In nurseries with inadequate facilities and insufficient staff, cohorting and isolation arrangements may be impossible, and the only way to cope with an escalating rate of staphylococcal infection is to close the units temporarily to new admissions.

Outbreaks of nursery staphylococcal disease frequently are caused by unrelated strains and presumably result from lapses in technique rather than the presence of a carrier on the obstetric or neonatal staff. Unfortunately, as noted previously, results of strain typing are seldom available immediately, and pressure may mount to treat all nasal carriers. This is understandable and perhaps unavoidable, since there may be few epidemiologic clues in a busy nursery in which most of the staff have contact with most of the infants. Because few nursery staphylococcal outbreaks have been shown to be caused by shedders on the staff, however, it may be more prudent to stress good aseptic technique and other standard infection control measures than to jump immediately to wholesale treatment of nasal carriers [146].

Methicillin-Resistant *S. Aureus*

Staphylococcus aureus resistant to methicillin and a number of other front-line antibiotics has emerged as a major nosocomial pathogen. Data from the NNIS System indicate that the incidence of MRSA infections continues to increase progressively; MRSA has penetrated hospitals of virtually all sizes and types, including the smallest community hospitals [147] and even the community in some locales [148,149]. The result has been a resurgence of interest in staphylococcal epidemiology, as literally hundreds of published papers and several comprehensive reviews attest [150–152]. These intensive studies have yielded few epidemiologic surprises, but it has been interesting to watch a new crop of epidemiologists reaffirming the observations made by their mentors who investigated methicillin-sensitive staphylococci years ago. Nonetheless, control (or preferably eradication) of MRSA is a high priority for hospital epidemiologists, since these strains are just as virulent as their more susceptible relatives but much more difficult and expensive to treat.

In hospitals with major methicillin resistance problems, vancomycin, a relatively expensive and toxic agent that requires costly monitoring, has become the antibiotic of choice for empiric coverage of *S. aureus* as well as for therapy of documented infections. Other agents—for example, trimethoprim-sulfamethoxazole, minocycline, the quinolones, and new glycopeptides such as teicoplaninmay have therapeutic potential, but vancomycin is the last commercially available antibiotic that has activity against all strains of *S. aureus* isolated to date and has demonstrated efficacy in animal models and patients as well. With the emergence of vancomycin-resistant enterococci and *S. haemolyticus*, the specter of vancomycin-resistant *S. aureus* looms large. In fact, transfer of vancomycin resistance from enterococci to *S. aureus* has been accomplished in the laboratory [153], and clinical *S. aureus* isolates with intermediate resistance to vancomycin (through a mechanism different than that seen in the enterococci) have been reported in both Japan and the United States [154]. In response, the Centers for Disease Control and Prevention has published interim guidelines for the prevention and control of staphylococcal infection with reduced susceptibility to vancomycin [155].

Once MRSA has become established in a hospital, it is exceedingly difficult to eradicate. Accurate laboratory identification of methicillin resistance is therefore of paramount importance not only to the physician treating the patient but to the hospital epidemiologist as well. Appropriate susceptibility testing methods are described in standard laboratory references and recent reviews [150,156,157]. Cultures should be incubated at 35°C for a full 24 hours. Particular caution is required when using certain automated microdilution instruments, although some of these systems perform satisfactorily when appropriate media and cations are employed. As an additional screening measure, it may be advisable to inoculate isolates on Mueller-Hinton agar dilution plates containing 4% sodium chloride plus 6 g/ml of oxacillin [156]. These antibiotic-containing plates can also be used to screen patients rapidly and efficiently for colonization with MRSA. In the author's experience, sensitivity of skin cultures can be enhanced by incubating the swab in broth media and then inoculating the plate directly with a portion of this overnight culture. Similar findings have been reported by others [159].

It is now clear that there are several types of methicillin resistance in *S. aureus*, and these developments have added further complexities to an already confusing field (see Chapters 14–16). The strains of MRSA that have caused nosocomial headaches throughout the world are highly resistant to methicillin and related agents because they have altered penicillin-binding proteins (PBPs) with reduced affinity for these antibiotics. Specifically, these intrinsically resistant strains contain a 78-kd PBP 2a or 2b′ [160] and a genetic determinant that can be detected with a *mec*-specific DNA probe. They are often called *heteroresistant* because only a small fraction (one in 10^4 to 10^8) of bacterial cells in a culture population actually expresses methicillin resistance. In addition to these highly methicillin-resistant strains of *S. aureus*, other strains have been recognized to have borderline resistance to methicillin, with minimum inhibiting concentrations in the range of 4 μg/ml [161].

Some of these isolates have the typical characteristics of heteroresistant strains in that they contain PBP 2a and are positive with the *mec* probe. Others do not react with the *mec* probe, do not have PBP 2a, and do not have any highly resistant subpopulations on culture. It has been hypothesized that the apparently normal PBPs of these isolates have lower affinity for methicillin and related compounds. Finally, some borderline resistant strains express large amounts of β-lactamase, particularly when grown under the high salt concentrations used to enhance detection of heteroresistance [162]. Most authorities believe that the β-lactamase hyper-producing strains can be treated successfully by oxacillin and related agents and should be considered susceptible for therapeutic and epidemiologic purposes.

The initial introduction of MRSA into a hospital population usually goes undetected, but in many cases the organism is brought in by a patient transferred from another institution in which MRSA already is endemic [63,164]. Nursing homes and other chronic-care facilities are major reservoirs for MRSA, and the transfer of chronically colonized patients to acute-care settings requires particular vigilance [65,166]. However, MRSA is circulating increasingly in the community at large, particularly within such subpopulations as injection drug users [167,168] or the previously hospitalized [148,149]. Community colonization has even been noted in patients with no demonstrable risk factors [148].

Colonized hospital personnel can also be responsible for interhospital spread of MRSA [70,74,169], although this sort of spread probably occurs relatively rarely. In one outbreak, transmission was traced to a member of the surgical house staff who had nasal colonization following a paronychia [74]. In another outbreak, a pediatric resident introduced a strain of rifampicin-resistant MRSA into a special-care nursery [69]. This physician had previously worked in a hospital where rifampicin-susceptible MRSA was endemic and had subsequently been treated with rifampicin for pulmonary tuberculosis, presumably leading to the selection of rifampicin resistance in the strain of MRSA he had acquired. Hospitalized patients are at greater risk of becoming colonized with MRSA if they undergo prolonged hospital stays, have received a large number of antibiotics or lengthy antibiotic courses, or have invasive devices [74,163,164,170,172]. Colonized patients, particularly those with chronic diseases, may remain carriers for months or even years [173]. Thus, patients should be screened upon any readmission to a healthcare facility so that appropriate precautions may be instituted [64,74,163,164,170,171].

In general, MRSA is transmitted in the hospital by personnel who have contaminated their hands while providing direct care for colonized patients [159]. Patients with tracheostomies, contaminated wounds or decubitus ulcers, and extensive skin disease or burns tend to be colonized with exceptionally large numbers of staphylococci and are especially likely to contribute to the cycle of person-to-person transmission. The role of carriers on the hospital staff in the nosocomial dissemination of MRSA is less clear. Personnel appear to be less likely to become persistent nasal carriers of MRSA than of methicillin-susceptible strains [151]. Carrier rates as low as 0.4% have been reported, even after extensive contact with colonized patients [148,174]. In a review of 49 studies involving 7,129 patients, Reboli and colleagues [70] found an average colonization rate of only 2.5%. Nonetheless, some of these studies reported much higher carrier rates, and nasal carriers have been implicated in a few outbreaks [74,169].

Environmental contamination probably plays a minor role in most institutions, and it is difficult to recover MRSA outside the immediate environment of most patients [159]. However, colonized patients with burn wounds or severe dermatologic conditions can heavily contaminate their environment [174–176], and other colonized persons, such as those with endotracheal tubes or tracheostomies, probably require special consideration as well. To determine whether patients are likely to be heavy dispersers, settling plates may be placed in the room as a simple and inexpensive screening procedure, although the reproducibility and predictive value of this technique have not been validated.

Hospitals faced with the daunting task of trying to contain the spread of MRSA have adopted a wide variety of strategies, but almost all have found the effort inordinately expensive, in terms of both time and resources. The proper approach to take is a matter of considerable controversy. A working party of the Hospital Infection Society and the British Society for Antimicrobial Chemotherapy has issued [177] and revised [178] extraordinarily tough, comprehensive, and expensive recommendations for MRSA control. In essence, these guidelines suggest isolation of known carriers or patients admitted from hospitals where MRSA is endemic until screening culture results are available. If a colonized patient has been in a critical care area, all patients and staff who cared for the patient should be cultured; in other areas of the hospital, only patients in the vicinity of the colonized persons need be screened. Suggested sites for screening cultures include nose, perineum, fingers, and axilla for personnel, with the addition of wounds, tracheostomy sites, catheter sites, and indwelling for patients.

If more than one case is detected, the net should be widened to include screening of all staff caring for colonized patients, and the ward may have to be closed to new admissions. Antiseptic hand-washing agents are recommended, and the use of agents other than chlorhexidine gluconate should be considered, since some MRSA strains seem to have reduced susceptibility to this antiseptic [179]. Hospitalization in a customized isolation unit is suggested, but single rooms at negative pressure are deemed acceptable; barrier precautions are considered inadequate. Terminal cleaning of rooms with a phenolic disinfectant is recommended. Carriers among patients and staff should be treated vigorously, as discussed previously, and application of mupirocin to colonized lesions, or even total body bathing with an agent such as triclosan [180], is considered an adjunct to the treatments for nasal colonization cited earlier. Carriers are not considered cured until three sets of screening cultures show negative results. Personnel with MRSA confined to the nose may return to clinical work after 1 day of intranasal mupirocin, but those with more widespread colonization are kept off the wards until treatment is completed and three cultures give negative results.

While they provide a framework for an aggressive approach to this vexing problem, the necessity of such draconian measures has been questioned [181]. More feasible guidelines have been provided in the U.S. literature [115,182], with recommendations that include identifying previously colonized patients upon hospital readmission, assigning patients to private rooms or cohorting colonized patients, the use of gloves for contact with colonized patients (plus gowns if soiling is likely), and strict isolation for burn patients with MRSA colonization. Mulligan et al. [182] recommend meticulous room cleaning plus the use of dedicated equipment for colonized persons, while Boyce and colleagues [115] contend that special housekeeping practices are not warranted since environmental surfaces have not proved to be an important reservoir for MRSA. Both reviews advise against indiscriminant culturing of personnel or decolonization therapy without a compelling epidemiologic rationale, such as investigation or control of an outbreak.

REFERENCES

1. Perry WD, Siegel AC, Rammelkamp CH, et al. Transmission of group-A streptococci. I. The role of contaminated bedding. *Am J Hyg* 1957;66:85–95.
2. Perry WD, Siegel AC, Rammelkamp CH. Transmission of group-A streptococci. II. The role of contaminated dust. *Am J Hyg* 1957; 66:96–101.
3. Wannamaker LW. The epidemiology of streptococcal infections. In: McCarthy M, ed. *Streptococcal infections*. New York: Columbia University Press, 1954:157.
4. Rammelkamp CH Jr., Mortimer EA Jr., Wolinsky E. Transmission of streptococcal and staphylococcal infections. *Ann Intern Med* 1964; 60:753–758.
5. Burnett IA, Norman P. *Streptococcus pyogenes*: an outbreak on a burns unit. *J Hosp Infect* 1990;15:173–176.
6. Viglionese A, Nottebart VF, Bodman HA, Platt R. Recurrent group A streptococcal carriage in a healthcare worker associated with widely separated nosocomial outbreaks. *Am J Med* 1991;91:329S–333S.
7. Willson R, Bollinger CC, Ledger WJ. *Am J Obstet Gynecol* 1964; 90:726–736.
8. Berkelman RL, et al. Streptococcal wound infections caused by a vaginal carrier. *JAMA* 1982;247:2680–2682.
9. McIntyre DM. An epidemic of *Streptococcus pyogenes* puerperal and postoperative sepsis with an unusual carrier—the anus. *Am J Obstet Gynecol* 1968;101:308.
10. McKee WM, DiCaprio JM, Roberts CE Jr, Sherris JC. Anal carriage as the probable source of a streptococcal epidemic. *Lancet* 1966;1: 1007–1009.
11. Richman DD, Breton SJ, Goldmann DA. Scarlet fever and group A streptococcal surgical wound infection traced to an anal carrier. *J Pediatr* 1977;90:387.
12. Schaffner W, Lefkowitz LB, Goodman JS. Hospital outbreak of infections with group-A streptococci traced to an asymptomatic anal carrier. *N Engl J Med* 1969;280:1224.
13. Stamm WE, Feeley JC, Facklam RR. Wound infections due to group-A streptococcus traced to a vaginal carrier. *J Infect Dis* 1978;138:287.
14. Voelker R. Making sense of group A streptococcus scare. *JAMA* 1994;272:190–191.
15. Demers B, Simon AE, Vellend H, et al. Severe invasive group A streptococcal infections in Ontario, Canada: 1987–1991. *Clin Infect Dis* 1993;16:792–800.
16. Hosier DM, Crachen JM, Teske DW, et al. Resurgence of acute rheumatic fever. *Am J Dis Child* 1987;141:730.
17. Barrter T, Dascal A, Carroll K, Curley FJ. "Toxic strep syndrome": a manifestation of group A streptococcal infection. *Arch Intern Med* 1988;148:1421–1988.
18. Stollerman GH. Variation in group A streptococci and the prevalence of rheumatic fever: a half-century vigil. *Ann Intern Med* 1993;118: 467–469.
19. Wheeler MC, Roe MH, Kaplan EL, et al. Outbreak of group A streptococcus septicemia in children: clinical, epidemiologic, and microbiological correlates. *JAMA* 1991;266:533–537.
20. Bisno AL, T SS, Dajani AS. The rise and fall (and rise?) of rheumatic fever. *JAMA* 1988;259:728–729.
21. Hoge CW, Schwartz B, Talkington DF, et al. The changing epidemiology of invasive group A streptococcal infections and the emergence of streptococcal toxic shock–like syndrome: a retrospective population-based study. *JAMA* 1993;269:384–389.
22. Bisno AL. The resurgence of acute rheumatic fever in the United States. *Annu Rev Med* 1990;41:319–329.
23. Gunzenhauser JD, Longfield JN, Brundage JF, et al. Epidemic streptococcal disease among army trainees, July 1989 through June 1991. *J Infect Dis* 1995;172:124–131.
24. Stevens DL, Tanner MH, Winship J, et al. Severe group A streptococcal infections associated with a toxic shock–like syndrome and scarlet fever toxin A. *N Engl J Med* 1989;321:1–6.
25. Strobaek S, Jepsen OB, Zimakoff J, Ronne T. Increased number of sporadic nosocomial group A streptococcal bacteraemias during a community epidemic. *J Hosp Infect* 1991;19:129–136.
26. Christie CD, Havens PL, Shapiro ED. Bacteremia with group A streptococci in childhood. *Am J Dis Child* 1988;142:559–561.
27. Bradley JS, Schlievert PM, B SP. Streptococcal toxic-shock-like syndrome as a complication of primary varicella. *Pediatr Infect Dis J* 1991;10:77–78.
28. Stollerman GH. Changing group A streptococci: the reappearance of streptococcal toxic shock. *Arch Intern Med* 1988;148:1268.
29. Defining the group A streptococcal toxic shock syndrome: rationale and consensus definition. The Working Group on Severe Streptococcal Infections. *JAMA* 1993;269: 390–391.
30. Forni AL, Kaplan EL, Schlievert PM, Roberts RB. Clinical and microbiological characteristics of severe group A streptococcus infections and streptococcal toxic shock syndrome. *Clin Infect Dis* 1995;21: 333–340.
31. Lee PK, Schlievert PM. Molecular genetics of pyrogenic exotoxin "superantigens" of group A streptococci and *Staphylococcus aureus*. *Curr Top Microbiol Immunol* 1991;174:1.
32. Lee PK, Schlievert PM. Quantification and toxicity of group A streptococcal pyrogenic exotoxins in an animal model of toxic shock syndrome–like illness. *J Clin Microbiol* 1989;27:1890.
33. Musser JM, Hauser AR, Kim MH, et al. *Streptococcus pyogenes* causing toxic-shock-like syndrome and other invasive diseases: clonal

diversity and pyrogenic exotoxin expression. *Proc Natl Acad Sci USA* 1991;88:2268–2672.
34. Hauser AR, Stevens DL, Kaplan EL, et al. Molecular analysis of pyrogenic exotoxins from *Streptococcus pyogenes* isolates associated with toxic shock–like syndrome. *J Clin Microbiol* 1991;29:1562–1567.
35. Schlievert P. Role of superantigens in human disease. *J Infect Dis* 1993;167:997–1002.
36. Stevens DL. Invasive group A streptococcus infections. *Clin Infect Dis* 1992;14:2–11.
37. Holm SE, Norrby A, Bergholm AM, Norgren M, et al. Aspects of pathogenesis of serious group A streptococcal infections in Sweden, 1988–1989. *J Infect Dis* 1992;166:31–37.
38. Congeni B, Rizzo C, Congeni J, Sreenivasan VV. Outbreak of acute rheumatic fever in northeast Ohio. *J Pediatr* 1987;111:176–179.
39. Veasy LG, Weidmeier SE, Orsmond GS, et al. Resurgence of acute rheumatic fever in the intermountain area of the United States. *N Engl J Med* 1987;316:421–427.
40. Wallace MR, Garst PD, Papadimos TJ, Oldfield EC 3rd., et al. The return of acute rheumatic fever in young adults. *JAMA* 1989;262: 2557–2561.
41. Westlake RM, Graham TP, Edwards EM. An outbreak of acute rheumatic fever in Tennessee. *Pediatr Infect Dis J* 1990;9:97.
42. Veasy LG, Tani LY, Hill HR. Persistence of acute rheumatic fever in the intermountain area of the United States. *J Pediatr* 1994;124:9–16.
43. Denny FW. A 45-year perspective on the streptococcus and rheumatic fever: the Edward H. Kass Lecture in infectious disease history. *Clin Infect Dis* 1994;19:1110–1122.
44. Johnson DR, Stevens DL, Kaplan EL. Epidemiologic analysis of group A streptococcal serotypes associated with severe systemic infections, rheumatic fever, or uncomplicated pharyngitis. *J Infect Dis* 1992;166:374–382.
45. Kaplan EL, Johnson DR, Cleary PP. Group A streptococcal serotypes isolated from patients and sibling contacts during the resurgence of rheumatic fever in the United States in the mid-1980's. *J Infect Dis* 1989;159:101–103.
46. Wessels MR, et al. Hyaluronic acid capsule is a virulence factor for mucoid group A streptococci. *Proc Natl Acad Sci USA* 1991;88: 8317–8321.
47. Wessels MR, Goldberg JB, Moses AE, DiCesare TJ, et al. Effects on virulence of mutations in a locus essential for hyaluronic acid capsule expression in group A streptococci. *Infect Immun* 1994;62:433–441.
48. Maxted WR, Widdowson JP, eds. The protein antigens of group-A streptococci. In: Wannamaker LW, Matsen SM, eds. *Streptococci and streptococcal diseases*. New York: Academic Press, 1972:251.
49. Musser JM, Kapur V, Peters JE, et al. Real-time molecular epidemiologic analysis of an outbreak of *Streptococcus pyogenes* invasive disease in U.S. Air Force trainees. *Arch Pathol Lab Med* 1994;118: 128–133.
50. Jamieson FB, Green K, Low DE, et al. A cluster of surgical wound infections due to unrelated strains of group A streptococci. *Infect Control Hosp Epidemiol* 1993;14:265–267.
51. Goldmann DA, Breton SJ. Group-C streptococcal surgical wound infections transmitted by an anorectal and nasal carrier. *Pediatrics* 1978;61:235.
52. Ridgway EJ, Allen KD. Clustering of group A streptococcal infections on a burns unit: important lessons in outbreak management. *J Hosp Infect* 1993;25:173–182.
53. Chaudhary S, Bilinsky SA, Hennessey JL. Penicillin V and rifampin for the treatment of group A streptococcal pharyngitis: a randomized trial of 10 days penicillin vs 10 days penicillin with rifampin during the final 4 days of therapy. *J Pediatr* 1985;106:481.
54. Tanz RR, et al. Penicillin plus rifampin eradicates pharyngeal carriage of group A streptococci. *J Pediatr* 1985;106:876.
55. Auerbach SB, Schwartz B, Williams D, et al. Outbreak of invasive group A streptococcal infections in a nursing home: lessons on prevention and control. *Arch Intern Med* 1992;152:1017–1022.
56. Walter CW, Kundsin RB. The airborne component of wound contamination and infection. *Arch Surg* 1973;107:588.
57. Wells WF. *Airborne contagion and air hygiene*. Cambridge: Harvard University Press, 1955.
58. Williams REO. Epidemiology of airborne staphylococcal infection. *Bacteriol Rev* 1966;30:660–672.
59. Lidwell OM, et al. Effect of ultraclean air in operating rooms on deep sepsis in the joint after total hip or knee replacement: a randomized study. *Br Med J* 1982;285:10.
60. Howard JM, Barker WF, Culbertson WR, et al. Postoperative wound infections: the influence of ultraviolet irradiation of the operating room and of various other factors. *Ann Surg* 1964;160(suppl):1.
61. Wheat LJ, Kohler RB, White A. Treatment of nasal carriers of coagulase-positive staphylococci. In: Maibach HI, Aly R, eds. *Skin microbiology: relevance to clinical infection*. New York: Springer, 1981:55–58.
62. Tuazon CV, Perez A, Kishaba T, Sheagren JN. *Staphylococcus aureus* among insulin-injecting diabetic patients: an increased carrier rate. *JAMA* 1975;231:1272.
63. Yu VL, Goetz A, Wagener M. *Staphylococcus aureus* nasal carriage and infection in patients on hemodialysis: efficacy of antibiotic prophylaxis. *N Engl J Med* 1986;315:91.
64. Luzar MA, Coles GA, Faller B, et al. *Staphylococcus aureus* nasal carriage and infection in patients on continuous ambulatory peritoneal dialysis. *N Engl J Med* 1990;322:505–509.
65. Tuazon CV, Sheagren JN. Increased risk of carriage of *Staphylococcus aureus* among narcotics addicts. *J Infect Dis* 1974;129:725.
66. Kirmani N, Tuazon CV, Alling D. Carriage rate of *Staphylococcus aureus* among patients receiving allergy injections. *Ann Allergy* 1980;45:235.
67. Raviglione MC, et al. High *Staphylococcus aureus* nasal carriage rate in patients with acquired immunodeficiency syndrome or AIDS-related complex. *Am J Infect Control* 1990;18:64.
68. Bethune DW, Blowers R, et al. Dispersal of *Staphylococcus aureus* by patients and surgical staff. *Lancet* 1965;1:480.
69. Hare R, Thomas CGA. The transmission of *Staphylococcus aureus*. *Br Med J* 1958;1:69–73.
70. Reboli AC, John J Jr, Platt CG, Cantey JR. Methicillin-resistant *Staphylococcus aureus* outbreak at a Veterans' Affairs Medical Center: importance of carriage of the organism by hospital personnel. *Infect Control Hosp Epidemiol* 1990;11:291–296.
71. Ehrenkranz NJ. Person-to-person transmission of *Staphylococcus aureus*: quantitative characterization of nasal carriers spreading infection. *N Engl J Med* 1964;271:225–230.
72. Boyce JM, Opal SM, Potter-Byn G, Medeirose AA. Spread of methicillin-resistant *Staphylococcus aureus* in a hospital after exposure to a healthcare worker with chronic sinusitis. *Clin Infect Dis* 1993;17: 496–504.
73. Belani A, Sheretz RH, Sullivan ML, et al. Outbreak of staphylococcal infection in two hospital nurseries traced to a single nasal carrier. *Infect Control Hosp Epidemiol* 1986;7:487–490.
74. Ward TT, Winn RE, Hartstein AI, Sewell DL. Observations relating to an interhospital outbreak of methicillin-resistant *Staphylococcus aureus*: role of antimicrobial therapy in infection control. *Infect Control Hosp Epidemiol* 1981;2:453.
75. White A. Relation between quantitative nasal cultures and dissemination of staphylococci. *J Lab Clin Med* 1961;58:273–277.
76. Hill RLR, Duckworth GJ, Casewell MW. Elimination of nasal carriage of methicilin-resistant Staphylococcus aureus with mupirocin during a hospital outbreak. *J Antimicrob Chemother* 1988;22:377.
77. Sherertz RJ, Reagan DR, Hampton KD, Robertson KI. A cloud adult: the *Staphylococcus aureus*–virus interaction revisited. *Ann Intern Med* 1996;124:539–547.
78. Fournier JM, et al. Predominance of capsular polysaccharide type 5 among oxacillin-resistant *Staphylococcus aureus*. *J Clin Microbiol* 1987;25:1932.
79. Karakawa WW, et al. Method for serological typing of the capsular polysaccharides of *Staphylococcus aureus*. *J Clin Microbiol* 1985; 22: 445.
80. Kosarsky PE, Rimland D, Terry PM, Wachsmuth K. Plasmic analysis of simultaneous nosocomial outbreaks of methicillin-resistant *Staphylococcus aureus*. *Infect Control Hosp Epidemiol* 1986;7:577.
81. Boyce JM, Bouvet A. Epidemiologic markers for epidemic strain and carrier isolates in an outbreak of nosocomial oxacillin-resistant *Staphylococcus aureus*. *J Clin Microbiol* 1990;28:1338.
82. Branger C, Goullet PH. Genetic heterogeneity in methicillin-resistant strains of *Staphylococcus aureus* revealed by esterase electrophoretic polymorphism. *J Hosp Infect* 1989;14:125.
83. Stolz SM, Maki DG. The use of Western blotting to subtype nosocomial isolates of methicillin-resistant *Staphylococcus aureus* [Abstract A25]. Proceedings of *The Third Decennial International Conference on Nosocomial Infections*. Atlanta:July 31–August 3, 1990.
84. Sands KE, Pursley D, Kalaidjian R, et al. Clinical and molecular epidemiology of *Staphylococcus aureus* in a neonatal intensive care unit [Abstract]. *Infect Control Hosp Epidemiol* 1995;16(suppl):P29.

85. Maslow JN, E MM, Arbeit RD. Molecular epidemiology: application of contemporary techniques to the typing of microorganisms. *Clin Infect Dis* 1993;17:153–164.
86. Prevost G, Jaulhac B, Premont Y. DNA fingerprinting by pulsed-field gel electrophoresis is more effective than ribotyping in distinguishing among methicillin-resistant *Staphylococcus aureus* isolates. *J Clin Microbiol* 1992;30:967–973.
87. Back NA, Linnemann CC, Pfaller MA, et al. Recurrent epidemics caused by a strain of erythromycin-resistant *Staphylococcus aureus*: the importance of molecular epidemiology. *JAMA* 1993;270: 1329–1333.
88. Kreisworth BN, Kravitz GR, Schlrevert PM, Novick RP. Nosocomial transmission of a strain of *Staphylococcus aureus* causing toxic shock syndrome. *Ann Intern Med* 1986;105:704.
89. Archer GL, Mayhall CG. Comparison of epidemiological markers used in the investigation of an outbreak of methicillin-resistant *Staphylococcus aureus* infections. *J Clin Microbiol* 1983;18:395.
90. Licitra CM, et al. Use of plasmid analysis and determination of aminoglycoside-modifying enzymes to characterize isolates from an outbreak of methicillin-resistant *Staphylococcus aureus*. *J Clin Microbiol* 1989;27:2535.
91. McGowan JE Jr., et al. Nosocomial infections with gentamicin-resistant *Staphylococcus aureus*: plasmid analysis as an epidemiologic tool. *J Infect Dis* 1979;140:864.
92. Rhinehart E, Shlaes DM, Keyes TF, et al. Nosocomial clonal dissemination of methicillin-resistant *Staphylococcus aureus* infections. *Arch Intern Med* 1987;147:521–524.
93. Fang FC, McClelland M, Guiney DG, et al. Value of molecular epidemiologic analysis in a nosocomial methicillin-resistant *Staphylococcus aureus* outbreak. *JAMA* 1993;270:1323–1328.
94. Wheat LJ, Kohler RB, White AL. Effect of rifampin on nasal carriers of staphylococci. *J Infect Dis* 1977;144:177.
95. Boyce JM. Methicillin-resistant *Staphylococcus aureus* in hospitals and long-term care facilities: microbiology, epidemiology, and preventive measures. *Infect Control Hosp Epidemiol* 1992;13:725–737.
96. Mulligan ME, Ruane PJ, Johnston L, et al. Ciprofloxacin for eradication of methicillin-resistant *Staphylococcus aureus* colonization. *Am J Med* 1987;82:215–219.
97. Walsh TJ, Standiford HC, Reboli AC, et al. Randomized double-blinded trial of rifampin with either novobiocin or trimethoprim-sulfamethoxazole against methicillin-resistant *Staphylococcus aureus* colonization: prevention of antimicrobial resistance and effect of host factors on outcome. *Antimicrob Agents Chemother* 1993;37: 1334–1342.
98. Ellison RT III, et al. Oral rifampin and trimethoprim/sulfamethoxazole therapy in asymptomatic carriers of methicillin-resistant *Staphylococcus aureus* infections. *West J Med* 1984;140:735.
99. Fekety R. The management of the carrier in methicillin-resistant *Staphylococcus aureus*. In: Remington JS, Swartz MN, eds. *Current clinical topics in infectious diseases*, vol. 8. New York: McGraw-Hill, 1987:169.
100. Roccaforte JS, Bittner MJ, Stumpt CA, Preheim LC. Attempts to eradicate methicillin-resistant *Staphylococcus aureus* colonization with the use of trimethoprim-sulfamethoxazole, rifampin, and bacitracin. *Am J Infect Control* 1988;16:141.
101. Bryan CM, Wilson RS, Meade P, Sill LG. Topical antibiotic ointments for staphylococcal nasal carriers: survey of current practices and comparison of bacitracin and vancomycin ointments. *Infect Control Hosp Epidemiol* 1981;1:153–156.
102. Barrett SP. The value of mupirocin in containing an outbreak of methicillin-resistant *Staphylococcus aureus* in an orthopaedic unit. *J Hosp Infect* 1990;15:137.
103. Casewell MW, Hill RL. The carrier state: methicillin-resistant *Staphylococcus aureus*. *J Antimicrob Chemother* 1986;18:1.
104. Cederna JE, et al. *Staphylococcus aureus* nasal colonization in a nursing home: eradication with mupirocin. *Infect Control Hosp Epidemiol* 1990;11:13.
105. Doebbeling BN, Breneman DL, Neu HC, et al. Elimination of *Staphylococcus aureus* nasal carriage in healthcare workers: analysis of six clinical trials with calcium mupirocin ointment. *Clin Infect Dis* 1993;17:466–474.
106. Doebbeling BN, Reagan DR, Pfaller MA, et al. Long-term efficacy of intranasal mupirocin ointment: a prospective cohort study of *Staphylococcus aureus* carriage. *Arch Intern Med* 1994;154:1505–1508.
107. Layton MC, Perez M, Heald P, Patterson JE. An outbreak of mupirocin-resistant *Staphylococcus aureus* on a dermatology ward associated with an environmental reservoir. *Infect Control Hosp Epidemiol* 1993;14:369–375.
108. Rahman M, Noble WC, Cookson B. Transmissible mupirocin resistance in *Staphylococcus aureus*. *Epidemiol Infect* 1989;102:261–270.
109. Bradley S, Ramsey M, Morton TM, Kauffman CA. Mupirocin resistance: clinical and molecular epidemiology. *Infect Control Hosp Epidemiol* 1995;16:354–358.
110. Smith GE, Kennedy CTC. *Staphylococcus aureus* resistant to mupirocin. *J Antimicrob Chemother* 1988;21:141.
111. Kauffman CA, Terpenning MS, He X, et al. Attempts to eradicate methicillin-resistant *Staphylococcus aureus* from a long-term-care facility with the use of mupirocin ointment. *Am J Med* 1993;94: 371–378.
112. Cookson BD, et al. Mupirocin-resistant *Staphylococcus aureus*. *Lancet* 1990;335:1095.
113. Shinefield HR, Ribble JC, Boris, M. Bacterial interference between strains of *Staphylococcus aureus*, 1960–1970. *Am J Dis Child* 1971; 121:148.
114. Steele RW. Recurrent staphylococcal infection in families. *Arch Dermatol* 1980;116:189.
115. Boyce JM, Jackson MM, Pugliese G, et al. Methicillin-resistant *Staphylococcus aureus* (MRSA): a briefing for acute care hospitals and nursing facilities. The AHA Technical Panel on Infections Within Hospitals. *Infect Control Hosp Epidemiol* 1994;15:105–115.
116. Garner RN. Guideline for isolation precautions in hospitals. *Infect Control Hosp Epidemiol* 1996;17:53.
117. Calia FM, Wolinsky E, Mortimer EA, et al. Importance of the carrier state as a source of *Staphylococcus aureus* in wound sepsis. *J Hyg Camb* 1969;67:49.
118. Williams REO, et al. Nasal staphylococci and sepsis in hospital patients. *Br Med J* 1959;2:658–663.
119. Weinstein HJ. The relation between the nasal-staphylococcal-carrier state and the incidence of postoperative complications. *N Engl J Med* 1959;260:1303.
120. Kluytmans JA, Mouton JW, Ijzerman EP, et al. Nasal carriage of *Staphylococcus aureus* as a major risk factor for wound infections after cardiac surgery. *J Infect Dis* 1995;171:216–219.
121. Morales E, et al. *S. aureus* carriage and saphenous vein harvest site infection following coronary artery bypass surgery. Presented at the 34th Interscience Conference on Antimicrobial Agents and Chemotherapy, Orlando, October 4–7, 1994.
122. Lye WC, Leong SO, vanderStraaten J, Lee ESJ. *Staphylococcus aureus* CAPD-related infections are associated with nasal carriage. *Adv Perit Dial* 1994;10:163–165.
123. Kluytmans JA, Mouton JW, Vandenberg FQ, et al. Reduction of surgical site infections in cardiothoracic surgery by elimination of nasal carriage of *Staphylococcus aureus*. *Infect Control Hosp Epidemiol* 1996;17:780.
124. Boelaert JR, et al. Nasal mupirocin ointment decreases the incidence of *Staphylococcus aureus* bacteraemias in haemodialysis patients. *Nephrol Dial Transplant* 1993;8:235–239.
125. Kluytmans JA, Manders MJ, Bommel EV, Verbrugh HA. Elimination of nasal carriage of *Staphylococcus aureus* in hemodialysis patients. *Infect Control Hosp Epidemiol* 1996;17:793–797.
126. Perez-Fontan M, Garcia-Falcon T, Rosales M, et al. Treatment of *Staphylococcus aureus* nasal carriers in continuous ambulatory peritoneal dialysis with mupirocin: long-term results. *Am J Kidney Dis* 1993;22:708–712.
127. Boyce JM. Preventing staphylococcal infections by eradicating nasal carriage of *Staphylococcus aureus*: proceeding with caution. *Infect Control Hosp Epidemiol* 1996;17:775.
128. Fairchild JP, Graber CD, Vogel EH. Flora of the umbilical stump: 2,479 cultures. *J Pediatr* 1958;53:538.
129. Jellard J. Umbilical cord as reservoir of infection in maternity hospital. *Br Med J* 1957;1:925.
130. Haley RW, Bregman DA. The role of understaffing and overcrowding in recurrent outbreaks of staphylococcal infection in a neonatal special care unit. *J Infect Dis* 1982;145:875.
131. Gillespie WA, Simpson K, Tozer RC. Staphylococcal infection in maternity hospital: epidemiology and control. *Lancet* 1958;2:1075.
132. Light IJ, Sutherland JM, Cochran ML, Soitorius J, et al. Ecological relationship between *Staphylococcus aureus* and *Pseudomonas* in a nursery population. *N Engl J Med* 1968;278:1243.
133. Shinefield HR. Staphylococcal infections. In: Remmington JS, Klein JO, eds. *Infectious diseases of the fetus and newborn infant*, 3rd ed. Philadelphia: WB Saunders, 1990:866.

134. Gezon HM, et al. Hexachlorophene bathing in early infancy: effect on staphylococcal disease and infection. *N Engl J Med* 1964;270:379.
135. Kimbrough RD, Gaines TB. Hexachlorophene effects on the rat brain: study of high doses by light and electron microscopy. *Arch Environ Health* 1971;23:114.
136. Shuman RM, Leech RW, Alvord EC. Neurotoxicity of hexachlorophene in the human. I. A clinicopathologic study of 248 children. *Pediatrics* 1974;54:689–695.
137. Powell H, Swarmer O, Gluck L, Lampert P. Hexachlorophene myelinopathy in premature infants. *J Pediatr* 1973;82:976.
138. Kaslow RA, et al. Staphylococcal disease related to hospital nursery bathing practices: a nationwide epidemiologic investigation. *Pediatrics* 1973;51(suppl):418.
139. Garland JS, Buck RK, Maloney P. Comparison of 10% povidone-iodine and 0.5% chlorhexidine gluconate for the prevention of peripheral intravenous catheter colonization in neonates: a prospective trial. *Pediatr Infect Dis J* 1995;14:510–516.
140. Pildes RS, Ramamurthy RS, Vidyasagar D. Effect of triple dye on staphylococcal colonization in the newborn infant. *J Pediatr* 1973; 82:907.
141. Haley RW, Cushion NB, Tenover FC, et al. Eradication of endemic methicillin-resistant *Staphylococcus aureus* infections from a neonatal intensive care unit. *J Infect Dis* 1995;171:614–624.
142. Davies EA, et al. An outbreak of infection with methicillin-resistant *Staphylococcus aureus* in a special care baby unit: value of topical mupirocin and of traditional methods of infection control. *J Hosp Infect* 1987;10:120.
143. Back NA, Linnemann CC Jr, Staneck JL, Kotagal UR. Control of methicillin-resistant *Staphylococcus aureus* in a neonatal intensive-care unit: use of intensive microbiologic surveillance and mupirocin. *Infect Control Hosp Epidemiol* 1996;17:227–231.
144. Zafar AB, Butler RC, Reese DJ. Use of 0.3% triclosan (Bacti-Stat) to eradicate an outbreak of methicillin-resistant *Staphylococcus aureus* in a neonatal nursery. *Am J Infect Control* 1995;23:200–208.
145. Eichenwald HF, Kotsevalov O, Fasco LA. The "cloud baby": an example of bacterial viral interactions. *Am J Dis Child* 1960;100:161.
146. Jernigan JA, Titus MG, Grosch DH, et al. Effectiveness of contact isolation during a hospital outbreak of methicillin-resistant *Staphylococcus aureus*. *Am J Epidemiol* 1996;143:496–504.
147. Gaynes RP, Culver DH, Horan TC, et al. Trends in methicillin-resistant *Staphylococcus aureus* in United States hospitals. *Infect Dis Clin Pract* 1993;2:452–455.
148. Lugeon C, Blanc DS, Wenger A, et al. Molecular epidemiology of methicillin-resistant *Staphylococcus aureus* at a low-incidence hospital over a 4-year period. *Infect Control Hosp Epidemiol* 1995; 14:29.
149. Trilla A, et al. Restriction endonuclease analysis of plasmid DNA from methicillin-resistant *Staphylococcus aureus*: clinical application over a three-year period. *Infect Control Hosp Epidemiol* 1993;14:29.
150. Boyce JM. Methicillin-resistant *Staphylococcus aureus*: detection, epidemiology, and control measures. *Infect Dis Clin North Am* 1989; 3:901.
151. Brumfitt W, Hamilton-Miller J. Methicillin-resistant *Staphylococcus aureus*. *N Engl J Med* 1989;320:1188.
152. Casewell MW. Epidemiology and control of the "modern" methicillin-resistant *Staphylococcus aureus*. *J Hosp Infect* 1986;7(suppl A):1.
153. Noble WC, Virani Z, Cree RG. Co-transfer of vancomycin and other resistance genes from *Enterococcus faecalis* NCTC 12201 to *Staphylococcus aureus*. *FEMS Microbiol Lett* 1992;72:195.
154. Centers for Disease Control and Prevention. Staphylococcus aureus with reduced susceptibility to vancomycin—United States, 1997. *MMWR* 1997;46:765–766.
155. Centers for Disease Control and Prevention. Interim guidelines for prevention and control of staphylococal infection associated with reduced susceptibility to vancomycin. *MMWR* 1997;46:626–628.
156. Pfaller M, Wakefield DS, Stewart B, et al. Evaluation of laboratory methods for the classification of oxacillin-resistant and oxacillin-susceptible *Staphylococcus aureus*. *Am J Clin Pathol* 1988;89:120–125.
157. Jorgensen JH. Mechanisms of methicillin resistance in *Staphylococcus aureus* and methods for laboratory detection. *Infect Control Hosp Epidemiol,* 1991;12:14–19.
158. Thornsberry C, McDougal LK. Successful use of broth microdilution in susceptibility tests for methicillin-resistant (heteroresistant) staphylococci. *J Clin Microbiol* 1983;18:1084.
159. Cookson BD, et al. Staff carriage of epidemic methicillin-resistant *Staphylococcus aureus*. *J Clin Microbiol* 1989;27:1471.
160. Hartman BJ, Tomasz A. Low affinity penicillin-binding protein associated with beta-lactam resistance in *Staphylococcus aureus*. *J Bacteriol* 1984;158:513.
161. Tomasz A, et al. New mechanisms for methicillin resistance in *Staphylococcus aureus*: clinical isolates that lack the PBP 2a gene and contain normal penicillin-binding proteins with modified penicillin-binding capacity. *Antimicrob Agents Chemother* 1989;33:1869.
162. McDougal LK, Thornsberry C. The role of β-lactamase in staphylococcal resistance to penicillinase-resistant penicillins and cephalosporins. *J Clin Microbiol* 1986;23:832.
163. Locksley RM, et al. Multiply antibiotic-resistant *Staphylococcus aureus*: introduction, transmission and evolution of nosocomial infection. *Ann Intern Med* 1982;97:317.
164. Guiguet M, Rekacewiez C, Leclercq B, et al. Effectiveness of simple measures to control an outbreak of nosocomial methicillin-resistant *Staphylococcus aureus* infections in an intensive care unit. *Infect Control Hosp Epidemiol* 1990;11:23–26.
165. Hsu CCS, Macaluso CP, Special L. High rate of methicillin resistance in *Staphylococcus aureus* isolated from hospitalized nursing home patients. *Arch Intern Med* 1988;148:28.
166. Thomas JC, et al. Transmission and control of methicillin-resistant *Staphylococcus aureus* in a skilled nursing facility. *Infect Control Hosp Epidemiol* 1989;10:106.
167. Craven DE, Rixinger AI, Goularte TA, et al. Methicillin-resistant *Staphylococcus aureus* bacteremia linked to intravenous drug abusers using a "shooting gallery." *Am J Med* 1986;80:770–776.
168. Saravolatz LD, Pohlod DJ, Arking LM. Community-acquired methicillin-resistant *Staphylococcus aureus* infections: a new source for nosocomial outbreaks. *Ann Intern Med* 1982;97:325.
169. Coovadia YM, et al. A laboratory-confirmed outbreak of rifampin-methicillin resistant *Staphylococcus aureus* (RMRSA) in a newborn nursery. *J Hosp Infect* 1989;14:303.
170. Longfield JN, et al. Methicillin-resistant *Staphylococcus aureus* (MRSA): risk and outcome of colonized vs. infected patients. *Infect Control Hosp Epidemiol* 1985;6:445.
171. Lentino JR, Hennein H, Krause S. A comparison of pneumonia caused by gentamicin, methicillin-resistant and gentamicin, methicillin-sensitive *Staphylococcus aureus*: epidemiologic and clinical studies. *Infect Control Hosp Epidemiol* 1985;6:267.
172. Rimland D. Nosocomial infections with methicillin and tobramycin resistant *Staphylococcus aureus*: implications of physiotherapy in hospital-wide dissemination. *Am J Med Sci* 1985;290:91.
173. Sanford MD, Widmer F, Bale MJ, et al. Efficient detection and long-term persistence of the carriage of methicillin-resistant *Staphylococcus aureus*. *Clin Infect Dis* 1994;110:1123–1128.
174. Thompson RL, Cabezudo I, Wenzel RP. Epidemiology of nosocomial infections caused by methicillin-resistant *Staphylococcus aureus*. *Ann Intern Med* 1982;97:309.
175. Layton MC, Hierholzer W Jr., Patterson JE. The evolving epidemiology of methicillin-resistant *Staphylococcus aureus* at a university hospital. *Infect Control Hosp Epidemiol* 1995;16:12.
176. Crossley K, Landesman B, Zaska D. An outbreak of infections caused by strains of *S. aureus* resistant to methicillin and aminoglycosides II. Epidemiological studies. *J Infect Dis* 1979;139:280.
177. Report of a combined working party of the Hospital Infections Society and the British Society for Antimicrobial Chemotherapy. Guidelines for the control of epidemic methicillin-resistant *Staphylococcus aureus*. *J Hosp Infect* 1986;7:193.
178. Report of a combined working party of the Hospital Infection Society and the British Society for Antimicrobial Chemotherapy, prepared G. Duckworth. Revised guidelines for the control of epidemic methicillin-resistant *Staphylococcus aureus*. *J Hosp Infect* 1990;16: 351.
179. Reboli AC, John JJ Jr, Levkoff AH. Epidemic methicillin-gentamicin-resistant *Staphylococcus aureus* in a neonatal intensive care unit. *Am J Dis Child* 1989;143:34.
180 Bartzokas CA, et al. Control and eradication of methicillin-resistant *Staphylococcus aureus* on a surgical unit. *N Engl J Med* 1984;311: 1422.
181. Hartstein AI, Denny MA, Morthland VH, et al. Control of methicillin resistant *Staph. aureus* in a hospital and an intensive care unit. *Infect Control Hosp Epidemiol* 1995;16:405–1411.
182. Mulligan ME, Murray-Leisure KA,Ribner BS, et al. Methicillin-resistant *Staphylococcus aureus*: a consensus review of the microbiology, pathogenesis, and epidemiology with implications for prevention and management. *Am J Med* 1993;94:313–328.

Hospital Infections, Fourth Edition,
edited by John V. Bennett and Philip S. Brachman.
Lippincott–Raven Publishers, Philadelphia © 1998

CHAPTER 42

Selected Viruses of Nosocomial Importance

William M. Valenti

Viral infections probably account for more nosocomial infections than has been realized; 5% of all nosocomial infections in hospitals are due to viruses [1], and this figure is probably an underestimate. Although much of the data on nosocomial viral infections comes from pediatric services [2–4], adults, especially the elderly and chronically ill, appear to be at risk as well [5,6]. There are scant data on viral infections outside the hospital, such as in ambulatory or home care settings [7,8] (see Chapter 28).

healthcare facilities bring together a great variety of workers of all ages with a wide range of educational and clinical backgrounds, which have an impact on the implementation of infection control procedures. In addition, the numbers of pregnant women working in healthcare facilities are probably greater than in any other workplace, which requires additional strategies for protecting workers from potential infections. Medical facilities are a challenge in terms of prevention of infection in both patients and personnel. Infection control professionals must be familiar with the potential for nosocomial transmission of viruses and must be aware of their modes of transmission and possible methods of control and prevention. healthcare workers are an integral part of the chain of transmission of viral infections in healthcare facilities. Vaccination programs for personnel and the widespread adoption of precautions systems, such as universal precautions and body substance isolation, are important ways of interrupting this chain of transmission (see Chapters 3, 13). In addition, the Centers for Disease Control and Prevention (CDC) has proposed a four-category system for isolation, which includes precautions for most of the viruses discussed in this chapter.

As the move to managed care shifts healthcare delivery toward ambulatory settings, rapid methods of diagnosing viral infections, new and improved vaccines, and antiviral chemotherapy become increasingly important components in the control of viral infections in healthcare facilities. In this chapter, the following viral diseases and agents will be discussed: influenza, respiratory syncytial virus, parainfluenza virus, rhinovirus, adenovirus, herpesviruses (varicella zoster, herpes zoster, and herpes simplex), cytomegalovirus, Epstein-Barr virus, hepatitis (A, B, and C), rubella, measles, mumps, parvovirus B19, Creutzfeldt-Jakob disease, rotavirus, Norwalk agent, picornaviruses, nonpolio enteroviruses, polioviruses, rabies, arenaviruses, papillomaviruses, and viral hemorrhagic fevers.

RESPIRATORY VIRUSES

Transmission of respiratory viruses in healthcare facilities is an annual event in temperate climates (see Chapter 32). Both patients and personnel are at special risk during the winter season, and large numbers of healthcare personnel with acute respiratory illnesses become a major concern. In addition to pediatric patients [2], patients who seem to be at greatest risk of acquiring nosocomial viral respiratory disease are those in closed or semiclosed populations, such as psychiatric units [1] and patients in extended-care facilities [5]. Despite the current shift in delivery of care away from hospitals, the risk of respiratory viral transmission in ambulatory facilities has not been studied.

The two major mechanisms of transmission of respiratory viruses are by means of droplet nuclei (small-particle aerosol) and droplets (large-particle spread). Droplet nuclei aerosols (median diameter < 5 μm) containing infectious virions are produced by coughing, sneezing, or talking and are capable of transmitting infectious virus over considerable distances (> 3 feet). Smallpox provides the classic example of this type of spread, but influenza virus and varicella virus exhibit this pattern of spread. With droplet spread, viral agents may be transmitted over

W. M. Valenti: Community Health Network, Rochester, New York 14620.

shorter distances by mechanisms requiring close person-to-person contact, generally at a distance of < 3 feet separating two persons. This method of transmission may occur when droplets produced by coughing or sneezing either directly infect the susceptible host (e.g., mucous membranes of the eye or nose) or contaminate the donor's hands or when a fomite transfers infectious virus indirectly to the skin or mucous membranes of a susceptible host. Infection in the susceptible host may also result from autoinoculation, with transfer of virus from hands to mucous membranes of the eye or nose. Rhinoviruses and respiratory syncytial virus are spread by close-contact transmission. In the absence of viral diagnostic facilities, it may be possible to establish a presumptive viral diagnosis based on the predominant site of involvement in the respiratory tract, such epidemiologic data as season of the year, geographic location, type of population, and data from area surveillance activity.

INFLUENZA VIRUS

Influenza A and B viral infections are among the most communicable diseases of humans. They are characterized by explosive epidemics, and nosocomial transmission of influenza A [5,9] and B [6] has been well documented (see Chapter 32). Person-to-person transmission is believed to take place primarily by droplet nuclei. These aerosols help account for the explosive nature of influenza outbreaks, since, in a closed environment, one infected person can potentially infect large numbers of susceptible persons.

Most nosocomial outbreaks are reported from nursing homes and chronic care facilities [1,5,6], in part because of a low rate of vaccine in these closed populations (see Chapter 29). In addition to underuse of vaccine, many persons at high risk fail to develop an adequate protective antibody response despite vaccination [2,5,6]. Outbreaks have also occurred in general hospitals, psychiatric units, and medical and pediatric services [7,9]. This underuse of vaccine is a major factor contributing to outbreaks of influenza in healthcare facilities and its associated morbidity, including primary influenza pneumonia, secondary bacterial pneumonia, cardiopulmonary complications, and exacerbations of other chronic diseases. In terms of mortality, the CDC has estimated that > 10,000 excess deaths occurred during each of seven different U.S. epidemics during the 1978 to 1988 respiratory disease season [10].

Precautions

Graman and Hall have described the components of a comprehensive approach to preventing nosocomial influenza infection [11]. It includes immunization of healthcare workers and patients at high risk in the fall of each year; early identification and isolation or cohorting of infected patients and personnel; and the flexibility to offer vaccine later when cases of influenza are first identified in the community or hospital. In addition, isolation in private rooms with negative pressure, if possible, is best for known or suspected cases of influenza.

The infection control isolation strategy of cohort isolation (cohorting) may also be useful when larger numbers of patients or personnel are infected with influenza [11,12]. Cohort isolation attempts to separate different groups of people in an effort to reduce disease transmission [12]. In this case, cohorts of infected and uninfected persons are identified and separated as a means of reducing the spread of influenza. Since most facilities will have only a limited supply of private or negative-pressure-equipped rooms, more than one patient with proven influenza may be cohorted or isolated together. Depending on the severity of the outbreak, it may also be necessary to restrict from patient contact healthcare workers who are ill, curtail visitation, and reschedule some elective admissions and surgical procedures. Shedding of virus may persist for as long as 5 days after the onset of symptoms in adults [13] and for 7 days in children [14]. Maintain droplet precautions for patients with influenza viral infection for 7 days or the duration of clinical illness, whichever is longer.

Immunization

Control of influenza requires herd immunity to have some degree of protection for influenza. Large numbers of people in a particular group at risk must be immune to infection [15,16]. There are two approaches to reducing the impact of influenza infection: immunoprophylaxis with inactivated influenza vaccine and chemoprophylaxis with amantadine or other influenza-specific antiviral drugs. Amantadine is a useful adjunct when herd immunity is not present because of underuse of vaccine and/or inadequate response to vaccination [16]. Vaccination is also important for staff in ambulatory settings, since patients are not usually isolated as such, and staff may have short-term, but intense exposure to influenza virus during the respiratory season.

At least one new vaccine preparation is pending licensure. This live attenuated intranasal influenza A vaccine was compared with standard inactivated influenza vaccine in a randomized, double-blind placebo-controlled trial in 523 persons (mean age, 84 years) from three nursing homes. Results showed that the addition of live intranasal vaccine provided additional protection from confirmed influenza (6% vs. 14%), respiratory illnesses (8% vs. 20%), and influenza-like illnesses (4% vs. 11%) [17]. A genetically engineered vaccine that has been shown to be as effective as the live attenuated preparations now in use is under investigation. The CDC has published a helpful document for managing influenza vaccination programs in nursing homes. While the focus is on long-term care, this information is applicable to other healthcare facilities and is a useful adjunct to the Advisory Committee on Immunization Practices' (ACIP) recommendations for planning and implementing a vaccine program [18]. Figure 42-1 shows a timetable and work plan from the CDC handbook.

Chemoprophylaxis

The antiviral drugs amantadine hydrochloride (Symmetrel) and rimantidine hydrochloride (Flumidine) are effective against influenza A. Neither drug is effective against influenza B. As treatment, these drugs lessen the severity of influenza illness and shorten the duration of illness among healthy adults. However, we do not know if amantadine treatment plays a role in preventing the complications of influenza A in high-risk patients. It is recommended that amantadine be started as soon as possible after the onset of clinical illness [11,16,18,19]. Since so many high-risk patients and healthcare workers are not vaccinated each year, it is inevitable that clusters and outbreaks of influenza will occur and require additional prevention and control activities, including prophylaxis with amantadine or rimantidine for influenza A. Use of these drugs is an appropriate outbreak control measure [11,18, 19] but difficult to implement [16].

For outbreak control, however, it is also recommended that in closed populations such as nursing homes, patients with influenza who are taking amantadine for treatment be isolated or cohorted from the asymptomatic patients who are taking amantadine for prophylaxis [12,16,19,20]. Patients at high risk can still be vaccinated after an outbreak of influenza A has begun. Since the development of antibodies in adults after vaccination takes 2 weeks, amantadine should be administered during the 2 weeks after vaccination, while waiting for maximum vaccine antibody production. Children being vaccinated for the first time may need 6 weeks for antibodies to develop after vaccination or 2 weeks after the second vaccine dose. In either case, amantadine does not interfere with the antibody response after vaccination with killed influenza antigens.

Outbreak-initiated use of amantadine or rimantidine is usually associated with problems. The spread of influenza among patients and healthcare workers can often outpace the best intentions and efforts to provide prophylaxis and

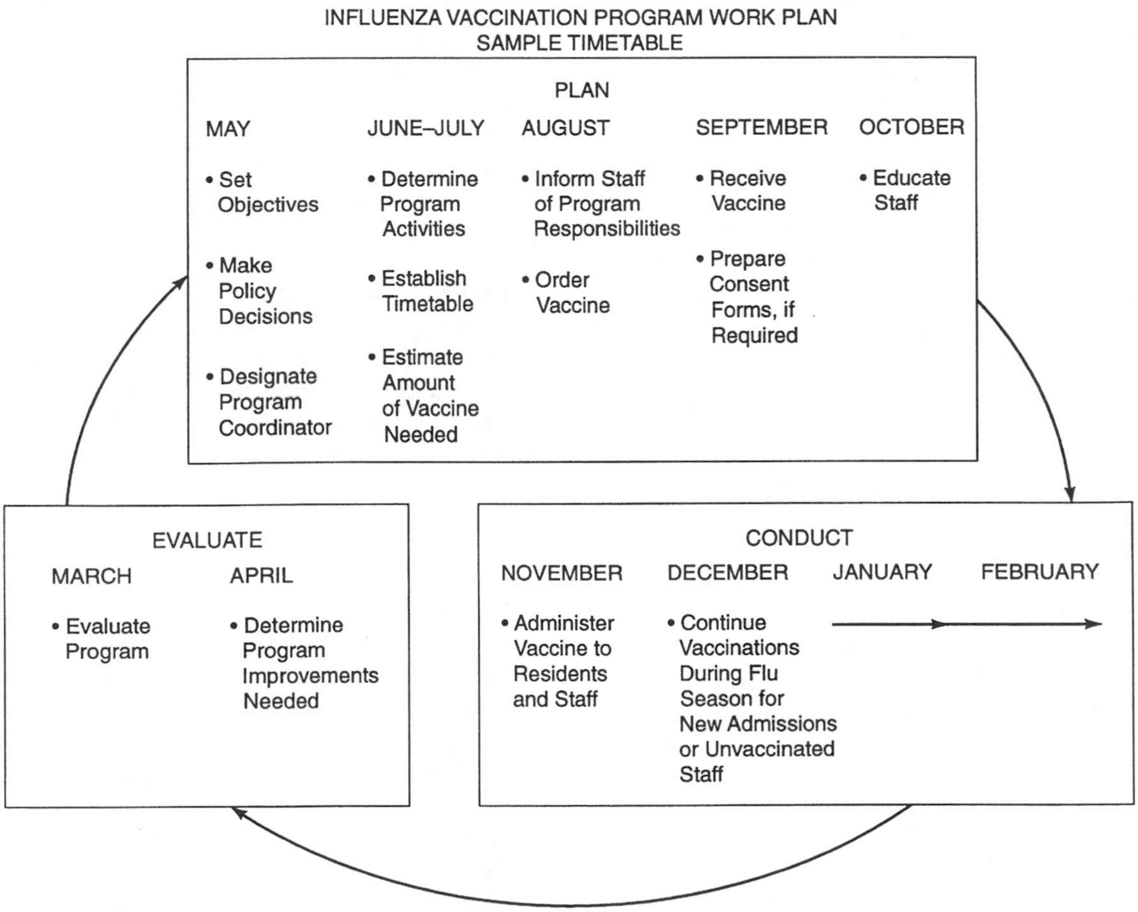

FIGURE 42-1. Influenza vaccination program work plan. (Reproduced from Centers for Disease Control and Prevention. *Managing an influenza vaccination program in the nursing home*. Atlanta: Centers for Disease Control and Prevention, 1987.)

treatment to those who might benefit from it [11,16]. Additional problems involve drug distribution, staff education, compliance, and financial considerations. It is not known whether amantadine or rimantidine is effective if given > 48 hours after the onset of illness. This means that unless rapid diagnostic techniques (e.g., rapid antigen detection for influenza A or virus isolation) are readily available, amantadine will be started for treatment based on clinical and/or epidemiologic impressions of influenza, since it may take several days to weeks to establish a diagnosis of influenza A based on laboratory tests.

Side effects, which tend to be less severe in young and healthy adults at the usual adult dose of either drug (200 mg/day), are mild central nervous system symptoms (nervousness, anxiety, insomnia, difficulty concentrating) or gastrointestinal symptoms (anorexia and nausea). These side effects often improve after several days to a week on the drug or can be lessened by decreasing the dose to 100 mg/day [15,18,19]. The recommended dose for patients 65 years of age or older is 100 mg per day because of the potential for the drug to accumulate in patients with decreased renal clearance [18].

In recent years, there have been reports of amantadine-resistant influenza virus strains emerging during hospital outbreaks [16,20]. The frequency with which resistant isolates arise and the extent of transmission are unknown. There is no evidence that amantadine-resistant viruses are more easily transmitted or more virulent than amantadine-sensitive isolates. These resistant isolates play a role in outbreaks and can create more problems when patients being treated are not separated from those who are receiving amantadine for prophylaxis [16,19]. It is recommended that when it is used for treatment, amantadine be discontinued as soon as clinically warranted [19,20] (usually after 3 to 5 days), which will reduce the risk of developing resistance,

Strategies to Increase Vaccination Rates

Despite the efficacy of vaccine and greater emphasis on childhood and adult immunization, < 30% of persons aged 65 are vaccinated with influenza vaccine each year [10,16]. Immunization has been reported in higher numbers of people in some nursing home populations [5,6]. The collective experiences of public health and infection control experts is that promoting influenza vaccination, or any other kind of vaccination for that matter, requires more than just posters announcing the availability of vaccine [10,21].

Strategies have been developed and studied that are effective in increasing influenza vaccination rates and reducing influenza-related morbidity and mortality rates. According to the Influenza and Pneumonia Action Group of the National Coalition for Adult Immunization, components of a successful vaccination program are education for healthcare workers, a plan for identifying people at risk (often by review of medical records), and efforts to remove administrative and financial barriers that prevent people from receiving vaccine [10,16]. In the case of healthcare workers, vaccine should be administered in the workplace to maximize compliance. While making a vaccine available to employees is no guarantee of acceptance, free and accessible vaccine is one less barrier to an effective program for healthcare workers.

Vaccine is also cost effective [21,22]. Patriarca et al. developed a model to project morbidity and mortality rates and costs associated with type A influenza illness in nursing homes [15]. Assuming 100 residents and a 60% rate of vaccination in the fall of the previous year, the combined use of previous vaccination and amantadine during outbreaks was associated with significantly fewer cases of influenza than vaccination alone, probably owing to the < 100% efficacy of vaccine to induce protective antibody. The authors predicted an increase in herd immunity if more patients than 60% were to be vaccinated. They conclude that influenza control programs in nursing homes are highly beneficial, cost-effective, and clinically sound. There was only a modest increase in program costs with the addition of amantadine. Overall indexes of cost-effectiveness used by the researchers continued to justify vaccination. When vaccine use reached 70%, the risk of an outbreak approached zero. When taken together with the ACIP's recommendations, an 80% vaccine rate in populations at risk is still a good target [15,16]. Finally, influenza vaccination of healthy adults has been shown to reduce time lost from work and to lead to fewer physician office visits for upper respiratory illnesses, with a cost savings of $46.88 per person vaccinated [22].

RESPIRATORY SYNCYTIAL VIRUS

Respiratory syncytial virus (RSV) is the most common cause of lower respiratory tract disease in children < 2 years old [2] (see Chapter 32). In recent years, RSV infections have accounted for ~ 45% of all hospital admissions for acute respiratory disease in children < 2 years old [23]. It is also the most common nosocomial infection on pediatric wards [6,24]. In addition, people in all age groups are potentially susceptible to RSV infection and, because immunity is incomplete and not permanent, reinfections may occur throughout life [25]. RSV infections have also been documented in hospital personnel [24], in elderly chronically ill patients [5], and in immunocompromised adults [26]. In general, RSV infections occur in annual epidemics of 2 to 3 months' duration, often beginning in late December.

The primary mode of transmission of RSV appears to be by close person-to-person contact, probably through the unwashed hands of hospital personnel. Studies by Hall and co-workers [23,27] have demonstrated that patients infected with RSV shed large amounts of virus in their respiratory secretions, with a mean duration of shedding of 6 to 7 days and a range of 1 to 21 days. The virus can be recovered from the immediate environment of infected patients for prolonged periods of time. For example, RSV in nasal secretions from infected infants can be recovered for ≤ 30 minutes from contaminated skin, gowns, or paper tissues [27]. The virus appears to survive best on non-porous surfaces, such as counter tops, and has been recovered for ≤ 6 hours from these surfaces [27]. Infectious virus can then be transferred from these environmental surfaces to hands and from hand to hand [27].

Studies among volunteers have also demonstrated that infection can be transmitted by RSV-containing fluid inoculated into the mucous membranes of the eyes or nose but not the mouth. Therefore, spread by direct inoculation of drops or large particles or by self-inoculation after touching contaminated surfaces, such as skin or fomites, seems feasible. Spread by small-particle aerosols is less likely, since nosocomial outbreaks are not as explosive as those due to influenza virus; studies in volunteers show that only persons cuddling infected infants and touching contaminated surfaces became infected with RSV. Persons did not become infected if they kept > 6 feet away from an infected baby, suggesting that small-particle aerosol transmission is not a major route of dissemination of RSV.

The risk of nosocomial RSV infection has been correlated with the duration of hospitalization; the risk increases with each subsequent week of hospitalization during the respiratory disease season. In one study, RSV infection was acquired by 45% of contact infants hospitalized for 1 week. The rate of RSV acquisition increased with each subsequent week of hospitalization until all infants hospitalized 4 weeks became infected. The rate of infection was not related to underlying illness or age of the patient. In addition, healthcare workers are an important link in nosocomial transmission of RSV. Each year, ~50% of the adult staff working on the pediatric service (nurses, house staff, and medical and nursing students) become infected with RSV. Conventional infection control measures, such as hand washing, wearing gowns, isolation or cohorting of infected infants, and cohorting of staff to infants, have lowered the rate of nosocomial acquisition of RSV in patients but not in hospital personnel [24].

Precautions

Graman and Hall's [11] recommendations for prevention of nosocomial RSV mirror the CDC's proposed contact precautions category: hand washing before and after all patient contacts, isolation or cohorting of infected patients whenever possible, cohorting of personnel so that a single staff member does not care for both infected and uninfected patients during the same shift, gowning for close contact with infected infants, postponement of elective admissions of high-risk patients, protective isolation of high-risk patients, and use of gloves for contact with mucous membranes and when handling respiratory secretions (see Chapter 13). However, these experts warn that gloves must be changed faithfully between patients, since RSV can survive longer on gloves than on skin [11, 27].

Immunization

There is no effective vaccine for RSV.

Treatment

Aerosolized ribavirin has been shown to be effective treatment for infants with lower respiratory tract infection with RSV. Although ribavirin decreases both the quantity and duration of RSV shedding, it is not known whether treatment reduces the risk of nosocomial infection [28]. Ribavirin's role in the treatment of adult patients is still not clear, and limited use in outbreaks among adults has not produced noticeable benefit [26,29].

Special Considerations

Additional strategies to minimize nosocomial transmission of RSV should include education of patient care staff on both the mode of transmission of RSV and the role of personnel in the chain of infection. Efforts should be made to curtail visits from family and friends who have respiratory illness, especially during periods of increased RSV prevalence in the community. In the absence of locally generated data on RSV prevalence, one can assume its occurrence from December through March in the United States and Europe.

PARAINFLUENZA VIRUS

Nosocomial transmission of parainfluenza virus on pediatric services has been documented [30]. In one study, Mufson et al. report that 18% of infants who are well or infected with another respiratory pathogen at the time of admission to a children's hospital subsequently acquire nosocomial infections with parainfluenza type 3. Infections in hospitals have also been reported in adult renal transplant patients [31] and in elderly institutionalized patients [32]. Details of transmission of parainfluenza virus have still not been fully elucidated, but dissemination is believed to take place by contact spread, either direct (person to person) or indirect (via fomite) [32]. Infections with parainfluenza types 1 and 2 are seasonal, with the greatest activity occurring during the fall months. Community epidemics with types 1 and 2 occur approximately every 2 years, whereas infections with parainfluenza virus type 3 tend to occur throughout each year. In a simultaneous outbreak of parainfluenza type 3 and respiratory syncytial virus in a newborn nursery, the clinical illnesses were indistinguishable [33].

Isolation Precautions

The importance of careful hand washing cannot be overemphasized, especially in view of the proposed mechanism of transmission of parainfluenza virus. Precautions are the same contact precautions used for RSV, with patients placed in a private room or cohorted together (see Chapter 13). Hand washing and gown changes after each contact are the most effective means of minimizing nosocomial transmission of parainfluenza viruses [32]. Precautions should be maintained for the duration of illness.

RHINOVIRUS

Rhinovirus infections are ubiquitous during the winter and spring months. Rhinovirus was a cause of significant morbidity in premature infants in an outbreak of rhinovirus infection in an intensive care nursery [4]. The affected infants had significant respiratory decompensation. The outbreak also involved respiratory syncytial virus, and the two illnesses were indistinguishable. Rhinovirus has also caused clinically consequential disease in an extended care facility [34].

Large quantities of virus are present in nasal secretions and readily contaminate the hands of the infected person. Virus transmission appears to take place directly from hand to hand or indirectly via fomites. Virus may be inoculated from the recipient's hands via touching of the mucous membranes of the nose and eyes [35,36]. More recent studies have shown that aerosols also play a role in adult rhinovirus transmission [37].

Hand washing appears to be the most effective way of minimizing transmission of rhinovirus. In outbreak situations, droplet precautions are the best infection control strategy, especially in view of the possibility of aerosol transmission in addition to droplet spread. Dilute solutions containing 1% iodine are effective skin antiseptics [38]. Since rhinoviruses are remarkably resistant to drying and survive for long periods of time on hard surfaces and plastic and synthetic fabrics [36], iodinated compounds may be useful as disinfectants on surfaces contaminated with rhinovirus-containing secretions (see Chapter 20). Generally, precautions other than hand washing are not recommended for patients with rhinovirus infection (see Chapter 13). However, cohorting of patients with rhinovirus infection may be necessary in outbreak situations [34].

ADENOVIRUS

Adenovirus infections occur in the general population throughout the year. These viruses are highly stable, can be transmitted via a number of routes, and cause a wide spectrum of illnesses. Adenoviruses are associated with conjunctivitis, keratoconjunctivitis, pharyngoconjunctival fever, pneumonia, and a pertussis-like syndrome. Respiratory transmission via aerosols occurs in all age groups [39], and volunteer studies have shown that inhalation of small doses of virus can initiate acute respiratory illness, including pneumonia [39]. Fecal-oral transmission takes place but probably is more important in children than in adults [39]. Adenoviruses are a frequent cause of sporadic diarrhea in children [40] and immunocompromised adults [41].

Hospital-acquired adenovirus infection has been reported in both patients and personnel [42,43]. Infections in neonates [44] and in pediatric patients [43] account for many of the reported cases of nosocomial adenovirus infections. One recently described outbreak in an intensive care nursery affected patients, staff, and parents, resulting in the deaths of two neonates and closure of the nursery for 3 weeks [44]. Although adenovirus pneumonia has been reported more frequently among military recruits, adenovirus can be the cause of sporadic cases of pneumonia in ≤ 10% of pediatric patients admitted with pneumonia [39]. Transmission of adenovirus from patients with pneumonia to hospital personnel has occurred in these situations, with personnel developing conjunctivitis and pharyngoconjunctival fever [45]. The finding of adenovirus infections in immunocompromised hosts (e.g., acquired immunodeficiency syndrome, or AIDS) and in transplant recipients suggests that adenoviruses, like herpesviruses, may be reactivated after primary infection [41,46,47] (see Chapter 45). All of these infections may have resulted from endogenous reactivation of adenovirus. Nosocomial transmission from staff with mild upper respiratory illness to immunocompromised patients may also have been involved.

An outbreak has been reported of epidemic keratoconjunctivitis due to adenovirus type 8, originating in an ophthalmology clinic, where 63 patients became infected in 1 month [17]. healthcare workers served as a major source of virus, with transmission to susceptible patients occurring by direct transfer of virus from hands and by indirect transfer via a Schiötz tonometer. A similar outbreak of keratoconjunctivitis was associated with a contaminated ophthalmic solution in an industrial health clinic [48].

Precautions

Droplet precautions, in addition to standard precautions, should be used. Patients with adenovirus infection should be placed in private rooms if possible (see Chapter 13). Personnel should wear gowns and gloves when direct contact with skin and mucous membranes or feces is anticipated. Care must also be taken when handling secretions, contaminated articles, and contaminated linens. Because shedding of adenovirus may be highly variable and prolonged, these precautions should be maintained for the duration of clinical illness.

Immunization

A live attenuated trivalent vaccine containing adenovirus types 3, 4, and 7 has been used for immunizing military personnel and has been found to be safe and effective. However, this vaccine is not available for routine civilian use.

Special Considerations

Adenoviruses are very stable and survive for long periods of time. Special care must be given to the decontamination and sterilization of contaminated instruments, such as reusable tonometers (see Chapter 20). Thorough cleaning followed by steam sterilization consisting of 15 pounds per square inch (psi) for 15 minutes at 121°C (250°F), or 15 psi for 10 minutes at 126°C (259°F), or 29 psi for 3 minutes at 134°C (273°F) is recommended. The use of a disposable tonofilm to cover and preserve sterility of the tonometer has also been suggested [49]. Equipment for ocular pressure measurement without direct contact may be considered for use as well. Personnel with conjunctivitis present a hazard to patients; it is recommended that employees with infectious conjunctivitis have no contact with patients in nurseries, obstetric units, or operating rooms until all drainage ceases.

HERPESVIRUSES

The members of the family *Herpesviridae* include varicella zoster virus (VZV), herpes simplex virus (HSV) types I and II, cytomegalovirus (CMV), and Epstein-Barr virus (EBV). Herpesvirus infections become latent or inactive after primary infection and can reactivate at a time remote from the primary infection. Infectious virus can be isolated in both primary and reactivated infections due to herpesviruses. Often primary infection is symptomatic, whereas reactivation infection is asymptomatic [50]. In the United States, most persons have come in contact with all the human herpesviruses (except herpesvirus type II) by age 50 [50]. Thus, infection is usually endogenous, and nosocomial infection occurs relatively infrequently.

Transmission of the herpesviruses occurs primarily by direct-contact spread (person to person) and, except for VZV, requires close personal contact. Varicella zoster virus is the most capable of nosocomial transmission because of its airborne route of dispersal as well as direct-contact spread. In addition, because of immunosuppression due to underlying diseases, transplantation, or chemotherapy, many hospitalized patients are susceptible to reactivation of herpesvirus infections. Nosocomial transmission of herpesviruses may be difficult to establish, since all but HSV types I and II have prolonged incubation periods, and illness often develops after discharge.

Before the era of the human immunodeficiency virus (HIV), during a 17-month period of careful viral surveillance, 20 cases of reactivation infection with herpesviruses were documented based on clinical criteria [1]. These infections, all due to CMV, were classified as endogenous nosocomial infections because signs and symptoms of infection were not apparent at the time of admission. During this same period, only one episode of primary CMV infection was detected; this was associated with virus from a transplanted kidney [1]. The epidemiology of the herpesvirus infections has not changed significantly during the HIV era, since the most common viral opportunistic infection in this group of patients is a form of reactivated CMV.

VARICELLA ZOSTER VIRUS

The most communicable of the herpesviruses, VZV is the causative agent of chickenpox and herpes zoster (shingles). Nosocomial transmission of chickenpox is well recognized [51–54] and is a cause of mortality and serious morbidity in immunocompromised patients [51,55] (see Chapter 45). The mechanisms of transmission of varicella are either via direct contact with infectious lesions or by the airborne route [56,57]. Epidemiologic evidence suggests that patients shed varicella virus in respiratory secretions as early as 2 days before the onset of rash [58], but this has never been proved by virus isolation. Whenever possible, patients with uncomplicated chickenpox should not be admitted to the hospital because they present a hazard to susceptible patients and personnel. In addition, patients in whom chickenpox develops or who are exposed to chickenpox while hospitalized should be discharged, if possible. Of course, severely ill patients are exceptions to these rules.

Precautions

As the newly licensed varicella vaccine comes into use, infection control strategies for chickenpox will change from reacting to exposures to a focus on pre-exposure intervention for both patients and employees (discussed later herein). In the meantime, nonimmune patients exposed to chickenpox or patients with chickenpox should be isolated in a private room or cohorted (see Chapter 13). Precautions that prevent contact with both respiratory secretions and secretions from patients' vesicles are required (see Chapter 13). The period of contagion of varicella virus from vesicles appears to decline ~5 days after the onset of rash. Because this period is somewhat variable, isolation precautions should be continued until all skin lesions are completely dried and crusted.

The susceptible patient exposed to chickenpox who cannot be discharged from the hospital presents a difficult problem in terms of restriction of activity and isolation precautions. Because of the high degree of communicability of chickenpox, personnel and patients in the same unit as a patient with chickenpox should be considered exposed [59]. Furthermore, patients with negative or unknown histories of chickenpox should be considered susceptible and will require isolation precautions beginning 10 days after exposure and continuing until 21 days after the last exposure. Since communicability of disease before the onset of the rash is not accurately predictable, precautions or cohorting of exposed persons should be initiated on the 10th day after exposure. Unless immunity can be proved, these patients should remain isolated until discharged from the hospital or for 21 days, whichever occurs first.

An important part of a varicella control program involves assessing the immunity of healthcare workers at the time of employment and vaccination of those staff members who are susceptible (see Chapter 3). Screening can be done by asking employees if they have ever had chickenpox. If the employee answers in the affirmative, the history of having had disease is thought to be reliable. However, hospital healthcare workers who have negative or unknown histories of previous varicella infection should be tested serologically.

Employees who show negative results on serologic testing should receive two doses of the Oka vaccine 4 to 8 weeks apart (see later herein). Susceptible healthcare workers who are exposed to persons with active varicella should not work with susceptible patients from the 10th to the 21st day after exposure [60]. If employee immunity to varicella can be proved, employees need not be sent home from work. If large numbers of employees are affected, these precautions may result in a significant expense to the hospital in time lost from work. In general, a history of chickenpox or herpes zoster in an adult or child is a reliable indication of immunity. In an attempt to control nosocomial transmission of chickenpox, the immune status in exposed persons with negative or unknown histories of chickenpox should be determined by a sensitive and reliable assay, such as the fluorescent antibody to membrane antigen test, enzyme immunoassay, or the immune adherence hemagglutination test; these tests are more sensitive than the older complement fixation test, since they measure antibodies that are believed to persist indefinitely [61]. Employees should be notified of their antibody status and offered vaccination if their results are negative [62].

Immunization

The best strategy to avoid sending employees home from work unnecessarily is to vaccinate with varicella vaccine those who are susceptible by serologic testing [63]. Now that the varicella vaccine is available, health facilities need to review their varicella control policies to address vaccine usage. A live attenuated varicella vaccine (Oka/Merck; Varivax) has been approved for marketing in the United States. This long-awaited vaccine, named for the Japanese child from whom virus was derived, has been studied extensively over the past 10 years. Clinical trials in the United States in children, adolescents, and adults have shown a variety of benefits and cleared the way for the vaccine's approval and use as a public health, clinical, and infection control tool. It has been found that 98.8% of children and 97.2% of adolescents and adults still had varicella antibodies 1 year after vaccination. The likelihood of natural varicella developing after vaccination declined with detectable postvaccine titer. Among adolescents and adults, after 2 years of follow-up there was still a 70% reduction in breakthrough infections after household exposure. The duration of protection from vaccination is still unknown, and it is also not known how the Oka vaccine will perform when given immediately after exposure or what its effect may be on herpes zoster [64].

The indication for vaccination is broad; the vaccine can be used against varicella in anyone 12 months of age. The recommended dose for children 12 months to 12 years is a single dose, given subcutaneously in the deltoid muscle or the anterolateral surface of the thigh. For those 13 years of age (adolescents and adults), two doses given 4 to 8 weeks apart are recommended. For varicella control to succeed, vaccination needs to be directed to susceptible people and not used narrowly. This is the same strategy that has ultimately emerged for rubella. From a public health perspective, immunization of children would shift the age distribution of cases to older patients, who are more likely to have serious varicella-related complications. Vaccine could save the national economy almost $350 million per year in healthcare and work loss savings [65,66]. At a cost to the consumer of $35.00 a dose, the vaccine should save more than $5.00 for every vaccine dollar spent [66].

Postexposure Prophylaxis

Varicella zoster immune globulin (VZIG) is licensed for passive immunization of susceptible immunocompromised children after significant exposure to chickenpox or herpes zoster [67]. When VZIG is administered within 96 hours of exposure, chickenpox can be prevented or modified in children with impaired immunity. It is readily available through the regional Red Cross network [67].

HERPES ZOSTER VIRUS

Transmission of virus from patients with herpes zoster to produce chickenpox has been described [68]; it happens occasionally, but less frequently than transmission of virus from patients with chickenpox. This is probably owing to the lower incidence of VZV in oral secretions of patients with herpes zoster than patients with chickenpox. Localized herpes zoster requires standard precautions to guard against acquisition of infection by direct contact with secretions from vesicles and from secretion-contaminated articles (see Chapter 13). A private room is desirable but not required. Patients with disseminated herpes zoster should be cared for in the same way as patients with chickenpox. They require the stricter isolation precautions used for varicella, including a private room with negative air pressure. Susceptible healthcare personnel should avoid contact with patients with either localized or disseminated herpes zoster.

Gershon and colleagues [69] have shown that > 95% of American-born women of childbearing age have detectable antibody to VZV. Ross [70] noted a low attack rate of 8% in adults with household exposure to chickenpox whose histories indicate they are susceptible. The conclusion is that a negative or unknown history of chickenpox in adults is often unreliable. These data suggest that the risk to hospital personnel for varicella acquisition from patients is small but measurable. The pool of susceptible persons, however small, represents a potential hazard for transmission of varicella to both susceptible patients and personnel.

HERPES SIMPLEX VIRUS

Reactivation of HSV type I infection frequently occurs spontaneously in healthy patients or personnel as well as in immunocompromised hosts (see Chapter 45). Persons with reactivated HSV type I infection rarely have intraoral lesions and often do not have labial lesions. Therefore, asymptomatic personnel potentially can transmit HSV type I to susceptible patients. Persons with herpes simplex labialis (fever blisters) do not transmit virus efficiently in respiratory secretions [52]. However, virus has been recovered from the hands of two thirds of the patients with herpes labialis [52]. This form of transmission may explain the clusters of infections that have been described in burned patients [71] and in immunocompromised patients [72]. Transmission of infection from hospital patients to personnel is well documented. Direct inoculation of HSV type I can take place on the fingers or hands of personnel after contact with the infected patient's mouth [73]. Herpetic whitlow infection of the fingers is the most common and can easily be mistaken for pyogenic paronychia; it is often quite disabling to hospital personnel [73]. Herpetic whitlow can infect immune or nonimmune persons [74]. In addition, primary herpes simplex stomatitis and pharyngitis can develop in hospital personnel [75]. A cluster of cases of primary HSV stomatitis and pharyngitis has been documented due to transmission of HSV type I to patients in a dental office from a dental hygienist with herpetic whitlow [76]. It is hoped that with increased attention to glove use, many of these infections can be prevented.

Herpes simplex virus type II and its potential for transmission from mother to newborn infant has long been a concern on obstetric and newborn services (see Chapter 26). When genital herpes is active in a mother at term, 40% to 60% of vaginally delivered infants will have clinically apparent infection with HSV type II [77]. Approximately 50% of these infants will have severe or fatal illness. The risk of neonatal infection can be minimized, but not eliminated, if delivery is by cesarean section and membranes remain unruptured or have been ruptured for < 6 hours [77]. The risk of infection at birth is also lessened if the mother's infection is reactivated rather than primary [77]. Although transmission of infection from mother to infant at the time of birth is well documented, evidence for transmission in the postpartum period is only indirect. Infection control policies under these circumstances are often ambiguous and confusing, and there is lack of uniformity from one institution to another [78]. It is generally agreed, however, that certain precautions may be indicated, depending on the clinical status of the mother.

Precautions

Infection control recommendations for mothers with known, suspected, or inactive HSV have been described in detail in the past; they involve strategies to reduce the risk of transmitting herpes simplex to the neonate without over-isolating either the mother or the baby, yet still offering protection to other infants in the nursery [79] (see Chapter 13). Women with proved or clinically suspected genital herpes simplex at term may transmit virus postnatally to their offspring as well as to other close contacts. Therefore, personnel should observe standard precautions, using gloves for direct contact with wet lesions containing virus (see Chapter 13). Perineal pads and dressings can be discarded in the regular trash unless they are blood soaked; in that case they should be discarded in red bag trash. There are no special precautions for linen. The mother may care for her baby, but she should be out of bed, with hands thoroughly washed before contact with the baby and wearing a clean cover gown. The infant should be observed after birth for signs and symptoms of illness, and personnel should follow contact precautions for direct contact with the infant. At present, there are no data regarding use of the observation or isolation nursery for such infants after birth. However, an observation nursery for these infants is recommended, whenever possible, even though nursery outbreaks of herpes simplex are uncommon.

Standard precautions are reasonable for women with active nongenital herpes simplex at term. A private room is not indicated. Mothers may care for their infants using the same precautions as noted for mothers with known or suspected genital herpes simplex, with the addition of a mask or dressing to cover the active lesions. The infant may be kept in the general newborn nursery without isolation after birth if there has been no maternal contact. After the first contact with the mother, the infant should be placed in the observation nursery, if possible, using precautions noted previously for babies born to mothers with active genital herpes simplex. Women with clinically inactive herpes simplex at term require no special precautions other than standard precautions, for either the mother or infant.

Special Considerations

The issue of work restrictions is raised frequently. When assessing the need for work restrictions for employees with herpes simplex infection, it is useful to distinguish between covered and uncovered (exposed) active lesions of herpes simplex. Personnel who have either uncovered or active lesions of herpes simplex should not work with newborn infants (term or preterm), burned patients, or immunocompromised hosts until all lesions have dried and crusted. Personnel with herpetic whitlow should be excluded from any patient care until the lesions are dried and crusted. Wearing a glove on the involved hand has been suggested as an alternative, but it is not known if this is a truly effective barrier to disease transmission. Early treatment with one of the antiherpes antivirals (acyclovir, valacyclovir, famcyclovir) may shorten the period of contagion and restriction. Personnel who have active genital herpes simplex or covered lesions of herpes simplex are not restricted from patient contact, but careful hand washing is required before and after contact with patients.

Measures to prevent herpetic whitlow include wearing gloves on both hands for direct contact with oral or pharyngeal secretions [73,79]. Gloves are especially important when suctioning patients and should be worn on both hands routinely during this procedure. Also, patients with proved or suspected herpes simplex labialis who require intensive nursing care should be placed on precautions that require the use of gloves whenever contact with these lesions is anticipated [50,69].

Although the virus has been found to survive for short periods of time outside the human body, the geometric mean titer of virus on plastic and skin surfaces declines rapidly during the first hour Figure 42-2 provides the scientific documentation for this [52]. Transmission of herpes simplex from inanimate surfaces, such as plastic and cloth, has not been documented. The consensus of epidemiologists is that such transmission is nonexistent and that HSV is transmitted via direct contact with infectious lesions.

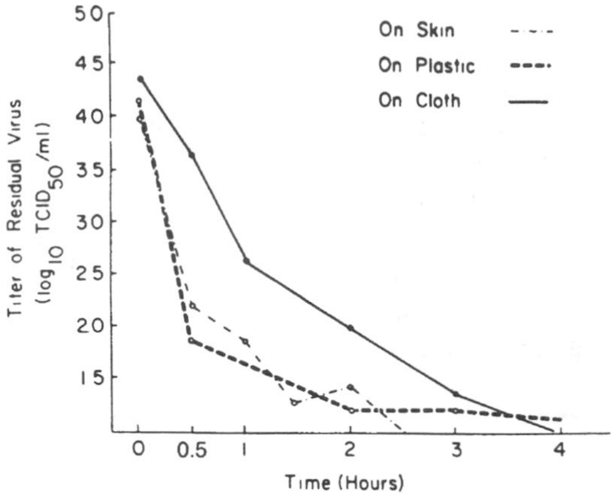

FIGURE 42-2. Geometric mean titers of residual herpesvirus in saliva. TCID, tissue culture infective dose. (Reprinted from Turner R, Shehab Z, Osborne K, Hendley O. Shedding and survival of herpes simplex virus from "fever blisters." *Pediatrics* 1982;70:547–549.)

CYTOMEGALOVIRUS

Cytomegalovirus, like other herpesviruses, requires direct contact for spread. Infection is most often via a sexually transmitted disease. The virus is found in cervical and vaginal secretions and in semen. In addition, the prevalence of CMV antibody has been found to be greater in homosexual (96%) than in heterosexual (57%) men [80]. It has also been shown to increase with years of sexual activity [81].

Occupational transmission of CMV has long been a concern of healthcare personnel because of its role in congenital malformations. Yeager [82] showed that there was no statistically significant difference in antibody conversion in pediatric nurses working with children who were shedding CMV, compared with personnel without such patient contact. One study of dialysis personnel failed to find any seroconversion after 2 years of follow-up [83]. More recently, it has been shown that pediatric healthcare workers are not at increased risk of acquiring CMV infection compared with women in the community [84,85]. Case reports have also confirmed lack of transmission of CMV from patients to healthcare personnel by using restriction endonuclease (DNA fingerprinting) techniques [86,87].

Cytomegalovirus transmission via blood transfusion has decreased considerably since 1972 [88]. This risk can also be eliminated by screening potential blood donors for antibody to CMV and by eliminating those with antibody, especially for transfusion to transplant recipients [89]. Patients undergoing renal transplantation are an important source of CMV [90] (see Chapter 45). The majority of such patients have reactivation of endogenous CMV as a result of the transplant process or from associated immunosuppressive therapy, so-called endogenous nosocomial infections [1]. A small number of transplant patients acquire CMV exogenously from the transplanted kidneys or from circulating cells present in the transplanted kidney. The use of CMV immune globulin has been effective in preventing or minimizing CMV acquisition in both renal transplant and bone marrow transplant patients [91].

Patient-to-patient transmission, although rare, has been documented by the restriction endonuclease method. Transmission probably occurred in these cases by horizontal dissemination due to close contact between children in a pediatric chronic care unit [92]. These contacts more closely resemble those in group day-care settings, where children and day-care staff seem to be at higher risk of acquiring CMV horizontally than in the traditional hospital setting [93,94]. The parents of children in group day care also show an increased risk of acquiring CMV when compared with the parents of children who stayed at home [93,94].

Precautions

Standard precautions, with frequent hand washing, represent the most important infection control barrier for patients with congenital or acquired CMV infection. Because the risk of transmission of CMV to hospital personnel is low, hospital personnel do not need to be screened for CMV antibody. Personnel should be educated regarding the mode of transmission of CMV, but pregnant personnel need not be discouraged from having contact with patients with known or suspected CMV infection, nor is transfer to an alternative assignment necessary or practical [95]. Even though many patients with HIV infection and AIDS also shed CMV, it is not necessary or practical to restrict pregnant healthcare workers from caring for these patients.

Special Considerations

Routine screening for antibody to CMV of healthcare personnel is not recommended.

EPSTEIN-BARR VIRUS

Epstein-Barr virus is shed in high concentration from the oropharynx of infected patients. Nosocomial person-to-person spread has not been documented. However, EBV is associated with several post-transplant infection syndromes and has been described after liver and renal transplantation [53] (see Chapter 45). Since transmission of EBV from the respiratory tract has not been documented in hospitals, isolation precautions other than standard precautions for patients with EBV infections are not indicated.

HEPATITIS

Hepatitis A

Nosocomial hepatitis A has been known for many years to occur in institutions for the developmentally disabled [96]. Fecal-oral transmission due to crowded conditions and the poor hygienic practices of many patients appear to be predisposing factors. Up to 80% of susceptible institutionalized patients may develop hepatitis A virus (HAV) infection, as measured by seroconversion of antibody to HAV within 3 years of admission [97]. This rate of seroconversion is considerably higher than the rate of seroconversion in noninstitutionalized adults or in child controls. Hepatitis A virus has a short incubation period of 15 to 45 days (mean, 30 days). Immunoglobulin M antibodies appear early, at about the time of onset of jaundice; peak at 4 to 6 weeks; and persist for 3 to 6 months. Hepatitis A virus does not cause chronic illness or produce side effects.

Transmission of HAV in general hospitals is relatively uncommon. Because of the very short period of viremia, transfusion of HAV by blood and blood products is rare, although it has been reported [98]. Nosocomial transmission from personnel to patients has rarely been documented. Transmission of HAV infection from patients to personnel has occurred, usually owing to breaks in technique [99,100]. Foodborne outbreaks have also taken place, primarily involving hospital workers but also small numbers of patients [101].

Precautions

Maximum fecal shedding of HAV occurs before the onset of symptoms [102]. Once the symptomatic patient with hepatitis A is admitted to the hospital, the time for maximal shedding should have passed. On the other hand, some patients who are incubating hepatitis A and shedding large amounts of virus might be admitted to ambulatory and inpatient facilities for other reasons. Also, because viral shedding can be variable, especially in infants and children [100], standard isolation precautions should be used for all patients with the addition of contact precautions for handling of feces, bedpans, and equipment or instruments contaminated with feces. Measures such as wearing gowns, gloves, and masks are not required routinely, but they should be used whenever necessary to minimize contact with feces or material contaminated with feces. Isolation in a private room is not mandatory unless the patient is incontinent of feces (see Chapter 13).

Prophylaxis

An inactivated vaccine for HAV has been licensed in the United States. The vaccine is recommended primarily for use in travelers to areas endemic for HAV [103]. However, the vaccine should be considered for patients and personnel in healthcare settings where hepatitis A is endemic, such as facilities for the developmentally disabled. Still unresolved at the time of this writing is the vaccine's more widespread use in populations who experience recurrent epidemics (e.g., among food service workers, sexually active populations, and injection drug users) [104]. Although outside of the recommendations of the Advisory Committee on Immunization Practices, vaccination of food service workers makes good sense when one considers the haphazard use of gloves on the part of food handlers and the potential for HAV transmission (see Chapter 22). Immune serum globulin (IG) is also effective in preventing or modifying hepatitis A both before exposure and early in the incubation period. If given within 2 weeks of exposure, IG will prevent 80% to 90% of HAV infections.

Hepatitis B

Nosocomial transmission of hepatitis B virus (HBV) is believed to occur most often by parenteral exposure to blood positive for hepatitis B surface antigen (HBsAg). The virus can pass from an acutely ill patient or, more likely, from an asymptomatic person who is positive for HBsAg and is unaware of it. The HBsAg carrier state accounts for the prolonged period of potential HBV infectivity of some patients even after the acute infection has resolved. The infectivity of blood is best correlated with the presence of either DNA polymerase or hepatitis B e antigen. For infection control purposes, however, all blood positive for HBsAg should be considered infectious. Although HBsAg has been detected in all body fluids, the frequency with which fluids other than blood contribute to hospital infection is probably low. The mechanisms of dissemination are by either overt or inapparent parenteral transmission [106], cited here from the lowest to the highest risk.

Overt parenteral transmission takes place via direct percutaneous inoculation by needles contaminated with serum or plasma (e.g., transfusion of contaminated blood or blood products, contaminated needle stick). Inapparent parenteral transmission happens four ways: (a) percutaneous inoculation of infective serum or plasma without overt needle puncture (e.g., contamination of cutaneous cuts, abrasions, or lacerations), (b) contamination of mucosal surfaces by infected serum or plasma (e.g., pipetting accidents, accidental ingestion, other direct contact with mucous membranes of the eye or mouth), (c) contamination of mucosal surfaces by infective secretions other than serum or plasma (e.g., sexual activity), or (d) transfer of infective material via fomites (e.g., toothbrushes, toys, drinking cups, horizontal surfaces in hospitals). Clearly, ample opportunity exists for transmission of hepatitis B to both patients and personnel in healthcare settings.

Work restrictions for the HBsAg-positive worker are the subject of controversy (see Chapter 3). The CDC Guidelines for Infection Control in Hospital Personnel states that employees who are chronic carriers of HBsAg need not be restricted from patient contact unless they have been implicated in disease transmission [60]. This recommendation is paradoxical and points out the complexity of the problem. All available evidence suggests that the greatest risk of nosocomial transmission of HBV takes place from patients to personnel [60,106,107], hence the Occupational Safety and Health Administration's (OSHA) final rule outlining the use of hepatitis B vaccine for healthcare workers [107]. Transmission of HBV from personnel to patients happens much less often. Epidemiologic data are available that show both transmission [54,108] and lack of transmission of hepatitis B [109,110] from HBsAg-positive personnel to their patients. Factors contributing to transmission of HBV from personnel to patients are probably the level and duration of antigenemia in the employee and the type of contact the employee has with the patient. Routine care of patients that does not afford contact with the blood of infected personnel does not present a risk to patients [109,110].

The physician-surgeon or dental surgeon who is HBsAg-positive may present a different degree of risk to patients when performing surgical procedures. It is not possible to make general recommendations regarding restrictions for these personnel in the operating room, since this type of evaluation should be made on an individual basis. Because high-risk personnel are vaccinated with the hepatitis B vaccine, the dilemma of the HBsAg-positive healthcare worker can be avoided through reduction in HBV transmission to healthcare workers [111].

Isolation Precautions

A private room is not required routinely for patients with acute hepatitis B (see Chapter 13), although the patient who is incontinent of feces or is bleeding is best placed in a private room. Gowns, gloves, and masks should be worn if contact with patients may also involve contact with blood or other body fluids. Gloves should be used for direct contact with blood or blood-contaminated equipment such as intravenous catheters, drains, or soiled dressings. Precautions should also be taken to avoid contact with feces or body fluids that have been contaminated with blood (see Chapter 13).

Prophylaxis

Pre-exposure Prophylaxis

The hepatitis B vaccine should be used as pre-exposure prophylaxis in high-risk persons. The vaccine is recommended for personnel at high risk owing to their regular contact with blood [107] (see Chapter 3). The high-risk groups should be selected based on the frequency of their contact with blood or needles. Other data sources from the facility include results of serologic screening done on an ongoing basis in some institutions, prevalence studies of hepatitis B markers in certain groups of employees, and records of needle punctures. Once the high-risk groups are identified in an institution, prevaccination screening for all vaccinated persons may not be necessary and will depend on the expected prevalence of hepatitis B markers and the cost of screening [105,107]. Groups of workers who were formerly screened periodically owing to their high risk of hepatitis B exposure (e.g., dialysis and laboratory workers) are automatically candidates for vaccination. In these cases, the vaccine is more cost-effective than routine screening because it offers the additional benefit of protection from hepatitis B and makes further screening unnecessary in those who respond with hepatitis B surface antibody (anti-HBs).

The OSHA standard for protection of healthcare workers from bloodborne pathogens incorporates free hepatitis B vaccine for healthcare workers who have blood contact. The key points for a hepatitis B vaccination program are [107] the following:

1. Under the OSHA final rule, all employees who have blood contact as part of their employment must be informed of the risk of hepatitis B and offered the hepatitis B vaccine at the expense of the employer. This instruction must be repeated and documented annually. This educational component must also include training on proper handling and disposal of blood, bloody instruments, sharp instruments and objects.
2. Voluntary vaccination of high-risk persons is an option under the OSHA final rule. However, employees must sign a waiver if they choose not to be vaccinated. They may be vaccinated at a later time if they choose.
3. The vaccine has been shown to be immunogenic (> 90% response with anti-Hbs after three injections of vaccine) and effective in preventing hepatitis B [112]. Clinical trials in large numbers of homosexual men have shown that the vaccine is 100% effective in preventing hepatitis B infection in those who respond with anti-HBs [112]. The rates of seroconversion have not been as high in the experience of most hospital infection control professionals. The site of injection has been suggested as one reason for variable response rates, and the deltoid muscle is now the recommended site of injection [113]. Even with response rates of 80% to 85%, however, vaccination clearly offers protection against hepatitis B in the majority of people who receive it and is an important infection control and employee health maintenance activity. The earlier plasma-derived vaccine is no longer manufactured, in favor of the two different recombinant vaccine preparations.

Postexposure Prophylaxis

Hepatitis B immune globulin (HBIG) and the hepatitis B vaccine are recommended for use as post-exposure prophylaxis for hepatitis B. These agents should be used together for the following types of contact [105]: parenteral inoculation of HBsAg-containing material, such as a needle stick or contamination of open skin with a large inoculum of HBsAg-positive blood; accidental ingestion of HBsAg-positive blood (e.g., pipetting accident); or accidental splash of HBsAg-positive blood on the mucous membranes of the eye or mouth. Ideally, prophylaxis should be given as soon as possible but certainly within 7 days of exposure. HBIG is given once at a dose of 0.06 ml/kg, at the same time as the first dose of hepatitis B vaccine. Additional doses of vaccine are given 1 and 6 months after the first dose. A second dose of HBIG is not given with this regimen. Workers who refuse the hepatitis B vaccine should be given two doses of HBIG (0.06 ml/kg each dose) 1 month apart (see Chapters 3, 23).

One of the most difficult aspects of postexposure hepatitis B prophylaxis is to determine whether the exposure was significant, that is, whether it actually involved parenteral inoculation of HBsAg-positive material. It is also important that the HBsAg status of the source be determined as soon as possible. Infection control and employee health professionals should try to apply uniform and consistent criteria when evaluating the need for prophylaxis after a hepatitis B exposure. However, the final evaluation may need to be done on an individual basis in some cases.

Infants born to mothers who are HBsAg-positive at the time of delivery should also be given hepatitis B prophylaxis to prevent development of the HBsAg carrier state. Both HBIG and the hepatitis B vaccine should be given at the time of birth. One dose of HBIG (0.5 ml) should be given along with the first dose of vaccine (0.5 ml). The additional doses of vaccine should be given 1 month and 6 months after the first [105,114]. Hepatitis B vaccine has become part of the recommended childhood vaccination strategy in the United States. This ambitious undertaking has met with slow acceptance initially, but it has the potential to change the approach to hepatitis B prevention in healthcare settings for generations to come.

Special Considerations

Postvaccination Screening

Screening for antibody (anti-HBs) should be done within 1 to 6 months after the third dose of vaccination. While postvaccine screening is not necessary for all vaccinees, it is important to establish a baseline for healthcare workers, who will need this information should an exposure to HBsAg occur. The employee who responded initially with protective levels of anti-HBs (i.e., > 10 SRU) will not need additional prophylaxis for an HBsAg exposure. Employees who fail to respond with protective levels of anti-HBs should be given two doses of HBIG following the standard protocol.

Revaccination: Booster Doses

Some vaccinees who have responded to vaccine may lose antibody over time. Since immunologic memory persists for 10 years, the current recommendation is not to revaccinate. However, many employee health professionals have chosen a more conservative stance, which uses a single booster dose of vaccine 10 years after the initial series of three injections. Employees who were originally vaccinated with the plasma-derived vaccine should be given a booster with a recombinant formulation. Others will not respond to the primary series of three injections at all. These people should be considered for revaccination with all three injections. About 15% to 25% of nonresponders will respond with anti-HBs after one injection and 30% to 50% will respond after repeating the entire series of three injections.

Interrupted Schedules

If the vaccine series is interrupted after the first dose, the second dose should be given as soon as possible and the third dose given on schedule 6 months after the first, whenever feasible. The second and third doses should be separated by an interval of 2 months.

Compliance with the OSHA Bloodborne Pathogens Rule

Hepatitis B in Hemodialysis Units

Historically, HBV has been an infection control hazard to both patients and personnel in many units [105] (see Chapters 24, 45). Hepatitis B was often introduced into the dialysis unit by HBsAg- positive patients, who probably acquired the infection from transfusion of HBsAg-positive blood. Screening of blood for HBsAg before transfusion was the first step toward a shift in our approach to dialysis-associated hepatitis. This was followed by use of hepatitis B vaccine and adoption of universal precautions [105,115]. More recently, OSHA's final rule on bloodborne pathogens, an emphasis on home dialysis, and the evolution of free-standing dialysis centers have changed the approach and risk of hepatitis B among dialysis patients and workers. These newer approaches to dialysis care have allowed dialysis settings to be handled more like other healthcare settings and less like the isolation fortresses of the past. Transmission of HBV infection from hemodialysis personnel to patients has not been reported. Transmission to personnel from either HBsAg-positive patients or contaminated equipment or environmental surfaces, on the other hand, is well documented. The greatest risk in such instances has been shown to be contact with blood or blood-contaminated materials and instruments.

Regular hepatitis screening for dialysis patients and staff has been an important component of hepatitis B prevention programs in dialysis units for many years. However, this activity has served only to monitor the introduction or transmission of HBV in dialysis units (see Chapters 3 and 24). Ideally, all dialysis candidates should be screened for hepatitis B markers (HBsAg, anti-HBs, and anti-HBc) before admission to the dialysis unit [105]. Similarly, all dialysis workers should be screened for hepatitis B markers before their employment in the unit. Vaccination, and not screening alone, offers the added advantage of providing immunity to infection, rather than merely monitoring the introduction of hepatitis B into the hemodialysis unit [116], and is cost-effective as well [117]. Once dialysis patients and personnel have been vaccinated, those who respond with protective levels of anti-HBs can be screened less frequently (e.g., yearly) to check for persistence of antibody.

Hepatitis C and Other Forms of Non-A, Non-B Hepatitis

The group of diseases called non-A, non-B hepatitis are caused by more than one agent [105]. In 1989, hepatitis C was identified as the primary cause of what previously had been called non-A, non-B hepatitis. Available data suggest that transmission in the United States is primarily parenteral, representing a significant problem among injection drug users. It is not yet possible to isolate hepatitis C virus in cell culture. However, there is one recently developed assay for hepatitis C antibody detection by polymerase chain reaction (quantitative PCR). The PCR test is more sensitive than the older hepatitis C antibody test (anti-HVC), which tends to show positive results later in the illness and is associated with a higher rate of false positivity [118]. While the PCR test does not distinguish between acute and chronic infection, it is a marker of infectivity [118].

Since the advent of donor blood testing for hepatitis C, nosocomial transmission of hepatitis C to patients has happened rarely; when it has been thought to occur, it is not easily explained [119]. Occupational risk is low, but not absent. Recent estimates of incidence come from the Italian Multicenter Study Group, which documented a rate of HCV seroconversion of 1.2% after hollow-bore needle sticks. No seroconversions were found among healthcare workers who sustained injuries with solid, sharp objects or contamination of nonintact skin or mucous membranes [120]. The same group found a hepatitis C seroconversion rate of 4% among dialysis workers with percutaneous injuries [121].

Isolation Precautions

Isolation precautions for patients with hepatitis C and other forms of non-A, non-B hepatitis are standard precautions. These precautions are the same as those for patients with hepatitis B, with an emphasis on care in handling blood or blood-contaminated articles.

Prophylaxis

There is no passive or active immunization for hepatitis C prevention. Currently available IG preparations lack appreciable hepatitis C antibody because of hepatitis C screening of the blood supply [122]. As of this writing, IG is not recommended for prophylaxis for hepatitis C [123].

RUBELLA

The introduction of rubella vaccine in 1969 has resulted in a marked decrease in the number of cases of rubella in school-aged children. The vaccine has not lowered the incidence of rubella in older age groups as dramatically, however [124,125]. From 1976 to 1979, > 70% of reported cases occurred in persons 15 years of age [125,126], and in 1980, 46.6% of patients were > 15 years [127]. Overall seronegativity among hospital employees has been reported to be as high as 14% [124]. Outbreaks of rubella in hospitals have also been reported [124,128–130]. These outbreaks emphasize the potential for transmission of rubella in institutional settings and underscore the importance of immunity against rubella to protect patients and personnel. In general, efforts to vaccinate susceptible hospital personnel on a voluntary basis, especially physicians, have been disappointing [130].

Isolation Precautions

Congenital Rubella

In congenitally acquired infection, virus may persist in pharyngeal secretions for many months after birth and may be shed for ≤ 4 years [131]. In general, these infants are not believed to be hazardous to others after ~2 to 3 years of age because little virus is shed after that time [131]. Infants with congenital rubella syndrome should be placed in private rooms and remain on precautions for the duration of hospitalization (see Chapter 13). Infants with congenital rubella who are < 2 years of age should be placed on precautions when readmitted to the hospital.

Acquired Rubella

Patients with acquired rubella or susceptible patients who have been exposed to rubella should be isolated for 21 days after exposure or for 5 days after the onset of rash.

Screening and Immunization

The current rubella strategy in the United States involves elimination of the congenital rubella syndrome, replacing an earlier narrower approach to rubella, which involved vaccination only of children or women of child-bearing age. A rubella program should be designed to prevent the introduction and spread of rubella in health-care facilities [132]. Screening for immunity is not enough. All healthcare workers, male or female, should be immune to rubella. Immunity to rubella is defined as laboratory evidence of a protective titer for rubella or evidence of vaccination with live rubella vaccine after 12 months of age [60]. Previous history of disease is not acceptable, since many exanthematous diseases can be confused with rubella [60,125]. Also, the trivalent mumps-measles-rubella (MMR) vaccine should be used whenever possible. Vaccination with MMR of persons who are already immune to one of its components is not associated with significant adverse effects [125].

Special Considerations

To prevent the transmission of rubella in outbreaks, those susceptible should be vaccinated promptly [125]. It is not recommended that pregnant women be vaccinated [125]. McLaughlin and Gold [128] have outlined restrictions during outbreaks. Personnel with rubella should not work in any area of the hospital because of the risk of transmitting disease to susceptible persons. Immune or nonexposed staff should care for pregnant patients at least during their first trimester and, whenever possible, all pregnant patients regardless of gestational stage [128]. Immune serum globulin may modify the disease in exposed persons, but its use is generally not recommended during pregnancy [128].

MEASLES (RUBEOLA)

Large hospital outbreaks of measles have been uncommon in recent years, but susceptible young healthcare workers are a potential reservoir of measles infection [129,133]. Measles has the potential to become a nosocomial pathogen again if programs are not in place to ensure immunity of healthcare workers. The public health goal of measles eradication has not been reached because of the numbers of unvaccinated preschool- and school-aged children and owing to vaccine failure. The previous recommendation of universal vaccination with one dose of live measles vaccine at 15 months of age provides long-lasting immunity for 95% of children. In recent years, however, measles outbreaks have occurred in the United States among the following groups: unvaccinated preschool-aged children, previously vaccinated school-aged children, and students and personnel on college campuses.

Isolation Precautions

Placing patients in a single room (or cohorting) and airborne precautions are required (see Chapter 13). Maintain precautions for the duration of illness.

Screening and Immunization

The currently recommended immunization schedule, an attempt to increase the pool of immune persons, calls for two doses of live measles vaccine, the first at 15 months of age for most children and the second at the time the child enters school. As with rubella, healthcare facilities should adopt policies that require immunity to measles: evidence of two live measles vaccinations, documentation of physician-diagnosed measles disease, or laboratory evidence of measles immunity for staff who will have direct contact with patients. Personnel who were born before 1957 can be considered immune. Personnel who were born in 1957 or later who have no documentation of immunity should be vaccinated at the time of employment and revaccinated 1 month later. Trivalent MMR vaccine for both injections will ensure adequate immunity to all three viruses. However, to contain costs when large numbers of personnel are vaccinated, the first injection could be given as MMR, and the second dose can be given as monovalent measles.

Mild reactions after live measles vaccination have occurred in 4% to 55% of recipients of killed vaccine. The reactions were generally a local reaction, with or without fever. These reactions are much milder than those seen with atypical measles, which occurs after killed vaccine recipients are exposed to natural measles (discussed later herein). Vaccine should be given 14 days before or deferred for 3 months after a person has received IG, blood, or blood products containing antibody.

"Modified Measles"

Measles modified by IG may be overlooked or result in delays in diagnosis. Respiratory shedding of virus does occur in patients given IG, and the isolation precautions mentioned previously should be instituted and maintained.

Atypical Measles

The atypical measles syndrome arises after exposure to wild measles virus in persons who have been vaccinated with the inactivated measles vaccine used before 1965 [134]. The illness is characterized by fever; an unusual skin rash that, like the measles rash, is maculopapular but is more likely to become petechial or hemorrhagic; and pulmonary manifestations. It appears to be caused by an altered immune response in a previously sensitized host [135]. The illness has also been recorded in persons vaccinated after 1965 with live attenuated vaccine [136]. Measles virus has not been isolated from patients with atypical measles. These patients are not believed to be infectious, and special isolation precautions, other than standard precautions, are not recommended.

Outbreak Management

In the event of an outbreak of measles in a healthcare facility, employees born in or after 1957 should be vaccinated if they have direct contact with patients and do not have proof of immunity to measles. Susceptible personnel who have been exposed should be relieved from direct patient contact from the 5th to the 21st day after exposure or, if they become ill, for 7 days after the onset of the rash.

MUMPS

Mumps virus is less communicable than either measles or varicella (chickenpox), and infections in compromised hosts have not been associated with the serious consequences that may follow measles or varicella [137]. Although nosocomial transmission has been documented [138,139], outbreaks are usually confined to families, schools, and military personnel. The use of the more expensive trivalent MMR vaccine for either rubella or measles prevention programs for healthcare workers, as noted earlier, also has its advantages in mumps prevention. Droplet precautions and placement of the patient in a private room are recommended for 9 days after the onset of parotitis, at which time infectiousness appears to decline (see Chapter 13).

PARVOVIRUS B19

Parvovirus B19 has been associated with five clinical entities: erythema infectiosum, adult arthritis, aplastic crisis in patients with diseases of increased red cell turnover (e.g., sickle cell anemia and hereditary spherocytosis), chronic anemia in immunocompromised patients, and fetal death in pregnant women. Most parvovirus B19 infections occur in children > 5 years. By age 18, 30% to 60% of adults have B19 antibodies in their serum. Parvovirus B19 transmission is not completely understood. The virus has been detected in respiratory secretions of patients with erythema infectiosum, and close contact seems to transmit the virus effectively. Spread may occur via large-particle aerosols, fomites (secretion-contaminated objects), or direct contact [140]. For example, teachers and other day-care providers were shown to be at high risk of acquiring B19 infection during outbreaks [141,142].

Erythema infectiosum is the classic B19 illness, characterized in children by a flulike illness followed by a maculopapular or erythematous macular eruption on the face, torso, and extremities. The facial rash has been described as resembling a slapped cheek. Parvovirus B19 infection usually produces a mild, self-limited illness with no serious long-term side effects in normal children and adults. The disease generally consists of a viremic phase with constitutional symptoms (myalgias, pyrexia, headache, malaise). This phase occurs 5 to 6 days after exposure and continues for 2 to 3 days. An asymptomatic period lasting 5 to 10 days follows, after which the second stage of infection occurs. This second phase continues for 1 to 2 weeks more and consists of rash and joint pains. By the time the rash appears, viremia has resolved and the patient is no longer considered infectious. The incidence of secondary transmission among healthcare workers may be as high as 50%.

The diagnosis is best made primarily through a high level of vigilance. In recent years, several diagnostic laboratory techniques have been developed to help establish the presence of acute infection. The most sensitive techniques involve detection of parvovirus B19 nucleic acids by direct DNA hybridization or PCR. Serologic techniques for IgM and IgG antibodies are thought to be less reliable, especially in compromised hosts, such as people with HIV/AIDS [143]. IgM antibody detection is done by a Western blot method. Viral-specific IgM antibodies appear in normal hosts within 3 days of infection, persist for as long as 3 weeks, and decline over several months afterward [144]. IgG antibodies indicating previous infection and immunity to parvovirus B19 may persist for several years after infection.

Parvovirus B19 infection during pregnancy has been a concern because of the potential risk to the fetus. In actuality, infants born to B19-infected women have not shown an increase in congenital malformations [145]. However, it has been recommended that pregnant healthcare workers not care for patients with known B19 infection [146,147]. The problem with this type of restriction, of course, is that most patients will be identified during the second, or rash, phase of the illness, after the period of maximum contagion. The best approach to prevention of B19 transmission involves staff education and droplet precautions in addition to standard infection control precautions, which emphasize frequent hand washing and wearing of gloves and other protective clothing when needed [60].

CREUTZFELDT-JAKOB DISEASE

Creutzfeldt-Jakob disease (CJD) is believed to be of viral origin with a long incubation period of 15 to 24 months. It is not contagious in the usual sense and does not appear to present excessive risks to hospital personnel. Sufficient concern in dealing with the transmission of CJD in hospitals has arisen in the past few years, because the diagnosis has been proved or suspected to exist in more patients. The disease has been reported to occur after corneal transplantation [148], through contaminated stereotactic electrodes used in neurosurgical procedures [149], from allogeneic dura mater graphs [150], and from injections of growth hormone of human pituitary gland origin [151].

Isolation Precautions

Precautions are recommended for patients suspected of having CJD until the diagnosis has been ruled out [152,153] (see Chapter 13). If a diagnosis is established by brain biopsy, patients are maintained on standard precautions that emphasize care in handling of all body fluids and tissue, especially blood, cerebrospinal fluid, and brain tissue [152,153]. To facilitate understanding of this disease on the part of hospital personnel, it should be stressed that these precautions are similar to those used for patients with bloodborne diseases, such as hepatitis B and HIV. Once a diagnosis of CJD has been confirmed, precautions are maintained for the duration of hospitalization and for subsequent hospitalizations.

Special Considerations

A policy should be established to ensure additional precautions in handling specimens from CJD patients and equipment and instruments used for these patients [57]. Policies and procedures for CJD should involve proper handling and sterilization of equipment and instruments used in invasive procedures before reuse. Flash sterilization should be discouraged in favor of a more rigorous process of mechanical cleaning followed by sterilization. Steam sterilization for 1 hour at 132°C is the preferred method. Soaking in one N sodium hydroxide is an alternative, but it is caustic to fragile instruments. Otherwise, high-level disinfection after thorough cleaning is acceptable for instruments with sensitive optics, such as endoscopes. Environmental surfaces can be disinfected with household bleach (undiluted or 1:10 dilution) (see Chapter 20). The widespread use of universal precautions as well as close attention to handling blood, body fluids, and instruments have made some of the precautions described previously a routine part of operations [152,153] (see Chapter 13).

GASTROENTERITIS VIRUSES

The rotaviruses are a major cause of viral diarrhea in infants and children [154]. The calicivirus-like agents (Norwalk gastroenteritis-like agents) generally cause gastroenteritis in older children and adults [154–159].

Rotavirus

The human rotavirus (human reovirus-like agent or infantile gastroenteritis virus) is a major case of gastroenteritis in infants and children during the winter in temperate climates [155]. Rotavirus disease is discussed in detail in Chapter 34.

Norwalk Gastroenteritis Virus and Related Agents

Included in this group are the Norwalk, Hawaii, W, and Montgomery County agents. These agents are major causes of viral gastroenteritis in children and adults and are associated with school, family, and community outbreaks; they probably are transmitted by fecal-oral spread (discussed later herein).

Isolation Precautions

Precautions for Norwalk gastroenteritis-like agents should be the same as for rotavirus. The period of shedding appears to be somewhat shorter than that of rotavirus [154]; therefore precautions should be maintained at least for the duration of illness. Additional precautions may be required because of explosive vomiting and the possibility of droplet spread of Norwalk and similar agents, as demonstrated in one hospital outbreak [160,161] and another on a cruise ship [162].

Special Considerations

Like rotavirus, the Norwalk gastroenteritis-like agents cannot be isolated on viral culture. The only laboratory test presently available for identifying infected materials is immune electron microscopy, which is tedious and not widely available. When rotavirus and nonbacterial pathogens have been ruled out, patients may be classified as having nonbacterial gastroenteritis other than rotavirus. Other agents, such as coronavirus-like agents, astrovirus, and mini-reovirus agents, also may be involved.

PICORNAVIRUSES

Of the three genera of the *Picornaviridae* family (enterovirus, rhinovirus, and calicivirus), the enteroviruses are the most common causes of nosocomial infection. Included in the enterovirus group are coxsackieviruses A and B, echoviruses, polioviruses, and enterovirus types 68 to 71. Enteroviruses cause sporadic disease throughout the year but are most prevalent in the community during the summer and fall in temperate climates [163]. Transmission of the virus is via the fecal-oral route, but droplet transmission has been described for coxsackie A21 and probably occurs with other enteroviruses as well [163]. Virus can be recovered easily from the oropharynx and rectum and may be shed for 1 month or more after infection. Transmission takes place among hosts with or without preexisting antibody [163].

Nonpolio Enteroviruses

Infection is common in the general population, particularly among children, and results in a variety of illnesses. Patients may be asymptomatic or have mild illness with fever, rash, and upper respiratory or gastrointestinal symptoms. Symptomatic enteroviral syndromes include severe disease in newborn infants, particularly in full-term infants, who may develop meningitis, encephalitis, myocarditis, or pericarditis in addition to the other symptoms mentioned. In older children, infection often is asymptomatic or benign. For these reasons, most of the reported nosocomial enterovirus infections have been outbreaks in neonatal units [164,165], whereas nosocomial enterovirus acquisition among older children often goes undetected.

Most nursery outbreaks involve the nonpolio enteroviruses. Often the virus is introduced into the nursery by an infected infant and is transmitted by indirect contact (i.e., from infant to infant via the hands of personnel). Infection also has been found in nursery personnel, suggesting that they may serve as sources of infection [164,165]. The most consistent mode of acquisition of nonpolio enteroviruses among infants is transmission from the mother [163,164]. Transmission may take place before, during, or after delivery. Up to 60% of the mothers whose children develop echovirus infection in the first 3 days of life have had an acute febrile illness during the last week before delivery [166]. Researchers have reported the endemic occurrence of enterovirus infection in nurseries [166]. Additional epidemiologic studies are needed, however, to determine the frequency with which infected infants are introduced into the nursery and the risk they pose to other babies and personnel.

Precautions

Because of the potentially serious consequences of enterovirus infection in newborn infants, precautions for the control of nosocomial enterovirus infection in the nursery are especially important. Infants with suspected or proved infection should be isolated in a private room or cohorted together (see Chapter 13). The cohort method of isolation may be useful in situations involving several infants and has proved to be an effective control measure in containing nursery outbreaks [166] (see Chapter 26). Contact precautions should be taken for isolating infants, using gowns and gloves for direct contact. Gowns should be changed after each contact with a patient.

The decision to close a nursery to new admissions, although difficult to make, may be necessary, especially in the case of prolonged outbreaks or if adequate cohort programs cannot be maintained. Hand washing before and after each contact with patients is required, and its importance cannot be overemphasized. Unless a particularly virulent enterovirus has been identified in the community (e.g., poliovirus or certain strains of enterovirus 71), such rigorous isolation precautions generally are not necessary for adults or for children beyond the neonatal period. Careful handling of feces and secretions and soiled objects and instruments should be the rule for all patients with enterovirus infection.

Prevention

A thorough maternal history is the best way to identify the infant at risk during the enterovirus season. A mild febrile illness in the mother during the summer may warn of infection in the infant. Any infant born to a mother who is known to have had a recent febrile illness should be placed in an observation nursery rather than the main nursery area (see Chapter 26). In addition, nursery personnel should be aware of their potential for infecting the newborn. Although it may not be possible or necessary to identify employees with these nonspecific illnesses, the importance of reporting febrile, respiratory, or diarrheal illnesses to the employee health service and the necessity for careful hand washing as part of an in-service program for nursery personnel must be emphasized (see Chapter 3).

Polioviruses

Poliovirus infection has become rare since the institution of widespread immunization programs, and wild virus transmission has been curtailed in the Western hemisphere. Nosocomial transmission of poliovirus is no longer a problem. Virus shedding may follow vaccination with live oral polio vaccine for a brief period of time. In general, paralytic poliovirus infection today is associated with the use of live oral vaccine, but this is rare [167]. Cases have occurred in recipients of live vaccine (recipient cases) or in their contacts (contact cases). The incidence of vaccine-induced paralysis in recipients is about 2.6 cases per million doses used [167].

Isolation Precautions

Children identified as having unspecified enterovirus infections should be isolated using contact precautions pending identification of the specific agent. Asymptomatic children subsequently found to be shedding poliovirus present a potential risk to certain high-risk patients, especially children with congenital immunodeficiency diseases (e.g., agammaglobulinemia, hypogammaglobulinemia, combined immunodeficiency states). It is recommended that as a precaution, unimmunized children or children with congenital or acquired immunodeficiency states not be placed in the same room as children who are known to be shedding poliovirus. However, routine screening of hospitalized children for poliovirus is not recommended.

Immunization

Routine vaccination of adults is not recommended. However, unvaccinated adults should receive primary vaccination with 3 doses of inactivated polio vaccine (IPV) because the risk of vaccine-associated paralysis (VAPP) with oral polio vaccine (OPV) is higher in adults than in children [125].

The risk for VAPP caused by OPV is now judged less acceptable because of the diminished risk for wild-virus-associated disease (indigenous or imported). Consequently, ACIP recommends a transition policy that will increase use of IPV and decrease use of OPV during the next 3 to 5 years. For overall public health benefit, ACIP recommends a sequential vaccination schedule of two doses of IPV followed by two doses of OPV for routine childhood vaccination.

In some situations, exclusive use of IPV or OPV alone is recommended, including IPV alone for children who are immunosuppressed; OPV alone for children who begin the primary vaccination schedule after 6 months of age, and IPV alone for immunization of unvaccinated adults.

Implementation of these recommendations should reduce the risk for vaccine-associated paralytic poliomyelitis in OPV recipients by 95% and facilitate a transition to exclusive use of IPV following further progress in global polio eradication [125].

Special Considerations

Enteroviruses are unusually stable and resist many commonly used disinfectants (e.g., 70% alcohol, 5% Lysol, and 1% quaternary ammonium compounds). The most effective virucidal agent is 5% sodium hypochlorite solution, which may be used for surface decontamination but is corrosive to metal, including stainless steel (see Chapter 20).

RHABDOVIRUS: RABIES

Although nosocomial rabies is uncommon, two cases have been documented of human-to-human transmission of rabies from corneal transplantation [167]. Both donors had obscure neurologic illnesses, one resembling Guillain-Barré syndrome and the other a flaccid paralysis. Because of this atypical presentation, the diagnosis of rabies was not suspected before the death of either donor, and their tissues were considered acceptable for transplantation.

Hospital personnel also are theoretically at risk when exposed to patients with rabies in whom the diagnosis may not be suspected before death [168,169]. In an investigation of hospital personnel exposed to one such patient, many employees were unable to recall the extent of exposure 15 to 43 days earlier. Because of this and because of the long duration of hospitalization of the index case, 198 of 371 hospital employees were believed to have had significant rabies exposure and were advised to receive postexposure rabies prophylaxis [169]. Laboratory personnel working with bat colonies and other potentially rabid animals also are at increased risk of this disease. Laboratory-associated rabies, presumably transmitted by aerosolization of laboratory virus strains, has been reported, resulting in revised safety recommendations for laboratory personnel working with rabies virus [170].

Isolation Precautions

Standard isolation precautions are recommended for the duration of illness in patients with proved or suspected rabies (see Chapter 13).

Immunization

Human diploid cell rabies vaccine (HDCV) [170] is recommended for persons with documented rabies exposure, for those who have had probable or possible exposure, and for pre-exposure prophylaxis of laboratory workers working with bats or other potentially rabid animals. Postexposure prophylaxis of hospital personnel should be handled according to established recommendations [170]. In addition, local wounds should be cleansed with soap and water [171]. Pre-exposure prophylaxis of laboratory workers at high risk also should be undertaken. Personnel should not work with potentially rabid animals until a complete series of vaccine has been administered.

Another vaccine preparation—rabies vaccine, adsorbed—is also licensed and available for pre- and postexposure prophylaxis. This vaccine is limited to use in the state of Michigan and was developed and is produced and distributed by the Biologics Products Program of the Michigan Department of Public Health. The dosing schedule is the same as with HDCV. This vaccine may cause less serum-sickness-like reactions because its preparation does not involve the use of the small amount of human serum albumin used in the HDCV preparation [172].

Special Considerations

The potential for transmission of rabies and other viral pathogens in transplanted tissues presents problems in evaluating potential donors. In general, corneas from patients who have died with a diagnosis of dementia, encephalopathy, undiagnosed neurologic illness, multiple sclerosis, conjunctivitis, or other viral diseases, including hepatitis B, rabies, or Creutzfeldt-Jakob disease, should not be used for the purposes of corneal transplantation. Corneas in such cases may be accepted for research purposes if they are labeled a biohazard.

ARENAVIRUSES

Lymphocytic choriomeningitis has been implicated as a cause of outbreaks of flulike illness with aseptic meningitis in laboratory workers and other hospital personnel [173]. It is not known to be transmitted from person to person in hospitals other than after contact with laboratory animals. Standard isolation precautions are required for patients with lymphocytic choriomeningitis infection.

PAPILLOMAVIRUSES

The human papillomaviruses (HPVs) are small, double-stranded DNA viruses that affect the skin and mucous membranes and cause warts and other benign tumors. The natural history of these tumors is variable, with some regressing spontaneously and others becoming malignant. There is good evidence to show that HPVs are sexually transmitted viruses. There is also a high prevalence of HPV-associated malignancies in the male sexual partners of women with genital cancers [174]. Other studies have shown an association between squamous cell carcinomas and genital warts [175]. Clinically, these associations point to the importance of early detection and treatment of HPV-associated genital lesions.

Laser therapy or vaporization has become a popular way of treating HPV condyloma, warts, and associated growths. Patients with laryngeal, cervical, and skin lesions may benefit from carbon dioxide laser therapy. The carbon dioxide laser generates a vapor or plume as it destroys these HPV-associated growths, and intact viral DNA has been shown to be liberated into the air with the vapor of laser-treated warts [176]. There are anecdotal reports of healthcare workers using lasers who have developed warts on their hands and fingers, suggesting work-related transmission.

Therefore, as a first step, infection control and employee health personnel need to be trained in laser safety programs in their facilities. With the widespread availability of the laser, current safety practices are probably variable. The most practical solution for now is proper maintenance of equipment, including the suction and exhaust apparatus. Lasers should also be operated in well-ventilated areas. It also makes sense for laser operators to wear masks, gowns, gloves, and protective eyewear in the universal precautions mode, as they would for any procedure that generates an aerosol [176].

VIRAL HEMORRHAGIC FEVERS

Ebola virus and Marburg virus are the two known members of the filovirus family. Ebola viruses were first isolated from humans during concurrent outbreaks of viral hemorrhagic fever (VHF) in northern Zaire and southern Sudan in 1976. An earlier outbreak of VHF caused by Marburg virus occurred in Marburg, Germany, in 1967, when laboratory workers were exposed to infected tissue from monkeys imported from Uganda. Two subtypes of Ebola virus, Ebola-Sudan and Ebola-Zaire, previously have been associated with disease in humans. In 1994, a single case of infection from a newly described Ebola virus was documented in a person from Cote d'Ivoire (Ivory Coast), Africa. In 1989, an outbreak among monkeys imported into the United States from the Philippines was caused by another Ebola virus but was not associated with human disease.

Initial clinical manifestations of Ebola hemorrhagic fever include fever, headache, chills, myalgia, and malaise; subsequent manifestations include severe abdominal pain, vomiting, and diarrhea. Maculopapular rash may occur in some patients within 5 to 7 days of onset. Hemorrhagic manifestations with presumptive disseminated intravascular coagulation usually accompany fatal cases. In reported outbreaks, 50% to 90% of cases have been fatal.

The natural reservoirs for these viruses are not known. Although nonhuman primates were involved in the 1967 Marburg outbreak, the 1989 U.S. outbreak, and the 1994 Cote d'Ivoire case, their role as virus reservoirs is unknown. Transmission of the virus to secondary cases occurs through close personal contact with infectious blood or other body fluids or tissue. In previous outbreaks, secondary cases developed among persons who provided medical care for patients; secondary cases also appeared among patients exposed to reused needles. Although aerosol spread has not been documented among humans, this mode of transmission has been confirmed among nonhuman primates. Based on this information, the high fatality rate, and the lack of specific treatment or a vaccine, work with this virus in the laboratory requires biosafety level 4 containment [177,178]. More recently, an outbreak of viral hemorrhagic fever caused by Ebola virus occurred in Zaire [177–179]. Of the almost 100 patients, none were found who did not have direct contact with another known infected patient.

The necessary precautions outlined by the CDC are in keeping with universal or standard precautions and should prevent delays or denial of medical care while maximizing the safety of hospital staff and patients (see Chapter 13). The recommendations apply only to patients who, within 3 weeks of onset of fever, have traveled in an area of a country where cases of VHF have recently been noted; who have had direct contact with blood or other body fluids, secretions, or excretions of a person or animal with VHF; or who have worked in a laboratory or animal facility that handles hemorrhagic fever viruses. The recommendations note that the likelihood of acquiring VHF is considered extremely low in persons who do not meet any of these criteria. The cause of fever in persons who have traveled in areas where VHF is endemic is more likely to be a different infectious disease, such as malaria or typhoid fever.

Pending testing for Ebola antigen and Ebola antibody by enzyme-linked immunosorbent assay and reverse transcription polymerase chain reaction for viral RNA, the recommendations for patients with suspected VHF are summarized briefly.

1. In the early stages of disease, most ill persons undergoing pre-hospitalization evaluation would not be expected to have symptoms that increase the likelihood of contacts' exposure to infectious body fluids (vomiting, diarrhea, hemorrhage), and universal or standard precautions are considered sufficient.
2. A private, negative-pressure room should be used, and nonessential staff should not enter the room. Caretakers should use contact barrier precautions, which include the wearing of gowns and gloves by those entering the room. Other barriers should be used (e.g., face shields or masks) if there is a possibility of coming in contact with blood or vomitus.
3. Additional precautions to prevent exposure to airborne particles should be taken if there is prominent cough, vomiting, or diarrhea. In addition to placing the patient in a negative-pressure room, personal protective respirators similar to those used for pulmonary tuberculosis should be used.
4. Care should be taken with the use and disposal of sharp objects and needles.
5. Clinical laboratory specimens should be limited to those needed for diagnosis and good patient care. Specimens should be placed in plastic bags that are sealed and transported in clearly labeled, durable, leakproof containers. Specimens should be handled in class II biological safety cabinets using biosafety level 3 practices. Serum used in laboratory tests should be pretreated with 10 μl of 10% Triton X-100

per ml of serum for 1 hour to reduce (but not eliminate) the titer of hemorrhagic fever virus in serum. Autoanalyzers should be disinfected as recommended by the manufacturer.

6. Environmental surfaces can be disinfected with an Environmental Protection Agency (EPA)-registered hospital disinfectant or a 1:100 dilution of household bleach.
7. Soiled linens should be placed in clearly labeled leakproof bags at the site of use. Linens can be decontaminated in a gravity displacement autoclave, incinerated, or washed in a washing machine with bleach.
8. Before bulk blood, suctioned fluids, secretions, or excretions are disposed of, they should be decontaminated by autoclave, processed in a chemical toilet, or treated with several ounces of undiluted household bleach for > 5 minutes.
9. If a patient dies, the body should be handled minimally after death. The corpse should be wrapped in leakproof material and either cremated or buried promptly in a sealed casket.
10. Persons with percutaneous or mucocutaneous exposures to blood or body fluids should immediately wash the affected skin surfaces with soap and water. Mucous membranes, such as conjunctivas, should be irrigated with copious amounts of water or eyewash solution.

For further information, the CDC has established a hot line for public inquiries about Ebola virus infection and prevention—(800) 900–0681.

METHODS OF PREVENTING SPREAD OF VIRUSES

Cohort Isolation Precautions

Cohort isolation generally consists of two groups of people, an infected group and an uninfected group, that are separated from each other. Occasionally a third group, an exposed group, is separated from the uninfected group and cared for separately from both of the other groups. This method of separation may involve the use of geographically distinct rooms or, if they are not available, physical separation in the same room. To ensure complete separation of cohorts, geographically separate rooms are preferable and should be used whenever possible. The separation of hospital staff often is overlooked, but this also is essential to a successful cohort program. Although it is not always possible to separate house staff and support personnel, the nursing staff caring for infected and noninfected cohorts should be separated as much as possible without disrupting staffing or services to patients. If possible, those caring for infected patients should be immune to the disease in question or receiving prophylactic treatment or vaccine. This immunity may be determined by previous infection or vaccination and may be identified by appropriate history of illness, vaccination, or antibody testing.

In cohort programs for viral illness, especially respiratory viruses, the same groups of personnel ideally should care for the same cohort for the duration of isolation. This plan minimizes the risk of transmission of infection to the uninfected cohort. Personnel who have recently recovered from the viral illness under consideration also may care for the infected cohort. In other cohort programs (e.g., staphylococcal outbreaks in nurseries), personnel may work with different cohorts on different days but not during the same day. In many instances, groups of personnel, such as house staff and support personnel, cannot be restricted as easily. In these situations, personnel should see patients in the "clean" area first, then go to the "dirty" area.

Separation of groups on the basis of symptoms alone will not guarantee that all members of the cohort have the same illness. It is important to take appropriate steps to confirm the suspected diagnosis as quickly as possible, to ensure proper cohorting of patients. More detailed guidelines for the use of cohort programs are presented in Table 42-1.

The cohort method of isolation may involve small numbers of patients or hospital staff, such as in clusters of infections in intensive care units. Other uses of cohorting may call for restriction of larger groups of patients and personnel, for example, in outbreaks of viral respiratory infections, such as RSV [24]. In general, however, cohort programs using geographically separate areas of the same room are not recommended for the control of viral respiratory infections.

Communicable Disease Survey ("Contagion Check")

The purpose of the communicable disease survey (contagion check) is to screen pediatric patients and visitors quickly to determine whether they are currently infected or have been exposed to and are incubating any communicable diseases. The main concern of the survey is to prevent the introduction of varicella into the hospital, but other illnesses, such as measles, mumps, and viral respiratory illnesses, also should be considered. A contagion check should be done for every pediatric patient and child visitor and is especially important during periods of peak virus activity in the community.

Before the admission of a pediatric patient to the hospital, information regarding the child's immunization history, susceptibility to chickenpox, and history of recent exposure to chickenpox should be obtained. A staff mem-

TABLE 42-1. *General guidelines for use of cohort isolation*

1. Patients should be separated into cohorts of infected ("dirty") and noninfected ("clean") patients.
2. Only persons with proved or suspected infection should be admitted to the infected cohort.
3. All exposed (potentially infected) persons should be included with the cohort of infected patients; in some instances, the potentially infected cohort may be separated into a third cohort.
4. The infected cohort should be closed to new, uninfected admissions, and all new, uninfected admissions should be placed with the uninfected cohort.
5. Personnel working with the infected cohort should be immune to the illness in question by either history of illness or vaccination *whenever possible.*
6. Personnel should be assigned so that separate groups work with the infected and uninfected cohorts *whenever possible*; crossover between cohorts should be discouraged to minimize the risk of cross-infection of the uninfected cohort.
7. Ideally, personnel should be separated for the duration of the cohort program, especially when viral illnesses are proved or suspected.
8. When personnel must work in both areas, they should work in the "clean" area first, then in the "dirty" area.
9. The infected cohort area should be closed as patients are discharged from the hospital and may be used for new uninfected admissions after thorough cleaning of the area and its equipment.

(Reproduced from Valenti WM, Menegus MM. Nosocomial virus infections. IV. Guidelines for cohort isolation, communicable disease survey, collection and transport of specimens for virus isolation. *Infect Control* 1981;2:236–245.)

ber should ask these questions. For child visitors, screening could be done by a volunteer stationed at the entrance to the unit, the unit secretary, or nursing staff. For patients being admitted to the hospital, the contagion check should be done by the nurse admitting the patient to the unit or by the admitting physician.

Questions that may yield additional helpful information, shown in Table 42-2, may be included in the communicable disease survey, especially for child visitors. This survey is relatively uncomplicated and assists in screening patients who present potential hazards to susceptible patients and personnel. Susceptible pediatric patients who have been exposed to proved or suspected viral illnesses are placed on precautions, as previously noted.

Infection Control and the Pregnant Healthcare Worker

Employee health personnel and infection control personnel are often consulted by the pregnant employee regarding contact with patients who have various infectious diseases (see Chapter 3). In these situations, the concern is not only for the pregnant employee but also for the fetus, who may be at risk of infection in the perinatal period. To counsel patients effectively in these matters, employee health personnel should be familiar with the mode of transmission of the various infectious agents as well as their risk to the pregnant employee. The educational gain from these visits may be all that is required to resolve the employee's concerns. The infectious processes that generate the most concern among pregnant employees include viral agents, such as HIV, CMV, HSV, hepatitis B, rubella, and VZV [95].

Work Restrictions for the Pregnant Employee

It may sometimes be advisable to restrict particular types of contact between infected patients and pregnant personnel. However, the transfer of pregnant employees to other areas of the hospital or other positions is proba-

TABLE 42-2. *Items to include in a communicable disease survey ("contagion check")*

Essential components for patients
- Immunization history
  - Measles, mumps, rubella
  - Polio
  - Diphtheria, pertussis, tetanus
  - Hepatitis B
  - Varicella
- Has the child had or recently been exposed to chickenpox?

Other considerations, especially for child visitors
- Has the child had or recently been exposed to the following?
  - Measles
  - Mumps
  - German measles
  - Hepatitis
- Does the child have any of the following now or has the child had any recently?
  - Streptococcal infection
  - Cough, cold, or upper respiratory infection of any kind
  - Diarrhea
  - Vomiting
  - Fever
  - Rash
  - Infection of any kind

(Adapted from Valenti WM, Menegus MM. Nosocomial virus infections. IV. Guidelines for cohort isolation, communicable disease survey, collection and transport of specimens for virus isolation. *Infect Control* 1981;2:236–245.)

TABLE 42-3. *Recommendations for work restriction for pregnant employees*

Disease	Restriction: No contact	Restriction: Follow isolation precautions	Comment
Cytomegalovirus			
Congenital		X	Risk of transmission very low in health care settings
Acquired		X	
Herpes simplex			
Genital		X	
Other		X	
Varicella zoster virus	X[a]	If immune	If history of chickenpox is negative or unknown, employee should not have contact with patients with chickenpox or herpes zoster until immunity is proved or employee is vaccinated.
Parvovirus B19	X		
Rubella	X[a]	If immune	Ideally, employee should be immune to rubella according to testing at employment or via vaccination.
Hepatitis B		X	Employees at risk should be vaccinated against hepatitis B.

[a]Until immunity is proved by serologic testing.

bly not necessary and is difficult to manage in most situations. A practical approach should be developed to deal with the issue of the pregnant healthcare worker in much the same way that the infection control personnel deal with work restriction in other infection control situations, taking into consideration the safety of the employee as well as the protection of the patient.

Pregnancy by itself does not usually make an employee more susceptible to acquiring infectious diseases from patients. Transferring employees during pregnancy may not be realistic, since the same infectious hazards may be present throughout the healthcare facility. In addition, routine movement of personnel may create an unnecessary burden on the departments

TABLE 42-4. *Interaction of factors in nosocomial transmission of viruses*

Virus	Transmissibility	Susceptibility of staff or other patients	Resultant nosocomial risk
Respiratory viruses			
Influenza	High	Variable[a]	High
Respiratory syncytial virus	High	High	High
Rhinovirus	Moderate	Moderate[a]	Moderate
Other (e.g., adenovirus, coronavirus)	Moderate	Moderate[a]	Moderate
Hepatitis B			
Needle sticks	High	High	High
Other exposure	Low	High	Low
Herpesviruses			
Herpes simplex I	Low	Moderate[a]	Low
Herpes simplex II	Very low	Moderate[a]	Very low[b]
Varicella (chickenpox) or disseminated zoster	High	Very low[a]	Low[a]
Herpes zoster (localized)	Moderate	Very low[a]	Very low
Epstein-Barr virus	Very low	Very low[a]	Very low
Cytomegalovirus	Low	Moderate[a]	Very low[c]
Human immunodeficiency virus	Very low	Low	Very low
Parvovirus	Moderate	Moderate	Moderate
Rubella	High	Moderate[a]	High

[a]High in pediatric age groups.
[b]Except to newborn during delivery or after rupture of membranes.
[c]Except for blood transfusion or organ transplantation.
(Adapted from Valenti WM, Menegus MM. Nosocomial virus infections. IV. Guidelines for cohort isolation, communicable disease survey, collection and transport of specimens for virus isolation. *Infect Control* 1981;2:236–245.)

involved. Recommendations for work restriction for pregnant employees are noted in Table 42-3 and have been reviewed previously [95].

Special Considerations

It is important to emphasize that some viral agents are more easily transmitted than others. Personnel may respond with extraordinary concern when caring for patients with CMV infection, whereas influenza vaccination programs and precautions for other more highly contagious viruses are often overlooked. Table 42-4 reviews briefly the relative risk of transmission to hospital personnel and patients of commonly encountered viruses.

Notification of Emergency Response Employees

An obscure amendment to the Ryan White CARE Act [180], effective April 1994, mandates that healthcare facilities must provide information to emergency response employees of exposure to potentially infectious diseases. Under this amendment, health facilities are required to provide this information to a so-called designated officer of the emergency response organization if the organization requests it. The list of potentially hazardous infectious diseases includes a number of viruses and is given in Table 42-5. The importance of this legislation is that it addresses an often troublesome area in infection control and outlines a process for communication between healthcare facilities and emergency response organizations. This federal regulation also says that it is the responsibility of the states to ensure that all reporting falls within their codes for confidentiality of medical information. Reporting and notification of infectious diseases exposure by the facility should be given to a designated officer of the emergency response organization.

TABLE 42-5. *Notification of emergency response employees: notifiable diseases by mode of transmission*

Airborne
Infectious pulmonary tuberculosis
Bloodborne
Hepatitis B
HIV
Uncommon or rare diseases
Diphtheria (*Corynebacterium diphtheriae*)
Meningococcal disease (*Neisseria meningitides*)
Plague (*Yersinia pestis*)
Hemorrhagic fevers
Lassa, Marburg, Ebola, Crimean-Congo, and others yet to be identified
Rabies

The healthcare facility presents a unique challenge to virologists and infection control professionals as they attempt to develop comprehensive programs for the control and prevention of viral infections. The continued development of antiviral chemotherapy, rapid viral diagnostic techniques, and new strategies for vaccine use and the ongoing evolution of our approach to isolation precautions provide opportunities to manage this important aspect of infection control.

Acknowledgment

The significant contributions of Paul F. Wehrle in preparing the chapters on nosocomial viral infections for the previous editions are gratefully acknowledged.

REFERENCES

1. Valenti WM, Menegus MA, Hall CB, et al. Nosocomial viral infections. I. Epidemiology and significance. *Infect Control* 1980;1:33–37.
2. Hall CB. Nosocomial viral respiratory infections: perennial weeds on pediatric wards. *Am J Med* 1981;70:670.
3. Mintz L, Ballard RA, Sniderman SH, et al. Nosocomial respiratory syncytial virus infections in an intensive care nursery: rapid diagnosis by immunofluorescence. *Pediatrics* 1979;64:149–153.
4. Valenti WM, Clarke TA, Hall CB, et al. Concurrent outbreaks of rhinovirus and respiratory syncytial virus in an intensive care nursery: epidemiology and associated risk factors. *J Pediatr* 1982;100:722–726.
5. Mathur U, Bentley DW, Hall CB. Concurrent respiratory syncytial virus and influenza A infections in the institutionalized elderly and chronically ill. *Ann Intern Med* 1980;93:49.
6. VanVoris LP, Belshe RB, Shaffer JL. Nosocomial influenza B in the elderly. *Ann Intern Med* 1982;96:153.
7. Valenti WM. Infection control, HIV, and home healthcare. I. Risk to the patient. *Am J Infect Control* 1994;22:371–372.
8. Valenti WM. Infection control, HIV, and home healthcare. II. Risk to the caregiver. *Am J Infect Control* 1995;23:78–81.
9. Valenti WM. Influenza viruses. In: Mayhall CG, ed. *Hospital epidemiology and infection control*. Baltimore: Williams and Wilkins, 1996.
10. Centers for Disease Control and Prevention. National Coalition for Adult Immunization: activities to increase influenza vaccination levels, 1989–1991 *MMWR* 1992;41:772–776.
11. Graman PS, Hall CB. Epidemiology and control of nosocomial infections. *Infect Dis Clin North Am* 1989;3:815.
12. Valenti WM, Menegus MM. Nosocomial virus infections. IV. Guidelines for cohort isolation, communicable disease survey, collection and transport of specimens for virus isolation. *Infect Control* 1981;2: 236–245.
13. Douglas RG Jr. Influenza in man. In: Kilbourne ED, ed. *The influenza viruses and influenza*. New York: Academic Press, 1975.
14. Hall CB, Douglas RG Jr. Nosocomial influenza as a cause of intercurrent fever in infants. *Pediatrics* 1975;55:673.
15. Patriarca PA, Arden NH, Koplan JP, Goodman RA. Prevention and control of type A influenza infections in nursing homes. *Ann Intern Med* 1987;107:732–740.
16. Centers for Disease Control and Prevention. Prevention and control of influenza. I. Vaccines: recommendations of the Advisory Committee on Immunization Practices (ACIP). *MMWR* 1994;43(RR-9):1–12.
17. Treanor J, Mattison HR, Dumyati G, et al. Protective efficacy of combined live intranasal and inactivated influenza A virus vaccines in the elderly. *Ann Intern Med* 1992;117:625–633.
18. Centers for Disease Control and Prevention, *Managing an influenza vaccination program in the nursing home*. Atlanta: Centers for Disease Control and Prevention, 1987.
19. Centers for Disease Control and Prevention. Control of influenza A outbreaks in nursing homes: amantadine as adjunct to vaccine, 1989–1990. *MMWR* 1991;40:841–844.

20. Degelau J, Somani SK, Cooper SL, Guay DR, Crossley KB. Amantadine-resistant influenza A in a nursing facility. *Arch Intern Med* 1992; 152:390–392.
21. Barton MB, Schoenbaum SC. Improving influenza vaccination performance in an HMO setting: the use of computer generated reminders. *Am J Public Health* 1990;80:534–536.
22. Nichol KL, Lind A, Margolis KL, et al. The effectiveness of vaccination against influenza in healthy, working adults. *N Engl J Med* 1995; 333:890–893.
23. Hall CB. The shedding and spreading of respiratory syncytial virus. *Pediatr Res* 1977;11:236.
24. McCarthy CA, Hall C. Prevention of nosocomial respiratory syncytial virus in the pediatric patient. *Infect Med* 1990;7:4.
25. Henderson FW, Collier AM, Clyde WA Jr, Denny FW. Respiratory syncytial virus infections, reinfections, and immunity: a prospective longitudinal study in young children. *N Engl J Med* 1979;300: 530–534.
26. Takimoto CH, Cram DL, Root RK. Respiratory syncytial virus infections, reinfections on an adult medical ward. *Arch Intern Med* 1991; 151:706–708.
27. Hall CB, Douglas RG Jr., Geiman JM. Possible transmission by fomites of respiratory syncytial virus. *J Infect Dis* 1980;141:98.
28. Hall CB, McBride, JT, Walsh EE, et al. Aerosolized ribavirin treatment of infants with respiratory syncytial viral infection. *N Engl J Med* 1983;308:1443–1447.
29. Liss HP, Bernstein J. Ribavirin aerosol in the elderly. *Chest* 1988;93: 1239–1241.
30. Mufson MA, Mocega HE, Krause HE. Acquisition of parainfluenza 3 virus infection by hospitalized children. I. Frequencies, rates, and temporal data. *J Infect Dis* 1973;128:141.
31. DeFabritis AM, et al. Parainfluenza type 3 in a transplant unit. *JAMA* 1979;241:384.
32. Centers for Disease Control. Parainfluenza outbreaks in extended-care facilities. *MMWR* 1978;27:475.
33. Meissner HC, Murray SA, Kiernan, MA, et al. A simultaneous outbreak of respiratory syncytial virus and parainfluenza virus 3 in a newborn nursery. *J Pediatr* 1984;104:680–684.
34. Wals TG, Shult P, Krause P, et al. A rhinovirus outbreak among residents of a long term care facility. *Ann Intern Med* 1995;123:588–593.
35. Gwaltney JM, Mosalski PB, Hendley JO. Hand-to-hand transmission of rhinovirus. *Ann Intern Med* 1978;88:453.
36. Hendley JP, Wenzel RP, Gwaltney JM. Transmission of rhinovirus colds by self-inoculation. *N Engl J Med* 1973;288:1362.
37. Dick EC, Jennings LC, Mink KA, et al. Aerosol transmission of rhinovirus colds. *J Infect Dis* 1987;156:442–448.
38. Hendley JO, Mika LA, Swaltney JM. Evaluation of virucidal compounds for inactivation of rhinovirus on hands. *Antimicrob Agents Chemother* 1978;14:690.
39. Foy HM, Grayston JT. Adenoviruses. In: Evans AS, ed. *Viral infections of humans: epidemiology and control*, 2nd ed. New York: Plenum Press, 1982:67–84.
40. Middleton PJ, Azymanski MT, Petric PJ. Viruses associated with acute gastroenteritis in young children. *Am J Dis Child* 1977;131:233.
41. Hierholzer JC. Adenovirus in the immunocompromised host. *Clin Microbiol Rev* 1992;5:262–274.
42. Centers for Disease Control and Prevention. Epidemic keratoconjunctivitis in an ophthalmology clinic California. *MMWR* 1990;39:598.
43. Straube RC, Thompson MA, Van Dyke RB, et al. Adenovirus type 7b in a children's hospital. *J Infect Dis* 1983;147:814–819.
44. Finn A, Anday E, Talbot GH. An epidemic of adenovirus 7a in a neonatal nursery: course, morbidity, and management. *Infect Control Hosp Epidemiol* 1988;9:398–404.
45. Larsen RA, Jacobson JT, Jacobson JA, et al. Hospital-associated epidemic of pharyngitis and conjunctivitis caused by adenovirus (212/H21-35). *J Infect Dis* 1986;154:706–709.
46. Maddox A, Frances N, Moss J, et al. Adenovirus infection of the large bowel in HIV-positive patients. *J Clin Pathol* 1992;45:684–688.
47. Ambinder RF, Burns W, Forman M, et al. Hemorrhagic cystitis associated with adenovirus infection in bone marrow transplantation. *Arch Intern Med* 1986;146:1400–1401.
48. Sprague JB, et al. Epidemic keratoconjunctivitis. *N Engl J Med* 1977;289:1341.
49. Jawetz E, et al. Laboratory infection with adenovirus type 8: laboratory and epidemiologic observations. *Am J Hyg* 1979;69:13.
50. Wentworth BB, Alexander ER. Seroepidemiology of infections due to members of the herpes virus group. *Am J Epidemiol* 1971;94:496.
51. Meyers JD, MacQuarrie MB, Merigan TC, Jennison MH. Nosocomial varicella. I. Outbreak in oncology patients at a children's hospital. *West J Med* 1979;130:196.
52. Turner R, Shehab Z, Osborne K, Hendley JO, et al. Shedding and survival of herpes simplex virus from "fever blisters." *Pediatrics* 1982;70:547.
53. Morrison VA, Dunn DL, Manivel JC, et al. Clinical characteristics of post-transplant lymphoproliferative disorders. *Am J Med* 1994;89: 14–24.
54. Welch J, Webster M, Tilzey AJ, et al. Hepatitis B infections after gynaecological surgery. *Lancet* 1989;1:205–207.
55. Morens DM, et al. An outbreak of varicella-zoster virus infection among cancer patients. *Ann Intern Med* 1980;93:414.
56. Gustafson JL. An outbreak of nosocomial airborne varicella. *Pediatrics* 1982;70:550.
57. Leclair JM, et al. Airborne transmission of chickenpox in a hospital. *N Engl J Med* 1980;302:450–453.
58. Gershon AA, LaRussa P. Varicella-zoster virus infections. In: Krugman S, et al., eds. *Infectious diseases of children*, 9th ed. St. Louis: Mosby Year Book, 1993:587–614.
59. Hayden CF, Meyers JD, Dixon RE. Nosocomial varicella. II. Suggested guidelines for management. *West J Med* 1979;130:300.
60. Department of Health and Human Services, Centers for Disease Control and Prevention. Draft Guideline for infection control in healthcare personnel, 1997. *Fed Reg* 1997;62:47275–47327.
61. Zaia JA, Oxman MN. Antibody to varicella-zoster-virus-induced membrane antigen: immunofluorescence assay using monodisperse glutaraldehyde target cells. *J Infect Dis* 1977;136:519.
62. Haiduven DJ, Hench, CP, Stevens DA. Postexposure varicella management of nonimmune personnel: an alternative approach. *Infect Control Hosp Epidemiol* 1994;15:329–334.
63. Centers for Disease Control and Prevention. *Varicella prevention: recommendations of the Immunization Practices Advisory Committee* (in press).
64. Gershon AA. Human responses to live attenuated varicella vaccine. *Rev Infect Dis* 1991;13(suppl):957–959.
65. Preblud SR. Varicella: complications and costs. *Pediatrics* 1986;78 (suppl):728–735.
66. Feldman S, Moffitt JE. Varicella vaccine. *Pediatr Ann* 1990;19: 721–726.
67. Centers for Disease Control and Prevention. Recommendation of the Immunization Practices Advisory Committee (ACIP): Varicella-zoster immune globulin for the prevention of chickenpox. *MMWR* 1984;33:84.
68. Berlin BS, Campbell T. Hospital-acquired herpes zoster following exposure to chickenpox. *JAMA* 1970;211:1831.
69. Gershon AA, Kalter ZG, Steinberg S. Detection of antibody to varicella-zoster virus by immune adherence hemagglutination. *Proc Soc Exp Biol Med* 1976;151:762.
70. Ross AH. Modification of chickenpox in family contacts by administration of gamma globulin. *N Engl J Med* 1962;267:369.
71. Foley FD, Greenwald KA, Nash MC, Pruitt BA. Herpes virus infection in burned patients. *N Engl J Med* 1970;282:652.
72. Naragi S, Jackson GG, Jonasson OM. Viremia with herpes simplex type 1 in adults. *Ann Intern Med* 1976;85:165.
73. Greaves WL, et al. The problem of herpes whitlow among hospital personnel. *Infect Control* 1980;1:381.
74. Blank H, Haines HG. Experimental reinfection with herpes simplex virus. *J Invest Dermatol* 1973;61:223.
75. Linneman CC Jr., et al. Transmission of herpes simplex virus type I in a nursery for the newborn: identification of viral isolates by DNA fingerprinting. *Lancet* 1978;1:964.
76. Manzella J, et al. An outbreak of herpes simplex virus stomatitis in a dental practice. *JAMA* 1984;252:2019.
77. Nahmias AN, et al. Perinatal risk associated with maternal genital herpes simplex virus infection. *Am J Obstet Gynecol* 1971;110:825.
78. Kibrick S. Herpes simplex infection at term: what to do with mother, newborn, and nursery personnel. *JAMA* 1980;243:157.
79. Valenti WM, et al. Nosocomial viral infections. II. Guidelines for prevention and control of respiratory viruses, herpesviruses, and hepatitis viruses. *Infect Control* 1980;1:165.
80. Drew WL, et al. Prevalence of cytomegalovirus infection in homosexual men. *J Infect Dis* 1981;143:188.
81. Weller TH. The cytomegaloviruses: ubiquitous agents with protean manifestations. *N Engl J Med* 1971;285:203.
82. Yeager AS. Longitudinal serological study of cytomegalovirus in nurses and personnel without patient contact. *J Clin Microbiol* 1975; 2:448.

83. Tolkoff-Rubin NE, et al. Cytomegalovirus infection in dialysis patients and personnel. *Ann Intern Med* 1978;89:625.
84. Balcarek KB, Bagley R, Cloud GA, et al. Cytomegalovirus infection among employees of a children's hospital: no evidence for increased risk associated with patient care. *JAMA* 1990;263:840.
85. Dworskey ME, Welch K, Cassady G, Stagno S. Occupational risk for primary cytomegalovirus infection among pediatric healthcare workers. *N Engl J Med* 1983;309:950.
86. Wilfert CM, Huang E, Stagno S. Restriction endonuclease analysis of cytomegalovirus deoxyribonucleic acid as an epidemiologic tool. *Pediatrics* 1982;70:717.
87. Yow MD, et al. Use of restriction enzymes to investigate the source of primary cytomegalovirus infection in a pediatric nurse. *Pediatrics* 1982;70:713.
88. Wilhelm JA, Matter L, Schopfer K, et al. The risk of transmitting cytomegalovirus to patients receiving blood transfusions. *J Infect Dis* 1986;154:169–171.
89. Preiksaitis JK. Indications for the use of cytomegalovirus seronegative blood products. *Transfus Med Rev* 1991;5:1–17.
90. Chou S. Acquisition of donor strain cytomegalovirus by renal transplant recipients. *N Engl J Med* 1986;314:11418–1423.
91. Meyers JD, Lesszczynski J, Zaia JA, et al. Prevention of cytomegalovirus infection by cytomegalovirus immune globulin after marrow transplantation. *Ann Intern Med* 1983;98:442–447.
92. Demmler GJ, Yow MD, Spector SA, et al. Nosocomial cytomegalovirus infections within two hospitals caring for infants and children. *J Infect Dis* 1987;156:9–16.
93. Adler SP. Cytomegalovirus and child day care: evidence for increased infection rate among day-care workers. *N Engl J Med* 1991;321:1290–1296.
94. Murph JR, Baron JC, Ebelhack CL, et al. The occupational risk of cytomegalovirus infection among day care providers. *JAMA* 1991;265:603–608.
95. Valenti WM. Infection control and the pregnant healthcare worker. *Nurs Clin North Am* 1995;28:673–686.
96. Matthew EB, et al. A major epidemic of infectious hepatitis in an institution for the mentally retarded. *Am J Epidemiol* 1973;98:199.
97. Szmuness W, Purcell RH, Dienstag JL, Stevens CE. Antibody to hepatitis A antigen in institutionalized mentally retarded patients. *JAMA* 1977;237:1702.
98. Hollinger FB, Khan NC, Oefinger PE. Postransfusion hepatitis A. *JAMA* 1984;250:2313–2317.
99. Centers for Disease Control. Outbreak of viral hepatitis in the staff of a pediatrics ward—California. *MMWR* 1977;26:77.
100. Rosenblu LS, Villarino ME, Nainan OV, et al. Hepatitis A outbreak in a neonatal intensive care unit: risk factors for transmission and evidence of prolonged viral excretion among preterm infants. *J Infect Dis* 1991;164:476–482.
101. Meyers JD, Romm FJ, Then WS, Bryan JA. Food-borne hepatitis A in a general hospital. *JAMA* 1975;231:1049.
102. Dienstag JL, et al. Fecal shedding of hepatitis A antigen. *Lancet* 1975;1:765.
103. Centers for Disease Control and Prevention. Prevention of hepatitis A through active or passive immunization practices (ACIP). *MMWR Morb Mortal Wkly Rep* 1996;45:1–30.
104. Margolis HS, Alter MJ. Will hepatitis A become a vaccine-preventable disease? *Ann Intern Med* 1995;122:464–465.
105. Centers for Disease Control and Prevention. Recommendation of the Immunization Practices Advisory Committee (ACIP): protection against viral hepatitis. *M.M.W.R* 1990;39(52):1.
106. Favero MS, Alter MA, Bland LA. Nosocomial infections associated with hemodialysis. In: Mayhall CG, ed. *Hospital epidemiology and infection control.* Baltimore: Williams and Wilkins, 1996.
107. Department of Labor. Occupational exposure to bloodborne pathogens: final rule. *Federal Register* Dec. 6, 1991:64175. (Amendment of part 1910 of Title 29 of the Code of Federal Regulations.)
108. Rimland D, et al. Hepatitis B traced to an oral surgeon. *N Engl J Med* 1977;296:953.
109. Meyers JD, et al. Lack of transmission of hepatitis B after surgical exposure. *JAMA* 1978;240:1725.
110. Gerber MA, et al. The lack of transmission of type B hepatitis in a special care nursery. *J Pediatr* 1977;91:120.
111. Thomas DL, Factor S, Kelen G, et al. The declining risk of hepatitis B and C in healthcare workers at the Johns Hopkins Hospital. *Arch Intern Med* 1993;153:1705–1712.
112. Szmuness W, Stevens CE, Jarley EJ, et al. Hepatitis B vaccine: demonstration of efficacy in a controlled clinical trial in a high risk population in the United States. *N Engl J Med* 1980;303:833.
113. Centers for Disease Control and Prevention. Suboptimal response to hepatitis B vaccine given by injection into the buttock. *MMWR* 1985;34:105.
114. Tada H, et al. Combined passive and active immunization for preventing perinatal transmission of hepatitis B virus carrier state. *Pediatrics* 1982;70:613.
115. Moyer LA, Alter MJ, Favero MS. Hemodialysis-associated hepatitis B: revised recommendations for serologic screening. *Semin Dial* 1990;3:201–204.
116. Szmuness W, Stevens CE, Jarley EJ, et al. Hepatitis B vaccine in medical staff of hemodialysis units: efficacy and subtype cross protection. *N Engl J Med* 1982;307:4181.
117. Alter MJ, Favero MS, Francis DP. Cost benefit of vaccination for hepatitis B in hemodialysis centers. *J Infect Dis* 1983;148:770–771.
118. Tedeschi V, Seef LB. Diagnostic tests for hepatitis C: Where are we now? *Ann Intern Med* 1995;123:383–385.
119. Allander T. Frequent patient-to-patient transmission of hepatitis C virus in a haematology ward. *Lancet* 1995;345:603–607.
120. Puro V, Petrosillo N, Ippolito M, and the Italian Study Group. Risk of hepatitis C seroconversion after occupational exposures. *Am J Infect Control* 1995;23:273–277.
121. Petrosillo N, Puro V, Jagger J, et al. The risks of occupational exposure and infection by HIV, hepatitis B virus, and hepatitis C virus in the dialysis setting. *Am J Infect Control* 1995;23:278–285.
122. Miller MA, Orenstein P, Amihod B. Administration of immune serum globulin following the exposure to hepatitis C virus. *Clin Infect Dis* 1993;16:35.
123. Pugliese G. Data lacking for postexposure prophylaxis with immune serum globulin following HCV exposure. *Infect Control Hosp Epidemiol* 1994;15:212.
124. Centers for Disease Control and Prevention. Rubella in hospitals in California. *MMWR* 1983;32:37.
125. Centers for Disease Control and Prevention. Poliomyelitis prevention in the United States: introduction of a sequential vaccination schedule of inactivated poliovirus vaccine followed by oral poliovirus vaccine. Recommendations of the Advisory Committee on Immunization Practices. *MMWR* 1997;46(no. RR-3):1–25.
126. Centers for Disease Control and Prevention. Recommendations for rubella prevention. *MMWR* 1990;39(no. RR-15):1.
127. Hethcote HW. Measles and rubella in the United States. *Am J Epidemiol* 1983;117:2.
128. McLaughlin MC, Gold LH. The New York rubella incident: a case for changing hospital policy regarding rubella testing and immunization. *Am J Public Health* 1979;69:287.
129. Poland GA, Nichol K. Medical students as sources of rubella and measles outbreaks. *Arch Intern Med* 1990;150:44.
130. Polk BF, White JA, DeGirolami PC, Modlin JF. Outbreak of rubella among hospital personnel. *N Engl J Med* 1980;303:541.
131. Shewmon DA, Cherry JD, Kirby SE. Shedding of rubella virus in a four–five-year-old boy with congenital rubella. *Pediatr Infect Dis* 1982;1:342.
132. Weiss KE, et al. Evaluation of an employee health service as a setting for a rubella screening and immunization program. *Am J Public Health* 1979;69:281.
133. Atkinson WL. Measles and healthcare workers. *Infect Control Hosp Epidemiol* 1994;15:5–7.
134. Nadar PR, Horowitz MS, Rousseau J. Atypical exanthem following exposure to natural measles: eleven cases in children previously inoculated with killed vaccine. *J Pediatr* 1968;72:22.
135. Fulginiti VA, Arthur JM. Altered reactivity to measles virus: skin test reactivity and antibody response to measles virus antigens in recipients of killed measles virus vaccine. *J Pediatr* 1979;75:604.
136. Cherry JD, et al. Atypical measles in children previously immunized with attenuated measles virus vaccine. *Pediatrics* 1973;50:712.
137. Feldman HA. Mumps. In: Evans AS, ed. *Viral infections of humans: epidemiology and control*, 3rd ed. New York: Plenum, 1989: 471–491
138. Sparling D. Transmission of mumps [Letter]. *N Engl J Med* 1979;280:276.
139. Wharton M, et al. Mumps transmission in hospitals. *JAMA* 1990;150:47.
140. Cossart YE, Field AM, Cant B, Widdows D. Parvo-like particles in human sera. *Lancet* 1975;1:72.
141. Adler SP, Manganello AM, Koch WC, et al. Risk of human parvovirus

B19 infections among school and hospital employees during endemic periods. *J Infect Dis* 1993;168:361–368.
142. Gillespie SM, Cartter ML, Asch S, et al. Occupational risk of human parvovirus B19 infection for school and day care personnel during an outbreak of eytema infectiosum. *JAMA* 1990;263:2062–2065.
143. Chernak E, Dubin G, Henry D, et al. Infection due to parvovirus B19 in patients infected with the human immunodeficiency virus. *Clin Infect Dis* 1995;20:170–173.
144. Jones M, Wold AD, Espy MJ, Smith TF. Serologic diagnosis of parvovirus B19 infection. *Mayo Clin Proc* 1993;68:1107–1108.
145. Anderson L, Hurwitz E. Human parvovirus B19 infection and pregnancy. *Clin Perinatol* 1988;15:273.
146. Committee on Infectious Diseases. Parvoviruses, erythema infectiosum and pregnancy. *Pediatrics* 1990;85:131.
147. Centers for Disease Control and Prevention. Risks associated with human parvovirus B19 infection. *MMWR* 1989;38:81.
148. Duffy P, Wolf J, Collins G, et al. Possible person-to-person transmission of Creutzfeldt-Jakob disease [Letter]. *N Engl J Med* 1974;290:692.
149. Benoulli C, et al. Danger of accidental person-to-person transmission of Creutzfeldt-Jakob disease by surgery. *Lancet* 1977;1:478.
150. Marx RE, Carlson ER. Creutzfeldt-Jakob disease from allogeneic dura: a review of risks and safety. *J Oral Maxillofac Surg* 1991;49:272.
151. Fradkin JE, et al. Creutzfeldt-Jakob disease in pituitary growth hormone recipients in the United States. *JAMA* 1991;265:880.
152. American Neurological Association. Precautions in handling tissues, fluids, and other contaminated materials from patients with documented or suspected Creutzfeldt-Jakob Disease. *Ann Neurol* 1986;19:75–77.
153. Greenlee JE. Containment precautions in hospitals for cases of Creutzfeldt-Jakob disease. *Infect Control* 1982;3:222.
154. Kapikian AZ, Chanock RM. Viral gastroenteritis. In: Evans AS, ed. *Viral infections in humans: epidemiology and control*, 3rd edition. New York and London: Plenum Press, 1991:293–340.
155. Le Baron CW, et al. Annual rotavirus epidemic patterns in North America. *JAMA* 1990;264:983.
156. Meurman OH, Laine MJ. Rotavirus epidemic in adults. *N Engl J Med* 1977;296:1289.
157. Marrie TJ, Lee SH, Faulkner RS, et al. Rotavirus infection in a geriatric population. *Arch Intern Med* 1982;142:313–316.
158. Hildreth C, Thomas M, Ridgway GL. Rotavirus infection in an obstetric unit. *Br Med J* 1981;282:231–232.
159. Bolivar R, et al. Rotavirus in travelers' diarrhea: study of an adult student population in Mexico. *J Infect Dis* 1978;137:324.
160. Sawyer LA, Murphy JJ, Kaplan JE, et al. 25-to-30 nm virus particle associated with a hospital outbreak of acute gastroenteritis with evidence for airborne transmission. *Am J Epidemiol* 1988;127:1261–1271.
161. Caul EO. Small round structured viruses: airborne transmission and hospital control. *Lancet* 1994;343:1240–1242.
162. Ho MS, Glass RI, Monroe SS. Viral gastroenteritis aboard a cruise ship. *Lancet* 1989;2:961–965.
163. Melnick JL. Enteroviruses. In: Evans AS, ed. *Viral infections in humans: epidemiology and control*, 3rd ed. New York: Plenum, 1991: 191–263.
164. Modlin JF. Perinatal echovirus and group B coxsackievirus infections. *Clin Perinatol* 1988;15:233–246.
165. Casolane DJ, Long AM, McKeever PA, et al. Prevention of spread of echovirus 6 in a special care baby unit. Arch Dis Child 1985;60: 674–676.
166. Modlin JF. Perinatal echovirus infection: insights from a literature review of 61 cases of serious infection and 16 outbreaks in nurseries. *Rev Infect Dis* 1986;8:919–926.
167. Nkowane BM, Wassilak SG, Orenstein WA, et al. Vaccine-associated paralytic poliomyelitis. United States: 1973–1984. *JAMA* 1987;257: 1335–1340.
168. Helmick CG, Tauxe RV, Vernon AA. Is there risk to contacts of patients with rabies? *Rev Infect Dis* 1987;9:511–518.
169. Centers for Disease Control and Prevention. Human rabies—Pennsylvania. *MMWR* 1979;28:75.
170. Centers for Disease Control and Prevention. Recommendation of the Immunization Practices Advisory Committee (ACIP): rabies prevention United States. *MMWR* 1991;40:1(no. RR-3):1–16.
171. Anderson LJ, Winkler WG. Aqueous quaternary ammonium compounds and rabies treatment. *J Infect Dis* 1979;139:494.
172. Centers for Disease Control and Prevention. Rabies vaccine, adsorbed: a new vaccine for use in humans. *MMWR* 1988;37:217–218,223.
173. VanZee BE, et al. Lymphocytic choriomeningitis in university hospital personnel. *Am J Med* 1975;58:803.
174. Barrasso R, et al. High prevalence of papillomavirus-associated penile intraepithelial neoplasia in sexual partners of women with cervical intraepithelial neoplasia. *N Engl J Med* 1987;317:916.
175. Rando R. Human papillomaviruses: implications for clinical medicine. *Ann Intern Med* 1988;108:628.
176. Garden JM, et al. Papillomavirus in the vapor carbon dioxide laser-treated verrucae. *JAMA* 1988;259:1199.
177. Centers for Disease Control and Prevention. Outbreak of Ebola viral hemorrhagic Fever—Zaire, 1995. *MMWR* 1995;44:381–382.
178. Centers for Disease Control and Prevention. Reemergence of Ebola virus in Africa. *Emerging Infect Dis* 1995;1:1–13.
179. Centers for Disease Control and Prevention. Update: management of patients with suspected viral hemorrhagic fever—United States. *MMWR* 1995;44:475–479.
180. Centers for Disease Control and Prevention. Implementation of provisions of the Ryan White Comprehensive AIDS Resources Emergency Act Regarding Emergency Response Employees. *Federal Register* March 21, 1994;59(54):13418–13428.

Hospital Infections, Fourth Edition,
edited by John V. Bennett and Philip S. Brachman.
Published by Lippincott–Raven Publishers, Philadelphia, 1998

CHAPTER 43

Human Immunodeficiency Virus Infection

Mary E. Chamberland and David M. Bell

In this chapter, we review available data on the risk of human immunodeficiency virus (HIV) transmission in healthcare settings, current strategies to reduce this risk, and some unresolved issues and prospects for the future. Unless otherwise specified, all data pertain to HIV-1. Few data are available regarding nosocomial transmission of HIV-2, which is uncommon outside of Africa, but has the same modes of transmission as HIV-1 [1].

TRANSMISSION FROM PATIENTS TO HEALTHCARE WORKERS

Monitoring Occupationally Acquired HIV Infection

The National HIV/AIDS Surveillance System of the Centers for Disease Control and Prevention (CDC) has monitored reports of healthcare workers (HCWs) with AIDS (acquired immunodeficiency syndrome) and occupationally acquired HIV infection. As of June, 1995, the CDC had received reports from state and local health departments of over 300,000 adults with AIDS, for whom occupational information was known; 4.8% had been employed in healthcare settings. In comparison, ~ 5.7% of the U.S. labor force is employed in health services. Of the HCWs with AIDS, 93% reported one or more nonoccupational risks for acquiring HIV. The remaining 7% did not report a nonoccupational risk; for many of these, it will not be possible to determine whether infection was acquired occupationally because of incomplete information [2].

In 1991, the CDC expanded surveillance to include reports of cases of occupationally acquired HIV infection, regardless of whether the AIDS case definition is met. HCWs with AIDS or HIV infection are classified as "documented" or "possible" cases of occupational transmission. With two exceptions, people classified as having documented cases have evidence of HIV seroconversion (i.e., from documented HIV seronegative to seropositive status) temporally associated with an occupational percutaneous, mucous membrane, or cutaneous exposure. The two exceptions are people who worked with concentrated HIV and were determined by HIV DNA sequence analysis to be infected with these HIV strains, although the time of exposure was not determined (Metler R, CDC, personal communication). People classified as having possible cases of occupational infection have been investigated by state or local health departments and are without identifiable behavioral or transfusion risks. Each of these HCWs reported percutaneous or mucocutaneous occupational exposure to blood or body fluids or laboratory solutions containing HIV. However, HIV seroconversion temporally associated with an occupational exposure was not documented.

As of December, 1995, 49 documented and 102 possible cases of occupationally acquired infection among HCWs in the United States were reported to the CDC (Table 43-1). Of the 49 people with documented cases, 44 were exposed to HIV-infected blood, 1 was exposed to visibly bloody fluid from a patient with HIV infection, 1 to an unspecified fluid (through an unknown sharp object in a waste container), and 3 to concentrated HIV in a laboratory. Forty-two (86%) workers sustained percutaneous, five (10%) mucocutaneous, and one (2%) both percutaneous and mucocutaneous exposures; one HCW (2%) had an unknown route of exposure to concentrated virus. Hollow-bore needles caused 39 (91%) of the 43 percutaneous injuries [3]. At least 27 documented and 40 possible cases of occupationally acquired HIV infection have been reported from other countries; the circumstances of these cases are similar to those in the United States [4]; also, see Heptonstall et al., Occupational transmission of HIV:

M. E. Chamberland: Division of Viral and Rickettsial Diseases
D. M. Bell: Office of the Director, Division of Antimicrobial Resistance, National Center for Infectious Diseases, Centers for Disease Control and Prevention, Atlanta, Georgia 30333.

TABLE 43-1. *U.S. healthcare workers with documented and possible occupationally acquired HIV infection, reported through December, 1995*

Occupation	Documented occupational transmission no.	Possible occupational transmission no.
Dental worker, including dentist	—	7
Embalmer/morgue technician	—	3
Emergency medical technician/paramedic	—	9
Health aide/attendant	1	12
Housekeeper/maintenance worker	1	7
Laboratory technician, clinical	15	15
Laboratory technician, nonclinical	3	0
Nurse	19	24
Physician, nonsurgical	6	10
Physician, surgical	—	4
Respiratory therapist	1	2
Technician, dialysis	1	2
Technician, surgical	2	1
Technician/therapist, other than those listed above	—	4
Other healthcare occupations	—	2
Total	49	102

(From Centers for Disease Control and Prevention. *HIV/AIDS surveillance report.* 1995;7(2):15.)

Summary of Published Reports to July 1995 (London: Public Health Laboratory Service, in press). In addition, home caregivers, such as friends and relatives, have occasionally acquired HIV infection while providing nursing and custodial care to HIV-infected patients [5].

Seroprevalence surveys have supplemented national surveillance in assessing the extent of occupationally acquired HIV infection (Table 43-2). Multiple HIV seroprevalence studies among surgical, medical, and dental HCWs have had similar findings, with HIV infection

TABLE 43-2. *HIV seroprevalence in selected groups of healthcare workers*

Worker Group	No. tested	No. positive (%)	No. positive with nonoccupational risk	Prevalence, (%) excluding seropositives with nonoccupational risk	Reference
Orthopedic surgeons	3,420	2 (0.06)	2	0.00	[6]
Surgeons in high AIDS incidence areas (USA)	770	1 (0.13)	0	0. 14	[7]
Medical personnel in U.S. Army Reserve	58,394	138 (0.24)	N/A	N/A	[8]
Dentists					
San Francisco	304[a]	0 (0)	—[a]	0	[9]
USA 1986 annual meeting and New York City	1,132[a]	1 (0.09)	—[a]	0.09	[10]
USA 1987 annual meeting	1,195	0 (0)	0	0	[11]
USA 1988 annual meeting	1,165	1 (0.09)	0	0.09	[11]
USA 1989 annual meeting	1,480	0 (0)	0	0	[11]
USA 1990 annual meeting	1,466	0 (0)	0	0	[11]
USA 1991 annual meeting	1,642	0 (0)	0	0	CS[b]
USA 1992 annual meeting	1,812	0 (0)	0	0	CS[b]
USA 1993 annual meeting	2,035	0 (0)	0	0	CS[b]
USA 1994 annual meeting	1,687	0 (0)	0	0	CS[b]
Dental assistants and hygienists (New York City and Sacramento)	343	0 (0)	0	0	[10,12]
Hemodialysis staff (New York, Paris, Chicago, Brussels, Florence)	356	0 (0)	0	0	[13 –17]
Blood donors (USA, six urban regions)	8,519	3 (0.04)	0 –1	0 – 0.01	[18]
Morticians					
Massachusetts	133	1 (0. 75)	1	0	[19]
Maryland	130	1 (0. 77)	1	0	[20]

N/A, not available.
[a]Persons with community risk not included.
[b](C. Siew American Dental Association, personal communication.)

rates of < 1 per 1,000 workers tested [6–20]. Relatively few seroprevalence surveys have been conducted among HCWs in developing countries, where the HIV seroprevalence among patients is high and resources for infection control are limited. In the few studies that have been conducted, rates of HIV infection in medical workers were generally similar to those in the community [21,22].

Human immunodeficiency virus seroprevalence studies have limitations. Rates of infection may be underestimated if workers who knew or suspected that they might be positive declined to be tested. The extent of occupational or community exposure to HIV is often not known or poorly characterized. Nevertheless, these studies are helpful in that they do not suggest a high rate of HIV infection among the HCWs studied.

Risk of Occupational HIV Infection

Several investigators have estimated the cumulative risk of occupational HIV infection. For example, The U.S. General Accounting Office estimated that in the 130 Department of Veterans Affairs acute care medical centers, one HCW would acquire HIV infection from a work-related needle injury every 3.5 years [23]. Gerberding and coworkers estimated that one occupational HIV infection may occur among surgical personnel at San Francisco General Hospital every 8 years [24]. The annualized risk of occupational HIV infection has been estimated to range from 0.0005% to 0.002% for a hospital emergency department physician or nurse in a low–HIV-seroprevalence area [25] and from 0.027% to 0.046% for a resident physician or medical student in Los Angeles [26]. In comparison, the annual risk of death due to a motor vehicle accident among 25- to 30-year-old people is 0.032% [26]. These estimates are subject to many limitations, including simplified assumptions and incomplete data.

The risk of occupational acquisition of HIV by a HCW is likely related to multiple factors; three of the more important include the prevalence of HIV among patients treated by the HCW; the risk of transmission after a single contact with blood; and the nature and frequency of blood contact.

HIV Seroprevalence Among Patients

In the United States, patient HIV seroprevalence varies widely. In the CDC Sentinel Hospital Study, leftover blood specimens from patients treated in 1989 to 1991 in 20 acute care hospitals in 15 U.S. cities were tested anonymously for HIV antibody [27]. Of 195,829 blood specimens tested, 4.7% were positive. HIV seroprevalence ranged from 0.2% in hospitals in Nebraska and Utah to 14.2% in a hospital in New York City. HIV seroprevalence was highest among men 25 to 44 years of age, and among patients presenting with pneumonia, other infections, or drug-related conditions. Only 32.4% of the HIV-positive patients presented with symptoms attributable to HIV infection. In this study, patient HIV seroprevalence was approximately 10.4 times the hospital's AIDS diagnosis rate (the number of new cases of AIDS diagnosed per 1,000 discharges) in 1990.

Similarly, seroprevalence studies among patients presenting to emergency departments, operating rooms, and obstetric suites have demonstrated considerable variation. For example, among patients in hospital emergency departments, HIV seroprevalence has ranged from 0.2 per 100 patient visits in a suburban hospital to 6% of patients at Johns Hopkins Hospital; most of these infections were unknown to HCWs treating them [25,28]. Many patients in these studies were coinfected with another bloodborne pathogen [28,29]. Montecalvo and associates at Westchester County Medical Center in Valhalla, New York, surveyed 1,062 surgical procedures, and determined that if patients had been tested for HIV alone, 76% of patients with a potentially infectious bloodborne pathogen (e.g., hepatitis B and C) would not have been detected [29].

Risk of HIV Infection After Exposure

The risk of HIV infection after a documented exposure to HIV-infected blood has been estimated in prospective studies conducted worldwide. In a CDC surveillance project in the United States, as of March, 1995, 1373 workers were enrolled after a percutaneous exposure to HIV-infected blood and tested at least 6 months later; 4 (0.29%) seroconverted to HIV [30]. Aggregating data from this and 22 other studies, 6135 HCWs were followed prospectively after a percutaneous exposure to HIV-infected blood, and 20 (0.33%; 95% confidence interval (CI) = 0.20% to 0.50%) became infected [4,30–33]. The risk estimate of 0.3% represents an average of many types of percutaneous exposures to blood from patients in various stages of HIV infection. There are undoubtedly subsets of exposures for which the risk is higher, and lower, than 0.3%. In vitro studies suggest that the volume of blood transferred in needlestick injuries is greater for more deeply penetrating injuries; for hollow-, compared with solid-bore, needles; and when the needle does not pass through glove material [34,35]. Because these differences in volume are generally within one order of magnitude, Gerberding and coworkers have noted that the most important determinant of transmission risk is likely to be the titer of HIV in the source patient's blood, which may vary by several orders of magnitude over the course of HIV infection [34,36]. It is also possible that the HCW's immune response may be important [37].

More recently, retrospective case–control methods have been used to identify risk factors for HIV seroconversion among HCWs after a percutaneous exposure to HIV-infected blood. In a collaborative study involving investigators in the United States, France, and the United Kingdom, 31 HCWs who seroconverted after exposure were compared with 679 HCWs who did not [38]. Multivariate analysis identified several risk factors, including a "deep" injury, visible blood on the device causing the injury, injury by a device previously placed in the source patient's vein or artery (e.g., a needle used for phlebotomy), the source patient being in the terminal stage of AIDS (i.e., death due to AIDS within 60 days postexposure), and lack of postexposure zidovudine (ZDV) use by the HCW (Table 43-3). Limitations of this study include its retrospective nature, the fact that cases and control subjects came from different sources, inability to exclude the possibility of biased reporting of exposures and infections to national surveillance systems, and that ZDV was not offered according to a standard protocol. Despite these limitations, the risk factors identified appear to be biologically plausible.

Assessment of the risk of HIV transmission after a mucous membrane or skin exposure has been more difficult because of the low number of seroconversions among workers with such exposures enrolled in prospective studies. In a report from Italy, a HCW seroconverted after extensive contact of eyes, mouth, and hands with a large amount of blood from a patient with asymptomatic HIV infection; aggregating this study with five others, Ippolito et al. estimated the risk after a mucous membrane exposure at 0.09% (1/1107; 95% CI = 0.006% to 0.50%) [33].

The risk after a skin exposure to HIV-infected blood is believed to be less than after other types of exposure, but has not been precisely quantified because no HCWs enrolled in prospective studies have seroconverted after an isolated skin exposure. In the largest study of HCWs with skin contact with HIV-infected blood, none of 2,712 workers at the National Institutes of Health (NIH) Clinical Center who recalled such contact seroconverted (0%; upper limit of 95% CI = 0.11%) [32]. At the same institution, Fahey and colleagues reported no HIV seroconversions among HCWs who estimated having had 20,028 skin contacts with blood from all patients, including an estimated 6,528 contacts with HIV-infected blood [39].

Although HIV has been detected in a variety of body fluids [40], occupational transmission to HCWs has been documented only for blood and visibly bloody fluids. There are insufficient data to estimate precisely the risk of HIV infection after occupational exposure to body fluids other than blood. There are, however, considerable data to indicate that HIV transmission does not occur through casual contact [41,42] and that the risk after occupational exposure to secretions and excretions not containing visible blood, if present at all, is extremely low [4]. For example, in questionnaire surveys, employees at the NIH Clinical Center reported 2,856 skin exposures to fluids other than blood (804 sputum, 912 urine, 300 feces, and 840 other fluids) from HIV-infected patients; none resulted in HIV transmission [32]. In addition, HIV transmission through saliva and respiratory secretions has not been demonstrated in epidemiologic studies among household contacts of people with HIV infection [41–43] or in (a relatively small number of) HCWs after exposure to saliva of infected patients [32,44,45]. HIV transmission from bites involving blood-contaminated saliva or extensive tissue trauma has been reported [46] (Metler R, CDC, unpublished data).

Although inhalation of particles of aerosolized blood (i.e., particles < 50 to 100 μm in diameter that, unlike droplets, may remain suspended in air for an extended period of time) may pose a theoretical risk of bloodborne pathogen transmission, no case of such transmission has been documented (see Chapter 1). Aerosols of blood require considerable mechanical energy to generate (e.g., power equipment) and are unlikely to be present in most clinical settings. Hepatitis B surface antigen (HBsAg) could not be detected in the air of dental operatories during treatment of hepatitis B carriers, including during procedures known to generate aerosols [47]. In a laboratory study using blood to which HIV had been added, certain surgical power instruments produced vapors that in some instances contained infective HIV [48]. The clinical significance of this experiment is uncertain, because HIV sero-

TABLE 43-3. *Risk factors for HIV infection in health care workers after percutaneous exposure to HIV-infected blood, based on a case–control study (France, United Kingdom, and United States, January, 1988–August, 1994)*

Risk factor	Adjusted odds ratio[a]	(95% confidence interval)
Deep injury	16.1	(6.1–44.6)
Visible blood on device	5.2	(1.8–17.7)
Procedure involving needle placed directly in source-patient's vein or artery	5.1	(1.9–14.8)
Terminal illness in source patient	6.4	(2.2–18.9)
Postexposure use of zidovudine	0.2	(0.1–0.6)

[a]All were significant at $p < 0.01$.

(From Centers for Disease Control and Prevention. Case–control study of HIV seroconversion in health-care workers after percutaneous exposure to HIV-infected blood: France, United Kingdom, United States, January 1988—August 1994. *MMWR Morb Mortal Wkly Rep* 1995;44:929–933.)

surveys of orthopedic surgeons and dentists do not suggest a risk of HIV transmission by aerosol [6] (see Table 43-2).

Epidemiology of Blood Contact

Surveillance and epidemiologic studies have described the nature and frequency of blood exposures involving HCWs and patients, defined risk factors for exposure and infection transmission, and, more recently, evaluated preventive measures. Many of these studies used trained observers who had no other duties (e.g., in operating rooms) than prospectively to collect exposure data, or, for procedures that could not be readily observed, interviewed HCWs or asked them (e.g., physicians and nurses on medical services) to record exposures on a daily or weekly basis. Such approaches have been necessary because self-reporting of blood exposures by HCWs is often incomplete or biased [49,50]. For example, one study found that the proportion of percutaneous injuries that were reported to the hospital ranged from 89% for phlebotomists to 30% for residents [50].

Based on prospective studies of the frequency of blood exposure per procedure performed or per shift worked by an individual HCW, annual rates of blood contact have been estimated for workers in various occupational groups in the United States [25,51–56] (Table 43-4). These figures are crude estimates that are not applicable to every worker in each occupational group. Also, all exposures may not be comparable. For example, most of the surgeons' exposures are due to solid-bore suture needles, as discussed later. Solid needles inject a smaller quantity of blood and so are probably less likely to transmit infection than hollow-needle exposures, which are more likely to be sustained by other HCWs, such as physicians and nurses on medical wards.

Several observational studies have found at least one sharp injury in 1.3% to 15.4% of surgical procedures [57]. These results vary with the study methodology and the procedures observed. For example, Tokars et al. observed 99 percutaneous injuries during 95 (6.9%) of 1,382 operations in 5 surgical specialties (general, orthopedic, gynecologic, cardiac, and trauma) [51]. Injury rates were highest on the gynecology service (10%); residents and attending surgeons had the highest rates (2.5 and 2.1 per 100 person-procedures, respectively). In terms of targeting preventive measures, there were some interesting observations. Most injuries in surgeons occurred during suturing; injuries in scrub nurses and technicians usually involved exchange of sharp instruments to and from the surgeon or self-inflicted injury while loading or disposing of needles and blades; and 24% involved a sharp object held by a coworker. Of the 99 injuries, 80% were caused by suture needles. Forty-six percent were associated with the surgeon's use of fingers rather than an instrument to hold tissue being sutured; 63% affected the nondominant hand, primarily the distal index and middle fingers.

In the surgical studies, overall rates of mucocutaneous blood contact ranged from 6.4% to 50.4% of procedures, depending on the study methodology, the definition of a blood contact, procedures observed, and the use of infection control precautions [57]. Blood–hand contacts represent at least half of all blood exposures in the operating room; the principal risk factor is the duration of the case [58,59]. The likelihood of blood–body contact is related to the amount of blood lost by the patient, and markedly increases with blood losses exceeding 500 ml [58,59]. Blood–body contacts occur primarily in two sites: the abdomen in surgeons facing the operating table, and the forearm. Forearm contacts are particularly common in procedures in which personnel reach inside the abdominal or pelvic cavity, such as abdominal procedures and obstetric deliveries [58–60]. Face and eye splashes are also most common in surgeons, but can also affect other people near the field in certain procedures. Irrigation,

TABLE 43-4. *Annual estimates of frequency of blood contact[a] in health care workers*

Authors	Occupation studied	Total no. of blood contacts[a] per year	No. of percutaneous blood contacts per year	References used to derive annual estimate
Tokars et al.	Surgeon	81–135	8–13	[51]
Panlilio et al.	Obstetrician	77	4	[52]
Cleveland et al.	Dentist	N/A	4	[53,54]
Wong et al.	Physician on medical ward	31.2	1.8	[55]
Aiken	Nurse on medical ward	N/A	0.98	LA[b]
Tokars et al.	Surgical scrub assistant	7–12	0.6–1.0	[51]
Marcus et al.	Hospital emergency department worker	24.2	0.4	[25]
Marcus et al.	Prehospital emergency medical worker	12.3	0.2	[56]

N/A, not available.
[a]Percutaneous, mucous membrane, or skin contact, based on prospective studies.
[b]L. Aiken (University of Pennsylvania, personal communication.)

orthopedic procedures requiring power saws or drills, and cardiovascular procedures were the factors most often associated with face and eye splashes [58,59]. Manipulating arterial lines and tubing that contains blood under pressure has resulted in blood exposures and also documented HIV seroconversions [33,61].

These data suggest that many percutaneous injuries in surgical and obstetric procedures may be preventable by using techniques that reduce the need for suturing, using safer suture needles, avoiding holding tissue with fingers, and improving coordination among members of the surgical team. Changes in personal protective equipment must also be considered, including double gloves, face shields, and, particularly during obstetric procedures, the routine use of gowns for the deliverer and measures such as reinforced gowns or elbow-length gloves to prevent soakage through gowns at the forearm [62].

Prospective studies of blood exposure have also been conducted in a variety of other settings, including emergency departments [25,28], anesthesiology [63], hemodialysis [64], radiology [65], clinical laboratories [66], hospital dental clinics [53], and among prehospital emergency medical services workers [56].

Because most documented cases of HIV seroconversion have involved injuries with hollow-bore needle devices used in frequently performed procedures (e.g., phlebotomy), the study of injuries involving these devices has received major attention. In a landmark paper reflecting the perspective of injury epidemiology, Jagger and colleagues analyzed 326 needlestick injuries reported to the employee health service at the University of Virginia Hospital [67]. They found that 17.8% occurred before or during use of the needle-bearing device, 69.6% occurred after use but before disposal, and 13.2% occurred during or after disposal. One third of injuries involved recapping, which was often reportedly done to avoid a competing hazard, such as disassembling a device with an exposed needle or carrying uncapped items to a disposal box. When injury rates were estimated based on number of devices purchased, the highest rates of injury were for items that required disassembly after use. These and similar observations in subsequent studies [68,69] led to an emphasis on redesign of needle devices to reduce needlestick injuries [70,71].

Prevention of Occupational Exposures

General Principles

Prevention of transmission of bloodborne pathogens to HCWs has traditionally relied on principles of infection control that were developed primarily for the prevention of nosocomial infections to patients. The HIV epidemic and the resurgence of tuberculosis have introduced HCWs to an alternative approach, based on long-standing principles of industrial hygiene and occupational medicine. This approach emphasizes a "hierarchy" of control strategies to prevent occupational injuries and exposures [72]. Control strategies include 1) elimination or modification of a hazard (e.g., needle or other sharp instrument) through the use of engineering controls or safety devices; 2) work practice controls (i.e., modification of techniques or practices to make them safer; 3) use of personal protective equipment; and 4) administrative controls. Integration of the principles of both infection control and occupational medicine offers the best chance to prevent occupational exposures and transmission of bloodborne pathogens without adverse consequences to patient care [73].

Infection Control Practices Based on the Principles of Universal Precautions

In the 1980s, recognizing that a patient's infection with HIV or other bloodborne pathogens is often unknown to HCWs providing care, the CDC recommended *universal precautions* to prevent the transmission of bloodborne pathogens in healthcare settings (see Chapter 13). Under universal precautions, blood, certain other body fluids, and tissues of *all* patients are considered potentially infectious and measures are recommended to prevent contact with these fluids, including 1) the routine use of appropriate barrier precautions (e.g., gloves, gowns, and facial protection to prevent mucocutaneous contact; 2) minimal manual manipulation of needles, scalpels, and other sharp instruments and devices (e.g., needles should not be recapped by hand); and 3) disposal of these items in puncture-resistant containers [74,75]. The concept of universal precautions formed the basis for the Occupational Safety and Health Administration (OSHA)'s standard for occupational exposure to bloodborne pathogens in hospitals and healthcare settings, which was finalized in 1991 [76]. The principle that certain barrier precautions should apply to all patients was expanded by many hospitals to include precautions for non-bloodborne pathogens. An example of this approach is *body substance isolation* (see Chapter 13) [77,78].

In 1995, the CDC's Hospital Infection Control Practices Advisory Committee published a new guideline for isolation precautions in hospitals [79]. This new system has two tiers of precautions. The first, termed "Standard Precautions," synthesizes the major features of universal precautions and body substance isolation into a single set of precautions to be used for the care of all patients in hospitals regardless of their presumed infection status. Intended to prevent transmission of many non-bloodborne, as well as bloodborne pathogens, Standard Precautions applies to blood; all body fluids, secretions, and excretions; nonintact skin; and mucous membranes. A second tier of precautions, termed "Transmission-based Precautions," applies to patients who are infected or colonized with highly transmissible or epidemiologically significant pathogens that require additional measures to prevent nosocomial transmission (e.g., airborne precautions for patients with infectious pulmonary tuberculosis) [79]. These isolation precautions are discussed further in Chapter 13.

At the time of this writing, there is little experience with the implementation of Standard Precautions. Because Standard Precautions incorporate the principles of universal precautions, much of the last decade's experience with universal precautions is likely to be applicable in the future as well. The remainder of this section summarizes experience with universal precautions.

Efficacy of Universal Precautions

Implementation of universal precautions has resulted in unprecedented efforts to train and educate HCWs regarding the epidemiology, modes of transmission, and prevention of HIV and other bloodborne infections, and appropriate postexposure management of percutaneous injuries and other blood exposures. It has been speculated that increases in the number of needlestick injuries reported to hospital surveillance and reporting systems, which are largely passive in nature, reflect better reporting and workers' increased awareness of the hazards and consequences of occupational blood contact [80,81].

Several investigators have attempted to assess the efficacy of universal precautions, as measured by the frequency of reported injuries and other blood contacts [39,82,83]. One study that was conducted at the NIH Clinical Center found a significant and sustained decrease in percutaneous injuries that was temporally associated with the implementation of universal precautions [82]. Injury rates declined regardless of which denominators were used to assess the possible effect of changes in patient acuity, patient days, and number of employees. Similarly, a decline in self-reported nonpercutaneous exposures to blood and other body substances was also temporally associated with implementation of the NIH's universal precautions policy and training protocol [39]. Using a prospective approach, Wong et al. had physicians on medical wards complete a daily questionnaire and found that the rate of exposure to blood and body fluids decreased from 5.07 to 2.66 per physician per patient care month [55]. This decline was primarily due to an increase in glove use after the implementation of universal precautions. In this study, the self-reported needlestick injury rate also declined from 0.39 to 0.15 per physician per patient care month, a change that the authors speculated may have been due to the presence of a sharps disposal unit in every patient room.

In conjunction with the implementation of universal precautions, many hospitals installed sharps disposal container systems. Several studies have reported a 70% or greater reduction in percutaneous injuries related to recapping of needles after the installation of sharps disposal boxes [81,84–87]; however, a reduction in overall injury rates has not been consistently observed [81,85,86, 88]. Disposal-related injuries associated with overfilled, poorly designed, or inconveniently located sharps containers remain a hazard [85,87,89]. To minimize these injuries, criteria for the design, selection, placement, and use of sharps containers have been developed [90].

Training, the use of barrier precautions to prevent predictable contact with blood and body fluids, and improved access to needle disposal containers have been important advances associated with the implementation of universal precautions. However, universal precautions alone are not sufficient to effect consistent and long-term reductions in occupational injuries and blood contacts [91,92]. First, low rates of compliance with universal precautions have been reported [88,93,94], underscoring the need to understand better the variables likely to affect HCWs' compliance and to develop possible behavior modification strategies [95]. Second, even when HCWs adhere to universal precautions, percutaneous injuries with conventional sharps still occur because HCWs often must use hazardous devices [91]. Third, data from several studies suggest that when safety devices or engineering controls are used, many injuries related to phlebotomy [96,97], intravenous (IV) catheter insertion and manipulation [98–101], and intraoperative suturing [102] may be prevented. Essential underpinnings to successful implementation of universal precautions and engineering controls must include comprehensive and continuing training and education, administrative support, and an understanding of HCWs' beliefs and attitudes about risk and risk reduction behavior [92].

Safety Devices: General Principles for Selection, Implementation, and Evaluation

Many new or modified products to prevent percutaneous injuries have been developed and marketed, which has presented hospitals with new challenges in their selection, implementation, and evaluation.

Before selecting a new device, several issues should be considered, including 1) the epidemiology of percutaneous injuries in the institution; 2) the risk of infection transmission posed by different percutaneous injuries (e.g., hollow-bore vs. solid-bore needles); 3) design features of the device; 4) availability of the device; and 5) relevant costs [70,103–106].

A number of desirable design features for safer needle devices have been proposed [67]. Ideally, devices should have safety features that function reliably and are an integral part of the device, automatically activated (i.e., a passive feature), and unable to be deactivated. In addition, devices that are easy to assemble and disassemble, permit the needle to be covered for as long as possible before and after use, and let the worker's fingers, hands, and body remain behind the exposed needle, are preferable. Finally, the device should not introduce new risks to workers or to patients. In addition to the incremental cost of the device itself, other costs must be considered, such as those for accessory equipment used with the device, changes in storage, inventory, and disposal practices, and education and training of personnel [107].

Three important outcome measurements should be considered when evaluating safety devices: 1) the efficacy of the device in preventing percutaneous injuries, 2) the occurrence of device-associated patient care complications (e.g., bacteremia, phlebitis, trauma to the artery or vein, hemolysis of blood samples), and 3) the acceptability of the device to the user.

Several studies have found an increased risk of bloodstream infections associated with needleless IV infusion systems used with central venous catheters or infection control practices related to these needleless systems [108–110] (see Chapter 44). In one investigation, home infusion therapy patients who received total parenteral nutrition and intralipid therapy through a central venous catheter with a needleless device were significantly more likely to acquire a bloodstream infection than other home infusion therapy patients [108]. A culture survey found that infusate from the lumens of preslit latex injection caps of needleless devices was more likely to be culture positive than fluid from lumens of conventional latex injection caps of protected-needle devices. The authors hypothesized that during routine manipulations, the injection caps of the needleless systems became contaminated, and during the 7 days before caps were routinely changed, contaminating bacteria proliferated in the nutrient-rich total parenteral nutrition and intralipid therapy fluids. These findings highlight the importance of infection control considerations in the design and use of devices and the need to conduct surveillance for adverse patient outcomes after the introduction of new devices.

No matter how effective a device may be in reducing percutaneous injuries, it must be acceptable to those who use it. In a study of various needlestick prevention devices that was conducted by the New York State Department of Health, three factors were found to influence the acceptability of a device: length of time needed for workers to become comfortable with the device, relative ease or difficulty of use, and the extent and type of changes in technique [111].

Safety Devices: Evaluation Studies

Despite the ever-growing number and diversity of safety devices, there are few data regarding their efficacy, the feasibility of wide-scale implementation, and their acceptability to HCWs. A CDC study evaluated a blunt-tip suture needle and found that increasing use of the blunt needle during gynecologic surgery procedures was associated with a consistent and significant reduction in the rate of injuries related to standard suture needles [102] (Figure 43-1). No injuries were observed for over 6,000 blunted needles. In contrast, the rates of injury for

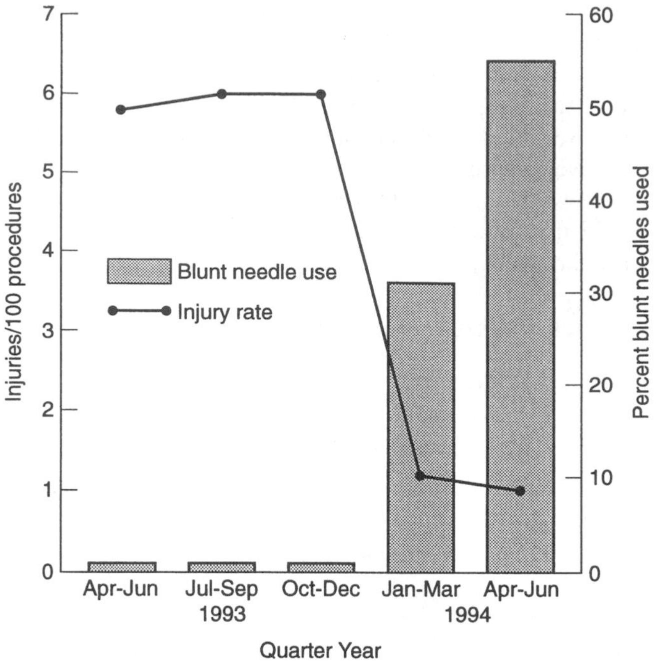

FIGURE 43-1. Rate of injury associated with use of curved suture needles during gynecologic surgical procedures and percentage of suture needles used that were blunt; by quarter, three hospitals, New York City, April 1993–June 1994. (From Centers for Disease Control and Prevention. Evaluation of blunt suture needles in preventing percutaneous injuries among health-care workers during gynecologic surgical procedures: New York City, March 1993–June 1994. *MMWR Morb Mortal Wkly Rep* 1997;46:25–29.)

conventional curved and straight suture needles were 1.9 and 14.2 per 1,000 needles used, respectively.

In contrast to injuries with solid suture needles, percutaneous injuries associated with phlebotomy may actually inject blood into the HCW and likely carry a higher risk of bloodborne pathogen transmission. In a study conducted among phlebotomists, nurses, medical students, and residents in six hospitals, several vacuum tube and winged steel blood collection phlebotomy needles with safety features that required the worker to activate them were evaluated [96]. After adjusting for underreporting and the level of device use, phlebotomy-associated injuries decreased from 3.8 to 2.4 injuries per 100,000 phlebotomy procedures after the introduction of safety devices. Billiet and associates compared a standard device with two safety devices for phlebotomy procedures performed by laboratory workers during three 9-month consecutive periods [97]. Compared with the preintervention rate of 9.1 needlestick injuries per 100,000 venipunctures, use of a recapping-type safety device and a needle-sheathing device that eliminated recapping and disassembly decreased the rates to 8.3 and 2.9 injuries per 100,000 venipunctures, respectively.

Access to IV lines with alternatives such as stopcocks and Luer-Loks can eliminate the use of needles for piggyback connections and intermittent IV therapy. Some of these injuries (e.g., injuries due to needles from peripheral IV lines and distal ports of central lines) likely represent a lower risk for transmission of bloodborne pathogens because blood may be undetectable, present in very small amounts, or greatly diluted [112]. Nonetheless, because IV tubing–needle assembly injuries are very common and preventable, many hospitals in the United States have introduced "needleless" IV delivery systems. During a pilot study by the New York State Department of Health, reported IV-related injuries decreased 75% to 94% in three of four hospitals that implemented needleless IV delivery systems; in the fourth hospital, the reported number of such injuries increased, which was attributed to improper use of the safety system [98]. Other studies have reported similar reductions, ranging from 72% to 100%, in IV-related percutaneous injuries that were temporally related to the introduction of a needleless system [99–101]. The greatest reductions were seen with those systems that did not permit needles to access IV lines. Two studies prospectively compared the incidence of various patient-related adverse outcomes for conventional and needleless intermittent peripheral IV access systems; needleless systems posed no greater risk of insertion site complications (e.g., phlebitis), nosocomial bacteremia, or positive cultures of catheter tips or adapter fluid [113,114]. In all of these studies, successful implementation and maintenance of the IV safety system was facilitated by comprehensive and innovative training and education programs, including written instructions, videotapes, posters, lectures, and display equipment for "hands-on" learning.

Work Practice Controls

Modification of techniques and practices is another approach to occupational injury prevention that is particularly applicable in surgical settings. For example, some open surgical procedures can be replaced by less invasive approaches such as laparoscopy that virtually eliminate the possibility of a percutaneous injury, yet do not appear adversely to affect patient outcomes [115]. During open surgical procedures, modification of standard techniques and use of alternatives to sharp instruments (e.g., electrocautery and staplers) can result in a nearly sharp-free procedure; such alternatives may decrease operative time, result in less blood loss, and reduce hospital stay [116].

Many intraoperative injuries occur during suturing, particularly when fingers are used to hold tissue [51]. Hence, alternative techniques and practices that minimize opportunities for the worker's fingers and a needle or sharp to come into contact have been proposed. These include "no-touch" suturing and tying techniques that use instruments instead of fingers to hold tissues and needles; avoidance of simultaneous suturing of a wound by two or more surgeons; and creation of a "neutral" or "safety" zone to avoid hand-to-hand passage of instruments, coupled with verbal announcements when sharps are placed in the safety zone [57,117,118]. Finally, periodic inspection of personal protective equipment may detect soakage or glove perforations.

Personal Protective Equipment

Gloves

The U.S. Food and Drug Administration regulates the quality of medical gloves and has established standards for latex gloves marketed in the United States [119]. Glove integrity can be evaluated using a variety of methods, including leak tests, immersion tests, and electrical conductivity [120–122]. Studies of the penetrability of various glove materials under conditions of use and with a variety of test probes, including viral particles, bacteria, blood, and water, have been difficult to interpret related in part to variations in test methods and the effect of latex and chemicals on the recovery of virus [123]. Although unused gloves may have detectable leaks [24,124–126], glove integrity is more likely to be compromised over time during actual use [120,127–130].

Although gloves do not offer absolute protection against blood contact, they greatly reduce the frequency of blood contact, and hence infection transmission [25,55]. Several studies have evaluated the effect of wearing more than one pair of gloves and have consistently found reduced rates of blood–hand contact [59,102,131, 132] or glove perforations [120,133–137] of the inner gloves among double- or triple-gloved surgical personnel. Further, wearing gloves may reduce the volume of blood that is injected during a percutaneous injury [34,35]. Although the acceptability of double gloving among surgeons varies [120,132,134], targeted educational campaigns can assist in improving acceptance.

Protective Gowns

The selection of appropriate protective gowns, particularly for the surgical setting, can be complex because there are many different types of reusable and disposable gowns available with varying fabric materials and type and extent of reinforcement. Neither OSHA nor the CDC have specific recommendations regarding gown design, gown fabric, or methods to assess a barrier's effectiveness. However, voluntary user guidelines for gown selection have been developed by various professional organizations [138,139]; in addition, consensus standards for evaluating the liquid and microbial barrier properties of protective clothing under laboratory conditions have been developed [140,141].

Selection of gowns should be guided by an understanding of the epidemiology of intraoperative blood contact. Telford and Quebbeman have developed a scheme for suggested attire (i.e., type of gown and need for leg protection) based on the anatomic site of the surgical procedure, estimated blood loss, and expected duration of the procedure [58]. Other factors to consider may include the occupation, skill, level of training and experience, and blood exposure history of the worker; comfort; cost; medical waste generated; and potential adverse effects on patient safety [58,118,142]. Blood soakage through the gown at the forearm, common during vaginal and cesarean deliveries, may be prevented by elbow-length gloves, a protective arm sleeve [143], or other approaches (e.g., changes in gown design) that prevent leakage of blood between the glove and the sleeve [144].

Masks and Protective Eyewear

Masks and protective eyewear such as goggles, glasses with solid side shields, or a face shield should be worn during procedures that are likely to generate splashes of blood or other body fluids to prevent exposure of mucous membranes of the mouth, nose, and eyes [74]. Facial mucocutaneous contacts appear to be largely preventable; in one study, the rate of contact was significantly lower among surgeons using eyeglasses (2/1,930 [0.1%]) or face shield or goggles (0/418) compared with those using no facial protection other than a surgical mask (15/1,166 [1.3%]) [59]. In contrast to intraoperative glove and gown blood contamination, which is usually grossly evident, contamination of face shields may not be readily evident to the wearer, and hence the need for such protection is underappreciated [145].

Administrative Controls

Administrative controls are the critical overarching controls in the hierarchy to reduce the risk of occupational blood exposure and affect the largest number of workers. Administrative controls figure prominently in the CDC's guidelines, which recommend that employers have policies for 1) initial orientation and continuing education of HCWs on the epidemiology and prevention of occupational bloodborne infections, 2) provision of necessary equipment and supplies, and 3) monitoring adherence to recommended protective measures [74]. Administrative controls are among the key provisions of OSHA's Bloodborne Pathogen Standard, and mandate that employers 1) develop exposure control plans (i.e., identify tasks, procedures, and job classifications that can result in occupational blood exposure); 2) provide and require workers to use appropriate personal protective equipment; 3) make hepatitis B virus (HBV) vaccine available to all workers who have occupational exposure to blood (see Chapters 3 and 42); 4) have postexposure evaluation and follow-up policies and procedures for all workers who have had an exposure; 5) provide relevant training and education at the time of initial assignment and annually; and 6) maintain worker medical and training records [76].

Developing comprehensive, integrated, and effective administrative control programs often requires coordination of multiple hospital departments and the active participation of knowledgeable and experienced HCWs. For example, an operating room committee with representatives from surgery, anesthesiology, nursing departments, and infection control can 1) identify tasks, procedures, and equipment that may result in blood exposures; 2) recommend specific interventions (i.e., engineering controls, work practice controls or protective equipment) or other approaches, such as changes in workers' assignments or limiting the number of consecutive hours worked; and 3) develop and enforce relevant policies [117,118].

Sterilization, Disinfection, and Environmental Control

Most laboratory studies have indicated that HIV is readily susceptible to a wide variety of disinfectants [146]. HIV titer is reduced by 90% to 99% within several hours after drying and then further diminishes with time [74,147]. The length of time that viable HIV can be detected depends on the conditions of the experiment, including the initial concentration of HIV, whether organic or other foreign material is present that may protect HIV from inactivation, and other factors.

Recommendations for sterilization, disinfection, waste disposal, and other aspects of environmental control have been published [148,149] and are discussed more fully in Chapters 20 and 21. Standard sterilization and disinfection procedures recommended for patient care equipment are adequate to sterilize or disinfect items contaminated with blood or other body fluids from people infected with bloodborne pathogens, including HIV. Because soil or other foreign material may interfere with the sterilization or disinfection procedure, these devices must first be adequately cleaned. Cleaning before disinfection is particularly important for devices such as endoscopes that may become heavily soiled and cannot tolerate heat sterilization [150].

There is no epidemiologic evidence for HIV transmission by walls, floors, countertops, or other environmental surfaces. Therefore, aside from routine cleaning, extraordinary attempts to disinfect or sterilize environmental surfaces are unnecessary. All spills of blood and blood-contaminated fluids should be promptly cleaned up by a person wearing gloves and using an Environmental Protection Agency-approved disinfectant or a 1 : 100 solution of household bleach. Visible material should first be removed with disposable towels or other means to prevent direct contact with blood. The area should then be decontaminated with an appropriate disinfectant [74].

Routine Testing of Patients for HIV Antibody

The U.S. Public Health Service (PHS) has recommended that routine voluntary testing of hospitalized patients be considered (for benefit of the patients) in groups with a high prevalence of HIV infection [151]. Personnel in some hospitals have also advocated testing of patients to protect HCWs in settings where exposure of HCWs to large amounts of patients' blood may be anticipated. For surgical patients who test positive, additional precautions have been advocated [152,153]. The efficacy of these and other measures in protecting workers and their effect on patient care are uncertain. Studies have not shown that testing patients, in addition to implementing universal precautions, is helpful for protecting HCWs [24,51,154].

Decisions regarding the need to establish routine voluntary testing programs for patients should be made by individual institutions in consultation with public health authorities and based, in part, on the HIV seroprevalence in patients in their institutions. For example, some investigators have reported that, among low-prevalence patient populations, routine HIV testing of patients is not cost effective [155] and can be associated with considerable logistic difficulties [154]. Patient testing should include provisions for obtaining informed consent, providing appropriate counseling, ensuring confidentiality of results, and providing optimal care for infected patients [74]. HCWs whose infection control practices are based on a patient's HIV test result should clearly understand that they risk a false sense of security with patients who test negative because these patients may, nevertheless, be infected with HIV or another bloodborne pathogen [29].

Management of an Occupational Exposure to HIV

Employers of workers for whom occupational exposure to blood or bloodborne pathogens may be reasonably anticipated should adopt an appropriate postexposure management plan [76,156–159]. This plan should include an explanation of what constitutes an occupational exposure that may place a worker at risk of HIV infection,[1] procedures for rapidly reporting and evaluating such exposures, and follow-up management of the exposed worker, including the possible use of chemoprophylaxis. Workers should be familiarized with these procedures before the exposure occurs.

Immediately after exposure, routine measures for the local treatment of the exposed site (e.g., irrigation) should be followed; extraordinary measures (e.g., application of bleach or other caustic agents) may be harmful and have not been shown to be of value in preventing the transmission of bloodborne pathogens. Evaluation and management of possible exposure to HBV and hepatitis C virus (HCV) are discussed elsewhere [159] (see Chapters 3, 42).

The source patient should be informed of the incident and tested for HIV infection after consent is obtained in accordance with state and local laws. If consent cannot be obtained from the source patient (e.g., because the patient is unconscious), policies should be developed for testing source patients in compliance with applicable laws. Confidentiality of the source patient and the exposed worker should be maintained [156].

If the source patient is infected with HIV or refuses testing, the worker should be evaluated clinically and serologically for evidence of HIV infection as soon as possible after the exposure (baseline), and, if seronegative, should be retested periodically for a minimum of 6 months after exposure (e.g., at 6 weeks, 12 weeks, and 6 months after exposure). During the follow-up period, especially the first 6 to 12 weeks after the exposure, when most infected people are expected to seroconvert, exposed workers should follow PHS recommendations for preventing transmission of HIV. These include refraining from blood, semen, or organ donation and abstaining from, or using measures to prevent HIV transmission during, sexual intercourse. When safe and effective alternatives to breastfeeding are available, exposed women should not breastfeed infants during the follow-up period to prevent possible exposure of the infant to HIV in breast milk [156]. Psychological counseling of the worker and, in some cases, the worker's family members is frequently beneficial.

If the source patient is HIV seronegative and has no clinical manifestations of AIDS or HIV infection, no further HIV follow-up of the exposed worker is necessary unless there is epidemiologic evidence to suggest that the source individual may have recently been exposed to HIV or if testing is desired by the worker or recommended by the healthcare provider. If the source individual cannot be identified, decisions regarding appropriate follow-up should be individualized, based on factors such as whether potential sources are likely to include an individual at increased risk of HIV infection.

If the HCW is subsequently found to be HIV seropositive, medicolegal and financial compensation issues may be simplified if seroconversion is temporally associated with an occupational exposure. Consequently, obtaining a serum specimen from the HCW promptly after exposure for testing or storage should be considered, regardless of the follow-up that is decided on.

---

[1] A percutaneous injury, contact of mucous membranes, or contact of skin (especially when the exposed skin is chapped, abraded, or afflicted with dermatitis or the contact is prolonged or involving an extensive area) with blood, tissues, or other body fluids to which universal precautions apply, including: 1) semen, vaginal secretions, or other body fluids contaminated with visible blood, because these substances have been implicated in the transmission of HIV infection; 2) cerebrospinal fluid, synovial fluid, pleural fluid, peritoneal fluid, pericardial fluid, and amniotic fluid, because the risk of transmission of HIV from these fluids has not yet been determined; and 3) laboratory specimens that contain HIV (e.g., suspensions of concentrated virus), during the performance of job duties [156].

Duration of Follow-up

Of the 49 documented cases of occupationally acquired HIV infection reported in the United States as of December, 1995, 46 workers became HIV seropositive within 6 months (usually within 3 months) postexposure; the date of exposure was unknown for one laboratorian whose occupational infection was confirmed by DNA sequencing. The remaining two cases tested HIV seronegative at 6 months and tested seropositive at 9.5 and 10 months, respectively, postexposure. Both HCWs had percutaneous exposures to HIV-infected blood; neither took ZDV postexposure [160].

For one HCW, specimens were not available for DNA sequencing to assess the degree of relatedness between HIV strains from the HCW and source patient. In the second case, HIV strains from the HCW and source patient were confirmed by DNA sequencing as being closely related. This HCW became infected with HIV and HCV during the same percutaneous exposure, had delayed seroconversions to both viruses, and died 29 months after exposure from HCV-induced chronic hepatitis and hepatorenal failure [161]. The possibility cannot be ruled out that the delayed antibody responses and severe course of HCV disease in this HCW may have been due to an underlying immunologic abnormality or to co-infection with HIV and HCV. Poorly documented assertions of delayed seroconversion in HCWs have also been published [162] and refuted [163].

Several sources of data indicate that HIV seroconversion later than 6 months after an occupational exposure is very unusual. These include surveillance data on 78 cases of occupationally acquired infection in the United States and abroad; only the two cases cited previously had documented negative HIV antibody tests at 6 months [4,160]. In addition, prospective follow-up of several hundred HCWs for 2 or more years after exposure to HIV-infected blood has not identified any cases of delayed seroconversion [31,32,44]. Several investigators also used the polymerase chain reaction (PCR) to examine specimens from HIV-seronegative HCWs > 6 months after exposure [30,164,165]. In one study, 3 of 133 HCWs with a history of parenteral exposure to HIV-infected blood had one or more positive PCR test results; after 3 or 4 years, all three were PCR negative and all remain seronegative, p24 antigen negative, culture negative, and clinically healthy [31]. Finally, statistical analyses using Markov models to analyze cases of HIV infection whose dates of exposure are known, but for whom follow-up testing was done at varying intervals, have estimated that at least 95% of seroconversions occurred within 6 months after exposure [166]. Based on these data, the PHS has recommended that HCWs be followed for a minimum of 6 months after exposure. Some hospitals, however, have elected to follow exposed workers for a longer period of time (e.g., 1 year).

Postexposure Prophylaxis

In 1996, the PHS and the International AIDS Society (USA) recommended chemoprophylaxis after certain types of occupational exposure to HIV [157,158]. The recommendations were developed based on information from a variety of sources suggesting that postexposure prophylaxis (PEP) is likely to be protective, although its efficacy has not conclusively established [167].

Zidovudine PEP was associated with a decrease of ~ 79% in the risk of HIV seroconversion after percutaneous exposure to HIV-infected blood in a case–control study among HCWs [38] (see Table 43-3). Although this study has several limitations largely because of its retrospective nature, it may represent the only approach to assessment of clinical efficacy; an earlier prospective trial was terminated prematurely because of inability to enroll the large number of HCWs needed for sufficient statistical power to assess ZDV efficacy in reducing a relatively low average risk (0.3%) [30,168].

In a placebo-controlled trial of the efficacy of ZDV in reducing the risk of maternal–infant HIV transmission, a regimen consisting of ZDV given antepartum and intrapartum to the mother and to the newborn for 6 weeks reduced the risk of transmission by ~ 67% [169]. The mechanism of ZDV protection may have included a direct prophylactic effect on the fetus or infant, because protection in the ZDV treatment group was only partly explained by reduction of the HIV titer in maternal blood [170].

Postexposure prophylaxis also prevented or ameliorated retroviral infection in some studies in animals [171–173], although in general, attempts to assess the efficacy of postexposure chemoprophylaxis in animals have yielded mixed results [174]. Studies in animals are difficult to interpret, in part because there is not a good animal model for HIV-1 infection in humans. Accordingly, most animal studies have been conducted using simian immunodeficiency virus or other nonhuman retroviruses that have different pathogenetic mechanisms than HIV-1 in humans. Another difficulty is that to ensure an adequate viral challenge, as manifested by infection of all control animals, animals are often injected with high-titer virus, sometimes intravenously; these exposures bear little resemblance to most occupational exposures. In the animal studies in which PEP appeared effective, efficacy was greatest when prophylaxis was begun before or within a few hours after exposure; there was no apparent effect when drugs were begun later than 24 to 36 hours postexposure.

Failure of ZDV to prevent HIV infection in humans when administered postexposure has been reported in at least 16 instances [175]. In five instances, the exposures involved injection of a larger quantity of HIV-infected blood than would be expected from a needlestick. They include two instances of accidental IV inoculation of HIV-infected blood or other body fluid during nuclear medicine procedures [176,177], a blood transfusion

[156], a suicidal self-inoculation [178], and an assault on a prison guard with a needle syringe [179].

Eleven other instances involved HCWs who became infected with HIV despite ZDV treatment after percutaneous exposure to HIV-infected blood. In these cases, summarized by Jochimsen, ZDV was begun 30 minutes to 8 days (median, 1.5 hours) after exposure and was used in doses of 600 to 1,200 mg/day (median, 1,000 mg/day) for 8 to 54 days (median, 21 days). Seven episodes involved source patients who had a history of ZDV use and may therefore have been infected with ZDV-resistant HIV. In 2 of the 11 cases, laboratory studies were conducted to assess possible ZDV resistance of the infecting strain. In one case, a phenotypic assay revealed decreased sensitivity; in the second case, genotypic assays did not suggest ZDV resistance, but phenotypic assays were not performed [175]. These case reports indicate that if ZDV is protective, any protection afforded is not absolute.

Antiretroviral agents more potent than ZDV have also been developed. Information on the potency and toxicity of these drugs is available from studies of HIV-infected patients, although it is uncertain to what extent these results apply to PEP. Passive immunization with HIV hyperimmune globulin has also been proposed as a possible option for PEP; its use for this purpose awaits evaluation in animal models. In HIV-infected patients, combination therapy with the nucleosides ZDV and lamivudine (3TC) has greater antiretroviral activity than ZDV alone and is active against many ZDV-resistant HIV strains without significantly increased toxicity [180]. Adding a protease inhibitor provides even greater increases in antiretroviral activity; among protease inhibitors, indinavir (IDV) is more potent than saquinavir at currently recommended doses and appears to have fewer drug interactions and short-term adverse effects than ritonavir [180]. Few data exist to assess possible long-term (i.e., delayed) toxicity resulting from use of these drugs in people not infected with HIV.

Zidovudine is usually well tolerated by HCWs as PEP in the currently recommended dose of 200 mg three times a day. With higher doses (1,000–1,200 mg/day), short-term toxicity consisted primarily of gastrointestinal symptoms, fatigue, and headache; mild decreases of hemoglobin and absolute neutrophil count were also observed [30,181,182]. Isolated cases of peripheral neuropathy, seizures, hepatic dysfunction, and rash have been reported [156,183,184].

The toxicity of other antiretroviral drugs in people not infected with HIV has not been well characterized. In HIV-infected adults, 3TC can cause gastrointestinal symptoms and, in rare instances, pancreatitis. IDV toxicity includes gastrointestinal symptoms and, usually after prolonged use, mild hyperbilirubinemia (10%) and kidney stones (4%); the latter may be limited by drinking at least 48 oz (1.5 L) of fluid per 24-hour period [180]. During the first 4 weeks of IDV therapy, the reported incidence of kidney stones was 0.8% (Merck Research Laboratories, unpublished data, 1996). As stated in the package insert, the concurrent use of IDV and certain other drugs, including some nonsedating antihistamines, is contraindicated. ZDV use in the second and third trimesters of pregnancy and early infancy was not associated with serious adverse effects in mothers or in 333 uninfected infants followed up to 78 months of age [169,185]; data are limited regarding the safety of ZDV during the first trimester of pregnancy or of other antiretroviral agents during pregnancy. Although 3TC has been associated with pancreatitis in HIV-infected children [180], whether 3TC causes fetal toxicity is unknown. Few data exist to assess possible long-term (delayed) toxicity of antiretroviral agents in uninfected people.

Public Health Service Recommendations

The recommendations published in June, 1996 are provisional because they are based on limited data regarding efficacy and toxicity of PEP and risk of HIV infection after exposure. Periodic updates are anticipated as additional data are obtained. Because the great majority of occupational exposures to HIV do not result in infection transmission, potential toxicity must be carefully considered when prescribing PEP. When possible, these recommendations should be implemented in consultation with people having expertise in antiretroviral therapy and HIV transmission. Changes in drug regimens may be appropriate, based on factors such as the probable antiretroviral drug resistance profile of HIV from the source patient; local availability of drugs; and medical conditions, concurrent drug therapy, and drug toxicity in the exposed worker. These recommendations were not developed to address nonoccupational (e.g., sexual) exposures.

1. Chemoprophylaxis should be recommended to exposed workers after occupational exposures associated with the highest risk for HIV transmission. For exposures with a lower, but nonnegligible risk, PEP should be offered, balancing the lower risk against the use of drugs having uncertain efficacy and toxicity. For exposures with negligible risk, PEP is not justified (Table 43-5). Exposed workers should be informed that 1) knowledge about the efficacy and toxicity of PEP is limited; 2) for agents other than ZDV, data are limited regarding toxicity in people without HIV infection or who are pregnant; and 3) any or all drugs for PEP may be declined by the exposed worker.
2. At present, ZDV should be considered for all PEP regimens because ZDV is the only agent for which data support the efficacy of PEP in the clinical setting. 3TC should usually be added to ZDV for increased antiretroviral activity and activity against many ZDV-resistant strains. A protease inhibitor (preferably IDV because of its high antiretroviral

TABLE 43-5. *Provisional Public Health Service recommendations for chemoprophylaxis after occupational exposure to HIV, by type of exposure and source material—1996*

Type of exposure	Source material[a]	Antiretroviral prophylaxis[b]	Antiretroviral regimen[c]
Percutaneous	Blood[d]		
	Highest risk	Recommend	ZDV + 3TC + IDV
	Increased risk	Recommend	ZDV + 3TC, ± IDV[e]
	No increased risk	Offer	ZDV + 3TC
	Fluid containing visible blood, other potentially infectious fluid,[f] or tissue	Offer	ZDV + 3TC
	Other body fluid (e.g., urine)	Not offer	
Mucous membrane	Blood	Offer	ZDV + 3TC, ± IDV[e]
	Fluid containing visible blood, other potentially infectious fluid,[f] or tissue	Offer	ZDV ± 3TC
	Other body fluid (e.g., urine)	Not offer	
Skin, increased risk[g]	Blood	Offer	ZDV + 3TC, ± IDV[e]
	Fluid containing visible blood, other potentially infectious fluid,[f] or tissue	Offer	ZDV ± 3TC
	Other body fluid (e.g., urine)	Not offer	

[a]Any exposure to concentrated HIV (e.g., in a research laboratory or production facility) is treated as percutaneous exposure to blood with highest risk.

[b]Postexposure prophylaxis (PEP) should be recommended to the exposed worker with counseling (see text). PEP should be offered to the exposed worker with counseling (see text). PEP should not be offered because these are not occupational exposures to HIV [156].

[c]Regimens: zidovudine (ZDV), 200 mg three times a day; lamivudine (3TC), 150 mg twice daily; indinavir (IDV), 800 mg three times a day (if IDV is not available, saquinavir may be used, 600 mg three times a day). Prophylaxis is given for 4 wk. For full prescribing information, see package inserts.

[d]*Highest risk*: BOTH larger volume of blood (e.g., deep injury with large-diameter hollow needle previously in source patient's vein or artery, especially involving an injection of source patient's blood) AND blood containing high titer of HIV (e.g., source with acute retroviral illness or end-stage acquired immunodeficiency syndrome; viral load measurement may be considered, but its use in relation to PEP has not been evaluated). *Increased risk*: exposure to larger volume of blood or blood with high titer of HIV. *No increased risk*: exposure to larger volume of blood nor blood with high titer of HIV (e.g., solid suture needle injury from source patient with asymptomatic HIV infection).

[e]Possible toxicity of additional drug may not be warranted (see text).

[f]Includes semen; vaginal secretions; cerebrospinal, synovial, pleural, peritoneal, pericardial, and amniotic fluids.

[g]For skin, risk is increased for exposures involving high titer of HIV; prolonged contact, an extensive area, or an area in which skin integrity is visibly compromised. For skin exposures without increased risk, the risk of drug toxicity outweighs the benefit of PEP.

(From Centers for Disease Control and Prevention. Update: provisional Public Health Service recommendations for chemoprophylaxis after occupational exposure to HIV. *MMWR Morb Mortal Wkly Rep* 1996;45:468–472.)

activity and apparently relatively low toxicity in short-term use) should be added for exposures with the highest risk for HIV transmission (see Table 43-5). Adding a protease inhibitor also may be considered for lower-risk exposures if ZDV-resistant strains are likely, although it is uncertain whether the potential additional toxicity of a third drug is justified for lower-risk exposures. For HIV strains resistant to both ZDV and 3TC or resistant to a protease inhibitor, or if these drugs are contraindicated or poorly tolerated, the optimal PEP regimen is uncertain; expert consultation is advised. An HIV strain is more likely to be resistant to a specific antiretroviral agent if it is derived from a patient who has been exposed to the agent for a prolonged period of time (e.g., 6 to 12 months or longer). In general, resistance develops more readily in people with more advanced HIV infection (e.g., CD4+ T-lymphocyte count < 200 cells/mm^3), reflecting the increasing rate of viral replication during later stages of the illness.

3. Postexposure prophylaxis should be initiated promptly, preferably within 1 to 2 hours postexposure. Although animal studies suggest that PEP probably is not effective when started later than 24 to 36 hours postexposure [171,173], the interval after which there is no benefit from PEP for humans is undefined. Initiating therapy after a longer interval (e.g., 1 to 2 weeks) may be considered for the highest-risk exposures; even if infection is not prevented, early treatment of acute HIV infection may be beneficial [186]. The optimal duration of PEP is unknown; because 4 weeks of ZDV appeared protective [38], PEP should probably be administered for 4 weeks, if tolerated.
4. If the source patient or the patient's HIV status is unknown, initiating PEP should be decided on a case-by-case basis, based on the exposure risk and

likelihood of HIV infection in known or possible source patients. If additional information becomes available, decisions about PEP can be modified.

5. Workers with occupational exposures to HIV should receive follow-up counseling and medical evaluation, including HIV antibody tests at baseline and periodically ≥ 6 months postexposure (e.g., 6 weeks, 12 weeks, and 6 months), and should observe precautions to prevent possible secondary transmission [156]. If PEP is used, drug toxicity monitoring should include a complete blood count and renal and hepatic chemical function tests at baseline and 2 weeks after starting PEP. If subjective or objective toxicity is noted, dose reduction or drug substitution should be considered with expert consultation, and further diagnostic studies may be indicated. HCWs who become infected with HIV should receive appropriate medical care.
6. Healthcare providers in the United States are encouraged to enroll all workers who receive PEP in confidential registry developed by the CDC, Glaxo Wellcome, Inc., and Merck & Co., Inc., to assess toxicity (toll-free: (888) PEP-4HIV). CDC expects to publish PEP recommendations in late 1997 or in early 1998.

HIV TRANSMISSION FROM HEALTHCARE WORKERS TO PATIENTS DURING INVASIVE PROCEDURES

The risk of HIV transmission from infected HCWs to patients during invasive procedures is very small; precise assessment has been complicated by lack of data to answer completely three critical scientific questions: 1) what event(s) result in HIV transmission from HCWs to patients, 2) what is the magnitude of the risk, and 3) what factors increase or decrease the risk [187].

Available data to assess this risk include surveillance of cases of HIV infection and AIDS, retrospective investigations of patients of HIV-infected HCWs, reports of transmission of other bloodborne pathogens (HBV and HCV) from HCWs to patients, and studies of blood exposure among HCWs and patients during surgical and dental procedures.

Reports of Transmission

As of February, 1997, HIV transmission from two infected HCWs to patients during invasive procedures has been reported. The first case involved a dentist in Florida. After a young woman reported with AIDS was determined to have most likely acquired HIV infection from the dentist, further investigation disclosed that HIV was transmitted during dental care to 6 of ~ 1,100 patients tested in the dental practice. Although the specific events responsible for HIV transmission in this practice remain unknown, findings of the epidemiologic and laboratory investigations support dentist-to-patient, rather than patient-to-patient transmission as the most likely route. No deficiency of infection control that would readily explain HIV transmission to these six patients was identified, nor was there evidence that the dentist intentionally transmitted HIV to the patients. However, the investigation was limited by the fact that the dentist could be interviewed only once before his death, which occurred early in the investigation, and the dental practice had been closed before the investigation began [188–191].

The second case involved an orthopedic surgeon in St. Germain-en-Laye, a suburb of Paris, France. In January, 1997, the French Ministry of Health announced the results of a retrospective investigation of the surgeon's patients, initiated when his diagnosis of AIDS became public knowledge. According to the summary of the official report disseminated on the World Wide Web, the surgeon is believed to have acquired HIV in 1983; he was diagnosed with HIV infection and AIDS simultaneously in March, 1994. HIV test results were ascertained for 968 patients (32% of the patients on whom the surgeon had performed an invasive procedure); one was HIV seropositive. This patient was a woman who reportedly had no risks for HIV infection. She had had a 10-hour orthopedic procedure performed by the surgeon in 1992, and had tested HIV seronegative preoperatively. Genetic sequencing performed at the Institut Pasteur indicated that HIV strains from the surgeon and patient were closely related [192].

The summary further states that assessment of surgical practices indicated that the surgeon experienced wounds or cuts during operations that may have subsequently exposed patients to his blood. The surgeon's exposures seemed to be related more to orthopedic surgical techniques than to the practices of the surgeon himself. The infection control procedures in effect in the operating suite are in accordance with recommendations for prevention of accidental exposures to blood, for the organization of operations, and for treatment and sterilization of medical and surgical material [192].

Additional Data From Surveillance and Retrospective Investigations

No additional cases of HIV transmission from HCWs to patients have been documented, although, because of the inherent limitations of surveillance data, it is possible that unrecognized cases may have occurred [187]. Direct evidence that the risk is small comes from retrospective investigations of patients of additional HIV-infected HCWs. Excluding the Florida dental practice and the French surgeon, as of February 18, 1997, the CDC was aware of investigations in which HIV test results were known for ~ 22,759 patients treated by 53 HIV-infected HCWs, including 29 dentists and dental students, 8

TABLE 43-6. *Epidemiologic and laboratory follow-up of patients infected with HIV who were treated by HIV-infected healthcare workers, January, 1995*

Follow-up status	No. of patients		
	Total	With viral strains sequenced	With viral sequences related to that of the healthcare worker
Infected before treatment	28	0	—
Established risk factors	62	14	0
Other potential for exposure to HIV	15	13	0
No identified risk	5	3	0
Investigation in progress	3	0	—
Total	113	30	0

(From Robert LM, Chamberland ME, Cleveland JL, et al. Investigations of patients of health care workers infected with HIV: the Centers for Disease Control and Prevention database. *Ann Intern Med* 1995;122:653–657.)

physicians and medical students, 15 surgeons or obstetricians, and 1 podiatrist. Of 113 HIV-infected patients identified, follow-up investigations have been completed for 110; no additional cases of HIV transmission to patients were documented [193] (Campbell S, CDC, personal communication) (Table 43-6).

Although data from these retrospective investigations are reassuring, they have limitations. HIV test results are available for only about 17% of patients of these HIV-infected HCWs. It is not known how many of the patients tested underwent invasive procedures and which procedures these were. In most cases it is not known what stage of infection the HCWs were in when the procedures were performed (e.g., whether they had developed AIDS, in which the titer of HIV in blood is highest and transmission may be more likely) [193].

Data from retrospective studies are consistent with estimates, derived by modeling techniques, that the average risk of HIV transmission from a surgeon to a patient due to percutaneous injury during an invasive procedure is 2.4 to 24 per million [194]. In contrast, the risk of HBV transmission to a patient from a surgeon positive for hepatitis B e antigen (HBeAg) has been estimated to be 100-fold higher (240 to 2,400 per million) [194]. The theoretical models used to derive these patient risk estimates have many limitations, including that they are broad averages that do not account for variations in practice or technique by individual surgeons. Also, the models do not apply to clusters of transmission in which the risk, for unclear reasons, is much higher [195].

Lessons From Reports of Hepatitis B and C Virus Transmission From Healthcare Workers to Patients

Transmission of HBV from HCWs to patients during invasive procedures is well documented and has occurred in some cases without evidence of inadequate infection control [187,196,197] (see Chapter 42). Recently, HCV transmission from an infected cardiac surgeon to patients has been reported in the United Kingdom and Spain [198,199]. Although the magnitude of risk for HIV transmission from HCWs to patients cannot be estimated based on data for HBV or HCV, recognized instances of HBV and HCV transmission can offer potentially useful information about risk factors for transmission of bloodborne pathogens.

The CDC is unaware of reports of HBV transmission from dentists to patients since 1987. This decrease in reports is likely due to increased use of gloves and HBV vaccine by dentists. In contrast, about one cluster per year of HBV transmission from surgeons to patients has been recognized worldwide (in developed countries) since 1978. The specialties involved have included obstetrics and gynecology (11 surgeons), general surgery (10), cardiac surgery (9), orthopedics (1), and urology (1) [187,197].

Although percutaneous transfer of blood was believed to be the most likely mechanism of HBV transmission in the surgical clusters, investigations did not identify the specific events that resulted in transmission. In some instances, surgeons reported having received only an occasional percutaneous injury. Of the HCWs whose HBeAg status was known, nearly all were positive, indicating that these HCWs had a high titer of circulating HBV. The exceptions involved viruses that were precore mutants (i.e, genetically unable to make HBeAg) [197]. In several investigations, risk depended on the degree of invasiveness of the procedure performed; for example, HBV transmission was more likely during hysterectomy than during dilatation and curettage. In some cases in which where HCWs resumed practice after counseling to modify techniques, no further clinically apparent HBV transmission was recognized, although serologic testing of patients to detect asymptomatic HBV infection was not routinely done. In other instances, however, HBV transmission occurred even after such changes were made, including the use of double gloves [187].

Blood Contact Studies

The mechanism of HIV transmission to patients presumably requires exposure of the patient, either directly or indirectly, to the blood of the infected HCW. Few data are available on the proportion of surgical or dental procedures in which such exposures may occur. In four observational studies conducted since 1990, a sharp object injured a surgeon and subsequently recontacted the patient's wound, thus potentially exposing the patient to the surgeon's blood, in 1.0% to 2.5% of operations and 0.1% of deliveries [51,200 to 202]. The risk of HIV transmission due to these injuries and recontacts is undoubtedly small because most injuries involved small, solid-bore suture needles. Nevertheless, in these studies, the specialties and procedures with increased injury and recontact rates tended to be the same as those most commonly implicated in HBV transmission to patients (e.g., gynecologic surgery procedures).

Surgeons have anecdotally reported skin lesions after exerting traction on suture material. In a single laboratory simulation conducted by the CDC, an HBeAg-positive cardiothoracic surgical resident described previously tied surgical knots continuously for 1 hour; this resulted in visible skin separations on his index fingers. HBsAg was detected in saline used to rinse out the surgeon's gloves; however, it is not known whether the HBsAg was associated with infective HBV or whether HBsAg was present on the outside of the gloves [196].

Strategies to Prevent Healthcare Worker-to-Patient Transmission of HIV

In 1991, the CDC published recommendations for preventing transmission of HIV and HBV to patients during "exposure-prone" invasive procedures [203]. The CDC recommended that HCWs who perform exposure-prone procedures should know their HIV antibody status and that HIV-infected HCWs should not perform exposure-prone procedures unless they sought counsel from an expert review panel and were advised under what circumstances, if any, they may continue to perform these procedures. Such circumstances would include notifying prospective patients of the HCW's seropositivity before they undergo exposure-prone invasive procedures. Mandatory testing of HCWs for HIV antibody was not recommended. The guidelines specified that HCWs who do not perform invasive procedures pose no risk of transmitting HIV to patients and that there is no basis to restrict the job duties of HCWs who perform invasive procedures not identified as exposure prone.

After publication of the recommendations, many professional organizations and other groups indicated that determination of the potential for exposure of the patient to the HCW's blood must include consideration of the HCW's technique, skill, and medical status, in addition to the procedures performed. In June, 1992 the CDC Director wrote to all state and territorial health departments that it would be appropriate to determine whether a procedure is exposure prone "on a case-by-case basis, taking into consideration the specific procedure as well as the skill, technique, and possible impairment of the infected HCW" [187].

In October, 1991, Public Law 102-141 was enacted, requiring that each state certify that it had implemented the CDC recommendations or their equivalent for preventing transmission of HIV and HBV to patients. The state guidelines certified to the CDC as being equivalent contain diverse mechanisms and criteria for evaluation of HIV- and HBV-infected HCWs; all have provisions for voluntary or mandatory review of the HCW's practice by a third party, such as an expert review panel. Relatively few of the state guidelines include the provision that patients undergoing exposure-prone procedures by infected HCWs should be prospectively notified of the HCW's HIV positive status [187].

In summary, evaluation of the appropriate job duties of HIV-infected HCWs is governed by state laws and regulations. In addition, HIV-infected HCWs have legal protection against discrimination under the Americans with Disabilities Act [204,205]. Several professional societies have also developed recommendations for the management of HIV-infected HCWs [206–210].

Current guidelines were developed before the advent of potent antiretroviral therapy that can reduce the HIV viral load in blood to very low or undetectable levels, as documented by sensitive and reliable assays widely available for clinical use [211,212]. At the time of this writing, the impact of these new developments on HIV transmission in the healthcare setting is uncertain, but they may be potentially useful in the management of HIV-infected HCWs.

Notification of Patients of Infected Healthcare Workers

Hospital officials who become aware that an HCW on their staff who has performed invasive procedures is infected with HIV have faced the difficult decision as to whether previous patients should be notified. The CDC recommends that such notifications should not be done routinely, but should be considered on a case-by-case basis in consultation with state public health officials, taking into consideration an assessment of specific risks, confidentiality issues, and available resources. Others have also recommend that such notifications not be done routinely [213,214].

PATIENT-TO-PATIENT TRANSMISSION

Because HIV is not transmitted by casual contact or fomites, patient-to-patient transmission of HIV in healthcare settings should be entirely preventable. Most reported instances of such transmission have occurred in countries that have few resources for infection control. HIV transmission in Mexico between plasmapheresis donors was attributed to reuse of IV tubing among different donors [215]. Large outbreaks in Russia and Romania were attributed to reuse of contaminated needles and syringes [216,217]. HIV transmission between patients in hemodialysis units (see Chapter 24) in developing countries was attributed to inadequate disinfection practices; in some cases, reuse of dialyzers, needles, and syringes for different patients was also suspected [218,219]. When standard infection control procedures are followed, nosocomial transmission of HIV in hemodialysis units should be rare [220].

Several incidents of nosocomial HIV transmission have been reported in the United States and other developed countries. In three published reports, patients undergoing nuclear medicine procedures were inadvertently injected with material that had been withdrawn from a different patient [176,177]. In Australia, four patients who had minor outpatient surgery after a patient with AIDS on the same day in the same office contracted HIV infection. No specific breach in technique could be identified in the investigation that was done 4 years later [221]. In a report from New York City, AIDS was diagnosed in a 9-month-old infant who had no known risks for HIV infection. When the infant was hospitalized at age 11 days for treatment of chlamydial conjunctivitis, two children with AIDS were on the same inpatient unit. Investigators hypothesized that the child was exposed to the HIV-infected blood or other body fluids of one of these two children during a medical procedure, but no specific exposure incident was identified [222].

Recommendations for preventing HIV transmission by blood transfusion, artificial insemination, and bone and organ donation include screening potential donors for HIV antibody and for a history of risk factors for HIV infection [223,224]. As a result of these preventive measures, the risk of HIV transmission in a unit of screened blood has been reduced to ~ 1 in 450,000 to 660,000 donations [225].

FUTURE DIRECTIONS

Future directions include more systematic surveillance of occupationally acquired HIV infection; better definition of the epidemiology of blood contact and the efficacy of preventive measures; development and evaluation of new devices and protective barriers; and evaluation of PEP.

Progress will be facilitated by development and implementation of surveillance and data management systems in healthcare institutions that facilitate case management of exposed workers, permit assessment of a variety of occupational hazards, and help to evaluate preventive interventions on both a local and national basis. A sustained commitment to the occupational health of HCWs will ensure maximum protection for HCWs and patients and the availability of optimal medical care for all who need it.

Acknowledgment

Connie G. Alfred assisted in the preparation of this chapter.

REFERENCES

1. De Cock KM, Adjorlolo G, Ekpini E, et al. Epidemiology and transmission of HIV-2: why there is no HIV-2 pandemic. *JAMA* 1993;270: 2083–2086.
2. Chamberland ME, et al. Health-care workers with AIDS: national surveillance update. *JAMA* 1991;266:3459.
3. Centers for Disease Control and Prevention. HIV/AIDS surveillance report, Table 16. 1995;7(2):21.
4. Fitch KM, Alvarez LP, Medina RD, et al. Occupational transmission of HIV in healthcare workers: a review. *Europ J Pub Health* 1995; 5:175–186.
5. Centers for Disease Control and Prevention. Human immunodeficiency virus transmission in household settings-United States. *MMWR Morb Mortal Wkly Rep* 1994;43:347–356.
6. Tokars JI, Chamberland ME, Schable CA, et al. The American Academy of Orthopaedic Surgeons Serosurvey Study Committee: A survey of occupational blood contact and HIV infection among orthopedic surgeons. *JAMA* 1992;268:489–494.
7. Panlilio AL, Shapiro CN, Schable CA, et al. Serosurvey of human immunodeficiency virus, hepatitis B virus, and hepatitis C virus infection among hospital-based surgeons. *J Am Coll Surg* 1995;180: 16–24.
8. Cowan DN, et al. HIV infection among members of the US Army Reserve Components with medical and health occupations. *JAMA* 1991;265:2826.
9. Gerberding JL, et al. Risk to dental professionals from occupational exposure to human immunodeficiency virus: follow-up [Abstract 698]. In: *Program and abstracts of the twenty-seventh interscience conference on antimicrobial agents and chemotherapy, New York, 1987*. Washington, DC: American Society for Microbiology; 1987.
10. Klein RS, et al. Low occupational risk of human immunodeficiency virus infection among dental professionals. *N Engl J Med* 1988;318: 86.
11. Gruninger SE, Siew C, Chang S-B, et al. Human immunodeficiency virus type 1 infection among dentists. *J Am Dent Assoc* 1992;123: 57–64.
12. Flynn NM, et al. Absence of HIV antibody among dental professionals exposed to infected patients. *West J Med* 1987;146:439.
13. Goldman M, et al. Markers of HTLV-III in patients with end stage renal failure treated by hemodialysis. *Br Med J* 1986;293:161.
14. Peterman TA, et al. HTLV-III/LAV infection in hemodialysis patients. *JAMA* 1986;255:2324.
15. Comodo N, et al. Risk of HIV infection in patients and staff of two dialysis centers: seroepidemiological findings and prevention trends. *Eur J Epidemiol* 1988;4:171.
16. Assogba U, et al. Prospective study of HIV 1 seropositive patients in hemodialysis centers. *Clin Nephrol* 1988;29:312.
17. Chirgwin K, Rao TKS, Landesman SH. HIV infection in a high prevalence dialysis unit. *AIDS* 1989;3:731.
18. Chamberland M, Petersen LR, Munn VP, et al. Human immunodeficiency virus infection among healthcare workers who donate blood. *Ann Intern Med* 1994;121:269–273.
19. Turner SB, Kunches LM, Gordon, et al. Occupational exposure to human immunodeficiency virus (HIV) and hepatitis B virus (HBV) among embalmers: a pilot seroprevalence study. *Am J Public Health* 1989;79:1425–1426.
20. Gershon RRM, Vlahov D, Farzedegan H, Alter MJ. Occupational risk of human immunodeficiency virus, hepatitis B virus, and hepatitis C virus infections among funeral service practitioners in Maryland. *Infect Control Hosp Epidemiol* 1995;16:194–197.
21. Mann JM, et al. HIV seroprevalence among hospital workers in Kinshasa, Zaire: lack of association with occupational exposure. *JAMA* 1986;256:3099.
22. N'Galy B, et al. Human immunodeficiency virus among employees in an African hospital. *N Engl J Med* 1988;319:1123.

23. General Accounting Office. *VA healthcare: purchases of safer devices should be based on risk of injury*. Washington, DC: General Accounting Office, 1994.
24. Gerberding JL, et al. Risk of exposure of surgical personnel to patients' blood during surgery at San Francisco General Hospital. *N Engl J Med* 1990;322:1788.
25. Marcus R, Culver DH, Bell DM, et al. Risk of human immunodeficiency virus infection among emergency department workers. *Am J Med* 1993;94:363–370.
26. O'Neill TM, Abbott AV, Radecki SE. Risk of needlesticks and occupational exposures among residents and medical students. *Arch Intern Med* 1992;1452–1456.
27. Janssen RS, St. Louis ME, Satten GA, et al. HIV infection among patients in U.S. acute-care hospitals: strategies for the counseling and testing of hospital patients. *N Engl J Med* 1992;327:445–452.
28. Kelen GD, et al. Human immunodeficiency virus infection in emergency patients: epidemiology, clinical presentations and risk to healthcare workers. The Johns Hopkins experience. *JAMA* 1989;262:516.
29. Montecalvo MA, Lee MS, DePalma H, et al. Seroprevalence of human immunodeficiency virus-1, hepatitis B virus and hepatitis C virus in patients having major surgery. *Infect Control Hosp Epidemiol* 1995;16:627–632.
30. Tokars JI, Marcus R, Culver DH, et al, for the Centers for Disease Control and Prevention Cooperative Needlestick Surveillance Group. Surveillance of HIV infection and zidovudine use among health-care workers after occupational exposure to HIV-infected blood. *Ann Intern Med* 1993;118:913–919.
31. Gerberding JL. Incidence and prevalence of HIV, hepatitis B virus, hepatitis C virus, and cytomegalovirus among healthcare personnel at risk for blood exposure: final report from a longitudinal study. *J Infect Dis* 1994;170:1410.
32. Henderson DK, et al. Risk for occupational transmission of human immunodeficiency virus type 1 (HIV-1) associated with clinical exposures: a prospective evaluation. *Ann Intern Med* 1990;113:740.
33. Ippolito G, Puro V, De Carli G, Italian Study Group on Occupational Risk of HIV Infection. The risk of occupational human immunodeficiency virus infection in healthcare workers. *Arch Intern Med* 1993; 153:1451–1458.
34. Mast ST, Woolwine JD, Gerberding JL. Efficacy of gloves in reducing blood volumes transferred during simulated needlestick injury. *J Infect Dis* 1993;168:1589–1592.
35. Bennett NT, Howard RJ. Quantity of blood inoculated in a needlestick injury from suture needles. *J Am Coll Surg* 1994;178:107–110.
36. Ho DD, Moudgil T, Alam M. Quantitation of human immunodeficiency virus type 1 in the blood of infected persons. *N Engl J Med* 1989;321:1621–1625.
37. Pinto LA, Sullivan J, Berzofsky JA, et al. ENV-specific cytotoxic T lymphocyte responses in HIV seronegative healthcare workers occupationally exposed to HIV-contaminated body fluids. *J Clin Invest* 1995;96:867–876.
38. Centers for Disease Control and Prevention. Case–control study of HIV seroconversion in health-care workers after percutaneous exposure to HIV-infected blood: France, United Kingdom, United States, January 1988—August 1994. *MMWR Morb Mortal Wkly Rep* 1995; 44:929–933.
39. Fahey BI, Koziol DE, Banks SM, Henderson DK. Frequency of nonparenteral occupational exposures to blood and body fluids before and after universal precautions training. *Am J Med* 1991;90:145.
40. Levy JA. Pathogenesis of human immunodeficiency virus infection. *Microbiol Rev* 1993;57:183–289.
41. Castro KG, et al. Transmission of HIV in Belle Glade, Florida: lessons for other communities in the United States. *Science* 1988;239:193.
42. Lifson AR. Do alternate modes for transmission of human immunodeficiency virus exist? *JAMA* 1988;259:1353.
43. Simonds RJ, Chanock S. Medical issues related to caring for human immunodeficiency virus-infected children in and out of the home. *Pediatr Infect Dis J* 1993;12:845–852.
44. Marcus R, Centers for Disease Control and Prevention Cooperative Needlestick Study Group. Surveillance of health-care workers exposed to blood from patients infected with the human immunodeficiency virus. *N Engl J Med* 1988;319:1118.
45. Richman KM, Rickman LS. The potential for transmission of human immunodeficiency virus through human bites. *Journal of Acquired Immune Deficiency Syndromes* 1993;6:402–406.
46. Vidmar L, Poljak M, Tomazic J, Seme K, Klavs I. Transmission of HIV-1 by human bite. *Lancet* 1996;347:1762–1763.
47. Petersen NJ. An assessment of the airborne route in hepatitis B transmission. *Ann NY Acad Sci* 1980;353:157.
48. Johnson GK, Robinson WS. Human immunodeficiency virus-1 (HIV-1) in the vapors of surgical power instruments. *J Med Virol* 1991; 33:47.
49. Mangione CM, Gerberding JL, Cummings SR. Occupational exposure to HIV: frequency and rates of underreporting of percutaneous and mucocutaneous exposures by medical housestaff. *Am J Med* 1991; 90:85.
50. Short L, Chamberland M, Culver D, et al. Underreporting of needlestick injuries among health-care workers [Abstract]. *Infect Control Hosp Epidemiol* 1994;15(4, part 2):P20.
51. Tokars JI, Bell DM, Marcus R, et al. Percutaneous injuries during surgical procedures. *JAMA* 1992;267:2899–2904.
52. Panlilio AL, Welch BA, Bell DM, et al. Blood and amniotic fluid contact sustained by obstetric personnel during deliveries. *Am J Obstet Gynecol* 1992;167:703–708.
53. Cleveland JL, Lockwood SA, Gooch BF, et al. Percutaneous injuries in dentistry: an observational study. *J Am Dent Assoc* 1995;126: 745–751.
54. Siew C, Gruninger SE, Miaw CL, Neidle EA. Percutaneous injuries in practicing dentists: a prospective study using a 20 day diary. *J Am Dent Assoc* 1995;126:1227–1234.
55. Wong ES, et al. Are universal precautions effective in reducing the number of occupational exposures among healthcare workers? A prospective study of physicians on a medical service. *JAMA* 1991; 265:1123.
56. Marcus R, Srivastava PU, Bell DM, et al. Occupational blood contact among pre-hospital providers: a prospective study. *Ann Emerg Med* 1995;25:776–779.
57. Short LJ, Bell DM. Risk of occupational infection with blood-borne pathogens in operating and delivery room settings. *Am J Infect Control* 1993;21:343–350.
58. Telford GL, Quebbeman EJ. Assessing the risk of blood exposure in the operating room. *Am J Infect Control* 1993;21:351–356.
59. Tokars JI, Culver DH, Mendelson MH, et al. Skin and mucous membrane blood contacts during surgical procedures: risk and prevention. *Infect Control Hosp Epidemiol* 1995;16:703–711.
60. Rudnick J, Chamberland M, Panlilio A, et al. Blood contacts during obstetrical procedures. *Infect Control Hosp Epidemiol* 1994;15:349.
61. Centers for Disease Control and Prevention. Update: human immunodeficiency virus infections in health-care workers exposed to blood of infected patients. *MMWR Morb Mortal Wkly Rep* 1987;36:285.
62. Rhodes RS, Bell DM, eds. Prevention of transmission of bloodborne pathogens. *Surg Clin North Am* 1995;75:1046–1217.
63. Greene ES, Berry AJ, Arnold WP, et al. Percutaneous injuries in anesthesia personnel. *Anesth Analg* 1996;83:273–278.
64. Ippolito G, Petrosillo N, Puro V, et al. The risk of occupational exposure to blood and body fluids for healthcare workers in the dialysis setting. *Nephron* 1995;70:180–184.
65. Hansen ME, Miller GL III, Redman HC, McIntire DD. Needle-stick injuries and blood contacts during invasive radiologic procedures: frequency and risk factors. *American Journal of Radiology* 1993:160:1119–1122.
66. Jagger J, Bentley M. Clinical laboratories: reducing exposures to bloodborne pathogens. *Advances in Exposure Prevention* 1996;2:1–2, 6–8.
67. Jagger J, Hunt EH, Brand-Elnaggar J, Pearson RD. Rates of needlestick injury caused by various devices in a university hospital. *N Engl J Med* 1988;319:284.
68. Ippolito G, De Carli G, Puro V, et al. Device-specific risk of needlestick injury in Italian healthcare workers. *JAMA* 1994;272:607–610.
69. Cardo D, Marcus R, McKibben P, et al. Preventability of hollow-bore needle exposures to HIV-infected blood among healthcare workers [Abstract]. *Infect Cont Hosp Epidemiol* 1994;15(4, Part 2):P20.
70. Chiarello L. Selection of needlestick prevention devices: a conceptual framework for approaching product evaluation. *Am J Infect Control* 1995;23:386–395.
71. Benson JS. *FDA safety alert: needlestick and other risks from hypodermic needles on secondary I.V. administration sets and piggyback and intermittent I.V.* Washington, DC: Food and Drug Administration; April 16, 1992.

72. Olishifski JB. Methods of control. In: Plog BA, ed. *Fundamentals of industrial hygiene.* 3rd ed. Chicago: National Safety Council, 1988: 457–474.
73. Gerberding JL. Occupational infectious diseases or infectious occupational diseases? Bridging the views on tuberculosis control. *Infect Control Hosp Epidemiol* 1993;14:686–688.
74. Centers for Disease Control and Prevention. Recommendations for prevention of HIV transmission in health-care settings. *MMWR Morb Mortal Wkly Rep* 1987;36(Suppl 2S):1S–18S.
75. Centers for Disease Control and Prevention. Update: universal precautions for prevention of transmission of human immunodeficiency virus, hepatitis B virus, and other bloodborne pathogens in health-care settings. *MMWR Morb Mortal Wkly Rep* 1988;37:377–382, 387–388.
76. Department of Labor, Occupational Safety and Health Administration. 29 CFR Part 1910,1030 Occupational exposure to bloodborne pathogens; final rule. *Federal Register* 1991;56(235):64004–64182.
77. Lynch P, Jackson MM, Cummings J, et al. Rethinking the role of isolation practices in the prevention of nosocomial infections. *Ann Intern Med* 1987;107:243–246.
78. Jackson MM, Lynch P. An attempt to make an issue less murky: a comparison of four systems for infection precautions. *Infect Control Hosp Epidemiol* 1991;12:448–450.
79. Garner JS, the Hospital Infection Control Practices Advisory Committee. Guideline for isolation precautions in hospitals. *Infect Control Hosp Epidemiol* 1996;17:54–80.
80. McCormick RD, Meisch MG, Ircink FG, et al. Epidemiology of hospital sharps injuries: a 14-year prospective study in the pre-AIDS and AIDS eras. *Am J Med* 1991;91(Suppl 3B):301S–307S.
81. Linnemann CC Jr, Cannon C, DeRonde M, et al. Effect of educational programs, rigid sharps containers, and universal precautions on reported needlestick injuries in healthcare workers. *Infect Control Hosp Epidemiol* 1991;12:214–219.
82. Beekmann SE, Vlahov D, Koziol DE, et al. Temporal association between implementation of universal precautions and a sustained, progressive decrease in percutaneous exposures to blood. *Clin Infect Dis* 1994;18:562–569.
83. Saghafi L, Raselli P, Farncillon C, et al. Exposure to blood during various procedures: results of two surveys before and after the implementation of universal precautions. *Am J Infect Control* 1992;20:53–57.
84. Haiduven DJ, DeMaio TM, Stevens DA. A five-year study of needlestick injuries: significant reduction associated with communication, education, and convenient placement of sharps containers. *Infect Control Hosp Epidemiol* 1992;13:265–271.
85. Sellick JA Jr, Hazamy PA, Mylotte JM. Influence of an educational program and mechanical opening needle disposal boxes on occupational needlestick injuries. *Infect Control Hosp Epidemiol* 1991;12:725–731.
86. Ribner BS, Ribner BS. An effective educational program to reduce the frequency of needle recapping. *Infect Control Hosp Epidemiol* 1990; 11:635–638.
87. Makofsky D, Cone JE. Installing needle disposal boxes closer to the bedside reduces needle-recapping rates in hospital units. *Infect Control Hosp Epidemiol* 1993;14;140–144.
88. Edmond M, Khakoo R, McTaggart B, et al. Effect of bedside needle disposal units on needle recapping frequency and needlestick injury. *Infect Control Hosp Epidemiol* 1988;9:114–116.
89. Weltman AC, Short LJ, Mendelson MH, et al. Disposal-related sharps injuries at a New York City teaching hospital. *Infect Control Hosp Epidemiol* 1995;16:268–274.
90. ECRI. Sharps disposal containers. *Health Devices* 1993;22:359–412.
91. Jagger J, Pearson RD. Universal precautions: still missing the point on needlesticks [Editorial]. *Infect Control Hosp Epidemiol* 1991;12: 211–213.
92. Gerberding JL. Needlestick prevention: new paradigms for research [Editorial]. *Infect Control Hosp Epidemiol* 1992;13:257–258.
93. Becker MH, Janz NK, Band J, et al. Noncompliance with universal precautions policy: why do physicians and nurses recap needles? *Am J Infect Control* 1990;18:232–239.
94. Henry K, Campbell S, Collier P, et al. Compliance with universal precautions and needle handling and disposal practices among emergency department staff at two community hospitals. *Am J Infect Control* 1994;22;129–137.
95. Williams CO, Campbell S, Henry K, et al. Variables influencing worker compliance with universal precautions in the emergency department. *Am J Infect Control* 1994;22;138–148.
96. Centers for Disease Control and Prevention. Evaluation of safety devices for preventing percutaneous injuries among health-care workers during phlebotomy procedures: Minneapolis-St. Paul, New York City, and San Francisco, 1993–1995. *MMWR Morb Mortal Wkly Rep* 1997;46:21–25.
97. Billiet LS, Parker CR, Tanley PC, et al. Needlestick injury rate reduction during phlebotomy: a comparative study of two safety devices. *Lab Med* 1991;22:120–123.
98. Chiarello L. Summary: New York State Department of Health pilot study of needlestick prevention devices. In: American Hospital Association, ed. *Implementing safer needle devices.* Chicago: American Hospital Association, 1992:29–32.
99. Skolnick R, LaRocca J, Barba D, et al. Evaluation and implementation of a needleless intravenous system: Making needlesticks a needless problem. *Am J Infect Control* 1993;21:39–41.
100. Gartner K. Impact of a needleless intravenous system in a university hospital. *Am J Infect Control* 1992;20:75–79.
101. Terrell F, Williams B. Implementation of a customized needleless intravenous delivery system. *Journal of Intravenous Nursing* 1993;16: 339–344.
102. Centers for Disease Control and Prevention. Evaluation of blunt suture needles in preventing percutaneous injuries among health-care workers during gynecologic surgical procedures: New York City, March 1993–June 1994. *MMWR Morb Mortal Wkly Rep* 1997;46: 25–29.
103. Owens-Schwab E, Fraser VJ. Needleless and needle protection devices: a second look at efficacy and selection. *Infect Control Hosp Epidemiol* 1993;14:657–660.
104. ECRI. Needlestick-prevention devices. *Health Devices* 1994;23: 359–369.
105. American Hospital Association, ed. *Implementing safer needle devices.* Chicago: American Hospital Association, 1992.
106. Quebbeman EJ, Short LJ. How to select and evaluate new products on the market. *Surg Clin North Am* 1995;75:1159–1165.
107. Laufer FN, Chiarello LA. Application of cost-effectiveness methodology to the consideration of needlestick-prevention technology. *Am J Infect Control* 1994;22:75–82.
108. Danzig LE, Short LJ, Collins K, et al. Bloodstream infections associated with a needleless intravenous infusion system in patients receiving home infusion therapy. *JAMA* 1995;273:1862–1864.
109. Maki DG, Stolz S, McCormick R, et al. Possible association of a commercial needleless system with central venous catheter-related bacteremia [Abstract J201]. In: *Abstracts of the 34th interscience conference on antimicrobial agents and chemotherapy, Orlando, 1994.* Washington, DC: American Society for Microbiology, 1994.
110. Kellerman S, Shay D, Howard J, et al. Bloodstream infections associated with needleless devices used for central venous catheter access in children receiving home healthcare [Abstract J11]. In: *Abstracts of the 35th interscience conference on antimicrobial agents and chemotherapy, San Francisco, 1995.* Washington, DC: American Society for Microbiology, 1995.
111. Chiarello LA. Reducing needlestick injuries among healthcare workers. *AIDS Clinical Care* 1993;5:77–79.
112. Manian FA, Meyer L, Jenne J. Puncture injuries due to needles removed from intravenous lines: should the source patient routinely be tested for bloodborne infections? *Infect Control Hosp Epidemiol* 1993;14:325–330.
113. Mendelson MH, Short L, Schechter C, et al. Comparative cross-over study of a needleless heparin lock system vs. a conventional heparin lock: impact on complications, sharps injuries, and cost [Abstract 1189]. In: *Abstracts of the 32nd interscience conference on antimicrobial agents and chemotherapy, Anaheim, CA, 1992.* Washington, DC: American Society for Microbiology; 1992.
114. Adams KS, Zehrer CL, Thomas W. Comparison of a needleless system with conventional heparin locks. *Am J Infect Control* 1993;21: 263–269.
115. Summitt RL, Stovall TG, Lipscomb GH, et al. Randomized comparison of laparoscopy-assisted vaginal hysterectomy with standard vaginal hysterectomy in an outpatient setting. *Obstet Gynecol* 1992;80: 895–901.
116. Lewis FR Jr, Short LJ, Howard RJ, et al. Epidemiology of injuries by needles and other sharp instruments: minimizing sharp injuries in gynecologic and obstetric operations. *Surg Clin North Am* 1995;75: 1105–1121.

117. Gerberding JL. Procedure-specific infection control for preventing intraoperative blood exposures. *Am J Infect Control* 1993;21: 364–367.
118. Short LJ, Benson DR. Special considerations for surgeons. In: Devita VT, Hellman H, Rosenberg S, eds. *AIDS: etiology, diagnosis, treatment, and prevention*. 4th ed. Philadelphia: Lippincott–Raven; 1997: 665–673.
119. Department of Health and Human Services, Food and Drug Administration. 21CFR Part 800 medical devices; patient examination and surgeons gloves; adulteration; final rule. *Federal Register* 1990;55(239): 51254–51258.
120. Gerberding JL, Quebbeman EJ, Rhodes RS. Hand protection. *Surg Clin North Am* 1995;75:1133–1139.
121. Stampfer JF, Kissane RJ, Martin LS. Electrical conductivity as a test for the integrity of latex gloves. *J Clin Eng* 1994;19:476–489.
122. Lytle CD, Cyr WH, Carey RF, et al. Standard quality control testing and virus penetration. In: Mellstrom GA, Wahlberg JE, Maibach HI, eds. *Protective gloves for occupational use.* Boca Raton, FL: CRC Press, 1994:109–127.
123. Lytle CD, Truscott W, Budacz AP, et al. Important factors for testing barrier materials with surrogate viruses. *Appl Environ Microbiol* 1991;57:2549–2554.
124. Otis LL, Cottone JA. Prevalence of perforations in disposable latex gloves during routine dental treatment. *J Am Dent Assoc* 1989;118: 321–324.
125. Yangco BG, Yangco NF. What is leaky can be risky: a study of the integrity of hospital gloves. *Infect Control Hosp Epidemiol* 1989;10: 553–556.
126. DeGroot-Kosolcharoen J, Jones JM. Permeability of latex and vinyl gloves to water and blood. *Am J Infect Control* 1989;17:196–201.
127. Arena B, Maffulli N, Vocaturo I, et al. Incidence of glove perforation during caesarean section. *Ann Chir Gynaecol* 1991;80:377–380.
128. Serrano CW, Wright JW, Newton ER. Surgical glove perforation in obstetrics. *Obstet Gynecol* 1991;77:525–528.
129. Rhoton-Vlasak A, Duff P. Glove perforations and blood contact associated with manipulation of the fetal scalp electrode. *Obstet Gynecol* 1993;81:224–226.
130. Chapman S, Duff P. Frequency of glove perforations and subsequent blood contact in association with selected obstetric surgical procedures. *Am J Obstet Gynecol* 1993;168:1354–1357.
131. Cohn GM, Seifer DB. Blood exposure in single versus double gloving during pelvic surgery. *Am J Obstet Gynecol* 1990;162:715–717.
132. Quebbeman EJ, Telford GL, Wadsworth K, et al. Double gloving: protecting surgeons from blood contamination in the operating room. *Arch Surg* 1992;127:213–217.
133. Bennett B, Duff, P. The effect of double gloving on frequency of glove perforations. *Obstet Gynecol* 1991;78:1019–1022.
134. Doyle PM, Alvi, S, Johanson R. The effectiveness of double-gloving in obstetrics and gynaecology. *Br J Obstet Gynaecol* 1992;99:83–84.
135. Cohen MS, Do JT, Tahery DP, et al. Efficacy of double gloving as a protection against blood exposure in dermatologic surgery. *J Dermatol Surg Oncol* 1992;18:873–874.
136. Dodds RDA, Barker SGE, Morgan NH, et al. Self protection in surgery: the use of double gloves. *Br J Surg* 1990;77:219–220.
137. Rose DA, Ramiro N, Perlman J, et al. Usage patterns and perforation rates for 6396 gloves from intra-operative procedures at San Francisco General Hospital [Abstract]. *Infect Control Hosp Epidemiol* 1994;15: 349.
138. Association for the Advancement of Medical Instrumentation. *Selection of surgical gowns and drapes in healthcare facilities*. TIR11-006-MM. Arlington, VA: Association for the Advancement of Medical Instrumentation; September, 1994.
139. Association of Operating Room Nurses. Recommended practices: protective barrier materials for surgical gowns and drapes. *AORN J* 1992;55:832–835.
140. American Society for Testing and Materials. *Emergency standard test method for resistance of protective clothing materials to synthetic blood*. Philadelphia: American Society for Testing and Materials, 1992.
141. American Society for Testing and Materials. *Emergency standard test method for resistance of protective clothing materials to penetration by bloodborne pathogens using viral penetration as a test system.* Philadelphia: American Society for Testing and Materials, 1992.
142. Belkin NI. Gowns: selection on a procedure-driven basis. *Infect Control Hosp Epidemiol* 1994;15:713–716.
143. Kabukoba JJ, Pearce JM. The design, effectiveness and acceptability of the arm sleeve for the prevention of body fluid contamination during obstetric procedures. *Br J Obstet Gynaecol* 1993;100:714–716.
144. Meyer KK, Beck WC. Gown–glove interface: a possible solution to the danger zone. *Infect Control Hosp Epidemiol* 1995;16:488–490.
145. Kouri DL, Ernest JM. Incidence of perceived and actual face shield contamination during vaginal and cesarean delivery. *Am J Obstet Gynecol* 1993;169:312–316.
146. Sattar SA, Springthorpe VS. Survival and disinfectant inactivation of the human immunodeficiency virus. *Rev Infect Dis* 1991;13: 430–447.
147. Van Bueren J, Simpson RA, Jacobs P, Cookson BD. Survival of human immunodeficiency virus in suspension and dried onto surfaces. *J Clin Microbiol* 1994;32:571–574.
148. Favero MS, Bond WW. Sterilization, disinfection, and antisepsis in the hospital. In: *Manual of clinical microbiology.* Washington, DC: American Society for Microbiology, 1991:183–200.
149. Garner JS, Favero MS. *Guideline for handwashing and hospital environmental control, 1985*. HHS publication no. (CDC) 99-1117. Atlanta: Department of Health and Human Services, Public Health Service, Centers for Disease Control, 1985.
150. Martin MA, Reichelderfer M, Association for Professionals in Infection Control and Epidemiology Inc, 1991, 1992, and 1993 APIC Guidelines Committee. APIC guideline for infection prevention and control in flexible endoscopy. *Am J Infect Control* 1994;22:19–38.
151. Centers for Disease Control and Prevention. Recommendations for HIV testing services for inpatients and outpatients in acute care hospital settings. *MMWR Morb Mortal Wkly Rep* 1993;42(RR-2):1–6.
152. American Academy of Orthopaedic Surgeons Task Force on AIDS and Orthopaedic Surgery. *Recommendations for the prevention of human immunodeficiency virus (HIV) transmission in the practice of orthopaedic surgery.* Park Ridge, IL: American Academy of Orthopaedic Surgeons, 1989.
153. Quebbeman EJ, Telford GL, Condon RE. Should patients or healthcare workers be screened for human immunodeficiency and hepatitis viruses? In: Howard RJ, ed. *Infectious risks in surgery.* Norwalk, CT: Appleton and Lange, 1991:117–123.
154. Harris RL, Boisaubin EV, Salyer PD, Semands DF. Evaluation of a hospital admission HIV antibody voluntary screening program. *Infect Control Hosp Epidemiol* 1990;11:628.
155. Mullins JR, Harrison PB. The questionable utility of mandatory screening for human immunodeficiency virus. *Am J Surg* 1993;166: 676–679.
156. Centers for Disease Control and Prevention. Public Health Service statement on management of occupational exposure to human immunodeficiency virus, including considerations regarding zidovudine postexposure use. *MMWR Morb Mortal Wkly Rep* 1990;39(RR-1):1.
157. Centers for Disease Control and Prevention. Update: provisional Public Health Service recommendations for chemoprophylaxis after occupational exposure to HIV. *MMWR Morb Mortal Wkly Rep* 1996;45:468–472.
158. Carpenter CJ, Fischl MA, Hammer SM, et al. Antiretroviral therapy for HIV infection in 1996: recommendations of an international panel. *JAMA* 1996;276:146–154.
159. Gerberding JL. Management of occupational exposures to bloodborne viruses. *N Engl J Med* 1995;332:444.
160. Ciesielski CA, Metler RP. Duration of time between exposure and seroconversion in healthcare workers with occupationally acquired infection with human immunodeficiency virus. *Am J Med* 1997; 102 (suppl 5B):115–116.
161. Ridzon R, Gallagher K, Ciesielski C, et al. Simultaneous transmission of human immunodeficiency virus and hepatitis C virus from a needle-stick injury. *N Engl J Med* 1997;336:919–922.
162. Meyohas MC, Morand-Jubert L, Van de Wiel P, Mariotti M, Lefrere JJ. Time to HIV seroconversion after needlestick injury. *Lancet* 1995; 345:1634–1635.
163. Heptonstall J, Gill ON. HIV, occupational exposure, and medical responsibilities. *Lancet* 1995;346:578–580.
164. Wormser GP, et al. Polymerase chain reaction for seronegative healthcare workers with parenteral exposure to HIV-infected patients. *N Engl J Med* 1989;321:1681.
165. Henry K, et al. Long-term follow-up of healthcare workers with work site exposure to human immunodeficiency virus. *JAMA* 1990;263: 1765.

166. Busch M, Satten G. Time course of viremia and antibody seroconversion following human immunodeficiency virus exposures. *Am J Med* 1997;102 (suppl 5B):117–124.
167. Bell DM, Gerberding JL, eds. HIV post-exposure management of healthcare workers: report of a workshop. *Am J Med* 1997;102 (suppl 5B):1–30.
168. LaFon SW, et al. A double-blind, placebo-controlled study of the safety and efficacy of Retrovir (zidovudine, ZDV) as a chemoprophylactic agent in healthcare workers exposed to HIV [Abstract 489]. In: *Proceedings of the 30th interscience conference on antimicrobial agents and chemotherapy, Atlanta, 1991*. Washington, DC: American Society for Microbiology, 1991.
169. Connor EM, Sperling RS, Gelber R, et al. Reduction of maternal-infant transmission of HIV type 1 with zidovudine treatment. *N Engl J Med* 1994;331:1173.
170. Sperling RS, Shapiro DE, Coombs R, et al. Maternal plasma HIV-1 RNA and the success of zidovudine in the prevention of mother–child transmission [Abstract LB1]. In: *Program and abstracts of the 3rd conference on retroviruses and opportunistic infections*. Alexandria, Virginia: Infectious Diseases Society of America, 1996:161.
171. Shih CC, et al. Postexposure prophylaxis with zidovudine suppresses human immunodeficiency virus type 1 infection in SCID-hu mice in a time-dependent manner. *J Infect Dis* 1991;163:625.
172. Van Rompay KK, Marthas ML, Ramos RA, et al. Simian immunodeficiency virus (SIV) infection of infant rhesus macaques as a model to test antiretroviral drug prophylaxis and therapy: oral 3′-azido-3′-deoxythymidine prevents SIV infection. *Antimicrob Agents Chemother* 1992;36:2381.
173. Tsai CC, Follis KE, Sabo A, et al. Prevention of SIV infection in macaques by (R)-9-(2-phosphonylmethyoxypropyl)adenine. *Science* 1995;270:1197–1199.
174. Black R. Animal studies of prophylaxis. *Am J Med* 1997;102 (suppl 5B):39–44.
175. Jochimsen E. Failures of zidovudine post-exposure prophylaxis. *Am J Med* 1997;102 (suppl 5B):52–55.
176. Lange JMA, et al. Failure of zidovudine prophylaxis after accidental exposure to HIV-1. *N Engl J Med* 1990;322:1375.
177. Centers for Disease Control and Prevention. Patient exposures to HIV during nuclear medicine procedures. *MMWR Morb Mortal Wkly Rep* 1992;41:575–578.
178. Durand E, Le Jeune C, Hugues FC. Failure of prophylactic zidovudine after suicidal self-inoculation of HIV-infected blood. *N Engl J Med* 1991;324:1062.
179. Jones PD. HIV transmission by stabbing despite zidovudine prophylaxis. *Lancet* 1991;338:884.
180. Anonymous. New drugs for HIV infection. *The Medical Letter on Drugs and Therapeutics* 1996;38:35–37.
181. Puro P, Ippolito G, Guzzanti E, et al. Zidovudine prophylaxis after accidental exposure to HIV: the Italian experience. *AIDS* 1992;6:963.
182. Fahrner R, Beekman S, Koziol DE, Gerberding JL, Henderson DK. Safety of zidovudine administered as post-exposure chemoprophylaxis to healthcare workers sustaining occupational exposures to HIV [Abstract I154]. *Abstracts of the 34th interscience conference on antimicrobial agents and chemotherapy, Orlando, 1994*. Washington, DC: American Society for Microbiology, 1994.
183. D'Silva M, Leibowitz D, Flaherty JP. Seizure associated with zidovudine. *Lancet* 1995;346:452.
184. Henry K, Acosta EP, Jochimsen E. Hepatotoxicity and rash associated with zidovudine and zalcitabine chemoprophylaxis. *Ann Intern Med* 1996;124:855.
185. Connor E, Sperling R, Shapiro D, et al. Long term effect of zidovudine exposure among uninfected infants born to HIV-infected mothers in pediatric AIDS Clinical Trials Group protocol 076. In: *Abstracts of the 35th interscience conference on antimicrobial agents and chemotherapy, San Francisco, 1995*. Washington, DC: American Society for Microbiology, 1995.
186. Kinloch-de Loës S, Hirschel BJ, Hoen B, et al. A controlled trial of zidovudine in primary human immunodeficiency virus infection. *N Engl J Med* 1995;333:408–413.
187. Bell DM, Shapiro CN, Ciesielski CA, Chamberland ME. Bloodborne pathogen transmission from healthcare workers to patients: the CDC perspective. *Surg Clin North Am* 1995;75:1189–1203.
188. Ciesielski C, Marianos D, Ou CY, et al. Transmission of human immunodeficiency virus in a dental practice. *Ann Intern Med* 1992; 116:798–804.
189. Ou CY, Ciesielski CA, Myers G, et al. Molecular epidemiology of HIV transmission in a dental practice. *Science* 1992;256:1165–1171.
190. Gooch B, Marianos D, Ciesielski C, et al. Lack of evidence for patient-to-patient transmission in a dental practice. *J Am Dent Assoc* 1993;124:38–44.
191. Ciesielski CA, Marianos DW, Schochetman G, Witte JJ, Jaffe HW. The 1990 Florida dental investigation: the press and the science. *Ann Intern Med* 1994;121:886–888.
192. Reseau National de Sante Publique. *HIV transmission from an infected surgeon to one patient in France*. World Wide Web (http://www. b3e.jussieu.fr:80/rnsp/sida/surgeon.html) January 20, 1997. St Maurice, France.
193. Robert LM, Chamberland ME, Cleveland JL, et al. Investigations of patients of healthcare workers infected with HIV: the Centers for Disease Control and Prevention database. *Ann Intern Med* 1995;122: 653–657.
194. Bell DM, Shapiro CN, Culver DH, Martone WJ, Curran JW, Hughes JM. Risk of hepatitis B and human immunodeficiency virus transmission to a patient from an infected surgeon due to percutaneous injury during an invasive procedure: estimates based on a model. *Infect Agents Dis* 1992;1:263–269.
195. Mishu B, Schaffner W. HIV-infected surgeons and dentists: looking back and looking forward. *JAMA* 1993;269:1843–1844.
196. Harpaz R, Von Seidlin L, Averhoff FM, et al. Transmission of hepatitis B virus to multiple patients from a surgeon without evidence of inadequate infection control. *N Engl J Med* 1996;334:549–554.
197. The Incident Investigation Teams and Others. Transmission of hepatitis B to patients from four infected surgeons without hepatitis B e antigen. *N Engl J Med* 1997;336:178–184.
198. Esteban JI, Gomez J, Martell M, et al. Transmission of hepatitis C virus by a cardiac surgeon. *N Engl J Med* 1996;334:555–560.
199. Public Health Laboratory Service Communicable Disease Surveillance Centre. Hepatitis C virus transmission from healthcare worker to patient. *CDR (London)* 1995;5:121.
200. Gerberding JL, Rose DA, Ramiro NZ, et al. Intraoperative provider injuries and potential patient recontacts at San Francisco General Hospital [Abstract]. *Infect Control Hosp Epidemiol* 1994;15:344.
201. Rudnick J, Chamberland ME, Panlilio A, et al. Blood contacts during obstetrical procedures [Abstract]. *Infect Control Hosp Epidemiol* 1994;15:349.
202. Robert L, Short L, Chamberland M, et al. Percutaneous injuries sustained during gynecologic surgery [Abstract]. *Infect Control Hosp Epidemiol* 1994;15:349.
203. Centers for Disease Control and Prevention. Recommendations for preventing transmission of human immunodeficiency virus and hepatitis B virus to patients during exposure-prone invasive procedures. *MMWR Morb Mortal Wkly Rep* 1991;40(RR-8):1.
204. Americans with Disabilities Act. *Public Law 101-336, 104 Stat. 327, 42 U.S.C., 12101 et seq. 101st Congress*.
205. Rhodes RS, Telford GL, Hierholzer WJ, Barnes M. *Bloodborne pathogen transmission from health-care worker to patients: legal issues and provider perspectives.* Surg Clin North Am 1995;75:1205–1217.
206. American Medical Association. *HIV and physicians.* AMA Policy Compendium (No. 20. 948). Chicago: American Medical Association, 1995.
207. American College of Surgeons. Statement on the surgeon and HIV infection. *Bulletin of the American College of Surgeons* 1991;76: 28–31.
208. American Academy of Orthopaedic Surgeons. *Advisory statement: HIV-infected orthopaedic surgeons*. Park Ridge, IL: American Academy of Orthopaedic Surgeons, 1991.
209. AIDS/TB Committee of the Society for Healthcare Epidemiology. Position paper: management of healthcare workers infected with hepatitis B virus, hepatitis C virus, human immunodeficiency virus, or other bloodborne pathogens. *Infect Control Hosp Epidemiol* 1997;18:349–363.
210. American College of Obstetricians and Gynecologists, Committee on Ethics. Human immunodeficiency virus infection: physician's responsibilities. *Obstet Gynecol* 1990;75:1043.
211. Gulick RM, Mellors J, Havlir D, et al. Potent and sustained antiretroviral activity of indinavir (IDV), zidovudine (ZDV), and lamivudine (3TC). In: *Abstracts of the XI international conference on AIDS, Vancouver 1996*. 1996:Th.B.931, Vol 2.
212. Saag MS, Holodniy M, Kuritzkes DR, et al. HIV viral load markers in clinical practice. *Nature Med* 1996;2:625–629.

213. AIDS Committee for the Society for Hospital Epidemiology of America. "Lookback" notification for HIV/HBV positive healthcare workers. *Infect Control Hosp Epidemiol* 1992;13:482–484.
214. Danila RN, et al. A look-back investigation of patients of an HIV-infected physician: public health implications. *N Engl J Med* 1991; 325:1406.
215. Avila C, Stetler HC, Sepulveda J, et al. The epidemiology of HIV transmission among paid plasma donors, Mexico City, Mexico. AIDS 1989;3:631–633.
216. Pokrovsky W. *Localization of nosocomial outbreak of HIV infection in southern Russia in 1988–1989.* Presented at the VIII International Conference on AIDS, Amsterdam, July, 1992.
217. Hersch BS, et al. Acquired immunodeficiency syndrome in Romania. *Lancet* 1991;338:645.
218. Velandia M, Fridkin SK, Cardenas V, et al. Transmission of HIV in a dialysis centre. *Lancet* 1995;345:1417–1422.
219. Dyer E. Argentinian doctors accused of spreading AIDS. *Br Med J* 1993;307:584.
220. Marcus R, et al. Prevalence and incidence of human immunodeficiency virus among patients undergoing long-term hemodialysis. *Am J Med* 1991;90:614.
221. Chant K, Lowe D, Rubin G, et al. Patient-to-patient transmission of HIV in private surgical consulting rooms. *Lancet* 1993;342:1548–1549.
222. Blank S, Simonds RJ, Weisfuse I, et al. Possible nosocomial transmission of HIV. *Lancet* 1994;344:512–514.
223. Centers for Disease Control and Prevention. Provisional Public Health Service recommendations for screening donated blood and plasma for antibody to the virus causing acquired immunodeficiency syndrome. *MMWR Morb Mortal Wkly Rep* 1985;34:1–5.
224. Centers for Disease Control and Prevention. Guidelines for preventing transmission of human immunodeficiency virus through transplantation of human tissue and organs. *MMWR Morb Mortal Wkly Rep* 1994;43:(RR-8):1–17.
225. Lackritz EM, Satten GA, Aberle-Grasse J, et al. Estimated risk of transmission of human immunodeficiency virus by screened blood in the United States. *N Engl J Med* 1995;333:1721–1725.

Hospital Infections, Fourth Edition,
edited by John V. Bennett and Philip S. Brachman.
Lippincott–Raven Publishers, Philadelphia © 1998

CHAPTER 44

Infections Due to Infusion Therapy

Dennis G. Maki and Leonard A. Mermel

Reliable intravascular access for administration of fluids and electrolytes, blood products, drugs, and nutritional support, and for hemodynamic monitoring is now one of the most essential features of modern medical care (Table 44-1). Each year in the United States, ~ 150 million intravascular devices are purchased by hospitals and clinics. The vast majority are peripheral venous catheters; however, >5 million central venous devices of various types are sold in the United States annually.

More than one half of all epidemics of nosocomial bacteremia or candidemia reported in the world literature between 1965 and 1991 derived from vascular access in some form [1,2]. One third to one half of episodes of nosocomial endocarditis have been traced to infected intravascular catheters [3–5], and nosocomial intravascular device-related bloodstream infection is associated with a 12% to 28% attributable mortality [6–9]. Yet, infusion therapy generally has an underappreciated potential for producing iatrogenic disease. For example, less than half of the intensive care units (ICUs) in the United Kingdom have a written policy concerning the care of central venous catheters after insertion [10].

Infusion-related bloodstream infection is too frequently unrecognized, in great measure due to its relative infrequency. The percentage of infusions identified as producing bloodstream infection is sufficiently low— < 1% on the average—that an average physician or nurse is unlikely to encounter more than an occasional case. But even a low incidence of infection applied to the estimated 30 million patients who receive infusion therapy in U.S. hospitals annually translates to an estimated 50,000 to 100,000 bloodstream infections nationwide each year [1,2], with 55,000 due to central venous catheters in U.S. ICUs [11]. Because neither the device nor the infusate is routinely cultured, the source of the bloodstream infection in a large proportion of cases is never recognized.

Intravascular device-related bloodstream infection is largely preventable. This premise forms the thesis for this review: the primary goal must not be simply to identify and treat these iatrogenic infections, but rather to prevent them. By critically scrutinizing existing knowledge of the pathogenesis and epidemiology of device-related infec-

D. G. Maki: Section of Infectious Diseases, University of Wisconsin Medical School, Center for Trauma and Life Support, Clinical Sciences Center, Madison, Wisconsin 53792.

L. A. Mermel: Department of Medicine, Brown University School of Medicine, Infection Control Department, Division of Infectious Diseases, Rhode Island Hospital, Providence, Rhode Island 02903.

TABLE 44-1. *Applications of infusion therapy in the 1990s*

Fluid and electrolyte replacement
Transfusion therapy
Blood products
Exchange transfusion
Plasmapheresis and apheresis
IV drug administration
Immediate circulatory access for critically ill patients
High blood and tissue levels
Drugs that cause tissue necrosis
Drugs that cause thrombolysis
Hemodialysis
Hemodynamic monitoring
Central venous catheters
Central venous pressure
Pulmonary artery Swan-Ganz catheters
Pulmonary artery pressure
Pulmonary artery occlusion (left atrial filling) pressure
Thermodilution cardiac output
Arterial catheters
Continuous arterial blood pressure
Total parenteral nutrition
Hyperalimentation (central venous catheters)
Peripheral parenteral nutrition (peripheral IV catheters)
Special nutritional support regimens for:
Acute renal failure
Hepatic failure
Cardiac cachexia
Pancreatitis
Acquired immunodeficiency syndrome
Intraarterial cancer chemotherapy

IV, intravenous.

tion—the reservoirs of nosocomial pathogens and modes of transmission to patients' infusions—rational and effective guidelines for prevention can be formulated [12].

SOURCES AND FORMS OF INFUSION-RELATED INFLAMMATION AND BLOODSTREAM INFECTION

There are three major sources of bloodstream infection associated with any intravascular device: 1) colonization of the cannula wound, 2) colonization of the cannula hub, and 3) contamination of the fluid (i.e., infusate) administered through the cannula. Cannulas, which cause most *endemic* device-related infections, produce bloodstream infection far more frequently than contaminated infusate, the source of most *epidemics* of infusion-associated bloodstream infection [1].

It is important to understand the different stages and forms of device-related inflammation or infection, which range from infusion phlebitis—usually unrelated to infection—to asymptomatic colonization of the intravascular device—usually by skin commensals with little intrinsic virulence—to overwhelming septic shock originating from an infected thrombus in a cannulated great central vein or from infusate heavily contaminated by gram-negative bacilli.

Infusion Phlebitis

Infusion phlebitis, defined as inflammation of the cannulated vein—pain, erythema, tenderness, or an inflamed, palpable, thrombosed vein—is a frequent cause of pain and discomfort to the millions of patients who receive infusion therapy through peripheral intravenous (IV) cannulas each year in U.S. hospitals. Most investigators have concluded that infusion phlebitis is primarily a physicochemical phenomenon, and prospective studies have shown that the cannula material, length, and bore size; operator skill on insertion; the anatomic site of cannulation; the duration of cannulation; the frequency of dressing changes; the character of the infusate; and host factors such as patient age, Caucasian race, female gender, and the presence of underlying diseases significantly influence the risk of infusion phlebitis (Table 44-2).

In a prospective clinical study of 1,054 peripheral IV catheters, the Kaplan-Meier risk for phlebitis exceeded 50% by the fourth day after catheterization. IV antibiotics (relative risk (RR), 2.0), female gender (RR, 1.9), catheterization beyond 48 hours (RR, 1.8), and catheter material (polyetherurethane (Vialon), tetrafluoroethylene-hexafluoropropylene (Teflon), RR, 0.7) were strong predictors of phlebitis in a Cox proportional hazards model (each, $p < 0.003$) [13]. The best-fit model for severe phlebitis identified the same predictors plus catheter-related infection (RR, 6.2), phlebitis with the

TABLE 44-2. *Risk factors for infusion phlebitis in peripheral IV therapy identified in prospective studies by multivariate discriminant analysis or in prospective, randomized, controlled trials*[a]

Catheter material
Polypropylene > Teflon
Silicone elastomer > polyurethane
Teflon > polyetherurethane
Teflon > steel needles
Catheter size
Large bore > smaller bore
8″ > 2″ Teflon
Insertion in emergency room > inpatient units
Disinfection of skin with antiseptic before catheter insertion
Experience, skill of person inserting catheter
House officers, nurses > hospital IV Team
House officers, nurses > decentralized unit IV nurse educator
Increasing duration of catheter placement in site
Subsequent catheters beyond the first infusate
Low-pH solutions (e.g., dextrose-containing)
Potassium chloride
Hypertonic glucose, amino acids, lipid for parenteral nutrition
Antibiotics (especially β-lactams, vancomycin, metronidazole)
High rate of flow of IV fluid (>90 ml/hr)
Disinfection of insertion site before catheter insertion
None > chlorhexidine–alcohol
Frequent IV dressing changes
Daily > every 48 hr
Catheter-related infection
Host factors
"Poor-quality" peripheral veins
Insertion site
Upper arm, wrist > hand
Age
Children: older > younger
Adults: younger > older
Sex
Female > male
Race
White > African American
Underlying medical disease
Individual biologic vulnerability

IV, intravenous.

Factors shown not to increase risk in well controlled, prospective, randomized trials include catheters made of polyethylene versus siliconized elastomer or of Teflon versus siliconized elastomer; type of antiseptic solutions used for cutaneous disinfection; use of topical antimicrobial ointment or spray on catheter insertion sites; type of dressing (e.g., gauze vs. transparent polyurethane dressing); dressing change every 48 hr versus not at all; administration of infusate by gravity flow versus pump; administration of IV antibiotics by slow infusion versus "IV push" over 2 min; maintenance of heparin locks with saline versus heparinized saline); and frequency of routine change of IV delivery system.

[a]Denotes significantly greater risk of phlebitis; factors found to be significant predictors of risk in a prospective study of 1,054 peripheral IV catheters at the University of Wisconsin Hospital and Clinics.

(From Maki DG, Ringer M. Risk factors for infusion-related phlebitis with small peripheral venous catheters. A randomized controlled study. *Ann Intern Med* 1991;114:845–854.)

previous catheter (RR, 1.5), and anatomical site (hand: forearm, RR, 0.7; wrist: forearm, RR, 0.6).

Although not all studies have identified an association between phlebitis and catheter-related infection [14,15], this large, prospective study showed a strong statistical association, as have other studies [16–20]. Phlebitis can also be produced by contaminated infusate. Patients with bloodstream infection from intrinsically contaminated fluid in a large nationwide epidemic traced to the contaminated products of one U.S. manufacturer in 1970 to 1971 had a much higher incidence of phlebitis than patients receiving IV fluids who did not develop bloodstream infection [21].

Only a small proportion of patients with IV cannula-associated peripheral vein phlebitis have infusion-related infection, and fewer than one half of patients with peripheral IV catheter-related bloodstream infection show phlebitis; however, the presence of phlebitis connotes a substantially increased risk of infection and indicates the need for immediate removal of the catheter to reduce the severity of phlebitis, for symptomatic relief, and to prevent catheter colonization from progressing to bloodstream infection.

Cannula-Related Infections

Between 5% and 25% of intravascular devices are *colonized* by skin organisms at the time of removal, as reflected by semiquantitative or quantitative cultures showing large numbers of organisms on the intravascular portion of the removed catheter or its tip. Colonization, which in most instances is asymptomatic, provides the biologic setting for systemic infection to occur and can be considered synonymous with localized infection. However, colonized cannulas are more likely than noncolonized ones to show phlebitis or local inflammation, especially purulence—pus spontaneously draining or expressable from the insertion site—and are far more likely to cause systemic infection (i.e., *cannula-related bacteremia or fungemia*) [17,22,23].

One of the most serious forms of intravascular device-related infection occurs when intravascular thrombus surrounding the cannula becomes infected. This causes *septic (suppurative) thrombophlebitis* when it occurs in association with peripheral IV cannulas [24,25], or *septic thrombosis of a great central vein* when associated with centrally placed catheters [26,27]. With suppurative phlebitis, the vein becomes an intravascular abscess, discharging myriads of microorganisms into the bloodstream, even *after the cannula has been removed*. The clinical picture is predictable: overwhelming bloodstream infection with high-grade and often unremitting bacteremia or fungemia. This syndrome is most likely to be encountered in burned patients or other ICU patients who have heavy cutaneous colonization and develop a cannula-related infection that goes unrecognized, permitting microorganisms to proliferate to high levels within the intravascular thrombus. The catheter insertion site is devoid of signs of inflammation more than half the time, and the clinical picture may not present until several days after the catheter has been removed. *In any patient with an intravascular catheter who develops high-grade bloodstream infection that persists after an infected cannula has been removed, it is likely the patient has infected thrombus in the recently cannulated vein, and may even have secondary endocarditis or seeding to other distant sites* [28].

The microorganisms most frequently implicated in suppurative phlebitis are predominantly *Staphylococcus aureus*, and *Candida* [24–27]. Although coagulase-negative staphylococci commonly cause catheter-related bloodstream infection, they rarely cause suppurative thrombophlebitis, possible because of their lesser tendency to bind to host-derived protein components of thrombus compared with other pathogens such as *S. aureus* [29,30].

Suppurative phlebitis of peripheral IV catheters is now rare, and the syndrome of IV suppuration is predominantly a complication of central venous catheters, characteristically catheters that have been left in place for many days in heavily colonized ICU patients.

Bloodstream Infection From Contaminated Infusate

It is also important to recognize that the infusate—parenteral fluid, blood products, or IV medications—administered through an intravascular device can also become contaminated and produce infusion-related bloodstream infection, which is more likely than cannula-related infection to culminate in frank septic shock. Contaminated fluid is a rare cause of endemic infection with short-term peripheral IV devices, but the infusate is more commonly associated with infections of catheters used for hemodynamic monitoring, central venous catheters, and, possibly, surgically implanted cuffed Hickman or Broviac catheters [31–34]. Most nosocomial *epidemics* of infusion-related bloodstream infection, however, have been traced to contamination of infusate by gram-negative bacilli, introduced during its manufacture (*intrinsic contamination*) [21] or during its preparation and administration in the hospital (*extrinsic contamination*) [1,2,35,36].

DIAGNOSIS OF INFUSION-RELATED BLOODSTREAM INFECTION

Clinical Features

Although meticulous aseptic technique during cannula insertion and good follow-up care greatly reduce the risk of device-related bloodstream infection, sporadic cases and even epidemics can still be expected occasionally to occur because of human error, intrinsically contaminated products, or the undue susceptibility to infection of many patients. If affected patients are to survive, the causal relationship between an infusion and a picture of bloodstream infection must be recognized as early as possible.

The general clinical features of infusion-related bacteremia or fungemia are nonspecific and indiscernible from bloodstream infections arising from any local site of infection, such as urinary tract or an infected surgical wound (Table 44-3). There also appears to be a poor correlation between clinical judgment and microbiologic confirmation of catheter-related bloodstream infection [37]. Infusion-related bloodstream infection occurring in ICU patients can be particularly insidious: bacteremia or fungemia is usually identified by positive blood cultures but is attributed to nosocomial pneumonia, urinary tract or surgical wound infection, or is simply accepted as "cryptogenic" and treated empirically.

Certain clinical, epidemiologic, and microbiologic findings can be extremely helpful to the clinician evaluating a hospitalized patient with a picture of nosocomial bloodstream infection or cryptogenic bacteremia or candidemia, and point toward an intravascular device as the source (see Table 44-3):

1. The patient is an unlikely candidate for bloodstream infection, being healthy and without underlying predisposing diseases [21,38].
2. No local infection to account for a picture of bloodstream infection [21,38].
3. An intravascular device in place, *especially a central venous catheter*, at the outset of bloodstream infection [38].
4. Local inflammation [17,22,23,39], especially purulence at the insertion site [23,39], which while present in only a minority of cases, is strongly suggestive of catheter-related infection.
5. Abrupt onset, associated with fulminant shock—suggestive of massively contaminated infusion [40].
6. Nosocomial bloodstream infection caused by staphylococci [38], especially coagulative-negative staphylococci, *Corynebacterium* (especially JK-1) or *Bacillus* species, or *Candida* [38], *Fusarium*, *Trichophyton*, or *Malassezia* species, suggests catheter-related infection. In contrast, bacteremia caused by streptococci, aerobic gram-negative bacilli—especially *Pseudomonas aeruginosa*—or anaerobes is very unlikely to have originated from an infected intravascular device [38].
7. Bloodstream infection refractory to antimicrobial therapy or dramatic improvement with removal of the cannula or discontinuation of the infusion [21,38].

During a large, nationwide outbreak in 1970 to 1971 due to intrinsic contamination of one U. S. manufacturer's products, patients treated with antibiotics to which the epidemic organisms were susceptible remained clinically septic, continued to have positive blood cultures after 24 hours or more of appropriate therapy, and did not improve clinically until their infusions were serendipitously or intentionally removed [21].

Focal retinal lesions—cotton wool spot patches—may be seen in patients with disseminated *Candida* infection deriving from central catheters, even in those without positive blood cultures [41]. Careful ophthalmologic examination should be a routine feature of the evaluation of patients with central venous catheters with suspected catheter-related bloodstream infection, especially patients receiving total parenteral nutrition (TPN). Bloodstream infection from arterial catheters may be heralded by embolic lesions that manifest as tender, erythematous papules, 5 to 10 mm in diameter, appearing in the distal distribution of the involved artery, usually in the palm or sole—Osler's nodes [42,43]. Arterial bleeding from the insertion site is often the harbinger of bloodstream infec-

TABLE 44-3. *Clinical, epidemiologic, and microbiologic features of intravascular device-related bloodstream infection*

Nonspecific	Suggestive of device-related etiology
Fever	Patient unlikely candidate for bloodstream infection (e.g., young, no underlying diseases)
Chills, shaking rigors[a]	Source of bloodstream infection inapparent
Hypotension, shock[a]	No identifiable local infection
Hyperventilation	Intravascular device in place, especially central venous catheter
Respiratory failure	Inflammation or purulence at insertion site
Gastrointestinal[a]	Abrupt onset, associated with shock[a]
Abdominal pain	Bloodstream infection refractory to antimicrobial therapy, or dramatic improvement with removal of cannula and infusion[a]
Vomiting	
Diarrhea	Bloodstream infection caused by staphylococci (especially coagulase-negative staphylococci), *Corynebacterium* (especially JK-1) or *Bacillus* species, *Candida*, *Trichophyton*, *Fusarium*, or *Malassezia* species
Neurologic[a]	
Confusion	
Seizures	

[a]Commonly seen in overwhelming gram-negative bloodstream infection originating from contaminated infusate, peripheral suppurative phlebitis, or septic thrombosis of a central vein.

tion caused by an infected arterial catheter and may denote an infective pseudoaneurysm [42,44,45]. Endocarditis, particularly right sided, is a rare but well documented complication of flow-directed pulmonary artery catheters [46–48].

Blood Cultures

Blood cultures are essential to the diagnosis of device-related bloodstream infection (see Chapter 9), and in any patient suspected of infusion-related infection, two or three separate 10-ml blood cultures should be drawn [49–51], ideally from peripheral veins, by separate venipunctures. If the patient is receiving antimicrobial therapy, blood cultures obtained immediately before a dose is due to be administered and blood antibiotic levels are likely to be low, may provide a higher yield. Use of resin-containing media to adsorb and remove any antibiotic present in the blood specimen [52], adsorb serum factors detrimental to the growth of Enterobacteriaceae [53], and lyse the cell wall of neutrophils, thereby releasing intracellular pathogens [54], may also increase the yield [55].

The use of a biphasic system, such as the Isolator® (E. I. DuPont, Nemours and Co., Wilmington, DE), or systems with selective high blood volume fungal media (BACTEC; Becton Dickinson Diagnostic Instrument Systems, Sparks, MD) appear significantly to enhance the laboratory detection of fungemia [56,57].

The volume of blood cultured is critical to maximize the yield of blood cultures for diagnosis of bacteremia or candidemia: in adults, obtaining at least 20 ml, ideally 30 ml, per drawing—each specimen containing 10 or 15 ml, inoculated into aerobic and anaerobic media—significantly improves the yield, compared with obtaining only 10 ml at each drawing and culturing a smaller total volume [58,59]. It is rarely necessary to obtain > two 15-ml cultures or three 10-ml cultures in a 24-hour period. If at least 30 ml of blood is cultured, 99% of detectable bacteremias should be identified [58].

It is common practice in many ICUs to draw blood cultures through central venous or arterial catheters or, in neonates, through umbilical catheters. Comparative studies of standard blood cultures drawn through central venous or arterial catheters in adults have usually shown good concordance with cultures drawn by percutaneous peripheral venipuncture [60–62], but rates of false-positive (contaminated) cultures can be considerably higher with catheter-drawn specimens [63]. The practice of drawing nonqualitative blood cultures through indwelling vascular catheters probably ought not to be encouraged because of the risk of introducing contamination during the manipulation [64]. If, however, to preserve dwindling superficial veins it is considered unavoidable to use a vascular catheter to obtain blood cultures, an attempt should be made to use a newly inserted catheter [60–62] and to draw at least every other specimen by percutaneous venipuncture.

If the laboratory is prepared to do pour-plate blood cultures or has available an automated quantitative system for culturing blood, such as the Isolator® system, catheter-drawn blood cultures can permit the diagnosis of device-related bloodstream infection to be made with reasonable sensitivity and specificity (both in the range of 90%), without removing the catheter [65–71]. With infected catheters, a quantitative blood culture drawn through the catheter usually shows a marked step-up—often > 10-fold—in the concentration of organisms compared with quantitative blood cultures drawn at the same time percutaneously through a peripheral vein. Quantitative catheter-drawn blood cultures probably have their greatest utility in diagnosis of device-related infection with surgically implanted cuffed Hickman or Broviac catheters and subcutaneous central venous ports [65–68].

Finding microbes on Gram stain or acridine orange stain of blood drawn through central venous catheters has been shown to be highly sensitive and specific for diagnosing catheter-related bloodstream infection [73,74]. If confirmed by others using the same and other intravascular devices, these may be the methods of choice for the rapid diagnosis of serious intravascular catheter-related infections. Intracellular bacteria have been found on Wright-stained peripheral smears in asymptomatic patients with occult central venous catheter-related bloodstream infection [75].

Microbiology of Device-Related Bloodstream Infection

The microbiologic profile of bloodstream infection (see Table 44-3) can strongly suggest an infusion-related source. Cryptogenic staphylococcal bacteremia, particularly with coagulase-negative staphylococci, bacteremia caused by *Bacillus* or *Corynebacterium* (especially JK-1) species or *Enterococcus*, or fungemia caused by *Candida*, *Fusarium*, *Trichophyton*, or *Malassezia* species, especially in a patient with a central venous catheter, is most likely to reflect catheter-related infection [1,2,38].

Bacteremias caused by *Enterobacter cloacae* or, especially, *Pantoea* (formerly *Enterobacter*) *agglomerans*, *Burkholderia cepacia*, *Stenotrophomonas maltophilia*, or *Citrobacter* species, in the setting of infusion therapy, may signal an epidemic and should prompt studies to rule out contaminated infusate [76]. A cluster of cases should mandate a full-scale investigation, which may include culturing of large numbers of in-use infusions and informing the local, state, and Federal public health authorities. Such actions averted a large, nationwide epidemic in 1973, when, prompted by five unexplained bacteremias in three hospitals, intrinsic contamination of one

U.S. company's products was identified and a recall put into effect so rapidly that the outbreak was limited to the five initially recognized cases [77]. It must be emphasized, however, that for surveillance of bacteremias to be maximally effective, all blood isolates must always be fully identified—that is, speciated. Failure to do so during the 1970 to 1971 nationwide epidemic traced to the contaminated products of one U.S. manufacturer resulted in preeminent hospitals experiencing large numbers of cases that were recognized as infusion-related only in retrospect [21].

Cryptogenic nosocomial bacteremia caused by psychrophilic (cold-growing) organisms, such as non-*aeruginosa* pseudomonads, Ochrobactrum *anthropi* (formerly *Achromobacter*) *Flavobacterium*, *Enterobacter*, or *Serratia* species [78,79], or by *Salmonella* [80] or *Yersinia* species [81], with a picture of overwhelming bloodstream infection, may indicate a contaminated blood product.

Cultures of Intravascular Devices

Some laboratories still culture vascular catheters qualitatively, amputating the tip aseptically and immersing it in liquid media. Unfortunately, a positive culture by this technique is diagnostically nonspecific because a single organism picked up from the skin as the catheter is removed can produce a positive—false-positive—culture [82]. Many catheter-related bloodstream infections derive from local infection of the transcutaneous cannula tract (see discussion later). Culture of the external surface of the withdrawn cannula should reflect the microbiologic status of the wound, and quantitative culture should more accurately distinguish infection from contamination. A standardized, semiquantitative method for culturing vascular cannulas in solid media was developed in 1977 [17]. Colony counts on semiquantitative culture are bimodally distributed, as they are in quantitative urine cultures. The method provides excellent discrimination between colonization and insignificant contamination acquired during catheter removal. Fifteen or more colony-forming units (cfu) growing on a semiquantitative plate is regarded as a positive culture, and denotes significant growth or colonization [17]. Based on experience with > 10,000 devices, positive cultures found using this technique have shown a 15% to 40% association with concordant bloodstream infection. Cannulas positive on semiquantitative culture are also strongly associated with local inflammation [17].

Good correlation between high colony counts and catheter-related bloodstream infection have been demonstrated with cultures of catheter segments semiquantitatively on solid media [83–85] or quantitatively in liquid media—removing organisms from the catheter by vortexing or sonication [83,86,87]. The latter techniques appear to have the greatest sensitivity and specificity for the diagnosis of vascular catheter-related infection [72,88]. However, a negative catheter culture may not rule out a catheter-related bloodstream infection [33,37,72,88,89]. Utilizing more than one catheter culture technique increases the yield [88], as does bedside plating of catheters for semiquantitative culture [90]. Direct Gram stains [91] or acridine orange stains [92] of intravascular segments of removed catheters also show excellent correlation with quantitative techniques for culturing catheters and can permit rapid diagnosis of catheter-related infection.

Given the strong evidence implicating cutaneous microorganisms in the genesis of most bloodstream infections caused by short-term, noncuffed intravascular catheters, a number of studies have shown that a quantitative culture [22,93] or Gram stain [94] of skin at the insertion site can also identify infected catheters with reasonable sensitivity and specificity, greatly exceeding an assessment based solely on clinical signs of infection. The combination of culturing both skin at the insertion site and the catheter hub has been reported to provide even better sensitivity for diagnosis of catheter-related infection, without removing the catheter [33,95,96].

To diagnose reliably infection caused by contaminated infusate requires a sample of fluid to be aspirated from the line and cultured quantitatively [76]. A variety of techniques are now available for culturing or processing parenteral admixtures and fluid medications in the laboratory for microbial contamination [97,98]. Because there is no evidence that anaerobic bacteria can grow in parenteral crystalloid admixtures, anaerobic culture techniques are not necessary unless blood or another biologic product is involved.

Definitions for Infusion-Related Infection

Using the results of semiquantitative or quantitative culture of the catheter and cultures of the hub of the catheter and of infusate aspirated from the line at the time the catheter is removed, and concomitant blood cultures, it is possible to formulate rigorous definitions for intravascular device-related infection [99]:

I. Catheter colonization: Significant growth of a microbial pathogen from the catheter tip, subcutaneous segment of the catheter, or catheter hub

II. Localized Intravascular Catheter-Related Infection

  A. Microbiologically Proven Exit Site Infection: Purulent exudate within 2 cm of the catheter exit site, in the absence of concomitant bloodstream infection

  B. Clinically Suspected Exit Site Infection: Erythema or induration within 2 cm of the catheter exit site, in the absence of concomitant bloodstream infection and without concomitant purulence

C. Tunnel Infection: Tenderness, erythema, or induration > 2 cm from the catheter exit site along the subcutaneous tract of a tunneled (e.g., Hickman or Broviac) catheter, in the absence of concomitant bloodstream infection
D. Pocket Infection: Purulent fluid in the subcutaneous pocket of a totally implanted intravascular catheter that may or may not be associated with spontaneous rupture and drainage or necrosis of the overlying skin, in the absence of concomitant bloodstream infection

III. Systemic Infection
A. Intravascular Catheter-Related Bloodstream Infection: Concordant microbial growth between a catheter segment or hub, infusate, or exit site exudate, and percutaneously drawn blood cultures or concordant microbial growth between catheter-drawn and percutaneously drawn quantitative blood cultures (catheter-drawn blood cultures : percutaneously drawn blood cultures ≥ 4 : 1)
   1. Primary Hub-Related Bloodstream Infection: Concordant growth from the catheter hub and a percutaneously drawn culture, regardless of the catheter tip results, with negative cultures or growth of a different microbe from the exit site and/or subcutaneous catheter segment culture by the roll-plate method. A negative culture or discordant growth from the catheter tip by the roll plate method [17] supports the diagnosis
   2. Primary Skin-Related Bloodstream Infection: Concordant growth from the exit site and/or subcutaneous catheter segment by the roll-plate method, and a percutaneously drawn blood culture with negative cultures or growth of a different microbe from the hub and infusate; concordant growth from the catheter tip by the roll-plate method further supports the diagnosis
   3. Primary Infusate-Related Bloodstream Infection: Concordant growth from the infusate and a percutaneously drawn blood culture with negative cultures or discordant growth from the hub, exit site, and/or subcutaneous catheter segment by the roll-plate method
B. Definite Intravascular Catheter-Related Sepsis: Catheter-related bloodstream infection in the setting of sepsis-defining symptoms [100]
C. Probable Intravascular Catheter Sepsis: Sepsis in the setting of negative blood cultures, resolution of sepsis-defining symptoms shortly after catheter withdrawal, and a catheter component with significant growth of a microbial pathogen or growth from purulent material at the exit site or subcutaneous pocket, or erythema and induration extending along the tunnel tract of a Hickman or Broviac catheter

The term "catheter sepsis" appears frequently in the literature but lacks stringent criteria. Although sepsis has been defined by a consensus panel [100], the term as applied to catheter-related infections may be insensitive because many of these infections are due to coagulase-negative staphylococci, and in some studies, only 55% to 71% of patients with bacteremia due to this pathogen had leukocytosis [101,102]. Also, the maximal body temperature is < 38°C in many patients with coagulase-negative staphylococcal bacteremia [102,103]. This term should likely not be further promulgated in the literature, especially in those prospective, comparative studies involving intravascular devices [99].

In addition, the definitions listed previously may be unnecessarily rigorous for use in clinical nosocomial infection surveillance because very few clinicians obtain cultures of catheter hubs or infusate, even if the cannula is cultured. Moreover, patients with disseminated candidiasis originating from an infected catheter often have negative blood cultures. It is also important to realize that multiple sites are often colonized when cultures are performed at the time of catheter withdrawal and it may be difficult to distinguish with certainty the source of many catheter-bloodstream infections. Therefore, for routine surveillance, use of the Centers for Disease Control and Prevention (CDC) definitions is recommended [104]. Updated definitions are also available [105].

CANNULA-ASSOCIATED INFECTION

Incidence of Cannula-Related Bloodstream infection

Intravascular device-related bloodstream infection is perhaps the least frequently recognized nosocomial infection. The true incidence of vascular catheter-related bloodstream infection is underestimated in most centers because a catheter is often not suspected as a source of the patient's clinical picture of nosocomial bloodstream infection, and is not cultured. Prospective studies in which every device enrolled is cultured at the time of removal indicate clearly that every type of intravascular device carries some risk of causing bloodstream infection, but the magnitude of risk *per device* varies greatly, depending on its type [2].

Table 44-4 shows representative rates of infection for various types of intravascular devices. The lowest rates are with small peripheral IV steel needles and Teflon or polyurethane catheters: large prospective studies have shown rates of approximately 0.2 bloodstream infections per 100 peripheral IV catheters [13–16,19,105–109]; two large, comparative trials have shown that if IV cannulas are inserted under scrupulous aseptic conditions, plastic catheters probably pose no greater risk of device-related

TABLE 44-4. *Approximate risks of bloodstream infection associated with various types of devices for intravascular access[a]*

Type of device	Representative rate	Representative range
Short-term temporary access[b]		
Peripheral IV cannulas		
Winged steel needles	< 0.2	0–1
Peripheral IV catheters		
Percutaneously inserted	0.2	0–1
Cutdown	6	0–1
Midline catheters	0.7	0.7–0.8
Arterial catheters	1	—
Central venous catheters		
All-purpose, multilumen	3	1–7
Pulmonary artery	1	0–5
Hemodialysis	10	3–18
Long-term indefinite access[c]		
Peripherally inserted, central venous catheters (PICCs)	0.20	—
Cuffed central catheters (e.g., Hickman, Broviac)	0.20	0.10–0.53
Subcutaneous central venous ports (e.g., Infusaport®, Port-a-cath®, Landmark®)	0.04	0.00–0.10

IV, intravenous.
[a]Based on data from recently published, prospective studies.
[b]Number of bloodstream infections per 100 devices.
[c]Number of bloodstream infections per 100 device-days.

bacteremia or candidemia than steel needles [106]. Prospective studies of arterial catheters used for hemodynamic monitoring have found rates of infusion-related bacteremia in the range of 1% [110].

The device that poses the greatest risk of iatrogenic bloodstream infection is the central venous catheter in its numerous forms [9,111–113]. Numerous prospective studies of short-term, noncuffed, single- or multilumen catheters inserted percutaneously into the subclavian or internal jugular vein have found rates of catheter-related bloodstream infection in the range of 2% to 5% [9,83, 114–119]. Percutaneously inserted, noncuffed central venous catheters used for hemodialysis have been associated with the highest rates of bloodstream infection, > 10% [120–122]; however, cuffed hemodialysis catheter use appears to be associated with a lower incidence of bloodstream infection [123,124]. *Peripherally inserted* central venous catheters pose a substantially lower risk of catheter-related bloodstream infection (0.04 to 0.4 per 100 catheter days), comparable to Hickman catheters [125, 126]. Swan-Ganz pulmonary artery catheters used for hemodynamic monitoring are associated with a 1% rate of bloodstream infection or 0.3 per 100 catheter-days [110]. The lowest rates of infection with central venous devices have been with surgically implanted Hickman or Broviac catheters that incorporate a Dacron cuff, which have been associated with rates of infection in the range of 0.1 bacteremias or fungemias per 100 catheter-days [127,128], and surgically implanted subcutaneous central venous ports, associated with a rates of bloodstream infection of < 0.05 per 100 device-days [127,128]. In prospective studies, the incidence of bloodstream infection has been demonstrated to be lower in patients who have subcutaneously implanted ports compared with those with tunneled catheters with a Dacron cuff [129–134].

It has been estimated that 90% of intravascular device-related bloodstream infections originate from central venous catheters of various types [2], leading to 55,000 bloodstream infections in U.S. ICUs each year [11]. Data from the CDC's National Nosocomial Infections Surveillance Study (NNIS) have shown that the incidence of secondary bloodstream infections, deriving from identifiable local infections such as of the urinary tract, postoperative surgical wounds, or pneumonias, has remained stable over the past decade; in contrast, the incidence of primary nosocomial bloodstream infections, the largest proportion of which derive from intravascular devices, has increased more than twofold over this same period [2,135], reflecting the great increase in the use of infusion therapy and, especially, the use of central venous devices of all types. It seems clear that the greatest hope for reducing the risk of intravascular device-related bloodstream infection will come from better understanding of infection with central venous catheters, which will form the basis for more effective strategies for prevention.

Epidemiology

The first and perhaps most important question that must be addressed to develop effective strategies for prevention is to determine the major source or sources of microorganisms that can colonize a percutaneous intravascular (Figure 44-1) device and cause invasive infection leading to bacteremia or candidemia. An intravascular catheter can easily become colonized extraluminally by organisms from the patient's cutaneous microflora. Contamination may occur during catheter insertion [136] or shortly thereafter [137]. Microorganisms can also contaminate the catheter hub where the administration set attaches to the catheter, or they may gain access to the fluid column and be infused directly into the patient's bloodstream; the device can also become infected hematogenously from remote sources of local infection; or the device might even be contaminated from its manufacture—which fortunately is very rare.

A large body of clinical and microbiologic data indicates that most intravascular device-related bloodstream infections caused by *short-term*, percutaneously inserted, noncuffed catheters are caused by extraluminal microorganisms of cutaneous origin that invade the transcutaneous insertion wound at the time the catheter is inserted or in the days after insertion:

1. Numerous prospective studies of intravascular device-related infection have shown that coagulase-negative staphylococci, the predominant aerobic species on the human skin, are now the most common agents of catheter-related bacteremia [1,2,9,48,105–109,111, 117,127,135]. The vast majority of vascular catheter-related bloodstream infections are caused by microorganisms that colonize the skin of hospitalized patients: staphylococci, both coagulase-negative and coagulase-positive (*S. aureus*); *Candida*, *Corynebacterium*, and *Bacillus* species; and, to a lesser degree, aerobic gram-negative bacilli (Table 44-5).
2. Prospective studies have also shown strong concordance between organisms present on skin surrounding the catheter insertion site and organisms recovered from central venous catheters producing bloodstream infection [22,34,48,93,94,114–116, 136]. There appears to be a direct parallel between the level and profile of cutaneous colonization at the insertion sites of short-term central venous, arterial, and peripheral IV catheters and the risk of catheter-related bloodstream infection [138,139].
3. Intensive care unit and hemodialysis patients with cutaneous colonization by *S. aureus* experience four- to sixfold higher rates of vascular access-related bacteremia [140,141]. Use of recombinant interleukin-2, with or without lymphokine-activated killer (LAK) cells for cancer immunotherapy, which is associated with frequent dermatotoxicity (desquamation) and heavy cutaneous colonization by *S. aureus*, has been associated with a prohibitively high incidence of central venous catheter-related *S. aureus* bacteremia [142].
4. Burned patients, who have huge populations of microorganisms on the skin surface, experience very high rates of catheter-related bloodstream infection [143,144] (see Chapter 38).
5. Numerous outbreaks of intravascular catheter-related bloodstream infection have been traced to contaminated cutaneous antiseptics [145–148].
6. High counts of microorganisms on semiquantitative culture of the external surface of a removed catheter are strongly associated with bacteremia caused by the catheter [17,22,83–85,95,121,143,149].

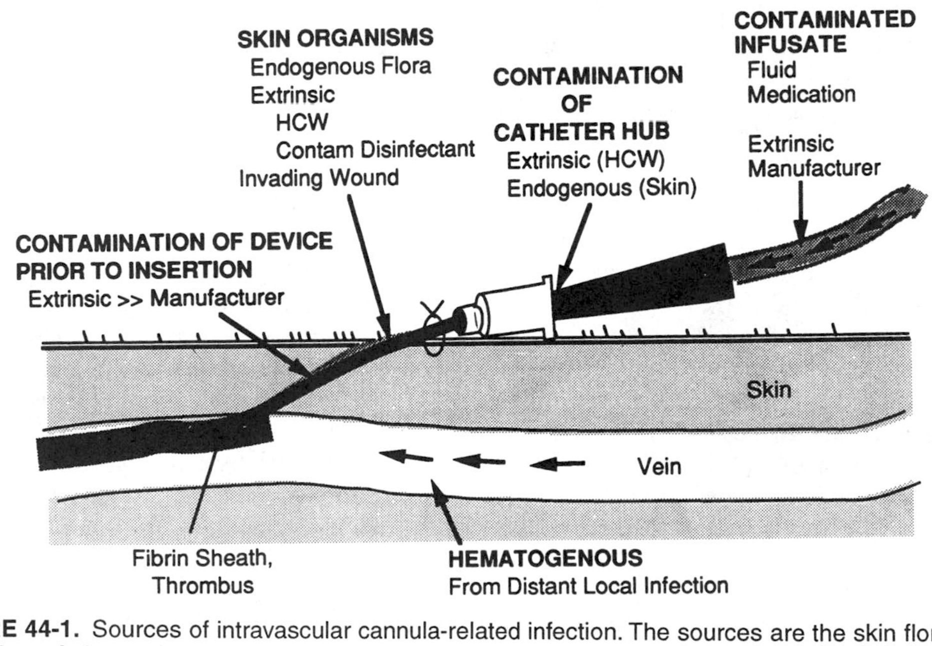

FIGURE 44-1. Sources of intravascular cannula-related infection. The sources are the skin flora, contamination of the catheter hub, contamination of infusate, and hematogenous colonization of the intravascular device and its fibronectin–fibrin sheath. (HCW, healthcare worker.)

TABLE 44-5. *Microorganisms most frequently encountered in various forms of intravascular line-related infection*

Source	Pathogens
Catheter-related	
Peripheral IV catheter	Coagulase-negative staphylococci[a]
	Staphylococcus aureus
	Candida spp[a]
Central venous catheters	Coagulase-negative staphylococci
	S. aureus
	Candida spp
	Corynebacterium spp (especially JK-1)
	Klebsiella and *Enterobacter* spp
	Mycobacterium spp
	Trichophyton beiglii
	Fusarium spp
	Malassezia furfur[a]
Contaminated IV infusate	Tribe Klebsielleae
	Enterobacter cloacae
	Enterobacter agglomerans
	Serratia marcescens
	Klebsiella spp
	Burkholderia cepacia
	Burkholderia acidivorans, Burkholderia pickettii
	Stenotrophomonas maltophilia
	Citrobacter freundii
	Flavobacterium spp
	Candida tropicalis
Contaminated blood products	*E. cloacae*
	S. marcescens
	Ochrobactrum anthropi
	Flavobacterium spp
	Burkholderia spp
	Yersinia spp
	Salmonella spp

IV, intravenous.
[a]Also seen with peripheral IV catheters in association with the administration of lipid emulsion for parenteral nutritional support.

7. Microscopic examination of infected central venous catheters has shown heavy colonization of the external surface [91,92], especially with short-term catheters [150].
8. Prospective studies have shown that use of a more effective cutaneous disinfectant, such as chlorhexidine, for disinfection of the insertion site at the time of catheter insertion and in follow-up care of the catheter greatly reduces the risk of infusion-related bloodstream infection [32,151–153].
9. Prospective trials have shown that antiseptics or antimicrobials applied topically to the intravascular catheter insertion site can reduce the risk of catheter-related bloodstream infection [122,154].
10. Surgically implanted Broviac or Hickman catheters, which have a subcutaneous Dacron cuff that becomes ingrown by tissue and poses a mechanical barrier against invasion of the tract by skin organisms, have been associated with considerably lower rates of catheter-related bacteremia (~ 0.20 cases per 100 catheter-days) [155–157] than short-term, noncuffed central venous catheters (~ 0.6 to 1.0 per 100 catheter days) [22,91,111,114,115,117] (see Table 44-4). However, in a clinical trial, nonsurgically implanted, nontunneled, noncuffed Silastic catheters were inserted for prolonged periods of time with a very low risk of infection [125]. These data suggest that with careful follow-up, insertion of noncuffed central venous catheters with the Seldinger technique outside of the operating room may be an acceptable alternative to Hickman or Broviac cuffed catheters. With one exception [158], prospective, randomized, clinical trials of a subcutaneous silver-impregnated cuff that can be attached to a short-term (< 10 to 14 days) central venous catheter at the time of insertion can also reduce the risk of catheter colonization and catheter-related bloodstream infection [115,116,159]. However, with more prolonged catheterization (> 14 days), this device does not appear to be efficacious [160–162]. Studies have shown that novel short-term (~ 7 days) central venous catheters with an externally antimicrobial [163,164] or antiseptic or heparin [165–169]

greatly reduce the incidence of catheter colonization and, in some instances, catheter-related bloodstream infection. Again, efficacy of these novel devices has not been demonstrated with more prolonged catheterization [170,171]. This may reflect the greater importance of the catheter hub as a source of invading pathogens, compared with the skin at the insertion site, with more prolonged catheterization [72,150]. A number of studies have shown that the colonized hubs of intravascular catheters are an important source of pathogens causing catheter-related bloodstream infections [34], particularly with more prolonged duration of catheterization [33,72,95,150,172–174].

Central venous and arterial catheters can also become colonized hematogenously, from remote, unrelated sites of infection, but the evidence suggests that this occurs relatively less frequently than colonization from microbes at the insertion site or catheter hub [32,34,48,115,175,176] (Table 44-6), except in patients with short bowel syndrome [177].

Although infusate not infrequently becomes contaminated by small numbers of organisms, mainly skin commensals such as coagulase-negative staphylococci, with the exception of arterial catheters used for hemodynamic monitoring [31,32], endemic bacteremic infections originating from contaminated infusate also appear to be uncommon [32,109,115]. In contrast, contaminated infusate is the single most common identified cause of epidemic nosocomial bacteremia [1,2], caused predictably by microorganisms capable of multiplying in parenteral glucose-containing admixtures, members of the tribe Klebsielleae (*Klebsiella*, *Enterobacter* and *Serratia*), *B. cepacia*, *Burkholderia pickettii*, or *Citrobacter* species [76]. Nearly 100 epidemics of infusion-related bloodstream infection since 1965 have been traced to contaminated infusate or IV medications, with microorganisms most frequently introduced during preparation or administration in the hospital (*extrinsic* contamination) or during its manufacture (*intrinsic* contamination).

Analysis of risk factors predisposing to intravascular catheter-related infection by stepwise logistic regression of data from large, prospective studies of peripheral IV catheters [109], arterial catheters used for hemodynamic monitoring [31], multilumen central venous catheters used in ICU patients [32], and Swan-Ganz pulmonary artery catheters [175] shows that heavy cutaneous colonization of the insertion site is one of the most powerful predictors of catheter-related infection with all types of short-term, percutaneously inserted catheters (Table 44-7).

Pathogenesis

Examination of an infected intravascular device by scanning electron microscopy characteristically shows the surface covered by an amorphous film [150,176,189], presumably representing host proteins, with microcolonies of the infecting organism encased in a thick matrix of glycocalyx (slime), all comprising a "biofilm" [190] (Figure 44-2). Studies of the pathobiology of prosthetic device-related infection have shown considerable differences in the capacity of microorganisms to adhere to various prosthetic materials. In vitro, catheters made of Teflon or polyurethane are more resistant to bacterial adherence, especially by staphylococci, than catheters made of polyethylene, polyvinylchloride, or, especially, silicone [191,192]. These differences are maintained if the experiments are done with previously implanted catheters or catheters precoated with specific plasma pro-

TABLE 44-6. *Potential sources of Swan-Ganz pulmonary artery (PA) catheter-related bloodstream infection, based on a prospective study of 442 Swan-Ganz pulmonary artery catheters*

	Gauze (2 days)	Conventional polyurethane (5 days)	Highly permeable polyurethane (5 days)	Overall
Total no. of catheter-related bloodstream infections	2	1	2	5
Microbiologic				
Concordance with source				
Intravascular segment of introducer or PA catheter	2	1	2	5
Skin	1	—	1	2
Hub	1	1	1	3
Infusate	1	1	1	3
Extravascular portion of PA catheter, beneath external protective sleeve	—	—	1	1
Hematogenous from remote source	—	1	1	—

(From Maki DG, Stolz SS, Wheeler S, Mermel LA. A prospective, randomized trial of gauze and two polyurethane dressings for site care of pulmonary artery catheters: implications for catheter management. *Crit Care Med* 1994;22:1729–1737.)

TABLE 44-7. *Risk factors for intravascular catheter-related infection based on multivariate analysis of data from large, prospective studies*

Type of catheter [ref.]	No. catheters studied	Risk factors	Relative risk
Peripheral IV [109]	2,050	Cutaneous colonization of site > 10^2 cfu	3.9
		Contamination of catheter hub	3.8
		Moisture on site, under dressing	2.5
		Placement > 3 days	1.8
		Systemic antimicrobial therapy	0.5
Peripheral IV [153] (pediatric patients)	826	Heavy colonization of insertion site	3.6
		Catheterization for ≥72 hr	2.0
		Gestational age ≤ 32 wk	1.8
		Ampicillin infusion	0.4
		Cutaneous antisepsis with chlorhexidine	0.2
Arterial [31]	491	Cutaneous colonization of site > 10^2 cfu	10.0
		Second catheter in site, placed over guidewire	—
Umbilical artery [178] (pediatric patients)	189	Very low birth weight	—
		Prolonged antibiotic therapy	—
		Antibiotic therapy at time of catheter removal	—
Umbilical vein [178] (pediatric patients)	144	High birth weight	—
		Hyperalimentation in high-birthweight patients	—
Central venous [179]	345	Exposure of catheter to unrelated bacteremia	9.4
		Cutaneous colonization of site > 10^2 cfu	9.2
		Placement > 4 days	—
Central venous [193]	188	Catheter-related thrombosis	—
Central venous [181]	1,258	Respiratory tract colonization or infection	—
		Hypoalbuminemia	—
Central venous [182]	76	Heavy insertion site colonization	13.2
		Difficult catheter insertion	5.4
		Female gender	0.2
		Underlying secondary diagnosis	0.2
Central venous [183]	1,212	Internal jugular vein insertion	3.3
		Patient transfer within the hospital	3.0
		Disease of the gastrointestinal tract	2.4
		Prolonged hospital length of stay before catheter insertion	1.0
		Concomitant antibiotic use	0.3
		Polyurethane catheter	0.2
Central venous [22]	140	Insertion site colonized with organisms other than coagulase-negative staphylococci	14.9
		Insertion site erythema	4.4
		Insertion site colonized with > 50 cfu of coagulase-negative staphylococci or > 1 cfu of any other microbe	6.4
Pulmonary artery [175]	297	Cutaneous colonization of site > 10^3 cfu	5.5
		Internal jugular vein cannulation	4.3
		Duration > 3 days	3.1
		Placement in operating room under less stringent barrier precautions	2.1
Pulmonary artery [184]	86	Catheterization > 5 days	14.4
		Antibiotic use	0.2
Hemodialysis [120]	53	Chronic renal failure	7.2
Peripheral, central venous, arterial, and pulmonary artery (pediatric patients) [185]	1,649	Age < 1 yr	—
		Dwell time = 3 days	—
		Inotropic support	—
Peripheral, central venous, arterial [186]	353	Distant focus of infection	8.7
		Inappropriate catheter care	5.3
		Prolonged hospitalization > 14 days	3.5
Peripheral, central venous, arterial (burn patients) [144]	101	Insertion site colonization at catheter removal	6.2
Peripheral, central venous, pulmonary artery, arterial [174]	623	Duration of catheterization 7–14 days	3.9
		Duration of catheterization > 14 days	5.1
		Coronary care unit	6.7
		Surgery service	4.4
		Second catheterization	7.6
		Insertion site colonization	56.6
		Hub colonization	17.9
Hickman [187]	690	Double-lumen catheter	2.1
		Obesity	1.7
		Granulocytopenia	1.6
Implantable port [188]	1,550	Increased number of line breaks/day	—

cfu, colony-forming units.

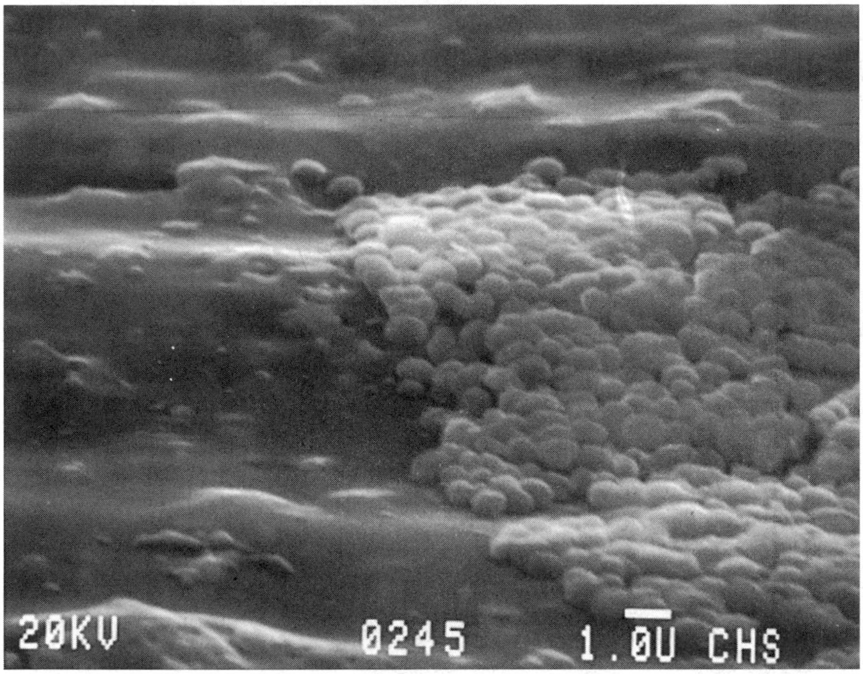

FIGURE 44-2. Scanning electron micrograph of an infected central venous catheter (×6,000). The amorphous matrix encasing the microcolonies of *Staphylococcus epidermidis* is glycocalyx (slime).

catheters or catheters precoated with specific plasma proteins [193–196].

Initial attachment of *Staphylococcus epidermidis* directly to a catheter is mediated, in part, by the hydrophobicity of the strain [197] and by specific adhesins [198–202]. Initial attachment of *S. aureus* to catheters appears to be more dependent on the presence of preadsorbed plasma or tissue proteins such as fibronectin, thrombospondin, fibrin, vitronectin, and laminin [29,30,196,203]. Because many of these proteins are an integral part of thrombus formation, the presence of thrombus on the catheter surface also appears to promote adherence and catheter-associated infection [88,180,204,205]. Persistence of bacteria and fungi attached to the catheter surface appears to be promoted by surface exoglycocalyx [206,207]. Whereas subtherapeutic levels of antibiotics reduce microbial adherence [195,208], once microorganisms such as coagulase-negative staphylococci colonize a prosthetic surface, host defenses become secondarily impaired and are unable to eradicate spontaneously the infection [209,210]. Moreover, once associated with a foreign surface, microorganisms exhibit increased resistance to antimicrobials [211–216]. It should be no surprise that infections of prosthetic implants are difficult to cure with antimicrobial therapy alone, even with prolonged administration of high doses of bactericidal drugs.

BLOODSTREAM INFECTION FROM CONTAMINATED INFUSATE

It took > 10 years after the introduction of intravascular plastic catheters before they were ultimately recognized as an important source of serious iatrogenic infection; however, it required > 40 years and the occurrence of epidemic gram-negative bacteremias in hospitals across the United States in 1970 and 1971 [21] to bring about awareness that fluid given in intravascular infusions—infusate—also was vulnerable to contamination. It has become clear that although the majority of intravascular device-related bloodstream infections derive from infection of the percutaneous infection wound or contamination of the catheter hub, contamination of infusate is the most common cause of epidemic device-related bloodstream infection [1]. From 1965 to 1978, 28 (85%) of the 30 reported epidemics of infusion-related bacteremia were traced to contaminated infusate, with the organisms introduced during its manufacture (intrinsic contamination, which accounted for 7 of the 20 epidemics) or during its preparation and administration in the hospital (extrinsic contamination, which accounted for the remaining 21 outbreaks) [1,2].

Growth Properties of Microorganisms in Parenteral Fluids

The pathogens implicated in nearly all reported bloodstream infections linked to contaminated infusate have been aerobic gram-negative bacilli capable of rapid growth at room temperature (25°C) in the solution involved [76]: for example, certain members of the family Enterobacteriaceae in 5% dextrose-in-water, and pseudomonads or *Serratia* in distilled water. It must be emphasized that microbial growth in most parenteral solutions—the exception being lipid emulsion—is actually quite limited.

In 1970, we evaluated the ability of 105 clinical isolates from human nosocomial infections, representing 9 genera and 13 species, to grow at room temperature (25°C) in 5% dextrose-in-water, the most frequently used commercial parenteral solution [217]. Of 51 strains of the tribe Klebsielleae—*Klebsiella*, *Enterobacter*, and *Serratia*—50 attained concentrations of at least 100,000 cfu/ml within 24 hours, beginning with washed organisms at an initial concentration of 1 cfu/ml. In contrast, only 1 of 54 strains of other bacteria, including staphylococci, *Escherichia coli*, *P. aeruginosa*, and *Acinetobacter*, and *Candida*, showed any growth in 5% dextrose-in-water. With most microorganisms, even with a level of contamination exceeding 10^6 cfu/ml of fluid, evidence of microbial growth was not visible to the unaided eye.

Review of studies of the growth properties of microorganisms in various commercial parenteral products has shown [76] that rapid multiplication in 5% dextrose-in-water appears limited mainly to the tribe Klebsielleae and *B. cepacia*; in distilled water, *P. aeruginosa*, *B. cepacia*, *Acinetobacter*, and *Serratia*; and in lactated Ringer's solution, *P. aeruginosa*, *Enterobacter*, and *Serratia*. Normal (0.9%) sodium chloride solution allows growth of most bacteria while supporting the growth of *Candida* rather poorly. *Candida* species can grow in the synthetic amino acid–25% glucose solutions used for TPN, but only very slowly; most bacteria are greatly inhibited [218]. Most microorganisms grow rapidly in commercial 10% lipid emulsion for infusion (Intralipid®) [219,220]; in a study of 57 strains, we found that 12 of 13 bacterial species tested and *Candida* multiplied in Intralipid almost as rapidly as in bacteriologic media [219]. Infections with *Malassezia furfur* have also been associated with administration of lipids [221–223]. This is not surprising because this dimorphic, lipophilic yeast cannot synthesize medium- and long-chain fatty acids and uses exogenous lipids, such as those found in supplemented TPN, for growth [220]. Use of TPN supplemented with lipids has also been shown significantly to increase the risk of bloodstream infection by coagulase-negative staphylococci [224,225]. Epidemics have also been reported due to extrinsic contamination of a lipid-based anesthetic, propofol (Diprivan; Stuart Pharmaceuticals, Wilmington, Delaware, U.S.A.) [36]. This anesthetic agent supports the exuberant growth of several gram-negative, gram-positive bacteria and *Candida albicans* [226].

The growth properties of most microorganisms in commercial parenteral admixtures and the vast aggregate experience with epidemic and endemic bloodstream infections traced to contaminated infusate have shown that the identity of an organism causing nosocomial bloodstream infection can point strongly toward contaminated fluid as the plausible source: *P. agglomerans, E. cloacae, Serratia marcescens, B. cepacia*, or *Citrobacter* cultured from the blood of a patient receiving infusion therapy should prompt strong suspicion of contaminated infusate—parenteral fluid or an IV drug (see Table 44-5). Conversely, recovery of organisms such as *E. coli*, *Proteus*, *Acinetobacter*, or staphylococci, all of which grow poorly if at all in parenteral admixtures, suggests strongly that the bloodstream infection is unlikely to be due to contaminated infusate.

Mechanisms of Fluid Contamination

As noted, the vast majority of nosocomial bloodstream infections traced to contaminated infusate and reported in the literature occurred in an epidemic setting [1,2]. Parenteral fluids do, however, commonly become contaminated during administration in the hospital. Culture surveys of in-use IV fluids in the hospital have shown contamination rates in the range of 1% to 2% [227–229]. However, most of the organisms recovered from positive in-use cultures are common skin commensals that are generally considered of low virulence and grow poorly, if at all, in the parenteral admixture; the level of contamination (<10 cfu/ml) is usually far too low to produce clinical illness, even in the most compromised host. When contamination occurs with gram-negative bacilli capable of proliferation in the product to concentrations $>10^2$ to 10^3 cfu/ml, however, the risk of bloodstream infection and even septic shock becomes substantial.

The likelihood of fluid becoming contaminated during use is directly related to the duration of uninterrupted infusion through the same administration set and the frequency with which the set is manipulated. Microorganisms gain access from air entering bottles as they evacuate, from entry points into the administration set—during injections into the line or aspiration of blood specimens from the intravascular device through the line—or at the junction between the administration set and the catheter hub. Microorganisms capable of growth in fluid, once introduced into a running infusion, may persist in an administration set for many days despite multiple replacements of the bottle or bag and high rates of flow [21]; it appears more likely, however, that the majority of introduced contaminants are rapidly cleared from the running infusion by the continuous flow [227–230], especially if the organisms grow poorly in the fluid.

A healthcare worker may rarely encounter a filmy cloud in a glass IV bottle. Microscopic examination of the material reveals it is a filamentous fungus, such as *Penicillium* or *Aspergillus*. Molds usually gain access to glass IV bottles through microscopic cracks long before the bottle is hung for use, and over the course of weeks or months grow to produce visible cloudiness or filmy precipitates. Fortunately, "fungus balls" in IV bottles have rarely resulted in systemic infection in patients receiving a mold-contaminated infusion [233].

The incidence of endemic nosocomial bacteremia caused by extrinsically contaminated IV fluid is not precisely known, but based on studies of the pathogenesis of device-related infection, is 5- to 10-fold lower than the incidence of endemic cannula-related bloodstream infection. Moreover, prospective studies of the optimal interval for periodic replacement of administration sets [227–233] (Table 44-8), which have involved cultures of infusate from large numbers of in-use infusions in an institution, have shown low rates of contamination and a very low risk of related bloodstream infection: meta-analysis of five studies in which more than 9,000 infusions in 5 hospitals were prospectively cultured, with no associated episodes of bacteremia or candidemia identified, yields an incidence of endemic bloodstream infection due to contaminated infusate of less than 1 case per 2,000 IV infusions. It must be emphasized, however, that IV infusate can be identified as the source of bloodstream infection only if it is cultured. Because this rarely occurs in most hospitals, unless a cluster of cases—an epidemic—occurs, it is likely that most sporadic (endemic) bloodstream infections caused by contaminated fluid go unrecognized or are attributed to the intravascular cannula.

Approximately one half of the bloodstream infections caused by arterial infusions used for hemodynamic monitoring stem from contamination of fluid in the infusion [31], perhaps because these infusions consist of a stagnant column of fluid subjected to frequent manipulations, including frequent drawing of blood specimens. However, more recent studies have demonstrated that infusate contamination of hemodynamic pressure monitoring equipment is rare [234]. Over the past 20 years, there have been 28 epidemics of nosocomial bloodstream infection traced to contaminated fluid in arterial infusions used for hemodynamic monitoring [235–238]. Nearly all of these epidemics have involved gram-negative bacilli, particularly *S. marcescens*, pseudomonads, or *Enterobacter* species that are able to multiply rapidly in the 0.9% saline commonly used in these infusions.

Endemic bloodstream infections deriving from transfusion of contaminated blood products have been rare, presumably because most blood products are routinely refrigerated, because contamination is low level, and because of universal awareness that blood products must be used promptly after removal from refrigeration [79,239]. Bloodstream infection from contaminated whole blood is associated with adverse reactions in half of cases, including fever (80%), rigors (53%), hypotension (37%), and nausea or vomiting (26%), with an associated mortality of 35% [79]. Overwhelming shock is usually due to contamination with massive numbers of psychrophilic (cold-growing) organisms such as *Serratia*, *B. cepacia*, *S. maltophilia*, *Yersinia*, and other uncommon, nonfermentative gram-negative bacilli, such a *Flavobacterium* species, in the contaminated unit [79–81, 241]. Bacteria have often been visible on a direct Gram-stained smear of the product. Blood products should be infused immediately after they are removed from refrigeration. On completion of the transfusion, the entire delivery system should be replaced. If bloodstream infection is suspected of being related to a contaminated blood product, the entire infusion should be removed. Aliquots of the remaining product should be cultured aerobically *and* anaerobically on solid media at both 35° to 37°C and 16° to 20°C [76]. Platelet units may be stored at room temperature for ≤ 5 days prior to use and may be more prone to contamination with large numbers of microbial

TABLE 44-8. *Studies of replacing intravenous administration sets at periodic intervals as an infection control measure*

Reference	Location of patients	Types of infusion	No. of sets cultured	Prevalence of contamination in sets changed at intervals			
				24 Hr	48 Hr	72 Hr	Indefinite
[229]	Ward	Mainly peripheral[a]	2,537	0.4	0.6	—	—
[231]	Ward, ICU	Peripheral	694	0.5	1.0	0.7	—
		Central, access[a,b] plus TPN	119	0	0	0	—
[232]	ICU	Peripheral (62%) plus central, access (38%)[a]	676	2.0	4.0	—	—
[230]	Ward	Peripheral	219	—	0.8	—	0.8
[227]	ICU	Peripheral, plus central, access[a]	1,194	—	5.0	4.4	—
[228]	Ward, ICU	Peripheral	878	—	0.2	1.0	—
		Central, access	331	—	1.9	1.2	—
		Central, TPN	165	—	2.7	4.4	—
	Ward	All types	1,168	—	0.5	1.4	—
	ICU	All types	204	—	3.2	1.8	—

ICU, intensive care unit; TPN, total parenteral nutrition.

[a]Infusions for TPN excluded; contamination rates with different types of infusions not given.

[b]"Access" refers to a central venous infusion used for administering fluids, blood products, delivery of drugs, or hemodynamic monitoring, but not TPN.

(From Maki DG, Botticelli JT, LeRoy ML, Thielke TS. Prospective study of replacing administration sets for intravenous therapy at 48- vs 72-hour intervals: 72 hours is safe and cost effective. *JAMA* 1987;258:1777–1781.)

pathogens. As many as 10% of platelet pools used for transfusion are contaminated with bacteria [239]. Although most contaminants are skin flora [242], contamination with gram-negative bacilli has been reported [79,80].

The most important measures to prevent rare sporadic bloodstream infections from contaminated in-use infusate are stringent asepsis during the preparation and compounding of admixtures in the hospital central pharmacy or on individual patient care units, and good aseptic technique when infusions are handled during use, such as during injections of medications or changing bags or bottles of fluids. It also appears that replacing the administration set at periodic intervals can prevent the buildup of dangerous introduced contaminants and further reduce the risk of related bloodstream infection; during the large, nationwide U.S. epidemic in 1971 due to the contaminated products of one manufacturer, the empiric recommendations that the entire delivery system be routinely changed every 24 hours and that at every change of the cannula all equipment be totally replaced resulted in a substantial reduction in epidemic bloodstream infections [21]. Since that time, routinely replacing the delivery system at periodic intervals has been practiced in most North American hospitals as an important measure for reducing the hazard of contaminated infusate. However, in some instances, routine replacement at more prolonged intervals may be associated with epidemics, particularly in vulnerable patient populations and when the fluids infused promote microbial growth [243].

EPIDEMIC INFUSION-RELATED BLOODSTREAM INFECTIONS

Outbreaks Due to Intrinsic Contamination

Since 1970, there have been more than a dozen reported epidemics of infusion-related bloodstream infection caused by intrinsically contaminated infusate—blood products, IV drugs, or vacutainer tubes (Table 44-9)—illustrating the potential iatrogenic hazards of infusion therapy. The frequency and size of these outbreaks have declined since the late 1980s [2], reflecting appreciation of the importance of stringent quality control during the manufacturing process.

The first and largest epidemic—and the outbreak that more than any other factor brought about wide-scale appreciation of the iatrogenic hazards of infusion therapy—had its onset several years ago when one U.S. manufacturer of large-volume parenterals began to distribute bottles of fluid with a new elastomer-lined screw cap closure [21]. By early 1970, the first cases of infusion-related bloodstream infection caused by biologically characteristic strains of *E. cloacae* and *P. agglomerans* (designated *Erwinia* at the time) were reported to the CDC, although retrospective review subsequently showed that numerous hospitals had been experiencing epidemic bacteremias for a number of months. Although it was established very early, virtually at the outset of the investigation, that epidemic bacteremias derived from contaminated IV fluids, the ultimate source of contamination—*intrinsic* contamination of the new closures—was not conclusively established until March, 1971. Between July, 1970 and April, 1971, 25 U.S. hospitals reported nearly 400 cases of infusion-related bloodstream infection to the CDC (Figure 44-3). It is likely that there were more than 10,000 cases nationwide. More than 20 microbial species, including *P. agglomerans*, were isolated from the closures of previously unopened bottles. Organisms were readily dislodged from the cap liner and introduced into IV fluid when bottles were handled under con-

TABLE 44-9. *Reported sources of epidemics of intravascular device-related bloodstream infection*

Extrinsic contamination
Antiseptics or disinfectants
Arterial pressure monitoring infusate
Disinfectants
Transducers
Heparin
Ice for chilling blood gas syringes
Aneroid pressure calibration device
Hand carriage by medical personnel
Hemodialysis related
Inadequate decontamination of reused dialyzer coils
Contaminated dialysate water
Contaminated disinfectants
Parenteral crystalloid solutions
Lipid emulsion
Hyperalimentation solutions in central pharmacy
IV medications, multidose vials
Theft of fentanyl and replacement by (contaminated) distilled water
Blood products
Whole blood
Platelet packs
Blood donor with silent transient bacteremia
Intravenous radiologic contrast media
Sclerosing solution for injecting esophageal varices
Central venous catheter hubs
Leaking catheter hub administration set connections
Adhesive tape used in IV site dressings
Warming bath for blood products
Green soap
Hand carriage by medical personnel
Heart–lung machines
Intraaortic balloon pumps
Inordinately prolonged intravascular catheterization in intensive care unit patients
Intrinsic (manufacturer-related) contamination
Commercial IV crystalloid solutions, container closures
Blood products
Platelet packs
Human albumin
Plasma protein fraction (PPF)
IV drugs
Vacutainer® tubes

IV, intravenous.

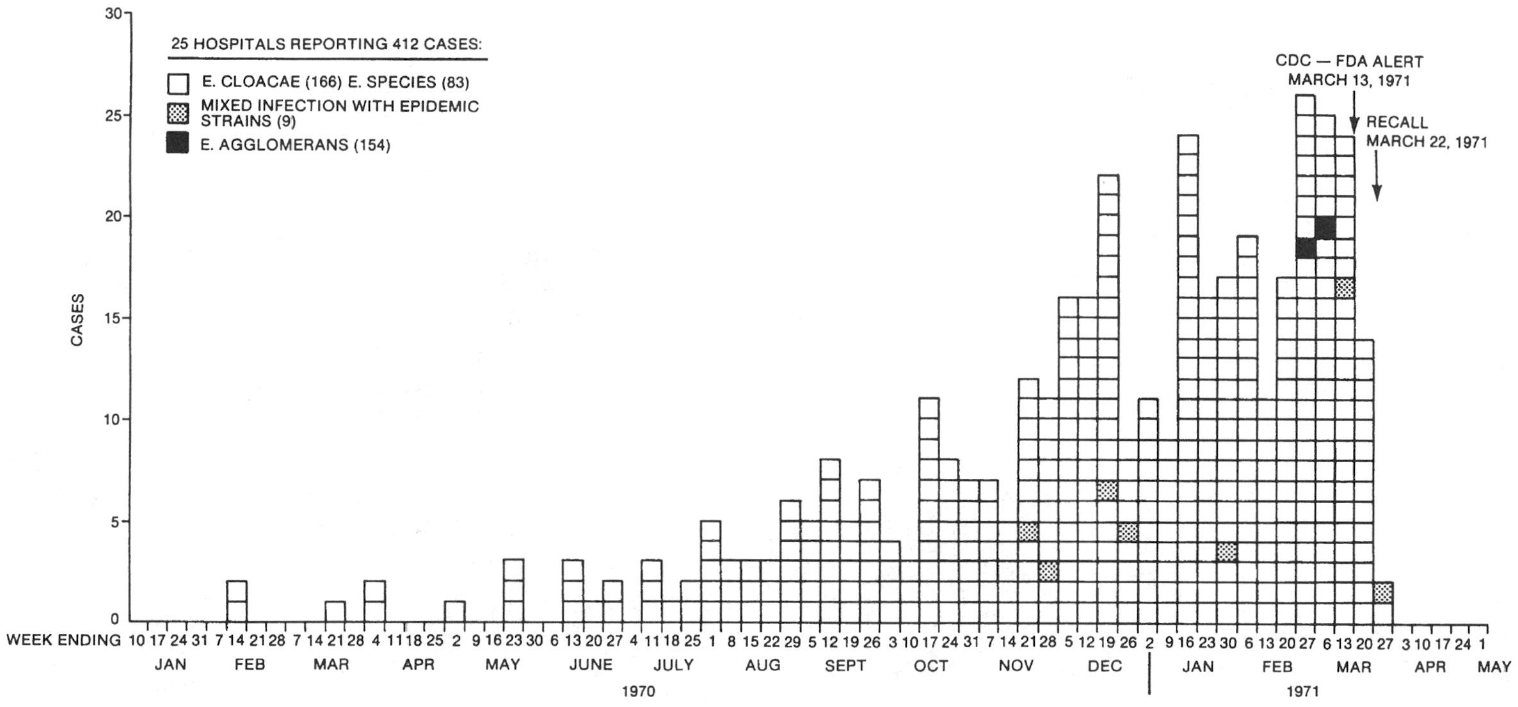

FIGURE 44-3. Nationwide outbreak of nosocomial bacteremias due to intrinsic contamination of one U.S. manufacturer's large-volume parenteral products. Three hundred ninety-seven cases of IV-associated bloodstream infection in 25 tabulated U.S. hospitals, occurring between July 1, 1970, and April 27, 1971, fulfilled criteria for epidemic cases. The epidemic was curtailed immediately in individual hospitals and nationally by a nationwide recall of the manufacturer's products. (From Maki DG, Rhame FS, Mackel D, Bennett JV. Nationwide epidemic of bloodstream infection caused by contaminated intravenous products. *Am J Med* 1976;60:47–485, with permission.)

ditions duplicating normal in-hospital use. The appearance of epidemic bloodstream infections in individual hospitals paralleled the distribution of the company's product with the new closures, and the epidemic was terminated only by a nationwide product recall in early April, 1971.

Since 1975, numerous additional outbreaks have been reported from hospitals in a number of countries, all involving gram-negative bacilli and parenteral products shown to have been contaminated during manufacture [76,77,244–256]. Most have been of national scope. A large outbreak in Greece in 1981 [245] reaffirmed the findings of the large 1970 to 1971 U.S. outbreak [21] that screw-cap closures are not microbiologically safe for fluids used in medical care that must remain sterile. Outbreaks of pyrogenic reactions [248] and epidemic *Pseudomonas* species bloodstream infection [249] have been traced to intrinsically contaminated normal serum albumin, and an epidemic of bloodstream infection with *Ochrobactrum anthropi* has been traced to organisms from contaminated rabbit anti-thymocyte globulin [250]. Most notably, during the past decade outbreaks of *Pseudomonas* infection have been traced to intrinsic contamination of 10% povidone–iodine [251], the most widely used cutaneous antiseptic in North American hospitals for preparation of the insertion site of central venous catheters [252]. Dilute chlorhexidine solution, which is coming into more widespread use in this regard [32,151–153], may support the growth of bacteria, leading to epidemic bloodstream infection [148].

All of these outbreaks illustrate how subtle and insidious the factors that influence sterility can be. In many instances, there was no documented failure of the sterilization process. Instead, seemingly minor alterations in the manufacturing process resulted in contamination of individual units in the manufacturing plant after the sterilization stage [253].

Although intrinsic contamination is, fortunately, exceedingly rare, its potential for producing harm is great because of the large numbers of patients in multiple hospitals who may be affected. Also, direct contamination of infusate at the manufacturing level gives contaminants an opportunity to proliferate to dangerously high concentrations.

It seems likely that intrinsic contamination is a continuous source of infusion-related bloodstream infection, but of such low magnitude that the resulting bloodstream infections are never identified as related to intrinsic contamination. Only when infusion-associated bloodstream infections occur in epidemic numbers is intrinsic contamination likely to be suspected and proven. A substantial increase in the incidence of cryptogenic infusion-associated bloodstream infection, particularly with *Enterobacter* species, pseudomonads, *Burkholderia* species, or *Citrobacter*, should prompt immediate, in-depth studies to exclude intrinsic contamination. There are no clinical clues reliably to differentiate intrinsic from extrinsic contamination. Bacteremia from contaminated fluid has the same manifestations and signs as catheter-related bloodstream infection and other nosocomial bloodstream infections. The few clues to infusion-related bloodstream infection—absence of an obvious source of infection, its common occurrence in patients without a predilection to systemic infection, and the dramatic clinical response to discontinuing the infusion (see Table 44-3)—do not differentiate between intrinsic and extrinsic sources of contamination. The distinction must be made epidemiologically.

If intrinsic contamination of a commercially distributed product is identified, or even strongly suspected, especially if clinical infections have occurred as a consequence, the local, state, and Federal (CDC and the Food and Drug Administration (FDA)) public health authorities must be immediately contacted. Unopened samples of the suspect lot or lots should be quarantined and saved for their analysis.

Outbreaks Due to Extrinsic Contamination

Even when commercially manufactured products are sterile on arrival in the hospital, circumstances of hospital use can compromise that initial sterility. As previously noted, most sporadic infections deriving from infusion therapy, whether due to the cannula or contaminated infusate, are of extrinsic origin. Similarly, most reported epidemics have originated from exposure of multiple patients' infusions to a common source of contamination in the hospital [2,36,235,254–258].

Numerous outbreaks of infusion-related bacteremia have been caused by use of unreliable chemical antiseptics, or antiseptics such as aqueous benzalkonium and aqueous chlorhexidine used for cutaneous disinfection [145–148] or, in more recent years, for decontaminating transducer components used in hemodynamic monitoring [235] (see Table 44-9).

Despite the numerous reports of epidemic gram-negative bloodstream infections deriving from contaminated disinfectants used for decontaminating reusable transducer components in hemodynamic monitoring during the 1970s, one third of all outbreaks of nosocomial bacteremia investigated by the CDC between 1977 and 1987 were traced to contamination of infusions used for arterial pressure monitoring [256]. Since 1980, there have been 28 outbreaks of nosocomial bloodstream infection associated with arterial pressure monitoring reported in the literature, nearly all caused by gram-negative bacilli, most frequently *S. marcescens* and *Burkholderia* species [235,236–238]. Two thirds of these epidemics were linked to failed decontamination of reusable transducer components. Epidemic organisms were most commonly found on metal transducer heads, in the interface between transducers and disposable chamber domes. Eight epidemics were traced to introduction of organisms into closed monitoring systems from external sources of contamination in the hospital, such as contaminated ice used to chill syringes for drawing arterialized blood for blood gas measurements, heparinized saline from multidose vials, and contaminated external devices to calibrate pressure-monitoring systems. The epidemic organisms were found on the hands of healthcare providers in at least nine outbreaks; however, most of the reports do not provide sufficient data to establish the precise mechanism of fluid contamination.

With all forms of infusion therapy, the connection between the administration set and the catheter must be secure. This is especially important with central venous catheters, where accidental disconnections can result in exsanguination or life-threatening air embolus or blood loss. In TPN, a faulty connection may also increase the risk of iatrogenic infection: one reported outbreak of 23 catheter-related bloodstream infections caused by different strains of coagulase-negative staphylococci was linked to a manufacturing defect that resulted in hyperalimentation solution leaking from administration set–catheter connections and seeping under dressings, where it resulted in heavy bacterial overgrowth [259]. Another outbreak of coagulase-negative staphylococcal bacteremia has been associated with excessive manipulation of a catheter delivery system because of air appearing in the IV pump tubing. This resolved when the IV pump was placed at or below the heart level of the patients and air entry into the tubing ceased [260].

During the 1970s, numerous outbreaks of gram-negative bloodstream infection, particularly with pseudomonads other than *P. aeruginosa*, were traced to contamination of dialysate in patients' hemodialysis machines [261] (see Chapter 24); however, improved quality control, the decontamination of reused dialyzer coils, and the widespread use of disposable dialyzers have resulted in a marked decline in the incidence of nosocomial outbreaks traced to contaminated dialysate [2].

Compounding of admixtures is another important means by which contamination can be introduced [262]. The greatest concern about this mode of contamination, especially if it occurs in the central pharmacy, is that a large number of patients may be exposed. Moreover, the delay between compounding and use provides opportunity for proliferation of introduced microorganisms to levels that can cause overwhelming septic shock when administered. Two large outbreaks of candidemia have been traced to contaminated solutions used for IV hyperalimentation [263,264]; in each outbreak, a vacuum system in the hospital's pharmacy used to evacuate fluid from bottles before introducing other admixture components was shown to be heavily contaminated by the epidemic strain of *Candida*. Presumably, organisms refluxed into bottles during compounding of the admixtures. In outbreaks traced to contaminants introducing during compounding, after compounding, bottles were permitted to stand at room temperature for up to 48 hours before use. The necessity for stringent attention to a bloodstream infection in central admixture programs cannot be overemphasized. Fluid admixtures should be used within 6 hours or immediately refrigerated.

Investigations of > 100 epidemics over the past 2 decades [1,2] have documented contamination of in-use infusate or contamination of cannula insertion sites, deriving from a myriad of extrinsic sources in the hospital (see Table 44-9). In many outbreaks, the hospital reservoir of the epidemic pathogen and even the mode of transmission eluded detection, but the microorganism was found in large numbers on the hands of healthcare providers caring for patients receiving infusion therapy and handling their infusions. Manipulations of the delivery system, especially the administration set, appear to provide a highly effective means for access of microorganisms to in-use infusate, as illustrated by a spate of nosocomial outbreaks across the United States traced to in-use contamination of the IV anesthetic, propofol (Diprivan®). The solution provides a rich medium for rapid microbial proliferation [226], and outbreaks of primary bacteremia or surgical wound infection with a variety of gram-positive and gram-negative organisms and yeasts were traced to in-use contamination of propofol administered in the operating room, because of poor aseptic technique, storage of opened vials at room temperature, and use of single vials for multiple patients [36,264,265]. Similarly, a veritable explosion of hospital outbreaks of nosocomial candidemia in the past decade [265–267], primarily in ICUs, has been linked to carriage of the epidemic strain on the hands of nurses handling vulnerable patients' intravascular devices and infusions.

Approach to an Epidemic

If an epidemic is suspected, the epidemiologic approach must be methodical and thorough, yet expeditious. It is directed toward establishing the *bona fide* nature of the putative epidemic infections [269] and existence of an epidemic, defining the reservoirs and modes of transmission of the epidemic pathogens, and, most importantly controlling the epidemic quickly and completely. Control measures are obviously predicated on accurate delineation of the epidemiology of the causative pathogen (see Chapter 6).

The essential steps in dealing with a suspected outbreak of nosocomial bloodstream infection can be found in Table 44-10. To illustrate the approach to an epidemic of infusion-related bacteremia, the epidemiologic investigation of an extraordinary outbreak that occurred in the University of Wisconsin Hospital and Clinics is recounted [35].

> During a 2-week period in late March, 1985, three patients in our university hospital acquired primary nosocomial bacteremia with a similar nonfermentative gram-negative bacil-

TABLE 44-10. Evaluation of a suspected epidemic of nosocomial bloodstream infections

Administrative preparedness
Immediately retrieve putative epidemic blood isolates for confirmation of identity through spaces and subtyping by one or more methods:
Biotyping
Antimicrobial susceptibility pattern (antibiogram)
Serotyping
Phage typing
Bacteriocin typing
SDS-PAGE protein electrophoresis
Polymerase chain reaction
Pulsed-field gel electrophoresis
Immunoblot pattern
Multifocus enzyme electrophoresis
Restriction enzyme digestion and restriction fragment polymorphism patterns
DNA probes
Preliminary evaluations and control measures
Identify and characterize individual cases in time, place, risk factors
Strive to identify source of bloodstream infections
Ascertain if cases represent true bloodstream infections, rather than "pseudobacteremias"
Ascertain if cases represent a true epidemic, rather than a "pseudoepidemic"
Provisional control measures
Intensify surveillance, to detect every new case
Review general infection control policies and procedures
Determine need for assistance, especially extramural (local, state, Centers for Disease Control and Prevention)
Epidemiologic investigations
Clinicoepidemiologic studies, especially case–control studies
Microbiologic studies
Definitive control measures
Confirm control of epidemic by intensified follow-up surveillance
Report the findings

SDS-PAGE, sodium dodecyl sulfate–polyacrylamide gel electrophoresis.

lus. All three patients had had open heart surgery between March, 11 and March, 25 and became bacteremic 48 to 148 hours after operation.

The bloodstream pathogen in each case was shown to be *B. pickettii* biovariant 1. The organism was also cultured from the IV fluid of two of the patients at the time because, serendipitously, during the outbreak most adult patients in the hospital receiving IV fluids were participating in a study of IV catheter dressings [109]; as part of the study protocol, specimens were routinely obtained from patients' IV fluid when the catheter was removed. Review of nearly 1000 cultures of IV fluid from the infusions of participants in the study since its outset 3 months earlier showed that three additional surgical patients operated on in March had had IV fluid cultures positive for *B. pickettii* biovariant 1, even though none had shown clinical signs of bacteremia. Molecular subtyping by restriction enzyme digestion and pulsed-field electrophoresis to delineate restriction polymorphism patterns showed all six isolates to be the same. Three more patients who had been operated on in January had had IV fluid cultured positive for a similar nonfermentative gram-negative bacillus; although the three isolates were no longer available, the results of screening by AP-20E biochemical panel (API Analytab, Inc., Plainville, New York, U.S.A.) at the time were identical to those of the six patients with *B. pickettii* contamination of IV fluid, with or without associated bacteremia.

All of the patients had had multiple positive blood cultures and were in septic shock. *B. pickettii* had not been isolated from any local site of infection, such as the urinary tract, lower respiratory tract, or an surgical wound, in any of the patients.

Review of nosocomial bacteremias over the past 7 years showed that *B. pickettii* had not previously been identified in blood cultures from our institution, indicating that the cluster of three cases and six instances of contaminated infusate without bacteremia represented a true epidemic, and with the results of the subtyping, a common-source epidemic.

The CDC and the manufacturer were contacted: none of more than 70 NNIS hospitals had reported *B. pickettii* bacteremias in the past year, and the manufacturer had never identified contamination with *B. pickettii* in its quality-control microbiologic sampling of fentanyl before distribution, or received any complaints from users about suspected contamination of their fentanyl. Moreover, survey of surrounding hospitals that also used the manufacturer's fentanyl revealed none experiencing nosocomial bacteremias with *B. pickettii*.

A case–control study comparing the 9 infected patients, all of whom had had recent surgery, and 19 operated patients who had had negative IV fluid cultures in the IV dressing study, showed that all 9 cases but only 9 of the 19 operated control cases had received fentanyl intravenously in the operating room ($p = 0.05$); the mean total dose given to the 9 cases was far greater than that given to control patients who received the drug (3,080 vs. 840 μg, $p < 0.001$).

At the time, fentanyl was used at the University of Wisconsin Hospital only in the operating rooms as part of balanced anesthesia. The drug was received in 20-ml ampules from the manufacturer and each week, one of three pharmacy technicians, by rotation, predrew into sterile syringes all fentanyl likely to be needed the following week in the operating rooms. Each day, one of the technicians delivered enough predrawn syringes to the operating rooms to meet the needs of the cases being done that day. Cultures of predrawn fentanyl in syringes in the central pharmacy, prompted by the findings of the case–control study, showed that 20 (40%) of 50 30-ml syringes sampled were contaminated by *B. pickettii* in a concentration of more than 10^4 cfu/ml; none of 35 5-ml or 2-ml syringes showed contamination ($p < 0.001$).

Extensive culturing in the central pharmacy was negative for evidence of environmental contamination by *B. pickettii*, with one exception: *B. pickettii* biovariant 1, with an identical antimicrobial susceptibility pattern and restriction enzyme fragment pattern to the epidemic strain recovered from blood cultures or patients' IV infusions, was cultured in a concentration of 28 to 80 cfu/ml from five specimens of distilled water drawn from a tap in the central pharmacy. The epidemic strain was shown to multiply well in the fentanyl solution, attaining concentrations exceeding 10^4 cfu/ml within 48 hours.

A second case–control study suggested strongly that the epidemic was caused by theft of fentanyl from 30-ml syringes by a pharmacy staff member and replacement with distilled water that the individual thought was sterile but that, unfortunately, was contaminated by *B. pickettii*. The pharmacy member resigned early in the investigation. On April 29, the hospital's system for providing fentanyl and other narcotics to the operating rooms was changed; narcotics were no longer predrawn into syringes in the central pharmacy but were delivered to the operating rooms in unopened vials or ampules; anesthesiologists' orders for narcotics are filled by a staff pharmacist assigned to the operating room. There have been no further bacteremias with *B. pickettii* since March 25, 1985, and cultures of > 6,000 samples of hospitalized patients' IV fluid in research studies since that time have shown no further contamination by *B. pickettii*.

This outbreak illustrates the power of case–control analyses to identify the probable cause of an epidemic. It further illustrates the potential for contamination of parenteral drugs or admixtures and the extraordinary range of epidemiologic mechanisms of nosocomial bloodstream infection deriving from such contamination.

STRATEGIES FOR PREVENTION

Extensive guidelines for prevention of catheter-related infection have been published [12]. Specific interventions are discussed in the following sections.

Aseptic Technique

To accord it due respect, any device for vascular access must be thought of in fundamental terms as a direct conduit between the external world, with its myriad of microorganisms, and the bloodstream of the patient. Vigorous handwashing, ideally with an antiseptic-containing preparation, and gloving must always precede the insertion of a peripheral IV cannula and should also precede later handling of the device or the administration set [270]. It is further recommended that sterile gloves be routinely used during the insertion of peripheral IV cannulas in high-risk patients, such as those with severe burns. Sterile gloves are strongly recommended for placement of all other types of intravascular devices—arterial and all central venous catheters—which are associated with a higher risk of associated bloodstream infection [12].

Although there has been considerable controversy as to the level of barrier precautions necessary during insertion of a central venous catheter, in a study of Swan-Ganz pulmonary artery catheters, the use of maximal barrier precautions—sterile gloves, a long-sleeved sterile surgical gown, a surgical mask, and a large, sterile sheet drape, as contrasted to the use of sterile gloves, a surgical mask, and a small, fenestrated drape—was associated with a twofold lower risk of infection [175]. Despite the fact that Swan-Ganz catheters inserted in the ICU using maximal barrier precautions remained in place an average of 22 hours longer than catheters inserted in the operating room (inserted with lesser barrier precautions), were more frequently placed in infected patients, and were used more frequently for TPN, catheters inserted in the ICU using maximal barrier precautions were much less likely to be contaminated under the external protective sheath or infected than catheters inserted in the operating room by anesthesiologists using lesser barrier precautions. The efficacy of maximal barrier precautions in the prevention of nontunneled central venous catheter-related infection has been demonstrated [271,272]. In this investigation, the incidence of catheter-related bloodstream infection was 6.3 times higher in those patients who were prospectively randomized to have their catheters inserted with only sterile gloves and small sterile drapes, compared with those patients whose catheters were inserted with maximal barrier precautions (mask, cap, sterile gloves, gown, and large, sterile drape) [272]. In another study, use of maximal barrier precautions with central venous catheter insertion, in addition to a mandatory 5-minute scrub of the insertion site, reduced the incidence catheter colonization from 36% to 17% [273]. Considering that of all intravascular devices, central venous catheters are most likely to produce nosocomial bloodstream infection, a strong case can be made for mandating maximal barrier precautions during the insertion of such devices, particularly the use of a long-sleeved surgical gown and large, sterile sheet drape, to minimize touch contamination, in addition to sterile gloves, the use of which should be routine [12,272].

Inappropriate catheter care is an independent risk factor for catheter-related infections [186]. Not surprisingly, the use of special IV therapy teams, consisting of trained nurses or technicians to ensure a high level of aseptic technique during catheter insertion and in follow-up care of the catheter, has been associated with substantially lower rates of catheter-related infection [108,273–282] (Table 44-11). Such teams are highly cost effective, reducing the costs of complications of infusion therapy nearly 10-fold [281,282].

In the absence of a dedicated IV team, some investigators have carried out intensive educational programs in catheter care. In one study, this led to improved care overall and a concomitant reduction of colonization of the catheter insertion site; however, the incidence of catheter hub colonization was unchanged [283]. In some U.S. hospitals, all central venous catheters, particularly those dedicated to TPN, are cared for by such teams. Other investigators have also shown that institutions can greatly reduce their rate of catheter-related bloodstream infection by scrutiny of catheter care protocols and more intensive education and training of nurses and physicians [284]. The importance of adequate staffing of nurses to care for patients with central venous catheters has recently been demonstrated [286]. After controlling for other risk factors associated with catheter-related infection in a logistic regression model, as the patient-to-nurse ratio doubled due to nurse understaffing in an ICU, the risk of central venous catheter-related bloodstream infection increased dramatically (OR 62). This seminal observation suggests that in this era of fiscal restraint in healthcare, cost-cutting measures which lead to understaffing of personnel aimed at caring for intravascular devices will ultimately

TABLE 44-11. Impact of a dedicated IV team on the rate of catheter-related bloodstream infection

Type of study [reference]	Type of catheter	Care given by	No. catheters	Incidence IV-related bloodstream infection (per 100 catheters)	*p*-value
		Concurrent but not randomized			
[274]	PIV	House officers	4,270	0.40	
		IV team	470	0.04	< 0.001
[275]	CVC-TPN	Ward nurses	33	21.2	
		IV nurses	78	2.3	< 0.001
[276]	CVC-TPN	Ward nurses	391	26.2	
		IV team	284	1.3	< 0.001
[277]	CVC-TPN	Ward nurses	179	24.0	
		IV team	377	3.5	< 0.001
[278]	CVC-TPN	House officers	45	28.8	
		IV nurses	30	3.3	< 0.001
		Historical controls			
[279]	CVC-TPN	Ward nurses	335	28.6	
		IV team	172	4.7	< 0.001
[280]	CVC-TPN	Ward nurses	51	33.0	
		IV nurses	48	4.0	< 0.001
[281[a]]	PIV and CVC	House officers	—	—	0.001
		IV team	—	—	
		Randomized, concurrent controls			
[108]	PIV	House officers	427	2.1	
		IV team	433	0.2	< 0.05
[282]	PIV	House officers	453	1.5	
		IV team	412	0.0	< 0.02

IV, intravenous; PIV, peripheral IV catheter; CVC, central venous catheter; TPN, total parenteral nutrition.
[a]Catheter-related bacteremia with house officers (4.5/1,000 patient discharges) vs. with IV team (1.7/1,000 patient discharges).

increase cost and increase the risk of nosocomial infection in today's hospitalized patients.

Cutaneous Antisepsis

Given the evidence for the important role of cutaneous microorganisms in the genesis of many intravascular device-related infections, measures to reduce cutaneous colonization of the insertion site would seem of the highest priority, particularly the use of chemical antiseptics for disinfection of the site. In the United States, an iodophor such as 10% povidone–iodine is used most widely [252]. The lack of published comparative trials of cutaneous antiseptics to prevent catheter-related infection prompted the following prospective investigation: 668 patients' central venous and arterial catheters in a surgical ICU were randomized to 10% povidone–iodine, 70% alcohol, or 2% aqueous chlorhexidine for disinfection of the site before insertion and site care every other day thereafter [32]. Chlorhexidine was associated with the lowest incidence of infection; of the 14 infusion-related bloodstream infections, 1 was in the chlorhexi-

TABLE 44-12. Results of a prospective, randomized trial of three cutaneous antiseptics for prevention of intravascular device-related bloodstream infection

Source of bloodstream infection	10% Povidone–iodine (n = 227)	70% Alcohol (n = 227)	2% Chlorhexidine (n = 214)
Catheter related	6	3	1
From contaminated:			
Infusate		3	
Hub	1		
All sources (%)	7 (3.1)	6 (2.6)	1 (0.5)[a]

[a]Compared with the other two groups combined, odds ratio, 0.16, $p = 0.04$.
(From Maki DG, Alvarado CJ, Ringer M. A prospective, randomized trial of povidone–iodine, alcohol and chlorhexidine for prevention of infection with central venous and arterial catheters. *Lancet* 1991;338:339–343.)

dine group and 13 were in the other two groups (odds ratio, 0.16; $p = 0.04$; Table 44-12). This study suggests that the use of 2% chlorhexidine, rather than 10% povidone–iodine or 70% alcohol, for cutaneous disinfection before insertion of an intravascular device and in postinsertion site care can substantially reduce the incidence of device-related infection. Of note, there was no difference in the incidence of catheter-related infection when povidone–iodine was used for cutaneous antisepsis compared with alcohol. Other investigators have also found that use of aqueous chlorhexidine to prepare the catheter insertion site is associated with a lower incidence of catheter-related infection compared with povidone–iodine [151–153].

In a historical analysis of the impact on the incidence of catheter-related bloodstream infection of using different antiseptics for site care and disinfection of tubing connections in a home TPN program, 0.58 cases per catheter-year were observed during use of 10% povidone–iodine as contrasted to 0.26 to 0.28 cases per catheter-year during use of a 0.5% to 2% tincture of iodine or 0.5% tincture of chlorhexidine [287]. Prospective, randomized studies comparing the blood culture contamination rate using povidone–iodine vs. iodine tincture to prepare the puncture site, use of iodine tincture was associated with a contamination rate one-half that of the povidone–iodine group [288]. Thus, iodine tincture may be the cutaneous antiseptic of choice in the United States until an FDA-approved chlorhexidine-based preparation becomes available [11].

"Defatting" the skin with acetone is still widely practiced in many centers as an adjunctive measure for disinfecting central venous catheter sites, especially in TPN; however, it was found to be of no benefit whatsoever in a prospective, randomized trial [114]. In contrast, the use of acetone was associated with greatly increased inflammation and discomfort to the patient.

Topical Antimicrobial Ointments

In theory, application of topical antimicrobial agents to the catheter insertion site should confer some protection against microbial invasion. Clinical trials of topical polyantibiotic ointments (polymyxin, neomycin, and bacitracin) on peripheral venous catheters have shown only moderate or no benefit [154,290], and the use of polyantibiotic ointments has been associated with an increased frequency of *Candida* infections [116,154]. In prospective, randomized trials, application of the topical antibacterial, mupirocin, which is active primarily against gram-positive organisms, to catheter insertion sites has been associated with a significant reduction in central venous catheter colonization, but not arterial or peripheral catheter colonization. Without colonization by *Candida*, the impact on catheter-related bloodstream infection could not be assessed [291]. However, widespread use of mupirocin at catheter insertion sites may lead to resistance [292], and for this reason it is not recommended for routine application to the insertion site of central venous catheters.

There have been two prospective studies of topical povidone–iodine ointment applied to central venous catheter sites; one large, randomized trial in a surgical ICU showed no benefit [293], but a more recent comparative trial with subclavian hemodialysis catheters showed a fourfold reduction in the incidence of hemodialysis catheter-related bloodstream infection [122].

Dressings

The importance of the cutaneous microflora in the pathogenesis of device-related infection might suggest that the dressing applied to the catheter insertion site could have considerable influence on the incidence of catheter-related infection. When used on vascular catheters, transparent dressings permit continuous inspection of the site, secure the device reliably, and are generally more comfortable than gauze and tape. Moreover, transparent dressings permit patients to bathe and shower without saturating the dressing. Clinical trials of these dressings have been prompted by the knowledge that cutaneous occlusion with tape or impervious plastic films results in an explosive increase in cutaneous microflora, with overgrowth of gram-negative bacilli and yeasts [293]. Although polyurethane dressings are semipermeable—impervious to extrinsic microbial contaminants and liquid-phase moisture, and variably permeable to oxygen, carbon dioxide, and water vapor—and studies in healthy volunteers have shown little effect of these dressings on the cutaneous flora [294], a meta-analysis has raised concern that these dressings could increase cutaneous colonization and the risk of catheter-related infection [295].

Transparent polyurethane dressings are more expensive than gauze and tape, and to obviate the issue of greater cost and to increase convenience, many users leave transparent dressings on for prolonged periods, for up to 7 days or even longer. It has been questioned whether transparent dressings left on for prolonged periods might increase the risk of catheter-related infection. There have been a number of trials comparing polyurethane dressings with gauze and tape on peripheral venous catheters [14,15,107,109, 296–300]. Three trials [296–298] have found significantly higher rates of catheter colonization with transparent dressings left on indefinitely. Other investigators also found a higher rate in catheters dressed with a transparent dressing, but only during the summer months [107]. In additional studies, however, significant differences were found [14,15,109,299,300]. Rates of catheter colonization in all of these trials have been low with all dressings, in the range of 1.6% to 8.5%. Only 3 catheter-related bloodstream infections were identified among the nearly 4,000 catheters studied in all of the reported trials.

In a prospective, randomized trial of various dressings used with 2,088 Teflon peripheral IV catheters [109], the transparent polyurethane dressing studied, left on for the lifetime of the catheter, was not associated with increased cutaneous colonization under the dressing or an increased rate of catheter colonization, compared with the control gauze and tape dressing; however, there were no catheter-related bloodstream infections. Cutaneous colonization was not heavier under transparent dressings during the spring and summer months, as previously described [107], perhaps because the hospital was air conditioned. Multivariate analysis showed cutaneous colonization of the insertion site (relative risk of infection, 3.9) and moisture under the dressing (relative risk, 2.5) to be significant risk factors for catheter-related infection (see Table 44-7). These data indicate that it is probably not cost effective to redress peripheral IV catheters at periodic intervals, and that for most patients either sterile gauze or a transparent dressing can be used and left on until the catheter is removed [12].

Studies of transparent dressings on short-term, noncuffed central venous and/or pulmonary artery catheters have yielded conflicting results [34,182,300–308], in part reflecting differences in study protocols (e.g., the use of topical antimicrobial ointments under the dressing in the control gauze group, but not in the transparent dressing group) and different dressings studied. One group of investigators [302] reported a threefold increase in infectious complications associated with subclavian catheters using transparent dressings for ≤ 7 days compared with gauze replaced three times weekly, but the difference did not achieve statistical significance. Others [182] have found a much higher rate of catheter-related bloodstream infection using transparent dressings compared with gauze and tape (16% vs. 0%). In a similar trial performed in an ICU, there were no significant differences in catheter-related infection with transparent dressings compared with gauze dressings when the transparent dressing was changed every 2 days [305]; however, in these high-risk ICU patients, we observed a significant buildup of skin flora, associated with a 50% increase in catheter-related infection, when transparent dressings were left on for up to 7 days between changes, suggesting that if used on central venous catheters in ICU patients, the dressing studied may need to be replaced more frequently. Other prospective trials, which in aggregate studied hundreds of central venous catheters in high-risk patients, many of whom were receiving TPN through the catheter, did not find an increased risk of catheter-related infection associated with transparent dressing left on for a prolonged duration, as compared with gauze and tape replaced more frequently [34,300,301,303,304,306–308]. In a large, prospective, randomized clinical trial, we found no difference in the incidence of catheter colonization or catheter-related bloodstream infection in patients whose catheters were covered with gauze and tape dressing changed every 2 days, conventional polyurethane dressing, or a polyurethane dressing with a high moisture vapor transmission rate, both replaced every 5 days [34]. However, at the time of catheter withdrawal, insertion site colonization was greater under both polyurethane dressings compared with the gauze and tape dressing group. There was no significant difference in colonization between the polyurethane dressing groups. Similarly, the incidence of central venous catheter-related bloodstream infection was no different for patients whose catheters were dressed with gauze and tape every 2 days compared with transparent dressing every 5 days in a multicenter trial however, colonization was significantly more common in the polyurethane dressing group [308].

Two randomized studies of the use of transparent dressings on surgically implanted, cuffed Hickman or Broviac catheters have been reported in which microbiologic data were provided [305,309]; in both trials, one in renal transplant patients [305] and the other in bone marrow transplant recipients [309], the transparent dressing studied provided satisfactory cover, and even when left on for prolonged periods, for up to 5 to 7 days, was not associated with a significantly increased risk of exit site or tunnel infection, or of catheter-related bloodstream infection. These studies of central venous, pulmonary artery, and long-term tunneled catheters suggest that either transparent or gauze and tape dressings can be safely used to cover the insertion site of these devices.

There have been only two reported studies of transparent polyurethane dressings with arterial catheters [15,305]. In one prospective study of dressings for arterial catheters used for hemodynamic monitoring in a surgical ICU, the use of the transparent dressing, even replaced every other day, was associated with a fivefold increased incidence of catheter-related bloodstream infection, compared with gauze and tape [305]. The greatly increased risk of infection associated with transparent dressings used on arterial catheters found in this study may reflect the presence of macroscopic blood in the puncture wound, under arterial pressure, which is common under transparent dressings on arterial catheters; if the blood cannot be cleared, it may provide a rich medium for microbial proliferation, which can result in infection of the catheter. As a consequence, gauze and tape is preferred to transparent dressings for arterial catheters.

Changing Catheters Over a Guidewire

The Seldinger technique, in which the vessel is identified and entered percutaneously with a fine-gauge needle and cannulated with a guidewire passed through the needle, after which the cannula is guided into the vessel over the guidewire, has been a major advance, permitting vessels to be cannulated with large catheters with much less risk of vascular injury and, in the case of subclavian or internal jugular central venous catheters, pneumothorax, and with less manipulation and potential for contamination. To avoid iatrogenic pneumothorax and other mechanical complications associated with percutaneous insertion of a new cannula, particularly a central venous catheter, new catheters are commonly placed over a guidewire in the site of an old catheter [118]. Prospective, randomized clinical trials have shown that routinely replacing central venous catheters over guidewires is unnecessary [118,158,310]. In the largest of these studies [118], the incidence of catheter-related bloodstream infection per 1,000 catheter days was nearly twofold higher in patients randomized to the guidewire groups, and 75% of catheter-related bacteremias and fungemias occurred within 72 hours of guidewire exchange or catheter insertion. In a study performed in a pediatric ICU, central venous catheters were left in place without routine guidewire exchange [311]. Despite prolonged catheterization, the incidence density of catheter-related infection did not increase with the duration of time the catheters were left in situ. Similar results were found in a study of adult oncology patients whose noncuffed, nontunneled central venous catheters were left in place for a mean of 136 days [125]. These data suggest that routine guidewire exchange of central venous catheters is unnecessary in patients who are without unexplained fever and without induration or drainage from the catheter insertion site. In two prospective studies of central venous and Swan-Ganz pulmonary artery catheters, the incidence of catheter-related infection was not significantly different among patients whose catheters were routinely changed over guidewires or left in place [118,310]. However, the data derived from all prospective clinical trials of Swan-Ganz pulmonary artery catheters demonstrate that the incidence of bloodstream infection rises sharply on the fifth day of catheterization [48]. Because of these conflicting results, firm recommendations regarding the safe duration of Swan-Ganz pulmonary artery catheters cannot be made at this time.

One prospective study of arterial catheters found that there was a greater incidence of catheter-related bloodstream infection when catheters were routinely exchanged over guidewires compared with catheters removed after 7 days and inserted into a new site [31]. Other studies have shown that the incidence density of arterial catheter-related infection did not increase with the duration of time the catheters were left in place [312,313], and in three prospective studies in which the catheters, transducers, and plasticware were not routinely changed [314–316], the incidences of catheter colonization (2.9%) and catheter-related bloodstream infection (0.2%) were quite low and comparable with those in other prospective studies. Therefore, these data suggest that arterial catheters, similar to central venous catheters, may not need to be replaced at routine intervals as long as signs of localized infection are absent and the patient is without unexplained fever. It is important to remember that all invasive devices, including intravascular catheters of any type, increase the risk of infection, and their need should be assessed on a daily basis. In one study, nearly 20% of patients on medical wards had idle catheters for 2 or more consecutive days, and 20% of all patient-days of IV catheter use were idle and unnecessarily increasing the risk of catheter infection in these patients [317]. In a follow-up study, intensive educational efforts reduced the incidence of idle catheters [318].

If it is considered desirable to replace a central venous or arterial catheter because it has been in place for a prolonged period and there is suspicion of infection (e.g., unexplained fever) it is not unreasonable to replace the catheter in the same site over a guidewire *if* the patient has limited sites for new access or would be at high risk for the percutaneous puncture required for placement of a new catheter in a new site (e.g., has coagulopathy or is morbidly obese). However, it is imperative that the same meticulous aseptic technique that should be mandatory during insertion of any new catheter must be employed, including the routine use of sterile gloves and a sterile drape, and for central venous catheters, a sterile gown as well. After vigorously cleansing the site and the old catheter with the antiseptic solution, inserting the guidewire, removing the old catheter, and cleansing the guidewire and site once more with the antiseptic solution, the operator should *reglove and redrape the site* because the original gloves and drapes are likely to be contaminated from manipulation of the old catheter. After regloving and repreparing the site, the new catheter can be inserted over the guidewire.

It is also important *routinely* to culture the old catheter after guidewire exchange and, if the patient is febrile or shows other signs of bloodstream infection, to obtain blood cultures. If these cultures demonstrate that the old catheter was colonized, the new catheter just placed in the old site should be immediately removed to prevent progression to catheter-related bloodstream infection (or perpetuation of ongoing catheter-related bloodstream infection) because the new catheter has been inserted into an infected tract. Need for continued access would mandate placement of a new catheter in a new site. If, on the other hand, culture of the old catheter is negative, it has been possible to preserve access and to examine the initial catheter microbiologically and exclude it as the cause of fever or bloodstream infection, without subjecting the patient to the hazards associated with percutaneous insertion of a new catheter.

If the old insertion site is inflamed at the outset, especially if it is purulent, or the patient shows signs of sepsis that might be originating from the catheter, or the catheter recently has been shown to be infected by quantitative blood cultures drawn through the catheter, it is strongly recommended that a new catheter not be inserted over a guidewire into an old, potentially infected site.

The Effect of Subcutaneous Tunnel Insertion of Central Venous Catheters

Subcutaneous tunnel insertion of central venous catheters has traditionally been carried out in an effort to reduce the risk of catheter-related infection. In a prospective, randomized study in immunocompromised patients, the incidence of catheter-related bloodstream infection was the same in those patients whose catheters were tunneled, compared to those whose catheters were not [318]. In a randomized trial of catheters used for administering TPN [279], the incidence of catheter sepsis was reduced with tunneling of catheters before, but not after, a trained IV nurse assumed complete responsibility for catheter care. In a more recent, prospective, randomized study, tunneling central venous catheters inserted into the internal jugular vein dramatically reduced the incidence of catheter-related bloodstream infection (RR 0.19 [320]). However, this may be difficult to extrapolate to the U.S. experience since most tunneled catheters in the U.S. are inserted in the subclavian, rather than the internal jugular vein. Also, no blood was drawn through the catheters in this study, which is common practice in the U.S. This may have led to a lower incidence of hub-related bloodstream infection, further magnifying the difference in tunneled and non-tunneled catheter groups with regards to bloodstream infection. In another study [125], nontunneled central venous catheters in immunocompromised patients inserted for prolonged periods of time also had a very low incidence of associated bloodstream infection when the catheters were cared for by specialized IV nurses. Therefore, central venous catheters cared for by specialized IV nurses may not need to be tunneled in an attempt to reduce the incidence of catheter-related infection. The utility of tunneled subclavian central venous catheters in situations without specialized IV nursing teams requires further study.

Measures Aimed at the Delivery System

Numerous studies have shown that most catheter-related bloodstream infection are caused by infections contaminated infusate [1,2]; however, infusate can occasionally become contaminated and cause endemic bacteremia or fungemia [32,33,34,115,175]. If an infusion runs continuously for an extended period, the cumulative risk of contamination increases, and further, there is increased risk that the contaminants can grow to dangerously high concentrations that will result in bloodstream infection in the recipient of the fluid. For nearly 20 years, most U.S. hospitals have routinely replaced the entire delivery system of patients' IV infusions at 24- or 48-hour intervals [1,2], to reduce the risk of bloodstream infection from extrinsically contaminated fluid. Prospective studies (see Table 44-8), however, now indicate that IV delivery systems do not need to be replaced more frequently than every 72 hours, including infusions used for TPN or any infusions in ICU patients [227,228,230]; extending the duration of use allows considerable cost savings to hospitals [228]. Other prospective studies have demonstrated that replacement of the IV delivery system every 96 to 120 hours did not increase the incidence of catheter-related infection [312,321]. It is important to remember that replacement of the IV delivery system at more prolonged intervals may predispose to epidemic bloodstream infection, particularly when the fluids infused promote microbial growth [243].

Three clinical settings might be regarded as exceptions to using 72 hours as an interval for routine set change: 1) during administration of blood products or 2) lipid emulsions, and 3) if an epidemic of infusion-related bloodstream infections is suspected. In these circumstances, it is most prudent that administration sets be changed routinely at 24- or 48-hour intervals. Minute amounts of blood buffers acidic solutions and provides organic nutrients that greatly enhance the ability of most microorganisms to grow in parenteral fluids [217]. Moreover, most hospital pathogens, including coagulase-negative staphylococci, some gram-negative bacilli, *Candida*, and *M. furfur*, grow rapidly in commercial lipid emulsion [219,220,225,243], and outbreaks of bloodstream infection have been associated with administration of lipid emulsion [243,246,323].

Studies suggest that the infusion system, including the administration set and other delivery components, for hemodynamic monitoring may not need routine replacement as long as the catheter insertion site is without induration or discharge and the patient is without an unresolved source of fever [234,314–316].

The type of infusion pump and delivery system used may affect the incidence of catheter-related infection. Line breaks associated with some infusion pumps and delivery systems appear to be susceptible to air entry into the tubing, leading to greater manipulation, and at one institution this was associated with an outbreak of coagulase-negative staphylococcal bacteremia [260]. Some systems require significantly fewer line breaks than others [324], and this may lessen the risk of catheter-related infection because an excessive number of line breaks per day has been demonstrated to be an independent risk factor for catheter-related infection [188].

Needleless IV systems have come into widespread use in an effort to reduce the risk of exposure to bloodborne pathogens. However, the risk of catheter-related bloodstream infection associated with use of these systems has not been systematically addressed in prospective, randomized trials. A number of studies have found that these systems may actually increase the risk of catheter-related infection [258,325–329]. A unifying problem is the inability to clean the inner components of these systems; once they become contaminated, bacteria and fungi can proliferate to large numbers, leading to intraluminal seeding of the blood [325,326]. Prospective studies are needed to determine the safety of needleless systems with regard to needlestick injury, catheter hub colonization, and bloodstream infection.

Terminal in-use membrane filters continue to be advocated as a means of reducing the hazard of contaminated infusate. However, filters must be changed at periodic intervals and can become blocked, leading to added manipulations of the system and, paradoxically, greater potential for contamination [330,331]. Some commercial in-line filters may also permit the passage of endotoxin [331,332]. The increased risk for phlebitis associated with the administration of IV antibiotics may be reduced by removing the microparticulates that are associated with compounding these drugs with 0.22 or 0.44 μm in-line filters [334]; however, not all randomized trials have shown a substantial reduction in phlebitis with the use of in-line filters [335]. Moreover, filters are expensive, and their use adds substantially to the costs of phlebitis from microparticulates. Few controlled, prospective clinical trials have been done to assess the effect of in-line filters on the incidence of serious catheter-related infections. In these studies, small numbers of patients were enrolled and the outcomes were variable [336,337]; however, studies carried out in animals suggest that with heavily contaminated infusate, in-line filters reduce mortality [337]. Large, prospective, double-blind clinical studies establishing their efficacy and cost effectiveness are needed before their routine use can be advocated, especially as a control measure for prevention of rare sporadic bloodstream infections deriving from extrinsic contamination of infusate [12].

Innovative Technology

The development and application of novel technology holds the greatest promise for a quantum reduction in the risk of infusion-related bloodstream infection, especially infection due to the percutaneous device used for intravascular access: innovations in the design or construction of the infusion apparatus that implicitly deny access of microorganisms to the system or that prevent organisms that might gain access from proliferating to high concentrations or colonizing the implanted cannula can obviate poor aseptic technique or undue patient vulnerability.

In a burn model, silver-coated dressings reduced the tissue penetration of *P. aeruginosa* in animals and may reduce the risk of catheter-related infections [339]. Previous studies of incorporating an antiseptic, namely povidone–iodine into a transparent catheter dressing to suppress cutaneous colonization under the dressing have been disappointing [109]. However, in view of the superiority of chlorhexidine over povidone–iodine for cutaneous disinfection of vascular catheter sites [32,151–153], incorporation of chlorhexidine into a dressing's adhesive might prove more effective. A chlorhexidine-impregnated urethane sponge composite (Biopatch; Johnson & Johnson, Arlington, Texas, U.S.A.) has been shown significantly to reduce epidural catheter colonization, from 29% to 4% [340]. In a nonrandomized clinical trial using historical controls, use of the composite sponge reduced the incidence of central venous catheter-related bloodstream infections from 21 to 13 per 1,000 catheter-days [341]. Prospective, randomized studies are needed to prove the efficacy of this device.

A tissue–interface barrier (VitaCuff; Vitafore Corporation, San Carlos, California, U.S.A.) has been developed that incorporates aspects of the technology of Hickman and Broviac catheters; the device consists of a detachable cuff made of biodegradable collagen to which silver ion is chelated (Figure 44-4). The cuff can be attached to central venous catheters immediately before insertion. After insertion, subcutaneous tissue grows into the collagenous matrix, anchoring the catheter and creating a barrier against invasive organisms from the skin. The silver ion provides an additional chemical barrier against introduced contamination, augmenting the mechanical barrier. However, this device affords protection against extraluminal, not intraluminal, migration of microbial pathogens into the bloodstream. In most prospective, randomized clinical trials of short-term central venous catheters, the incidence of catheter colonization and catheter-related bloodstream infection was reduced with use of the cuff [116,117,159]

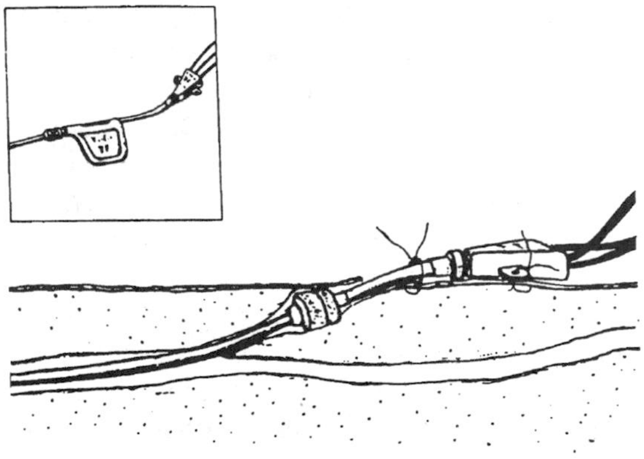

FIGURE 44-4. Schematic depiction of a silver-impregnated, tissue barrier cuff (VitaCuff) and the cuff attached to a central venous catheter in situ. It is important for the cuff to be positioned at least 0.5 to 1.0 cm below the surface of the skin and for the catheter to be well immobilized, preferably with a skin suture, to prevent extrusion. (From Maki DG, Cobb L, Garman JK, Shapiro J, Ringer M, Helgerson RB. An attachable silver-impregnated cuff for prevention of infection with central venous catheters. A prospective randomized multicenter trial. *Am J Med* 1988; 85:307–314.)

TABLE 44-13. Efficacy of the silver-impregnated cuff (VitaCuff) catheter colonization in preventing catheter-related bloodstream infection (CRBSI)

Catheter colonization (%)		CRBSI (%)		
Cuff	Control	Cuff	Control	Reference
9	29[a]	1	4	[115]
8	36[a]	0	14	[116][b]
13	28	—	—	[159][b]
15	18	5	0	[158][b]
5	5	12	14	[342][c]
—	—	36	32	[161][c]
15	20	4	4	[162][c]

[a] $p < 0.05$.
[b] Catheterization (mean) ≤ 14 days.
[c] Catheterization (mean) ≥ 14 days.

(Table 44-13). The cuff did not confer protection, however, against infection with catheters inserted over a guidewire to old sites [116]. A cost–benefit analysis shows that if an institution's rate of short-term central venous catheter-related bacteremia is in the range of 2% to 3%, use of the cuff should prove cost effective [116]. In prospective studies of patients in whom the duration of central venous catheterization was > 2 weeks [161,162,342], cuff use was not found to reduce the incidence of catheter colonization or catheter-related bloodstream infection. This may be due to the greater importance of hub colonization as a source of catheter-related infections with more prolonged catheterization [72,150]. Therefore, use of the cuff should be considered in patients with an expected duration of catheterization of < 2 weeks.

Given the multiplicity of potential sources for infection of an intravascular device and the importance of adherence of microorganisms to the catheter surface in the pathogenesis of infection, it would seem logical that the best strategy for prevention might be to develop a catheter material implicitly resistant to colonization. It has been demonstrated that hydrophilic catheters are less likely to become colonized by bacteria in in vitro assays [343,344]. Binding a nontoxic antiseptic or antimicrobial to the catheter surface or incorporating such a substance into the catheter material itself might prove to be the most effective technologic innovation for preventing device-related infection. In a prospective, randomized clinical trial of central venous and arterial catheters in a surgical ICU, catheters coated with cefazolin bonded to the surface with a cationic surfactant were associated with a sevenfold reduction in colonization of the catheter; however, there were no catheter-related bacteremias identified in the study population [163]. More recently, catheters coated with minocycline and rifampin have been shown significantly to reduce the incidence of catheter colonization and catheter-related bloodstream infection [164]. Widespread use of these devices is also tempered by the risk of the development of resistance to these valuable antibiotics [345]. We have studied a novel central venous catheter in which the catheter material itself, polyurethane, is impregnated with minute quantities of silver sulfadiazine and chlorhexidine (Arrowgard; Arrow International, Reading, Pennsylvania, U.S.A.); in a randomized, comparative trial in 402 patients in a surgical ICU, antiseptic catheters were twofold less likely to be colonized and fourfold less likely to produce bacteremia [168]. Adverse effects from the test catheter were not seen. In a prospective, randomized study, other investigators have also found that this device reduced the incidence of catheter-related infection [169]; however, with more prolonged catheterization, efficacy appears to wane [170,171] (Table 44-14). Silver-coated catheters have also been shown to reduce the incidence of catheter-related infection [165], as have catheters bound with benzalkonium or heparin [166,167]. Strategies that hold the greatest promise are those that will change the intravascular device itself in a novel way that is unlikely to promote resistance to antibiotics or antiseptics. One innovative approach is to apply an electric current to the catheter [346,347]. In vitro studies with these catheters demonstrate that they inhibit the growth of bacteria and fungi [346] and are resistant to colonization, and that application of an electric current sterilizes colonized catheters [345]. In an animal model of *S. aureus* catheter-related infection, these catheters were more effective in preventing infection than the silver sulfadiazine–chlorhexidine-impregnated catheters [347].

Strategies aimed at reducing hub-related bloodstream infection have been devised, and in a clinical trial, a novel hub incorporating an iodine tincture reservoir reduced the incidence of bloodstream infection fourfold [348].

The addition of a nontoxic, biodegradable or easily metabolized antiseptic to IV fluid or IV admixtures [349–353] might eliminate the hazard of fluid contamination altogether and, further, reduce the risk of hub contamination, obviating the need for periodic replacement of the delivery system.

TABLE 44-14. Efficacy of the chlorhexidine–silver sulfadiazine catheter (CHSS) [Arrowgard™] in preventing catheter colonization and catheter-related bloodstream infection (CRBSI)

Catheter colonization (%)		CRBSI (%)			
CHSS	Control	CHSS	Control	Duration (days)	Reference
13.5	24.1[a]	1.0	7.6[a]	6	168
18.1	30.8[a]	0	2.6	~8	169
—	—	6.3	7.5	10–11	171
10.9	12.1	8.7	8.1	12–13	170

[a] $p < 0.05$.

THE FUTURE

We believe that the future is very hopeful for continued progress in the prevention of device-related infection. A great deal of progress has been made over the past decade, with studies showing reduced rates of infection with the use of more stringent barrier precautions during insertion of central venous catheters, with IV teams, with the use of more effective cutaneous antiseptics, and with the results of the first studies of innovative technologies, such as contamination-resistant hubs, attachable cuffs, and catheters with colonization-resistant surfaces. We are optimistic that future intravascular devices will be highly resistant to thrombosis and infection, and that it will be possible to allow percutaneously inserted catheters safely to remain in place in high-risk patients nearly indefinitely.

Scientia est potentia

Acknowledgments

We express our appreciation to our colleagues in the studies cited from the University of Wisconsin research group, particularly Drs. Jeffrey Band and Lazaro Velez, and Carla Alvarado, Rita McCormick, Marilyn Ringer, Sue Stolz, Sue Wheeler, and Lorna Will; and Kimberly and Gail Maki and Ann Cappali, for secretarial assistance in preparation of the manuscript.

REFERENCES

1. Maki DG. Nosocomial bacteremia. *Am J Med* 1981;70:183–196.
2. Maki DG. The epidemiology and prevention of nosocomial bloodstream infections [Abstract]. In: *Program and abstracts of the third international conference on nosocomial infections, August 1990, Atlanta, Georgia*. Centers for Disease Control, The National Foundation for Infectious Diseases and the American Society for Microbiology, 1990:20.
3. Friedland G, von Reyn CF, Levy B, et al. Nosocomial endocarditis. *Infect Control* 1984;5:284–288.
4. Terpenning MS, Buggy BP, Kauffman CA. Hospital-acquired infective endocarditis. *Arch Intern Med* 1988;148:1601–1603.
5. Fang G, Keys TF, Gentry LO, et al. Prosthetic valve endocarditis resulting from nosocomial bacteremia: a prospective, multicenter study. *Ann Intern Med* 1993;111:560–567.
6. Martin MA, Pfaller MA, Wenzel RP. Coagulase-negative staphylococcal bacteremia: mortality and hospital stay. *Ann Intern Med* 1989; 110:9–16.
7. Smith RL, Meixler SM, Simberkoff MS. Excess mortality in critically ill patients with nosocomial bloodstream infections. *Chest* 1991;100: 164–67.
8. Pittet D. Nosocomial bloodstream infections in the critically ill. *JAMA* 1994;272:1819–1820.
9. Collignon PJ. Intravascular catheter associated sepsis: a common problem. *Med J Aust* 1994;161:374–378.
10. Inglis TJJ, Sproat LJ, Hawkey PM, et al. Infection control in intensive care units: U.K. national survey. *Br J Anaesth* 1992;68:216–220.
11. Mermel LA. Prevention of intravascular catheter-related infections. *Infect Dis Clin Pract* 1994;3:391–398.
12. Pearson ML. The Hospital Infection Control Advisory Committee. Guideline for prevention of intravascular-device-related infections. *Infect Control Hosp Epidemiol* 1996;17:438–473.
13. Maki DG, Ringer M. Risk factors for infusion-related phlebitis with small peripheral venous catheters. *Ann Intern Med* 1991;114: 845–854.
14. Gantz NM, Presswood GM, Goldberg R, et al. Effects of dressing type and change interval on intravenous therapy complication rates. *Diagn Microbiol Infect Dis* 1984;2:325–332.
15. Hoffman KK, Western SA, Kaiser DL, et al. Bacterial colonization and phlebitis-associated risk with transparent polyurethane film for peripheral intravenous site dressings. *Am J Infect Control* 1988;16: 101–106.
16. Collin J, Collin C, Constable FL, et al. Infusion phlebitis and infection with various cannulas. *Lancet* 1975;2:150–153.
17. Maki DG, Weise CE, Sarafin HW. A semiquantitative culture method for identifying intravenous-catheter-related infection. *N Engl J Med* 1977;296:1305–1309.
18. Smallman L, Burdon DW, Alexander-Williams J. The effect of skin preparation on the incidence of infusion thrombophlebitis. *Br J Surg* 1980;67:861–862.
19. Larson E, Hargiss C. A decentralized approach to maintenance of intravenous therapy. *Am J Infect Control* 1984;12:177–186.
20. Adams SD, Killien M, Larson E. In-line filtration and infusion phlebitis. *Heart Lung* 1986;15:134–140.
21. Maki DG, Rhame FS, Mackel DC, et al. Nationwide epidemic of septicemia caused by contaminated intravenous products. *Am J Med* 1976;60:471–485.
22. Armstrong CS, Mayhall CG, Miller KB, et al. Clinical predictors of infection of central venous catheters used for total parenteral nutrition. *Infect Control Hosp Epidemiol* 1990;2:71–78.
23. Pittet D, Churad C, Rae AC, et al. Clinical diagnosis of central venous catheter line infections: a difficult job [Abstract]. In: *Program and abstracts of the thirty-first interscience conference on antimicrobial agents and chemotherapy, October 1991, Chicago, Illinois*. Washington, DC: American Society for Microbiology; 1991:174.
24. Torres-Rohas JR, Stratton CW, Sanders CV, et al. Candidal suppurative peripheral thrombophlebitis. *Ann Intern Med* 1982;96:431–435.
25. Johnson RA, Zajac RA, Evans ME. Suppurative thrombophlebitis: correlation between pathogen and underlying disease. *Infect Control* 1986;7:582–585.
26. Strinden WD, Helgerson RB, Maki DG. *Candida* septic thrombosis of the great veins associated with central catheters: clinical features and management. *Ann Surg* 1985;202:653–658.
27. Verghese A, Widrich WC, Arbeit RD. Central venous septic thrombophlebitis: the role of medical therapy. *Medicine* 1985;64:394–400.
28. Raad II, Sabbagh Mouin F. Optimal duration of therapy for catheter-related *Staphylococcus aureus* bacteremia: a study of 55 cases and review. *Clin Infect Dis* 1992;14:75–82.
29. Herrmann M, Vaudaux PE, Pittet D, et al. Fibronectin, fibrinogen, and laminin act as mediators of adherence of clinical staphylococcal isolates to foreign material. *J Infect Dis* 1988;158:693–701.
30. Herrmann M, Suchard SJ, Boxer LA, et al. Thrombospondin binds to *Staphylococcus aureus* and promotes staphylococcal adherence to surfaces. *Infect Immun* 1991;59:279–288.
31. Maki DG, Ringer M. Prospective study of arterial catheter-related infection: incidence, sources of infection and risk factors [Abstract]. In: *Programs and abstracts of the twenty-ninth interscience conference on antimicrobial agents and chemotherapy, September 1989, Houston, Texas*. Washington, DC: American Society for Microbiology, 1989:284.
32. Maki DG, Alvarado CJ, Ringer M. A prospective, randomized trial of povidone–iodine, alcohol and chlorhexidine for prevention of infection with central venous and arterial catheters. *Lancet* 1991;338: 339–343.
33. Segura M, Llado L, Guirao X, et al. A prospective study of a new protocol for "in situ"' diagnosis of central venous catheter related bacteraemia. *Clin Nutr* 1993;12:103–107.
34. Maki DG, Stolz SS, Wheeler S, et al. A prospective, randomized trial of gauze and two polyurethane dressings for site care of pulmonary artery catheters: Implications for catheter management. *Crit Care Med* 1994;32:1729–1737.
35. Maki DG, Klein BS, McCormick RD, et al. Nosocomial *Pseudomonas pickettii* bacteremias traced to narcotic tampering: a case for selective drug screening of healthcare personnel. *JAMA* 1991;265: 981–986.
36. Bennett SN, McNeil MM, Bland LA, et al. Postoperative infections traced to contamination of an intravenous anesthetic, propofol. *N Engl J Med* 1995;333:147–154.
37. Schmitt S, Hall G, Knapp C, et al. Poor correlation between clinical

judgement and microbiologic confirmation of catheter-related bacteremia (CRB) due to coagulase-negative staphylococci (CNS) [Abstract]. In: *Programs and abstracts of the ninety-fourth general meeting of the American Society for Microbiology, May 1994, Las Vegas, Nevada*. Washington, DC: American Society for Microbiology, 1994:615.

38. Mermel LA, Velez LA, Zilz MA, et al. Epidemiologic and microbiologic features of nosocomial bloodstream infection (NSBI) implicating a vascular catheter source: a case–control study of 85 vascular catheter-related and 101 secondary NBSIs [Abstract]. In: *Program and abstracts of the thirty-first interscience conference on antimicrobial agents and chemotherapy, October 1991, Chicago, Illinois*. Washington, DC: American Society for Microbiology, 1991:174.
39. Band JD, Maki DG. Infections caused by indwelling arterial catheters for hemodynamic monitoring. *Am J Med* 1979;67:735–741.
40. Maki DG. Sepsis arising from extrinsic contamination of the infusion and measure for control. In: Phillips I, ed. *Microbiologic hazards of infusion therapy*. Lancaster, England: MTP Press, 1977:99–141.
41. Henderson DK, Edwards JE, Montgomerie JZ. Hematogenous *Candida* endophthalmitis in patients receiving parenteral hyperalimentation fluids. *J Infect Dis* 1981;143:655–661.
42. Maki DG, McCormick RD, Uman SJ, et al. Septic endarteritis due to intra-arterial catheters for cancer chemotherapy: I. Evaluation of an outbreak. II. Risk factors, clinical features and management. III. Guidelines for prevention. *Cancer* 1979;44:1228–1240.
43. Cohen A, Reyes R, Kirk B, et al. Osler's nodes, pseudoaneurysm formation, and sepsis complicating percutaneous radial artery cannulation. *Crit Care Med* 1984;12:1078–1079.
44. Arnow PM, Costas CO. Delayed rupture of the radial artery caused by catheter-related sepsis. *Rev Infect Dis* 1988;10:1035–1037.
45. Falk P, Scuderi PE, Sherertz RJ, et al. Infected radial artery pseudoaneurysms occurring after percutaneous cannulation. *Chest* 1992;101: 490–495.
46. Ehrie M, Morgan AP, Moore FD, et al. Endocarditis with the indwelling balloon-tipped pulmonary artery catheter in burn patients. *J Trauma* 1978;18:664–666.
47. Rowley KM, Clubb KS, Smith GJW, et al. Right-sided infective endocarditis as a consequence of flow-directed pulmonary-artery catheterization: a clinicopathologic study of 55 autopsied patients. *N Engl J Med* 1984;311:1152–1156.
48. Mermel LA, Maki DG. Infectious complications of Swan-Ganz pulmonary artery catheters. *Am J Respir Crit Care Med* 1994;149: 1020–1036.
49. Aronson MD, Bor DH. Blood cultures. *Ann Intern Med* 1987;106: 246–253.
50. Weinstein MP. Current blood culture methods and systems: clinical concepts, technology, and interpretation of results. *Clin Infect Dis* 1996;23:40–46.
51. Mermel LA, Maki DG. Detection of bacteremia in adults: consequences of culturing an inadequate volume of blood. *Ann Intern Med* 1993;119:270–272.
52. Crepin O, Roussel-Delvallez M, et al. Effectiveness of resins in removing antibiotics from blood cultures. *J Clin Microbiol* 1993;31:734–735.
53. Reimer LG, Barth Reller L, et al. Controlled comparison of a new Becton Dickinson agar slant blood culture system with Roche Septichek for the detection of bacteremia and fungemia. *J Clin Microbiol* 1989;27:2637–2639.
54. Jungkind D, Thakur M, Dyke J. Evidence for a second mechanism of action of resins in BACTEC NR16A aerobic blood culture medium [Abstract]. In: *Programs and abstracts of the eighty-ninth general meeting of the American Society for Microbiology, May 1989, New Orleans, Louisiana*. Washington, DC: American Society for Microbiology, 1989:431.
55. Tegtmeier BR, Vice JL. Evaluation of the BACTEC 16B medium in a cancer center. *Am J Clin Pathol* 1984;81:783–786.
56. Tarrand JJ, Guillot C, Wenglar M, et al. Clinical comparison of the resin-containing BACTEC 26 Plus and the Isolator 10 blood culturing systems. *J Clin Microbiol* 1991;29:2245–2249.
57. Wilson M, Davis TE, Mirrett S, et al. Controlled comparison of the BACTEC high-blood-volume fungal medium, BACTEC Plus 26 aerobic blood culture system for detection of fungemia and bacteremia. *J Clin Microbiol* 1993;31:865–871.
58. Weinstein MP, Reller LB, Murphy HR et al. The clinical significance of positive blood cultures: a comprehensive analysis of 500 episodes of bacteremia and fungemia in adults: I. laboratory and epidemiological observations. *Rev Infect Dis* 1983;5:35–53.
59. Koontz FP, Flint KK, Reynolds JK, et al. Multicenter comparison of the high volume (10 ml) NR Bactec Plus system and the standard (5 ml) NR bactec system. *Diagn Microbiol Infect Dis* 1991;14:111–118.
60. Wormser GP, Onorato IM, Preminger TJ, et al. Sensitivity and specificity of blood cultures obtained through intravascular catheters. *Crit Care Med* 1990;18:152–156.
61. Isaacman DJ, Karasic RB. Utility of collecting blood cultures through newly inserted intravenous catheters. *Pediatr Infect Dis J* 1990;9: 815–818.
62. Pourcyrous M, Korones SB, Bada HS, et al. Indwelling umbilical arterial catheter: a preferred sampling site for blood culture. *Pediatrics* 1988;81:821–825.
63. Bryant JK, Strand CL. Reliability of blood cultures collected from intravascular catheter vs. venipuncture. *Am J Clin Pathol* 1987;88: 113–116.
64. Maki DG, Hassemer CH. Endemic rate of fluid contamination and related septicemia in arterial pressure monitoring. *Am J Med* 1981;70: 733–738.
65. Weightman NC, Simpson EM, Speller DCE, et al. Bacteraemia related to indwelling central venous catheters: prevention, diagnosis and treatment. *Eur J Clin Microbiol Infect Dis* 1988;7:125–129.
66. Flynn PM, Shenep JL, Stokes DC, et al. In situ management of confirmed central venous catheter-related bacteremia. *Pediatr Infect Dis J* 1987;6:729–734.
67. Raucher HS, Hyatt AC, Barzilai A, et al. Quantitative blood cultures in the evaluation of septicemia in children with Broviac catheters. *J Pediatr* 1984;104:29–33.
68. Benezra D, Kiehn T, Gold JWM, et al. Prospective study of infections in indwelling central venous catheters using quantitative blood cultures. *Am J Med* 1988;85:495–498.
69. Ascher DP, Shoupe BA, Robb M, et al. Comparison of standard and quantitative blood cultures in the evaluation of children with suspected central venous line sepsis. *Diagn Microbiol Infect Dis* 1992;15: 499–503.
70. Capedevila JA, Planes AM, Palomar M, et al. Value of differential quantitative blood cultures in the diagnosis of catheter-related sepsis. *Eur J Clin Microbiol Infect Dis* 1992;11:403–407.
71. Douard MC, Clementi E, Arlet G, et al. Negative catheter-tip culture and diagnosis of catheter-related bacteremia. *Nutrition* 1994;10: 397–404.
72. Siegman-Igra Y, Anglim AM, Shapiro DE, et al. Diagnosis of vascular catheter-related bloodstream infection: a meta-analysis. *J Clin Microbiol* 1997;35:928–936.
73. Rushforth JA, Hoy CM, Kite P, Puntis JW. Rapid diagnosis of central venous catheter sepsis. *Lancet* 1993;342:402–403.
74. Moonens F, EL Alami S, Van Gossum A. Usefulness of Gram staining of blood collected from total parenteral nutrition catheter for rapid diagnosis of catheter-related sepsis. *J Clin Microbiol* 1994;32: 1578–1579.
75. Torlakovic E, Hibbs JR, Miller JS, et al. Intracellular bacteria in blood smears in patients with central venous catheters. *Arch Intern Med* 1995;155:1547–1550.
76. Anderson RL, Highsmith AK, Holland BW. Comparison of the standard pour plate procedure and the ATP and *Limulus* amoebocyte lysate procedures for the detection of microbial contamination in intravenous fluids. *J Clin Microbiol* 1986;23:465–468.
77. Centers for Disease Control and Prevention. Septicemias associated with contaminated intravenous fluids. *MMWR Morb Mortal Wkly Rep* 1973;22:99, 114, 124.
78. Braude AI, Carey FJ, Siemienski J. Studies of bacterial transfusion reactions from refrigerated blood: the properties of cold-growing bacteria. *J Clin Invest* 1955;34:311–325.
79. Morduchowicz G, Silvio D, Pitlik D, et al. Transfusion reactions due to bacterial contamination of blood and blood products. *Rev Infect Dis* 1991;3:307–314.
80. Heal JM, Jones ME, Chaudhry A, et al. Fatal *Salmonella* septicemia after platelet transfusion. *Transfusion* 1987;27:2–5.
81. Centers for Disease Control and Prevention. Red blood cell transfusions contaminated with *Yersinia enterocolitica*—United States, 1991–1996, and initiation of a national study to detect bacteria-associated transfusion reactions. MMWR 1997;46:553–555.
82. Nahass RG, Weinstein MP. Qualitative intravascular catheter tip cul-

tures do not predict catheter-related bacteremia. *Diagn Microbiol Infect Dis* 1990;13:223–226.
83. Kristinsson KG, Burnett IA, Spencer RC. Evaluation of three methods for culturing long intravascular catheters. *J Hosp Infect* 1989;14: 183–191.
84. Gutierrez J, Leon C, Matamoros R, et al. Catheter-related bacteremia and fungemia. *Diagn Microbiol Infect Dis* 1992;15:575–578.
85. Dooley DP, Garcia A, Kelly JW, et al. Validation of catheter semiquantitative culture technique for nonstaphylococcal organisms. *J Clin Microbiol* 1996;34:409–412.
86. Brun-Buisson C, Abrouk F, Legrand P, et al. Diagnosis of central venous catheter-related sepsis: critical level of quantitative tip cultures. *Arch Intern Med* 1987;147:873–877.
87. Sheretz RJ, Raad II, Belani A, et al. Three-year experience with sonicated vascular catheter cultures in a clinical microbiology laboratory. *J Clin Microbiol* 1990;28:76–82 .
88. Sherertz R, Heard S, Raad I, Gentry L. Culturing catheter (C) tips (T) is an insensitive method for diagnosing triple lumen vascular C infection [Abstract]. In: *Programs and abstracts of the thirty-second interscience conference on antimicrobial agents and chemotherapy, October 1992, Anaheim, California*. Washington, DC: American Society for Microbiology, 1992:247.
89. Collignon P. Quantitative blood cultures for catheter-associated infections. *J Clin Microbiol* 1989;27:1487–1488.
90. Hnatiuk OW, Pike J, Stoltzfus D, et al. Value of bedside plating of semiquantitative cultures for diagnosis of central venous catheter-related infections in ICU patients. *Chest* 1993;103:896–899.
91. Cooper GL, Hopkins CC. Rapid diagnosis of intravascular catheter-associated infection by direct gram staining of catheter segments. *N Engl J Med* 1985;18:1142–1150.
92. Zufferey J, Rime B, Francioli P, et al. Simple method for rapid diagnosis of catheter-associated infection by direct acridine orange staining of catheter tips. *J Clin Microbiol* 1988;26:175–177.
93. Raad II, Baba M, Bodey GP. Diagnosis of catheter-related infections: the role of surveillance and targeted quantitative skin cultures. *Clin Infect Dis* 1995;20:593–597.
94. McGeer A, Righter J. Improving our ability to diagnose infections associated with central venous catheters: value of Gram's staining and culture of entry site swabs. *Can Med Assoc J* 1987;137:1009–1021.
95. Fan ST, Teoh-Chan CH, Lau KF, et al. Predictive value of surveillance skin and hub cultures in central venous catheter sepsis. *J Hosp Infect* 1988;12:191–198.
96. Cercenado E, Ena J, Rodriguez-Creixems M, et al. A conservative procedure for the diagnosis of catheter-related infections. *Arch Intern Med* 1990;150:1417–1420.
97. Mayhall CG, Pierpaoli PG, Hall GO, et al. Evaluation of a device for monitoring sterility of infectable fluids. *Am J Hosp Pharm* 1981;38: 1148–1150.
98. Longfield JN, Charache P, Diamond EL, et al. Comparison of broth and filtration methods for culturing of intravenous fluids. *Infect Control* 1982;3:397–400.
99. Mermel LA. Defining intravascular catheter-related infections: a plea for uniformity. *Nutrition* 1996;12:1–3.
100. Bone RC, Balk RA, Cerra FB, et al. American College of Chest Physician/Society of Critical Care Medicine Consensus Conference: definitions for sepsis and organ failure and guidelines for the use of innovative therapies in sepsis. *Crit Care Med* 1992;20:864–874.
101. Sattler FR, Foderato JB, Aber RC. *Staphylococcus epidermidis* bacteremia associated with vascular catheters: an important cause of febrile morbidity in hospitalized patients. *Infect Control* 1984;5: 279–283.
102. Ponce DeLeon S, Wenzel RP. Hospital-acquired bloodstream infections with *Staphylococcus epidermidis*. *Am J Med* 1984;77:639–644.
103. Kirchhoff LV, Sheagren JN. Epidemiology and clinical significance of blood cultures positive for coagulase-negative staphylococcus. *Infect Control* 1985;6:479–486.
104. Garner JS, Jarvis WR, Emori TG, et al. CDC definitions for nosocomial infections, 1988. *Am J Infect Control* 1988;16:128–140.
105. Sheretz RJ. Surveillance for infections associated with vascular catheters. *Infect Control Hosp. Epidemiol* 1996;17:746–752.
106. Williams DN, Gibson J, Vos J, et al. Infusion thrombophlebitis and infiltration associated with intravenous cannulae: a controlled study comparing three different cannula types. *NITA* 1982;5:379–382.
107. Craven DE, Lichtenberg A, Kunches LM, et al. A randomized study comparing a transparent polyurethane dressing to a dry gauze dressing for peripheral intravenous catheter sites. *Infect Control* 1985;6: 361–366.
108. Tomford JW, Hershey CO, McLaren CE, et al. Intravenous therapy team and peripheral venous catheter-associated complications: a prospective controlled study. *Arch Intern Med* 1984;144:1191–1194.
109. Maki DG, Ringer M. Evaluation of dressing regimens for prevention of infection with peripheral intravenous catheters. *JAMA* 1987;258: 2396–2403.
110. Mermel LA, Maki DG. Infectious complications of Swan-Ganz pulmonary artery catheters and peripheral artery catheters. In: Seifert H, Jansen B, Farr BM, eds. *Catheter related infections*. New York: Marcel Dekker, 1997 (in press).
111. Nyström B, Olesen Larsen S, Dankert J, et al. Bacteraemia in surgical patients with intravenous devices: a European multicentre incidence study. *J Hosp Infect* 1983;4:338–349.
112. Trilla A, Gatell JM, Mensa J, et al. Risk factors for nosocomial bacteremia in a large Spanish teaching hospital: a case–control study. *Infect Control Hosp Epidemiol* 1991;2:150–156.
113. Wey SB, Mori M, Pfaller MA, et al. Risk factors for hospital-acquired candidemia: a matched case–control study. *Arch Intern Med* 1989; 149:2349–2353.
114. Maki DG, McCormack KN. Defatting catheter insertion sites in total parenteral nutrition is of no value as an infection control measure. *Am J Med* 1987;83:833–840.
115. Maki DG, Cobb L, Garman JK, et al. An attachable silver-impregnated cuff for prevention of infection with central venous catheters: a prospective randomized multi-center trial. *Am J Med* 1988;85:307–314.
116. Flowers RH III, Schwenzer KJ, Kopel RJ, et al. Efficacy of an attachable subcutaneous cuff for the prevention of intravascular catheter-related infection. *JAMA* 1989;261:878–883.
117. Richet H, Hubert B, Nitemberg G, et al. Prospective multicenter study of vascular-catheter-related complications and risk factors for positive central-catheter cultures in intensive care unit patients. *J Clin Microbiol* 1990;28:2520–2525.
118. Cobb DK, High KP, Sawyer RG, et al. A controlled trial of scheduled replacement of central venous and pulmonary-artery catheters. *N Engl J Med* 1992;327:1062–1068.
119. Hulliger S, Pittet D. Incidence and morbidity of central venous catheter-related infections in intensive care units [Abstract]. In: *Programs and abstracts of the thirty-second Infectious Diseases Society of America annual meeting, October 1994, Orlando, Florida*. Alexandria, VA: Infectious Diseases Society of America, 1994:28A.
120. Almirall J, Gonzalez J, Rello J, et al. Infection of hemodialysis catheters: incidence and mechanisms. *Am J Nephrol* 1989;9:454–459.
121. Rello J, Gatell JM, Almirall J, et al. Evaluation of culture techniques for identification of catheter-related infection in hemodialysis patients. *Eur J Clin Microbiol Infect Dis* 1989;8:620–622.
122. Levin A, Mason AJ, Jindal KK, et al. Prevention of hemodialysis subclavian vein catheter infections by topical povidone–iodine. *Kidney Int* 1991;40:934–938.
123. Schwab SJ, Buller GL, McCann RL. Prospective evaluation of a Dacron cuffed hemodialysis catheter for prolonged use. *Am J Kidney Dis* 1988;11:166–169.
124. Dryden MS, Samson A, Ludlam HA, et al. Infective complications associated with the use of the Quinton "Permcath" for long-term central vascular access in haemodialysis. *J Hosp Infect* 1991;19:257–262.
125. Raad I, Davis S, Becker M, et al. Low infection rate and long durability of nontunneled silastic catheters. *Arch Intern Med* 1993;153: 1791–1796.
126. Pauley SY, Vallande NC, Riley EN, et al. Catheter-related colonization associated with percutaneous inserted central catheters. *J Intraven Nurs* 1993;16:50–54.
127. Clarke DE, Raffin TA. Infectious complications of indwelling long-term central venous catheters. *Chest* 1990;97:966–972.
128. Mayhall G. Diagnosis and management of infections of implantable devices used for prolonged venous access. *Curr Clin Top Infect Dis* 1992;12:83–110.
129. Carde P, Cosset-Delaigue MF, LaPlanche A, et al. Classical external indwelling central venous catheter vs. totally implanted venous access systems for chemotherapy administration: a randomized trial in 100 patients with solid tumors. *Eur J Cancer Clin Oncol* 1989;25: 939–944.
130. Ingram J, Weitzman S, Greenberg ML, et al. Complications of

indwelling venous access lines in the pediatric hematology patient: a prospective comparison of external venous catheters and subcutaneous ports. *American Journal of Pediatric Hematology and Oncology* 1991;13:130–136.
131. Pegues D, Axelrod P, McClarren C, et al. Comparison of infections in Hickman and implanted port catheters in adult solid tumor patients. *J Surg Oncol* 1992;49:156–162.
132. Mueller BU, Skelton J, Callender DPE, et al. A prospective randomized trial comparing the infectious and noninfectious complications of an externalized catheter vs. a subcutaneously implanted device in cancer patients. *J Clin Oncol* 1992;10:1943–1948.
133. Groeger JS, Lucas AB, Thaler HT, et al. Infectious morbidity associated with long-term use of venous access devices in patients with cancer. *Ann Intern Med* 1993;119:1168–1174.
134. Pullyblank AM, Carey PD, Pearce SZ, et al. Comparison between peripherally implanted ports and externally sited catheters for long-term venous access. *Ann R Coll Surg Engl* 1994;76:33–38.
135. Banerjee SN, Emori G, Culver DH, et al. National Nosocomial Infections Surveillance System: secular trends in nosocomial primary bloodstream infections in the United States, 1980–1989. *Am J Med* 1991;91(Suppl 3B):86S–89S.
136. Elliott TSJ, Tebbs SE, Moss HM, et al. Nosocomial infections and surgical infections and related epidemiologic studies [Abstract]. In: *Programs and abstracts of the thirty-fifth interscience conference on antimicrobial agents and chemotherapy, September 1995, San Francisco, California*. Washington, DC: American Society for Microbiology, 1995:257.
137. Cooper GL, Schiller AL, Hopkins CC. Possible role of capillary action in pathogenesis of experimental catheter-associated dermal tunnel infections. *J Clin Microbiol* 1988;26:8–12.
138. Maki DG. Marked differences in insertion sites for central venous, arterial and peripheral IV catheters: the major reason for differing risks of catheter-related infection [Abstract]? In: *Program and abstracts of the thirtieth interscience conference on antimicrobial agents and chemotherapy, October 1990, Atlanta, Georgia*. Washington, DC: American Society for Microbiology, 1990:205.
139. Bertone SA, Fisher MC, Mortensen JE. Quantitative skin cultures at potential catheter sites in neonates. *Infect Control Hosp Epidemiol* 1994;15:315–318.
140. Yu VL, Goetz A, Wagener M, et al. *Staphylococcus aureus* nasal carriage and infection in patients on hemodialysis: efficacy of antibiotic prophylaxis. *N Engl J Med* 1986;315:91–96.
141. Pujol M, Pena C, Pallares R, et al. Nosocomial *Staphylococcus aureus* bacteremia among nasal carriers of methicillin-resistant and methicillin-susceptible strains. *Am J Med* 1996;100:509–516.
142. Snydman DR, Sullivan BS, Gill M, et al. Nosocomial sepsis associated with interleukin-2. *Ann Intern Med* 1990;112:102–107.
143. Maki DG, Jarrett F, Sarafin HW. A semiquantitative culture method for identification of catheter-related infection in the burn patient. *J Surg Res* 1977;22:513–520.
144. Franceschi D, Gerding RL, Phillips G, et al. Risk factors associated with intravascular catheter infections in burned patients: a prospective, randomized study. *J Trauma* 1989;29:811–816.
145. Dixon RE, Kaslow RA, Mackel DC, et al. Aqueous quaternary ammonium antiseptics and disinfectants: use and misuse. *JAMA* 1976;236: 2415–2417.
146. Frank MJ, Schaffner W. Contaminated aqueous benzalkonium chloride: an unnecessary hospital infection hazard. *JAMA* 1976;236:2418–2419.
147. Kahan A, Philippon A, Paul G, et al. Nosocomial infections by chlorhexidine solution contaminated with *Pseudomonas pickettii* (biovar VA-I). *J Infect* 1983;7:256–263.
148. Pein F, Lebbar A, Lecointe D, et al. Nosocomial outbreak of catheter related bacteremia due to *Pseudomonas pickettii* originated from a contaminated antiseptic solution [Abstract]. In: *Programs and abstracts of the thirty-fourth interscience conference on antimicrobial agents and chemotherapy, October 1994, Orlando, Florida*. Washington, DC: American Society for Microbiology, 1994:241.
149. Rello J, Coll P, Prats G. Laboratory diagnosis of catheter-related bacteremia. *Scand J Infect Dis* 1991;23:583–588.
150. Raad I, Costerton W, Sabharwal U, et al. Ultrastructural analysis of indwelling vascular catheters: a quantitative relationship between luminal colonization and duration of placement. *J Infect Dis* 1993; 168:400–407.
151. Sheehan G, Leicht K, O'Brien M, et al. Chlorhexidine vs. povidone–iodine as cutaneous antisepsis for prevention of vascular-catheter infection [Abstract]. In: *Programs and abstracts of the thirty-third interscience conference on antimicrobial agents and chemotherapy, October 1993, New Orleans, Louisiana*. Washington, DC: American Society for Microbiology, 1993:414.
152. Mimoz O, Pieroni L, Lawrence C, et al. Prospective trial of povidone–iodine (PI) and chlorhexidine (CH) for prevention of catheter-related sepsis (CRS) [Abstract]. In: *Programs and abstracts of the thirty-fourth interscience conference on antimicrobial agents and chemotherapy, October 1994, Orlando, Florida*. Alexandria, VA: Infectious Disease Society of America, 1994:68.
153. Garland JS, Buck RK, Maloney P, et al. Comparison of 10% povidone–iodine and 0.5% chlorhexidine gluconate for the prevention of peripheral intravenous catheter colonization in neonates: a prospective trial. *Pediatr Infect Dis J* 1995;14:510–516.
154. Maki DG, Band JD. A comparative study of polyantibiotic and iodophor ointments in prevention of catheter-related infection. *Am J Med* 1981;70:739–744.
155. Fuchs PC, Gustafson ME, King JT, et al. Assessment of catheter-associated infection risk with the Hickman right atrial catheter. *Infect Control* 1984;5:226–530.
156. Press OW, Ramsey PG, Larson EB, et al. Hickman catheter infections in patients with malignancies. *Medicine* 1984;63:189–200.
157. Wurzel CL, Halom C, Feldman JG, et al. Infection rates of Broviac-Hickman catheters and implantable venous devices. *American Journal of Diseases of Children* 1980;142:536–540.
158. Bonawitz SC, Hammell EJ, Kirkpatrick JR. Prevention of central venous catheter sepsis: a prospective randomized trial. *Am Surg* 1991; 57:618–623.
159. Rafkin HS, Hoyt JW, Crippen DW. Prevention of central venous catheter related infection with a silver-impregnated cuff [Abstract]. *Chest* 1990;98:117S.
160. Babycos CR, Barrocas A, Webb WR. A prospective randomized trial comparing the silver-impregnated collagen cuff with the bedside tunneled subclavian catheter. *JPEN J Parenter Enteral Nutr* 1993;17:61–63.
161. Groeger JS, Lucas AB, Coit D, et al. A prospective, randomized evaluation of the effect of silver impregnated subcutaneous cuffs for preventing tunneled chronic venous access catheter infections in cancer patients. *Ann Surg* 1993;218:206–210.
162. Dahlberg PJ, Agger WA, Singer JR, et al. Subclavian hemodialysis catheter infections: a prospective, randomized trial of an attachable silver-impregnated cuff for prevention of catheter-related infections. *Infect Control Hosp Epidemiol* 1995;16:506–511.
163. Kamal GD, Pfaller MA, Rempe LE, et al. Reduced intravascular catheter infection by antibiotic bonding. *JAMA* 1991;265:2364–2368.
164. Raad I, Darouiche R. Central venous catheters (CVC) coated with minocycline and rifampin (M/R) for the prevention of catheter-related bacteremia (CRB) [Abstract]. In: *Programs and abstracts of the thirty-fifth interscience conference on antimicrobial agents and chemotherapy, September 1995, San Francisco, California*. Washington, DC: American Society for Microbiology, 1995:258.
165. Goldschmidt H, Hahn U, Salwender H, et al. Prevention of catheter related infections by silver coated central venous catheters in oncological patients. Zbl Bakt 1995;283:215–223.
166. Mermel LA, Stolz SM, Maki DG. Surface antimicrobial activity of heparin-bonded and antiseptic-impregnated vascular catheters. *J Infect Dis* 1993;167:920–924.
167. Applegren P, Ransjo U, Bindsley L, et al. Does surface heparinisation reduce bacterial colonisation of central venous catheters? *Lancet* 1995;345:130.
168. Maki DG, Wheeler SJ, Stolz SM, et al. Clinical trial of a novel antiseptic central venous catheter. In: *Program and abstracts of the thirty-first interscience conference on antimicrobial agents and chemotherapy, September 1994, Chicago, Illinois*. Washington, DC: American Society for Microbiology, 1991:176.
169. Bach A, Schmidt H, Bottiger B, et al. Retention of antibacterial activity and bacterial colonization of antiseptic-bonded central venous catheters. *J Antimicrob Chemother* 1996;37:315–322.
170. Ciresi DL, Albrecht RM, Volkers PA, et al. Failure of antiseptic bonding to prevent central venous catheter-related infection and sepsis. *Am Surg* 1996;62:641–646.
171. Pemberton Beaty L, Ross V, Cuddy P, et al. No difference in catheter sepsis between standard and antiseptic central venous catheters. *Arch Surg* 1996;131:986–989.

172. deCicco M, Chiaradia V, Verones A, et al. Source and route of microbial colonisation of parenteral nutrition catheters. *Lancet* 1989;2: 1258–1261.
173. Salzman MB, Isenberg HD, Shapiro JF, et al. A prospective study of the catheter hub as the portal of entry for microorganisms causing catheter-related sepsis in neonates. *J Infect Dis* 1993;167:487–490.
174. Moro LM, Vigano EF, Lepri AC, et al. Risk factors for central venous catheter-related infections in surgical and intensive care units. *Infect Control Hosp Epidemiol* 1994;15:253–264.
175. Mermel LA, McCormick RD, Springman SR, et al. The pathogenesis and epidemiology of catheter-related infection with pulmonary artery Swan-Ganz catheters: a prospective study utilizing molecular subtyping. *Am J Med* 1991;91(Suppl 3B):197S–205S.
176. Anaissie E, Samonis G, Kontoyiannis D, et al. Role of catheter colonization and infrequent hematogenous seeding in catheter-related infections. *Eur J Clin Microbiol Infect Dis* 1995;14:134–137.
177. Kurkchubasche AG, Smith SD, Rowe MI: Catheter sepsis in short-bowel syndrome. *Arch Surg* 1992;127:21–25.
178. Landers S, Moise AA, Fraley JK, et al. Factors associated with umbilical catheter-related sepsis in neonates. *American Journal of Diseases of Children* 1991;145:675–680 .
179. Maki DG, Will L. Risk factors for central venous catheter-related infection within the ICU: a prospective study of 345 catheters [Abstract]. In: *Programs and abstracts of the thirtieth interscience conference on antimicrobial agents and chemotherapy, October 1990, Atlanta, Georgia*. Washington, DC: American Society for Microbiology, 1990:205.
180. Farkas JC, Timsit JF, Boyer JM, et al. Does catheter-related thrombosis (CRT) increase the risk of catheter-related sepsis (CRS) in ICU patients [Abstract]? In: *Programs and abstracts of the third international conference on the prevention of infection, April 1994, Nice, France*. 1994:52.
181. Ehrenkranz NJ, Eckert DG, Phillips PM. Sporadic bacteremia complicating central venous catheter use in a community hospital: a model to predict frequency and aid in decision-making for initiation of investigation. *Am J Infect Control* 1989;17:69–76.
182. Conly JM, Grieves K, Peters BA. A prospective, randomized study comparing transparent and dry gauze dressings for central venous catheters. *J Infect Dis* 1989;159:310–319.
183. Pittet D. Intravenous catheter-related infections: current understanding [Abstract]. In: *Programs and abstracts of the thirty-second interscience conference on antimicrobial agents and chemotherapy, October 1992, Anaheim, California*. Washington, DC: American Society for Microbiology, 1992:411.
184. Rello J, Coll P, Net A, et al. Infection of pulmonary artery catheters: epidemiologic characteristics and multivariate analysis of risk factors. *Chest* 1993;103:132–136.
185. Damen J, Van Der Tweel I. Positive tip cultures and related risk factors associated with intravascular catheterization in pediatric cardiac patients. *Crit Care Med* 1988;3:221–228.
186. Ena J, Cercenado E, Martinez D, et al. Cross-sectional epidemiology of phlebitis and catheter-related infections. *Infect Control Hosp Epidemiol* 1992;13:15–20.
187. Newman KA, Reed WP, Schimpff SC, et al. Hickman catheters in association with intensive cancer chemotherapy. *Support Care Cancer* 1993;1:92–97.
188. Duthoit D, Devleeshouwer C, Paesmans M, et al. Infection of totally implantable chamber catheters (TICC) in cancer patients: multivariate analysis of risk factors [Abstract]. In: *Programs and abstracts of the thirty-third interscience conference on antimicrobial agents and chemotherapy, October 1993, New Orleans, Louisiana*. Washington, DC: American Society for Microbiology, 1993:416.
189. Passerini L, Lam K, Costerton JW, et al. Biofilms on indwelling vascular catheters. *Crit Care Med* 1992;20:665–673.
190. Hoyle BD, Jass J, Costerton JW. The biofilm glycocalyx as a resistance factor. *J Antimicrob Chemother* 1990;26:1–6.
191. Sheth NK, Rose HD, Franson TR, et al. In vitro quantitative adherence of bacteria to intravascular catheters. *J Surg Res* 1983;34:213–218.
192. Ashkenazi S, Weiss E, Drucker MM. Bacterial adherence to intravenous catheters and needles and its influence by cannula type and bacterial surface hydrophobicity. *J Lab Clin Med* 1986;107:136–140.
193. Barrett SP. Bacterial adhesion to intravenous cannulae: influence of implantation in the rabbit and of enzyme treatments. *Epidemiol Infect* 1988;100:91–100.
194. Vaudaux P, Pittet D, Haeberli A, et al. Host factors selectively increase staphylococcal adherence on inserted catheters: a role for fibronectin and fibrinogen or fibrin. *J Infect Dis* 1989;160:865–875.
195. Pascual A, Fleer A, Westerdaal NAC, et al. Modulation of adherence of coagulase-negative staphylococci to Teflon catheters in vitro. *Eur J Clin Microbiol* 1986;5:518–522.
196. Vaudaux P, Pittet D, Haeberli A, et al. Fibronectin is more active than fibrin or fibrinogen in promoting *Staphylococcus aureus* adherence to inserted intravascular catheters. *J Infect Dis* 1993;167:633–641.
197. Hogt AH, Dankert J, De Vries JA, et al. Adhesion of coagulase-negative staphylococci to biomaterials. *J Gen Microbiol* 1983;129: 2959–2968.
198. Tojo M, Yamashita N, Goldmann DA,et al. Isolation and characterization of transposon mutants of *Staphylococcus epidermidis*. *J Infect Dis* 1988;157:713–722.
199. Christensen GD, Barker LP, Mawhinney TP. Identification of an antigenic marker of slime production for *Staphylococcus epidermidis*. *Infect Immun* 1990;58:2906–2911.
200. Timmerman CP, Fleer A, Besnier JM, et al. Characterization of proteinaceous adhesin of *Staphylococcus epidermidis* which mediates attachment to polystyrene. *Infect Immun* 1991;59:4187–4192.
201. Rupp ME, Archer GL. Hemagglutination and adherence to plastic by *Staphylococcus epidermidis*. *Infect Immun* 1992;60:4322–4327.
202. Mack D, Siemssen N, Laufs R. Parallel induction by glucose of adherence and a polysaccharide antigen specific for plastic-adherent *Staphylococcus epidermidis*: evidence for functional relation to intercellular adhesin. *Infect Immun* 1992;60:2048–2057.
203. Herrmann M, Lai QJ, Albrecht RM, et al. Adhesion of *Staphylococcus aureus* to surface-bound platelets: role of fibrinogen/fibrin and platelet integrins. *J Infect Dis* 1993;167:312–322.
204. Stillman RM, Soliman F, Garcia L, et al. Etiology of catheter-associated sepsis: correlation with thrombogenicity. *Arch Surg* 1977;112: 1497–1499.
205. Raad I, Luna M, Khalil SAM, et al. The relationship between the thrombotic and infectious complications of central venous catheters. *JAMA* 1994;271:1014–1016.
206. Muller E, Takeda S, Shiro H, et al. Occurrence of capsular polysaccharide/adhesin among clinical isolates of coagulase-negative staphylococci. *J Infect Dis* 1993;168:1211–1218.
207. Goldmann DA, Pier GB. Pathogenesis of infections related to intravascular catheterization. *Clin Microbiol Rev* 1993;6:176–192.
208. Schadow KH, Simpson WA, Christensen GD. Characteristics of adherence to plastic tissue culture plates of coagulase-negative staphylococci exposed to subinhibitory concentrations of antimicrobial agents. *J Infect Dis* 1988;157:71–77.
209. Zimmerli W, Lew PD, Waldvogel FA. Pathogenesis of foreign body infection: evidence for a local granulocyte defect. *J Clin Invest* 1984; 73:1191–1200.
210. Gristina AG. Biomaterial-centered infection: microbial adhesion vs. tissue integration. *Science* 1987;237:1588–1595.
211. Gristina AG, Jennings RA, Naylor PT, et al. Comparative in vitro antibiotic resistance of surface-colonizing coagulase-negative staphylococci. *Antimicrob Agents Chemother* 1989;33:813–816.
212. Widmer AF, Frei R, Rajacic Z, et al. Correlation between in vivo and in vitro efficacy of antimicrobial agents against foreign body infections. *J Infect Dis* 1990;162:96–102.
213. Widmer AF, Frei R, Rajacic Z, et al. Killing of nongrowing and adherent *Escherichia coli* determines drug efficacy in device-related infections. *Antimicrob Agents Chemother* 1991;35:741–746.
214. Vergeres P, Blaser J. Amikacin, ceftazidime, and flucloxacillin against suspended and adherent *Pseudomonas aeruginosa* and *Staphylococcus epidermidis* in an in vitro model infection. *J Infect Dis* 1992;165: 281–289.
215. Chuard C, Vaudaux P, Waldvogel FA, et al. Susceptibility of *Staphylococcus aureus* growing on fibronectin-coated surfaces to bactericidal antibiotics. *Antimicrob Agents Chemother* 1993;37:625–632.
216. Gander S. Bacterial biofilms: resistance to antimicrobial agents. *J Antimicrob Chemother* 1996;37:1047–1050.
217. Maki DG, Martin WT. Nationwide epidemic of septicemias caused by contaminated infusion products: IV. growth of microbial pathogens in fluids for intravenous infusion. *J Infect Dis* 1975;131:267–272.
218. Goldmann DA, Martin WT, Worthington JW. Growth of bacteria and fungi in total parenteral nutrition solutions. *Am J Surg* 1973;126: 314–318.
219. Maki DG. Growth properties of microorganisms in lipid for infusion

and implications for infection control [Abstract]. In: *Proceedings and abstracts of the twentieth interscience conference on antimicrobial agents and chemotherapy, September 1980, New Orleans, Louisiana.* Washington, DC: American Society for Microbiology, 1980:533.

220. Crocker KS, Noga R, Filibeck DJ, et al. Microbial growth comparisons of five commercial parenteral lipid emulsions. *JPEN J Parenter Enteral Nutr* 1984;8:391–394.
221. Redline RW, Redline SS, Boxerbaum B, et al. Systemic *Malassezia furfur* infections in patients receiving intralipid therapy. *Hum Pathol* 1985;16:815–822.
222. Aschner JL, Punsalang A, Maniscalco WM, et al. Percutaneous central venous catheter colonization with *Malassezia furfur*: incidence and clinical significance. *Pediatrics* 1987;80:535–539.
223. Shparago NI, Bruno PP, Bennett J. Systemic *Malassezia furfur* infection in an adult receiving total parenteral nutrition. *J Am Osteopath Assoc* 1995;95:375–377.
224. Freeman J, Goldmann DA, Smith NE, et al. Association of intravenous lipid emulsion and coagulase-negative staphylococcal bacteremia in neonatal intensive care units. *N Engl J Med* 1990;323:301–308.
225. Shiro H, Muller E, Takeda S, et al. Potentiation of *Staphylococcus epidermidis* catheter-related bacteremia by lipid infusions. *J Infect Dis* 1995;171:220–224.
226. Arduino MJ, Bland LA, McAllister SK, et al. Microbial growth and endotoxin production in the intravenous anesthetic propofol. *Infect Control Hosp Epidemiol* 1991;12:535–539.
227. Snydman DR, Reidy MD, Perry LK, et al. Safety of changing intravenous (IV) administration sets containing burettes at longer than 48 hour intervals. *Infect Control* 1987;8:113–116.
228. Maki DG, Botticelli JT, LeRoy ML, et al. Prospective study of replacing administration sets for intravenous therapy at 48- vs 72-hour intervals. *JAMA* 1987;258:1777–1781.
229. Buxton AE, Highsmith AK, Garner JS, et al. Contamination of intravenous fluid: effects of changing administration sets. *Ann Intern Med* 1979;90:764–768.
230. Josephson A, Gombert ME, Sierra MF, et al. The relationship between intravenous fluid contamination and the frequency of tubing replacement. *Infect Control* 1985;6:367–370.
231. Band JD, Maki DG. Safety of changing intravenous delivery systems at longer than 24-hour intervals. *Ann Intern Med* 1979;91:173–178.
232. Gorbea HF, Snydman DR, Delaney A, et al. Intravenous tubing with burettes can be safely changed at 48-hour intervals. *JAMA* 1984;251:2112–2115.
233. Daisy, JA, Abrutyn EA, MacGregor RR. Inadvertent administration of intravenous fluids contaminated with fungus. *Ann Intern Med* 1979;91:563–565.
234. O'Malley MK, Rhame FS, Cerra FB, et al. Value of routine pressure monitoring system changes after 72 hours of continuous use. *Crit Care Med* 1994;22:1424–1430.
235. Mermel LA, Maki DG. Epidemic bloodstream infections from hemodynamic pressure monitoring: signs of the times. *Infect Control Hosp Epidemiol* 1989;10:47–53.
236. Gahrn-Hansen B, Alstrup P, Dessau R, et al. Outbreak of infection with *Achromobacter xylosoxidans* from contaminated intravascular pressure transducers. *J Hosp Infect* 1988;12:1–6.
237. Hekker TAM, Overhage WV, Schneider AJ. Pressure transducers: an overlooked source of sepsis in the intensive care unit. *Intensive Care Med* 1990;16:511–512.
238. Thomas A, Lalitha MK, Jesudason MV. Transducer related *Enterobacter cloacae* sepsis in post-operative cardiothoracic patients. *J Hosp Infect* 1993;25:211–215.
239. Goldman M, Blajchman MA. Blood product-associated bacterial sepsis. *Transfus Med Rev* 1991;5:73–78.
240. Heal JM, Jones ME, Forey J, et al. Fatal *Salmonella* septicemia after platelet transfusion. *Transfusion* 1997;27:2–5.
241. Heltberg O, Skov F, Gerner-Smidt P, et al. Nosocomial epidemic of *Serratia marcescens* septicemia ascribed to contaminated blood transfusion bags. *Transfusion* 1993;33:221–227.
242. Centers for Disease Control and Prevention. Bacterial contamination of platelet pools. Ohio, 1991. *MMWR Morb Mortal Wkly Rep* 1992;41:36–37.
243. Sherertz RJ, Gledhill KS, Hampton KD, et al. Outbreak of *Candida* bloodstream infections associated with retrograde medication administration in a neonatal intensive care unit. *J Pediatr* 1992;120:455–461.
244. Roberts LA, Collignon PJ, Cramp VB, et al. An Australia-wide epidemic of *Pseudomonas pickettii* bacteraemia due to contaminated "sterile" water for injection. *Med J Aust* 1990;152:652–655.
245. Melin P, Struelens M, Mutsers J, et al. Nosocomial outbreak of *Pseudomonas pickettii* bacteremia originating from intrinsically contaminated sterile saline [Abstract]. In: *Programs and abstracts of the thirty-fifth interscience conference on antimicrobial agents and chemotherapy, September 1995, San Francisco, California.* Washington, DC: American Society for Microbiology, 1995:266.
246. Fernandez C, Wilhelmi I, Andradas E, et al. Nosocomial outbreak of *Burkholderia pickettii* infection due to a manufactured intravenous product used in three hospitals. *Clin Infect Dis* 1996;22:1092–1095.
247. Matsaniotis NS, Syriopolou VP, Theodoridou MC, et al. *Enterobacter* sepsis in infants and children due to contaminated intravenous fluids. *Infect Control* 1984;5:471–477.
248. Steere AC, Rifaat MK, Seligmann EB Jr, et al. Pyrogenic reactions associated with the infusion of normal serum albumin (human). *Transfusion* 1978;18:102–107.
249. Steere AC, Tenney JH, Mackel DC, et al. *Pseudomonas* species bacteremia caused by contaminated normal human serum albumin. *J Infect Dis* 1977;135:729–735.
250. Ezzedine H, Mourad M, Van Ossel C, et al. An outbreak of *Ochrobactrum anthropi* bacteraemia in five organ transplant patients. *J Hosp Infect* 1994;27:35–42.
251. Panlilio AL, Beck-Sague CM, Siegel JD, et al. Infections and pseudoinfections due to povidone–iodine solution contaminated with *Pseudomonas cepacia*. *Clin Infect Dis* 1992;14:1078–1083.
252. Clemence MA, Walker D, Farr BM. Central venous catheter practices: results of a survey. *Am J Infect Control* 1995;23:5–12.
253. Mackel DC, Maki DG, Anderson RL, et al. Nationwide epidemic of septicemia caused by contaminated intravenous products: mechanisms of intrinsic contamination. *J Clin Microbiol* 1975;2:486–497.
254. Jarvis WR, the Epidemiology Branch, Hospital Infections Program. Nosocomial outbreaks: the Centers for Disease Control's Hospital Infections Program experience, 1980–1991. *Am J Med* 1991;91(Suppl 3B):101S–106S.
255. Beck-Sague CM, Jarvis WR. Epidemic bloodstream infections associated with pressure transducers: a persistent problem. *Infect Control Hosp Epidemiol* 1989;10:54–59.
256. Pergues DA, Carson LA, Anderson RL, et al. Outbreak of *Pseudomonas cepacia* bacteremia in oncology patients. *Clin Infect Dis* 1993;16:407–411.
257. Goetz A, Muder RR, Rihs JP, et al. An outbreak of infusion-related *Klebsiella pneumoniae* bacteremia on a liver transplantation service [Abstract]. *Am J Infect Control* 1995;23:103.
258. Chodoff A, Pettis AM, Schoonmaker D, et al. Polymicrobial gram-negative bacteremia associated with saline solution flush used with a needleless intravenous system. *Am J Infect Control* 1995;23:357–363.
259. Deitel M, Krajden S, Saldanha CF, et al. An outbreak of *Staphylococcus epidermidis* bloodstream infection. *JPEN J Parenter Enteral Nutr* 1983;7:569–572.
260. Jackson S, Colligan M, Bender C. Increased nosocomial line-associated bacteremias in a neonatal intensive care unit related to a change in intravenous therapy administration [Abstract]. *Am J Infect Control* 1994;22:122.
261. Maki DG. Epidemic nosocomial bacteremias. In: Wenzel RR, ed. *Handbook of hospital infection*. West Palm Beach, FL: CRC Press, 1981:371–512.
262. Plouffe JF, Brown DG, Silva J, et al. Nosocomial outbreak of *Candida parapsilosis* fungemia related to intravenous infusions. *Arch Intern Med* 1977;137:1686–1689.
263. Solomon SL, Khabbaz RF, Parker RH, et al. An outbreak of *Candida parapsilosis* bloodstream infections in patients receiving parenteral nutrition. *J Infect Dis* 1984;149:98–102.
264. Centers for Disease Control and Prevention. Postsurgical infections associated with an extrinsically contaminated intravenous anesthetic agent: California, Illinois, Maine, and Michigan, 1990. *MMWR Morb Mortal Wkly Rep* 1990;39:426–433.
265. Veber B, Gachot B, Bedos JP, et al. Severe sepsis after intravenous injection of contaminated propofol. *Anesthesiology* 1994;80:712.
266. Solomon SL, Alexander H, Eley JW, et al. Nosocomial fungemia in neonates associated with intravascular pressure-monitoring devices. *Pediatric Infectious Disease* 1986;5:680–685.
267. Burnie JP, Matthews R, Lee W, et al. Four outbreaks of nosocomial systemic candidiasis. *Epidemiol Infect* 1987;99:201–211.

268. Reagan DR, Pfaller MA, Hollis RJ, et al. Characterization of the sequence of colonization and nosocomial candidemia using DNA fingerprinting and a DNA probe. *J Clin Microbiol* 1990;28:2733–2738.
269. Maki DG. Through a glass darkly: nosocomial pseudoepidemics and pseudobacteremias. *Arch Intern Med* 1980;140:26–28.
270. Maki DG. The use of antiseptics for handwashing by medical personnel. *J Chemother* 1989;1(Suppl 1):3–11.
271. Raad I, Hohn DC, Gilbreath BJ, et al. Prevention of central venous catheter-related infections by using maximal sterile barrier precautions during insertion. *Infect Control Hosp Epidemiol* 1994;15:237–238.
272. Maki DG. Yes, Virginia, aseptic technique is very important: maximal barrier precautions during insertion reduce the risk of central venous catheter-related bacteremia. *Infect Control Hosp Epidemiol* 1994;15: 227–230.
273. Bull DA, Neumayer LA, Hunter GC, et al. Improved sterile technique diminishes the incidence of positive line cultures in cardiovascular patients. *J Surg Res* 1992;52:106–110.
274. Bentley DW, Lepper MH. Septicemia related to indwelling venous catheter. *JAMA* 1968;206:1749–1752.
275. Freeman JB, Lemire A, MacLean LD. Intravenous alimentation and septicemia. *Surg Gynecol Obstet* 1972;135:708–712.
276. Nehme AE. Nutritional support of the hospitalized patient: the team concept. *JAMA* 1980;243:1906–1908.
277. Faubion WC, Wesley JR, Khalidi N, et al. Total parenteral nutrition catheter sepsis: impact of the team approach. *JPEN J Parenter Enteral Nutr* 1986;10:642–645.
278. Nelson DB, Kien CL, Mohr B, et al. Dressing changes by specialized personnel reduce infection rates in patients receiving central venous parenteral nutrition. *JPEN J Parenter Enteral Nutr* 1986;10:220–222.
279. Sanders RA, Sheldon GF. Septic complications of total parenteral nutrition: a five year experience. *Am J Surg* 1976;132:214–220.
280. Keohane PP, Jones BJM, Attrill H, et al. Effect of catheter tunnelling and a nutrition nurse on catheter sepsis during parenteral nutrition: a controlled trial. *Lancet* 1983;2:1388–1390.
281. Goetz A, Miller J, Squier C, et al. A comparison of nosocomial intravenous-related infections pre and post institution of an intravenous therapy team [Abstract]. *Am J Infect Control* 1993;82:xxx.
282. Tomford JW, Hershey CO: The I.V. therapy team: impact on patient care and costs of hospitalization. *NITA* 1985;8:387–389.
283. Soifer NE, Edlin BR, Weinstein RA, et al. A randomized IV team trial [Abstract]. In: *Program and abstracts of the twenty-ninth interscience conference on antimicrobial agents and chemotherapy, September 1989, Houston, Texas*. Washington, DC: American Society for Microbiology, 1989:284.
284. Parras F, Ena J, Bouza E, del Carmen Guerrero M, et al. Impact of an educational program for the prevention of colonization of intravascular catheters. *Infect Control Hosp Epidemiol* 1994;15: 239–242.
285. Puntis JWL, Holden CE, Smallman S, et al. Staff training: a key factor in reducing intravascular catheter sepsis. *Arch Dis Child* 1990;65: 335–337.
286. Fridkin SK, Pear SM, Williamson, et al. The role of understaffing in central venous catheter-associated bloodstream infections. *Infect Control Hosp Epidemiol* 1996;17:150–158.
287. Rannem T, Ladefoged K, Hegnhoj J, et al. Catheter-related sepsis in long-term parenteral nutrition with Broviac catheters: an evaluation of different disinfectants. *Clin Nutr* 1990;9:131–136.
288. Strand CL, Wajsbort RR, Sturmann K. Effect of iodophor vs iodine tincture skin preparation on blood culture contamination rate. *JAMA* 1993;269:1004–1006.
289. Little JR, Murray PR, Traynor S, et al. Blood culture contamination rates following venipuncture site disinfection with iodophor VS iodine tincture. *Infect Control Hosp Epidemiol* 1997;18:55.
290. Zinner SH, Denny-Brown BC, Braun P, et al. Risk of infection with intravenous indwelling catheters: effect of application of antibiotic ointment. *J Infect Dis* 1969;120:616–619.
291. Hill R, Salem RB, Casewell MW. Topical calcium mupirocin for the prevention of colonisation of intravascular cannulae: a randomized double-blind controlled trial [Abstract]. In: *Programs and abstracts of the thirty-third interscience conference on antimicrobial agents and chemotherapy, October 1993, New Orleans, Louisiana*. Washington, DC: American Society for Microbiology, 1993:341.
292. Zakrzewska-Bode A, Muytjens HL, et al. Mupirocin resistance in coagulase-negative staphylococci after topical prophylaxis for the reduction of colonization of central venous catheters. *J Hosp Infect* 1995;31:189–193.
293. Prager RL, Silva J. Colonization of central venous catheters. *South Med J* 1984;77:458–461.
294. Rhame FS, Feist JF, Mueller CL, et al. Transparent adherent dressings (TADs) do not promote abnormal skin flora [Abstract]. *Am J Infect Control* 1983;11:152.
295. Hoffmann KK, Weber DJ, Samsa GP, et al. Transparent polyurethane film as an intravenous catheter dressing: a meta-analysis of the infection risks. *JAMA* 1992;267:2072–2076.
296. Andersen PT, Herlevsen P, Schaumburg H. A comparative study of "Op-site" and "Nobecutan gauze" dressings for central venous line care. *J Hosp Infect* 1986;7:161–168.
297. Kelsey MC, Gosling M. A comparison of the morbidity associated with occlusive and non-occlusive dressings applied to peripheral intravenous devices. *J Hosp Infect* 1984;5:313–321.
298. Joseph P, Marzouk J. Transparent vs. dry gauze dressings for peripheral IV sites [Abstract]. In: *Program and abstracts of the general meeting of the American Society for Microbiology, March 1985, Las Vegas, Nevada*. Washington, DC: American Society for Microbiology, 1985:378.
299. McCredie KB, Lawson M, Marts K, et al. A comparative evaluation of transparent dressings and gauze dressings for central venous catheters [Abstract]. *JPEN J Parenter Enteral Nutr* 1984;8:96.
300. Ricard P, Martin R, Marcoux JA. Protection of indwelling vascular catheters: incidence of bacterial contamination and catheter-related sepsis. *Crit Care Med* 1985;13:541–543.
301. Pinheiro SMC, Starling CAF, Couto BRGM. Transparent dressing versus conventional dressing: comparison of the incidence of related catheter infection. *Am J Infect Control* 1997;25:148.
302. Powell C, Regan C, Fabri PJ, et al. Evaluation of opsite catheter dressings for parenteral nutrition: a prospective, randomized study. *JPEN J Parenter Enteral Nutr* 1982;6:43–46.
303. Palidar PJ, Simonowitz DA, Oreskovich MR, et al. Use of Op-Site as an occlusive dressing for total parenteral nutrition catheters. *JPEN J Parenter Enteral Nutr* 1982;6:150–151 .
304. Nehme AE, Trigger JA. Catheter dressings in central parenteral nutrition: a prospective randomized comparative study. *Nutrition Support Services* 1984;4:42–43.
305. Maki DG, Will L. Colonization and infection associated with transparent dressings for central venous, arterial, and Hickman catheters: a comparative trial [Abstract]. In: *Program and abstracts of the thirty-fourth interscience conference on antimicrobial agents and chemotherapy, October 1994, Orlando, Florida*. Washington, DC: American Society for Microbiology, 1984:253.
306. Powell CR, Traetow MJ, Fabri PJ, et al. Op-site dressing study: a prospective randomized study evaluating povidone iodine ointment and extension set changes with 7-day op-site dressings applied to total parenteral nutrition subclavian sites. *JPEN J Parenter Enteral Nutr* 1985;9:443–446.
307. Young GP, Alexeyeff M, Russell DM, et al. Catheter sepsis during parenteral nutrition: the safety of long-term OpSite dressings. *JPEN J Parenter Enteral Nutr* 1988;12:365–370.
308. Maki DG, Mermel LA, Martin M, et al. A highly-semipermeable polyurethane dressing does not increase the risk of CVC-related BSI: a prospective, multicenter, investigator-blinded trial [Abstract]. In: *Programs and abstracts of the thirty-sixth interscience conference on antimicrobial agents and chemotherapy, September 1996, New Orleans, Louisiana*. Washington, DC: American Society for Microbiology, 1996:230.
309. Shivnan JC, McGuire D, Freeman S, et al. Comparison of transparent adherent and dry sterile gauze dressings for long-term central catheters in patients undergoing bone marrow transplant. *Oncology Nurses Forum* 1991;18:1349–1356.
310. Eyer S, Brummitt C, Crossley K, et al. Catheter-related sepsis: prospective, randomized study of three methods of long-term catheter maintenance. *Crit Care Med* 1990;18:1073–1079.
311. Stenzel JP, Green TP, Fuhrman BP, et al. Percutaneous central venous catheterization in a pediatric intensive care unit: a survival analysis of complications. *Crit Care Med* 1989;17:984–988.
312. Pinilla JC, Ross DF, Martin T, et al. Study of the incidence of intravascular catheter infection and associated septicemia in critically ill patients. *Crit Care Med* 1983;11:21–25.
313. Leroy O, Billiau V, Beuscart C, et al. Nosocomial infections associated

with long-term radial artery cannulation. *Intensive Care Med* 1989;15:241–246.
314. Thomas F, Burke JP, Parker J, et al. The risk of infection related to radial vs. femoral sites for arterial catheterization. *Crit Care Med* 1983;11:807–812.
315. Shinozaki T, Deane RS, Mazuzan JE Jr, et al. Bacterial contamination of arterial lines. *JAMA* 1983;249:223–225.
316. Furfaro S, Gauthier M, Lacroix J, et al. Arterial catheter-related infections in children: a 1-year cohort analysis. *American Journal of Diseases of Children* 1991;145:1037–1043.
317. Lederle FA, Parenti CM, Berskow LC, et al. The idle intravenous catheter. *Ann Intern Med* 1992;116:737–738.
318. Parenti C, Lederle FA, Impola CL, et al. Reduction of unnecessary intravenous catheter use: internal medicine house staff participate in a successful quality improvement project. *Arch Intern Med* 1994;154: 1829–1832.
319. Andrivet P, Bacquer A, Vu Ngoc C, et al. Lack of clinical benefit from subcutaneous tunnel insertion of central venous catheters in immunocompromised patients. *Clin Infect Dis* 1994;18:199–206.
320. Timsit J-F, Sebile V, Farkas J-C, et al. Effect of subcutaneous tunneling on internal jugular cather-related sepsis in critically ill patients. A prospective randomized multicenter study. *JAMA* 1996;276:1416–1420.
321. Sitges-Serra A, Linares J, Perez JL, et al. A randomized trial on the effect of tubing changes on hub contamination and catheter sepsis during parenteral nutrition. *JPEN J Parenter Enteral Nutr* 1985;9: 322–325.
322. Alothman A, Scharf S, Bryce EA. Extending central venous catheters tubing changes to five days: safety and cost effectiveness. *Programs and Abstracts of the Thirty-Fourth Infectious Diseases Society of America Annual Meeting*, October 1994, Orlando, FL. Washington, DC: Infectious Diseases Society of America, 1994: 861.
323. Moro ML, Maffei C, Manso E, et al. Nosocomial outbreak of systemic candidosis associated with parenteral nutrition. *Infect Control Hosp Epidemiol* 1990;11:27–35.
324. Craver D, Hodges L, Hutchenson K, et al. Baxter infusion pumps and needleless tubings/devices have lower infection control risks and costs for intravenous therapy than Abbott infusion pumps and needleless tubings/devices [Abstract]. *Am J Infect Control* 1994;22:104.
325. Maki DG, Stolz S, McCormick R, et al. Possible association of a commercial needleless system with central venous catheter-related bacteremia [Abstract]. In: *Programs and abstracts of the thirty-fourth interscience conference on antimicrobial agents and chemotherapy, October 1994, Orlando, Florida*. Washington, DC: American Society for Microbiology, 1994:195.
326. Danzig LE, Short LJ, Collins K, et al. Bloodstream infections associated with needleless intravenous infusion system in patients receiving home infusion therapy. *JAMA* 1995;273:1862–1864.
327. Vassallo D, Blanc-Jouvan M, Bret M, et al. *Staphylococcus aureus* septicemia and a needleless system of infusion [Abstract]. In: *Programs and abstracts of the thirty-fifth interscience conference on antimicrobial agents and chemotherapy, September 1995, San Francisco, California*. Washington, DC: American Society for Microbiology, 1995:259.
328. Kellerman S, Shay D, Howard J, et al. Bloodstream infections associated with needleless devices used for central venous catheter access in children receiving home healthcare [Abstract]. In: *Programs and abstracts of the thirty-fifth interscience conference on antimicrobial agents and chemotherapy September 1995, San Francisco, California*. Washington, DC: American Society for Microbiology, 1995:258.
329. Do A, Ray B, Barnett B, et al. Evaluation of the role of needleless devices (ND) in bloodstream infections (BSIs) in home infusion therapy (HIT) [Abstract]. In: *Programs and abstracts of the thirty-sixth interscience conference on antimicrobial agents and chemotherapy, September 1996, New Orleans, Louisiana*. Washington, DC: American Society for Microbiology, 1996:229.
330. Miller RC, Grogan JB. Incidence and source of contamination of intravenous nutritional infusion systems. *J Pediatr Surg* 1973;8:185–190.
331. Freeman JB, Litton AA. Preponderance of gram-positive infections during parenteral alimentation. *Surg Gynecol Obstet* 1974;139: 905–908.
332. Baumgartner TG, Schmidt GL, Thakker KM, et al. Bacterial endotoxin retention by inline intravenous filters. *Am J Hosp Pharm* 1986;43:681–684.
333. Holmes CJ, Kundsin RB, Ausman RK, et al. Potential hazards associated with microbial contamination of in-line filters during intravenous therapy. *J Clin Microbiol* 1980;12:725–731.
334. Falchuk KH, Peterson L, McNeil BJ. Microparticulate-induced phlebitis: its prevention by in-line filtration. *N Engl J Med* 1985;312:78–82.
335. Maddox RR, John JF Jr, Brown LL, et al. Effect of inline filtration on postinfusion phlebitis. *Clin Pharm* 1983;2:58–61.
336. Quercia RA, Hills SW, Klimek JJ, et al. Bacteriologic contamination of intravenous infusion delivery systems in an intensive care unit. *Am J Med* 1986;80:364–368.
337. Ginies Jl, Joseph MG, Champion G, et al. Etude prospective de l'efficacite des diltres intibacteriens sur la prevention des complications de la nutrition parenterale centrale chez le nouveau-ne. *Agressologie* 1990;31:495–496.
338. Rapp RP, Brack A, Bivins A, et al. Sepsis in rabbits following administration of contaminated infusions through filters of various pore sizes. *Am J Hosp Pharm* 1979;36:1711–1713.
339. Heggers JP, Stabenau J, Listengarten D, et al. A new efficacious Ag-coated dressing: II. in vivo assay [Abstract]. *Am J Infect Control* 1995;23:135.
340. Shapiro JM, Bond EL, Garman JK. Use of a chlorhexidine dressing to reduce microbial colonization of epidural catheters. *Anesthesiology* 1990;73:625–631.
341. Keyserling H, Dykes F, Newsome P, et al. Pilot study of a chlorhexidine disc catheter dressing in a neonatal unit [Abstract]. *NAVAN* 19xx;1:12–13.
342. Clementi E, Marie O, Arlet G, et al. Usefulness of an attachable silver-impregnated cuff for prevention of catheter-related sepsis (CRS) [Abstract]. In: *Programs and abstracts of the thirty-first interscience conference on antimicrobial agents and chemotherapy, October 1991, Chicago, Illinois*. Washington, DC: American Society for Microbiology, 1991:175.
343. Tebbs SE, Sawyer A, Elliott TSJ. Influence of surface morphology on *in vitro* bacterial adherence to central venous catheters. *Br J Anaesth* 1994;72:587–591.
344. Francois P, Vaudaux P, Mathiue HJ, et al. Effects of surface treatment on the surface chemistry and topography of central venous catheters (CVC) and on protein-d adhesion of *Staphylococcus aureus* [Abstract]. In: *Programs and abstracts of the thirty-fourth interscience conference on antimicrobial agents and chemotherapy, October 1994, Orlando, Florida*. Washington, DC: American Society for Microbiology, 1994:194.
345. Neu HC. The crisis in antibiotic resistance. *Science* 1992;257: 1064–1072.
346. Liu WK, Tebbs SE, Byrne PO, et al. The effects of electric current on bacteria colonising intravenous catheters. *J Infect* 1993;27:261–269.
347. Raad I, Hachem R, Zermeno A. Silver iontophoretic catheter: a prototype of a long-term antiinfective vascular access device. *J Infect Dis* 1996;173:495–498.
348. Segura M, Alvarez-Lerma F, Ma Tellado J, et al. A clinical trial on the prevention of catheter-related sepsis using a new hub model. *Ann Surg* 1996;223:363–369.
349. Freeman R, Holden MP, Lyon R, et al. Addition of sodium metabisulfite to left atrial catheter infusate as a means of preventing bacterial colonization of the catheter tip. *Thorax* 1982;37:142–144.
350. Root JL, McIntyre OR, Jacobs NJ, et al. Inhibitory effect of disodium EDTA upon growth of *Staphylococcus epidermidis* in vitro: relation to infection prophylaxis of Hickman catheters. *Antimicrob Agents Chemother* 1983;32:1627–1631.
351. Elliot TSJ, Curran A. Effects of heparin and chlorbutol on bacterial colonisation of intravascular cannulae in an in vitro model. *J Hosp Infect* 1989;14:193–200.
352. Wiernikowski JT, Elder-Thornley D, Dawson S, et al. Bacterial colonization of tunneled right atrial catheters in pediatric oncology: a comparison of sterile saline and bacteriostatic flush solutions. *American Journal of Pediatric Hematology and Oncology* 1991;13:137–140.
353. Kropec A, Huebner J, Frank U, et al. In vitro activity of sodium bisulfite and heparin against staphylococci: new strategies in the treatment of catheter-related infection. *J Infect Dis* 1993;168:235–237.

Hospital Infections, Fourth Edition,
edited by John V. Bennett and Philip S. Brachman.
Lippincott–Raven Publishers, Philadelphia © 1998

CHAPTER 45

Infection in Transplant Recipients

Robert H. Rubin and Jay A. Fishman

Clinical transplantation has undergone an extraordinary transformation since the mid-1960s, evolving from an interesting experiment in human immunobiology to the most practical means of rehabilitating patients with end-stage kidney, liver, heart, and lung disease, as well as an increasing number of malignant conditions. Two closely linked processes, allograft rejection (and its equivalent in bone marrow transplantation, graft-versus-host disease (GVHD) and infection, remain the major barriers to successful transplantation. Both allograft rejection and GVHD are initiated by the immunologic recognition of major and minor histocompatibility differences between the donor and recipient. Much of the progress in transplantation has occurred because of success in limiting the extent of these processes with new forms of immunosuppressive therapy. In addition, a clearer understanding of the linkage between the immunologic processes that result in allograft rejection and GVHD, immunosuppressive therapy, and the infectious complications of transplantation has emerged, making possible a therapeutic strategy that has two components: an immunosuppressive one to prevent and treat the immunologic events that lead to failure of the transplant; and an antimicrobial one to make it safe. An important truism of transplantation is the following: Any manipulation or intervention that decreases the risk of infection will then permit the use of more intensive immunosuppression and allow better control of rejection or GVHD; conversely, any manipulation or intervention that decreases the risk of rejection or GVHD, and thus permits the use of lesser amounts of immunosuppression, will decrease the risk of infection [1,2].

R.H. Rubin: Division of Human Pharmacology and Experimental Therapeutics, Harvard–Massachusetts Institute of Technology Division of Health Sciences and Technology, Cambridge, Massachusetts 02142.

J.A. Fishman: Department of Infectious Disease and Transplantation, Massachusetts General Hospital, Boston, Massachusetts 02114.

The combination of rejection, immunosuppressive therapy, and exposures to a variety of potential microbial pathogens creates a unique set of challenges to the infectious disease clinician responsible for the care of the transplant recipient [1,2]:

1. The potential sources of infection are almost limitless, including endogenous organisms, the allograft itself, and the air, water, and food the patient encounters. Immunosuppressive therapy renders the transplant recipient susceptible to microbial species and inoculum sizes that would have little impact on the normal host.
2. Chronic immunosuppression, persistent infection with immunomodulating viruses (such as cytomegalovirus [CMV], Epstein-Barr virus [EBV], and the hepatitis viruses) that themselves are modulated by the exogenous immunosuppressive therapy, and the presence of foreign tissue in which the expression of a variety of surface antigens including histocompatibility antigens is modulated by infectious processes and by cytokines elaborated in response to these infectious processes, all combine to produce an array of unique clinical syndromes.
3. The cornerstone of effective therapy of infection in these immunosuppressed individuals is early recognition and prompt treatment. This is a particular challenge in patients whose impaired inflammatory response can greatly blunt the extent of symptoms, physical findings, and radiologic abnormalities generated by microbial invasion. This problem is further exacerbated by the fact that many of the important pathogens (e.g., *Cryptococcus neoformans*, *Pneumocystis carinii*, atypical mycobacteria) affecting these patients are comparatively bland, exciting minimal responses until the disease process is relatively far advanced.
4. The nature of the infections that occur in these patients, particularly those due to fungi, viruses, pro-

tozoans, and such bacteria as *Nocardia asteroides* and *Mycobacterium tuberculosis*, renders treatment difficult, in that prolonged courses of toxic antimicrobial therapy are usually required. Such prolonged therapy in patients receiving cyclosporine or FK-506 (tacrolimus) can be particularly challenging because of the chance of significant toxicity related to drug interactions.

5. Because the clinical impact of infection in these patients is so protean, and diagnosis and curative therapy so difficult, prevention of infection should be the major goal of the clinician.

The importance of these challenges is underlined by the following observations: clinically significant infection occurs in at least three fourths of all transplant recipients, and is still the leading cause of death. This chapter is devoted to answering these challenges so that the benefits of successful transplantation can be brought to a greater number of individuals.

FACTORS DETERMINING THE RISK OF INFECTION IN THE TRANSPLANT RECIPIENT

The occurrence of infection, particularly opportunistic infection, in the transplant patient, as in any patient, is largely due to the interaction between two factors—*the patient's net state of immunosuppression* and the *epidemiologic exposures* that he encounters. The relationship between these two factors is a semiquantitative one. Thus, if the patient's net state of immunosuppression is great enough, even trivial exposures to relatively avirulent organisms can produce life-threatening infection; conversely, if the exposure is great enough, even immunologically normal individuals can succumb to the infectious challenge [1,3].

The Net State of Immunosuppression

The net state of immunosuppression is a complex function determined by the interaction of a number of factors: host defense defects engendered by the underlying disease process that led to the need for transplantation; the dose, duration, and temporal sequence of immunosuppressive therapies administered; the presence or absence of damage to the mucocutaneous surfaces of the body (the primary host defense barrier to invasive infection, which is particularly important in these patients who may have profound defects in their secondary host defenses), foreign bodies that bypass these surfaces, and neutropenia; the presence of metabolic abnormalities such as malnutrition, uremia, and, perhaps, hyperglycemia; and the presence of infection with one of the immunomodulating viruses: CMV, EBV, the hepatitis viruses, or the human immunodeficiency virus (HIV). The major determinant of the net state of immunosuppression is the nature of the immunosuppressive therapy. However, two other observations underline the principle that other factors are important as well: > 90% of the opportunistic infections occur in individuals with preceding immunomodulating viral infection, with the 10% exceptions almost invariably due to excessive environmental exposures. If the transplant population is stratified into two groups on the basis of a serum albumin greater than or no more than 2.8 g/dl, those with the lower value have a 10-fold greater risk of life-threatening infection [1,3].

Epidemiologic Exposures

The epidemiologic exposures of importance for the transplant patient can be divided into two general categories—those occurring in the community and those taking place in the hospital environment. Community exposures of particular importance to the transplant recipient include the following: *M. tuberculosis*, the geographically restricted systemic mycoses (blastomycosis, coccidioidomycosis, and histoplasmosis), *Strongyloides stercoralis*, and such community-acquired respiratory viruses as influenza, parainfluenza, and respiratory syncytial virus. Many routine infections, including those due to *Streptococcus pneumoniae*, *Hemophilus influenzae*, *Listeria monocytogenes*, and staphylococci, are prevented by standard antimicrobial prophylaxis. In the case of *M. tuberculosis* (see Chapter 33) and the mycoses, three patterns of infection are observed: progressive primary infection with postprimary dissemination; reactivation infection with secondary dissemination; and superinfection, when previous immunity is attenuated by the exogenous immunosuppressive therapy and a new exposure results in reinfection, again with the possibility of systemic dissemination. Clinical syndromes suggestive of these events include fever of unknown origin, progressive pneumonia, and metastatic infection (not uncommonly involving the mucocutaneous surfaces of the body) [1,3].

Strongyloides stercoralis, because of its unique autoinfection cycle, can remain asymptomatically in the gastrointestinal tract of an individual for decades, only to be reawakened clinically by the initiation of immunosuppressive therapy. This reawakening can result in two clinical syndromes: a hyperinfestation syndrome, resulting in exacerbation of the usual manifestations of strongyloidiasis: hemorrhagic pneumonia and enterocolitis; or a disseminated infection, in which *Strongyloides* migrates through the bowel wall, accompanied by gut flora, producing a clinical syndrome of antimicrobial-unresponsive gram-negative sepsis or meningitis. Individuals with epidemiologic histories consistent with possible exposure to this organism need to be screened and effectively treated before the initiation of immunosuppressive therapy [4].

As far as the community-acquired respiratory viruses are concerned, there are important differences from the general population in terms of their clinical impact: the efficacy of such vaccines as the influenza vaccine is significantly less than in nonimmunosuppressed individuals, and there is a higher rate of both viral pneumonia and superinfecting bacterial pneumonia per episode of infection than is observed in the general population [5] (see Chapter 32).

In the hospital, outbreaks of invasive aspergillosis, legionellosis, and *Pseudomonas aeruginosa* (and other gram-negative bacillary) infection among transplant patients due to contaminated air or potable water have been well documented (see Chapter 20). Two epidemiologic patterns are recognized: a *domiciliary* pattern, in which the exposure occurs on the transplant ward, with clustering of cases in time and space; and a *nondomiciliary* pattern, in which the exposure occurs when the patient is taken to the radiology suite, the cardiac catheterization or bronchoscopy facility, or operating room for an essential procedure. Nondomiciliary outbreaks are more common, but more difficult to detect because of the frequent lack of recognizable clustering of cases. *The major clue to the existence of an excessive epidemiologic hazard is the occurrence of a significant infection at a point in time when the net state of immunosuppression is not, under normal circumstances, great enough to allow such an infection* [16]. The essential point to remember is that immunosuppressed patients such as transplant recipients are like "sentinel chickens," reflecting any excess traffic in microbes in the environment (particularly with agents that cause opportunistic respiratory infection) [7]. Constant surveillance of infections in any transplantation unit is essential (see Chapter 5). In addition, in institutions undergoing major reconstruction, transplant recipients may benefit greatly from being housed in areas where the air quality is maintained by high-efficiency particulate air filters [1] (see Chapter 20).

TIMETABLE OF INFECTION AFTER ORGAN TRANSPLANTATION

The general pattern of infection is the same in all forms of organ transplantation, reflecting the use of similar immunosuppressive programs in all of these patients. Thus, a timetable can be defined, delineating when in the posttransplantation course a particular form of infection is likely to occur; that is, although a given infectious disease clinical syndrome, such as pneumonia, can occur at any point in the posttransplantation period, the microbial etiologies are very different in the different time periods. Application of this timetable to the clinical management of transplant patients is useful in at least three different ways: in arriving at a differential diagnosis of the causes of a particular clinical presentation; in the design of directed, cost-effective antimicrobial preventative strategies; and in the recognition of epidemiologic hazards—exceptions to the timetable are invariably due to a hitherto unrecognized environmental exposure, often within the hospital environment. In the organ transplant patient, the timetable is conveniently divided into three different time periods: the first month posttransplantation, the period 1 to 6 months posttransplantation, and the late period, more than 6 months posttransplantation [1,3] (Figure 45-1).

Infection in the First Month Posttransplantation

In the first month posttransplantation, there are three major causes of clinically important infection: infection that was present in the recipient before the transplantation procedure and that is exacerbated by the surgery, anesthesia, and immunosuppressive therapy; active infection conveyed with the allograft; and the same wound-, catheter-, or vascular access-related infection and pneumonia seen in nonimmunosuppressed patients subjected to comparable amounts of surgery.

Importance of Infection in the Recipient Before Transplantation

A cardinal rule of clinical transplantation is that all infectious processes should be under control before the transplantation procedure and initiation of immunosuppressive therapy. Thus, before transplantation, every attempt must be made to identify and eradicate infection such as tuberculosis, localized and systemic fungal infection, and strongyloidiasis. As heart, lung, and liver transplantation are being used to treat an ever-increasing number of diseases, acute bacterial and fungal infection of clinical importance may be acquired during the wait for emergency transplantation. Examples include aspiration pneumonia in the patient with advanced hepatic encephalopathy; pneumonia and line sepsis in the patient with end-stage cardiac disease who is intubated and receiving life support from pressors delivered through central venous access and cardiac assist devices; and bronchopulmonary infection or colonization with antibiotic-resistant gram-negative bacilli in the patient with end-stage pulmonary disease. For the promise of transplantation to be fulfilled for these individuals, certain guidelines should be followed [1,3,8]:

1. For patients with chronically progressive disease of the liver, heart, and lungs, early transplantation should be considered, before the start of the terminal systemic downhill spiral that accompanies the infectious complications of intensive care unit interventions.
2. Metabolic derangements in patients with renal failure can, and should, be corrected by dialysis before

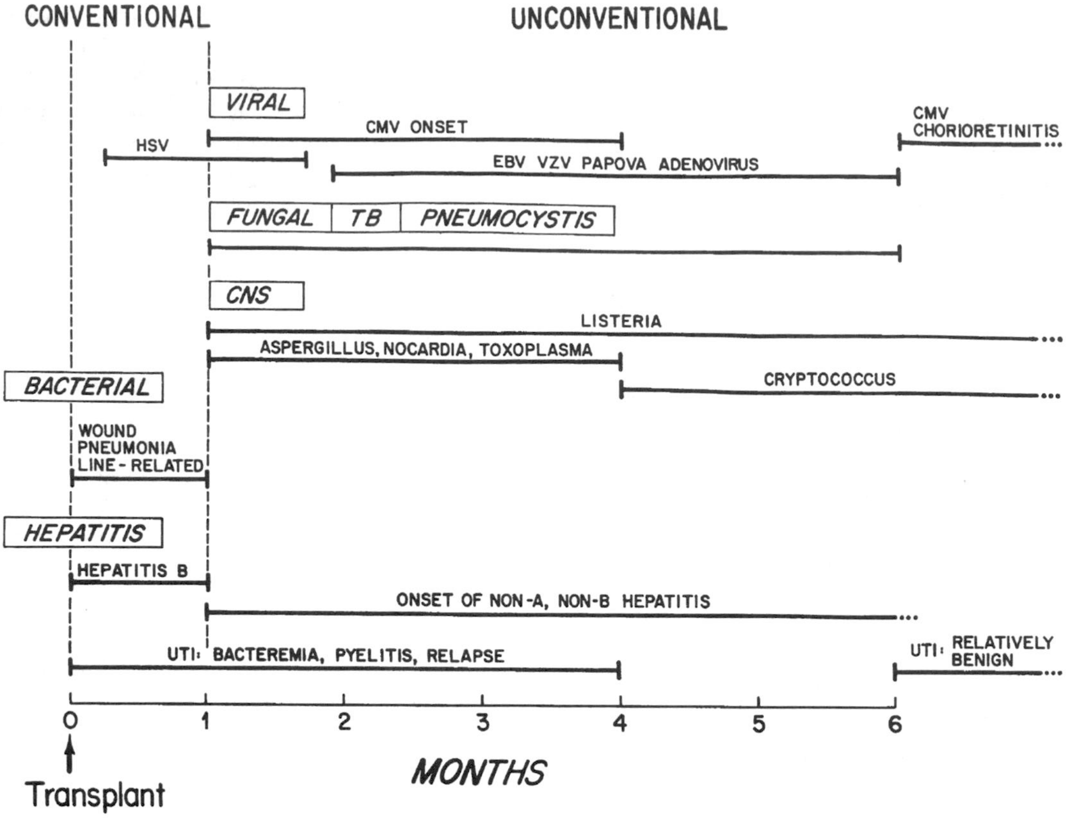

FIGURE 45-1. Timetable of infection after organ transplantation. (Reprinted with permission from Rubin RH, Wolfson JS, Cosimi AB, et al. Infection in the renal transplant recipient. *Am J Med* 1981;70:405–411.)

transplantation. Thus, infectious disease issues can be addressed by delaying surgery in patients with active infection. In the absence of equivalent options in patients with advanced hepatic, cardiac, or pulmonary failure or in patients with aggressive malignancy such as leukemia, prevention of infection is critical. Major concerns include airway protection in the patient with hepatic encephalopathy; wound care in the patient requiring the intraaortic balloon pump for cardiac support; ventilator care in the intubated patient; and mucosal care in the neutropenic patient preparing for bone marrow transplantation.

3. Transplantation of patients with active infection is fraught with great hazard. In particular, active pneumonia is a temporary contraindication (until the active inflammatory process has been effectively treated), as is active bloodstream infection (which carries a significant risk of seeding the allograft's vascular anastomosis, resulting in a mycotic aneurysm and the risk of catastrophic rupture).
4. Colonization of the transplant candidate with certain organisms pretransplantation requires antimicrobial intervention; in particular, colonization of the respiratory tract with *Aspergillus* species (as can be seen in patients with cystic fibrosis undergoing lung or liver transplantation or in debilitated, intubated patients in a contaminated environment) carries a > 65% risk of subsequent lung invasion posttransplantation. Accordingly, eradication of respiratory tract carriage of these organisms pretransplantation should be given a high priority.

Donor as a Source of Infection

To prevent transmission of active infection with the allograft itself, the prospective donor must undergo a careful evaluation for the presence of such long-standing infectious processes as HIV, hepatitis B virus (HBV), hepatitis C virus (HCV), and CMV as well as acute infectious complications associated with preterminal intensive care unit management. Transplantation of an organ from a donor infected with HIV, HBV, or HCV is an extremely efficient method of transmitting these viruses to the recipient [1,8–13]. In the case of such infectious agents as *M. tuberculosis*, *Histoplasma capsulatum*, and *C. neoformans*, transmission by an infected allograft has been documented to occur, but such an event is quite uncommon [1]. In contrast, the protozoan *Toxoplasma gondii* is a potential hazard primarily in patients undergoing cardiac transplantation. Transplantation of a heart from a donor seropositive for toxoplasmosis into a seronegative recipient is associated with a high incidence of *T. gondii* myocarditis and disseminated infection. Because of this risk, prophylaxis against toxoplasmosis (usually with pyrimethamine and a sulfonamide) is indicated for these individuals, although not for other categories of organ transplant patients [14–17].

A more difficult problem is the identification of immediately preterminal contamination of organs due to acute infection developing while the potential donor is in the intensive care unit. For example, our group reported a case of unsuspected *P. aeruginosa* bacteremia in an afebrile donor that resulted in seeding of both of the harvested kidneys. In both recipients, massive retroperitoneal bleeds developed that required emergency graft nephrectomy [18]. Both recipients were found to have ruptured mycotic aneurysms infected with *P. aeruginosa* at the site of the renal artery anastomosis. Less commonly, organs may be secondarily contaminated during the harvesting process or during handling before the transplant procedure [1,18–25]. Individuals receiving blood products before organ donation may have false-positive serologic tests for CMV or other pathogens that may confuse attempts at antiviral prophylaxis.

Technical Complications as a Risk Factor for Infection

The concept that technical complications lead to significant infectious problems is an important one because it applies to the perioperative period as well as the operation itself. Thus, poor management of the airway leads to aspiration pneumonia; inadequate attention to vascular access devices, particularly central venous catheters, leads to septicemia; and drainage catheters ultimately lead to infection of normally sterile sites. Infection occurring as a consequence of technical mishaps accounts for > 95% of the infections that occur in the first month posttransplantation. The consequences of such infections can be far greater than in the normal host; for example, although transient vascular access-related candidemia carries a risk of visceral seeding of < 10%, in the transplant patient the risk is > 50%, and all such episodes require systemic antifungal chemotherapy (in addition to removal of the contaminated vascular access device) [1,3,8].

Wound infection is the most important treatable infection occurring in the first month after transplantation (see Chapter 37). Its incidence is directly related to the success of the surgical team in performing a technically impeccable transplant operation that avoids vascular compromise and the creation of devitalized tissue, wound hematomas, fluid collections (blood, urine, bile, or lymph), and the need for reexploration or prolonged use of drainage catheters (see later). The particular technical challenges of liver transplantation, with a biliary anastomosis that is susceptible to ischemic injury, as well as four vascular anastomoses (superior and inferior vena cava, portal vein, and hepatic artery)—all performed in patients with coagulopathies—explains the high rate of intraabdominal infection that dominates the first month posttransplantation in these patients. Indeed, the major difference between liver transplant recipients and other allograft recipients is the higher occurrence of technically related infections in and around the allograft [1].

There is a consensus among many transplant surgeons that local irrigation of the wound with antibacterial solutions, such as bacitracin–neomycin, is beneficial in preventing wound infection. Another area of agreement, also in the absence of controlled studies, is the need to avoid using open drains because of the direct conduit to deep tissues that the open drain might provide to potential pathogens. Closed-suction drainage to eliminate dead space and prevent fluid collections is used in many centers, with attention being paid to meticulous aseptic care and early removal [1].

There is considerable variability in the use and choice of perioperative antibiotics to prevent wound infection among different transplant centers. Two principles apply, however: first, antibiotic prophylaxis is not a substitute for technically expert surgery; and second, antibiotic choice should be directed toward prevention of wound infection, not systemic sepsis. In our institution, cefazolin alone, begun on call to the operating room and continued for < 72 hours, has provided adequate protection without creating intensive pressure for the selection of highly resistant flora. In the special case of liver transplantation, some centers opt for the use of an elaborate program of nonabsorbable antimicrobials aimed at eliminating the aerobic gram-negative flora and yeast from the gastrointestinal tract, and then using a perioperative drug such as cefotaxime that leaves the anaerobic flora (and hence, "colonization resistance") intact. Our group does attempt to eliminate yeast from the gastrointestinal tract, but does not use the rest of the program. Both of these programs, probably more from the technical success of the operation than the antimicrobial strategy, have rates of posttransplantation intraabdominal infection of < 5% [1, 26–28].

Opportunistic Infection in the First Month Posttransplantation

Noteworthy in this discussion of infections in the first month after organ transplantation is the absence of any mention of opportunistic infections. Indeed, in this 1-month "golden period" the net state of immunosuppression should not be great enough to permit infection due to such organisms as *P. carinii*, *Aspergillus fumigatus*, or *Legionella pneumophila*. This observation leads to two important conclusions: the net state of immunosuppression is primarily determined by the duration of immunosuppression ("the area under the curve"), rather than the daily dose—because the daily dose of drugs is highest in the first month posttransplantation; the occurrence of opportunistic infection during this period is an important clue to the presence of an unsuspected environmental hazard or preexisting infection and requires immediate attention. The first of these observations, the importance of sustained immunosuppression in the pathogenesis of opportunistic infection, underlines the biggest challenge in immunosuppressive therapy: Increasing the dose of immunosuppressive drugs usually results in a discernible improvement in allograft function within 24 to 48 hours, whereas the infectious disease consequences may not be perceived for another 2 to 4 weeks. Balancing immediate benefits with long-term side effects is the secret of successful management of transplant recipients [1,3].

Infection 1 to 6 Months Posttransplantation

The beginning of the second posttransplantation month signifies the patient's entry into the period of greatest risk for life-threatening infection. Whereas in the first month, the major determinants of infection are the technical skill with which the surgery is performed and the nosocomial epidemiologic hazards encountered, the effects of sustained immunosuppressive therapy are now sufficient to affect adversely the patient's ability to resist microbial invasion. As a consequence of the immunosuppressive therapy, and directly related to its intensity and type, the immunomodulating viruses (CMV, EBV, the hepatitis viruses, and HIV) have their greatest clinical impact in this period.

Two aspects of the infections that occur in this time period merit special attention: 1) the range of clinical effects that these viruses have, which is far greater than those observed with the identical organisms in the nonimmunosuppressed host; and 2) the critical role of immunosuppressive therapy in modulating the clinical events that occur during this time [1,3].

Impact of Viral Infection on the Transplant Recipient

When clinical infection due to viral pathogens occurs in nonimmunosuppressed patients, the patient either recovers or succumbs to the direct consequences of the virus. In the transplant recipient, the direct consequences of viral infection are frequently superseded by the indirect effects. Thus, the possible clinical consequences of viral infection must be considered in four subgroups [1,3]:

1. The *direct* production of such infectious disease syndromes as fever, mononucleosis, pneumonia, hepatitis, and the like.
2. The *indirect* effects of viral infection include the following:
   A. The production of a state of immunosuppression *in addition to* that induced by the antirejection therapy being administered, such that the patient is at increased risk of invasive infection with such opportunistic pathogens as *P. carinii*, *L. monocytogenes*, and *Aspergillus* species in the absence of an excessive epidemiologic exposure.
   B. The initiation of a series of events that lead to diminished allograft function and permanent injury by processes other than direct infection or classical rejection.
   C. The participation of the virus in the process of oncogenesis.

Data suggest that the link between the direct effects of a particular virus and the indirect effects is the release of cytokines by the host in response to viral invasion (see later).

Effects of Immunosuppressive Therapy on the Occurrence of Infection

Since the first days of clinical transplantation in humans, it has been apparent that the main determinant of the pathogenesis of infection in these patients is the immunosuppressive therapy that is administered. Over the ensuing decades, important information has emerged regarding the relationship between immunosuppressive therapy and infection. This information may be summarized as follows:

1. Of all the immunosuppressive agents administered, the class of agents with the most global depressant effect on host defenses is corticosteroids. A second adverse effect of corticosteroids in these patients is that the antiinflammatory effects of corticosteroids can often mask clinical symptoms of invasive infection until late in the clinical course. For example, it is not uncommon for transplant patients with perforating sigmoid diverticulitis to continue to have bowel movements and to be without physical signs of peritoneal irritation up to the point when they lapse into septic shock. Thus, central to modern immunosuppressive therapy is the concept of *steroid sparing therapy*, using multiple alternative agents that allow the use of relatively low-dose steroid therapy (aiming for a maintenance dose no > 10–15 mg/day) while still controlling rejection [1].
2. Immunosuppressive regimens need to be scrutinized not just for the effects of individual components of the regimen but for the totality of effects produced by the entire regimen. Thus, when antithymocyte globulin (ATG) is added to azathioprine and prednisone, there is a marked increase in the incidence of clinical disease due to CMV. This adverse effect can be attenuated, while still maintaining the beneficial antirejection effects, by decreasing the doses of azathioprine and prednisone by > 50% for the duration of the ATG therapy [29]. A second example of this phenomenon was observed in cardiac transplant patients who received prolonged courses of OKT3, an anti–T-

cell monoclonal antibody, in addition to full doses of cyclosporine, azathioprine, and prednisone. These patients had an excessive incidence of EBV-related, posttransplantation lymphoproliferative disorder (PTLD) [30]. In contrast, patients in whom the doses of the other drugs were decreased in conjunction with the OKT3 therapy were spared the increased rate of PTLD. Thus, by manipulating each component of the immunosuppressive program, one can increase or decrease the incidence of important infection [1].

3. Studies carried out in a murine model of CMV, in which different immunosuppressive drugs were administered in dosage schedules that were equipotent in terms of their antirejection effects, have shed considerable light on the interactions of the different components of the immunosuppressive program. In these studies, the two major stages of CMV infection were studied—the reactivation of the virus from latency, and the systemic dissemination of the virus, which, in normal hosts, is prevented by major histocompatibility complex (MHC)-restricted, virus-specific, cytotoxic T cells. Whereas ATG and anti-CD3 antibodies were potent activators of latent virus, cyclosporine, FK-506, rapamycin, and prednisone had no ability to activate the virus. In contrast, once virus had been activated and was replicating, cyclosporine and FK-506 greatly amplified the spread of the virus because of their effects on the key anti-CMV host defense, the cytotoxic T cell. In contrast, ATG and anti-CD3 were only moderately active in this regard. Indeed, we refer to cyclosporine and FK-506 as "in vivo polymerase chain reactions (PCR) for CMV." Not surprisingly, then, the situation most calculated to cause serious clinical disease due to CMV (and to the closely related herpes group virus, EBV) is when ATG or OKT3 therapy is followed or accompanied by high-dose cyclosporine or FK-506 therapy [1,31].

Infection More Than 6 Months Post-transplantation

Patients with functioning allografts more than 6 months posttransplantation can be divided into three general categories in terms of their infectious disease problems:

1. Approximately 75% of patients have good allograft function and are being maintained on minimal immunosuppression. Their infectious disease problems are largely related to exposures within the community, and are of three types:
   A. Community-acquired respiratory infections, with influenza, respiratory syncytial virus, parainfluenza and others having a particular impact on these patients. In general, the rate of both viral pneumonia and secondary bacterial pneumonia associated with these infections is higher than the general population; that is, the etiology is the same, but the incidence of severe disease is increased [32].
   B. Community-acquired gastrointestinal infection after the ingestion of contaminated food or water, due to *Salmonella* species, *L. monocytogenes*, *Campylobacter jejuni*, and others. In general, the duration of disease and the incidence of bacteremia and metastatic infection is greater in the transplant patient than for individuals in the general population [1].
   C. Exposure in the community to one of the geographically restricted systemic mycoses or tuberculosis, which, as previously stated, have a greater incidence of systemic spread than in the general population.

   Because therapies of these infections are not ideal, transplant recipients are cautioned to avoid exotic travel or undue exposure to infection within the community. Disease prevention with vaccine administration is less successful in transplant patients as well, making the avoidance of exposure particularly important.
2. A few individuals, ~ 5% to 15% of the group, will acquire progressive organ dysfunction, malignancy, or full-blown acquired immunodeficiency syndrome (AIDS) due to chronic viral infection. Thus, CMV chorioretinitis (unless intensively treated with ganciclovir) proceeds inexorably to blindness, hepatitis B and C can cause end-stage liver disease and contribute to the development of hepatocellular carcinoma, EBV can initiate PTLD, and HIV infection progresses to AIDS—all occurring at a more rapid and higher rate than in any populations other than those individuals with progressive immune deficiency due to HIV infection unrelated to transplantation [1].
3. A few individuals, again ~ 5% to 15% of transplant patients, who have had a poor result from their transplant (relatively poor allograft function because of repeated episodes of acute or chronic rejection, hence requiring higher than normal doses of immunosuppressive drugs for prolonged periods, and often with chronic immunomodulating viral infection) are at the highest risk for life-threatening opportunistic infection. These "chronic n'er do wells" are at particular risk for *P. carinii* pneumonia, cryptococcosis, listeriosis, and nocardiosis. If their overall clinical state cannot be reversed, then consideration should be given to chronic prophylaxis with trimethoprim–sulfamethoxazole (TMP-SMX) and fluconazole (see later). Recurrent CMV infection, squamous cell carcinomas, or herpes simplex infections may necessitate long-term antiviral or chemotherapeutic approaches in these individuals [1].

INFECTIONS OF PARTICULAR IMPORTANCE IN THE TRANSPLANT RECIPIENT

Cytomegalovirus

Cytomegalovirus (see Chapter 42) is the single most important cause of infectious disease morbidity and mortality in transplant patients, with evidence of active viral replication being found in 50% to 75% of transplant recipients. Three patterns of CMV transmission, each with a different risk for clinically overt disease, may be observed [1,31]:

1. *Primary CMV infection* occurs when latently infected cells from a CMV-seropositive donor (D+) are administered to a CMV-seronegative recipient (R–). More than 90% of the time, those cells are contained in the allograft; occasionally, viable leukocytes in blood transfusions can transmit the virus. Approximately 60% of individuals at risk for primary CMV infection become clinically ill. D+R- transplants account for 10% to 15% of all transplants (D-R- transplants account for a similar number) [1,31–35].
2. *Reactivation CMV infection* occurs when a CMV-seropositive individual (D±R+) reactivates endogenous latent virus. When conventional cyclosporine (or FK-506)-based immunosuppression is used in transplant patients, the incidence of clinical disease is ~ 10%; when anti-lymphocyte antibody therapy is used in the first 5 to 7 days posttransplantation as "induction" therapy, the incidence of clinical disease is 24%; and when anti-lymphocyte antibody therapy (either ATG or OKT3) is used to treat allograft rejection, > 60% of seropositive individuals not receiving effective antiviral prophylaxis become ill from CMV infection. Approximately 70% to 80% of patients coming to transplantation are CMV seropositive [1,31, 36,37].
3. *Superinfection with CMV* occurs when a CMV-seropositive recipient (R+) receives an allograft from a seropositive donor (D+), and the virus that is reactivated is of donor origin. Although the data base for making this statement is quite incomplete, there is the general impression that the rate of clinical disease is somewhat higher in patients with superinfection as opposed to reactivation infection. An estimated 25% to 35% of transplant patients have CMV superinfection [1,31,38,39].

Whatever form of CMV infection is operative, clinically overt disease usually (> 90% of the time) presents in the time period 1 to 4 months posttransplantation. Two exceptions to this pattern may be observed: an individual who is still CMV seronegative after this period can acquire primary CMV disease because of acquisition of the virus in the community after intimate contact; an occasional seropositive patient with severe bacterial infection, such as urosepsis, can acquire symptomatic CMV disease 3 to 4 weeks later because of cytokine release, particularly tumor necrosis factor (TNF) or TNF release during the septic episode, and its subsequent effects on viral reactivation (see later).

The general pattern of clinical disease due to CMV is similar in all forms of organ transplantation, with one notable exception: the organ transplanted is far more vulnerable than are native organs; for example, CMV hepatitis is a significant problem only in liver transplant patients, CMV myocarditis in heart transplant patients, and CMV pancreatitis in pancreas transplant patients, whereas the attack rate for CMV pneumonia is many times higher in lung and heart–lung transplant patients [1,31]. The spectrum of clinical illness produced by CMV ranges from asymptomatic shedding of virus (most common in patients with reactivation infection), to a complex of symptoms that resembles infectious mononucleosis and has been termed the *CMV syndrome*, to life-threatening disease. The CMV syndrome typically refers to a prolonged episode of otherwise unexplained fever associated with constitutional symptoms in concert with such laboratory abnormalities as leukopenia (with or without thrombocytopenia), a mild atypical lymphocytosis (usually < 10% of the circulating leukocytes and often not seen), and a mild, usually transient hepatitis. Severe CMV disease consists of severe leukopenia and thrombocytopenia, pneumonia, gastrointestinal ulcerations and perforation, and, in the liver transplant patient, severe hepatitis. Not infrequently, opportunistic superinfection with other pathogens further complicates the course of severe CMV infection. CMV chorioretinitis is a late manifestation of systemic CMV infection, presenting 4 months or more posttransplantation. Chorioretinitis may follow earlier clinical manifestations of CMV infection or be the first manifestation of CMV disease [1,31]. A unique clinical syndrome of interstitial pneumonitis is observed in the bone marrow transplant recipient after marrow engraftment. Although many of these forms of pneumonitis are idiopathic, up to 50% are observed in CMV-seropositive recipients and are preventable with empiric antiviral therapy. This disease likely reflects both CMV infection and the emerging T-cell, cytotoxic response to CMV antigens. Both in bone marrow transplants and solid-organ transplants, the degree of MHC mismatch appears to contribute to the incidence and severity of disease [40].

The most valuable diagnostic test for managing clinical CMV disease is the demonstration of viremia (although invasive biopsies of tissue are even more specific, but are usually not available until relatively late in the disease course). Viremia is usually present as early as 5 to 7 days before the onset of clinical disease and continues until death or effective treatment. Demonstration of "shed" virus in respiratory secretions and urine may be found in most transplant patients, and hence correlates poorly with clinical events. Similarly, serial measurements of antibody not only correlate poorly with clinical events ("diagnostic rises" in antibody titers or the appearance of IgM antibody) but are too delayed to allow for use in clinical decision making. Hence, the major use of antibody testing is to characterize donor and recipient at the time of transplant in an effort to guide preventative strategies. The major question is how to demonstrate viremia: although the gold standard remains cell culture with cytopathic effect as an endpoint, this may require up to 6 weeks for definitive results, which is unacceptable in this era of antiviral chemotherapy; the shell vial technique is rapid, but has a sensitivity of < 50%; the CMV antigenemia assay and quantitative PCR are now the diagnostic tests of choice, with both yielding > 90% sensitivity and specificity [1,31,41–50].

Although still somewhat controversial, there is increasing evidence that CMV contributes to the pathogenesis of allograft injury (as well as to GVHD in bone marrow transplant patients). CMV infection has been particularly linked to accelerated coronary artery atherosclerosis in cardiac allograft recipients, to bronchiolitis obliterans in lung transplant recipients, to certain forms of hepatic injury in liver transplant patients, to an unusual glomerulopathy in renal transplant patients, as well as to more conventional patterns of rejection. The problem has been that each of these lesions has also been observed in patients without viral infection. Direct viral injury and immunologic mimicry (sequence homology and immunologic cross-reactivity between a portion of the immediate early antigen of CMV and the human leukocyte antigen-DR beta chain, and the production by CMV-infected cells of a glycoprotein homologous to MHC class I antigens) have been described. An immune response to CMV that could cross-react with the allograft and produce injury has, therefore, been suggested as a possible mechanism by which CMV could damage the allograft. A third hypothesis also accounts for the occurrence of such processes as bronchiolitis obliterans in patients without CMV: cytokines elaborated in the course of CMV infection (and other processes) affect the display of histocompatibility antigens and thus modulate the immune response to the allograft. Thus, CMV is not the only way to cause these reactions, it is just a common way [1]. A report in which allograft dysfunction was successfully treated with ganciclovir, and not increased immunosuppression, is particularly interesting in this regard [51].

As discussed previously, the nature of the immunosuppressive therapy administered has a major influence on the course of CMV infection. Relatively recent data have emphasized the role of TNF and other cytokines in the pathogenesis of CMV-related events. The excessive rate of CMV infection induced by anti-lymphocyte antibody administration has now been shown to be largely related to release of TNF. It is clear, as well, that the occasional cases of CMV disease that follow other circumstances in which TNF is released (e.g., severe allograft rejection and urosepsis) are due to the same mechanism [52–54].

The proposed linkage between rejection and CMV disease appears to be mediated by cytokines as well and seems to be *bidirectional*: in addition to the TNF–CMV activation mechanism, it is now apparent that gamma-interferon (and presumably other cytokines) elaborated in response to CMV infection upregulate the display of histocompatibility antigens on the allograft, thus promoting rejection [1]. Finally, CMV disease appears to be a significant risk factor in the occurrence of EBV-related PTLD, with a greater than sevenfold increase in PTLD in patients with CMV, probably because of the effects of growth factors and cytokines elaborated in the course of the CMV infection, but also because GVHD, allograft rejection, and immune suppression are major activators of latent viral infection [1,55].

Given the myriad of effects due to CMV, considerable effort has been directed at controlling it. Intravenous ganciclovir, at a dose of 5 mg/kg twice daily (with dosage correction in the face of renal dysfunction), for 2 to 3 weeks is quite effective in treating symptomatic disease. Because ganciclovir-resistant CMV has never been described in organ transplant patients, and because foscarnet is significantly more toxic, there appears to be little reason to recommend the latter's use. Relapse, which may develop several times after seemingly effective treatment, occurs in ~ 10% of seropositive individuals and in > 60% of those with primary infection. Based on apparent success in several cases with multiple relapses, we now routinely add oral ganciclovir at a dose of 2 to 3 g/day for 10 weeks to the conventional intravenous course of therapy for those with primary infection. Many clinicians add anti-CMV hyperimmune globulin to the treatment program in patients with severe disease [1,2].

Far less clear is the appropriate way to prevent CMV disease, which would be far preferable. As delineated in Table 45-1, both hyperimmune globulin and high-dose oral acyclovir are moderately effective in preventing disease in patients seropositive before transplantation, although this benefit is attenuated by antirejection anti-lymphocyte antibody therapy [1,3]. Prevention in those at risk for primary disease, particularly in the recipients of the extrarenal organs, is far more difficult. At present, only extended courses of intravenous ganciclovir have shown clear-cut efficacy in these patients [56]. An important question is whether intravenous ganciclovir followed by oral ganciclovir will offer adequate protection.

Two forms of *preemptive* therapy (see later) have been described: monitoring patients for preclinical viremia and treating on that basis without any prophylaxis [57]; and the administration of ganciclovir during anti-lymphocyte antibody therapy [36,37]. Both offer considerable protection, and the concept of linking a particular antimicrobial strategy to the type of immunosuppression used is especially appealing.

TABLE 45-1. *Estimated efficacies of different prophylactic antiviral strategies against cytomegalovirus (CMV) infection in different forms of organ transplantation*[a]

Type of transplant	Form of CMV infection	Antimicrobial strategy used	Estimated efficacy
Kidney	Primary	CMV hyperimmune globulin	2+
		High-dose acyclovir	2+
		CMV hyperimmune globulin + moderate-dose acyclovir	3+
	Secondary[b]	High-dose acyclovir	3+
		CMV hyperimmune globulin + moderate-dose acyclovir	3+
Heart or lung	Primary	High-dose ganciclovir (1 mo)	0
	Secondary[a]	High-dose ganciclovir (1 mo)	4+
Liver	Primary	CMV hyperimmune globulin	0
	Secondary[a]	CMV hyperimmune globulin	3+

[a]Unless otherwise noted, the regimens outlined were administered for a minimum of 3 mo. Only semi-quantitative assessments of efficacy are given, because of the recognition that the type of immunosuppression used will have a major effect on the efficacy of each of these regimens.

[b]Patients were not differentiated in the studies as to whether they had reactivation or superinfection; all patients seropositive for CMV before transplantation are grouped together.

(Modified from Rubin RH, Tolkoff-Rubin NE. Antimicrobial strategies in the care of organ transplant recipients. *Antimicrob Agents Chemother* 1993;37:619–624.)

Epstein-Barr Virus

Active EBV replication (see Chapter 42) is present in 20% to 30% of organ transplant patients on maintenance immunosuppression (slightly higher than the general population), rising to > 80% during anti-lymphocyte antibody therapy of acute rejection. Although a mononucleosis-like syndrome (usually heterophile negative in this patient population) comparable to that produced by CMV has been shown to be due to EBV in some patients, the critical impact of EBV is in its role in the pathogenesis of PTLD [1,55].

Posttransplantation lymphoproliferative disorder is a B-cell lymphoproliferative process that ranges in severity from a benign polyclonal process that responds to a decrease in immunosuppressive therapy (± antiviral therapy) to a highly malignant monoclonal process resistant to all forms of treatment. It is frequently totally extranodal in presentation, with brain involvement, invasion of the allograft, gastrointestinal tract disease, and liver invasion being not uncommon. The pathogenesis of this process is related to the effects of immunosuppressive therapy on the usual mechanisms for preventing the outgrowth of EBV-infected, immortalized B cells. As with CMV, the cornerstone of this defense is EBV-specific, MHC-restricted, cytotoxic T cells, which destroy the EBV-infected B cells. Cyclosporine and FK-506 have a dose-related inhibitory effect on this defense, and thus on the incidence of PTLD. OKT3 and ATG contribute to the pathogenesis of PTLD at two levels: they inhibit the surveillance mechanism, but, even more important, as with CMV, are their potent effects in reactivating latent EBV, thus increasing the potential for outgrowth of immortalized B cells. Other risk factors for PTLD include primary EBV infection, the level of virus replicating in the oropharynx, and, as previously discussed, preceding CMV disease [1,55].

Other than decreasing immunosuppression, which will result in regression of 20% to 30% of these processes, therapy of PTLD remains unclear. Most groups use high-dose acyclovir or ganciclovir in hopes that EBV is still driving the process, although evidence that infection susceptible to antiviral therapy is present at the time of development of PTLD is lacking. Patients not responding to these measures are usually treated with some combination of chemotherapy, radiation therapy, and surgery—with frequently disappointing results. Other experimental therapies include interferon, an anti–B-cell antibody, and, perhaps most interesting, the adoptive transfer of activated cytotoxic T cells [1,55].

Clearly, this process would best be prevented. Both antivirals commonly used in transplant patients, ganciclovir and acyclovir, can inhibit EBV replication. The critical question is whether this will interrupt the pathogenesis of PTLD, either directly through effects on EBV replication, or indirectly through effects on CMV [1,55].

Viral Hepatitis

The course of both HBV and HCV infection is accelerated in these immunosuppressed patients compared with the general population, with both progressive liver failure and cirrhosis with hepatocellular carcinoma occurring as consequences of these infections (see Chapter 42). With modern serologic testing, it is now uncommon for patients to acquire HBV infection at the time of transplantation from either the donor of the organ or from blood. This is fortunate, because the acquisition of HBV at the time of transplantation has a relatively high incidence of acute hepatic failure. The bigger problem clinically is the question of disease progression in HBV-infected individuals after transplantation. By 10 years posttransplantation, more than half of these individuals will have progressed to end-stage liver disease or hepatocellular carcinoma. Before that, the greatest impact of HBV infection on the transplant recipient is in increasing the net state of immunosuppression, with an increased incidence of extrahepatic infection occurring as a consequence [9].

Hepatitis B has a particularly detrimental effect on liver transplant recipients. Recurrent HBV infection occurs in 80% to 90% of patients undergoing liver transplantation, and 1-year survival in these patients has been 50% to 60% (significantly less than the 80% to 85% survival seen in other patient groups). Recurrent disease is rare in patients being transplanted for fulminant hepatic failure due to HBV or in those with simultaneous delta virus infection. The range of clinical disease that results from recurrent HBV infection is quite broad: mild, persistent hepatitis to aggressive, chronic hepatitis and fulminant liver failure. The administration of 10,000 units of hyperimmune anti-HBV immunoglobulin during the anhepatic phase, followed by daily administration for 6 days, and then administration at ~ 3- to 6-week intervals to maintain the anti-hepatitis B surface antigen titer at > 1 : 100 IU appears to provide significant protection against recurrent liver disease and to increase patient survival. However, the indefinite need for this therapy adds $15,000 to $25,000 to the first-year costs (and continues to be a significant cost thereafter). It is to be hoped that the advent of lamivudine therapy or of other antiviral therapies under development will achieve cost-effective management of this and other forms of HBV infection in the transplant patient [58].

Hepatitis C virus infection is the major cause of infection in transplant patients. It is the most common single cause of hepatic failure leading to liver transplantation, recurs almost universally after liver transplantation, and causes chronic infection in 5% to 15% of transplant recipients. In the first few years posttransplantation, the major impact of HCV infection is its contribution to the net state of immunosuppression. After that, there is slow progression of chronic liver disease such that by 10 years posttransplantation, an estimated 10% to 25% of these individuals have serious morbidity and some mortality from chronic liver disease (and, occasionally, hepatocellular carcinoma). Interferon therapy is far less effective in this patient population than in the nonimmunosuppressed patient population [10].

Approximately 5% of all donors are anti-HCV positive, with approximately half of these being positive by PCR assay for circulating viral RNA. Organs from PCR-positive individuals are extremely efficient at transmitting virus to the recipient. Given the relatively slow pace of HCV illness and the continuing shortage of donors, there has been great controversy about whether to accept anti–HCV-positive donors. Reserving these organs for anti–HCV-positive recipients appears not to be a viable alternative because superinfection with donor-strain HCV appears to occur commonly. Our policy is to reserve organs from anti–HCV-positive donors for critically ill heart and liver patients, for highly sensitized renal patients, and for older patients (with potentially shorter life spans during which the hepatitis would progress). Even in these circumstances, ethical considerations require full disclosure to the individuals involved regarding the potential consequences of such an action [10,11].

Mycobacterial Infections

Infection due to *M. tuberculosis* has been less of a problem after transplantation than might have been predicted (see Chapter 32). Despite immunosuppressive therapy, reactivation and dissemination of *M. tuberculosis* have been exceedingly uncommon in individuals whose only evidence of dormant tuberculosis is a positive tuberculin test. Conversely, patients with 1) a history of active tuberculosis (treated or untreated); 2) an abnormal chest radiograph; 3) nonwhite racial background; 4) protein-calorie malnutrition; or 5) another immunosuppressing illness, in addition to a positive tuberculin test, are at significant risk for reactivating their tuberculosis. It is our approach to reserve antituberculous prophylaxis for those with added risk factors, in addition to a positive tuberculin skin test, for several reasons: we have now followed more than 100 "low-risk" individuals posttransplantation for periods of up to 10 years, without a single case of reactivation despite the positive tuberculin reaction; the high background rate of hepatocellular dysfunction in these patients makes the use of isoniazid or rifampin challenging in these patients; and antituberculous drugs affect the pharmacokinetic profile of cyclosporine and FK-506, rendering the use of these drugs more difficult as well [1].

Atypical mycobacterial infection may also be observed in transplant recipients: Local or disseminated disease due to *Mycobacterium kansasii* and progressive skin infection due to *Mycobacterium marinum*, *Mycobacterium haemophilum*, and *Mycobacterium chelonei* has been reported. These infections typically present initially at sites of cutaneous injury. Management usually involves surgery and chemotherapy based on in vitro antimicrobial susceptibility testing [1].

Fungal Infections

The fungal infections that affect transplant recipients can be divided into two general categories: 1) disseminated primary or reactivated infection with one of the geographically restricted systemic mycoses (histoplasmosis, blastomycosis, and coccidioidomycosis), and 2) invasive opportunistic infections with such organisms as *Candida* species, *Aspergillus* species, *C. neoformans*, and the Mucoraceae. The first category of disease should be considered in patients with a history of recent or remote travel to an endemic region who present with one of the following clinical syndromes: subacute respiratory illness, with focal, disseminated, or miliary infiltrates on chest radiograph; a nonspecific, systemic, febrile illness; unexplained pancytopenia; and an illness in which metastatic aspects of the infection predominate (e.g., mucocutaneous manifestations in histoplasmosis and blastomycosis or central nervous system manifestations in coccidioidomycosis or histoplasmosis) [1,59,60].

The opportunistic fungal infections have a far greater impact on the transplant patient than do the endemic mycoses. Primary infection, usually of the lungs, but occasionally of the nasal sinuses, may occur in patients who inhale air contaminated with *Aspergillus* species, *C. neoformans* or, particularly in diabetic patients, Mucoraceae. In addition, secondary infection of wounds and hematomas and intravenous lines by *Candida* or *Aspergillus* species may occur. Evidence of metastatic infection may follow either primary or secondary fungal infection, with the skin and central nervous system being common sites of presentation. Fungal infection is a particular concern at the broncheal anastomotic site of lung transplant recipients, with chronic infection and occasional dehiscence [1,58,59].

In the past, the cornerstone of antifungal therapy has been amphotericin B. However, even in the precyclosporine era, use of this nephrotoxic agent in the transplant recipient was difficult. In the postcyclosporine era, the synergistic nephrotoxicity produced by amphotericin B and cyclosporine has become more complicated. Fortunately, the newer triazole antifungal agent fluconazole has been shown to be both effective and nontoxic in the treatment of many invasive candidal, cryptococcal, and dermatophytic infections in the transplant recipient concurrently treated with cyclosporine. Preliminary experience with another triazole, itraconazole, suggests that it may be an alternative agent to amphotericin B for the treatment of infections due to the *Aspergillus* species. However, experience suggests that this agent may be more appropriate for secondary therapy after amphotericin or in patients suffering amphotericin-related toxicities. Liposomal formulations of amphotericin may also allow further antifungal treatment in such patients intolerant of standard amphotericin [1,59–62].

Pneumocystis carinii

Long considered a protozoan, *P. carinii* (see Chapter 43) has been shown, by molecular taxonomic studies, to be more appropriately regarded as a fungus. Regardless of this detail of classification, effective therapy thus far has been provided by drugs having antiprotozoan (as opposed to antifungal) profiles. The incidence of *Pneumocystis* pneumonia in organ transplant patients not receiving anti-*Pneumocystis* prophylaxis is 10% to 15%, depending on the institution. Traditionally, such infection have been regarded as immunosuppression-induced reactivation of infection acquired in childhood. However, the possibility of immunosuppressed person-to-immunosuppressed person spread (possibly by an aerosolized route) exists. It is our policy, therefore, to isolate patients with *P. carinii* pneumonia from other immunosuppressed patients, including transplant recipients [1,4].

In transplant recipients, *P. carinii* infection typically occurs either in the period 1 to 6 months posttransplantation, often in association with CMV infection, or in the late period, typically in the subgroup of patients with poor allograft function, excessive immunosuppression, and chronic viral infection [1,4].

When *Pneumocystis* pneumonia does develop, it is a subacute disease characterized by fever, nonproductive cough, and progressive dyspnea with hypoxemia occurring over several days, and the presence of an interstitial infiltrate on chest radiograph. Administration of low-dose TMP-SMX (one single-strength tablet at bedtime) is effective in the prevention of *Pneumocystis* pneumonia and is routinely used in our transplant recipients. Alternative therapies are less effective but include monthly aerosolized or intravenous pentamidine, atovaquone, and clindamycin with pyrimethamine. Because treatment of confirmed *Pneumocystis* pneumonia with high-dose TMP-SMX or parenteral pentamidine in transplant recipients is associated with a high rate of side effects, particularly bone marrow and renal toxicity, the importance of prevention cannot be overemphasized [1,4].

PRINCIPLES OF ANTIMICROBIAL THERAPY IN TRANSPLANT RECIPIENTS

Problem-Directed Prophylactic Strategies

There are several challenges of antimicrobial therapy in transplant recipients: Many of the antimicrobial agents are themselves toxic and, frequently, that toxicity is exacerbated by cyclosporine, the cornerstone of current immunosuppressive regimens. Prolonged courses of therapy with these toxic agents are required to achieve adequate treatment of clinically overt disease. Once disease has occurred, the infected tissue may become vulnerable to infection with other organisms (secondary infections). The only way to avoid these difficulties is to shift the emphasis of infectious disease management of the transplant recipient to the prevention of infectious complications. This principle has led to development of prophylactic strategies directed toward specific problems, such as prevention of urinary tract infection in the renal transplant patient, prevention of procedure-related complications in the liver transplant recipient, prevention of toxoplasmosis in the heart transplant recipient, and prevention of *P. carinii* infection in all transplant recipients. All of these strategies have proved to be useful and cost-effective approaches to disease prevention [1,2].

The practice of routine prophylaxis is best illustrated by the use of TMP-SMX (one single-strength tablet daily) for 6 months after transplantation. As a result of this practice, a large series of common infections are prevented without perturbing the anaerobic flora of the gastrointestinal tract. Among the infections generally prevented are those due to *P. carinii*, *T. gondii*, *L. monocytogenes*, *N. asteroides*, susceptible organisms involved in urinary tract infections due to Enterobacteriaceae; sinopulmonary infections due to *S. pneumoniae* and *H. influenzae*; and gastrointestinal infections due to *Salmonella* and *Shigella* species. Four aspects of patient care are altered by the routine use of TMP-SMX: 1) infections, when they occur, are rarely due to these pathogens; 2) the presence of these pathogens in a compliant patient suggests an increased epidemiologic exposure or excessive immune suppression (e.g., high-dose steroids, drug-induced neutropenia, CMV infection); 3) in the absence of increased risk, mechanical factors (obstruction, hematoma, lymphocele, indwelling stent, anastomotic leak) must be considered; the mechanical factors may not be directly related to surgery; sinusitis or diabetic foot infections provide common sites of infection; and 4) infections, when they occur, are usually due to antibiotic-resistant, often nosocomially acquired, organisms. Initial clinical evaluations and therapies must be aggressive (e.g., invasive procedures, broad-spectrum antibiotics) to identify and reverse the infectious process and any predisposing factors, and to obtain appropriate microbiologic data to guide further therapies [1,2].

Two examples of the limitations of prophylaxis are relevant. The use of daily quinolone prophylaxis in renal transplant recipients successfully prevents urinary tract infections in the absence of mechanical obstruction. However, a 10% to 14% incidence of *P. carinii* pneumonia is observed in these individuals. The routine use of fluconazole prophylaxis successfully prevents infections due to susceptible yeasts. However, these patients and these institutions experience, over time, a shift to colonization and infection with resistant yeasts (e.g., *Candida glabrata*, *Candida krusei*) and filamentous fungi (e.g., *Aspergillus* and *Mucorales* species) Thus, individualized antifungal strategies (for those at greatest risk because of prolonged antibiotic use or those already colonized) may be preferred [1,2].

Preemptive Therapy

A newer mode of antimicrobial therapy, called preemptive therapy, has been described. Traditionally, antimicrobial therapy has been administered either prophylactically to a large number of patients at risk of disease, before there is evidence of infection, to prevent serious disease in a few, or therapeutically to the few in whom tissue invasion and clinically overt disease are present. Typically, prophylactic regimens involve the administration of a nontoxic drug, often with less-than-ideal antimicrobial activity, for a prolonged period of time, whereas therapeutic regimens use the most effective medications, often at toxic doses, for shorter periods of time. Preemptive therapy combines the most desirable aspects of these two options—administration of highly effective therapy over a short period of time to a relatively small number of patients who are at risk of serious infection. The short duration of therapy reduces the potential toxicity, and clinical and laboratory markers may be used to determine predictors of serious infection. For example, preemptive therapy with low-dose ganciclovir, administered in conjunction with OKT3 therapy, to CMV-seropositive renal transplant recipients appears to be a promising approach to the prevention of CMV disease. Similarly, the early use of fluconazole to eradicate asymptomatic candiduria in renal transplant recipients, to prevent progression to urinary tract obstruction and pyelonephritis, and use of fluconazole in association with surgical manipulation of a pulmonary nodule due to *Cryptococcus* to prevent cryptococcal meningitis, are other examples of preemptive therapy [1,36,37,63].

Future Trends

Given the therapeutic constraints imposed by the necessary immunosuppressive regimen and the devastation that infection may cause in the transplant recipient, appropriate emphasis is increasingly being placed on evaluation of predictors of serious infection. New technologies, including molecular hybridization and PCR, may allow the cost-effective screening and detection of "at-risk" individuals most in need of preemptive treatments. Development of clinical epidemiologic data bases and appropriate laboratory markers will permit further major advances beyond the preemptive approach to infection in this ever-increasing and challenging population of patients.

REFERENCES

1. Rubin RH. Infection in the organ transplant recipient. In: Rubin RH, Young LS, eds. *Clinical approach to infection in the compromised host.* 3rd ed. New York: Plenum Press; 1994:629–705.
2. Rubin RH, Tolkoff-Rubin NE. Antimicrobial strategies in the care of organ transplant recipients. *Antimicrob Agents Chemother* 1993;37: 619–624.
3. Rubin RH, Wolfson JS, Cosimi AB, et al. Infection in the renal transplant recipient. *Am J Med* 1981;70:405–411.
4. Fishman JA. *Pneumocystis carinii* and parasitic infections in transplantation. *Infect Dis Clin North Am* 1995;9:1005–1044.

5. Sable CA, Hayden FG. Orthomyxoviral and paramyxoviral infections in transplant patients. *Infect Dis Clin North Am* 1995;9:987–1003.
6. Hopkins C, Weber DJ, Rubin RH. Invasive *Aspergillus* infection: possible non-ward common source within the hospital environment. *J Hosp Infect* 1989;12:19–25.
7. Rubin RH. The compromised host as sentinel chicken. *N Engl J Med* 1987;317:1151–1153.
8. Fischer SA, Trenholme GM, Levin S. Fever in the solid organ transplant patient. *Infect Dis Clin North Am* 1996;10:167–184.
9. Davis CL, Gretch DR, Carithers RL Jr. Hepatitis B and transplantation. *Infect Dis Clin North Am* 1995;9:925–941.
10. Terrault NA, Wright TL, Pereira BJG. Hepatitis C infection in the transplant recipient. *Infect Dis Clin North Am* 1995;9:943–964.
11. Fishman JA, Rubin RH, Koziel M, Pereira BJG. Hepatitis C virus and organ transplantation. *Transplantation* 1996;62:147–154.
12. Rubin RH. Infectious disease complications of renal transplantation. *Kidney Int* 1993;44:221–236.
13. Rubin RH, Tolkoff-Rubin NE. The problem of human immunodeficiency virus (HIV) infection and transplantation. *Transplant Int* 1988; 1:36–42.
14. Luft BJ, Naot Y, Araujo FG, et al. Primary and reactivated *Toxoplasma* infection in patients with cardiac transplants. *Ann Intern Med* 1983;99: 27–31.
15. McGregor CG, Fleck DG, Nogington J, et al. Disseminated toxoplasmosis in cardiac transplantation. *J Clin Pathol* 1984;37:74–77.
16. Hakim M, Esmore D, Wallwork J, et al. Toxoplasmosis in cardiac transplantation. *Br Med J* 1986;292:1108.
17. Michaels MG, Wald ER, Fricker FJ, et al. Toxoplasmosis in pediatric recipients of heart transplants. *J Clin Infect Dis* 1992;14:847–851.
18. Nelson PW, Delmonicao FL, Tolkoff-Rubin NE, et al. Unsuspected donor *Pseudomonas* infection causing arterial disruption after renal transplantation. *Transplantation* 1984;37:313–314.
19. Gottesdiener KM. Transplanted infections: donor-to-host transmission with the allograft. *Ann Intern Med* 1989;110:1001–1016.
20. McCoy GC, Loening S, Braun WE, et al. The fate of cadaver renal allografts contaminated before transplantation. *Transplantation* 1975;20: 467–472.
21. Doig RL, Boyd PJR, Eykyn S. *Staphylococcus aureus* transmitted in transplanted kidneys. *Lancet* 1975;2:243–244.
22. McLeish KR, McMurray SD, Smith EJ, et al. The transmission of Candida albicans by cadaveric allografts. *J Urol* 1977;118:513–516.
23. Majeski JA, Alexander JW, First MR, et al. Transplantation of microbially contaminated cadaver kidneys. *Arch Surg* 1982;117:221–224.
24. Spees EK, Light JA, Oakes DD, et al. Experience with cadaver renal allograft contamination before transplantation. *Br J Surg* 1982;69: 482–485.
25. Vander Vliet JA, Tidow G, Koostra G, et al. Transplantation of contaminated organs. *Br J Surg* 1980;67:596–598.
26. Arnow PM. Prevention of bacterial infection in the transplant recipient: the role of selective bowel decontamination. *Infect Dis Clin North Am* 1995;9:849–862.
27. Wiesner RH, Hermans PE, Rakela J, et al. Selective bowel decontamination to decreased gram-negative aerobic bacterial and *Candida* colonization and prevent infection after orthotopic liver transplantation. *Transplantation* 1988;45:570–574.
28. Townsend TR, Rudolf LE, Westervelt FB Jr, et al. Prophylactic antibiotic therapy with cefamandole and tobramycin for patients undergoing renal transplantation. *Infect Control* 1980;1:93–96.
29. Rubin RH, Cosimi AB, Hirsch MS, et al. Effects of antithymocyte globulin on cytomegalovirus infection in renal transplant recipients. *Transplantation* 1981;31:143–145.
30. Swinnen LJ, Costanzo-Nordin MR, Fisher SG, et al. Increased incidence of lymphoproliferative disorder after immunosuppression with the monoclonal antibody OKT3 in cardiac transplant recipients. *N Engl J Med* 1990;323:1723–1728.
31. Rubin RH. Impact of cytomegalovirus infection on organ transplant recipients. *Rev Infect Dis* 1990;12(Suppl 7):S754–S766.
32. Ho M. *Cytomegalovirus: biology and infection*. 2nd ed. New York: Plenum Medical Book; 1991.
33. Cheeseman SH, Rubin RH, Stewart JA, et al. Controlled clinical trial of prophylactic human leucocyte interferon in renal transplantation. effect on cytomegalovirus and herpes simplex virus infection. *N Engl J Med* 1981;300:1345–1349.
34. Betts RF, Freeman RB, Douglas RH Jr, et al. Transmission of cytomegalovirus infection with renal allograft. *Kidney Int* 1975;8: 385–392.
35. Ho M, Suwansirikul S, Dowling JN, et al. The transplanted kidney as a source of cytomegalovirus infection. *N Engl J Med* 1975;293:1109–1112.
36. Hibberd PL, Tolkoff-Rubin NE, Cosimi AB, et al. Symptomatic cytomegalovirus disease in the cytomegalovirus antibody seropositive renal transplant recipient treated with OKT3. *Transplantation* 1992;53: 68–72.
37. Hibberd PL, Tolkoff-Rubin NE, Conti D, et al. Preemptive ganciclovir therapy to prevent cytomegalovirus disease in cytomegalovirus antibody-positive renal transplants recipients. *Ann Intern Med* 1995;123:18–26.
38. Grundy JE, Lui SF, Super M, et al. Symptomatic cytomegalovirus infection in seropositive patients. reinfection with donor virus rather than reactivation of recipient virus. *Lancet* 1988;2:132–135.
39. Chou S. Acquisition of donor strains of cytomegalovirus by renal-transplant recipients. *N Engl J Med* 1986;314:1418–1423.
40. Zaia JA, Forman SJ. Cytomegalovirus infection in the bone marrow transplant recipient. *Infect Dis Clin North Am* 1995;9:879–900.
41. van der Bij W, van Dijk RB, van Son WJ, et al. Antigen test for early diagnosis of active cytomegalovirus infection in heart transplant patients. *J Heart Transplant* 1988;7:106–110.
42. van den Berg AP, van der Bij W, van Son WJ, et al. Cytomegalovirus antigenemia as a useful marker of symptomatic cytomegalovirus infection after renal transplantation: a report of 130 consecutive patients. *Transplantation* 1989;48:991–995.
43. van den Berg AP, Klompmaker IJ, Haagsma EB, et al. Antigenemia in the diagnosis and monitoring of active cytomegalovirus infection after liver transplantation. *J Infect Dis* 1991;164:265–270.
44. Erice A, Holm MA, Gill PC, et al. Cytomegalovirus (CMV) antigenemia assay is more sensitive than shell vial cultures for rapid detection of CMV in polymorphonuclear blood leukocytes. *J Clin Microbiol* 1992;30:2822–2825.
45. Kosleinen PK, Nieminen MS, Mattila SP, et al. The correlation between symptomatic CMV infection and CMV antigenemia in heart allograft recipients. *Transplantation* 1993;55:547–555.
46. van Dorp WT, Vlieger A, Jiwa NM, et al. The polymerase chain reaction, a sensitive and rapid technique for detecting cytomegalovirus infection after renal transplantation. *Transplantation* 1992;54:661–664.
47. Jiwa NM, van Gemert GW, Raap AK, et al. Rapid detection of human cytomegalovirus DNA in peripheral blood leukocytes of viremic transplant recipients by the polymerase chain reaction. *Transplantation* 1989;48:72–76.
48. Olive DM, Simsek M, Al-Mufti S. Polymerase chain reaction assay for detection of human cytomegalovirus. *J Clin Microbiol* 1989;27: 1238–1242.
49. Fox JC, Griffiths PD, Emery VC. Quantification of human cytomegalovirus DNA using the polymerase chain reaction. *J Gen Virol* 1992;73:2405–2408.
50. Bitsch A, Kirchmer H, Dupke R, et al. Cytomegalovirus transcripts in peripheral blood leukocytes of actively infected transplant patients detected by reverse transcription-polymerase chain reaction. *J Infect Dis* 1993;167:740–743.
51. Reinke P, Fietze E, Ode-Hakim S, et al. Late acute renal allograft rejection and symptomless cytomegalovirus infection. *Lancet* 1994;344: 1737–1738.
52. Stein J, Volk HD, Liebenthal C, et al. Tumour necrosis factor alpha stimulates the activity of the human cytomegalovirus major immediate early enhancer/promoter in immature monocytic cells. *Transplantation* 1994;58:35–41.
53. Docke WD, Prosch S, Fietze E, et al. Cytomegalovirus reactivation and tumour necrosis factor. *Lancet* 1994;343:268–269.
54. Fietze E. Prosch S, Reinke P, et al. Cytomegalovirus infection in transplant recipients: the role of tumour necrosis factor. *Transplantation* 1994;58:675–680.
55. Basgoz N, Preiksaitis JK. Post-transplant lymphoproliferative disorder. *Infect Dis Clin North Am* 1995;9:901–923.
56. Winston DJ, Wirin D, Shaked A, Busuttil RW. Randomized comparison of ganciclovir and high dose acyclovir for long-term cytomegalovirus prophylaxis in liver transplant recipients. *Lancet* 1995; 346:69–74.
57. Singh NT, Yu VL, Mieles L, et al. High dose acyclovir compared with short course preemptive ganciclovir therapy to prevent cytomegalovirus

disease in liver transplant recipients: a randomized trial. *Ann Intern Med* 1994;120:375–381.
58. Dienstag JL, Perillo RP, Schiff ER, et al. A preliminary trial of lamivudine for chronic hepatitis B infection. *N Engl J Med* 1995;333:1657–1661.
59. Hadley S, Karchmer AW. Fungal infections in solid organ transplant recipients. *Infect Dis Clin North Am* 1995;9:1045–1074.
60. Hibberd PL, Rubin RH. Clinical aspects of fungal infection in organ transplant recipients. *Clin Infect Dis* 1994;19(Suppl 1):533–538.
61. Conti DJ, Tolkoff-Rubin NE, Baker GP Jr, et al. Successful treatment of invasive fungal infection with fluconazole in organ transplantation recipients. *Transplantation* 1989;48:692–695.
62. Tolkoff-Rubin NE, Conti DJ, Doran M, et al. Fluconazole in the treatment of invasive candidal and cryptococcal infections in organ transplant recipients. *Pharmacotherapy* 1990;10:1595–1655.
63. Rubin RH. Preemptive therapy in immunocompromised hosts. *N Engl J Med* 1991;324:1057–1059.

Hospital Infections, Fourth Edition,
edited by John V. Bennett and Philip S. Brachman.
Lippincott–Raven Publishers, Philadelphia © 1998

CHAPTER 46

Other Procedure-Related Infections

Robert A. Weinstein and Sharon F. Welbel

With yards of entrails, miles of vascular network, dozens of extravascular spaces, and several organ systems, any patient is a candidate for a staggering array of diagnostic and therapeutic procedures. Although many of these procedures provide information that is essential for sophisticated patient care or to supplant more traumatic intervention, or is critical for life support, most procedures also bypass natural host defenses and place patients at increased risk of nosocomial infection [1,2]. It is not surprising, then, that the introduction of any new procedure is often followed closely by case reports of procedure-associated infections. Occasionally, epidemiologic experiments of nature, in the form of nosocomial outbreaks, provide more detailed information on certain procedure-related hazards, and eventually such hazards may be subjected to prospective study. In this chapter, we discuss a variety of procedure-associated infections that have been highlighted by retrospective or prospective investigations and that have not been discussed elsewhere in this volume.

Because of the seemingly eclectic contents of this chapter, it is important to recognize from the outset that the procedures to be discussed have certain themes in common. First, all the procedures are exquisitely vulnerable to inexperienced operators, to breaks in aseptic technique, to contaminated, inadequately disinfected, or technically difficult-to-clean equipment, or to ineffective antiseptics. Second, many procedure-related infection problems unfortunately reemerge as new generations of healthcare workers rediscover these vulnerabilities—hence the importance of reviewing hazards that at first glance may appear remote. Third, various procedures involving many different sites have as a common site of infection the bloodstream, although the risk of infection differs depending on whether the bloodstream contamination is transient or persistent, as well as on host- and organism-specific factors. Finally, many procedures bear the burden that the specific risks have not been defined sufficiently to determine whether certain preventive measures, such as the use of prophylactic antimicrobial therapy, are mandated.

R.A. Weinstein, S.F. Welbel: Department of Medicine, Rush Medical College, Division of Infectious Diseases, Cook County Hospital, Chicago, Illinois 60612.

INFECTIONS FROM PROCEDURES INVOLVING THE VASCULAR SYSTEM

Phlebotomy

Phlebotomy is one of the oldest and certainly the most common invasive procedure practiced in hospitals and clinics and, ever since the leech was replaced by the sterile hypodermic needle, blood drawing has been regarded by most clinicians as totally safe and simple. In the 1940s, however, it became apparent that despite sterile needles, epidemic jaundice was being transmitted by nonsterile syringes that were used commonly for phlebotomy. With a mock venous system and methylene blue as a marker, investigators showed that reflux occurred from the syringe into the test system when tourniquet pressure was released. By sterilizing syringes between uses, clinic workers abruptly halted the transmission of phlebotomy-associated hepatitis [3].

Historically, the next major risk of phlebotomy to be recognized was staphylococcal septic arthritis of the hip in neonates [4]. In the early 1960s, it was noted that this complication occasionally followed 5 to 9 days after femoral venipuncture. Localized suppuration at the puncture site and thrombosis of the femoral vein, both unusual findings with isolated septic arthritis, suggested a causal relationship between pyoarthritis and a preceding femoral venipuncture. Because it is common to strike the femoral head during femoral venipuncture in neonates (which denotes that the joint capsule has been entered), femoral "sticks" demand the same aseptic conditions used for arthrocentesis, rather than the more lax conditions under which venipuncture is frequently performed. In light of the severe disability that may follow septic arthritis, many pediatricians now condemn the use of neonatal femoral venipuncture and recommend at least 10 other sites for pediatric phlebotomy. When heel punctures are used, the most medial or lateral portion of the heel's plantar surface should be used to avoid calcaneal puncture and osteochondritis [5].

The most recent innovation in blood drawing—the popular and ingeniously simple evacuated collection tube—has streamlined blood collection, but, unfortunately, it has also reintroduced the reflux, or backflow, hazard that was first recognized in the 1940s. When commercial evacuated tubes are not sterilized routinely, they may be a source of hospital-acquired sepsis. One hospital traced an outbreak of five cases of "primary" *Serratia* bacteremia to contaminated commercial vacuum tubes used for blood collection. This outbreak prompted a detailed study of the backflow phenomenon, and it was shown that reflux may occur not only when the tourniquet is released (after active flow of blood into the tube has ceased), but when the tube is tilted upward, when blood touches the stopper, when pressure on the end of the tube compresses the stopper, or when a "short draw" occurs because of insufficient vacuum [6]. Although practices that might increase the risk of backflow are proscribed in the package insert that accompanies many commercial vacuum tubes, such inserts are not always seen by those responsible for blood drawing, and many of the recommendations, particularly those concerning the positioning of patients for phlebotomy, are difficult to follow.

Even when a sterile syringe is used to draw blood, backflow during serial inoculation of vacuum tubes and blood culture bottles can result in cross-contamination and false-positive blood cultures. Although potentially avoidable, such serial inoculation is a convenient and common practice, particularly when blood is obtained in a single syringe for hemogram and culture, and it has resulted in two reported outbreaks of pseudobacteremia [7]. Although none of the patients was affected directly, false-positive cultures put them at risk of unwarranted antibiotic therapy.

More than 500 million commercial evacuated blood collection tubes are used annually in the United States and Canada. The problems cited previously, as well as culture surveys of evacuated blood collection tubes [8], have led to the routine marketing and use of sterile tubes in the United States. The preservative and diagnostic reagents present in many tubes may still pose a risk, one that is probably minimal but not fully evaluated. It is hoped that the major problem of backflow has been solved. Nevertheless, health workers should be aware of the hazard, particularly when investigating the source of an apparently primary bacteremia.

Needleless Intravenous Infusion Systems

Health care workers have always been at risk of needlestick injuries. Because of increased awareness of the transmission of bloodborne pathogens such as hepatitis B and C viruses and human immunodeficiency virus (HIV) secondary to such injuries, needleless systems have been introduced (see Chapters 3, 42, 43). In fact, there appears to have been a decrease in the rate of occupational needlestick exposures since the introduction of needleless systems [9]. The impact for the patient is less clear. In a study to determine risk factors for bloodstream infections in patients receiving home intravenous infusion therapy [10], receipt of total parenteral nutrition and intralipid therapy through a needleless system was a risk factor for bloodstream infection. A survey of injection caps demonstrated that positive cultures were significantly more common from needleless devices than from protected-needle devices. It was concluded that nutrient-rich solutions may remain in the injection caps of the needleless devices and become contaminated during the 7 days that injection caps are manipulated.

Another study that assessed needleless systems used with Hickman catheters suggested that such systems may be associated with increased rates of catheter-related bloodstream infections [11]. In this study, luminal fluid from Hickman catheters of hematology patients was cultured. Hickman catheters with the needleless system were twice as likely to show luminal contamination compared with catheters without the system. Four bloodstream infections in patients with the needleless device had peripheral blood and luminal fluid cultures that yielded concordant bacterial strains, based on results of pulsed-field electrophoresis and restriction fragment polymorphism studies. As needleless systems are used more widely, their risk–benefit ratio will be better defined.

Leeches

Despite the popular appeal of highly sharpened, disposable phlebotomy needles for diagnostic bloodletting, leeches have, in fact, resurfaced as a specialized part of the reconstructive and microvascular surgeons' armamentarium [12]. However, as with many other advances discussed in this chapter, there remains an infectious dark side [13]. *Aeromonas hydrophila*, normal gut flora of the leech, has caused wound infections after as many as 20% of microsurgical procedures using leeches [14]. Reuse of individual leeches also carries the theoretic risk of cross-infection.

Cardiac Catheterization

Serious local and systemic infections may result from cardiac catheterization procedures, particularly when contaminated instruments or ineffective antiseptics (e.g., dilute aqueous benzalkonium chloride) are used inadvertently or when breaks in technique occur in the cardiac catheterization laboratory. The major pathogens are staphylococci and gram-negative bacteria.

Up to 50% of patients undergoing cardiac catheterization experience an increase in temperature of more than 1°C (1.8°F) within 24 hours after catheterization. Their fever, however, has been attributed to the use of angiocardiographic contrast material rather than to infection [15]. In fact, bacterial endocarditis has been reported very rarely in large series evaluating the complications of cardiac catheterization, and individual examples may have been due to concurrent infection that was initially undetected.

In some studies, the febrile reactions after a cardiac catheterization have been traced to pyrogenic endotoxin present in sterile catheters [16]. Reusable cardiac catheters (and disposable catheters, which many institutions now reuse in efforts to contain costs) may be exposed to contaminated distilled water during the initial phases of cleaning. Despite subsequent sterilization, usually by ethylene oxide, residual bacterial endotoxin may be present in the lumen or on the surface of the catheters and lead to sporadic as well as epidemic cases of fever and hypotension after cardiac catheterization. Single-use disposable catheters may prevent this complication. If catheters are reused, rinsing with sterile water before sterilization may lessen the problem.

Pyrogen has also been noted on sterile latex surgical gloves [17]. The incidence of febrile reactions after catheterization was reduced in one study from 11.6% to 0.6% when rinsing of latex gloves before catheterization was made routine [18]. One lot of surgical gloves was called to our attention because of an offensive odor left on wearers' hands. The manufacturer attributed this to "sour" talc used in preparing the gloves. The Food and Drug Administration found high levels of endotoxin on the glove surfaces. However, there are no regulations requiring testing of gloves for endotoxin, and the frequency with which commercially available surgical gloves are contaminated with endotoxin, and its side effects, are unknown.

Transient bacteremia during cardiac catheterization has been observed to occur in 4% to 18% of patients. In the studies reporting such an incidence, however, blood cultures were obtained from the intravascular catheter or from the vessel from which the catheter had been removed; it is therefore possible that some of the isolates represented contamination of the external part of the catheter or the site of insertion and that bacteremia was actually less frequent. In a study designed to assess this possibility, blood for culture was obtained by standard techniques from a vein distant from the site of catheter manipulation [15]. Venous blood cultures of 106 patients, most whom had valvular heart disease, were obtained in this manner during cardiac catheterization, and all were sterile. Three of 38 samples that were drawn through the catheter that was placed in the heart or aorta during the procedure grew diphtheroids or microaerophilic streptococci. It was concluded that contamination of the hub end of the catheter with normal skin flora led to an overestimation of the incidence of bacteremia. Removal of organisms by lung filtration may also have accounted in part for the failure to isolate organisms from distal sites. In either case, it is clear that some contamination of the catheterization cutdown field has occurred. With rigorous application of strict aseptic technique and adoption of the working principle that cardiac catheterization is a surgical procedure, catheterization-associated infection should be very infrequent, and systemic antibiotic prophylaxis does not appear justified.

The most recently described cardiac catheterization problems relate to percutaneous transluminal angioplasty. Because catheter sheaths may be left in the catheterization site for 12 to 24 hours, there is increased risk of bacteremia and local infection.

Indwelling Arterial Catheters

Indwelling arterial catheters are used regularly in patients whose precarious cardiovascular status necessitates pressure monitoring or repeated blood gas determination (see Chapter 44). Even though they provide information that is essential for sophisticated patient care and eliminate the need for potentially traumatic repeated arterial punctures, such catheters also provide a continuing portal of entry for microbial invasion of the bloodstream.

The infectious complications of the use of arterial catheters have been studied most extensively in neonates. In different centers, the incidence of colonization of indwelling umbilical artery catheters varies from 6% to 60% [19–22]. Unexpectedly, however, the incidence of colonization fails to increase with duration of catheterization, which suggests that catheters become contaminated initially or soon after insertion through the umbilical stump, an area that is heavily colonized and impossible to sterilize completely by local or systemic antibiotics. Indeed, the same organisms usually are isolated from both the cord and catheter in any individual patient. The most frequent contaminants are staphylococci, streptococci, and gram-negative bacilli, particularly *Pseudomonas, Proteus, Escherichia coli*, and *Klebsiella*.

The clinical significance of umbilical catheter colonization is difficult to assess, because the incidence o
sepsis in most studies has been low. When serial prosp
tive blood cultures have been obtained from cathete
neonates, however, transient catheter-related bac
has been noted. In a prospective study of tempo
4 hours) umbilical catheterization for excha
sion, investigators showed a 60% inciden
contamination and a 10% incidence o
teremia due to *Staphylococcus epider*

case, *Proteus*) that occurred 4 to 6 hours after transfusion; this study suggests that the risk from umbilical catheterization may be greatest during the insertion and removal of catheters [23]. In this study and others, prophylactic systemic antibiotics failed to reduce the incidence of catheter contamination or bacteremia. At present, antibiotic prophylaxis does not appear to be beneficial during umbilical catheterization; instead, attention should be focused on meticulous cord preparation and care.

In adults, Gardner and coworkers [24] demonstrated positive arterial catheter tip cultures in 4% of 200 patients exposed to radial artery catheterization (the preferred site in adults). The source of these organisms was not evaluated, and no direct relation with patient disease was established, but the incidence of colonization of radial catheters (in contrast to umbilical catheters) did appear to be related to longer durations of catheterization (> 4 days) [25]. Inflammation at the catheter site and the use of a cutdown procedure to place the catheter also appear to be associated with an increased risk of infection [26] (see Chapter 44). More recent studies in adults have emphasized the risk of endemic infections caused by arterial catheters used for hemodynamic monitoring [26,27]. A prospective study of 95 patients (130 catheters) in a medical–surgical intensive care unit showed a 4% risk of arterial cannula-related septicemia; 12% of all sepsis in this unit was the result of intraarterial catheters [26]. These bacteremias were caused by gram-negative bacilli, enterococci, and *Candida* organisms.

Flow-directed pulmonary artery catheters carry the added risk of right-sided endocarditis related to endocardial trauma or septic thrombosis of the great vein or pulmonary artery. In one autopsy study, 7% of 55 patients had endocarditis in association with these catheters [28]. Studies that used multivariate analysis found a number of risk factors for infection associated with the use of pulmonary artery catheters [29]. The use of catheters in neonates and in younger children [30], placement of the catheter with less barrier precautions (sterile gloves, a surgical mask, and a small fenestrated drape as opposed to sterile gloves, a long-sleeved surgical gown, a surgical mask, and a large sterile drape) [30], placement in an internal jugular (rather than a subclavian) vein [30], ...neous colonization of the insertion site [30], ...theterization [30–32], particularly ...strong independent predic... olonization. ...ay create a greatly ...ntamination and sep... ...eak of *Flavobacterium* ...l hospital, the sterile, ...or clearing arterial lines ...lood samples were sub... ...w minutes before use. The ...tensive care unit was contaminated with *Flavobacterium* (an organism that can survive and grow at temperatures as low as −38°C (−36°F)), and contamination of in-use phlebotomy syringes with this ice resulted in 14 cases of *Flavobacterium* sepsis. Control of the outbreak depended on improved aseptic technique—that is, on discontinuing the practice of cooling syringes in ice before blood withdrawal and of reinjecting blood to clear the catheter system. Ice-related bacteremia is also a potential problem if open cardiac output injectate delivery systems are used [34].

Guidelines for prevention of infections related to intravascular pressure monitoring have been formulated by the Centers for Disease Control and Prevention (CDC) [35].

Transducers

Pressure-monitoring devices (transducers or gauges connected to a closed space by a length of fluid-filled tubing) are used regularly for monitoring cardiovascular pressures of critically ill patients. These devices can provide a portal of entry for microbial invasion. Although such devices frequently are used in the setting of arterial cannulation or cardiac catheterization, we believe that the threat posed by monitoring devices is so prominent and so frequently overlooked that a separate section on transducer-related infection is warranted.

Although many hospital personnel assume that a protective pressure gradient exists between patients and transducers, contaminated monitoring devices have been the source of nosocomial infection in outbreaks of gram-negative bacteremia, candidemia, and dialysis-associated hepatitis [36]. As electronic monitoring has been used increasingly to measure cerebrospinal fluid (CSF) and intrauterine pressure, there have been occasional reports of transducer-related infections in neurosurgical and obstetric patients. In one study, epidemiologic evidence and culture suggested that contaminated intrauterine pressure transducers used during labor were a nosocomial source of group B streptococcal colonization [37].

As in infusion-related sepsis, any organism that can survive in the fluid used in the monitoring system is capable of causing monitoring-related infection. *Pseudomonas* species and members of the tribe Klebsielleae (*Klebsiella, Enterobacter*, and *Serratia*) have caused most of the reported bacteremias. The *Pseudomonas* species—*P. cepacia* and *P. acidovorans*—that were implicated in three outbreaks may reflect an emphasis on unusual epidemics that are more readily recognized and evaluated. Pathogens such as *P. cepacia*, however, may have selective advantages in the hospital environment because of their ability to grow with minimal nutrients and to resist commonly used disinfectants, such as dilute aqueous benzalkonium chloride.

In the outbreaks that we investigated, pressure-monitoring devices were contaminated most frequently by an index patient. Just as organisms from a contaminated transducer may migrate (or be flushed) through fluid-filled monitoring lines to infect a patient, organisms in the bloodstream of a patient with preexisting bacteremia or viremia may migrate (or be refluxed) through the lines to contaminate a transducer. If the transducer is not sterilized after use, cross-infection can result.

Although we do not know how often personnel fail to sterilize transducers between uses, there are several reasons to believe that this is a relatively common error if reusable transducers are used. First, many hospital personnel, failing to recognize that transducers may be a source of infection, are loath to subject such expensive and relatively delicate instruments to adequate cleaning efforts. Second, many transducers cannot withstand autoclaving, and heavy patient loads frequently may not allow time for the more lengthy gas or chemical sterilization procedures that these devices require. Finally, even when an attempt at proper care is made, the many recesses in the traditional dome-and-diaphragm transducer may hamper cleaning and sterilizing efforts.

Once transducers are sterilized for use, the many manipulations involved in using a monitoring system make extrinsic contamination of the equipment easy. As anticipated [36], when unsterile mercury manometers are used for calibrating sterile transducers, contamination is likely [38]. Other potential vehicles for transducer contamination include cleaning solutions and intravenous fluids and medications, particularly those in multidose vials [39]. Infusion bacteremia caused by extrinsically contaminated intravenous fluid is rare (see Chapter 44); however, the fluid column in pressure-monitoring systems is at much greater risk of contamination (and sepsis) because it may be stagnant and subjected to frequent manipulations.

For reasons outlined previously, we suspect that transducer contamination is relatively common and that monitoring-related infections have been occurring sporadically since transducers were introduced into clinical medicine. As increasing use of invasive procedures places a large population at risk of monitoring-related infection, and as awareness of this problem increases, such sporadic cases and the means for preventing them should receive more attention. In each hospital, guidelines [40] need to be established for the care of transducers and for surveillance and management of monitoring-related infection.

Efforts are under way to improve the ease of transducer sterilization and to simplify the aseptic use of monitoring systems [41]. More recent innovations, not yet widely used, include miniature extravascular transducers that are built into the tips of standard Luer-Lok fittings and thus can be attached directly to monitoring lines (or designed for intravascular use), obviating the need for cumbersome domes; however, when sterilizing these miniature transducers, care must be taken to ensure that the area between the transducer and the Luer fitting is thoroughly cleaned and comes into full contact with the sterilizing medium.

The traditional reusable transducer dome has been largely replaced by the disposable chamber dome, which has a thin membrane that abuts the transducer diaphragm and keeps the monitoring fluid in a sterile, disposable circuit. The viability of this approach depends on the chamber dome not being reused and on the thin membrane reliably maintaining its integrity throughout a monitoring period [41]. Several outbreaks have documented the failure of disposable domes to prevent septicemia acquired from contaminated transducers [42–45]. The exact way that bacteria spread from contaminated transducers to the sterile circuit is not clear; however, hand transmission of organisms from transducer heads to dome fluid was shown experimentally during assembly, calibration, and manipulation of ports. Contamination is most likely to occur when glucose solutions are used between the transducer head and the chamber dome membrane and when transducers are not adequately disinfected between uses. Most outbreaks that have occurred since the introduction of the disposable chamber dome have been due to this type of contamination of the system [46]. Thus, sterilization, or at least high-level disinfection, of transducer heads appears necessary even when disposable chamber domes are used.

Finally, the most widely used advance in pressure monitoring is the totally disposable transducer system. Based on the results of a prospective, controlled trial of extended use of disposable pressure transducers, these devices can be safely used without change for 4 days, even in busy intensive care units [47]. In fact, since the publication of the CDC guidelines for preventing monitoring-related infections, a prospective study of 117 patients has called into question the need to change routinely any component of the monitoring circuit [48]. In this study, no contamination of monitoring system fluid was found despite prolonged use (25 to 439 hours). The researchers believed that by placing the continuous-flow device just distal to the transducer, they eliminated the static in-line fluid column that, in other studies [49], may have led to contamination. The researchers also commented on their meticulous care of stopcocks, which is a part of the transducer system most frequently manipulated and contaminated. Plugs were used for all stopcock sampling ports. The plugs were placed on a sterile sponge soaked with povidone–iodine whenever the stopcock was manipulated, and the port was cleaned with povidone–iodine before the plug was reinserted. Unless such stringent practices are adhered to uniformly, the best current approach appears to be use of the totally disposable transducer, with a 4-day change policy. The additive protective effect of using systems that use only truly closed sampling ports, as recently suggested [47] and studied [50], could potentially extend the microbe-free life of the disposable transducer. As of this publication, no outbreaks attributed to the use of disposable pressure transducers have been reported to the CDC [35].

Circulatory Assist Devices

A number of circulatory assist devices (CADs), either biventricular or univentricular (Figure 46-1), are used to maintain a patient's circulation while awaiting cardiac transplantation. These devices have supplanted the totally artificial heart because of morbidity and mortality associated with wound infection [51]. Although CADs may be life-saving, infection has been one of the most common CAD complications [52,53]. Infections associated with CADs include device-related bloodstream infections, mediastinitis, exit site infections, or infections at the entrance site of the transcutaneous power cables.

Infectious complications of CADs are particularly important because they may preclude subsequent heart transplantation [54]. In a retrospective analysis of experience with CADs over an 8-year period, 14 (32%) of 44 patients did not receive a donor organ because of CAD-related infection. However, in another retrospective analysis of 14 patients who required a CAD, despite 4 device-related infections in 3 patients, all 14 patients underwent transplantation that was not delayed because of infection [55]. Others have had the same experience [56].

Although duration of device use, host factors such as immunosuppression, and type of CAD may influence infection risk, the literature on CAD-related infections is all retrospective. Because CADs are being used more

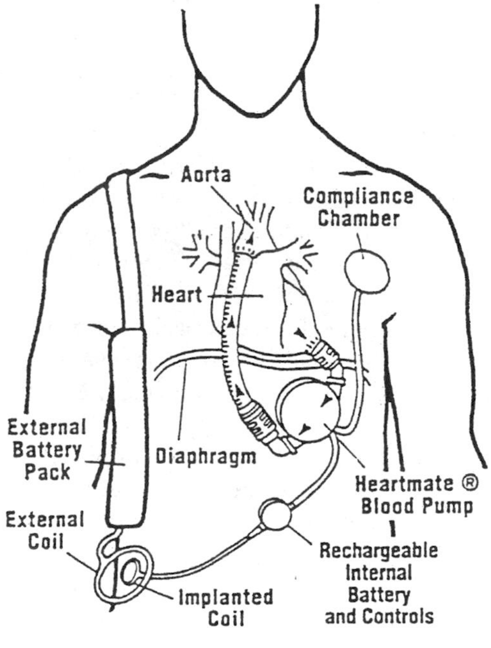

FIGURE 46-1. Electric ventricular device system. (With permission from the manufacturer of the HeartMate ventricular device, Thermo Cardiosystems, Inc., Woburn, Massachusetts, U.S.A.)

regularly, careful surveillance of device-related infections, with uniform definitions, is warranted to determine specific risk factors for infection and preventive measures.

TRANSFUSION-ASSOCIATED INFECTIONS

This section covers transfusion-associated infections [57] other than hepatitis, cytomegalovirus, and HIV infections, which are discussed elsewhere (see Chapters 42, 43).

Blood Transfusion and Bacteremia

The first case reports of transfusion-related sepsis appeared in the 1940s and 1950s and involved shock syndromes produced by transfusion of cold-stored blood contaminated with psychrophilic organisms able to survive and grow at 4°C (30°F), such as *Achromobacter* and some *Pseudomonas* species. Prospective microbiologic studies soon followed these reports and documented a contamination rate of 1% to 6% in banked blood [58]. Most contaminants were normal skin flora, presumably introduced with fragments of donor skin cored out during phlebotomy. Such contaminants were usually present in extremely low concentrations (several logarithmic factors below the level of ~ 100 organisms per milliliter of blood associated with transfusion sepsis), and additional multiplication of organisms during storage seemed unlikely because of the long lag phase produced by refrigeration and because of the antibacterial action of blood. Indeed, retrospective studies failed to document any clinical illness associated with the transfusion of blood that contained low-level contamination with skin flora [59].

In addition to the donor as a source of contamination, bacterial contamination of blood components can also come from contamination during collection or processing. For example, in a Scandinavian report, an outbreak of *Serratia marcescens* was traced to use of blood bags contaminated during manufacturing [60]. However, with the sterile, disposable, closed systems used at present for blood collection, with good collection technique, and with the prompt use of dated, refrigerated, banked blood, problems with blood transfusions should be minimal.

Nevertheless, asymptomatic patients or patients with non-specific gastrointestinal symptoms occasionally still may be a source of bacterial contamination. Approximately 21 cases of *Yersinia enterocolitica*-contaminated red blood cell transfusions have been reported and have been associated with a high mortality rate, particularly associated with units older than 25 days of storage at 1° to 6°C (34° to 43°F). Presumably the donors had asymptomatic bacteremia at the time of donation.

When an episode of transfusion-associated sepsis does occur, it is important to search for breakdowns in technique or a contaminated common source (e.g., collection sets, disinfectants, and anticoagulants [61]) that could put other patients at risk. Furthermore, the possibility of transfusion-associated sepsis should be investigated in any case of febrile transfusion reaction [62].

Blood Transfusion and Parasitemia

The increased use of blood transfusions and the increased travel to countries where malaria is endemic have led to an increased occurrence of transfusion-related malaria. It is estimated that during the period between 1911 and 1950, ~ 350 cases of transfusion-associated malaria were reported worldwide, but during the period 1950 to 1972, the number of reported cases exceeded 2,000 [64]. In the United States, 101 cases of transfusion-induced malaria were reported in the years 1957 to 1994 [65,66]. Currently, an average of three transfusions per year are complicated by transmission of a malaria infection [67]. This increase has been linked to imported cases of malaria; > 50% of the implicated donors had a history of recent military service in Southeast Asia [65].

Based on worldwide incidence data, *Plasmodium malariae* appears to be the most common cause of transfusion-associated malaria, accounting for almost 50% of cases. *Plasmodium vivax* and *Plasmodium falciparum* are second and third in worldwide incidence, respectively. This ordering probably reflects the fact that although *P. malariae* infection may persist in an asymptomatic donor for many years, the longevity of *P. vivax* malaria in humans rarely exceeds 3 years, and that of *P. falciparum*, rarely a year. Hence, there is greater chance for an asymptomatic donor infected with *P. malariae* to escape detection and become the source of an infected transfusion.

Recommended guidelines for the selection of blood donors to prevent transmission of malaria were adopted by the American Association of Blood Banks in 1970 and relaxed in 1974 [65,66]. In the amended guidelines and still in the January, 1994 guidelines, prospective donors who have a definite history of malaria are deferred for 3 years after becoming asymptomatic or ceasing therapy. Immigrants, refugees, citizens, or visitors from an endemic area are acceptable 3 years after departure from the area if they have been asymptomatic. Donors who have traveled to an endemic area but who have remained free of symptoms are acceptable one year after their return to the United States. Because platelet and leukocyte preparations also have been incriminated in the transmission of malaria, the guidelines must be applied to potential donors of any formed elements of blood.

Chagas' disease, or American trypanosomiasis, is prevalent through South and Central America, and there is a high potential for bloodborne transmission, because some infected individuals may become asymptomatic but still have persistent parasitemia for 10 to 30 years. Although the infectivity of blood contaminated with this parasite declines after 10 days of storage, this frequently is not a useful method for preventing transmission; moreover, the parasite is viable in whole blood and red blood cells stored at 4°C for ≥ 21 days [63]. Serologic screening has become mandatory for the acceptance of blood donors in many South American countries. The problem of transfusion-associated Chagas' disease has also become an issue for U.S. blood banks, secondary to increased emigration and to greater numbers of potentially infected blood donors in the United States (it has been estimated that about 100,000 infected people live in the United States) [68]; ≥ 2 cases of transfusion-acquired Chagas' disease have been documented in the United States, [69] and 1 unconfirmed case in Texas [70]. Anyone with a history of Chagas' disease must be deferred permanently from donating blood [71].

Toxoplasmosis is a disease that is receiving increasing clinical attention, particularly as a cause of opportunistic infection in patients with impaired host defenses. In one prospective survey of thalassemic patients who were frequently transfused, subclinical toxoplasmosis was detected at a rate comparable to that seen in a control group, and this was considered to be evidence against the transmission of toxoplasmosis by transfusion [73]. In another study, however, patients treated for acute leukemia acquired toxoplasmosis after leukocyte transfusions from donors with chronic myelogenous leukemia; serologic data retrospectively obtained from donors revealed elevated anti-*Toxoplasma* antibody titers [74]. This inferential evidence for transfusion-associated toxoplasmosis is supported by the findings that the disease can be transmitted between animals by transfusion, that *Toxoplasma* organisms retain their viability in stored blood for ≤ 50 days, and that organisms can be recovered from the blood buffy-coat layers of patients with toxoplasmosis. Because it seems likely that toxoplasmosis can be transmitted if large concentrations of leukocytes are transfused, and because all of the leukocyte donors had chronic myelogenous leukemia, it is recommended that blood or leukocytes from patients with leukemia not be used [63], particularly because the host defenses of recipients usually are severely compromised.

At least 18 cases of transfusion-transmitted babesiosis have been documented in the United States; however, symptoms can be mild in immunocompetent people and the true incidence of the infection is unknown. Donors with a history of babesiosis are indefinitely deferred from donating blood because of the possibility of ongoing asymptomatic parasitemia [71].

Platelet Transfusion

The incidence of bacterial contamination of platelet concentrates has been a source of controversy. Although many investigators have reported no contamination, others have consistently found bacterial contaminants in 1% to 6% of concentrates [75]. Because it is now recommended that platelets be stored at room temperature (rather than 4°C [39°F]) to increase in vivo half-life, there is justifiable concern over the true incidence of intrinsic contamination and the possible proliferation of contaminants during storage. It seems reasonable to assume that platelet concentrates are as susceptible to contamination during collection as is blood, which is routinely found to have a 1% to 6% incidence of low-level contamination. Moreover, platelet concentrates, unlike blood, have no protective antibacterial activity, and platelet transfusions are frequently obtained by pooling the contributions of several donors, which additionally increases the risk of contamination. Despite this seemingly negative picture, most bacterial contaminants isolated from platelet concentrates have been normal skin flora, such as *S. epidermidis* and diphtheroids, and they have been present in extremely low concentrations. Even in the highly susceptible patient populations that normally receive platelet transfusions, such contaminants have failed to produce any documented adverse reactions [76].

Although meticulous blood-banking techniques and the widespread use of closed collection systems have made platelet transfusion relatively safe, the occurrence of outbreaks emphasizes the possibility of sporadic, significant contamination of platelets. One outbreak involved seven cases of *Salmonella choleraesuis* sepsis that were traced to platelet transfusions from a blood donor with clinically inapparent *Salmonella* osteomyelitis and intermittent asymptomatic bacteremia [77]. A long incubation period in this outbreak—that is, a mean interval of 9 days between the transfusion with contaminated platelets and the signs of sepsis—was caused by coincidental administration of antibiotics at the time of platelet transfusion in several cases, and this initially delayed recognition of platelets as the vehicle of infection.

A second outbreak involved two cases of transfusion-induced *Enterobacter cloacae* sepsis [75]. An investigation prompted by the occurrence of these cases revealed that 20% of the platelet pools prepared in the affected hospital were contaminated. Although most of the contaminants were nonpathogens and present only in low concentrations, 6 of 258 platelet pools were shown to harbor *E. cloacae*. The source of these unusual contaminants was not discovered.

A third outbreak with *Serratia* was traced to contaminated evacuated tubes used after blood collection [61].

In a fourth outbreak [78], a cluster of four patients at a university hospital received platelets contaminated with *Bacillus cereus, Pseudomonas aeruginosa*, or *S. epidermidis* during a 34-day period. The patient with platelet transfusion-related *Pseudomonas* sepsis died; the remaining patients survived. The investigators thought that the most likely explanation for the outbreak was contamination of the platelets at the time of phlebotomy. In addition, the four contaminated platelet units were significantly older (mean age, 4.8 days) than 106 randomly selected individual platelet units (mean age, 3.7 days; $p = 0.04$). The hospital had increased its surveillance, probably after the one patient died, and increased surveillance may have fostered the discovery of the contaminated platelet pools. Prospective surveillance would help estimate the rate of infection due to platelet contamination.

Albumin Infusion

Because of faith in commercial manufacturing practices and the extremely low incidence of reactions to albumin infusion, most physicians consider commercial human serum albumin to be a completely safe product. A nationwide outbreak of albumin-related *P. cepacia* sepsis, however, emphasized that any commercial product, particularly any blood component, is susceptible to contamination [79]. The outbreak involved four lots of commercial 25% normal human serum albumin. One of the lots had an estimated 1% contamination rate and resulted in at least seven cases of albumin-associated sepsis in one Maryland hospital; the other three lots caused isolated cases of albumin-related disease in patients in four other states. The organisms most likely gained access to the albumin vials during a hand-filling procedure.

In addition to emphasizing the risk of infection associated with the infusion of a nonformed blood component, it is worthwhile noting that the albumin outbreak points up several general problems in the detection and evaluation of low-frequency contamination of commercial products. First, nosocomial infections caused by low-frequency contaminants may be difficult to distinguish from endemic problems in any one institution. In the Maryland hospital, the infusion-related infections became apparent only because of the enormous quantity of albumin that was used in the hospital. Second, because commercial products are usually prepared and sterilized in bulk lots, it is important to be able to trace the distribution of individual suspect lots. Although the Maryland hospital did not routinely record information on albumin distribution and use, an alert physician fortuitously noted the lot number and brand of albumin used in one case of suspected infusion-related sepsis. Third, sterility of an infusion product cannot be ascertained by visual inspection. Despite *P. cepacia* concentrations of approximately 100 organisms per milliliter, the contaminated albumin was completely clear. Finally, when present in low frequency, some contaminants can be missed by the sampling schemes currently used for product quality control, and endotoxin may escape terminal filtration and be missed by currently used pyrogen tests. To facilitate the monitoring of albumin-related reactions, some hospitals distribute this product through their blood banks.

Albumin-transmitted hepatitis is discussed elsewhere (see Chapter 42).

INFECTION HAZARDS ASSOCIATED WITH ANESTHESIA

As noted in previous chapters, severe bacterial infections have been well documented in association with the use of contaminated equipment for local or spinal anesthesia or the use of contaminated anesthesia machines for delivery of general anesthesia. An additional well recognized infectious complication of general anesthesia unrelated to the use of contaminated equipment is aspiration pneumonia attributable either to the passage of an endotracheal tube or to postoperative difficulties.

Anesthetic Agents

Propofol (Diprivan; Stuart Pharmaceutical, Wilmington, Delaware, U.S.A.) is an oil-based anesthetic agent, and although this drug does not contain any preservatives or antimicrobials, refrigeration is not recommended by the manufacturer (Diprivan injection, 1993 package insert). An investigation of seven outbreaks of postoperative infection or acute febrile illness revealed an association with the receipt of propofol. The extrinsic contamination of propofol due to poor aseptic technique by anesthesia personnel, compounded by the ability of the oil-based product to support growth of contaminants, or use of the same syringe for multiple patients, was thought to be the cause of these outbreaks [80]. Infection control practitioners must maintain surveillance for infections due to propofol, which also has been approved for use as a sedative agent in the intensive care unit. In addition, practitioners may have to investigate the manner in which such products are handled to ensure that aseptic technique is being used. Products that do not contain preservatives or antimicrobials, and have the ability to support microbial growth because of the properties of the product, should not be used in multidose vials.

Aspiration of Stomach Contents

Aspiration of stomach contents into the lungs during or after obstetric anesthesia was first described by Mendelson [81], who found the incidence of this complication to be 0.15% during the preantibiotic era. A common clinical pattern was that 2 to 5 hours after vomiting and aspiration, a dramatic onset of cyanosis, tachycardia, and shock was noted.

More recent investigations have shown a surprisingly high incidence of aspiration associated with general anesthesia. In one study, Evans blue dye was placed in the stomach preoperatively to be used as a marker for chemical aspiration; after anesthesia, the dye was sought by bronchoscopy [82]. Of 300 patients observed in this manner, 25% vomited, and aspiration was documented in 16% of the overall group. Interestingly, aspiration was "silent" and unnoticed by the entire operating team in one half of those patients who did aspirate (an overall rate of 8%), and there were no obvious clues to the time of occurrence. No incidence of pneumonia was reported in this series, but it seems that in normal patients the aspirated inoculum is usually cleared without sequelae. Patients who have significant retention of gastric contents and preexisting pulmonary disease may be at much higher risk for development of a chemical aspiration pneumonitis and subsequent bacterial infection.

Despite these studies documenting intraoperative aspiration, it seems likely that postoperative aspiration accounts for most aspiration pneumonias associated with general surgery. Surgical procedures involving the upper abdomen, thorax, or upper gastrointestinal tract have been the operations most commonly associated with aspiration pneumonia. The highest-risk patients include those undergoing emergency procedures with a full stomach and those whose condition prevents the stomach from emptying well (e.g., full-term pregnancy, marked obesity, ileus, or massive ascites).

Measures to prevent anesthesia-associated aspiration have included prolonged preoperative fasting, adequate sedation, attention to problems during anesthesia, insertion of a nasogastric tube before anesthesia, and careful monitoring of the patient in the early postoperative period. Such principles can be readily applied to elective surgical intervention. Although the insertion of a nasogastric tube is believed to reduce the incidence of aspiration during anesthesia, more than half the cases of postoperative aspiration occur in patients whose nasogastric tubes have been left in place, and a quarter of cases of postoperative aspiration pneumonia have also been associated with tracheostomy. It is difficult to interpret these data, however, because the most seriously ill and aspiration-prone patients have tracheostomies or nasogastric tubes left in place.

In emergency procedures and for the high-risk patients cited previously, measures used to prevent aspiration or ameliorate its effect include attempts to empty the stomach (with metoclopramide or a large nasogastric tube); to decrease stomach acid (with anticholinergic drugs, H_2 blockers, or antacids, although some common antacids are suspensions of particulate matter that may themselves incite pulmonary inflammation if aspirated); to use cricoid pressure to occlude the esophagus during induction of anesthesia; or to pass an endotracheal tube with an inflatable balloon under topical anesthesia with the patient awake (and empty the stomach after this).

Endotracheal Intubation

Aside from aspiration, another potential hazard of anesthesia may be the occurrence of bacteremia secondary to the passage of an endotracheal tube. The organisms isolated from the blood usually are α-hemolytic streptococci, both aerobic and anaerobic diphtheroids, and other anaerobic organisms that normally colonize the upper respiratory tract. There may, however, be a higher incidence of such bacteremia after the nasotracheal route of intubation than after the less traumatic orotracheal route [83], but antibiotic prophylaxis is not recommended for either route.

Prolonged nasotracheal (or nasogastric) intubation has been associated with a 2% to 5% incidence of sinusitis, which may be occult [84,85]. The maxillary and sphenoid sinuses are most commonly involved [84], and frequent pathogens include *Staphylococcus aureus, Enterobacter, P. aeruginosa, Hemophilus*, pneumococci, and anaerobes [85]. Sterile and occasionally infected middle ear effusions may also be common in patients receiving endotracheal intubation and mechanical ventilation [86].

INFECTIONS OF THE CENTRAL NERVOUS SYSTEM: RESERVOIRS AND SHUNTS

Serious infection can complicate the insertion or prolonged use of two very important neurosurgical devices: the Ommaya-type subcutaneous reservoir, which is used for administering intrathecal therapy for fungal or neoplastic meningitis, and the ventricular shunt, which is used for decompression of hydrocephalus (see Chapter 36).

Complications have been observed frequently after the insertion or chronic use of subcutaneous intraventricular reservoirs [87–89]. In one series involving 21 reservoirs, 9 patients acquired CSF bacterial infections as a result of reservoir use or insertion, and complications associated with 17 reservoirs in 12 patients either necessitated reservoir removal or prevented their later use for intrathecal therapy [87]. *S. epidermidis, Corynebacterium acnes*, and α-hemolytic streptococci were the major causes of the reservoir infections, and this predominance of normal skin flora suggests that the bacteria gained access to the CSF during repeated percutaneous injections of antifungal or antineoplastic agents into the reservoir. A more recent experience projected a 15% risk of infection during the first year after insertion of a reservoir [88]. Therapy of the bacterial superinfection usually is given systemically; the efficacy of antimicrobials added to the reservoir, either for prophylaxis or for treatment of superinfection, has not been established. Although in one study 80% of the patients who completed the treatment course were cured by systemic antimicrobial therapy alone [87], many believe that infected CSF devices should be removed.

The use of valved catheters for the treatment of hydrocephalus (i.e., to shunt CSF from the lateral ventricle of the brain to the superior vena cava, the right atrium, or the peritoneum) has also been complicated by a high incidence of infections. In a number of series, the overall incidence of shunt infections has ranged from 6% to 23%, with a median of ~ 14% [90]. Most of these infections are caused by *S. aureus* or *S. epidermidis* and occur within 2 weeks to 2 months after surgery, which stresses the importance of intraoperative and perioperative wound or shunt contamination in the pathogenesis of shunt infection. The equal risk of infection in patients with ventriculoatrial and ventriculoperitoneal shunts suggests that transient bacteremia is a less likely cause of such infections, because ventriculoperitoneal shunts are not exposed to the bloodstream [91].

Patients with infected ventricular shunts have several different clinical presentations. Some display a markedly toxic course with persistent pyrexia, progressive anemia, splenomegaly, and repeatedly positive blood cultures. More often there is a chronic, indolent course, and considerable clinical suspicion may be necessary before appropriate steps are undertaken. In certain cases, the clinical pattern may be related to the bacteriologic characteristics of the infection. Only one third or so of infected shunts, for example, exhibit visible wound infection and necrosis but, when these occur, they are important signs of underlying infection, usually with *S. aureus*. In contrast to cases with obvious local inflammation, *S. epidermidis* is found in most of the other cases, and this organism is most frequently associated with bacteremic infections.

The antimicrobial treatment of the shunt infections that complicate hydrocephalus is usually unsatisfactory unless the shunt is removed [92]. Adherence of slime-producing, coagulase-negative staphylococci to shunt material may be one reason for failure of antimicrobial therapy alone [93]. Although fewer than 10% of patients have their infection eradicated by systemic antimicrobial therapy alone, patients treated with combinations of systemic and intraventricular antibiotics may have 30% to 90% cure rates [94]. Repeated administration of intraventricular antibiotics has its own complications, however, and when infection is widespread, the treatment of choice appears to be the administration of appropriate systemic antibiotics and the complete removal of the shunt to a new site [95]. Preferably, some time should elapse between the removal of the infected shunt and the insertion of a new one. Despite this discouraging picture, it should be recognized that many of the antibiotics that were used to treat shunt infections in the past have been supplanted by newer agents that may prove to be more efficacious. In addition, the epidemiologic characteristics of shunt infections (e.g., perioperative acquisition of organisms) and the narrow spectrum of shunt pathogens suggest that the use of prophylactic antimicrobials at the time of shunt surgery may prove beneficial. Although one controlled study of relatively low-dose oxacillin prophylaxis failed to show that antibiotics had a significant protective effect [96], two meta-analysis studies [97,98] looking at the use of perioperative antimicrobial prophylaxis did suggest that use of prophylactic antibiotics was associated with a significant reduction in subsequent CSF shunt infection. Both studies demonstrated an ~ 50% reduction in infection risk. Only a few of the studies included in these two meta-analyses reached statistical significance by themselves, which may be, at least in part, due to lack of power.

Epidural catheters, used for anesthesia or pain management, and spinal cord or dorsal column simulators, used for pain management, also have the potential for device-related infections. A prospective, randomized, controlled trial [99] to assess the efficacy of a chlorhexidine dressing in reducing the microbial flora at the insertion site of epidural catheters found that the use of the antiseptic at the catheter wound site reduced catheter colonization. The authors hypothesized that this would possibly reduce the risk of epidural catheter-related infection. To evaluate the effectiveness of preventive measures, such as antiseptic dressings at the catheter site, it will be important to look at clinical end-points such as infection rates.

TRANSIENT BACTEREMIA FROM NONVASCULAR PROCEDURES

The occurrence of transient bacteremia associated with relatively noninvasive manipulation of colonized mucosa is well recognized [100]. Such bacteremia usually lasts no longer than 5 to 15 minutes, may shower at its peak 100 organisms per milliliter of blood (although the peak concentration is almost always much less), and is largely asymptomatic. Hundreds of studies have reported on bacteremia after oral treatments alone [101]. In this section, we discuss bacteremia after diagnostic gastrointestinal procedures, genitourinary instrumentation, and bronchoscopy; bacteremia after endotracheal intubation and invasive vascular procedures is covered earlier in this chapter. Table 46-1 presents a summary of the characteristics of bacteremia associated with selected nonvascular procedures.

Gastrointestinal Procedures

Bacteremia has been reported as a sequel to a variety of gastrointestinal procedures, including sigmoidoscopy, colonoscopy, barium enema, esophagoscopy, biopsy of mucosal masses, injection sclerotherapy of esophageal varices, endoscopic retrograde cholangiopancreatography (ERCP), liver biopsy, esophageal dilatation, and rectal examination. In one prospective study of sigmoidoscopy, transient asymptomatic bacteremia was noted in 19 of 200 procedures [102]. Most of the organisms isolated were enterococci, and bacteremia was observed more frequently 5 minutes after than 1 minute after the termination of the procedure. Of note in this study, serial blood cultures were obtained through an indwelling venous needle. Although this convenient approach may have distorted or amplified culture results and is thus open to some criticism, the temporal profile and magnitude of bacteremia, as well as the types of organisms isolated, are consistent with bacteremia arising from the site of instrumentation. Other investigators using similar methods, however, have found bacteremia to be a rare complication of their sigmoidoscopic examinations, and they have concluded that other factors, particularly the experience of the sigmoidoscopist, need to be evaluated before routine antibiotic prophylaxis can be advocated for patients undergoing sigmoidoscopy [103].

In a study of colonoscopy, careful anaerobic culturing and subsequent hourly temperature evaluation of patients showed a 27% incidence of transient bacteremia during the procedure and a 33% incidence of postprocedure fever in patients who had been bacteremic [104]. The greater trauma of colonoscopy compared with sigmoi-

TABLE 46-1 *Characteristics of transient bacteremia associated with selected procedures*

Involved system	Maximum incidence of bacterimia (%)
Dental	90
Urologic	80
Airway	30
Gastrointestinal	15
Obsteric-gynecologic	4
Concentration of bacteria (cfu) per milliliter:	< 20–130
Duration of bacteremia (min after procedure):	10–30
Predominant bacterias:	anaerobes, enterococci, enteric gram-negative bacilli; occasionally, *Streptococcus pneumoniae*
Symptoms:	usually none; fever more common with urologic-related bacteremia

cfu, Colony forming units.

doscopy may be responsible for the greater incidence of bacteremia and the more marked clinical response, although these are not consistently found [105]. Host factors may also influence the incidence and outcome of procedure-related bacteremia. In this regard, it is noteworthy that rare cases of symptomatic barium enema septicemia have been reported in patients with impaired host defenses (acute leukemia) and in patients with active inflammatory bowel disease.

Although the role of antibiotic prophylaxis for endoscopy procedures is not always certain, other preventive measures—particularly careful disinfection of endoscopes and good aseptic technique—are of definite importance. The importance of such measures is highlighted by many anecdotal reports and outbreaks [24, 106–114]. In one report, two cases of *Pseudomonas* sepsis in leukemic patients undergoing esophagoscopy with mucosal biopsy were traced to exogenous bacteria introduced at the time of biopsy. Cultures of the esophagoscope and of the endoscopy room revealed widespread contamination with enteric organisms, including *P. aeruginosa*, and it was shown that in the routine handling of the instruments, aseptic technique was ignored [112].

In addition, several series of ERCP-related cases of bacteremia or cholangitis [106–108,110] highlight the multiple sources of contamination in the endoscopy suite, particularly the lens irrigation bottles; the difficulty disinfecting the levers and many small-bore channels in these sophisticated instruments, even when automatic washes are used; the fact that some automatic endoscope "sterilizers," at times, are the source of endoscope contamination, particularly by *P. aeruginosa*; the fact that significant sporadic problems can be easily overlooked for prolonged periods, even with established infection control programs; and the poor level of endoscope disinfection in many hospitals, despite established guidelines [115] and the many reported outbreaks. Interestingly, almost all of the ERCP-related cases are due to *P. aeruginosa*, and most to one particular serotype, 010, which is either very prevalent or has an undisclosed source related to ERCP procedures.

Most of the ERCP patients are at particular risk because of obstructions in the biliary or pancreatic ducts that can trap contaminated injectate. Any patient undergoing ERCP who has suspected ductal obstruction should receive antimicrobial prophylaxis [116]. Large series of ERCP cases have also emphasized the better results obtained with experienced operators [117].

Percutaneous liver biopsy, although an invasive procedure, is not usually considered to be associated with infection risk. Two studies, however, have documented incidences of bacteremia of 6% and 14% after liver biopsy. In the first study, bacteremia was detectable in patients for several hours after biopsy, and it was associated in at least one patient with signs of gram-negative sepsis, but it may not have been attributable directly to the biopsy in all the cases [118]. In the second study, however, the bacteremias were transient, lasted for only 15 to 20 minutes after biopsy, and were asymptomatic [119]. In this study, cultures of liver biopsy specimens were positive in 7% of patients, and patients with positive specimens had a significantly higher incidence of bacteremia (83%) than did patients whose specimens were sterile (8.4%), which suggests a direct relationship between biopsy and bacteremia. One explanation of this relationship is that the hepatic reticuloendothelial cells that were in the process of "clearing" gut bacteria from the portal system were sampled, resulting in a culture-positive biopsy specimen, a temporary defect in the bacterial clearance mechanisms of the sampled area, and an associated transient bacteremia. The incidence and clinical significance of liver biopsy-associated bacteremia need additional evaluation, as does an association noted in the second study [119] between liver biopsy and transient pneumococcal bacteremia in patients with cirrhosis. Antibiotic prophylaxis with liver biopsy is not warranted at present.

Nasogastric feeding and enteral nutrition have been associated with bacteremia as well as with diarrhea and feeding intolerance, particularly in neonates, due to contamination introduced during collection, preparation, or administration of formula or human milk [120,121].

UROLOGIC AND GYNECOLOGIC INSTRUMENTATION

An association among urethral instrumentation, fever, and bacteremia has been recognized for many years. In various studies, the incidence of bacteremia associated with urologic procedures has been 2% to 80%, with the greatest risks of bacteremia occurring in patients with preexisting urinary tract infections, patients undergoing transurethral resection of the prostate, and patients with prostatitis that is evident on histologic section of biopsy specimens [122]. In 50% to 67% of patients in whom bacteremia develops after instrumentation, similar organisms are recovered from both preinstrumentation urine cultures and postinstrumentation blood cultures. The available evidence suggests that the sources of the other 33% to 50% of postinstrumentation bacteremias include occult prostatitis, the introduction of normal urethral flora, and the contamination of equipment or irrigating fluids before or during instrumentation. It is apparent that careful evaluation for genitourinary tract infection before instrumentation, treatment of any infection [123], appropriate disinfection of equipment, and careful aseptic technique are mandatory. Moreover, because of the relatively frequent occurrence of enterococcal bacteremia after urologic instrumentation and because of the association of instrumentation with gram-negative sepsis as well as with infection at distal sites (e.g., joints), a brief pulse of systemic prophylactic antibiotics at the time of surgical instrumentation may be warranted in high-risk patients, such as those with valvular heart disease, preexisting joint disease, or impaired host defenses [124].

Endometrial biopsy and chorionic villus sampling have been associated rarely with bacteremia [125,126].

Bronchoscopy

Although fever and bacteremia have been documented in patients after rigid-tube bronchoscopy [124], bacteremia has not yet been documented prospectively in patients undergoing flexible fiberoptic bronchoscopy. There are, however, case reports of bacteremia related to fiberoptic bronchoscopy, including one report of fatal *Pseudomonas* bacteremia in a patient with preexisting *Pseudomonas* bronchitis. Furthermore, in one series of 100 patients who were followed carefully after fiberoptic bronchoscopy, fever developed in 16, transient parenchymal infiltrates developed in 5, and rapidly fatal pneumonia developed in 1 [127]. Older patients (> 60 years of age) and those with abnormalities on bronchoscopy were at greatest risk of complications. With the exception of the one fatal pneumonitis, however, all complicating infections resolved without antibiotic therapy, and prospective culturing failed to demonstrate bacteremia in any of the 100 patients [127].

Conclusions

Two conclusions can be drawn from the studies of procedure-related bacteremia just cited: The equipment used for the procedures should be adequately disinfected or sterilized before every use, and proper aseptic technique should be observed by the operator (see Chapter 20). Beyond this, it is apparent that carefully planned, prospective, multicenter studies are needed to assess the incidence and clinical significance of procedure-related transient bacteremia, to determine which hosts are at risk of associated sepsis or infection at distal sites, to determine if specific risks for certain procedures can be sufficiently defined to justify preventive measures such as antibiotic prophylaxis, and to determine which prophylactic regimens would be most efficacious. Although such studies may not be available for some time (if ever), the procedures clearly will continue, and we have tried to note situations in which it seems reasonable to "cover" patients [100,124]. In this regard, it should be noted that for years dental patients with valvular heart disease have received endocarditis prophylaxis, largely on an empiric basis [128], although the specific regimens [129] and even the mechanisms by which prophylaxis may protect [130,131] have been called into question and recommendations have been relaxed in the 1997 guidelines of the American Heart Association [132].

ADDITIONAL PROCEDURES ASSOCIATED WITH INFECTIONS

Interventional Radiology

Percutaneous radiologically guided placement of biopsy needles, catheters, and stents for diagnosis and therapy has become commonplace since the mid 1980s [133]. Infectious complications—primarily bacteremia, organ perforation, and catheter site infection—vary with the particular procedure, patient risk factors, skill of the operator, and experience of the hospital, but are no more frequent than after more invasive procedures [133]. The use of prophylactic antibiotics for interventional radiographic procedures depends on the situation [134]. In addition, when infection is suspected clinically, therapeutic antibiotics should be administered before a procedure.

Laparoscopic Surgery

Laparoscopic surgery, particularly laparoscopic cholecystectomy, has received much attention from both the public and the medical community. Recovery is much faster than after conventional surgery. For cholecystectomy, infection rates (wound, 0.9% to 2.0%; lung, 0.2% to 0.5%; urinary tract, 0.4% to 1.0%) are comparable with those after open surgery [135]. Although there is a large body of literature that examines the surgical complications of therapeutic laparoscopy, very little information has been published on the infectious complications. Because the biliary tract is normally sterile, antimicrobial prophylaxis in biliary surgery has been recommended only for high-risk patients—defined as those who are older than 60 years of age or who have had common duct stones, bile duct obstruction, recent acute cholecystitis, or prior operations on the biliary tract. Until risk stratification data exist for patients undergoing laparoscopic cholecystectomy, antimicrobial prophylaxis standards that are used for the same procedure done through a traditional incision can be used [123].

Cystoscopy

In addition to the risk of bacteremia associated with cystoscopy, a significant risk of urinary tract infection is associated with this procedure. Several remarkably similar outbreaks have been reported in which the use of dilute aqueous quaternary ammonium compounds as cystoscope disinfectants was associated with procedure-related urinary tract infections with *Pseudomonas* species, particular *P. cepacia* (see Chapter 31). In these outbreaks, the quaternary ammonium compounds either were ineffective in decontaminating the equipment or were themselves actually harboring viable bacteria while in use as disinfectants [136].

Although the risk of infection associated with the use of dilute aqueous quaternary ammonium compounds has been known at least since the mid-1970s, many hospital personnel persist in using these compounds as antiseptics and disinfectants. Such use has most likely resulted in many outbreaks of nosocomial urinary tract infection, as well as outbreaks of nosocomial bacteremia and occasional outbreaks of nosocomial respiratory tract and wound infection. To help decrease the risk of nosocomial urinary tract infection after cystoscopy, it is important that the equipment be thoroughly cleaned and properly disinfected between uses.

Bronchoscopy and Endoscopy

In addition to the risks of bronchoscopy cited, several outbreaks have highlighted the problems of pulmonary infection and false-positive culture results due to inadequately cleaned fiberoptic bronchoscopes [137,138]. Especially worrisome is a report of the failure of povidone–iodine to kill *Mycobacterium tuberculosis* on bronchoscopes [139]. Preparations of this agent that are intended for skin degerming are often used inadvisably for decontaminating equipment. This experience has reemphasized the need for higher-level disinfection (e.g., with glutaraldehyde) or sterilization of these scopes, especially after use on patients who may have tuberculosis [140,141]. In addition, some parts of the bronchoscopes, such as reusable spring-operated suction valves, may require autoclaving if they become heavily contaminated with microbes that are relatively resistant to disinfection, such as mycobacteria [142].

We suspect that bronchoscopic or gastrointestinal endoscopic procedure-related infection and pseudoinfection is an ongoing problem whose full impact is yet to be defined. Because infection may be associated with an endoscope that has been exposed to microorganisms either from the environment or from a previous patient use (Figure 46-2), several organizations have published guidelines on infection control for flexible endoscopes [141,142,144]. In spite of the many adverse reports noted previously, and published guidelines, a variety of suboptimal procedures for disinfecting endoscopes are being practiced [145,146].

Even if institutions using endoscopes followed the manufacturer's guidelines for disinfecting endoscopes, it is becoming more evident that it may not always be possible to clean such devices, likely because of the complex nature of endoscopes (Figure 46-3). When inspection endoscopes were used to examine the conditions of the working and suction channels of 241 flexible gastrointestinal endoscopes at 80 healthcare facilities [147], it was found that 38 (47%) of 80 facilities had at least 1 patient-ready endoscope whose suction or biopsy channels were visibly encrusted with debris; 26 (11%) of 241 endoscopes had severely scratched channels that provided pockets for debris. Only 3 (5.4%) of 56 facilities that attempted to dry their endoscopes between procedures were successful. Because high-level disinfectants require clean surfaces, flexible endoscopes must be carefully cleaned of all mucus, blood, and other biologic materials before they are subject to a high-level disinfectant [141].

To further complicate endoscope care, automated machines, developed for endoscope reprocessing, have been flawed [148–151]. Users should adhere carefully to the manufacturer's protocols but also should be aware that colonization of the washer holding tanks may not be reversible despite use of the manufacturer's recommended disinfection protocol. Surveillance for endoscope-related infection and pseudoinfection is important, and infection control practitioners must educate their endoscope users about problems discussed in this section.

Arthrocentesis and Thoracentesis

Although septic arthritis is caused most commonly by hematogenous spread of organisms, sporadic cases of staphylococcal arthritis and, at times, gram-negative bacillary arthritis have followed several days after invasive joint manipulations. During the mid-1960s, CDC epidemiologists investigated a cluster of cases of staphylococcal arthritis in which the infections occurred 1 to 7 days after outpatient arthrocentesis or intraarticular injection of steroids. Epidemiologic evidence suggested that the physician who had performed these procedures was a disseminator of the epidemic strain, and microbiologic investigation showed that areas of chronic dermatitis on the physician's hands harbored the epidemic organism. A similar cluster of cases of staphylococcal arthritis, in which the infections occurred 5 to 6 days after arthrographic examination of the knee joint and 3 to 4 days after knee surgery, was traced epidemiologically to the surgeon who had performed these procedures, who was a nasal carrier of staphylococci. More recently, 10 cases of *Serratia* septic arthritis were traced to contaminated benzalkonium chloride antiseptic used in a physician's office [152].

Other diagnostic taps, such as thoracentesis [153], have also been associated with nosocomial infections,

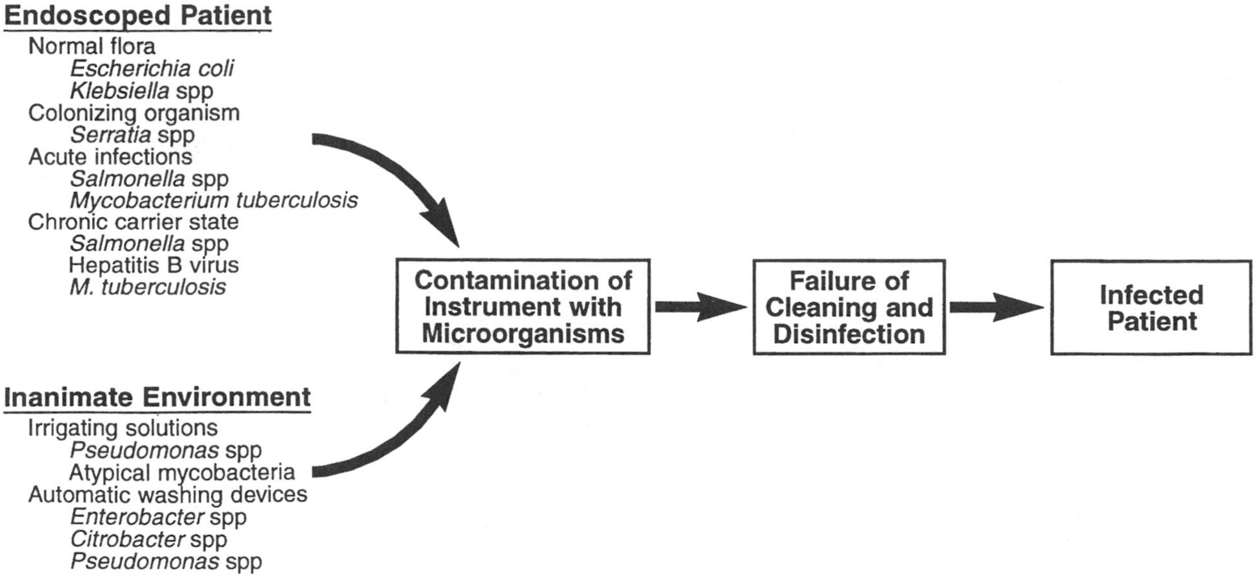

FIGURE 46-2. Nosocomial transmission of microorganisms by endoscopes. Flow diagram shows major routes and sources of nosocomial transmission of microorganisms by endoscopes. (With permission from Spach DH, et al. Transmission of infection by gastrointestinal endoscopy and bronchoscopy. *Ann Intern Med* 1993;118:118.)

which emphasizes the fact that all invasive procedures should be performed only under strict aseptic conditions, with careful skin preparation, by an appropriately scrubbed and gloved operator, and using sterile equipment. Although the relative rarity of centesis-associated infections may be considered testimony that good technique is usually observed in hospitals and clinics, the lack of such infections also may be evidence of the capacity of the local tissue response to limit bacterial invasion in uncompromised hosts [154]. When procedures are performed in patients with compromised host defenses or on tissues that may have diminished ability to limit bacterial invasion (e.g., rheumatoid joints), the risk of procedure-associated infections may be considerable, which emphasizes the need for continued vigilance.

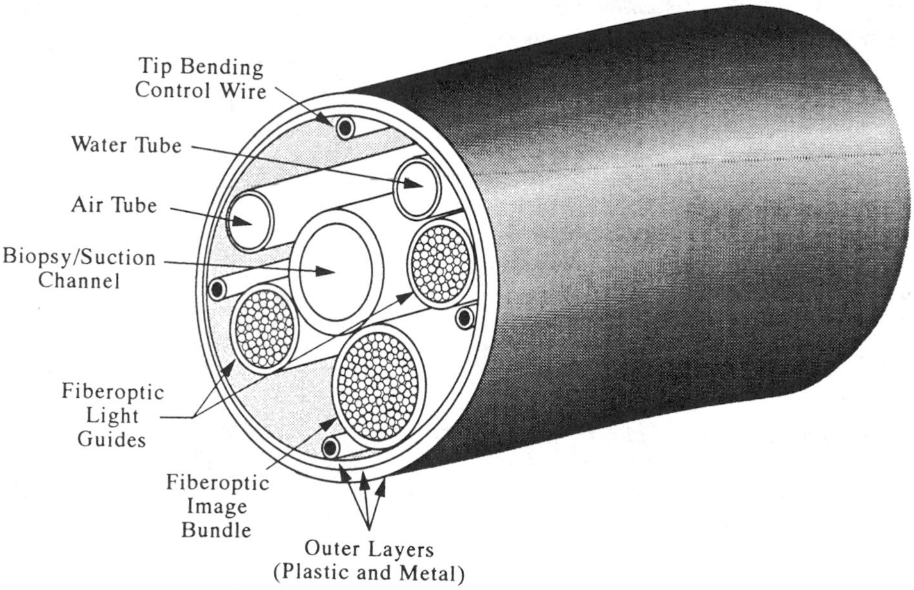

FIGURE 46-3. Cross-section of typical gastrointestinal endoscope. (With permission from Spach DH, et al. Transmission of infection by gastrointestinal endoscopy and bronchoscopy. *Ann Intern Med* 1993;118:120.)

Peritoneal Manipulation

Infectious complications of laparoscopy and amniocentesis are rare, presumably because of careful technique, sterile equipment, local host defense mechanisms, and the frequently healthy nature of the subjects. In fact, high-level disinfection of peritoneoscopes with glutaraldehyde instead of gas sterilization has appeared acceptable. In a retrospective analysis of polymicrobial bacterial ascites in 1,578 abdominal paracenteses, only 1 case of clinical peritonitis developed, presumably due to entry of the bowel by the paracentesis needle [155].

Artificial Insemination

A variety of infections have been transmitted by artificial insemination and mandate careful adherence to protocol for screening [156]. Artificial insemination may have resulted in HIV-1 infection of a woman inseminated with her HIV-infected husband's semen in spite of attempts to remove the virus from semen. The CDC recommends against insemination with semen from HIV-infected men [157].

Water Baths

Contaminated water baths have led to a large number of similar outbreaks. Warm water baths used to thaw packs of cryoprecipitate for intravenous use by hemophiliacs, to warm peritoneal dialysate, or to warm radiopaque contrast material have led to outbreaks of *P. cepacia* bacteremia, *Acinetobacter* peritonitis, and endotoxemia, respectively [158–160]. Cold ice baths used to chill the cardioplegia solution for open heart surgery or to cool blood gas syringes have been implicated in outbreaks of mediastinitis and bacteremia [161].

The exact mechanism of bacterial transfer in these situations is often unknown, but probably involves contamination of medication ports, splash onto operative fields, or hand transmission by staff. Possible preventive measures include using dry heat, using impermeable outer wraps or drying any immersed object before use, using sterile water or ice, and handwashing after contact with water baths. The use of disinfectants in water baths has been suggested but not widely attempted.

Ophthalmologic Examination

Manipulation of the conjunctiva and cornea may occur during tonometry, instillation of eye drops, and manual ophthalmologic examination, and it can result in transmission of conjunctivitis and other eye infections. The infection most commonly transmitted is epidemic keratoconjunctivitis, a highly contagious, frequently iatrogenic disease, which usually is caused by adenovirus type 8 [162] (see Chapter 42). Transmission of the virus occurs through fomites, such as inadequately disinfected tonometers and contaminated eye droppers, as well as by indirect person-to-person spread on the hands of healthcare workers. Similar modes of transmission have been implicated in outbreaks of other viral and bacterial eye infections. Although proper care of equipment and conscientious handwashing between patient contacts is remarkably effective in halting the transmission of such diseases, some manufacturer recommendations for disinfection may be inadequate [163], and ongoing community outbreaks may require extra-stringent triage and infection control to limit nosocomial spread [164].

Barium Enema

In addition to transient bacteremia, patients undergoing barium enema are at risk of two other infectious complications. First, infants may aspirate barium when faulty technique produces excessive retrograde flow of contrast material. Second, if the enema bag or tip is not replaced or is not adequately disinfected between uses, or if the barium is contaminated, the procedure may transmit enteric pathogens. This risk was highlighted by Meyers and Richards [165] when they demonstrated that attenuated poliovirus can be transferred by contaminated barium enema. At present, the use of disposable enema bags, tubing, and enema tips has largely controlled such risks.

REFERENCES

1. Schroeder SA, Marton KI, Strom BL. Frequency and morbidity of invasive procedures: report of a pilot study from two teaching hospitals. *Arch Intern Med* 1978;138:1809.
2. Wenzel RP, et al. Identification of procedure-related nosocomial infections in high-risk patients. *Rev Infect Dis* 1981;3:701.
3. Sherwood PM. An outbreak of syringe-transmitted hepatitis with jaundice in hospitalized diabetic patients. *Ann Intern Med* 1950;33:380.
4. Asnes RS, Arendar GM. Septic arthritis of the hip. *Pediatrics* 1966;38:837.
5. Blumenfeld TA, Turi GK, Blanc WA. Recommended site and depth of newborn heel skin punctures based on anatomical measurements and histopathology. *Lancet* 1979;1:230.
6. Katz L, Johnson DL, Neufeld PD, Gupta KG. Evacuated blood-collection tubes: the backflow hazard. *Can Med Assoc J* 1975;113:208.
7. Hoffman PC, et al. False-positive blood cultures: association with nonsterile blood collection tubes. *JAMA* 1976;236:2073.
8. Washington JA. The microbiology of evacuated blood collection tubes. *Ann Intern Med* 1977;86:186.
9. Ippolito G, De Carli G, Puro V, et al. Device-specific risk of needlestick injury in Italian healthcare workers. *JAMA* 1994;272:607–610.
10. Danzig LE, Short LJ, Collins K, et al. Bloodstream infections associated with a needleless intravenous infusion system in patients receiving home infusion therapy. *JAMA* 1995;273:1882–1884.
11. Maki DG, Stolz S, McCormick R, et al. Possible association of a commercial needleless system with central venous catheter-related bacteremia [Abstract]. In: *Programs and abstracts of the thirty-fourth interscience conference on antimicrobial agents and chemotherapy,*

October 1994, Orlando, Florida. Washington, DC: American Society for Microbiology, 1994:195.
12. Adams SL. The medicinal leech. *Ann Intern Med* 1988;109:399.
13. Abrutyn E. Hospital-associated infection from leeches. *Ann Intern Med* 1988;109:356.
14. Mercer NS, Beere DM, Bornemisza AJ, Thomas P. Medical leeches as sources of wound infection. *Br Med J* 1987;294:937.
15. Sande MA, Levinson ME, Lukas DS, Kaye D. Bacteremia associated with cardiac catheterization. *N Engl J Med* 1969;281:1104.
16. Reyes MP, et al. Pyrogenic reactions after inadvertent infusion of endotoxin during cardiac catheterizations. *Ann Intern Med* 1980;93:32.
17. Kundsin RB, Walter CW. Detection of endotoxin on sterile catheters used for cardiac catheterization. *J Clin Microbiol* 1980;11:209.
18. Kure R, Grendahl H, Paulssen J. Pyrogens from surgeons' sterile latex gloves. *Acta Pathol Microbiol Immunol Scand* 1982;90:85.
19. Adam RD, Edwards LD, Becker CC, Schrom HM. Semiquantitative cultures and routine tip cultures on umbilical catheters. *J Pediatr* 1982; 100:123.
20. Bard H, et al. Prophylactic antibiotics in chronic umbilical artery catheterization in respiratory distress syndrome. *Arch Dis Child* 1973; 48:630.
21. Krauss AN, Albert RF, Kannan MM. Contamination of umbilical catheters in the newborn infant. *J Pediatr* 1970;77:965.
22. Powers WF, Tooley WH. Contamination of umbilical vessel catheters. *Pediatrics* 1971;48:470.
23. Anagnostakis D, et al. Risk of infection associated with umbilical vein catheterization. *J Pediatr* 1975;86:759.
24. Gardner RM, Schwartz R, Wong HC, Burke JP. Percutaneous indwelling radial-artery catheters for monitoring cardiovascular function. *N Engl J Med* 1974;290:1227.
25. Raad I, Umphrey I, Khan A, Truett LJ, Bodey GP. The duration of placement as a predictor of peripheral and pulmonary arterial catheter infections. *J Hosp Infect* 1993;23:17–26.
26. Band JD, Maki DG. Infections caused by arterial catheters used used for hemodynamic monitoring. *Am J Med* 1979;67:735–741.
27. Michel L, et al. Infection of pulmonary artery catheters in critically ill patients. *JAMA* 1981;245:1032.
28. Rowley KM, Clubb KS, Smith GJW, Cabin HS. Right-sided infective endocarditis as a consequence of flow directed pulmonary artery catheterization. *N Engl J Med* 1984;311:1152.
29. Mermel LA, Maki DG. Infectious complications of Swan-Ganz pulmonary artery catheters. *Am J Respir Crit Care Med* 1994;149: 1020–1036.
30. Damen J, Ver Der Twell I. Positive tip cultures and related risk factors associated with intravascular catheterization in pediatric cardiac patients. *Crit Care Med* 1988;16:221–228.
31. Mermel LA, McCormick RD, Springman SR, Maki DG. The pathogenesis and epidemiology of catheter-related infection with pulmonary artery Swan-Ganz catheters: a prospective study utilizing molecular subtyping. *Am J Med* 1991;38:197S–205S.
32. Rello J, Coll P, Net A, Prats G. Infection of pulmonary artery catheters: epidemiologic characteristics and multivariate analysis of risk factors. *Chest* 1993;103;132–136.
33. Stamm WE, Colella JJ, Anderson RL, Dixon RE. Indwelling arterial catheters as a source of nosocomial bacteremia. *N Engl J Med* 1975; 292:1099.
34. Pien FD, Bruce AE. Nosocomial *Ewingella americana* bacteremia in an intensive care unit. *Arch Intern Med* 1986;146:111.
35. Pearson ML, Hospital Infection Control Practices Advisory Committee. Guideline for prevention of intravascular device-related infections. *Infect Control Hosp Epidemiol* 1996;17:438–473.
36. Weinstein RA, Stamm WE, Kramer L, Corey L. Pressure monitoring devices: overlooked source of nosocomial infection. *JAMA* 1976;236: 936.
37. Davis JP, et al. Nasal colonization of infants with group B streptococcus associated with intrauterine pressure transducers. *J Infect Dis* 1978;138:804.
38. Fisher MC, et al. *Pseudomonas maltophilia* bacteremia in children undergoing open heart surgery. *JAMA* 1981;246:1571.
39. Walton JR, Shapiro BA, Harrison RA. *Serratia* bacteremia from mean arterial pressure monitors. *Anesthesiology* 1975;43:113.
40. Centers for Disease Control and Prevention. Guideline for prevention of infections related to intravascular pressure-monitoring systems. *Infect Control* 1982;3:61.
41. Weinstein RA. The design of pressure monitoring devices. *Med Instrum* 1976;10:287–290.
42. Buxton AE, Anderson RL, Klimek J, Quintiliani R. Failure of disposable domes to prevent septicemia acquired from contaminated pressure transducers. *Chest* 1978;74:508.
43. Donowitz LG, Marsik FJ, Hoyt JW, Wenzel RP. *Serratia marcescens* bacteremia from contaminated pressure transducers. *JAMA* 1979;242:1749.
44. Villarino ME, Jarvis WR, O'Hara C, Bresnaham J, Clark N. Epidemic of *Serratia marcescens* bacteremia in a cardiac intensive care unit. *J Clin Microbiol* 1989;27:2433–2436.
45. Hekker TAM, Van Overhagen W, Schneider AJ. Pressure transducers: an overlooked source of sepsis in the intensive care unit. *Intensive Care Med* 1990;16:511–512.
46. Beck-Sague CM, Jarvis WR. Epidemic bloodstream infections associated with pressure transducers: a persistent problem. *Infect Control* 1989;10:54–59.
47. Luskin RL, et al. Extended use of disposable pressure transducers. *JAMA* 1986;255:916.
48. Shinozaki T, et al. Bacterial contamination of arterial lines: a prospective study. *JAMA* 1983;249:223.
49. Maki DG, Hassemer CA. Endemic rate of fluid contamination and related septicemia in arterial pressure monitoring. *Am J Med* 1981;733: 207.
50. Crow S, Conrad SA, Chaney-Rowell C, King JW. Microbial contamination of arterial infusions used for hemodynamic monitoring: a randomized trial of contamination with sampling through conventional stopcocks versus a novel closed system. *Infect Control Hosp Epidemiol* 1989;10:557.
51. Kormos RL, Borovetz HS, Armitage JM, et al. Evolving experience with mechanical circulatory support. *Ann Surg* 1991;214:471–477.
52. Pennington DG, McBride LR, Peigh PS, Miller LW, Swartz MR. Eight years' experience with bridging to cardiac transplantation. *J Thorac Cardiovasc Surg* 1994;107:472–481.
53. Farrar DJ, Hill DJ. Univentricular and biventricular Thoratec VAD support as a bridge to transplantation. *Ann Thorac Surg* 1993;55: 276–282.
54. Mill CA, Pae WE, Pierce WS. Combined registry for the clinical use of mechanical ventricular assist pumps and the total artificial heart in conjunction with heart transplantation: fourth official report. *J Heart Transplant* 9, 1989:453–458.
55. Myers TJ, McGee MG, Zeluff BJ, Radovancevic B, Frazier OH. Frequency and significance of infections in patients receiving prolonged LVAD support. *ASAIO Trans* 1991;37:M283–M285.
56. Fisher S, Trenholme G, Costanzo MR, Piccione W. Infectious complications of left ventricular assist device recipients. *Clin Infect Dis* 1997; 24:18–23.
57. Tabor E. *Infectious complications of blood transfusions*. New York: Academic, 1982.
58. James JD. Bacterial contamination of preserved blood. *Vox Sang* 1959; 4:177.
59. Braude AI, Sanford JP, Bartlett JE, Mallery OT. Effects and clinical significance of bacterial contaminants in transfused blood. *J Lab Clin Med* 1952;39:902.
60. Heltberg O, Skov F, Grener-Smidt P, et al. Nosocomial epidemic of *Serratia marcescens* septicemia ascribed to contaminated blood transfusion bags. *Transfusion* 1993;33:221–227.
61. Blajchman MA, et al. Platelet transfusion-induced *Serratia marcescens* sepsis due to vacuum tube contamination. *Transfusion* 1979;19:39.
62. Stenhouse MAE, Milner LV. *Yersinia enterocolitica*: a hazard in blood transfusion. *Transfusion* 1982;22:396.
63. Deleted in proof.
64. BruceChwatt LJ. Blood transfusion and tropical disease. *Tropical Disease Bulletin* 1972;69:825.
65. Dover AS, Schultz MG. Transfusion-induced malaria. *Transfusion* 1971;11:353.
66. Guerrero IC, Weniger BC, Schultz MG. Transfusion malaria in the United States, 1972–1981. *Ann Intern Med* 1983;99:221.
67. Turc JM. Malaria and blood transfusion. In: Westphal RG, Carlson KB, Ture JE, eds. *Emerging global patterns in transfusion transmitted infections*. Arlington, VA: American Association of Blood Banks, 1990: 31–43.
68. Schmunis GA. *Trypanosoma cruzi*, the etiological agent of Chagas' disease as a contaminant of blood supplies: a problem of endemic and non-endemic countries. *Transfusion* 1991;31:547–557.

69. Kirchhoff LV. Is *Trypanosoma cruzi* a threat to our blood supply? *Ann Intern Med* 1989;111:773.
70. Skolnick A. Deferral aims to deter Chagas' parasite. *JAMA* 1991, 265: 173.
71. Widmann FK, ed. *Standards for blood banks and transfusion services.* 15th ed. Arlington, VA: American Association of Blood Banks, 1993.
72. Deleted in proof.
73. Kimball AC, Kean BH, Kellner A. The risk of transmitting toxoplasmosis by blood transfusion. *Transfusion* 1965;5:447.
74. Siegel SE, et al. Transmission of toxoplasmosis by leukocyte transfusion. *Blood* 1971;37:388.
75. Buchholtz DH, et al. Bacterial proliferation in platelets stored at room temperature. *N Engl J Med* 1971;285:429.
76. Cunningham M, Cash JD. Bacterial contamination and platelet concentrates stored at 20°C. *J Clin Pathol* 1973;26:401.
77. Rhame FS, et al. *Salmonella* septicemia from platelet transfusions. *Ann Intern Med* 1973;78:633.
78. Zaza S, Tokars JI, Yomtovian R, et al. Bacterial contamination of platelets at a university hospital: increased identification due to intensified surveillance. *Infect Control Hosp Epidemiol* 1994;15:82–87.
79. Steere AC, et al. *Pseudomonas* species bacteremia caused by contaminated normal human serum albumin. *J Infect Dis* 1977;135:729.
80. Bennett SN, McNeil MM, Bland LA, et al. Postoperative infections traced to contamination of an intravenous anesthetic, propofol. *N Engl J Med* 1995;333:147–154.
81. Mendelson CL. The aspiration of stomach contents into the lungs during obstetric anesthesia. *Am J Obstet Gynecol* 1946;52:191.
82. Culver GA, Makel HP, Beecher HK. Frequency of aspiration of gastric contents by the lungs during anesthesia and surgery. *Ann Surg* 1951;133:289.
83. Berry FA, Blankenbaker WL, Ball CG. A comparison of bacteremia occurring with nasotracheal and orotracheal intubation. *Anesth Analg* 1973;52:873.
84. Fassoulaki A, Pamouktsoglou P. Prolonged nasotracheal intubation and its association with inflammation of paranasal sinuses. *Anesth Analg* 1989;69:50.
85. Linden BE, Aguilar EA, Allen SJ. Sinusitis in the nasotracheally intubated patient. *Arch Otolaryngol Head Neck Surg* 1988;114:860.
86. Lucks D, Consiglio A, Stankiewicz J, O'Keefe P. Incidence and microbiological etiology of middle ear effusion complicating endotracheal intubation and mechanical ventilation. *J Infect Dis* 1988;157: 368.
87. Diamond RD, Bennett JE. A subcutaneous reservoir for intrathecal therapy of fungal meningitis. *N Engl J Med* 1974;288:186.
88. Lishner M, et al. Complications associated with Ommaya reservoirs in patients with cancer. *Arch Intern Med* 1990;150:173.
89. Trump DL, Grossman SA, Thompson G, Murray K. CSF infections complicating the management of neoplastic meningitis. *Arch Intern Med* 1982;142:583.
90. Luthardt T. Bacterial infections in ventriculo-auricular shunt systems. *Dev Med Child Neurol Suppl* 1970;12:105.
91. Schoenbaum SC, Gardner P, Shillito J. Infections of cerebrospinal fluid shunts. J Infect Dis 1975;131:543.
92. James HE, et al. Prospective randomized study of therapy in cerebrospinal fluid shunt infection. *Neurosurgery* 1980;7:459.
93. Younger JJ, et al. Coagulase-negative staphylococci isolated from cerebrospinal fluid shunts: importance of slime production, species identification, and shunt removal to clinical outcome. *J Infect Dis* 1987;156:548.
94. McLaurin RL, Frane PT. Treatment of infections of cerebrospinal fluid shunts. *Rev Infect Dis* 1987;9:595.
95. Guertin SR. Cerebrospinal fluid shunts: evaluation, complications, and crisis management. *Pediatr Clin North Am* 1987;34:203.
96. Weiss SR, Raskind R. Further experience with the ventriculoperitoneal shunt. *Int Surg* 1970;53:300.
97. Langley JM, LeBlanc JC, Drake J, Milner R. Efficacy of antimicrobial prophylaxis in placement of cerebrospinal fluid shunts: meta-analysis. *Clin Infect Dis* 1993;17:98–103.
98. Haines SJ, Walters BC. Antibiotic prophylaxis for cerebrospinal fluid shunts: a metanalysis. *Neurosurgery* 1994;34:87–92.
99. Shapiro JM, Bond EL, Garman JK. Use of a chlorhexidine dressing to reduce microbial colonization of epidural catheters. *Anesthesiology* 1990;73:625–631.
100. Everett ED, Hirschmann JV. Transient bacteremia and endocarditis prophylaxis: a review. *Medicine* 1977;56:61.
101. Crawford JJ, et al. Bacteremia after tooth extractions studied with the aid of pre-reduced anaerobically sterilized culture media. *Appl Microbiol* 1974;27:927.
102. LeFrock JL, Ellis CA, Turchik JB, Weinstein L. Transient bacteremia associated with sigmoidoscopy. *N Engl J Med* 1973;289:467.
103. Engeling ER, et al. Bacteremia after sigmoidoscopy: another view. *Ann Intern Med* 1976;85:77.
104. Pelican G, Hentges D, Butt JH. Bacteremia during colonoscopy. *Gastrointest Endosc* 1976;22:233.
105. Schwesinger WH, Levine BA, Ramos R. Complications in colonoscopy. *Surg Gynecol Obstet* 1979;148:270.
106. Allen JI, et al. *Pseudomonas* infection of the biliary system resulting from use of a contaminated endoscope. *Gastroenterology* 1987;92:759.
107. Classen DC, et al. Serious *Pseudomonas* infections associated with endoscopic retrograde cholangiopancreatography. *Am J Med* 1988;84: 590.
108. Cryan EMJ, et al. *Pseudomonas aeruginosa* cross-infection following endoscopic retrograde cholangiopancreatography. *J Hosp Infect* 1984; 5:371.
109. Doherty DE, et al. *Pseudomonas aeruginosa* sepsis following retrograde cholangiopancreatography (ERCP). *Dig Dis Sci* 1982;27:169.
110. Earnshaw JJ, Clark AW, Thom BT. Outbreak of *Pseudomonas aeruginosa* following endoscopic retrograde cholangiopancreatography. *J Hosp Infect* 1985;6:95.
111. Elson CO, Hattori K, Blackstone MO. Polymicrobial sepsis following endoscopic retrograde and cholangiopancreatography. *Gastroenterology* 1975;69:507.
112. Greene WH, et al. Esophagoscopy as a source of *P. aeruginosa* sepsis in patients with acute leukemia: the need for sterilization of endoscopes. *Gastroenterology* 1974;67:912.
113. Low DE, Micflikier AB, Kennedy JK, Stiver HG. Infectious complications of endoscopic retrograde cholangiopancreatography: a prospective assessment. *Arch Intern Med* 1980;140:1076.
114. Spach DH, Silverstein FE, Stamm WE. Transmission of infection by gastrointrestinal endoscopy and bronchoscopy. *Ann Intern Med* 1993; 118:117–128.
115. Anonymous. Infection control during a gastrointestinal endoscopy. *Gastrointest Endosc* 1988;34:37S.
116. Anonymous. Preparation of patients for gastrointestinal endoscopy. *Gastrointest Endosc* 1988;34:32S.
117. Bilbao MK, Dotter CT, Lee TG, Katon RM. Complications of endoscopic retrograde cholangiopancreatography (ERCP). *Gastroenterology* 1976;70:314.
118. McCloskey RV, Gold M, Weser E. Bacteremia after liver biopsy. *Arch Intern Med* 1973;132:213.
119. LeFrock JL, et al. Transient bacteremia associated with percutaneous liver biopsy. *J Infect Dis* 1975;131(Suppl):104.
120. Botsford KB, et al. Gram-negative bacilli in human milk feedings: quantitation and clinical consequences for premature infants. *J Pediatr* 1986;109:707.
121. Levy J. Enteral nutrition: an increasingly recognized cause of nosocomial bloodstream infection. *Infect Control Hosp Epidemiol* 1989;10: 395.
122. Sullivan NM, et al. Bacteremia after genitourinary tract manipulation. *Appl Microbiol* 1972;23:1101.
123. Dellinger EP, Gross PA, Barrett TL, et al. Quality standard for antimicrobial prophylaxis in surgical procedures. Infectious Disease Society of America. *Clin Infect Dis* 1994;18:422–427.
124. Committee on the Prevention of Rheumatic Fever and Bacterial Endocarditis: Prevention of bacterial endocarditis. *Circulation* 1984;70: 1123A.
125. Barela AI, et al. Septic shock with renal failure after chorionic villus sampling. *Am J Obstet Gynecol* 1986;154:1100.
126. Livengood CH, Land MR, Addison WA. Endometrial biopsy, bacteremia, and endocarditis, risk. *Obstet Gynecol* 1985;65:678.
127. Pereira W, et al. Fever and pneumonia after flexible fiberoptic bronchoscopy. *Am Rev Respir Dis* 1975;112:59.
128. Durack D. Prevention of infective endocarditis. *N Engl J Med* 1995; 332:38–44.
129. Oakley C, Somerville W. Prevention of infective endocarditis. *Br Heart J* 1981;45:233.

130. Hess J, Holloway Y, Dankert J. Incidence of postextraction bacteremia under penicillin cover in children with cardiac disease. *Pediatrics* 1983;71:554.
131. Lowy FD, et al. Effect of penicillin on the adherence of *Streptococcus sanguis* in vitro and in the rabbit model of endocarditis. *J Clin Invest* 1983;71:668.
132. Dajani AS, Taubert KA, Wilson W, et al. Prevention of bacterial endocarditis. Recommendations by the American Heart Association. *JAMA* 1997;277:1794–1801.
133. Mueller PR, van Sonnenberg E. Interventional radiology in the chest and abdomen. *N Engl J Med* 1990;322:1364.
134. Hunter DW, Simmons RL, Hulbert JC. Antibiotics for radiologic interventional procedures. *Radiology* 1988;166:571.
135. White JV. Laparoscopic cholecystectomy: the evolution of general surgery. *Ann Intern Med* 1991;115:651.
136. Dixon RE, et al. Aqueous quaternary ammonium antiseptics and disinfectants: use and mis-use. *JAMA* 1976;236:2415.
137. Hoffman KK, Weber DJ, Rutala WA. Pseudoepidemic of *Rhodotorula rubra* in patients undergoing fiberoptic bronchoscopy. *Infect Control Hosp Epidemiol* 1989;10:511.
138. Bennett S, Peterson D, Johnson D, et al. Bronchoscopy-associated *Mycobacterium xenopi* pseudoinfections. *Am J Respir Crit Care Med* 1994;150:245–250.
139. Nelson KE, Larson PA, Schraufnagel DE, Jackson J. Transmission of tuberculosis by flexible fiberbronchoscopes. *Am Rev Respir Dis* 1983; 127:97.
140. Favero MS. Sterilization, disinfection and antisepsis in the hospital. In: *Manual of clinical microbiology.* 4th ed. Washington, DC: American Society for Microbiology, 1985:129–137.
141. Martin MA, Reichelderfer M, Association for Professionals in Infection Control and Epidemiology, Inc. 1991, 1992, and 1993 APIC Guidelines Committee. APIC guideline for infection prevention and control in flexible endoscopy. *Am J Infect Control* 1994;22:19–38.
142. Wheeler PW, Lancaster D, Kaiser AB. Bronchopulmonary cross-colonization and infection related to mycobacterial contamination of suction valves of bronchoscopes. *J Infect Dis* 1989;159:954.
143. British Society for Gastrointestinal Endoscopy. Cleaning and disinfection of equipment for gastrointestinal flexible endoscopy: interim recommendations of a working party. *Gut* 1988;29:1134–1151.
144. American Association of Operating Room Nurses. Proposed recommended practices: the use and care of endoscopes. *AORN J* 1993;57: 543–550.
145. Rutala WA, Clontz E, Weber DJ, Hoffmann KK. Disinfection practices for endoscopes and other semicritical items. *Infect Control Hosp Epidemiol* 1991;12:282–288.
146. Favero MS. Strategies for disinfection and sterilization of endoscopes: the gap between basic principles and actual practice [Editorial]. *Infect Control Hosp Epidemiol* 1991;12:279–281.
147. McCracken JE. Endoscopy revels debris, fluid, and damage in patient-ready GI endoscopes. *Infection Control and Sterilization Technology* 1995;1:32–43.
148. Maloney S, Welbel S, Daves B, et al. *Mycobacterium abscessus* pseudoinfection traced to an automated endoscope washer: utility of epidemiologic and laboratory investigation. *J Infect Dis* 1994;169: 1166–1169.
149. Centers for Disease Control and Prevention. Nosocomial infection and pseudoinfection from contaminated endoscopes and bronchoscopes: Wisconsin and Missouri. *MMWR Morb Mortal Wkly Rep* 1991;40:675–678.
150. Alvardo CJ, Stolz SM, Maki DG. Nosocomial infections from contaminated endoscopes: a flawed automated endoscope washer. An investigation using molecular epidemiology. *Am J Med* 1991;91(Suppl 3B): 272S–280S.
151. Fraser V, Jones M, Murray P, Medoff G, Zhang Y, Wallace R Jr. Contamination of flexible bronchoscopes with *Mycobacterium chelonae* linked to an automated bronchoscope disinfection machine. *Am Rev Respir Dis* 1992;145:853–855.
152. Nakashima AK, McCarthy MA, Martone WJ, Anderson RL. Epidemic septic arthritis caused by *Serratia marcescens* and associated with benzalkonium chloride antiseptic. *J Clin Microbiol* 1987;25:1014.
153. Bayer AS. Necrotizing pneumonia and empyema due to *Clostridium perfringens*. *Am J Med* 1975;59:851.
154. Dann TC. Routine skin preparation before injection: an unnecessary procedure. *Lancet* 1969;2:96.
155. Runyon BA, Hoefs JC, Canawati HN. Polymicrobial bacterascites: a unique entity in the spectrum of infected ascitic fluid. *Arch Intern Med* 1986;146:2173.
156. Mascola L, Guinan ME. Screening to reduce transmission of sexually transmitted diseases in semen used for artificial insemination. *N Engl J Med* 1986;314:1354.
157. Centers for Disease Control and Prevention. HIV-1 infection and artificial insemination with processed semen. *MMWR Morb Mortal Wkly Rep* 1990;39:249, 255–256.
158. Rhame FS, McCullough J. Follow-up on nosocomial *Pseudomonas cepacia* infection. *MMWR Morb Mortal Wkly Rep* 1979;28:409.
159. Rubin J, et al. Management of peritonitis and bowel perforation during chronic peritoneal dialysis. *Nephron* 1976;16:220.
160. Sharbaugh RJ. Suspected outbreak of endotoxemia associated with computerized axial tomography. *Am J Infect Control* 1980;8:26.
161. Kuritsky JN, et al. Sternal wound infections and endocarditis due to organisms of the *Mycobacterium fortuitum* complex. *Ann Intern Med* 1983;98:938.
162. Hendley JO. Epidemic keratoconjunctivitis and hand washing. *N Engl J Med* 1973;289:1368.
163. Koo D, et al. Epidemic keratoconjunctivitis in a university medical center ophthalmology clinic: need for re-evaluation of the design and disinfection of instruments. *Infect Control Hosp Epidemiol* 1989;10:547.
164. Warren D, et al. A large outbreak of epidemic keratoconjunctivitis. problems in control of nosocomial spread. *J Infect Dis* 1989;160:938.
165. Meyers PH, Richards M. Transmission of polio virus vaccine by contaminated barium enema with resultant antibody rise. *American Journal of Roentgenology, Therapy, and Nuclear Medicine* 1964;91:864.

Subject Index

Subject Index